Aicardi's Epilepsy in Children

Third Edition

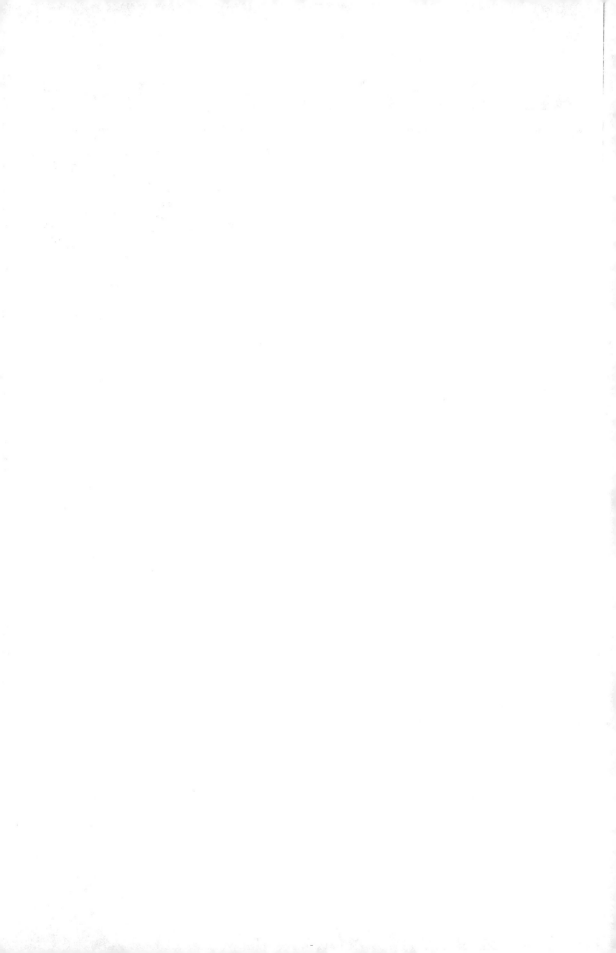

Aicardi's Epilepsy in Children

Third Edition

Alexis Arzimanoglou, M.D.

Head, Pediatric Epilepsy Unit
Department of Child Neurology and Metabolic Disorders
and
Institut National de la Santé et de la Recherche Médicale
University Hospital Robert Debré
Paris, France

Renzo Guerrini, M.D.

Professor of Child Neurology and Psychiatry
Head of the Epilepsy, Neurophysiology and Neurogenetics Unit
Department of Child Neurology and Psychiatry
University of Pisa and Research Institute Stella Maris Foundation
Pisa, Italy

Jean Aicardi, M.D., F.R.C.P.

Honorary Professor of Child Neurology
Institute of Child Health, University College London;
Research Director
Institut National de la Santé et de la Recherche Médicale;
Honorary Consultant
Department of Child Neurology and Metabolic Disorders
University Hospital Robert Debré
Paris, France

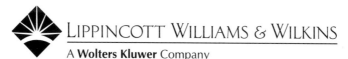

LIPPINCOTT WILLIAMS & WILKINS
A **Wolters Kluwer** Company
Philadelphia • Baltimore • New York • London
Buenos Aires • Hong Kong • Sydney • Tokyo

Acquisitions Editor: Anne M. Sydor
Developmental Editor: Jenny Kim
Production Editor: Christiana Sahl
Manufacturing Manager: Benjamin Rivera
Cover Designer: Christine Jenny
Compositor: Lippincott Williams & Wilkins Desktop Division
Printer: Maple Press

Library of Congress Cataloging-in-Publication Data

Arzimanoglou, A.
    Aicardi's epilepsy in children / Alexis Arzimanoglou, Renzo Guerrini, Jean Aicardi.—
    3rd ed.
      p. ; cm.
    Rev. ed. of: Epilepsy in children / Jean Aicardi. 2nd ed. c1994.
    Includes bibliographical references and index.
    ISBN 0-7817-2698-0
      1. Epilepsy in children. I. Title: Epilepsy in children. II. Guerrini, Renzo.
    III. Aicardi, Jean. IV. Aicardi, Jean. Epilepsy in children. V. Title.
    [DNLM: 1. Epilepsy—classification—Child. 2. Epilepsy—classification—infant. 3.
    Epilepsy—diagnosis—Child. 4. Epilepsy—diagnosis—Infant. 5. Epilepsy—therapy—
    Child. 6. Epilepsy—therapy—Infant. WL 385 A797a2004]
    RJ496.E6A43 2004
    618.92'853—dc22

                                            2003054693

10 9 8 7 6 5 4 3 2 1

Contents

**Section IV. Selected Aspects of Diagnosis, Prognosis, and Treatment
of Convulsive Disorders in Children**

Preface

Since the second edition of this book, an enormous amount of new knowledge on epilepsy has accumulated at an increasing pace on both its basic and clinical aspects. Novel techniques of investigation and new forms of therapy, both medical and surgical, have been developed. Advances in genetics have clarified the etiology of some forms of monogenic epilepsy, and they may shortly provide some understanding of the more common syndromes with a multifactorial inheritance. Genetics have been shown to play a major role in some cases of ionic channel dysfunction. New concepts about the mechanisms of seizures and their propagation have led to the development of the concept of the epileptic network. New antiepileptic agents, some of which have been rationally rather than empirically devised, have been introduced as a result of the better knowledge of the mechanisms of excitatory or inhibitory neurotransmission. Surgical treatment, which has benefitted immensely from the spectacular progress that has occurred in the techniques of structural and functional imaging, has become an established form of therapy, and new surgical methods such as stimulation are being tested.

Such remarkable technical developments have evolved in parallel with the refinements in diagnostic capabilities, leading to the more precise delineation of epilepsy syndromes and to a better knowledge of their natural history and sensitivity to drugs. The result has been the identification of more rational indications and contraindications for the use of antiepileptic agents on a syndromic basis, as well as the better overall management of the patients. The realizations that epilepsy may consist of more than simply having seizures and that cognitive or behavioral abnormalities or both may result from infraclinical paroxysmal neuronal activity, such as occurs in the Landau-Kleffner syndrome or the syndrome of continuous spike-waves of sleep, emphasize some of the peculiar aspects of epilepsy in childhood. They underline the probable role of paroxysmal epileptic brain dysfunction on the development of the brain, possibly as a result of the plastic changes induced by the epileptic process.

The incorporation of at least some of these recent findings while still retaining the clinical orientation of the book necessitated the development of a new edition. Collecting this mass of data and literature and reviewing them in an accessible manner proved to be a formidable challenge beyond the abilities of a single author, so a collective endeavor was required. The three authors of this edition have long shared a similar approach to the study of epilepsy in children, as well as having considerable experience in its clinical diagnosis and management. We hope this common experience maintains the homogeneity of the text and avoids discrepancies. We have reviewed, discussed, and amended all chapters together in an effort to achieve a degree of coherence analogous to that of a single-authored book.

The general structure of the book is the same as that of the previous two editions. The volume is divided into four parts. The first part discusses general notions about seizure disorders, including definitions of the basic terms that are necessary to the understanding of the subsequent chapters, and the problems of classification of epileptic seizures and epilepsies. The second part describes the major types of epileptic seizures and the epilepsy syndromes in which the particular seizures are the major manifestation. For each type of seizure, an attempt has been made to delineate the associated syndromes and to assess the validity and usefulness of these syndromes for prognosis and treatment. This conforms with the clinical approach that uses the symptom as a starting point for reaching the most precise diagnosis possible. The third part deals with those epileptic manifestations for which the age of occurrence or the precipitating factors are more informative than the clinical characteristics. General etiologies, both genetic and lesional, are also discussed in this section. The fourth part is concerned with the general aspects of diagnosis, prognosis, and treatment, while taking into account that the specific aspects of these problems are considered in the discussion of the individual syndromes.

Jean Aicardi
Alexis Arzimanoglou
Renzo Guerrini

Acknowledgments

The authors thank the persons who directly or indirectly contributed to this book. Many of the opinions and ideas expressed here were discussed over the years with our faithful collaborators, Jean-Jacques Chevrie, Françoise Goutières, Edouard Hirsch, Philippe Kahane, and Lucio Parmeggiani. Their contribution to our understanding of the many problems of epilepsy in children and their approach to dealing with them have been invaluable.

This book is also a tribute to the memory of Professor Henri Gastaut and to Dr. Joseph Roger, pioneers in the field of epilepsy, whose examples have been a constant stimulation to us. Thanks are also due to Drs. Pierre Thomas, Françoise Salefranque, Jeanne Misès, and Perrine Plouin for their contributions to the illustrations.

We also thank Brigitte Tricot, who, for the third time, did the considerable secretarial work for this text. In addition, we express our appreciation to the editorial team of Lippincott Williams & Wilkins, especially Anne Sydor, Jenny Kim, and Christiana Sahl for their support, help, and understanding.

Aicardi's Epilepsy in Children

Third Edition

1

Epilepsy: Overview and Definitions

The term *epilepsy* is loosely applied to a host of conditions that have in common only the propensity to the occurrence of paroxysmal clinical events known as epileptic seizures. The word *epilepsy* derives from the Greek word επιλαμβανειν, which means *to seize*. The word has a dual meaning. On the one hand, it refers to the ancient concept that diseases represent "attacks" or seizures by gods or demons (O'Donohoe, 1985). This concept applies especially to epileptic seizures, in which the victims are deprived of consciousness while their bodies are wildly agitated, almost as if someone else were in command of their movements. On the other hand, the words *to seize* have an objective justification in the case of epilepsy because the attacks occur suddenly, overwhelming the patient, who has no possibility of avoiding the fit and its consequences. The sudden, unexpected nature of epileptic attacks explains both the ancient magic concept that a seizure is caused by demonic possession and the more logical fear of the consequences of an event that is both unpredictable and repeated.

DEFINITIONS

Those disorders that are characterized by episodic attacks involving brain functions are *not* epilepsy. The realizations that have been slowly reached are that all seizures marked by loss of consciousness, involuntary movements, or disturbances of sensorium are not of the same origin, that they may be the result of different mechanisms, and that they have widely different outcomes and implications. Although such paroxysmal events as syncopes, hysterical fits, sleepwalking, and others were undoubtedly confused with epileptic attacks in the past, they are now considered completely separate from epileptic seizures. The latter term applies only to a particular type of attack that can be attributed to a specific neurophysiologic mechanism. According to Jackson's classic definition (Jackson, 1931), "epilepsy is the name for occasional, sudden, excessive, rapid, and local discharge of gray matter." That definition has remained the basic foundation to the modern understanding of epileptic phenomena even though the clinical differentiation may be difficult.

Epileptic seizures or attacks are transient clinical events that result from the abnormal, excessive activity of a more or less extensive population of cerebral neurons. As used by Jackson, the term *local* may not be appropriate for those many cases in which instantaneous or very rapid involvement of large areas of brain is seen without any demonstrable evidence of a local discharge. Epileptic seizures are usually brief, lasting from seconds to minutes, and they are marked by the sudden appearance of behavioral manifestations that may be purely motor or that may affect other brain functions (Gastaut and Broughton, 1972; Penfield and Jasper, 1954). The abnormal and excessive neuronal activity at the origin of the epileptic seizures is inferred from both the clinical events that constitute the attacks and the electroencephalogram (EEG) concomitants of the clinical seizures. The clinical events are not always obviously excitatory. Many seizures are characterized to a greater or lesser degree by negative phenomena, such as the loss of awareness, muscle tone, or language. However, in all cases, an epileptic seizure results in a paroxysmal *disorganization* of one or several brain functions (Bancaud et al., 1965, 1973).

The EEG events are essential for the characterization of attacks as epileptic seizures as opposed to one of the other types of paroxysmal attacks. These events constitute the *epileptic discharge* (Gastaut, 1973), which is defined as a temporary paroxysmal change in EEG activity, whether diffuse or localized. The epileptic discharge usually can be recorded on the scalp, but, on occasion, recording may occur only from the surface of the brain or even from the buried convolutions and other deep structures (Bancaud et al., 1973). This EEG recording is the most direct evidence of the abnormal, excessive neuronal activity postulated by Jackson. The main characteristics of the epileptic discharge are its high amplitude and its rhythmicity, both of which are caused by the excessive synchronization of an abnormal number of potentials in a neuronal aggregate; these therefore imply dysfunction in a *population* of neurons (Aird et al., 1989; Fenwick, 1983). The epileptic discharge may be related to the abnormal behavior of individual neurons, known as the paroxysmal depolarization shift (Prince and Connors, 1986), especially in focal seizures. In some models, a temporal and spatial correlation has been shown between the paroxysmal depolarization shift and the occurrence of EEG spikes on the cortex or the scalp (Aird et al., 1984). However, neither the paroxysmal depolarization shift nor the "epileptic spike" on the EEG can be equated with clinical epilepsy. The epileptic discharge is a complex phenomenon resulting from the interaction of excitatory and inhibitory influxes from a network formed by multiple diverse neuronal sources. In its most classic form, the epileptic discharge comprises an initial rapid activity of 10 to 20 Hz that increases progressively in amplitude, which is known as the *epileptic recruiting rhythm* (Gastaut et al., 1974a, 1974b; Gastaut and Broughton, 1972). As the seizure proceeds, the rapid rhythm is fragmented by the admixture of a slower rhythm—usually about 3 Hz in frequency—that progressively becomes more prominent until the discharge ends (Gastaut and Tassinari, 1975a). This latter rhythm is thought to reflect the activity of inhibitory elements that are within, around, or distant from the site of origin of the discharge. Many other patterns of epileptic discharges are possible (Gastaut and Tassinari, 1975a), depending on the type of epilepsy and the recording techniques. No pattern is general enough to apply to all of the types that are observed. These include fast rhythms of low amplitude or flattening of the EEG activity (*desynchronization*), rather than typical *hypersynchronous* discharges. In practice, the repertoire of EEG discharges that electroencephalographers and clinicians recognize as epileptic is limited (Blume, 1982). Theoretically, such discharges are a constant concomitant of epileptic seizures even though they are not necessarily detectable by conventional techniques of EEG recording in every case. Experience with depth electrodes and stereo-EEG has shown that discharges recorded from the depth of the brain do not necessarily appear on the overlying scalp or even on the nearby cortex (Bancaud and Talairach, 1975). Not all epileptic *discharges*, however, correspond to epileptic *seizures* (i.e., paroxysmal clinical events). Subjects who do not demonstrate any clinical evidence of paroxysmal brain dysfunction yet who have generalized (Eeg-Olofsson et al., 1971) or partial (Cavazzuti et al., 1980) paroxysmal abnormalities showing the typical EEG characteristics are not uncommon. In some such patients, minimal behavioral or cognitive changes can be demonstrated with the use of special tests performed at the time of the discharges, even if

they are brief, despite the absence of an overt clinical seizure (Kasteleijn-Nolst Trenité et al., 1988; Aarts et al., 1984; Fenwick, 1983; Gloor, 1979). Some authors refer to such cases as *subclinical* seizures (Gastaut, 1973). For those cases in which the same techniques of observation fail to detect any clinical change, the authors of this text sometimes use the terms *infraclinical* or *electrical* seizure. Such terms should be avoided because a seizure, by definition, is a clinical phenomenon (Gastaut, 1973).

Epileptic seizures are often difficult to distinguish from other paroxysmal events such as syncope and hysteria attacks. In theory, the distinction implies the presence or absence of an epileptic discharge. The epileptic discharge, however, is not recorded in most cases because seizures rarely occur at the time of the EEG recording. In addition, the discharge may be difficult to recognize, it may be obscured by muscular artifacts, or it may be altogether absent on the scalp. Such difficulties limit the practical usefulness of the epileptic discharge as a diagnostic tool. Even from a theoretical standpoint, the differentiation of an epileptic discharge from other paroxysmal activities may be difficult. For example, tonic seizures occurring with acute anoxia usually are interpreted as a release phenomenon that results from the interruption of the inhibitory influences from the cortex, which is more sensitive than the brainstem reticular formation to the lack of oxygen (Stephenson, 1990; Gastaut, 1974; Lombroso and Lerman, 1967). In such a situation, one must ask what the nature of the excessive activity of the brainstem neurons responsible for tonic contraction is. Could this activity be considered an excessive discharge in the gray matter? Other such examples could be given (e.g., the paroxysmal dyskinesias), but debate on that problem is beyond the scope of this book. However, the reader should understand that reasonable agreement does exist on which paroxysmal events should be regarded as epileptic seizures, even though borderline cases are undoubtedly encountered.

The clinical events that constitute epileptic seizures can be extremely diverse, and no single manifestation is essential. Seizures may appear as disturbances of consciousness only; they may be evinced by sensory, visceral, or motor signs; or they may present as perversions of ideation, emotion, or mood (Gastaut and Broughton, 1972). Some seizures may include a single symptom, while others may have a complex symptomatology. In such cases, analyzing the *temporal sequence* of events is important because this permits the construction of hypotheses regarding the origin and propagation of the discharge in various brain structures (Wieser, 1983b; Bancaud and Talairach, 1975) and it has possible consequences for surgical therapy. All the seizures of an individual patient do not have to be identical. The symptoms may be so slight or so trivial that a seizure may escape recognition unless it is authenticated by simultaneous EEG recording. Such an occurrence is common in neonatal seizures, but it may be present at any age. Concurrent video-EEG recording during seizures (Binnie, 1991; Mizrahi, 1984) is particularly useful in these difficult cases as it allows the detection of subtle clinical seizure phenomena and a better interpretation of the EEG phenomena, which can then be precisely correlated with the clinical changes.

Convulsions are attacks of involuntary muscle contractions, either sustained (tonic) or interrupted (clonic). The term does not imply a specific mechanism, and convulsions may be either epileptic or nonepileptic. However, the term is currently used primarily to designate attacks due to an epileptic mechanism.

Pediatricians have long been using the term *convulsion* to designate occasional seizures (e.g., febrile seizures) as opposed to recurrent attacks, or epilepsy. Thus, the term is traditionally associated with a favorable prognosis. As Chapter 15 discusses, most infantile convulsions are epileptic seizures, but some may have another mechanism (e.g., anoxic convulsions). Theoretically, separating epileptic from nonepileptic convulsions is desirable. However, the adjective *epileptic* is still frightening to many families as it is associated with the idea of a chronic incurable condition; therefore, it is better deleted. Nevertheless, the clinician must still remember that most infantile convulsions are indeed epileptic seizures. As this chapter discusses later, epileptic seizures may occur in nonepileptic persons, and they do not have a grave prognostic significance *per se*, unless complicating factors are associated.

Realizing that, under the right circumstances, the normal human brain is capable of producing epileptic seizures is essential. Many alterations in homeostasis that originate outside of the central nervous system (CNS) can provoke epileptic seizures, especially in children. Epileptic seizures also may occur in quasi-experimental or pathologic conditions such as electroconvulsive therapy, the injection or ingestion of convulsant drugs or toxins, head trauma, or other acute insults to the brain.

Seizures induced by acute cerebral pathology or by extracerebral disturbances are called *occasional seizures* because they occur only in response to pro-voking circumstances. These must be distinguished from epilepsy, which is a spontaneously recurring condition. The classic example of occasional epileptic seizures is that of *febrile convulsions* (see Chapters 14 and 15), which occur only in response to a rise in body temperature. Recurring convulsions that repeatedly occur in response to a known precipitating factor, such as recurrent hypoglycemia, are not regarded as epilepsy.

Epilepsy is an enduring condition, or rather a group of conditions, in which epileptic seizures occur repeatedly without a detectable extracerebral cause (Gastaut, 1973). An individual's tendency to recurrent paroxysmal dysfunction may result primarily from the presence of structural brain abnormalities or from an intrinsic constitutional propensity to have seizures. The nature of that propensity is determined, at least in part, by genetic factors (Hauser and Anderson, 1986) involved in the regulation of neuronal excitability. The current research suggests that changes in the ionic channels play an important role in this regard (see Chapter 20). Genetic (or constitutional) factors and structural abnormalities are often found in various proportions in the same patient, and a complete spectrum of epilepsies ranging from purely "lesional" to purely "functional" epilepsies is encountered. These definitions, however, imply that epilepsy is not an entity since it may result from many causes.

DIFFICULTIES AND LIMITS OF DEFINITIONS

The *definition of epilepsy* is fraught with many difficulties. First, the number of seizures and the duration necessary to satisfy the definition of a recurrent and enduring condition is an arbitrary determination. Most physicians would not make a diagnosis of epilepsy in an individual who has a cluster of seizures within a single episode over one or a few days, even if no obvious precipitant was found. Such episodes, however, may well be the first manifestation of a chronic seizure disorder. This also applies to the occurrence of an isolated seizure (see Chapter 15). On the other hand, most epileptologists do not hesitate to diagnose epilepsy in an individual after a single seizure as long as the attack has the typical features of those observed in well-defined epilepsy syndromes and it is associated with the typical EEG manifestations of that syndrome. For example, a single seizure occurring on awakening in a child who is 5 to 10 years of age that is marked by gurgling noises, drooling, and aphemia and that is associated with a spike focus in one centrotemporal area would be diagnosed as rolandic epilepsy (see Chapter 10). In recent epidemiologic studies (Sander and Sillanpää, 1998; Hauser et al., 1991; Hauser and Kurland, 1975), the occurrence of two seizures, provided they did not occur during the same morbid episode, was accepted as the operational definition of epilepsy. This definition, though convenient, is obviously arbitrary. In other studies (Todt, 1984), the threshold for a diagnosis of epilepsy was set at three attacks.

Thus, no single term such as *epilepsy* can adequately cover the extremely broad spectrum of clinical presentations and the innumerable possible patterns of seizure recurrences. Any single term that is used for so many clinical pictures is bound to be unsatisfactory.

Cases in which paroxysmal EEG activity (often intense) is not associated with clinical seizures in the conventional meaning of the term but with nonparoxysmal, lasting clinical changes pose a special problem, however. Such changes involve mainly cognitive functions or behavior, and the individual presents with intellectual dysfunction or deterioration, as well as learning difficulties, sometimes associated with psychiatric overtones (Gillberg et al., 1996). The deterioration may be global, or it may affect only specific functions, especially language; however, it may also manifest as disturbances in perception (*gnosias*) or executive functions. Chapter 11 provides examples of these conditions, including the Landau-Kleffner syndrome or the syndrome of continuous spike-waves of slow sleep (CSWS) or "electrical status epilepticus of slow sleep" (ESES). Increasing evidence indicates that such lasting changes can be regarded as the equivalent of a clinical seizure despite their nonparoxysmal expression. Deonna (1996) has proposed the use of the term *cognitive epilepsy* for such cases. The cognitive problems may be directly related to the interference of the paroxysmal activity with the normal function of the involved cortical areas, not to structural causes.

Fluctuation in the intensity of these cognitive or behavioral disturbances that varies with that seen in the EEG disturbances and the possible disappearance of these disturbances following the abatement of the EEG paroxysmal activity are arguments for a functional origin for these disturbances. However, the regression of abnormalities may be only partial, such that prolonged functional changes seem capable of inducing lasting, irreversible effects (Aicardi, 1999a).

Another difficulty with the definition of epilepsy is that it assumes that seizures in this condition are unprovoked events. Commonsense thinking indicates that, for all seizures, factors that precipitate the attack

and factors that contribute to arresting it must exist. Some of the precipitating factors, such as intermittent photic stimulation, certain sounds, or lack of sleep, are known (see Chapter 17). Many more precipitating factors are as yet unknown, or they are only imperfectly described, while still others are only suspected. Stress (Friis, 1990; Aird, 1988), psychologic factors, and fatigue are probably responsible for precipitating a sizeable proportion of epileptic seizures, but the exact nature of these stimuli and their mechanisms of action in producing epilepsy remain unexplored. Most seizures likely have a multifactorial origin. Patients with a focal brain lesion may convulse only when excessive or abnormal sensory stimulation is applied to the part of the body corresponding to the lesion (e.g., a stump after the amputation of one limb [Symonds, 1959]).

In general, the production of a seizure probably requires a brain lesion, a genetic predisposition, or both, with its resulting hyperexcitability on the one hand and afferent stimuli of either cerebral or extracerebral origin on the other. The state of the brain and its excitability is therefore influenced by both intrinsic factors, such as circadian rhythms, stress, or the state of vigilance, and extrinsic factors that may be neural or of another nature. The source of some of those extrinsic influxes may well be extracerebral. Therefore, a fever; a disturbance in an individual's water balance; or hormonal factors, especially those seen with the ovulatory cycle in women (Mattson et al., 1981; Schmidt, 1981) can provoke or inhibit the occurrence of seizures in certain patients with epilepsy. When observed from this perspective, the dividing line between occasional epileptic seizures and epilepsy becomes immaterial. In practice, the proper classification of a number of seizures is often arbitrary. An adolescent with two or three attacks occurring only in response to flickering lights or television receives a diagnosis of photogenic epilepsy, whereas, in a child with numerous febrile convulsions, the label of epilepsy is avoided. The issue with unprovoked events may become even more difficult for those patients who have both occasional and "unprovoked" epileptic attacks in succession. The most common example of such a combination is the child who has one or a few febrile convulsions and then who later has a limited number of afebrile seizures (see Chapters 9 and 14).

Such difficulties of classification indicate that *epilepsy is not necessarily an all-or-none phenomenon.* Rather, a continuous variation in the threshold for seizures exists, with the severe repeated type representing one end and the occasional seizure, the other. Occasional seizures, in turn, can have a recognized cause, or they can apparently be unprovoked. The latter case corresponds to the single-seizure problem (see Chapter 15). This absence of a precise borderline between epilepsy and convulsions is of practical importance, as labeling any individual as having *epilepsy* is better avoided in any dubious case because of the dread that is still attached to this word.

INFLUENCE OF AGE ON CHILDHOOD EPILEPSY

In children, the factors of age, growth, and development are of primary importance in determining not only whether epilepsy is developing (O'Donohoe, 1985) but also what the clinical and electrical manifestations of the seizures are and the type of seizure disorders that will be encountered. Age is generally recognized as an important determinant of the prognosis for the disorder (Sillanpää, 1990, 2000; Chevrie and Aicardi, 1978), although this is not universally accepted (Ellenberg et al., 1984). Even within the same epilepsy syndrome (e.g., infantile spasms), a young age at onset compared with the average for the syndrome is an unfavorable predictor of prognosis. In some syndromes (e.g., absence epilepsy), cases of early onset (before 3 years of age) or of late onset (after 8 to 9 years of age) have a substantially poorer prognosis than do those with an onset between 4 and 8 years of age (see Chapter 8). Similarly, age has a strong influence on the outcome of status epilepticus. Sequelae are more common in those younger than 2 to 3 years than they are in older patients.

The metabolism of anticonvulsant medication also depends on the patient's age (see Chapter 24). The absorption, protein binding, clearance, and apparent half-life of antiepileptic drugs vary at different periods of life. In general, neonates metabolize anticonvulsant drugs slowly, and they become easily intoxicated. After a few weeks, the rate of metabolism of most drugs increases such that optimum blood levels are difficult to attain, even with the use of large doses. Thereafter, the dose requirements progressively diminish as the metabolism of drugs slowly becomes less rapid. These changes, however, are not necessarily advantageous. For instance, at adolescence, a sudden slowing down of the metabolism may occur, resulting in the inadvertent overdosage of these patients (Morselli et al., 1983).

Four main periods of age can be distinguished in childhood epilepsy (Aicardi, 1985a). The *neonatal period* extends from birth to approximately 3 months of age, exceeding the conventional limit of 4 weeks.

This period is characterized by the predominance of seizures that are caused by structural pathology; consequently, these have a severe prognosis. Febrile seizures are *not* observed during the first 3 or 4 months of life. If a neonate has fits that are associated with fever, the clinician should search diligently for an intracranial infection. The clinical expression of neonatal seizures is different from that encountered in older patients; these seizures tend to be fragmentary and erratic, and bilateral tonic-clonic seizures are virtually never observed. *The period that extends between 3 months and 3 to 4 years of age* is remarkable because of the high susceptibility of the CNS to a number of extrinsic changes, particularly fever. The occurrence of occasional seizures is concentrated in this period. Certain specific types of seizures are limited to this period, or they may have their onset during this period; most notably, these include infantile spasms and most cases of myoclonic epilepsy and Lennox-Gastaut syndrome. Most of the chronic seizure disorders of this period are also associated with structural lesions, although this mainly applies to the epilepsies that evolve during the first or second year of life. *The third period*, which begins at 3 and 4 years and continues to early adolescence, is marked by the predominance of the epilepsies of cryptogenic origin. In most cases, genetic factors are important in the causation of these epilepsies, while structural brain damage is less common. This is the period during which certain well-defined epilepsy syndromes, such as absence epilepsy (petit mal) or benign rolandic epilepsy, make their appearance, and spike-wave complexes at 3 Hz are most commonly observed, although the latter may rarely evolve earlier (Aicardi, 1995). Complex partial seizures become well defined in children in this age bracket, and their apparent frequency increases. Occasional seizures, on the other hand, are rare, and those that occur are associated with major metabolic disturbances, not simply with fever. *The final period*, which includes children 9 to 10 years of age and older, is characterized by the emergence of "primary generalized epilepsy," with its tonic-clonic seizures that are often associated with myoclonic jerks (benign juvenile myoclonic epilepsy). In this period, the transient partial epilepsies of childhood and some of the epilepsies characterized by absence attacks disappear. Furthermore, the partial epilepsies associated with brain damage, especially those expressed by partial seizures, steadily increase in frequency as the result of exposure to a variety of insults, especially those that are traumatic. Such a division into four periods is clearly schematic, and broad overlap of the periods and numerous exceptions are encountered. However, the scheme is useful for general orientation in diagnosis, as well as for prognostic purposes.

The physiopathologic changes underlying the modifications in the clinical expression of seizures with age are poorly understood (Aicardi, 1980c). The increase in complexity of synaptic connections, the various degrees of development of inhibitory versus excitatory systems, and the changes in the synthesis of neurotransmitters with increasing age are certainly essential. For more details, see specialized reviews (Pierson and Swann, 1999; Moshé, 1993; Prince and Connors, 1986; Moshé and Albala, 1983).

SUMMARY

Epilepsy is a chronic condition that is characterized by the repeated occurrence of epileptic seizures. Epileptic seizures can occur in nonepileptic patients who have been subjected to a variety of stresses and stimuli, so the occurrence of solitary seizures or of seizures that are regularly induced by precipitating factors should not be diagnosed as epilepsy. Attacks provoked by extracerebral factors (occasional seizures) are extremely common in children, especially in those between the ages of 6 months to 4 years, in whom the main precipitant is fever. Epileptic seizures differ from other types of paroxysmal attacks by their clinical expression and mechanism. The latter is postulated to be an excessive and abnormal discharge of a more or less extensive assembly of neurons. This excessive activity is expressed on the EEG by the epileptic discharge, which generally is inferred more from clinical manifestations than from an actual recording. An epileptic discharge is not always associated with clinical manifestation, and it is not necessary for the diagnosis of epilepsy. Consequently, the diagnosis of both epileptic seizures and epilepsy is based primarily on clinical history, even though the EEG has been and still remains a powerful tool in the investigation of patients with epileptic seizures.

2

Classification of Epileptic Seizures and Epilepsies

The need for a comprehensive classification of epileptic phenomena has been increasingly recognized. According to Masland (1974), "the development of a uniform and generally accepted classification of disease is an essential step in the understanding of the underlying processes and in establishing communication through which the results of scientific investigation may be compared and evaluated." Classification of epileptic phenomena is also of practical importance, as medication should be prescribed according to seizure type and syndrome. However, no single code can cover the multiple aspects (e.g., clinical, electroencephalographic [EEG], etiologic, and anatomic) of the various epilepsies (Aicardi, 1986a), and the limited knowledge of the medical community regarding their basic mechanisms does not permit classification based on the physiopathology of the disorder.

Empiric classifications of epilepsies are possible only if they are limited to one aspect of the condition. For example, one might construct classifications based on the etiology of epilepsy (symptomatic versus idiopathic or genetic), the topographic origin of the seizures and the location of the responsible lesion (e.g., insular or occipital epilepsy), or the presumed mechanisms (e.g., corticoreticular or "centrencephalic" epilepsy) (Gloor et al., 1990; Gloor, 1979). Such classifications, however, are not mutually exclusive. Any classification used is inherently imperfect, reflecting primarily the need of its user. For instance, a neurosurgeon working with epilepsy requires a topographic classification, whereas pediatricians or neurologists prefer a system based on the clinical presentation of the attacks or on their course and outcome.

The empiric classification of *epileptic seizure types* has proven more accessible because it avoids the insuperable difficulties that are associated with the attempts to classify the multiple chronic disorders that are characterized by the recurrent seizures that comprise the epilepsies. An ad hoc committee of the International League Against Epilepsy (ILAE) accepted a first classification of epileptic seizures in 1969 (Gastaut, 1969a).

INTERNATIONAL LEAGUE AGAINST EPILEPSY SEIZURE CLASSIFICATIONS

The 1969 Classification

The 1969 ILAE seizure classification scheme was based on the following six criteria: clinical seizure type, EEG seizure type, EEG interictal expression, anatomic substrate, etiology, and age (Table 2.1). The four main groups that it included were partial seizures, generalized seizures, unilateral or predominantly unilateral seizures, and unclassified epileptic seizures. *Partial seizures* were defined as those in which the first clinical symptoms indicated the activation of an anatomic and/or functional system of neurons that was limited to a part of a single hemisphere with a correspondingly localized EEG discharge. Partial seizures were further subdivided into the following two subgroups: those with elementary (simple partial seizures) symptomatology and those with complex (complex partial seizures) symptomatology. The term *simple* or *elementary* referred to those seizures involving disturbances of the primary motor, sensory, or similar cortical areas. The term *complex* referred to those seizures involving higher level functions in the widest sense and arising in the so-called *association* or *interpretative cortex*, which subserves more elaborate functions than those supported by the primary areas. *Generalized seizures* were defined as those in which the first clinical changes indicated an initial involvement of both hemispheres. They included several subgroups involving either convulsive or nonconvulsive manifestations.

The 1981 Classification

The 1969 ILAE classification was revised in 1981 (Commission on Classification and Terminology of the International League Against Epilepsy, 1981). The 1981 revision (Table 2.2) classified seizures on the basis of only two criteria: the clinical features and the EEG features of the seizures. In this scheme, partial seizures were subdivided into simple and complex seizures, a division that depended exclusively on the

TABLE 2.1. *International League Against Epilepsy (1969) classification of epileptic seizures*

Partial seizures (or seizures beginning locally)
Partial seizures with elementary symptomatology (generally without impairment of consciousness)
    With motor symptoms: focal motor, jacksonian, versive, postural, somatic inhibitory (?), aphasic, phonatory
    With special sensory or somatosensory symptoms: somatosensory, visual, auditory, olfactory, gustatory, vertiginous
    With autonomic symptoms
    Compound forms
Partial seizures with complex symptomatology
    With impaired consciousness alone
    With cognitive symptomatology
        With dysmnesic disturbances (conscious amnesia, déjà vu, déjà vécu)
        With ideational disturbances (including "forced thinking"), dreamy state
    With affective symptomatology
    With psychosensory symptomatology
        Illusions (e.g., macropsia, metamorphopsia)
        Hallucinations
    With psychomotor symptomatology: automatisms
    Compound forms
Partial seizures secondarily generalized
Generalized seizures (bilateral symmetric seizures or seizures without local onset)
Absences
    Simple absences, with impairment of consciousness only
        Typical, with 3-Hz spike-wave discharge
        Atypical, with fast rhythms or slow spike-waves
    Complex absences, with other phenomena associated with impairment of consciousness; may be typical or atypical as in simple absences
        Myoclonic
        Hypertonic
        Atonic
        Automatic
        Autonomic
    Mixed forms
Bilateral massive epileptic myoclonus: myoclonic jerks
Infantile spasms
Clonic seizures
Tonic seizures
Tonic-clonic seizures: grand mal seizures
Atonic seizures, sometimes associated with myoclonic jerks (myoclonic-atonic seizures) (a) of a very brief duration (epileptic drop attacks); (b) of longer duration (including atonic absences)
Akinetic seizures
Unilateral or predominantly unilateral seizures
Unclassified epileptic seizures, including all seizures that cannot be classified because of inadequate data

state of consciousness during the attacks. Simple partial seizures are those during which "consciousness is preserved," while complex partial seizures are those during which consciousness is absent or disturbed.

The 1981 revision emphasized that different types of seizure may evolve in temporal succession in the same patient. For instance, a simple partial seizure (which may be motor or which may have cognitive or other psychic manifestations) can be followed by a complex partial one (i.e., with impairment of consciousness), a generalized seizure, or a sequence of both (Overweg et al., 1987; Porter, 1983a). The category of *unilateral seizures* was dropped from the 1981 revision because these only represented partial

seizures with more extensive diffusion. Akinetic seizures and compound, or mixed, seizures were also omitted. The 1981 revision further excluded infantile spasms from the category of generalized seizures. Infantile spasms were considered an epilepsy syndrome, rather than a type of seizure, even though the spasms, which may also occur in older patients, undoubtedly represent a peculiar type of seizure (Egli et al., 1985) with specific electroclinical features.

However, many criticisms have been directed at this scheme (Engel, 2001; Lüders et al., 1993a, 1998; Porter, 1983a). First, as Gloor (1986) emphasized, consciousness is a highly complex concept whose de-

TABLE 2.2. *International League Against Epilepsy (1981) revised classification of epileptic seizures*

Partial (focal, local) seizures
Simple partial seizures
    With motor signs: focal, motor, jacksonian, versive, postural, phonatory
    With autonomic symptoms and signs
    With somatosensory or special sensory symptoms (simple hallucinations [e.g., tingling, light flashes, buzzing]): somatosensory, visual, auditory, olfactory, gustatory, vertiginous
    With psychic symptoms (disturbances of higher cerebral functions): dysphasic, dysmnesic, cognitive, affective, illusions, structured hallucinations
Complex partial seizures (with impairment of consciousness; may sometimes begin with simple symptomatology)
    Simple partial: onset followed by impairment of consciousness
    With simple partial features (A_1-A_4) followed by impaired consciousness
    With automatisms
Partial seizures evolving to secondarily generalized tonic-clonic (GTC) seizures
    Simple partial seizures evolving to GTC
    Complex partial seizures evolving to GTC
    Simple partial seizures evolving to complex partial seizures, evolving to GTC
Generalized seizures[a]
Absence seizures with impairment of consciousness, with clonic, atonic, tonic, or autonomic components, or with automatisms occurring alone or in combination
Atypical absences, more pronounced changes of tone than in absence seizures; onset and/or cessation not abrupt
Myoclonic seizures (single or multiple)
Clonic seizures
Tonic seizures
Tonic-clonic seizures
Atonic seizures

[a]Combinations of the seizures listed here may occur.

finition and assessment are extremely difficult. In the glossary appended to the 1981 revision, *consciousness* was defined as "the degree of awareness and/or responsiveness of the patient to externally applied stimuli." *Responsiveness* was defined as "the ability of the patient to carry out simple commands or willed movements," and *awareness* as "the patient's contact with events during the period in question." These restricted definitions do not consider other important aspects of consciousness such as awareness of "self" or amnesic retention. In the new definitions, the term *complex* is used to designate those partial seizures that are associated with the impairment of consciousness, whether or not they begin with elementary symptoms (motor or otherwise) or with symptoms previously termed *complex*. Seizures with dysphasic, dysmnesic, cognitive, and affective manifestations are now classified as simple partial seizures as long as consciousness is not disturbed.

The second problem is that some of the concepts were derived from unproven assumptions. For example, labeling a seizure as *generalized* implies that it involves the whole of the cortex from onset, a concept that has yet to be proven; an apparently generalized seizure can result from the propagation of an initial focal discharge that is either too brief or too deeply located to be detected. Conversely, partial attacks may be related to temporary differences in excitability between the two hemispheres, which would thus explain the asymmetric expression of a seizure that, under other circumstances, would be symmetric (Gastaut et al., 1986a; Gastaut and Broughton, 1972).

Third, from the viewpoint of the pediatric neurologist, the classification neglects the all-important factor of age, which is essential for diagnosis and prognosis of seizure disorders in infancy and childhood.

Despite the controversy among epileptologists about the definitions of some seizure types in the 1981 revision of the ILAE classification of epileptic seizures (Bodensteiner et al., 1988; Aird et al., 1984; Parsonage, 1983), the general principles of this classification of seizures have been widely accepted.

New Proposals for Seizure Classification

As a result of recent progresses in epileptology, the need for a new approach to classification of seizures is understandable. Although no final classification of seizures has been universally accepted, both a revision of the terminology of seizures and a list of the generally recognized seizure types that avoids some of the dichotomous classifications previously used have been proposed (Engel, 2001).

A recently proposed classification scheme for epileptic seizures that is based exclusively on ictal clinical semiology has been presented (Noachtar and Lüders, 2000; Lüders et al., 1993a, 1998). The advantage of this scheme is that it avoids the need to establish a one-to-one relationship between a type of seizure and a particular EEG paroxysmal abnormality. It also provides a means for systematically describing seizures. Ictal symptoms can involve the following four "spheres" or domains: sensory domain, consciousness, autonomic sphere, and/or motor sphere. A simplified presentation of this proposal is given in Table 2.3. This scheme does not include any theoretical assumptions, and it constitutes a system for methodical and standardized descriptions of seizures and a descriptive glossary of the possible

types, rather than a classification proper. It allows the clinician to add somatotopic "modifiers" that, when appropriate, permit definition of the somatotopic distribution of ictal symptoms to the various types of seizures that are listed. This classification can also be applied to infantile seizures (Hamer et al., 1999).

EPILEPSY CLASSIFICATION

Classification of the *epilepsies*, not only of seizures, clearly is even more difficult than the classification of *seizures*. In addition to the descriptive elements in classification of seizures, a classification of epilepsies should incorporate some indication of the cause of the disorder, the age at occurrence, the features associated with the seizures, localization, and other aspects. In actuality, a classification that is adapted to the needs of the neurosurgeon cannot coincide with that aimed at the basic scientist. A classification of diseases is not possible as only a few epileptic disease entities have been identified (e.g.,

TABLE 2.3. *Proposed classification of epileptic seizures (Lüders et al., 1993a, 1998)*

Aura (consists exclusively of subjective symptoms)
  Somatomotor[a]
  Auditory[a] (includes complex hallucinations and illusions that affect other senses)
  Olfactory
  Visual[a] (includes complex multimodal hallucinations)
  Gustatory
  Autonomic[a] (purely subjective autonomic sensations)
  Psychic (includes complex hallucinations and illusions that affect other senses)
  Abdominal aura
Autonomic seizures (only with objective autonomic dysfunction)
Dialeptic seizures[b] (alteration of consciousness whatever electroencephalogram and mechanism)
Motor seizures[a]
  Simple motor[a] (unnatural movements resembling those produced by stimulation of areas 4 or 6)
  Myoclonic seizures[a]
  Epileptic spasms[a] (may occur after infancy)
  Tonic-clonic seizures
  Tonic seizures[a]
  Clonic seizures[a]
  Versive seizures[a] (contralateral or ipsilateral)
  Complex motor[b] (refers to movements that simulate natural movements)
  Hypermotor[b] (complex mostly proximal, often violent)
  Automotor[b] (refers to mostly distal, mouth or tongue, consciousness variable)
  Gelastic (those that cannot be included in the aforementioned categories)
Special seizures
  Atonic[a] (often preceded by short myoclonic seizure)
  Hypomotor[b] (decreased or total absence of motor activity; only when consciousness not assessable)
  Negative myoclonus[a]
  Astatic
  Akinetic[a] (inability to perform voluntary movement)
  Aphasic[b]
  Paroxysmal events (not sufficient evidence to assume epileptic nature)

[a]May be localized to left or right, axial, generalized, bilateral asymmetric.
[b]May rise from left or right hemisphere.

tuberous sclerosis, neuronal ceroid lipofuscinoses), so the classification of epilepsy must remain at the more accessible level of syndromes. Over the past two decades, the tendency to concentrate efforts on the delineation of recognizable *epilepsy syndromes,* rather than to try to construct a complete classification of the epilepsies has been growing.

The ILAE has adopted an International Classification of Epilepsies and Epileptic Syndromes (Table 2.4) that is based in large part on the delineation of

TABLE 2.4. *Proposed classification of epilepsies[a] and epilepsy syndromes*

Localization-related (focal, local, partial) epilepsies and epileptic syndromes
Idiopathic (with age-related onset)
    Benign childhood epilepsy with centrotemporal spikes
    Childhood epilepsy with occipital paroxysms
    Primary reading epilepsy
Symptomatic
    Chronic progressive epilepsia partialis continua of childhood (Kojewnikow syndrome)
    Syndromes characterized by seizures with specific modes of precipitation (include partial seizures
      following acquired lesions, usually involving tactile or proprioceptive stimuli; partial seizures precipitated
      by sudden arousal or startle epilepsy)
    Temporal lobe epilepsies
    Frontal lobe epilepsies
    Parietal lobe epilepsies
    Occipital lobe epilepsies
Cryptogenic[b]
Generalized epilepsies and syndromes
Idiopathic (with age-related onset)
    Benign neonatal familial convulsions
    Benign neonatal convulsions
    Benign myoclonic epilepsy in infancy
    Childhood absence epilepsy (pyknolepsy)
    Juvenile absence epilepsy
    Juvenile myoclonic epilepsy (impulsive petit mal[c])
    Epilepsy with grand mal seizures on awakening
    Other generalized epilepsies (not defined above)
    Epilepsies with seizures precipitated by specific modes of activation
Cryptogenic or symptomatic
    West syndrome (infantile spasms, Blitz-Nick-Salaam Krämpfe)
    Lennox-Gastaut syndrome
    Epilepsy with myoclonic-astatic seizures[d]
    Epilepsy with myoclonic absences
Symptomatic
    Nonspecific etiology
      Early myoclonic encephalopathy
      Early infantile epileptic encephalopathy with suppression-burst electroencephalogram
      Other symptomatic generalized epilepsies not defined above
    Specific syndromes (including diseases in which seizures are a presenting or predominant feature)
Epilepsies and epileptic syndromes undetermined whether focal or generalized
With both generalized and focal seizures
    Neonatal seizures
    Severe myoclonic epilepsy in infancy
    Epilepsy with continuous spike-waves during slow-wave sleep
    Acquired epileptic aphasia (Landau-Kleffner syndrome)
    Other undermined epilepsies not defined above
Without unequivocal generalized or focal features
Special syndromes: situation-related seizures
    Febrile convulsions
    Isolated seizures or isolated status epilepticus
    Seizures occurring only when there is an acute metabolic or toxic event

[a]Commission on Classification and Terminology of the International League Against Epilepsy (1989).
[b]Cryptogenic epilepsies are defined as "presumed to be symptomatic and the aetiology is unknown"; they differ from symptomatic epilepsies only by the lack of etiologic evidence. Etymologically, cryptogenic signifies that the cause is hidden, which also applies to so-called idiopathic epilepsies.
[c]The term *petit mal* would be better abandoned altogether.
[d]Probably identical to some myoclonic epilepsies. Criteria of definition are different (see Chapter 6).

epilepsy syndromes (Commission on Classification and Terminology of the International League Against Epilepsy, 1985, 1989).

Current Classification of Epilepsy Syndromes

Epilepsy syndromes are clusters of signs and symptoms customarily occurring together (Commission on Classification and Terminology of the International League Against Epilepsy, 1989; Aicardi, 1988b). The signs and symptoms may include the type of seizure, the mode of seizure recurrence, neurologic findings, and neuroradiologic or other findings of special investigations. A syndrome can have more than one cause, and, consequently, it may have different outcomes (e.g., West syndrome with both cryptogenic and symptomatic types).

Epilepsy syndromes may belong to different orders. Some of these represent rather broad concepts, while others are much more specific. Some syndromes, such as benign centrotemporal (rolandic) epilepsy, comprise not only common clinical and EEG signs and symptoms, but they also have a predictable course and, consistently, they are shown not to be associated with structural brain abnormalities. This syndrome likely has a single major genetic cause (see Chapter 10). Other syndromes, such as absence epilepsy, are less specific; these can variably be regarded as a single syndrome including all epilepsies that feature typical absences or as several subgroups with different outcomes and different associated features (see Chapter 8). Still other syndromes are actually rather loose collections of a few symptoms or signs that have relatively poor links (e.g., awakening grand mal). Overlap of one syndrome with, or the inclusion of one syndrome into, another syndrome frequently occurs. If the concept of epilepsy syndromes is to be practical and useful, it should be limited to those clusters of signs and symptoms that are characteristic enough to be agreed on by a majority of neurologists. Relatively heterogeneous syndromes such as typical absence epilepsy or West syndrome provide only limited indications as to a patient's prognosis. However, they do have practical significance in other areas because the identification of these syndromes is a guide to the likely causes of the epilepsy disorder, the investigations to be performed for diagnosis, and the drugs indicated for correction of the syndrome.

The ILAE classification uses two other sets of criteria concurrently. One set is topographic, which leads to a dichotomy between generalized and partial epilepsies; the latter were renamed as *localization-related* epilepsies. The other set of criteria is based on the etiology of the disorder; in its latest form, it separates the epilepsies of known causes (*symptomatic* or *secondary* epilepsies) from both those that are probably the results of some undetermined brain disorder (*cryptogenic epilepsy* [from the Greek word κρυπτος meaning *a hidden cause*]) and those that are not due to any brain lesion or disease other than a possible genetic propensity to generate seizures. This last type is termed *idiopathic* (from the Greek word ιδιος meaning *proper*), indicating that, in such cases, the epilepsy is a disease that is not secondary to any other condition. The terms *genuine, essential*, and *primary* epilepsy are sometimes used with the same meaning.

Merits and Problems of These Classifications

A classification based on syndromes has the advantage of dispensing with most assumptions that are necessary with other systems. It also has the following disadvantages:

1. It cannot cover all of the aspects of epilepsy because it systematically favors the clinical and EEG features of epileptic conditions at the expense of pathophysiology, etiologic factors, precipitating factors, or the rate of recurrence of seizures. A syndrome with similar EEG and clinical manifestations may have different causes, and the course, treatment, and prognosis, which may differ depending on the etiology, may thus require separate consideration.

2. Although some of the dichotomies proposed (e.g., generalized vs. partial or idiopathic vs. symptomatic) are of pragmatic value, they probably are not entirely justifiable from a pathophysiologic point of view; in some cases, they may also be difficult to use.

3. The number and the precise features of tentative syndromes inevitably cause disagreement. Some clinicians accept only the most specific syndromes. Such an approach does increase the practical usefulness in terms of prognosis or therapy of the syndromes delineated but leaves a larger number of cases unclassified. Others are less restrictive, with opposite results.

New Proposals

In the past few years, the difficulties associated with any classification of syndromes have been increasingly recognized, so a special task force of the ILAE was set up to tackle this problem. The proposals of this group were recently published (Engel,

2001). In addition, some changes to the previously used terms were made. For instance, the term *focal* is preferred to *partial* or *localization-related* seizures. The term *probably symptomatic* was proposed as a replacement to *cryptogenic* because the latter was rightly thought to be ambiguous. Furthermore, the words *convulsion* and *convulsive* were considered nonspecific, so the term *motor seizures* was substituted for these. However, the authors of this text believe that these terms are too deeply rooted among pediatricians to be easily eliminated at this time.

The new proposal recommends a complex system based on the construction of glossaries or lists of seizures, syndromes, and diseases, rather than on the previous dichotomous classification scheme. It is proposed as "a diagnostic scheme, rather than a fixed classification" that is intended to "provide the basis for a standardized description of individual patients." A single system was considered impossible, so the proposed system consists of the following five axes:

Axis 1: ictal phenomenology (glossary to describe ictal events)
Axis 2: seizure types (list of recognized seizure types)
Axis 3: syndromes (list of epilepsy syndromes with the realization that definite classification is not always possible)
Axis 4: etiology (list of diseases often associated with seizures or epilepsy)
Axis 5: impairment resulting from disease (optional)

However, the terms *generalized* and *idiopathic* or *symptomatic* are still included in the list of seizures and syndromes even though they are no longer the basis for fixed dichotomies. Indeed, although their pathophysiologic significance may be limited and differentiating epilepsies into these categories is not always possible, the practical value of these terms is difficult to contest. Individual syndromes are not meant to be "organized into a fixed dichotomous classification but rather categorized on various ways for various purposes" (Engel, 2001).

This proposed scheme is a major departure from the 1989 classification, and it introduces a flexibility that had been seriously compromised by the previous attempts. Clearly, as the current proposal acknowledges, any classification must remain open to dynamic changes and the lists mentioned should not be considered as definitive or exclusive. Furthermore, in no case should they be regarded as a substitute for scientific evidence that is presented in complete form with adequate discussion.

SUMMARY

The individualization and description of epilepsy syndromes is of great practical value for diagnosis, the choice of investigations to be performed, decisions about management, and prognostic purposes. Most of the following chapters contain a description of the major epilepsy syndromes of infancy, childhood, and adolescence. Each of these begins with the description of one major *type of seizure*, such as generalized seizures, typical absence seizures, or focal seizures. Following an overall description of the attacks and their incidence, diagnosis, and causes, the chapter describes the epilepsy syndromes that feature this particular type of seizure as their exclusive or predominant paroxysmal clinical manifestation. This approach conforms to clinical practice in which the first step is the identification of the type (or types) of seizure, followed by the classification of particular cases into epilepsy syndromes on the basis of any associated signs, the age at onset, the course of the disorder, and other clinical and EEG information. The various syndromes proposed are considered in a critical manner, and their significance is evaluated. Within each broad category of seizures, individual epilepsy syndromes are classified according to their age at emergence, cause, or peculiar clinical features. For example, for typical absence seizures, the childhood and juvenile types are dealt with in succession. In those cases where a single seizure type has a markedly different clinical significance depending on the age at onset (e.g., myoclonic seizures), separate sections are dedicated to each age group.

The descriptions of the various epilepsy syndromes in infancy, childhood, and adolescence are given in order of increasing age wherever possible because several epileptic syndromes are strongly age dependent and age is therefore an essential consideration in diagnosis.

Some important aspects of the epilepsies of childhood cannot be covered simply by a description of the seizure types or epilepsy syndromes. These include epilepsies resulting from brain tumors, abnormalities of cortical development, and other selected lesions; epilepsies occurring during the first 2 years of life; and the group of sensory-precipitated epilepsies. These epilepsies may present with different clinical syndromes; they are united by their cause, their age at occurrence, or provoking factors, rather than by their clinical or EEG manifestations. Their particular aspects are studied following the description of the main epilepsy syndromes (see Section III).

3

Infantile Spasms and Related Syndromes

Infantile spasms (ISs) are a unique form of seizure disorder, the occurrence of which is limited almost entirely to infants during the first year of life and that is refractory to conventional anticonvulsant drugs. ISs are usually associated with developmental retardation or deterioration and a characteristic electroencephalographic (EEG) pattern (*hypsarrhythmia*) that together configure a syndrome that is also known as *West syndrome*. The seizure type, regardless of the age and clinical context in which it is manifested, is defined as an *epileptic spasm* (Schwarztzkroin and Rao, 2002; Dulac et al., 1994); it may also occur in childhood or even in adult patients, although this is seen much more rarely than in infants (de Menezes and Rho, 2002; Cerullo et al., 1999; Bednarek et al., 1998; Egli et al., 1985; Ikeno et al., 1985).

In the 1969 international classification, *ISs* were classified as one type of generalized epileptic seizure (Gastaut, 1969a). The 1981 revision (Commission on Classification and Terminology of the International League against Epilepsy, 1981) dropped the use of the term both because various seizure patterns can occur with the syndrome and because the global picture, rather than the attacks themselves, was thought characteristic.

Often, ISs have been included in the group of myoclonic seizures as massive myoclonic attacks (Chariton, 1975) or in that of *minor motor seizures* (obsolete term) (Livingston et al., 1958). However, the typical muscle contraction in ISs reaches its maximum more slowly than in a myoclonic jerk, and it decreases in a manner that is equally as slow (Fusco and Vigevano, 1993), although it is not as slow and as sustained as that observed in tonic seizures. Moreover, by no means, are ISs of *minor* significance.

West syndrome is used synonymously with *ISs*. The use of this eponym calls attention to the unsurpassed description of the syndrome by West in his own son in 1841 (see Duncan, 2001).

CLINICAL AND ELECTROENCEPHALOGRAPHIC CHARACTERISTICS OF THE SYNDROME

Seizures

ISs involve a sudden, generally bilateral and symmetric contraction of the muscles of the neck, trunk,

and extremities. The type of seizure that occurs depends on what muscles (the flexor or extensor) are predominantly affected and on the extent of the contraction. *Flexor spasms* have long been regarded as the most characteristic type of seizure, and thus, they have been predominantly featured in naming the syndrome (*syndrome des spasmes en flexion, jackknife convulsions, salaam seizures, Grusskrämpfe*). They consist of a sudden flexion of the head, trunk, and legs, which are usually held in adduction. The arms, also in flexion, can be adducted or abducted. In three studies (Lombroso, 1983a; Kellaway et al., 1983; Lacy and Penry, 1976), flexor spasms represented 34%, 39%, and 42%, respectively, of the cases. Mixed flexor-extensor spasms, accounting for 42%, 47%, and 50% of the cases, were the most common type. These consist either of flexion of the neck, trunk, and arms with extension of the legs or, less commonly, of flexion of the legs and extension of the arms with varying degrees of flexion of the neck and trunk. *Extensor spasms*, which involve an abrupt extension of the neck and trunk accompanied by extension and abduction of the arms, are less common (23%, 24%, and 19%, respectively); only rarely do they represent the sole type of seizure in any particular infant (Lombroso, 1983b; Jeavons and Bower, 1974). Most infants with ISs have more than one type of spasm.

The intensity of the contractions and the number of muscle groups involved vary considerably both in different infants and in the same infant with different attacks. The spasms may consist of only slight head nodding, upward eye deviation, or elevation and adduction of the shoulders in a shrugging movement. In some cases, the spasms may be so slight that they can be felt but not seen, or they may be clinically unnoticeable, even though they do appear on polygraphic recordings (Kellaway et al., 1979, 1983; Gastaut et al., 1964). The number of spasms is vastly in excess of what parents record in these infants (Kellaway et al., 1979; Gaily et al., 2001). No apparent correlation exists between the overall prognosis and intensity of the spasms, although full-fledged attacks may tend to occur in cryptogenic cases (Dulac et al., 1986a). According to Kellaway et al. (1979), the muscle action tracing in an IS consists of an abrupt initial contraction lasting less than 2 seconds, followed by a more sustained contraction lasting 2 to 10 seconds. The second, or tonic, phase may be absent, with the spasm, in these cases, being limited to an initial phasic contraction lasting 0.5 seconds or less. The contraction may have a diamond shape on electromyographic records (Fusco and Vigevano, 1993; Egli et al., 1985). A cry is common at the time of, or just after, the spasm. Spasms are often followed by a brief episode of akinesia and diminished responsiveness that is termed *arrest*; this may also occur in the absence of a spasm (Donat, 1992; Lombroso, 1983b; Kellaway et al., 1979).

In 6% to 8% of patients (Lombroso, 1983a; Kellaway et al., 1979), the spasms may be unilateral, often with an adversive element, or they can be clearly asymmetric. Asymmetric spasms are associated with a symptomatic etiology; unilateral lesions, however, are often associated with symmetric attacks.

Asymmetric spasms may occur after a partial seizure that apparently triggers a series of spasms that are accompanied by special EEG concomitants (Yamamoto et al., 1988; Abou-Khalil et al., 1987) (see last paragraph of this section). Consistently asymmetric spasms were observed in 19% and 25% of children in two series (Gaily et al., 1995; Kramer et al., 1997).

Lateralized motor phenomena, including eye deviation, lateral upward eye deviation, eyebrow contraction, and abduction of one shoulder, may sometimes constitute the entire series of spasms, or they may initiate a series that eventually develops into bilateral phenomena. Such lateralized manifestations are usually accompanied by unilateral or asymmetric ictal EEG changes.

Individual spasms are grouped characteristically in series or clusters. The clusters can include as little as a few units to more than 100 individual jerks occurring from 5 to 30 seconds apart. The intensity of the jerks in a series may initially wax and wane, although not always regularly. Rare cases of status of ISs have been reported (Coulter, 1986). The repetitive character of the spasms is a highly important diagnostic clue. In a young infant, even very mild or atypical phenomena (e.g., head nodding, eye elevation, and movement of one limb) occurring repetitively should arouse the suspicion of ISs.

Brief interruptions of consciousness probably occur at the time of the jerks. Respiratory irregularities; crying at the end of a cluster; flushing; abnormal eye movements, such as nystagmus or tonic upward or lateral eye deviation; smiling; or grimacing are observed in one-third to one-half of the attacks. Laughter is occasionally noted (Matsumoto et al., 1981a; Fukuyama, 1960; Druckman and Chao, 1955). The number of series can vary from only 1 to 50 or more daily (Lacy and Penry, 1976; Jeavons and Bower, 1964). Clusters may occur during sleep, usually at the time of awakening or during the transition from slow to rapid eye movement (REM) sleep (Plouin et al., 1987). They are also frequent in drowsiness, and no obvious stimulus precipitates them. After a series of spasms, the infant may be exhausted and lethargic. Conversely, a brief period of increased alertness that appears to correlate with a brief period of improved background activity in the EEG may also be observed (Lombroso, 1983; Gastaut et al., 1964).

ISs may be infrequent at the onset of the disorder. Brief series or even single jerks are then common, and the spasms often go unnoticed; the disease then apparently presents as an isolated developmental deterioration in previously normal infants. The attacks eventually develop into typical clusters. After a period of months or, occasionally, of years, they tend to become less conspicuous. Spontaneously or as an effect of treatment, the spasms may also change their characteristics, becoming more subtle and difficult to detect. Video-EEG monitoring may be necessary to provide firm evidence demonstrating that the spasms have really disappeared in response to medication (Gaily et al., 2001). The total duration of the spasms is highly variable, depending, in part, on therapy. In rare cases, the spasms are present for only a few weeks, and they then disappear spontaneously (Dulac et al., 1986a; Aicardi and Chevrie, 1978). They disappear before 1 or 2 years of age in most patients. Cowan and Hudson (1991) indicate that spasms have disappeared by 3 years of age in 50% of patients and by 5 years in 90%. In a few patients, repetitive spasms can persist up to 10 to 15 years of age. The age at disappearance is difficult to determine when the spasms become longer and lose their repetitive character, resembling the tonic seizures of Lennox-Gastaut syndrome (Gastaut et al., 1964).

Other types of seizures commonly precede or accompany the spasms in the course of the disorder and sometimes during a series of spasms (Carrazana et al., 1993). Preceding seizures are often partial ones. They may occur as part of an acute episode that may be a cause of the syndrome or as isolated seizures (Velez et al., 1990). Concurrent seizures include focal motor atonic or tonic attacks; isolated myoclonic jerks; and, rarely, atypical absences (Yamamoto et al., 1988; Leestma et al., 1984; Gastaut et al., 1964).

Developmental Retardation or Deterioration

Developmental retardation may exist before the onset of the spasms. In different studies, this was the case in 68% to 85% of the patients (Riikonen, 1984; Kellaway et al., 1983; Matsumoto et al., 1981a; Kellaway, 1959). Associated neurologic abnormalities are often present (Aicardi and Chevrie, 1978). However, identifying mild degrees of cognitive delay retrospectively is difficult, and, even in patients who apparently developed normally before the onset of spasms, mild neurologic antecedents or subtle motor deficits have been found in up to 20% of cases (Lombroso, 1983a). In previously well infants, a definite behavioral regression is often observed. Social smile disappears; the infant becomes apathetic and hypotonic and no longer takes an interest in its surroundings to the point that blindness is at times suspected (Aicardi and Chevrie, 1978; Gastaut et al., 1964). A prospective study in children with perinatal brain injury (Guzzetta et al., 2002) showed that most of those who subsequently developed West syndrome lost previously acquired visual and cognitive abilities. In some cases, the deterioration of the child's visual attention abilities paralleled cognitive deterioration, even months before the onset of spasms. Defective visual attention was still present after the acute phase of the syndrome at the age of 2 years. Autistic withdrawal of variable intensity is common at the onset of West syndrome, and it may persist as a long-term sequela in a high proportion of children (Chugani and Conti, 1996). Motor regression is usually less profound, but voluntary reaching and grasping often disappear (O'Donohoe, 1985). These behavioral changes may appear before the spasms, but they usually are seen in association with a hypsarrhythmic EEG, or they may go unnoticed, thus leading to suspicion of a primary deteriorating disorder. Because West syndrome is one of the most common causes of mental deterioration in infants, a careful inquiry for mild seizures and an EEG recording should always be obtained in such patients. Even in children with abnormal development before the onset of ISs, the onset of the seizures is often marked by further obvious regression (Aicardi, 1989; Aicardi and Chevrie, 1978; Gastaut et al., 1964). Conversely, in some children, cognitive development may remain normal, at least for a period of time. In such patients, the mental outlook is probably more favorable (Jeavons et al., 1973). With the subsidence of the attacks, the child's development may begin to improve somewhat, but the resumption of mental functioning may lag for several weeks after the cessation of seizures.

Electroencephalographic Phenomena: Hypsarrhythmia

Hypsarrhythmia (Gibbs and Gibbs, 1952) is the most remarkable, but not the sole, EEG pattern associated with ISs, as it is observed in 40% to 70% of patients (Jeavons and Livet, 1992; Cowan and Hudson, 1991) and it is most common early in the course of the condition. The term refers only to the EEG aspect and it should not be used for designating West syndrome, in which the hypsarrhythmic pattern may not be seen. The pattern is one of very-high-voltage (up to 500 µV) slow waves that are irregularly interspersed with spikes and sharp waves occurring randomly in all cortical areas. The spikes vary from moment to moment in duration and location. They are not synchronous over both hemispheres, so the general appearance is that of a total chaotic disorganization of cortical electrogenesis (Fig. 3.1). However, the slow components may demonstrate some degree of organization, with rhythms that vary with age (Parmeggiani et al., 1990). Hypsarrhythmia is an interictal pattern observed mainly in the awake state. During slow sleep, the EEG recording often displays bursts of more synchronous, irregular polyspikes and waves that are separated by stretches of low-amplitude, poorly organized tracing. This pseudo-periodic pattern may be apparent as soon as the child is asleep, or it may take some time to set in (Kellaway et al., 1983; Lombroso, 1983a; Hoeffer et al., 1963). In addition, it may be seen in patients who do not exhibit a typical hypsarrhythmic pattern while they are awake or in those in whom full-blown hypsarrhythmia has not yet appeared. In such patients, it is of definite diagnostic value (Lombroso, 1983a). During REM sleep, the EEG tracings tend to be closer to normal (Kellaway et al., 1983; Lombroso, 1983a; Gastaut et al., 1964). Typical hypsarrhythmia is present mainly during the early stages of the disorder. It may precede the clinical phenomena by a few weeks. Conversely, in patients with previous EEG abnormalities, the hypsarrhythmic pattern may appear late or not at all.

As the disorder proceeds, the EEG pattern generally changes over weeks or months. Synchrony between the hemispheres and spike-wave complexes of long duration often appear in the late stages, a pattern that has been termed *modified hypsarrhythmia* by some investigators (Hrachovy et al., 1984; Druckman

FIG. 3.1. Hypsarrhythmic tracings in a 7-month-old girl with cryptogenic infantile spasms during wakefulness **(A)**, recorded spasm **(B)**, and during slow sleep **(C)**. Note the synchronization and fragmentation of paroxysmal activity during slow sleep. Note also the persistence of some sleep spindles in **(C)** and that of some normal background rhythm before spasm in **(B)**. (Calibration [**B** and **C**]: 1 second, 50 µV.)

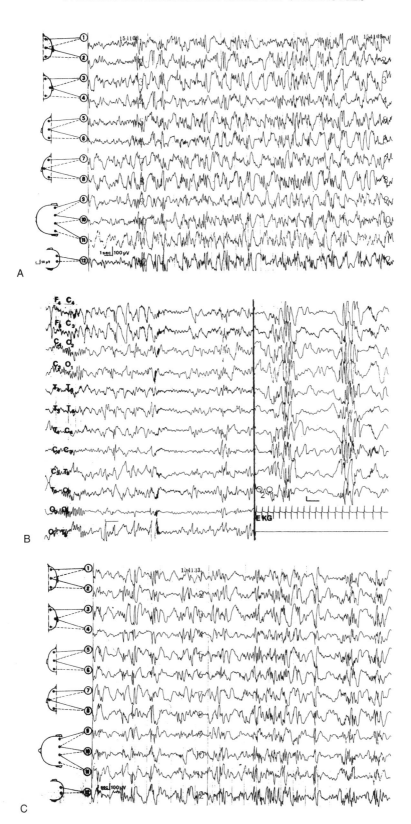

and Chao, 1955). The same term is used by other authors to denote the paroxysmal patterns that cannot be called *hypsarrhythmia* because of such atypical features as the background activity, partially preserved synchronous bursts of generalized spike-wave discharges, significant asymmetry, or a suppression-burst type of tracing (Aicardi and Ohtahara, 2002; Hrachovy et al., 1984; Lombroso, 1983a; Jeavons and Bower, 1974). These variants, which may be particularly common in younger children (Hrachovy et al., 1984) or in those with brain malformations, may be observed in up to 40% of patients with ISs (Dalla Bernardina and Watanabe, 1994; Jeavons and Livet, 1992; Lacy and Penry, 1976).

At least part of the cognitive and/or behavioral deterioration may result from the persistent diffuse hypsarrhythmic EEG activity that can be regarded as a variant of nonconvulsive status (Dulac, 2001); if this is so, maximal efforts at control are clearly in order (see "Treatment and Course").

The hypsarrhythmia tends to disappear in older patients, occasionally even when spasms may still be observed (Hrachovy and Frost, 1989; Jeavons et al., 1973). A typical hypsarrhythmic EEG is rare after the age of 3 years. The tracings may then become normal, or they may exhibit various abnormalities, especially focal spikes or slowing. The replacement of a hypsarrhythmic pattern with bilateral, symmetric slow spike-waves is common when Lennox-Gastaut syndrome develops following ISs (Watanabe et al., 1973; Gastaut et al., 1964).

The association of hypsarrhythmia with a constant focus of abnormal discharge is common (Riikonen, 1982; Gastaut et al., 1964), and, when focal discharges have a fixed topography, they often indicate focal pathology, especially when slow waves are prominent (Parmeggiani et al., 1990). Some investigators advise systematic use of intravenous diazepam to suppress the diffuse hypsarrhythmia, thus unmasking potential focal discharges (Dalla Bernardina and Watanabe, 1994; Dulac et al., 1986a). Asymmetric hypsarrhythmia is less common, while unilateral hypsarrhythmia is rare.

The hypsarrhythmic pattern may fail to appear for brief periods at onset of the disorder or after treatment, or it may always remain atypical. It does not appear with certain etiologies, such as lissencephaly or the Aicardi syndrome (see "Malformation of the Cerebral Cortex"). However, a consistently normal tracing, including sleep recording, virtually rules out the diagnosis of ISs (Lombroso, 1982, 1983a).

The ictal EEG patterns are variable (Dulac et al., 1986a; Kellaway et al., 1979; Gastaut et al., 1964).

The most common is a high-voltage, frontal-dominant, generalized slow-wave transient pattern with an inverse phase reversal over the vertex region (Fusco and Vigevano, 1993), followed by voltage attenuation. Bilateral and diffuse fast rhythms in the β-range (and occasionally in α-band) coincide with the clinical spasm and with the initial part of the low-voltage record, which lasts 2 to 5 seconds. In many patients, only voltage attenuation (decremental discharge) is present. Such electrical events may occur without apparent clinical concomitants (Hrachovy et al., 1984; Gastaut et al., 1964). Spasms with a more sustained tonic contraction are accompanied by the typical high-amplitude slow wave, followed by fast activity that is similar to that accompanying tonic seizures (Vigevano et al., 2001).

Other ictal patterns include generalized sharp-wave and slow-wave complexes, generalized slow-wave transients only, or fast rhythms occurring in isolation (Kellaway et al., 1979, 1983). Asymmetric and unilateral spasms are usually associated with contralateral EEG activity, suggesting a cortical generator for the spasms (Gaily et al., 1995; Donat and Wright, 1991a) and unilateral damage. Several ictal patterns may be combined, or they may vary from episode to episode. During a cluster, focal discharges may occur (Donat and Wright, 1991b). After the initial spasms of a series, transient suppression of the hypsarrhythmic pattern may be seen (Lombroso, 1983a; Gastaut et al., 1964) without a return of hypsarrhythmic activity between consecutive spasms. In other cases, hypsarrhythmia resumes between spasms. According to Dulac (1997), disappearance of hypsarrhythmia in the course of a series of spasms might indicate a symptomatic origin, whereas the resumption of hypsarrhythmia between serial spasms may indicate an "idiopathic" condition and may have a favorable prognosis. However, this finding has been disputed.

Children with organic lesional or severe encephalopathies, such as tuberous sclerosis, Aicardi syndrome, or lissencephaly, do not usually have typical hypsarrhythmia. Likely, only children with less severe brain impairment and better chances of less severe outcome are able to generate such an electrographic pattern.

DIAGNOSIS

The diagnosis of West syndrome is easy when the spasms are typical. At onset of the syndrome, however, single momentary head nods or jerks of the limbs may easily be missed by inexperienced parents or doctors. Indeed, in one series (Bobele and Bodensteiner, 1990) the diagnosis was made, on average, 3.5 months after the onset of spasms. Frost et al. (1978) used polygraphic and video recording to show that a vast number of attacks were missed by parents. The diagnosis of "colic" or *abdominal pain* is, however, made with surprising frequency, undoubtedly because of the cry that often accompanies the "doubling up" of the infant. The British National Childhood Encephalopathy Study indicated that a misdiagnosis of "colic" was made by 15% of primary care doctors, while only 12% made the correct diagnosis of ISs (28% made a diagnosis of some form of "convulsions") (Bellman, 1983). The repetitive character of the spasms is of great diagnostic value, especially when the seizures are fragmentary or of minor intensity, as frequently is the case (Hrachovy and Frost, 1989). The occurrence of clusters should lead the clinician to suspect that the observed phenomena are not simple colic, startles, Moro responses, or shoulder shrugs, and it should prompt the clinician to obtain an EEG, including a sleep recording.

Some other conditions may resemble ISs, but they do not have the same prognosis or EEG abnormalities. A few infants do experience repetitive jerks that closely mimic ISs, but these are unaccompanied by an EEG abnormality and they have a spontaneously favorable course. This curious syndrome, which is termed *benign myoclonus of early infancy* (Fejerman and Caraballo, 2002; Pachatz et al., 1999; Dravet et al., 1986; Lombroso and Fejerman, 1977), is apparently not an epileptic phenomenon; rather, it represents a sort of axial shudder that appears similar in nature to tics. In fact, the use of the term *myoclonus* is not entirely correct because the muscular contraction lasts longer than in myoclonic jerks and it closely resembles spasms (Pachatz et al., 1999). Another manifestation that may closely mimic ISs are the so called "repetitive sleep starts" that are sometimes observed in children with spasticity, with or without epilepsy (Fusco et al., 1999). These starts might represent a pathological enhancement of the hypnagogic jerks that are cyclically repeated while infants are falling asleep. Paroxysmal tonic upgaze deviation, which was described by Ouveier and Billson (1988), is repeated in clusters that occur every few seconds for several minutes. It represents *benign tonic upward gaze* (Guerrini et al., 1998a), a condition that is encountered in previously normal children between 6 and 20 months of age. During the attacks, the EEG recording is normal, and the child, who is conscious, may maintain visual fixation by bending the head downwards, a maneuver that produces vertical nys-

tagmus. This age-related condition disappears within 1 to 2 years from onset. *Compulsive masturbation* is a condition observed more frequently in girls during late infancy or early childhood. Some of these children may present with prolonged episodes of rhythmic contractions of the lower limbs and trunk that are accompanied by eye staring and adducted thighs, as well as an attitude of withdrawal that may mimic unresponsiveness.

Early forms of myoclonic epilepsy, especially benign myoclonic epilepsy (see Chapter 6), are not uncommonly mistaken for ISs (Aicardi, 1980a). The jerks are briefer than spasms, often having a saccadic appearance. As a rule, they are not repeated in series, and the EEG concomitant of the attacks is a short burst of irregular, fast polyspike-wave complexes that appears on a relatively normal background tracing. Because this form of epilepsy has a better prognosis than ISs and requires a different treatment, its recognition is important.

Differentiating ISs from the tonic seizures of Lennox-Gastaut syndrome may be difficult, especially when spasms are in extension and they are not repeated in clusters. Indeed, ISs and Lennox-Gastaut syndrome are closely related age-dependent responses to similar brain insults (Ohtahara and Yamatogi, 1990; Ohtahara et al., 1980; Niedermeyer, 1972a). A transition from typical brief spasms to episodes with a more sustained tonic contraction is often observed (Gastaut et al., 1964). Tonic seizures in series that are quite reminiscent of these spasms occur in many patients with Lennox-Gastaut syndrome, particularly those who had experienced ISs (Donat and Wright, 1991a). Failure to separate ISs from tonic seizures of early onset Lennox-Gastaut syndrome is likely responsible for the high incidence of cases of West syndrome with onset after the age of 1 year that has been reported in several series (Lacy and Penry, 1976). However, many cases of Lennox-Gastaut syndrome appear in patients who have never had ISs, and many types of epilepsy can occur following West syndrome (Lombroso, 1983a, 1983b).

ETIOLOGIC FACTORS

ISs have multiple causes, and their mechanism is, at best, incompletely understood. The incidence of the syndrome ranges between 0.25% and 0.42% in various series (Brna et al., 2001; Matsuo et al., 2001; Cowan and Hudson, 1991), and the cumulative incidence until 14 years of age was reported as 0.6% in children in a Finnish study (Riikonen and Donner, 1972). In the study by Trevathan et al. (1999), the cumulative incidence of IS was 2.9 per 10,000 live-births, and the age-specific prevalence was 2.0 per 10,000 among 10-year-old children. No evidence of a decrease in incidence of the disorder in Finland was seen from 1960 to 1991 (Riikonen, 2001). The small-for-gestational-age infants were more apt to develop ISs than were the preterm average-for-gestational-age infants. The number of small-for-gestational-age infants with neonatal hypoglycemia and ISs has decreased significantly. However, the number of cases of brain malformations, including tuberous sclerosis, has increased, probably as a consequence of improved neuroimaging detection.

Age, Sex, and Genetics

The *age dependency* of the syndrome is remarkable. Almost all cases have their onset during the first year of life. In a series of 78 cases (Chevrie and Aicardi, 1971), only 5% began after the age of 1 year. Corresponding figures of 3% in the series by Jeavons and Bower (1964) and 10% in the series of 277 patients by Lombroso (1983a) have been observed. The maximum incidence of onset is between 3 and 7 months of age (Lacy and Penry, 1976). Age at onset, however, depends on the proportion of symptomatic versus cryptogenic cases in any particular series, and some authors have reported a high proportion of cases with an onset before the age of 4 months (Kellaway et al., 1983). Cases with neonatal onset can be found in the literature, and ISs appearing before the age of 3 months may be more common than was previously thought (Lombroso, 1978). Seemingly, the location of the cortical lesions may influence the age of onset. Koo and Hwang (1996) analyzed the relationship of the site of the lesion with age at onset of spasms in 93 infants and observed that the earliest onset of spasms was seen in those infants with occipital lesions, whereas frontal lesions, which were rare, were associated with a latest onset.

Boys are affected more often than girls. Of the 594 patients discussed by Lacy and Penry (1976), 356 (60%) were boys, and the approximate ratio of boys to girls varied from 1.1:1 to about 2.8:1 in several large series (Riikonen, 1982; Matsumoto et al., 1981a; Livingston, 1972; Jeavons and Bower, 1964).

A family history of ISs is uncommon, being found in about 4% of the cases (Sugai et al., 2001; Riikonen, 1982; Fleiszar et al., 1977). A family history of epileptic seizures of any type is found in 6% to 17% of the cases (Chevrie and Aicardi, 1967; Cowan and Hudson, 1991), a proportion lower than that seen with most other types of epilepsy encountered in the first

year of life (Chevrie and Aicardi, 1977; Aicardi and Chevrie, 1978). However, Matsumoto et al. (1981a), Watanabe et al. (1976), and Millichap et al. (1962) found a positive family history of epilepsy in 40% of their cryptogenic cases and in 9.3% of the members of their "perinatal group." Familial cases of ISs probably represent the expression of several genetic disorders. Some such disorders are well characterized, including leukodystrophy (Coleman et al., 1977; Bignami et al., 1966), tuberous sclerosis (Riikonen, 1984), X-linked lissencephaly and band heterotopia (Guerrini and Carrozzo, 2001a), and X-linked mental retardation and ISs (Stromme et al., 1999; Claes et al., 1997) caused by mutations of the *ARX* gene (Stromme et al., 2002). Other genetic disorders are more rare, and these may be either recessive (Ciardo et al., 2001; Caplan et al., 1992; Fleiszar et al., 1977) or of undetermined inheritance (Reiter et al., 2000).

A syndrome of ISs of early onset, which is often both preceded by and followed by other types of seizures, hypsarrhythmia, facial dysmorphism, optic atrophy, and peripheral edema, has been reported from Finland and has been termed *PEHO syndrome* (progressive encephalopathy with edema, hypsarrhythmia, and optic atrophy) (Riikonen, 2001; Salonen et al., 1991). This syndrome is probably transmitted as an autosomal recessive trait. Cases have been found outside Finland. ISs have also been reported to occur in the costooculofacial syndrome (Harden et al., 1991) and the monosomy 1p36 microdeletion syndrome (Arzimanoglou et al., 2002).

Origin

ISs are traditionally divided into cases of *symptomatic* origin versus those that are *cryptogenic* (Dulac et al., 1994; Lombroso, 1983a; Matsumoto et al., 1981a; Jeavons and Bower, 1974; Chevrie and Aicardi, 1971; Gastaut et al., 1964). However, the definition of these terms varies among studies. Most authors place those cases in which a definite predisposing etiologic factor can be identified (Matsumoto et al., 1981a) or etiologic associations can be clearly specified (Kellaway et al., 1983) into the symptomatic group. Other investigators (Jeavons and Bower, 1974; Chevrie and Aicardi, 1971) classify symptomatic cases as those with one or both of the following: (a) abnormal mental and/or neurologic development before the onset of spasms and (b) evidence of a brain lesion by clinical or neuroradiologic examination. Clearly, novel techniques of investigation, especially structural and functional neuroimaging, tend to increase the apparent frequency of symptomatic cases. On the other hand, cryptogenic spasms are those for which no cause can be identified (Jeavons and Bower, 1974) or those cases that have developed normally before the onset of spasms (Lombroso, 1983a; Aicardi and Chevrie, 1978). These varying definitions of the terms may account for some of the differences in opinion about the prognostic significance of the cryptogenic or symptomatic origin of ISs. Some authors do not find a difference in outcome between symptomatic and cryptogenic cases (Matsumoto et al., 1981a, 1981b; Kurokawa et al., 1980), although the majority do (Lombroso, 1983a; Chevrie and Aicardi, 1971; Gastaut et al., 1964).

The distinction between symptomatic and cryptogenic ISs is of great practical significance because a poor prognosis is expected in patients with structural brain damage. However, the classification of a particular patient is always fraught with difficulties, especially if early development is accepted as a criterion, because historical data on infant development are often unreliable. Moreover, the classification depends heavily on the extent of the investigations performed and on the nature of the lesion, as well as the ease with which it may be detected. Furthermore, in ISs, the term *cryptogenic* does not necessarily mean that a lesion is not present; therefore, a difference of nature between cryptogenic and symptomatic cases has not been established. These uncertainties are reflected in the different proportions quoted for symptomatic ISs in the literature, which vary between 2% and 77% (Riikonen, 1996; Koo et al., 1993; Cowan and Hudson, 1991; Singer et al., 1982; Matsumoto et al., 1981b; Riikonen and Donner, 1972). According to some investigators (Vigevano et al., 1993; Dulac et al., 1986a), some of the cases that are not included in the symptomatic group may belong to a truly "idiopathic" group, related to other genetically determined epilepsies. This group could be recognized clinically because the syndrome occurs in a previously normal child, the hypsarrhythmic pattern is typical and symmetric, and it reappears between individual spasms during clusters (Plouin et al., 1987). However, these features may not be fully reliable, and Haga et al. (1995) were unable to differentiate etiologic groups and to predict short-term prognosis on the basis of clinical and ictal or interictal EEG features.

Specific Causes

Multiple causes of ISs are known (Table 3.1), and the statement that ISs are nothing but a response of the immature brain to multiple types of insults has often

TABLE 3.1. *Main causes of infantile spasms*

Neurocutaneous syndromes
  Tuberous sclerosis
  Neurofibromatosis
  Incontinentia pigmenti (Simonsson, 1972)
  Ito hypomelanosis
  Linear nevus sebaceus (Kurokawa et al., 1981)
Brain malformations (Riikonen, 1984)
  Spectrum of cortical dysplasias (Guerrini et al., 1996a)
  Aicardi syndrome
  Agyria-pachygyria (Dulac et al., 1983c)
  Congenital perisylvian syndrome
  Hemimegalencephaly (Tijam et al., 1978)
  Holoprosencephaly (Watanabe et al., 1973)
  Other migration disorders
  Down syndrome
  Fragile X syndrome (Guerrini et al., 1993a)
Metabolic and degenerative diseases
  Phenylketonuria (Poley and Dumermuth, 1968)
  Nonketotic hyperglycinemia (Seppälainen and Similä, 1971)
  Other organic acid disorders
  Mitochondrial disorders
  Menkes disease (Sfaello et al., 2002)
  Pyridoxine dependency (Krishnamoorthy, 1983)
  Biotinidase deficiency (Wolf, 1983)
  Congenital disorders of glycosylation (Stibler et al., 1993)
  PEHO syndrome (progressive encephalopathy with hypsarrhythmia, edema, and optic atrophy) (Salonen et al., 1991)
  X-linked infantile spasms (Claes et al., 1997)
  3-Phosphate-glycerate dehydrogenase (Pineda et al., 2000)
Infectious disorders
Fetal infections
  Cytomegalovirus infection (Riikonen, 1978)
Hypoxic-ischemic sequelae
  Prenatal, perinatal or postnatal (Jellinger, 1987; Watanabe et al., 2001)
  Periventricular leukomalacia (Okumura et al., 1999)
  Cerebral infarcts (Palm et al., 1988)
  Near-drowning (Hrachovy et al., 1987)
  Cardiac surgery with hypothermia (du Plessis et al., 1993)
Trauma and brain hemorrhage
Brain tumors (Branch and Dyken, 1979; Mimaki et al., 1983; Ruggieri et al., 1989)
Neonatal hemangiomatosis

been made. However, not all of the injuries incurred at an appropriate age give rise to the syndrome, and some causes are especially likely to result in ISs (Lombroso, 1983a). In actuality, the real causes of ISs are poorly known, and many of the often-quoted etiologic factors have not been demonstrated to have a convincing causal relationship to the syndrome. Primarily, this is because their frequency has not been studied in appropriate controls, except in a single study (Degen, 1978) that included only 13 cases.

Commonly, etiologic factors have been separated into the categories prenatal, perinatal, and postnatal (Jeavons and Livet, 1992; Aicardi and Chevrie, 1978). Although perinatal factors were considered prominent in earlier studies, prenatal factors, mainly malformations, now appear more significant (Riikonen, 2001; Dulac et al., 1994), as a consequence of the improvements in perinatal care and neuroimaging diagnosis.

Some earlier studies attributed a role to low birth weight, especially that caused by intrauterine growth retardation (Crichton, 1969), subsequent studies have not found an association of ISs with antecedents of low birth weight. Likewise, the role that had been attributed to neonatal hypoglycemia was not confirmed in later series (Riikonen, 2001), and the possible role of cytomegalovirus infection (Riikonen, 1978) is unlikely in view of the absence of an increased rate of cytomegalovirus infection in those with ISs over that of the controls (Cowan and Hudson, 1991). Toxoplasmosis (Kurokawa et al., 1981) and rubella have been implicated in few cases (Riikonen, 1984).

Anoxic Ischemic Encephalopathy

Traditionally, a prominent causative role had been attributed to anoxic-ischemic insults incurred either before or during birth. The incidence of such insults had variously been estimated at 18% to 80% of the cases (Lacy and Penry, 1976), and most of them had probably suffered during intrauterine life (Aicardi and Chevrie, 1978). However, the significance of the high figures quoted for anoxic-ischemic insults at birth is difficult to evaluate because a difficult birth or an abnormal perinatal period does not ensure a causal relationship. If only marked abnormalities of the birth process, followed by severe and persistent neurologic abnormalities in the neonatal period, were considered etiologically significant, the proportion of ISs due to a perinatal cause is about 15% (Aicardi and Chevrie, 1978). Abnormalities of both gestation and the perinatal period are significantly more common in infants with West syndrome than they are in those with febrile or other occasional seizures (Chevrie and Aicardi, 1977).

Malformations of the Cerebral Cortex

Malformations of the cerebral cortex or of cortical development (Barkovich et al., 2001) are a well-es-

tablished cause of ISs, and these appear operative in about 30% of patients (Guerrini et al., 1996b; Kuzniecky et al., 1994a; Robain and Vinters, 1994; Van Bogaert et al., 1993; Farrell et al., 1992; Vinters et al., 1992b).

Tuberous Sclerosis

Tuberous sclerosis is found in 7% to 25% of the patients (Curatolo et al., 2001; Riikonen and Simell, 1990; Bellman, 1983; Lombroso, 1983a; Matsumoto et al., 1981a; Aicardi and Chevrie, 1978; Pampiglione and Pugh, 1975). At the age at occurrence of ISs, tuberous sclerosis can be recognized by the presence of depigmented nevi (Aicardi, 1986a) and the detection of ocular phakomas (Gomez, 1988).

Intracranial calcifications can be demonstrated by computed tomography (CT) scan as early as at birth (Bellman, 1983; Gastaut et al., 1978) but not by conventional radiographs of the skull. Cortical tubers are usually well visualized as enlarged gyri with an atypical shape and an abnormal signal intensity that mainly involves the subcortical white matter (Barkovich, 1995) by magnetic resonance imaging (MRI). In the newborn, they are hyperintense with respect to the surrounding white matter on T1-weighted images and hypointense on T2-weighted images. Progressive myelination of the white matter in the older infant gives the tubers a hypointense center on T1-weighted images and a high-signal intensity on T2-weighted images. Tubers usually are multiple (Roach et al., 1991).

Some investigators believe that the location of the tubers is related to the type of associated neuropsychologic disturbance seen in the infant (Curatolo et al., 1987) and the severity of epilepsy (Jambaqué et al., 1991, 1993). However, some patients with multiple tubers can be cognitively normal, an occurrence that indicates that the relation between the number and location of tubers is complex. The special association of tuberous sclerosis with ISs is demonstrated by the following data: out of 32 patients with tuberous sclerosis and seizure onset before the age of 1 year, 27 (84%) had ISs and only 5 had other seizure types, even though only 230 (53%) of the 437 patients included in one study had ISs (Chevrie and Aicardi, 1977). Roger et al. (1984) observed that 63 (50%) of their 126 patients with tuberous sclerosis and epilepsy had experienced ISs.

The association of ISs with other neurocutaneous disorders is less clear. West syndrome has been observed in a few patients with neurofibromatosis, but the association may be coincidental (Millichap et al.,

1962; Crichton, 1966; Kurokawa et al., 1980). In one small series of children with neurofibromatosis, West syndrome was said to have a relatively good prognosis (Motte et al., 1993).

Other Brain Malformations

Other *brain malformations*, especially neuronal migration disorders and focal cortical dysplasia, increasingly are found to be a cause of ISs (Dulac et al., 1996; Guerrini et al., 1996a; Robain and Vinters, 1994). Different types of developmental brain defects were present in 13 of 32 autopsies of children in one series (Riikonen, 1984).

Some malformations have an elective association with ISs. *Aicardi syndrome* (Aicardi and Chevrie, 1993; Chevrie and Aicardi, 1986) consists of total or partial agenesis of the corpus callosum, chorioretinal lacunae in the fundi, and ISs. Spasms often are asymmetric and are associated with other seizures of early onset, especially focal (Donat and Wright, 1991a; Albright and Bruni, 1985). The syndrome occurs only in girls. In addition to callosal agenesis or dysgenesis, CT and MRI scans have demonstrated several brain defects, including periventricular heterotopia, abnormalities of gyration, cystic formations around the third ventricle, and gross hemispheral asymmetry (Aicardi and Chevrie, 1993). Abnormal neuronal migration with unlayered polymicrogyria is observed in histopathologic studies (Guerrini et al., 1993c). Vertebrocostal abnormalities are present in 50% of patients. The EEG recording rarely shows hypsarrhythmia; typically, the tracings are of the so-called "split-brain type," with a burst-suppression pattern that occurs independently over each of the two hemispheres. Prognosis is poor, with severe developmental delay, neurologic abnormalities, and persistence of the spasms being the rule. Aicardi syndrome is not a familial disorder, even though a single instance of a familial case has been recorded (Molina et al., 1989); therefore, it should be separated both from the few cases of familial agenesis of the corpus callosum associated with ISs (Cao et al., 1977) and from the rare X-linked lissencephaly with callosal agenesis and ambiguous genitalia, that is observed only in boys and that is often associated with spasms (Dobyns et al., 1999a).

Lissencephaly and pachygyria also have a special relationship with ISs (Guerrini and Carrozzo, 2001a, 2001b; Molaie et al., 1988; Jellinger, 1987; Gastaut et al., 1987a; Dulac et al., 1983c; Hakamada et al., 1979; Bignami et al., 1964). The dysmorphic features characteristic of the Miller-Dieker syndrome are present in a minority of patients. The diagnosis of this syndrome is based on neuroimaging showing the simplified gyral pattern with a decreased number of gyri, shallow sulci, thickened cortex, and rectilinear gray matter–white matter junction (Aicardi, 1991d; Barkovich, 1995). The presence of high-amplitude fast rhythms on EEG is highly suggestive. These may alternate with a mixture of high-amplitude theta and delta rhythms that may either suggest slow spike-waves or resemble hypsarrhythmia. About 75% of infants with lissencephaly-pachygyria have ISs (Guerrini et al., 1999a). Conversely, spasms are rarely observed in children with subcortical band heterotopia (Barkovich et al., 1994).

Hemimegalencephaly (Tijam et al., 1978), which is associated with abnormal gyration and neuronal dysplasia of one cerebral hemisphere, is a possible cause of ISs, and it may be amenable to hemispherectomy (King et al., 1985; Vigevano and Di Rocco, 1990). The EEG tracings may include unilateral fast rhythms, a suppression-burst pattern, or a slow spike-wave pattern (Paladin et al., 1989). *Holoprosencephaly* (Watanabe et al., 1973) may also be associated with ISs, but the number of reported cases is rather limited.

MRI may reveal anomalies, especially *focal dysplasia*, that do not appear on CT scans, but may give an abnormal signal in T2-weighted and fluid-attenuated inversion recovery sequences and an abnormal aspect and thickness of the cortex in T1-weighted sequences (Bergin et al., 1995; Sankar et al., 1995). The use of thin slices with multiplanar reconstruction (Chan et al., 1998) and other new techniques (Eriksson et al., 2001; Bastos et al., 1999) has enhanced the power of MRI investigations. Notwithstanding the use of these increasingly sophisticated structural imaging techniques, a number of children with ISs may harbor small areas of dysplasia that escape recognition by MRI. In addition, in children younger than 2 years of age, even macroscopic dysplasia may be overlooked as the typical blurring between gray and white matter may not be apparent because of incomplete myelination (Juhász et al., 2001a). Repeated MRI scanning is therefore advised in children with ISs in whom an initial early scan showed no abnormalities.

Interictal positron emission tomography (PET) with fluorine-18 fluorodeoxyglucose (^{18}F FDG) may demonstrate areas of hypometabolism that may correspond to areas of dysplasia that do not appear on MRI in about 20% of children with seemingly cryptogenic spasms (Chugani et al., 1990, 1996). Often, relatively good colocalization exists between hypometabolic areas and EEG abnormalities (Methahonkala et al., 2002; Chugani et al., 1990). However, hypometabolic foci in children with ISs may change localization, or they may even disappear during the course of the disorder. Such observations suggest that focal hypometabolism is not necessarily associated with an underlying structural abnormality (Methahonkala et al., 2002; Maeda et al., 1994). Multifocal or diffuse hypometabolic patterns may also be seen on ^{18}F FDG PET (Asano et al., 2001).

Single photon emission CT (SPECT) studies have shown focal defects in cerebral blood flow (Chiron et al., 1993; Dulac et al., 1987). That areas of reduced blood flow might correlate with specific neuropsychologic deficits at the time of onset of and following West syndrome has been proposed (Dulac et al., 1987). However, interpreting these data is difficult in a long-term perspective in view of the transient nature that cortical metabolic dysfunction may have in most children with ISs (Methahonkala et al., 2002).

Down Syndrome

ISs probably represent the most common seizure type observed in *Down syndrome* (trisomy 21). The early report of ISs in infants with Down syndrome treated with 5-hydroxytryptophan (5-HT) (Coleman, 1971) led to the hypothesis that these spasms might be secondary to altered serotonin metabolism (Silverstein and Johnston, 1984). However, ISs are not rare in patients with Down syndrome who are not treated with 5-HT (Cassidy et al., 1983). Stafstrom et al. (1991) found that 6 of 47 children with Down syndrome and seizures had West syndrome and that 4 of 18 children with Down syndrome without an obvious cause of epilepsy had ISs. In most children, the spasms have appeared despite no evidence of additional brain damage (Silva et al., 1996; Stafstrom and Konkol, 1994; Pueschel et al., 1991; Guerrini et al., 1989; Pollack et al., 1978), and remission has been obtained with use of conventional antiepileptic drugs, adrenocorticotropic hormone (ACTH) or steroids, without a relapse of seizures or with later onset of a mild age-related generalized seizure disorder (Silva et al., 1996). A recent study (Nabbout et al., 2001) suggests that vigabatrin (VGB) treatment for no longer than 6 months may produce long-lasting remission of spasms in children with Down syndrome.

Metabolic Disorders

Metabolic disorders are not a common cause of ISs. Phenylketonuria, however, is probably electively

related to West syndrome (Poley and Dumermuth, 1968), and series reported in the early 1960s did include such cases. A hypsarrhythmic EEG recording occurred in approximately one-third of the untreated phenylketonuric patients. However, phenylketonuria is now unlikely to be a cause of ISs because it is detected perinatally in industrialized countries.

Nonketotic hyperglycinemia (glycine encephalopathy) is a rare cause of ISs. In the neonatal period, the spasms are preceded by a myoclonic encephalopathy with a suppression-burst EEG and the hypsarrhythmia remains atypical (Seppäläinen and Similä, 1971). Rarely, pyridoxine dependency can first be manifested by ISs (Bankier et al., 1983; Krishnamoorthy, 1983), so a systematic trial of vitamin B_6 is justified. Carbohydrate-deficient glycoprotein disorders and abnormalities of serine metabolism are other rare, but important, causes because they are at least partly treatable.

Acquired Brain Disorders

West syndrome results from *acquired brain disorders* in 8% to 14% of the patients (Lacy and Penry, 1976). Many causes of diffuse brain damage, whether inflammatory (herpes simplex), traumatic (subdural hematomas), anoxic (Vinters et al., 1992b; Hrachovy et al., 1987), or ischemic, can be associated with the syndrome. Rare cases of tumors have also been shown as a cause (Asanuma et al., 1995; Ruggieri et al., 1989; Mimaki et al., 1983; Gabriel, 1980; Branch and Dyken, 1979). Some studies have implicated triple or quadruple immunization as an etiologic factor, with the pertussis component usually being incriminated (Bellman et al., 1983; Jeavons and Bower, 1964). Likely, the association between ISs and immunization is coincidental as the onset of spasms often occurs at the age at which infants are normally vaccinated. Melchior (1977) showed that a change in the immunization schedule in Denmark was not associated with a similar modification in the age at the onset of West syndrome. Similarly, Fukuyama et al. (1977) and Tsuchiya et al. (1978) demonstrated a wide variation in the interval between immunization and the onset of spasms and concluded that a chronologic association was due to chance, as did Bellman et al. (1983) in the largest controlled series to date.

Etiology and Clinical Picture

The question of whether the multiple etiologies of ISs give rise to different clinical pictures remains a controversial issue. Some of the causes are clearly associated with recognizable clinical and/or EEG patterns, the most obvious examples of which are Aicardi syndrome; hemimegalencephaly; and, to a lesser extent, the lissencephaly syndromes and some cases of tuberous sclerosis (Dalla Bernardina and Watanabe, 1994; Paladin et al., 1989). Suggestive features of idiopathic spasms have been proposed (see "Origin"). Currently, no firm evidence indicates that a subgroup that differs in nature from the rest of the ISs group exists.

Pathologic Studies

The multiplicity of causes of ISs is confirmed by *pathologic studies*, which have shown a large array of malformations, anoxic lesions, and metabolic disorders (Vinters et al., 1992b, 1993; Farrell et al., 1992; Jellinger, 1987). Negative findings also have been reported (Kellaway et al., 1979; Lacy and Penry, 1976; Gastaut et al., 1964); however, Meencke (1989) found no detectable pathology in only 12 (11%) of 107 cases. In most autopsied cases, ISs were due to prenatal factors (Jellinger, 1987; Meencke and Gerhard, 1985), and most were related to diffuse lesions, including developmental brain abnormalities. However, unilateral lesions, particularly cystic softening in the middle artery territory, may be responsible for ISs (Palm et al., 1988), and focal cortical dysplasia may be common (Robain and Vinters, 1994; Chugani et al., 1990). In rare cases, circumscribed inflammatory changes in the brainstem that may be of pathophysiologic interest have been found (Satoh et al., 1986; Kellaway, 1959).

These discrepant findings can be interpreted in two ways. Many authors believe that ISs are the result of certain patterns of diffuse brain damage when they occur in an immature brain at a certain susceptible stage of development (Riikonen, 1983). This view can be extended to cases without apparent lesions if the dendritic changes reported by Huttenlocher (1974) and the retarded myelination described by De Weerdt and Hooghwinkel (1976) are considered a special subtle type of diffuse brain insult. Other investigators suggest that localized lesions, especially of the brainstem (or a specific dysfunction of its structures), are responsible for ISs because of an imbalance among neurons of the gigantocellular area, the dorsal raphe, and the locus ceruleus (Kellaway et al., 1979). The finding that ISs were observed in a hydranencephalic infant (Neville, 1972) seems to support this hypothesis. Alternatively, the most recent view proposes that ISs should be regarded as a peculiar type of secondarily generalized seizure that, dur-

ing a critical developmental period, can be triggered by focal paroxysmal activity arising from limited or more diffuse areas of abnormal cortex (Asano et al., 2001). The results of epilepsy surgery unquestionably support the view that the abnormal cortex plays a key role in the initiation of seizures. Ictal ^{18}F FDG PET studies of ISs have shown that hypometabolism involves the focal cortical areas, as well as the lenticular nuclei and brainstem (Chugani et al., 1987). These findings could suggest an interaction between the cortical and subcortical structures during spasms. It has been suggested that activation of the raphe-striatal pathway, as well as of the descending spinal pathways, may be responsible for striatal activation and secondary generalization (Juhász et al., 2001a).

TREATMENT AND COURSE

ISs are resistant to most conventional antiepileptic drugs. Only ACTH, corticosteroids (Baram et al., 1996; Hrachovy et al., 1994), and vigabatrin (VGB) (Elterman et al., 2001; Aicardi, 1996; Chiron et al., 1991a) have conclusively demonstrated efficacy in the few controlled and the numerous uncontrolled trials conducted thus far. Because of the rarity of well-controlled comparative studies, considerable uncertainties remain regarding the best form of treatment (Hancok et al., 2002). The lack of evidence, however, may reflect objective limitations in both the performance of trials and outcome measures due to the nature of the disorder, rather than an actual lack of efficacy. The mode of action of these agents remains unknown, and their efficacy has been assessed through their short-term effects on the seizures and the EEG abnormalities. The long-term effects of various treatments on cognitive outcome have generally been studied retrospectively in an uncontrolled fashion, and no study of cognitive development is available for treatment with benzodiazepines or valproate. All of the treatments are difficult to assess because ISs usually disappear spontaneously. In patients receiving no effective therapy (only phenobarbital), Hrachovy et al. (1979) found that 25% were in remission by 11 months after the onset of ISs, and a small proportion (2%) became seizure free within 1 month.

Adrenocorticotropic Hormone and Steroids

Since 1958, *ACTH and steroids* have been the most popular treatment for ISs. The drugs and dosages employed and the duration and schemes of therapy have varied enormously. The most commonly used drug is ACTH in doses of 20 to 40 IU daily, a long-acting form of which is usually administered intramuscularly once daily. Lower doses on the order of 10 IU have been used by some (Sato et al., 1982a; Seki et al., 1976), while others have adopted very high doses of 60 to 240 IU (Lombroso, 1983a; Lerman and Kivity, 1982; Singer et al., 1980).

Corticosteroids are also effective (Lombroso, 1983a). Prednisolone (2 to 10 mg per kg per day), hydrocortisone (5 to 20 mg per kg per day), and dexamethasone (0.3 to 0.5 mg per kg per day) are most commonly recommended (Schlumberger and Dulac, 1994; Kellaway et al., 1983; Jeavons and Bower, 1964). Various combinations of corticotropin and steroids are often used, the most common of which is ACTH, followed by decreasing doses of corticosteroids. The recommended duration of treatment is no less variable; some investigators advocate short-term treatment (3 to 8 weeks) (Ohtahara et al., 1980; Aicardi and Chevrie, 1978), whereas others prolong therapy (often combination) for up to 6 or even 10 months (Lerman and Kivity, 1982; Singer et al., 1980). Some studies have concluded that steroids are as effective as ACTH (Riikonen and Donner, 1980; Hellström and Oberger, 1965), whereas others favored ACTH therapy (Farwell et al., 1984; Lombroso, 1983a; Snead et al., 1983; Riikonen and Donner, 1980). In actuality, no real comparison among these studies is possible because as many schemes as authors have been used, the groups were usually run at different times without concurrent controls, the criteria for the evaluation of the results were different or they were not indicated, and the factors capable of affecting treatment may have been distributed differently among the groups. In addition, antiepileptic drugs were combined with hormones in some studies.

A very few comparative studies have provided more reliable comparisons. In two randomized series, Hrachovy et al. (1979) and Glaze et al. (1988) found no difference between the effect of 20 IU of ACTH and that of 2 mg/kg of prednisone taken daily for 2 weeks. The group studied was small, however, and only a 50% difference in the response rate could have been ascertained. In a subsequent study, Hrachovy et al. (1994) found that the administration of high-dose, long-duration ACTH (150 U per m[2] for 3 weeks, followed by a progressive reduction over the following 9 weeks) was no more effective than low-dose short-duration treatment (20 to 30 IU per day for 2 to 4 weeks). A controlled study by Baram et al. (1996) that compared high-dose ACTH (150 U per m[2] per day) with prednisone (2 mg per kg per day) given for 2 weeks found ACTH to be clearly superior

in suppressing clinical spasms and hypsarrhythmic EEG. Thirteen of fifteen infants receiving ACTH went into remission, compared with only four of fourteen receiving prednisone. Heiskala et al. (1996) assessed the effects of an individualized therapeutic regimen of ACTH started at a dose of 3 IU per kg per day and progressively increased to a maximum of 12 IU per kg per day if no improvement was obtained. The total dose administered ranged from 58 to 373 IU per kg. Most cryptogenic cases responded to the smallest dose, whereas symptomatic cases required higher doses. Side effects, such as hypertension, brain shrinking, cardiac hypertrophy, and adrenocortical hyporesponsiveness, were related to the dose, and these were therefore minimized by this drug regimen.

From a practical viewpoint, the use of corticosteroids avoids the necessity of injections and their possible complications (e.g., abscesses, irregular absorption), shortens hospitalizations, and makes home treatment easier. However, ACTH treatment would be preferable if its superiority were confirmed in a larger series (Baram et al., 1996). Although synthetic ACTH (tetracosactin) has been said to produce more serious side effects than natural corticotropin (Riikonen and Donner, 1980), most authors have reported that it can be used regularly without major problems.

Side Effects

Corticotropin and steroids frequently cause *side effects* that at times are serious. Riikonen and Donner (1980) found that 60 (37%) of 162 patients had pronounced side effects, and the mortality was 4.9%. The facilitation of infections is probably the greatest hazard of hormonal treatment, and infections were responsible for most of the deaths reported in several series (Wong and Trevathan, 2001; Riikonen and Donner, 1980; Pinsard et al., 1976). Riikonen (1978, 1982) cautions against the use of hormonal treatment in patients with symptomatic congenital cytomegalovirus infection because the treatment can produce a reactivation of the disorder, which may then have a progressive course. Kusse et al. (1993) have suggested that non–depot-ACTH is as effective as depot-ACTH while causing fewer side effects, in particular significantly lower hypertension.

Minor infections, such as mucosal candidiasis and subcutaneous abscesses, are common with ACTH and steroid treatment. The incidence of infections can be lowered by short hospitalization periods, which result in a diminution of cross-infections, but pneumonia and sepsis remain a major hazard.

Arterial hypertension occurs in at least one-third of the patients (Kellaway et al., 1983). It is usually well tolerated, but at least two cases of intracranial hemorrhage have been recorded (Riikonen and Donner, 1980) and cardiac complications have also been reported. Treatment can generally be maintained with the use of antihypertensive drugs and a hyposaline diet.

Electrolyte imbalance is common but easily correctable. The possible harmful effects of massive and prolonged doses of ACTH or steroids on growth, especially brain growth, have not been fully assessed (Fitzhardinge et al., 1974). Several studies have demonstrated that hormonal treatment produces brain shrinkage (Ito et al., 1983; Hojo et al., 1981; Lagenstein et al., 1979a, 1979b), as demonstrated on CT or MRI scan (Konishi et al., 1992). This complication is reversible, and brain scans return to their previous appearance within 3 months of the discontinuation of therapy (Ito et al., 1983). A report of a complicating subdural effusion has been published (Sato et al., 1982a). The apathy, drowsiness, irritability, and the flattening of EEG records that are common with hormonal treatment may have a relationship to the structural changes seen on brain imaging (Lagenstein et al., 1979a). Adrenal unresponsiveness or hyporesponsiveness is a constant side effect following treatment with high-dose steroids. This has also been observed following ACTH therapy (Peerheentupa et al., 1986; Riikonen and Perheentupa, 1986). Clinical manifestations of acute adrenal insufficiency are, however, rare. The effects of hormonal treatment on sleep patterns include a reduction in total sleep time and in slow sleep duration (Rao and Willis, 1987; Hashimoto et al., 1981; Horita et al., 1980). In rare cases, benzodiazepines (Otani et al., 1991) or ACTH (Kanayama et al., 1989) have been reported to worsen ISs, but the practical significance remains uncertain.

Effectiveness and Relapses

Often, the short-term effect of the hormonal therapy on the spasms and the EEG abnormalities is dramatic (Table 3.2). Cryptogenic spasms improve more often than symptomatic ones (Aicardi, 1980c; Jeavons and Bower, 1964), even though this experience has not been universally shared (Hrachovy et al., 1983). The ameliorative effect of the hormone therapy on the spasms is often evident within the first week of use, but improvement in mentation and behavior may not be evident for several weeks. In fact, the infants are often rendered both irritable and depressed by the administration of high-dose steroids, and recovery of higher functions might be not occur immediately after the abatement of hypsarrhythmia.

In several series, the relapse rate after the discontinuation of hormone treatment is about 30% (Aicardi, 1986c; Riikonen, 1984), and most relapses occur within 2 months of the discontinuation of therapy. Relapses are preceded by the reappearance of EEG abnormalities, especially during sleep, with hypsarrhythmia being less common than other paroxysmal patterns. Regular monitoring with sleep EEG tracings is, therefore, advisable for 3 to 6 months after the end of treatment (Saltik et al., 2002). Low relapse rates have been reported with the prolonged use of high-dose ACTH (Lerman and Kivity, 1982; Singer et al., 1982). However, this may not be unexpected considering the early occurrence of most relapses. A second course of therapy is indicated in the

TABLE 3.2. *Initial effect of hormonal therapy on spasms and electroencephalogram abnormalities*

Number of Cases	Disappearance of Spasms	Disappearance of EEG Paroxysms	Treatment	Relapse	Reference
191	88 (46%)	44 (23%)	ACTH	?	Fois et al., 1988a
75	45 (60%)	49 (65%)	ACTH	15/45 (33%)	Harris and Tizard, 1960
56	39 (70%)	23 (41%)	ACTH	22/39 (56%)	Jeavons and Clark, 1974
			Prednisolone		Jeavons and Clark, 1974
			Dexamethasone		Jeavons and Clark, 1974
613	437 (71%)	162/512 (32%)	ACTH	?	Jeavons et al., 1973
			Hydrocortisone		Jeavons et al., 1973
100	62 (62%)	62 (62%)	ACTH	?	Pisani et al., 1987
			Hydrocortisone		Pisani et al., 1987
62	98 (60%)	73/74 (99%)	ACTH	33/98 (34%)	Riikonen, 1984
52	43 (83%)	42 (81%)	ACTH	22/43 (51%)	Snyder, 1984

Abbreviations: ACTH, adrenocorticotropic hormone; EEG, electroencephalogram; ?, data not available.

case of a relapse following an initial good response, as the rate of secondary response may be as high as 74%, although it is usually much lower (Riikonen, 1984).

Whatever the exact figures, the remarkable observation is that a sizable proportion of the patients seem to be definitively "cured" by courses of ACTH or steroid treatment that can be as brief as 2 weeks, a marked contrast with the results obtained by antiepileptic drugs in the other epilepsy syndromes. In view of the relative rapidity of the therapeutic response and the increased risk of side effects that accompany hormonal treatment, a short course of 4 to 6 weeks is advisable (Aicardi, 1998).

The *long-term effects* of ACTH or steroid therapy are much more difficult to evaluate than is its action on spasms and EEG. Normal or almost-normal cognitive level after follow-ups of variable durations has been reported in 6% to 29% of the patients (Riikonen, 1996; Pollack et al., 1979; Lacy and Penry, 1976). Better results are attained for cryptogenic cases, with a normal cognitive level being seen in 28% to 58% of the patients (Table 3.3).

Studies using strict selection criteria for inclusion in the cryptogenic group have reported good results (more than 80% with no sequelae) (Dulac et al., 1986a). The role of a strict selection process in such favorable outcomes is probably essential. Favorable mental results are rare for symptomatic patients, and, this may result in part from misclassification. Some patients with definite structural brain abnormalities (e.g., tuberous sclerosis) and IS eventually reach a normal mental status, whether with or without hormonal therapy (Yamamoto et al., 1987a).

The overall figures for normal mentality after hormonal treatment are not markedly better than the approximately 12% that was found in several series conducted before hormonal treatment was available (Lacy and Penry, 1976). Therefore, some doubt exists over the value of hormonal treatment in this regard. However, choosing not to use ACTH or steroid therapy is difficult, at least for those with cryptogenic ISs. No convincing proof indicating that these treatments have no effect on mental development exists, and their dramatic efficacy on seizures and hypsarrhythmia suggests that, if any drug is likely to have a long-term effect, these will. A short period of spasms has been associated with a favorable outcome (Riikonen, 1982; Seki et al., 1976; Jeavons et al., 1973), and hormones have a great probability of shortening the period during which spasms occur. However, in the British National Childhood Encephalopathy Study, among the infants not treated with steroids, those whose spasms spontaneously stopped within 1 month had a better prognosis than did those whose spasms persisted for longer periods. The spontaneous tendency of the spasms to remit is therefore an important prognostic factor that may be concealed by treatment (Bellman, 1983).

The authors' policy is to switch to ACTH rapidly after an initial trial of VGB has failed (see "Vigabatrin"). The authors prefer to adopt an individualized ACTH regimen, as Heiskala et al. (1996) suggests, the aim of which is to identify the lowest possible

TABLE 3.3. *Long-term mental outcome in patients with West syndrome receiving hormonal therapy*

Normal Mental Levels					
All Cases		Cryptogenic		Symptomatic		Duration of Follow-Up (Yr)	Reference
16/114	(14%)	16/36	(44%)	0/78	(0%)	?	Feldman, 1983a
20/139	(14%)	20/58	(34%)	0/81	(0%)	2–16	Cavazzuti et al., 1980
18/105	(17%)	18/55	(33%)	0/50	(0%)	2–12	Jeavons and Clark, 1974
16/90	(18%)	16/28	(58%)	0/62	(0%)	1–15	Pippenger and Rosen, 1975
21/100	(21%)	21/44	(48%)	0/56	(0%)	5–15	Offerman et al., 1979
42/240	(18%)	27/129	(21%)	11/111	(14%)	1 mo to 13 yr	Gibbs et al., 1937
30/124	(24%)	25/60	(42%)	5/64	(8%)	1–11	Chevrie and Aicardi, 1977
32/139	(23%)	—	(40%)[a]	—	(9.4%)[a]	>5	Matsumoto et al., 1983b
8/71	(11%)	8/20	(40%)	0/51	(0%)	14–207 mo	Sivenius et al., 1991b
21/162	(13%)	11/25	(44%)	10/137	(7%)	3–19	Riikonen, 1984
—	—	24/43	(56%)	—	—	?	Lerman and Kivity, 1986
—	—	36/90	(40%)	—	—	≥6	Lombroso, 1989

[a]Derived from the whole series (*n* = 159), not only from treated cases. The authors state that no difference was observed in results whether or not patients were treated with hormones.

Abbreviation: ?, data not available.

dose that is effective in minimizing side effects. The initial dose of 3 IU per kg per day is maintained for 3 to 4 weeks and is then tapered off in cases in whom complete control of the spasms has been achieved or is doubled every 2 weeks up to a maximum of 12 IU per kg per day if no improvement has been obtained.

Antiepileptic Drugs

Vigabatrin

VGB has been used in the treatment of ISs in Europe since 1990 (Chiron et al., 1990, 1991a). Chiron et al. (1991a) reported the first open add-on trial study of VGB in 70 children with ISs that had resisted previous medication, including steroids and ACTH. Complete suppression of spasms was observed in 43% of children. The best response was seen in symptomatic patients, especially those with tuberous sclerosis, and the withdrawal of all other medication was possible in a minority. In a large retrospective survey that included 190 infants with classic ISs, Aicardi et al. (1996) found that VGB at an average dose of 99 mg per kg per day suppressed spasms within 4 days in 68% of infants. The best responses were observed in infants with tuberous sclerosis and in those younger than 3 months of age at the onset of spasms. Several additional retrospective surveys and prospective open studies have confirmed these good results in ISs (Mackay et al., 2002; Gaily et al., 2001; Nabbout et al., 2001; Fejerman et al., 2000b; Jambaqué et al., 2000; Koo, 1999; Cossette et al., 1999; Hancock and Osborne, 1999; Siemes et al., 1998; Wohlrab et al., 1998; Gherpelli et al., 1997; Schmitt et al., 1994), although the rate of responders was lower when lower dosages were used (Granström et al., 1999).

A few controlled studies of the use of VGB have also been published. Appleton et al. (1999b) conducted a placebo-controlled parallel study in which 40 children with ISs were randomized to either VGB or a placebo for 5 days. At the end of the double-blind phase, the infants treated with VGB had a 78% reduction in spasms, compared with a 26% reduction in the group taking the placebo. On the final day of the short double-blind period, seven VGB-treated patients and two placebo-treated patients were spasm free, which demonstrates the difficulties in ruling out the possibility that some of the remissions observed in longer trials may be spontaneous. In a randomized study with a 2-week duration, the effects of low-dose VGB (18 to 36 mg per kg per day) were compared with those of high-dose VGB (100 to 148 mg per kg per day) (Elterman et al., 2001); subsequently, a 3-

year, open-label, dose-ranging follow-up was initiated on infants not previously treated with ACTH, steroids, or valproic acid. Of the 142 children who were evaluated for efficacy, 8 of 75 receiving low-dose VGB and 24 of 67 receiving high doses achieved complete control of the ISs. The response increased dramatically after 2 weeks of therapy, and it continued to increase over the 3-month follow-up, ultimately reaching 65%. Delayed responses, however, may actually represent spontaneous remissions. Significantly earlier responses were seen in those children treated with higher doses and in those with tuberous sclerosis.

A comparative study of VGB (100 to 150 mg per kg per day; 23 children) versus ACTH (10 IU per day; 19 children) (Vigevano and Cilio, 1997) indicated that VGB was slightly less effective, with cessation of spasms in 48% of infants randomized to VGB, compared with 74% in those randomized to ACTH. A response to VGB was observed within 1 to 14 days, with most responding within 3 days. The interictal EEG abnormalities disappeared sooner in those children randomized to ACTH. In a retrospective non-controlled survey of 51 consecutive children with ISs treated with either medication (Cossette et al., 1999), VGB was considered at least as effective as ACTH and it was better tolerated. From these comparative studies, the finding emerged that some of the children who resist either VGB or ACTH respond when they are switched to the other drug. A randomized trial comparing VGB and hydrocortisone monotherapy in two groups of 11 children with tuberous sclerosis and ISs (Chiron et al., 1997) showed complete cessation of spasms in the VGB group versus cessation in only 5 of 11 of the hydrocortisone-treated group. The non-responders were crossed to VGB, eventually becoming seizure free at 2 months. However, no sufficiently long follow-up was undertaken.

No complete agreement has been reached concerning the delay in the initial response to VGB and the relapse rates. A clinical response has been reported within 3 days in about two-thirds of the responders in some series (Granström et al., 1999; Vigevano and Cilio, 1997; Aicardi et al., 1996). Other authors suggest that the response may be scattered over 3 months, although most patients respond within the first month (Elterman et al., 2001). Consequently, in children who do not respond quickly, the suggestion is that treatment should be continued for up to 3 months, while increasing the dose to the highest tolerated (up to 200 mg per kg per day) (Elterman et al., 2001). However, in the authors' opinion, a maximum of 3 weeks should be allowed to elapse before switching to ACTH treatment (Granström et al., 1999). Relapse rates are also variable, ranging from about 16% to 21% at 3 to 4 months (Elterman et al., 2001; Aicardi et al., 1996) to 25% at 6 months (Cossette et al., 1999). The different studies do not agree about whether the most common seizure types at the time of relapse were spasms or other types.

The effects of VGB on the hypsarrhythmic or severely abnormal interictal EEG accompanying ISs seem less dramatic than those observed with steroids or ACTH (Vigevano and Cilio, 1997). Although a trend of marked EEG improvement is an almost constant feature in responders, the cessation of spasms may not be paralleled by EEG improvement and cognitive progress (Koo, 1999).

The tolerability and safety of VGB have been excellent in all of the controlled and retrospective reviews conducted. A small minority of children suffered from adverse events, including somnolence, hyperkinesia, insomnia, and agitation. Only rarely was the drug discontinued because of such events (Lewis and Wallace, 2001).

In the past, this excellent tolerability profile allowed clinicians not to establish strict criteria for treatment cessation. However, the recent report of irreversible concentric visual field defects in 30% to 50% of patients of all ages treated with VGB (Vanhatalo et al., 2002; Gross-Tsur et al., 2000; Lewis and Wallace, 2001) suggests a careful evaluation of the risks versus benefits of using this treatment. The visual defect is usually asymptomatic, and it is not ascertainable in the ISs age group. A mild defect could be of little clinical significance. However, some children may have additional risks of visual problems. The relationship between the duration of exposure to the drug and the development of a field defect has not yet been exactly established. The available information indicates a correlation with total VGB load (Vanhatalo et al., 2002; Lewis and Wallace, 2001; Manucheri, 2000). As most responses to VGB treatment are obtained within the initial 3 weeks, nonresponders probably have little risk, if any, of developing a visual field defect. In responders, the suggestion is that VGB could be discontinued after about 6 months (Vigabatrin Paediatric Advisory Group, 2000) but evidence for this is meager. Whether the infant is switched to an alternative treatment or treatment is stopped altogether should be decided according to the individual clinical and electrographic context. The fear of producing a visual field defect, however, should not overshadow the risks of reappearance of a severely disabling, sometimes life-threatening epilepsy.

The *long-term* effects of VGB treatment are largely unknown. None of the studies mentioned included data on the long-term outcome. Only one study that was conducted on a small number of children with ISs and tuberous sclerosis found that control of spasms was followed by a significant improvement in cognition and behavior, including recovery from autistic behavior (Jambaqué et al., 2000).

Benzodiazepines

The *benzodiazepines*, most notably nitrazepam (Chamberlain, 1996; Dreifuss et al., 1986), may be effective in bringing the spasms under control with relatively few side effects. However, their effect on the associated EEG abnormalities may be limited. Clonazepam has been found useful by some (Vassella et al., 1973), but others consider it inferior to nitrazepam. Most investigators consider the benzodiazepines to be less active than steroids (Kellaway et al., 1983; Lombroso, 1983a). Dreifuss et al. (1986) observed that nitrazepam and ACTH were both significantly effective in reducing spasms in a randomized study. However, the trial lasted only 4 weeks, a period that is too short to draw any firm conclusion.

Valproic Acid and Sodium Valproate

Valproic acid and *sodium valproate* appear to have some action on ISs. Bachman (1982) obtained control of ISs in 8 (40%) of 19 treated infants, and Pavone et al. (1981) reported excellent or good control in 12 (66%) of 18 infants. In a prospective study, Siemes et al. (1988) achieved satisfactory results with large doses of up to 100 mg per kg per day. Prats et al. (1991) treated 42 infants with doses of 100 to 300 mg per kg per day, and, according to their evaluation, the efficacy on both spasms and hypsarrhythmic EEG was similar to that of the corticosteroids. The side effects included somnolence, vomiting, and a reversible thrombocytopenia that led to the discontinuation of treatment in nine patients; however, in all cases, this was after a clinical response had been obtained. Fisher et al. (1992) reported favorable results (18 of 25 patients were seizure free) on valproate monotherapy, 100 mg per kg per day. In two infants, the presence of abnormal valproate metabolites was associated with evidence of reversible hepatotoxicity.

Pyridoxine

Pyridoxine is often employed as a first-line therapy by Japanese investigators (Toribe, 2001; Ohtsuka et al., 1987), and it has also been used in Europe (Blennow and Starck, 1986). Some investigators have reported good results with the combination of pyridoxine and valproate (Ito et al., 1991).

Other Drugs

Other drugs, including zonisamide (Suzuki et al., 1997, 2002; Yanai et al., 1999), felbamate (Hosain et al., 1997), lamotrigine (Veggiotti et al., 1994), and topiramate (Glauser et al., 1998, 2000a), have been used in a limited number of open-label studies conducted in small groups of children. Most authors use antiepileptic drugs, especially valproate, as maintenance therapy at the time of the discontinuation of steroids or ACTH even though no clear evidence indicates that this prevents recurrences. However, in the authors' opinion, antiepileptic therapy may be withheld in children who respond favorably to hormonal treatment.

Unconventional Treatments

Unconventional treatments include the ketogenic diet, which seems well tolerated but which has limited efficacy (Kossoff et al., 2002); barbiturate anesthesia (Riikonen et al., 1988), which is being abandoned because its effect is transient; and immunoglobulin therapy (Etzioni et al., 1991; Rapin et al., 1988; Arizumi et al., 1987), which has not been properly assessed (Wiles et al., 2002). Thyrotropin-releasing hormone treatment has also been tested in some children with West syndrome (Takeuchi et al., 2001), but the results await confirmation.

Treatment Recommendations

Pending definitive data, the authors' policy is to treat all patients, whether symptomatic or cryptogenic, with high doses of VGB. If a remission of spasms is obtained, the treatment is continued for a maximum of 6 months and is subsequently withdrawn. According to the clinical and etiologic context and EEG characteristics, a decision is then made on whether continued treatment with conventional antiepileptic drugs is needed. If the initial VGB treatment is ineffective within 3 weeks, ACTH is started in all patients, except those with very severe symptomatic conditions because these have very little hope of a reasonably favorable mental outcome and the risks associated with hormonal therapy are by no means negligible.

Surgical Treatment

Over the past decade, surgical resections for the treatment of ISs have been performed in several centers. About 50% to 60% of infants have been rendered seizure free (Asano et al., 2001; Chugani et al., 1990, 1996). Surgical treatment was initially proposed based on the observation that ISs are a special type of generalization of discharges involving the brainstem and deep gray matter (Chugani et al., 1990, 1992) that are triggered by partial, although extensive, cortical lesions that could be amenable to resection. This concept was elaborated after focal cortical lesions were detected with structural and functional neuroimaging in affected children and following demonstration that such lesions often correspond to the epileptogenic cortex (Henry and Chugani, 1997) (Fig. 3.2).

Large hemispheric abnormalities underlying ISs, such as hemimegalencephaly and extensive areas of cortical dysplasia, have been treated with anatomic or functional hemispherectomy or extensive multilobar resections (Asano et al., 2001; Shields et al., 1992a, 1992b; Chugani et al., 1990). Lobar resections have been performed in the presence of discrete dysplastic or neoplastic lesions (Asano et al., 2001; Wyllie et al., 1996; Mimaki et al., 1983). According to Asano et al. (2001), the resection should include the structural lesion and the contiguous electrographically-defined spiking cortex. The simple uncapping of a cystic brain lesion (Uthman et al., 1991; Palm et al., 1988) was reported to control spasms even though the mechanism of such an effect is difficult to understand.

Literature on the surgical treatment of epileptic spasms persisting beyond infancy includes 113 surgically treated children as part of small series or single case reports (Caplan et al., 1999; Wyllie et al., 1998; Arsanow et al., 1997; Kramer et al., 1997; Chugani and Conti, 1996a; Wyllie et al., 1996; Asanuma et al., 1995; Carrazana et al., 1993; Chugani et al., 1993; Uthman et al., 1991; Chugani et al., 1990; Duchowny et al., 1990; Gabriel, 1980; Branch and Dyken, 1979). Most of the children who underwent surgery had asymmetric clinical and EEG features or MRI-detectable structural lesions. Symptomatic patients comprised the large majority (95%), and the lesions included focal dysplasia (50%), hemimegalencephaly (10%), tuberous sclerosis (6%), tumors (10%), porencephaly (15%), and other miscellaneous rare lesions. The few cases initially diagnosed as "cryptogenic" were subsequently shown to harbor subtle areas of cortical dysplasia (Chugani et al., 1990, 1993). The child's age at operation varied from 4 months to 6

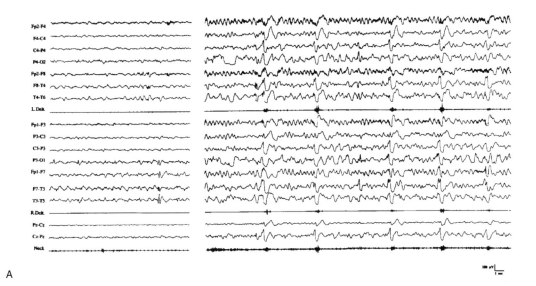

A

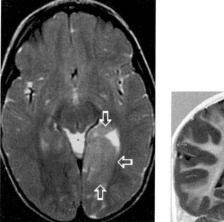

B

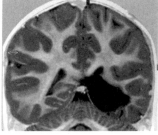

C

FIG. 3.2. A: Six-month-old girl with infantile spasms of recent onset. *Left:* The interictal electroencephalogram (EEG) shows slow-wave activity over both temporal regions that is much more prominent on the left where isolated spike-wave complexes are superimposed, showing equipotentiality on F7–T3. Independent sharp waves are seen over the left occipital area. *Right:* Ictal recording captured five spasms in about 25 seconds. During the series of spasms, slowing of background EEG activity occurs. The spasms are accompanied by rightward eye deviation. **B:** A magnetic resonance imaging scan of the same patient discussed in **(A)** shows an area of cortical dysplasia involving the left mesiobasal temporal lobe and the hippocampal region and extending back to the temporooccipital junction (*arrows*). **C:** Resection of most of the dysplastic cortex in the same patient, performed after stereoelectroencephalography at the age of 1 year (performed by Munari and his collaborators), was followed by the complete remission of spasms and by developmental recovery. Neuropathology showed Taylor type focal cortical dysplasia. No relapse of seizures had occurred during 4 years of follow-up.

years. The average rate of seizure-free cases as a result of surgery is about 50%, and, in some centers, it reaches about 65%. Whether children with bilateral but asymmetric clinical or imaging findings can be operated on remains unanswered (Asano et al., 2001). One study reported the results of callosotomy in 17 children with ISs and bilateral structural lesions or no lesion at all (Pinard et al., 1999). An improvement was observed in some of the older children whose spasms had caused drop attacks.

The developmental outcome of those children with ISs who had undergone surgical procedures was reviewed by Asarnow et al. (1997) at 2 years of follow-up. A remarkable improvement was seen in their communication, socialization, and daily living skills compared with their presurgical levels. Early surgery appeared to be followed by the best outcome. No clear correlation between developmental level and seizure frequency was apparent at postsurgical follow-up. The developmental level of children who had undergone surgery exceeded that of the ACTH-treated children with symptomatic spasms reported in a previous Finnish study (Riikonen, 1982). Such a comparative estimate has heavy methodologic limitations, however. In a further assessment of the same cohort of children, the improved social interaction was not paralleled by an improvement in their nonverbal communication skills (Caplan et al., 1999). On the whole, the outcome of children who had undergone surgery was considered worse than that of those children with cryptogenic spasms who responded to ACTH (Lombroso, 1989) or VGB (Fejerman et al., 2000b) in different studies.

PROGNOSIS IN INFANTILE SPASMS

The prognosis for children with ISs is strongly influenced, if not entirely determined, by the pathologic process underlying the syndrome. Different series have estimated the mortality to range between 5% and 31% (Koo and Trevathan, 2001; Trevathan et al., 1999; Riikonen, 1996). However, the higher rate reported in the study by Riikonen (1996) reflects cumulative data from a 20-year to 35-year-long follow-up. One-third of the patients died before 3 years of age and 50% before 10 years of age. Almost all of those who died were mentally retarded; often, they were living in institutions; and most had brain malformations.

In one-third to one-half of affected children, visual and auditory defects are present, and motor deficits are present (Riikonen, 1982; Pollack et al., 1979; Aicardi and Chevrie, 1978). In several series, mental retardation was observed in 71% to 90% of patients (Riikonen, 1996; Koo et al., 1993; Aicardi and Chevrie, 1978; Cavazzuti, 1973), and it was of a severe degree in more than 50% of patients. ISs of early onset (i.e., before 3 or 4 months of age) (Jeavons and Bower, 1974; Chevrie and Aicardi, 1971), those that are preceded by other types of seizures, or those that are associated with evidence of structural brain changes have a gloomy outlook. Koo et al. (1993) found that the average developmental quotient of cryptogenic cases at follow-up was significantly higher than that of the symptomatic group. A neurologic deficit was present in 23.5% of those in the cryptogenic group and in 75.0% of the symptomatic patients. Normal cognitive development was observed in two-thirds of the cryptogenic cases of Gaily et al. (1999) when assessed at the ages of 4 to 6 years.

A psychiatric disorder was diagnosed in 28% of the patients of Riikonen (1984), with autism and the hyperkinetic syndrome equally represented. Psychiatric abnormalities may be present even in patients of normal intelligence (Riikonen and Amnell, 1981; Thornton and Pampiglione, 1979), and ISs may play a significant role in the etiology of autism (Taft and Cohen, 1971; Chugani et al., 1996).

Epilepsy, in the form of other types of seizures following ISs, occurs in approximately 50% to 60% of children followed for several years. Lennox-Gastaut syndrome (see Chapter 4) and epilepsy with "complex partial seizures" are the most common forms observed (Riikonen, 1982; Riikonen and Amnell, 1981; Dravet et al., 1973). The late appearance of a temporal lobe focus has long been known (Gastaut et al., 1964), and systematic EEG studies have confirmed its frequency (Riikonen and Amnell, 1981).

A focal lesion is often, but not necessarily (Cusmai et al., 1988; Palm et al., 1988; Vining et al., 1987a; Alvarez et al., 1981), associated with a poor neurodevelopmental outcome. Early focal seizures are of ominous significance only if they occur repetitively, whereas those clustered in an acute episode may not indicate a poor prognosis (Ohtsuka et al., 1996; Velez et al., 1990; Chevrie and Aicardi, 1971, 1972). In a follow-up study of 92 children 3 years of age, Ohtsuka et al. (1996) noted that a stable clinical pattern of associated focal seizures predicted a significantly less favorable outcome.

For opposite reasons, patients with little or no neurodevelopmental regression, even after the spasms have appeared, seem to have a brighter outlook than those in whom a profound depression of mental functioning is observed (Jeavons et al., 1973).

Brain MRI has a high prognostic value that is closely linked to its diagnostic power. Infants with MRI scans showing no abnormalities have the best prognosis (Methahonkala et al., 2002; Saltik et al., 2002; Okumura et al., 1998). However, MRI scans may be normal in some metabolic disorders and dysplastic lesions that carry a poor prognosis.

Interictal *FDG PET* in children with ISs and normal MRI scans may show multifocal or diffuse hypometabolic patterns that may correspond to the developmental outcome (Chugani et al., 1996). For example, bilateral hypometabolism in the temporal lobes has been correlated with an autistic disorder and a poor long-term outcome (Chugani et al., 1996; Mimaki et al., 1983).

The influence of treatment lag has been variously reported. Kellaway et al. (1983) found that whether the patients were treated early or late made no difference in the outcome, and this conclusion was also reached by the British National Childhood Encephalopathy Study (Bellman, 1983). Most authors, however, believe that the earlier the treatment, whether medical (Lombroso, 1983a; Riikonen, 1982; Chevrie and Aicardi, 1971; Gastaut et al., 1964) or surgical (Asarnow et al., 1997; Asano et al., 2001), the better the ultimate outcome is. The association between a short treatment lag and a good prognosis is not necessarily one of cause and effect. Chevrie and Aicardi (1971) have shown that infants with cryptogenic spasms had an earlier medical treatment, on average, than those patients with symptomatic spasms, probably because any abnormal phenomenon is more obvious in previously normal babies. Thus, the effect of prompt treatment is difficult to separate from that resulting from the intrinsic severity of the disorder. Separation of these two factors was attempted in two studies, one after medical treatment (Chevrie and Aicardi, 1971) and one after surgical treatment (Asarnow et al., 1997); both concluded that a short treatment lag had a beneficial effect of its own. A rapid response to therapy, with disappearance of the spasms and the hypsarrhythmic pattern within a week, probably has a favorable prognostic significance (Wong and Trevathan, 2001; Riikonen, 1996; Rating et al., 1987).

The prognostic value of the initial EEG characteristics is uncertain. Unilateral and grossly asymmetric tracings predict an unfavorable outcome, whereas a typical hypsarrhythmic pattern may be associated with a more favorable prognosis (Saltik et al., 2002; Aicardi, 1980c). Some believe, however, that less abnormal patterns are indicative of a better outcome (Bellman, 1983; Friedman and Pampiglione, 1971;

Jeavons and Bower, 1964). Riikonen (1996) found no correlation between the presence of an EEG focus and a bad prognosis, but this has not been the universal experience.

LIMITS OF THE INFANTILE SPASMS SYNDROME AND RELATED SYNDROMES

Incomplete and atypical forms of West syndrome do occur, and agreeing on a minimal definition of the syndrome may be difficult (Jeavons and Livet, 1992). The classic form of West syndrome includes spasms, hypsarrhythmia, and mental retardation. Most authors would accept forms without hypsarrhythmia, provided that paroxysmal abnormalities of the EEG are present, and forms without mental retardation, at least temporarily. On the other hand, hypsarrhythmia and mental retardation that are unassociated with spasms are not included in West syndrome (Jeavons and Livet, 1992). Hypsarrhythmia without spasms is probably extremely rare if appropriate techniques are used to look for minimal spasms (Kellaway et al., 1979). West syndrome of early onset (i.e., before the age of 3 months) is often less typical than its later forms. The spasms are quite often associated with other types of seizures, especially partial ones, and typical hypsarrhythmia is rare before the age of 3 to 4 months. Conversely, focal EEG abnormalities are common in that age group, and, not uncommonly, a suppression-burst pattern precedes the appearance of a more typical hypsarrhythmia (Matsumoto et al., 1981b).

Early Infantile Epileptic Encephalopathy

Ohtahara et al. (1987, 1992) proposed that atypical ISs of early onset should be separated and placed in the category of early infantile epileptic encephalopathy. The syndrome is characterized by tonic spasms indistinguishable from those of West syndrome and by the suppression-burst pattern in the EEG. Some patients may have partial seizures, and myoclonic jerks have been reported by Clarke et al. (1987). The EEG pattern is composed of bursts of complex paroxysmal activity that are separated by periods of marked attenuation of activity or even by stretches of completely flat tracing. The paroxysmal bursts consist of an irregular mixture of spikes, sharp waves, and slow waves, which are irregularly intermingled. These bursts last from 1 to several seconds, and they may occur either synchronously or asynchronously over both hemispheres. Their individual components (spikes or sharp waves) are never bilaterally synchronous (Aicardi and Ohtahara, 2002). Ohtahara believes that early infantile epileptic encephalopathy is distinct from West syndrome and that it represents a specific age-related epileptic encephalopathy of the neonatal period and early infancy that is analogous to ISs in slightly older children and to Lennox-Gastaut syndrome in infants over 1 year of age (Yamatogi and Ohtahara, 1981). The syndrome apparently is caused by a great variety of early and extensive brain insults, especially brain malformations (Ohtahara et al., 1992). A few cases of metabolic origin, including glycine encephalopathy and mitochondrial disorders, have been reported (Aicardi and Ohtahara, 2002). Aicardi syndrome may be considered a subtype of early infantile epileptic encephalopathy in which the paroxysmal bursts occur independently over the two hemispheres (Chevrie and Aicardi, 1986). Early infantile epileptic encephalopathy often evolves into West syndrome at about 4 to 6 months of age. However, ISs do not follow in every case, and the nature and distribution of brain damage, as well as the age at emergence, may be responsible for the peculiar clinical picture (Aicardi, 1982a). Several clinicians do not consider early infantile epileptic encephalopathy a separate entity, regarding it merely as an early variant of ISs (Lombroso, 1990). A suppression-burst pattern has long been known to be commonly associated with

spasms occurring in the neonatal period (Lombroso, 1982, 1983a; Maheshwari and Jeavons, 1975), and the lesional nature and poor prognosis of ISs of very early onset are also well established. The fact that some of the cases do not evolve into ISs with hypsarrhythmia may indicate that these patients may have a syndrome that differs from West syndrome and that possibly has different causes.

Harding and Boyd (1991) found a similar suppression-burst pattern and various types of seizures (mainly tonic) that began at a few weeks of age in five infants with dentatoolivary dysplasia, a lesion that appears specific but that, thus far, is nonfamilial (Robain and Dulac, 1992). However, familial cases are known (Harding and Copp, 1997).

Neonatal (or Early) Myoclonic Encephalopathy

Neonatal myoclonic encephalopathy is a syndrome that is clinically characterized by the occurrence of erratic, fragmentary myoclonus of early onset, usually in association with other types of seizures, and, on EEG, by a stable suppression-burst pattern persisting after 2 weeks of age (Aicardi and Ohtahara, 2002; Aicardi, 1985a; Dalla Bernardina et al., 1983a; Aicardi and Goutières, 1973) (Fig. 3.3). Seizures associated with the myoclonus included partial motor

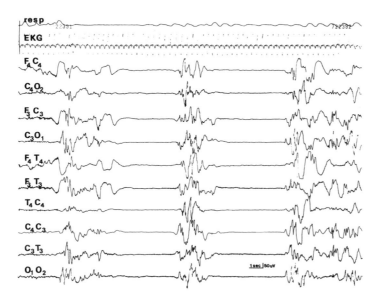

FIG. 3.3. Suppression-burst tracing of a 2-month-old girl with early myoclonic encephalopathy. Onset was at 48 hours of life, with erratic myoclonus and frequent partial seizures. Later (4 months), tonic spasms developed. The child was in a vegetative state when she was last seen at 19 months.

seizures, massive myoclonias, and tonic spasms that are not usually observed before 4 to 5 months of age. The onset was in the neonatal period in seven of the nine cases reviewed and before the age of 2 months in the remaining two patients (Aicardi, 1985a). All affected infants had severe neurologic impairment, and half of them died before the age of 6 months. Familial cases were common, and a recessive inheritance was considered probable in some of the cases.

This syndrome may result from undetermined metabolic defects or brain malformations (Aicardi and Ohtahara, 2002; Aicardi, 1986a). The clinical and EEG presentation of early myoclonic encephalopathy is remarkably similar to that of nonketotic hyperglycinemia, or glycine encephalopathy, a disorder in the metabolism of the amino acid glycine (Seppäläinen and Similä, 1971). Early myoclonic encephalopathy is the most common cause of nonketotic hyperglycinemia (glycine encephalopathy) (Aicardi, 1990b). Other metabolic errors occasionally present with myoclonic encephalopathy, including propionic acidemia, Menkes disease, encephalopathy with residual bodies, molybdenum cofactor deficiency, and a low γ-aminobutyric acid level in cerebrospinal fluid (CSF) that is probably due to a disturbance in the metabolism of this neurotransmitter (Aicardi and Ohtahara, 2002). Detailed metabolic studies are therefore warranted. A determination of both blood *and* CSF glycine levels is mandatory in the face of the clinical picture described.

The relationship of neonatal myoclonic encephalopathy with early infantile epileptic encephalopathy is not entirely clear. The two conditions have several clinical and EEG characteristics in common, including the occurrence of tonic spasms and a suppression-burst pattern. The prominence of erratic myoclonus and the late appearance of tonic spasms in neonatal myoclonic encephalopathy clearly separate it from early infantile epileptic encephalopathy on clinical grounds. However, cases have been reported in which the erratic myoclonus is only intermittent or in which it is replaced by massive myoclonus, so some overlap does exist between the two conditions and their separation may not be warranted (Aicardi, 1990b). Lombroso (1990), while accepting the premise that early myoclonic encephalopathy is distinct from Ohtahara syndrome, considers the latter only a variant of ISs.

Epileptic Spasms with an Onset Beyond Infancy

Epileptic spasms persisting or beginning beyond infancy probably represent a variant of ISs, rather than a related syndrome. Gobbi et al. (1987) described "periodic spasms" as the clinical and EEG features in a series of children with severe encephalopathies. The typical presentation included a frequent onset with a focal seizure or EEG discharge, followed by a series of spasms that were often asymmetric or even unilateral, each of which was marked on the EEG by a slow complex with superimposed, low-amplitude fast rhythms without a resumption of the interictal activity between individual spasms. Seizures occurred mainly on waking up or at the time of transition from REM to slow sleep. This electroclinical pattern has been repeatedly confirmed (Guerrini et al., 1992d; Donat and Wright, 1991a, 1991b; Gobbi et al., 1987; Bour et al., 1986), even in adults (Cerullo et al., 1999), and many considered it to be closely linked to developmental brain abnormalities (Cerullo et al., 1999; Pini et al., 1996). Although young children may present with clinical characteristics that closely resemble the syndrome of ISs, in older children and adults, the epileptic spasms are the only manifestation reminiscent of the syndrome, as the clinical context is quite different. Similar to the clinical appearance of spasms beginning in infancy, those with a later onset appear in series. However, the number of daily series is much lower than that observed in younger children.

Late-onset spasms are almost invariably resistant to treatment, including that with steroids and VGB, although this has not been fully assessed. Although the prognosis of late onset spasms is usually regarded as poor and most cases are due to brain malformations, that a number of cases are not associated with mental retardation or neurologic abnormalities has now been recognized. Apparently, the later the onset of spasms, the less the cognitive prognosis is influenced; aggressive treatment should therefore be limited to those cases in whom cognitive arrest or regression is manifest or to individuals who are severely disabled by spasms that cause drop attacks.

SUMMARY

ISs (West syndrome) are a remarkable age-dependent epilepsy syndrome. The syndrome occurs almost exclusively during the first year of life. In almost all patients, the spasms are associated with mental retardation or deterioration, and, in a majority, with a striking EEG pattern called *hypsarrhythmia*. This pattern consists of irregular, diffuse, asymmetric, high-voltage slow waves that are interspersed with sharp waves and spikes arising randomly throughout all scalp areas. A different, more periodic pattern occurs in slow sleep. Other paroxysmal EEG abnormalities may be seen in up to 40% of the patients.

West syndrome may have many causes. Tuberous sclerosis; certain brain malformations; and various diffuse, prenatal, or acquired encephalopathies are responsible for symptomatic cases. No cause can be determined in a variable proportion of patients with ISs. Such cases are called *cryptogenic*, and they have a better outlook than symptomatic ones. Some investigators reserve the term *cryptogenic* for those cases in which, in addition to the lack of detectable causes, cognitive and motor development are normal until the onset of the spasms. The distinction between cryptogenic and symptomatic ISs, although it undoubtedly has prognostic significance, may not be essential. The apparent absence of brain lesions does not preclude their existence, and undetectable brain damage might explain the poor outcome of apparently cryptogenic cases. A poor outcome also could be caused by diffuse epileptic activity in the absence of any detectable brain damage. Alternatively, mental deterioration in primary cases could result from a progressive, but self-limited, encephalopathy that is also responsible for the seizures and the EEG abnormalities.

ISs are notoriously resistant to conventional anticonvulsant drugs. Therapy with VGB, ACTH, or corticosteroids is effective for the spasms and, to a variable degree, the EEG abnormalities. The long-term efficacy of VGB or hormonal treatment on mental development and epilepsy of later onset has not been conclusively established. The reports of favorable results that have been published are based on clinical impressions and indirect evidence. In the face of such uncertainties, the selection of patients for either treatment depends on a subjective evaluation of the expected benefits and possible hazards, rather than on any firm evidence. From this perspective, VGB is considered a first-line drug in ISs by many authors, in spite of the risk of visual field constriction with its use. However, children who respond to VGB should be treated with this drug for no more than several months to limit this risk. Those who do not have a good response to VGB should be switched to hormonal therapy within a few weeks. The choice among the various modalities of hormonal therapy has been a matter of personal preference for many years, but some evidence indicates that ACTH is superior. Anticonvulsant treatment is indicated when VGB and hormonal treatment have failed or after VGB has been withdrawn if the risk of relapse is high. In the last 10 years, an increasing number of reports have indicated that ISs can be treated successfully with surgery, so this option should be considered early when the clinician faces resistance to VGB and hormonal treatment. Most infants have large multilobar or hemispheric lesions that require extensive resections. A discrete cortical epileptogenic lesion can only be identified in a minority of children, and the results in terms of their development are probably limited.

The long-term prognosis of West syndrome probably depends on the etiology of the syndrome and possibly on certain of its characteristics, more than on any form of therapy. Unfavorable prognostic factors include symptomatic spasms, an age at onset of earlier than 3 months, the occurrence of other types of seizures before the spasms, and the emergence of relapses after an initial response to therapy. A better outcome may be expected in cases with favorable clinical and etiologic factors, in those in whom deterioration at the onset of therapy is slight or altogether absent, and in children in whom the period during which spasms occur is short (less than 6 [preferably 3] months). Epileptic spasms may appear in older children and even in adults, and they are often indicative of a cortical malformation. In such cases, the actual level of the disability they produce, which can be limited, should be carefully weighed before vigorous treatment is initiated.

4

Lennox-Gastaut Syndrome

The definition of the Lennox-Gastaut syndrome (LGS) remains debated. The syndrome was originally described in 1966 by H. Gastaut, who proposed the use of the term *Lennox syndrome* to describe a childhood epileptic encephalopathy with diffuse spike-wave complexes and multiple types of attacks, including tonic seizures. The eponym was a tribute to the early work of Lennox and Davis (1950), who had described, in detail, the symptoms associated with slow spike-wave (SSW) activity in the electroencephalogram (EEG). The name *Lennox-Gastaut syndrome* was later adopted (Niedermeyer, 1969), and its use has gained wide acceptance even though the criteria for definition have been modified.

The term is often loosely used to denote severe epilepsy syndromes of childhood featuring several types of seizures, including falls, that are often medically intractable. Such a broad definition, however, encompasses several types of epilepsy for which the outcome and therapy differ. Recently, the tendency has been to limit the term *LGS* to a more narrowly defined syndrome from both the point of view of the seizures themselves and of the EEG characteristics (see Chapters 5 and 6).

Currently, LGS is defined as an epilepsy syndrome that is characterized by multiple types of seizures, including a nucleus of brief tonic or atonic seizures; atypical absences; and less characteristically, myoclonic attacks associated with an interictal EEG pattern of diffuse, slow (less than 2.5 Hz) spike-wave complexes (Commission on Classification and Terminology of the International League Against Epilepsy [ILAE], 1989). Several authors (Genton and Dravet, 1998; Beaumanoir, 1985; Beaumanoir et al., 1974) consider the presence of fast (10 Hz) rhythms associated with the tonic attacks or occurring with minimal or without associated clinical manifestations, especially during non–rapid eye movement (non-REM) sleep, an additional necessary criterion. Episodes of nonconvulsive status epilepticus are a common occurrence. Mental retardation is a highly common, but not an absolutely constant, feature (Aicardi and Gomes, 1991).

Even with this stricter definition, some disagreement still exists over the degree of subdivision that is desirable and the limits of accepted subsyndromes, and a fair proportion of cases resist precise classification because they display features of both LGS and myoclonic epilepsy; in some cases, the differentiation may rest on the quantitative proportions of the various types of seizures rather than on the specific features.

In addition to the suggestive types of seizures, other types of seizures and EEG features can occur with LGS; for example, focal seizures are often present either at the same time as or before the more typical types of attacks.

None of the aforementioned features is found in every case. Tonic seizures were present in 80% to 92% of patients (Gastaut et al., 1973a), and fast rhythms were seen during slow sleep in only 55% of those patients who had whole-night sleep recordings (Baldy-Moulinier et al., 1988). Moreover the "typical" seizures of LGS may have, in some patients, been preceded for prolonged periods by other types of attacks. This is especially true for myoclonic seizures, which may long be the prominent feature, leading some investigators to describe a "secondary type" of LGS that follows a phase of essentially myoclonic astatic epilepsy (Hoffmann-Riem et al., 2000).

As a result of these nosologic uncertainties, the features of LGS are variably described, depending on the definition that is accepted. In this chapter, the authors use the term *LGS* in the restrictive sense that is now accepted by most investigators (Beaumanoir and Dravet, 2003; Glauser and Morita, 2000; Genton and Dravet, 1998). The LGS syndrome is usually considered a secondary generalized epilepsy.

INCIDENCE AND ETIOLOGY

The frequency of LGS has been estimated as being between 1% and 10% of childhood epilepsies (Luna et al., 1988; Trevathan et al., 1997). The former figure is probably closer to reality, but a high incidence is observed in tertiary epilepsy centers that deal with intractable patients. The actual population incidence is poorly known because of the selection of patients for referral and the different definitions that are in use. Epidemiologic studies show that the proportion of LGS seems relatively consistent across various populations. The prevalence of LGS in mentally retarded children was reported as being 0.06 per 1,000 (Steffenburg et al., 1998), and the percentage of LGS in institutionalized patients with mental retardation may be as high as 16.3% (Mariani et al., 1993). Male children are affected more often than female children (54% to 63%). In the vast majority, onset is between 1 and 7 years of age. The peak age at onset is between 3 and 5 years. Up to 20% of cases have their onset before the age of 2 years. However, cases with onset in late childhood and adolescence or even adulthood are known to occur (Roger et al., 1987).

LGS can be preceded by other forms of seizures, especially infantile spasms (Beaumanoir and Dravet, 1992; Ohtahara and Yamatogi, 1990; Hodge et al., 1989; Chevrie and Aicardi, 1972), and timing the transition from brief "clonic" spasms to the longer tonic seizure of LGS precisely is difficult. Other types of epileptic seizures preceding the appearance of LGS include unilateral seizures, generalized tonic-clonic seizures, and episodes of convulsive status epilepticus. Focal seizures are relatively common (Aicardi, 1991c; Aicardi and Gomes, 1991; Gastaut and Zifkin, 1988; Gastaut et al., 1973a, 1974b). Primary generalized seizures, including typical absences, have been observed only rarely (Beaumanoir and Dravet, 1992; Roger et al., 1989). Some cases of myoclonic absences may evolve to LGS (Tassinari et al., 1992b). Focal and generalized seizures may also precede the appearance of the syndrome.

One-fourth to one-third of cases occur in children without previous developmental or neurologic abnormalities and without evidence of brain damage on imaging. In the 1989 Classification of Epilepsies and Epileptic Syndromes (Commission on Classification and Terminology of the ILAE, 1989), such cases were termed *cryptogenic* because of the usual presence of mental retardation. However, this mental retardation may not be the consequence of a lesion but rather the result of the epileptic activity itself, so the use of the term *idiopathic epilepsy*, which is sometimes encountered (Ohtahara, 1988; Boniver et al., 1987), may be acceptable even though LGS is classically considered a symptomatic or cryptogenic epilepsy.

The *etiology* of LGS is heterogeneous. Brain damage plays a major role, whereas genetic factors are generally regarded as less important. However, the frequency of a family history of epilepsy varies considerably from 2.5% to 47.8% (Dravet and Roger, 1988). This discrepancy is probably due to the different diagnostic criteria used, and it reflects the nosologic problems raised by the syndrome.

Two-thirds to three-fourths of cases result from a demonstrable brain abnormality or occur in patients with previous developmental delay (Ohtahara, 1988; Chevrie and Aicardi, 1972), and these are termed *symptomatic or secondary*.

Most lesions responsible for LGS are of developmental origin. Abnormalities of cortical development were the cause of 10 of 30 autopsy cases reported by Roger and Gambarelli-Dubois (1988). Multiple types of cortical malformations have been found, including bilateral perisylvian and central dysplasia (Kuzniecky et al., 1993a; Guerrini et al., 1992c, 1992d; Ricci et al., 1992), diffuse subcortical laminar heterotopias (Palmini et al., 1991a), and focal cortical dysplasias (Palmini et al., 1991c; Guerrini et al., 1996a). A few cases are due to Sturge-Weber syndrome (Chevrie et al., 1988; Roger and Gambarelli-Dubois, 1988) or tumors, especially of the frontal lobes (Angelini et al., 1979). LGS has also been reported in cases of hypothalamic hamartomas following a long period of focal gelastic seizures (Berkovic et al., 1988). The pathologic basis of cases of LGS not due to macroscopic lesions is poorly known. Biopsy studies (Renier, 1988; Renier et al., 1988b) have shown only relatively minor changes, such as poor dendritic arborizations and disturbed synaptic development of pyramidal cells in the inner layers of the cortex.

Major brain malformations are less commonly a cause of LGS than they are of infantile spasms (Aicardi, 1986a, 1994). LGS has not been reported in Aicardi syndrome or with the lissencephaly syndrome, which suggests that gross damage does not permit the organization of rhythmic discharges.

Acquired destructive lesions are also less common. Hypoxic brain damage has been reported (Ohtahara, 1988; Roger and Gambarelli-Dubois, 1988), and large porencephalic defects can also produce a picture of LGS (Ohtahara, 1988; Palm et al., 1988).

LGS can follow other epilepsy syndromes. The most common preceding syndrome is West syndrome, which was found prior to the onset of LGS in 17.5% to 41% of cases (Donat, 1992; Aicardi and Gomes, 1991; Ohtahara et al., 1988). Cases following infantile spasms may represent a special subgroup of LGS, with an early onset, a predominance of tonic seizures occurring in clusters, and a particularly poor prognosis (Aicardi and Gomes, 1992; Donat and Wright, 1991a; Ohtahara, 1988).

Cases of LGS following myoclonic astatic epilepsy (Hoffmann-Riem et al., 2000) are not included by all investigators. Many authors state that, although the late course of myoclonic astatic epilepsy is often marked by the appearance of nocturnal tonic seizures, usually the latter are not a prominent feature and they do not warrant the diagnosis of LGS. However, prominent tonic seizures may emerge after an initial history of myoclonic astatic seizures, and such cases are regarded by some investigators to fulfill the criteria for LGS because the differences, if any, are mainly quantitative and therefore are rather subjective. Such cases illustrate the difficulties in strictly delimitating LGS and differentiating it from some cases of related myoclonic epilepsy. Indeed, similar cases have been reported under the term *myoclonic variant of the LGS* (Dravet et al., 1982; Aicardi and Gomes, 1992).

CLINICAL AND ELECTROENCEPHALOGRAPHIC ICTAL FEATURES

Seizures

The seizures of LGS are usually repeated, occurring many times daily. They include a nucleus of "core" seizures, which are mainly atonic, tonic, and atypical absence seizures. They are often associated with other less characteristic types as well. They are particularly frequent during sleep. However, the frequency of seizures can change considerably, with the individual having both "bad" and "good" periods.

Tonic Seizures

Tonic seizures are the most characteristic type (Roger et al., 1989; Chevrie and Aicardi, 1972), although various estimates have placed their frequency from 17% of the cases (Niedermeyer, 1969) to 55% (Chevrie and Aicardi, 1972) and up to 95% (Gastaut et al., 1973a). The higher incidence has been found in series in which sleep tracings were systematically obtained. Tonic seizures occur frequently during non-REM sleep and less frequently during wakefulness, and they do not occur during REM sleep. They are usually brief, lasting from a few seconds to 1 minute, with an average duration of about 10 seconds. Consciousness is lost or obscured during the seizures, although arousal from light stages of sleep may occur (Erba and Cavazzuti, 1981). The *axial subtype* consists of a brief, but sustained, bilateral symmetric contraction of the axial muscles that results in a flexor movement of the head and trunk with apnea that occasionally is preceded by a brief cry. The eyes open and often deviate upwards. Clouding of consciousness and autonomic manifestations are usually associated with

this subtype. In *axorhizomelic seizures*, associated abduction and elevation of the arms occurs, whereas *global tonic attacks* involve most muscles and affect the distal parts of the limbs. When the child is standing, the flexion of the lower limbs and body axis may forcefully throw the patient to the ground. Patients who fall in a rigid posture, like a statue, are having a tonic seizure, whereas those who fall by collapsing may have either an atonic seizure or a global tonic seizure with triple flexion of the lower extremities (Erba and Browne, 1983). In all of the types, autonomic phenomena, including tachycardia, cyanosis, flushing of the face, salivation, and lacrimation, are common. Generally, eyelid retraction, staring, mydriasis, and cyanosis can be intense. Tonic seizures may be quite mild, especially in sleep, when they are often limited to a brief apnea, eye opening, an upwards deviation of the eyes, or a minimal stiffening, leading them to be easily mistaken for physiologic phenomena such as yawning or stretching. *Axial spasms* are very brief tonic seizures lasting 2 to 4 seconds that are a common cause of falls in patients with LGS (Egli et al., 1985; Ikeno et al., 1985). In infants, tonic seizures may tend to occur in clusters and to be followed by atonia, possibly making them difficult to distinguish from infantile spasms (Donat and Wright, 1991a; Roger et al., 1979). In older patients, episodes of automatic behavior may follow the tonic phase or may alternate with tonic contractions (Oller-Daurella, 1970). Such *tonic automatic seizures* have been found in 16% of patients (Roger et al., 1989).

The ictal EEG of tonic seizures may show a very fast discharge at a rhythm of 20 plus or minus 5 Hz that is usually of increasing amplitude or a discharge of 10 Hz with a high amplitude from onset; otherwise, it is similar to the "epileptic recruiting rhythm" (Brenner and Atkinson, 1982; Fariello et al., 1974; Gastaut et al., 1963, 1974a), lasting from 4 to 10 seconds in most cases. However, it may last from 30 to 60 seconds. Less commonly, a simple flattening of the tracing throughout the attack can be the only EEG manifestations (Fig. 4.1); the fast rhythm is followed by a brief discharge of spike-wave complexes or a burst of slow waves. The electromyographic (EMG) reading during tonic seizures resembles that of a normal tonic contraction.

Atypical Absence Seizures

Atypical absence seizures, which are observed in 13% to 100% of patients, are the second most common type of seizure in LGS (Aicardi and Gomes,

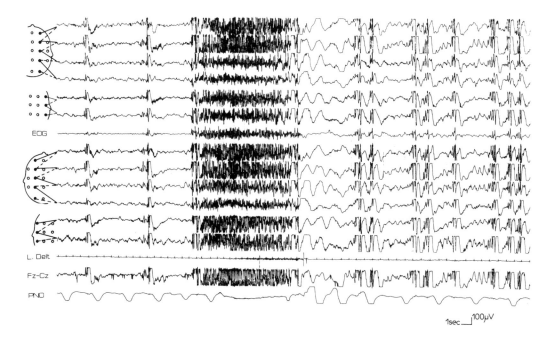

FIG. 4.1. A 12-year-old girl with Lennox-Gastaut syndrome experiences a tonic seizure during recording while asleep. A discharge of high-amplitude fast rhythms lasting about 10 seconds is accompanied by a slightly progressive tonic contraction that is apparent on the recorded muscle (left deltoid), and it is accompanied by apnea. The end of the seizure is characterized electrically by a discharge of polyspike and spike-wave complexes and a suppression burst and clinically by a short series of slow waves, followed by bursts of generalized multiple spike-wave complexes. Abbreviation: PNO, pneumogram.

1992; Gastaut et al., 1973a). They may closely resemble typical absences, although their onset and termination are said to be less abrupt or mild and they may be hardly detectable clinically because the loss of consciousness can be incomplete, allowing the child to continue his or her activities, albeit at a slower pace and imperfectly. The decreased consciousness is often associated with some loss of muscle tone, erratic myoclonic jerks, sialorrhea, or mild hypertonia of neck and back muscles. Relatively frequently, consciousness seems to be preserved. However, the execution of simple repetitive tasks is interfered with by the occurrence of the EEG discharge (Gastaut et al., 1974b; Porter et al., 1973; Goode et al., 1970). In some cases (Erba and Cavazzuti, 1977), a selective impairment of higher cortical functions in which responsiveness is maintained has been documented. The ictal EEG pattern of atypical absences is variable. The classic 3-Hz spike-waves are never observed (Beaumanoir and Dravet, 1992; Ohtahara, 1988; Porter and Penry, 1983; Goode et al., 1970), and this is often the only clear difference from typi-

cal absences. Often, a 10-Hz discharge that is similar to that recorded during tonic seizures is seen; in other cases, a burst of spike-waves, usually at 2.5 Hz or less, is recorded and is sometimes initiated by a brief phase of fast rhythm. A sudden voltage attenuation, sometimes with superimposed 20-Hz low-amplitude activity, may be present. Atypical absences are not precipitated by hyperventilation or photic stimulation. The duration of these discharges usually is 5 to 30 seconds. Identical discharges can be unassociated with clinical manifestations. The same applies to the discharges of fast rhythms that occur during slow sleep, although, in both situations, excluding the presence of minimal clinical phenomena can be difficult (Ohtsuka et al., 1982; Gastaut et al., 1963, 1974b).

Myoclonic Seizures

Myoclonic seizures are considered less characteristic and less common in LGS than tonic seizures or atypical absences. Their frequency has been variably estimated at 11% to 28% of cases (Beaumanoir and Dravet, 1992; Geoffroy et al., 1983; Dravet et al., 1982; Gastaut et al., 1973a; Chevrie and Aicardi, 1972). Myoclonic attacks are extremely brief, shocklike muscle contractions that may be isolated or repeated in a saccadic manner, usually for only a few seconds. The jerks are often bilateral and symmetric (massive myoclonus), and they preferentially involve the axial flexor muscles and the abductors of both arms. The involvement of the lower limbs can cause the patient to fall to the ground. No appreciable loss of consciousness occurs. However, myoclonias may be quite prominent in some patients with LGS (the so-called *myoclonic variant*). They are probably a common cause of the falls that constitute a major problem for children with LGS, although the mechanism of the fall may be impossible to determine without polygraphic recording. The EEG concomitants of most myoclonic seizures are bursts of generalized polyspike-waves that often have a frontal predominance. Recently, in a small group of patients, Bonanni et al. (2002) showed that the myoclonus in LGS is not really bilateral and synchronous, like that of idiopathic myoclonic epilepsies, but that it was constantly generated in one hemisphere with rapid generalization consistent with callosal transmission, which suggests that the origin of LGS may be focal in at least a proportion of cases.

A different type of myoclonus, termed *erratic* or *fragmentary*, is often associated with episodes of nonconvulsive status. It is not associated with EEG paroxysms.

Atonic Seizures

The frequency of atonic seizures is difficult to assess precisely. They are sometimes said to be the most common cause of falls, and they occur in 26% to 56% of patients (Livingston, 1988; Chayasirisobhon and Rodin, 1981; Schneider et al., 1970; Gastaut and Regis, 1961). However, most atonic seizures are probably associated with and are immediately preceded by a brief myoclonic jerk that may be difficult to detect because of its weak intensity, and myatonic seizures likely are much more common than are purely atonic ones. Indeed, a phase of resolution of muscular tone usually follows the myoclonic jerks, and it is the main cause of the fall, even though the jerk may be very mild or even absent. The EMG of a myoclonic jerk consists of a muscular spike lasting less than 100 ms that is followed by a period of electrical silence of variable duration, which corresponds to the clinical atonia that is responsible for a fall if its duration is of sufficient length. The EEG concomitants of most atonic seizures are similar to those of myoclonic jerks. In a few patients, atonic seizures are associated with a fast discharge that resembles that of tonic attacks.

Episodes of Nonconvulsive Status Epilepticus

Between 50% and 75% of patients with LGS suffer episodes of nonconvulsive status. The so-called "minor epileptic status" described by Brett (Brett, 1966) is most often a manifestation of LGS. The most typical form of status consists of subcontinuous atypical absences with variable degrees of altered consciousness that are periodically interrupted by recurring brief tonic seizures. On the EEG, the absences are marked by the occurrence of SSW complexes, whereas the tonic attacks are associated with a 10-Hz rhythm (Beaumanoir et al., 1988; Dravet et al., 1985). Such episodes may last hours and even days.

Episodes of *purely tonic status* can be accompanied by major autonomic disturbances that may become life threatening if they are prolonged because they may produce respiratory difficulties with apnea and bronchial hypersecretion even if the intensity of tonic contractions decreases to the point of almost complete disappearance. These episodes can be fatal.

Another common type of status is characterized by a variable degree of mental slowing, ranging from mild obtundation to coma, that is associated with dribbling and erratic myoclonus involving the perioral and distal limb muscles, with no tonic component. Twitching may be more easily palpable than seen (Doose, 1983). The facial expression is slack, and speech is slurred or altogether absent.

Episodes of nonconvulsive status in LGS often occur on awakening. They may last from a few minutes to hours or days. In up to one-half of the patients studied by Dravet et al. (1985), their duration exceeded 1 week. In fact, their exact duration may be difficult to determine because they can closely resemble the "bad" periods; they may have the same significance as these periods and they may precede or follow them with undetectable transitions. During bad periods, an apparent deterioration of mental performance and an increase in the EEG abnormalities often occur (Beaumanoir, 1981; Gastaut et al., 1963). According to Erba and Browne (1983), a distinctive feature of LGS may be the continuous fluctuation of response latencies to sensory stimuli. If sufficient time is allowed to process the information, the individual's ability to produce correct responses is preserved.

Not all the "core" types of seizures are present in all children with LGS, and, as was already indicated, one type (e.g., the "myoclonic variant") may predominate in a particular patient. In some children, only one type of seizure occurs, with the least unusual being tonic attacks. The nosologic situation of patients with only one type of attack (e.g., tonic seizures) remains uncertain because they do not fulfill the definition criterion for LGS of several types of attacks; these do, however, seem to be closely related to LGS.

The association of other types of attacks to the "core" seizures is common. They can precede the core attacks, but they may also accompany or follow them. These other types of attacks include generalized or focal tonic or tonic-clonic seizures, frequently at late stages; complex partial seizures (7% to 10%), which are also observed in children (Roger et al., 1987; Becker et al., 1989); and unilateral clonic seizures. The variable association of multiple seizure types in many patients is responsible for the considerable heterogeneity of clinical presentation, and it accounts for some of the difficulties in defining and diagnosing LGS. Underlining the role of drowsiness and inactivity in the precipitation of seizures is important.

CLINICAL AND ELECTROENCEPHALOGRAPHIC INTERICTAL FEATURES

Clinical Features

Mental retardation is the third component of the classic LGS triad. However, 7% to 10% of children with LGS remain within the accepted limits of normality (Chevrie and Aicardi, 1972; Aicardi and Gomes, 1988; Beaumanoir et al., 1988; Roger et al, 1989; Beaumanoir and Dravet, 1992; Offringa et al., 1992), even after long follow-up periods. However, even this small group of patients has difficulties in everyday life that seem to be due to a marked slowing of mental processing.

Many patients (20% to 60%) are already delayed at the onset of the syndrome (Beaumanoir and Dravet, 1992; Markand, 1977; Gastaut et al., 1973a; Oller-Daurella, 1973; Chevrie and Aicardi, 1972). Analogous to infantile spasms, such cases are called *secondary* or *symptomatic.* They are often associated with neurologic signs, abnormal antecedents, and neuroimaging abnormalities (Lagenstein et al., 1980; Zimmerman et al., 1977; Gastaut and Gastaut, 1976),

and psychomotor retardation tends to be particularly marked in such patients (Lagenstein et al., 1980). In primary cases (25% to 30%), the child's development seemed normal before the appearance of the first seizures. The proportion of mentally retarded patients increases to 75% to 93% at 5 years after onset (Livingston, 1988; Furune et al., 1986; Chevrie and Aicardi, 1972). Whether actual deterioration takes place after onset or whether the eventual cognitive defect results from a slowing of the child's normal mental progress is not clear because no precise neuropsychologic longitudinal study is available. The clinical impression, however, is that loss of skills clearly occurs in some children (Aicardi, 1994). Deterioration, if any, is self-limited, it is not associated with neurologic signs, and it may be partially reversible if the epileptic activity is better controlled. Likely, the epileptic activity itself plays a role in the mechanism of the cognitive and behavioral difficulties, which justifies the inclusion of LGS in the group of the *epileptic encephalopathies,* as they are defined by the new ILAE proposal for the classification of epilepsies (Engel, 2001). Some investigators (Hoffmann-Riem et al., 2000; Kaminska et al., 1999; Doose and Völzke, 1979) think that the occurrence of episodes of nonconvulsive status is causally related to the development of dementia, although other possible explanations may exist.

The ultimate degree of mental retardation is often severe—48 of 89 patients had an intelligence quotient (IQ) of less than 25 (Ohtsuka et al., 1987, 1990), and 21 of 40 children in another series had an IQ of less than 50 (Aicardi and Gomes, 1988). In addition, many patients have psychiatric problems, and they are hyperactive, insecure, and aggressive (Oller-Daurella, 1973); some may have autistic features (Gastaut et al., 1973a).

The resulting overall disability precludes normal school attendance and learning and later social insertion even when the cognitive deficit is of relatively mild degree.

Electroencephalographic Features

The classic interictal EEG feature of LGS is the SSW pattern, which was originally termed "petit mal variant pattern" because it was thought to be a variant of the 3-Hz spike-wave pattern of "true petit mal" (absence epilepsy) that had been reported a short time before. This pattern has no relationship, however, with true "petit mal."

The SSW complexes consist of a spike (less than 80 ms) or, more often, a sharp wave (80 to 200 ms), fol-

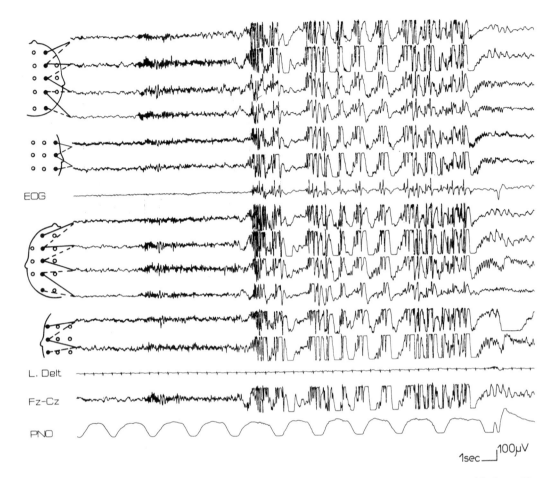

FIG. 4.2. Same 12-year-old patient as in Fig. 4.1. During sleep, a different ictal discharge occurs, this time with generalized low-voltage fast rhythms lasting about 10 seconds and remains subclinical; it is followed by quasi-rhythmic generalized multiple spike-wave complexes.

lowed by a sinusoidal electronegative slow wave of 350 to 400 ms in duration (Fig. 4.2). A prominent positive trough is present between the fast and the slow components (Blume, 1988; Blume et al., 1973). The SSW complexes may appear singly or in runs, with a repetition rate of 1.0 to 2.5 Hz. Runs of spike-waves at 3 Hz are not rare, but they do not predominate. They are bilateral and roughly symmetric, although shifting asymmetries are often evident. They are diffuse, but predominance over the frontocentral part of the scalp is usually present (Niedermeyer, 1969); they may be more obvious over the occipitotemporal area in a few patients (Blume, 1988). The SSWs are usually abundant, appearing as long sequences; but, in a few patients, they are rare and they may be visible only during slow-wave sleep, which increases their frequency

in all patients (Roger et al., 1989; Baldy-Moulinier et al., 1988). They are not necessarily symmetric, and, in some patients, same-side predominance is consistently present. The SSWs are not responsive to photic stimulation, and they show very little, if any, responsiveness to hyperventilation. Bursts of diffuse or bilateral fast (10 Hz) rhythms (or "polyspikes"), originally termed *grand mal pattern*, are often recorded during slow sleep. These usually last a few seconds but tend to recur at relatively brief intervals. These bursts are identical to those associated with clinical tonic seizures, although they are often of shorter duration (Fig. 4.3). Some are associated with minimal tonic attacks on polygraphic recording, which often demonstrates a brief apnea and/or mild EMG axial contraction (Baldy-Moulinier et al., 1988; Beaumanoir et al., 1988). Such

LGS : DIFFERENT TYPES OF ICTAL DISCHARGES DURING SLEEP

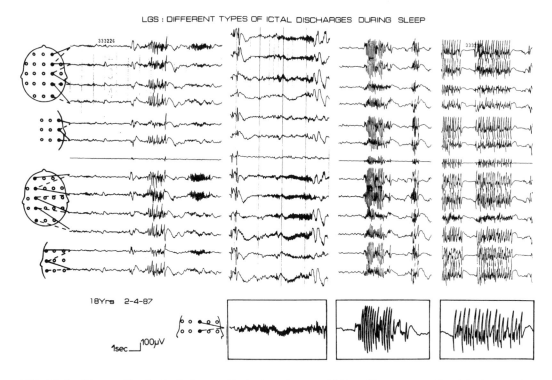

18Yrs 2-4-87

1sec ⌐100μV

FIG. 4.3. An 18-year-old patient with Lennox-Gastaut syndrome exhibiting different types of ictal discharges during sleep. The discharges are magnified on the bottom part of the figure corresponding to the Fz-Cz channel. The square on the left shows low-voltage fast rhythms; the central square, high-voltage fast rhythms; and the square on the right, a discharge of multiple spikes. All these types of discharges could be infraclinical, or they may accompany tonic seizures during sleep.

discharges are highly suggestive of LGS, and some investigators (Roger et al., 1989) considered them necessary for the diagnosis. However, they are not pathognomonic for the syndrome because they have been recorded in cases of focal epilepsy (Roger et al., 1989; Pazzaglia et al., 1985), and they are not found in all patients. Baldy-Moulinier et al. (1988) found them in 44 (55%) of 80 patients diagnosed with LGS who underwent all-night EEG recording. Fast-burst discharges disappear during REM sleep.

Time relationships between EEG and clinical events are rather inconsistent. Runs of SSWs may be ictal or interictal (Beaumanoir and Dravet, 1992; Dravet et al., 1985). Polyspike-waves may be correlated with myoclonus, but the precise relationship between spike and muscle activation is variable (Tassinari et al., 1971).

Other sleep discharges include polyspike-wave complexes (Degen and Degen, 1990; Roger et al., 1989), which are also common in slow-wave sleep, that may possibly include more than 10-Hz bursts.

Slowing of the background rhythms is present in more than one-half of patients, but it is not necessarily present on every recording. Focal paroxysmal activity (sharp waves or spikes) or focal slow activity are not uncommonly seen.

COURSE AND PROGNOSIS

The overall outcome of LGS is severe (Arzimanoglou, 2003). The short-term mortality has been estimated at 4.2% to 7% of those affected, in part as a result of tonic status (Erba and Browne, 1983). More than 80% of patients continue to have seizures (Gastaut et al., 1973a), and the repetition of absences and episodes of status, as well as the high-dose drug therapy, probably play a role in augmenting the mental deficiency by interfering with education and through latent anticonvulsant toxicity (Viani et al., 1977). Overall, reported remission rates range from nil (Beaumanoir and Dravet, 1992) to 4% (Roger et al., 1989) or 6.7% (Gastaut et al., 1973a), and the severity of the cognitive outcome roughly parallels that of the seizures. In general, studies that require strict criteria as defined by Beaumanoir and Dravet (1992) and Kaminska et al. (1999), including a complete clinical and EEG picture with tonic seizures, episodes of nonconvulsive status, and runs of 10-Hz discharges, report the most severe outcome. In such cases, the characteristic types of LGS seizures continue into adolescence and early adulthood, and the degree of mental deficit is severe. The heterogeneity of the syndrome and the variable criteria used by different authors account for the discrepancies among various studies. Chevrie and Aicardi (1972) found that the proportion of severely retarded patients was 72% of secondary cases, as opposed to 22% of primary cases. Patients with LGS occurring after infantile spasms fared significantly worse than did the rest of those in the series, whereas those patients in whom myoclonic seizures and atypical absences were prominent did significantly better. The differences were mainly explained by the following two interrelated factors: age at onset and primary and secondary etiology. An early age at onset was associated with a poor outcome (mean age at onset of 17.6 months in severely retarded patients and 48.5 in slightly retarded ones).

In patients with a less typical syndrome, with clear evidence of focal clinical and EEG manifestations, the characteristic LGS seizures often tend to be replaced by other types of seizure, mostly focal, simple, or complex (Beaumanoir and Dravet, 1992). In such cases, LGS may be only a transient phase in the course of a focal or multifocal epilepsy.

The degree of mental retardation following LGS is often severe. More than half the patients have an IQ of less than 50 at the end of follow-up. Similar results were found by other investigators (Markand, 1977; Blume et al., 1973; Gastaut et al., 1973a) Ohtahara et al. (1990) and Ohtsuka et al. (1990) defined three groups depending on the course. Forty-two of eighty-nine patients in the first group continued to display a typical electroclinical picture of LGS; nineteen patients in the second group developed other types of EEG discharges (mainly focal); and twenty-eight patients in the third group evolved into having a multifocal EEG recording. Only 40.5% of those in the second group were retarded, compared with 47.4% of those in the third group and over 90% in the first group. Patients in the first group more often belonged to the symptomatic cases and more frequently followed infantile spasms than those in the other groups.

The EEG abnormalities generally persist. The SSW pattern persisted over the entire follow-up in almost all the cases in the studies by Beaumanoir and Dravet (1992) and Roger et al. (1989). However, focal or multifocal spikes were superimposed in 75% of patients. In other series, focal abnormalities tended to replace the diffuse SSW pattern. Ohtsuka et al. (1990) found that diffuse spike-waves were replaced by independent multiple foci in 31 of their 89 patients. These patients tended to run an especially severe course, and they often had associated clinical or imaging evidence of cortical damage. Again, such differences probably reflect the use of different selection criteria.

Several possible *predictors of prognosis* have been proposed. According to Roger et al. (1989), a symptomatic etiology, an early age at onset (even in cryptogenic cases), a high frequency of tonic seizures, the occurrence of repeated episodes of nonconvulsive status epilepticus, and a constantly slow EEG background are strongly associated with a poor outcome. On the other hand, a late age at onset of seizures (after 4 years), a normal neuroimaging study result, a paroxysmal response to hyperventilation, and a relatively high proportion of fast (3-Hz) spike-wave complexes were associated with a less unfavorable outcome (Aicardi and Gomes, 1992). The predominance of myoclonic seizures was also found to have a relatively better prognosis (Dravet et al., 1982; Chevrie and Aicardi, 1972). The occurrence of multiple episodes of nonconvulsive status epilepticus has long been thought to be associated with mental deterioration (Doose and Völzke, 1979) in cases of myoclonic astatic epilepsy (see Chapter 6). Hoffmann-Riem et al. (2000) also found that such episodes were predictors of the secondary appearance of a picture of secondary LGS in cases of myoclonic epilepsy, as well as of a poor prognosis. Aicardi and Gomes (1988, 1992) did not find such episodes to be of prognostic significance, probably because their study included only cases of LGS defined by strict criteria and not those cases with prominent myoclonic attacks.

DIAGNOSIS AND NOSOLOGIC ISSUES

The diagnosis of LGS rests on the criteria previously defined, of which the predominance of tonic seizures and of runs of fast rhythms are probably the most suggestive. However, these features are not present in every patient, and many other types of seizures and EEG abnormalities may be present. Even if one accepts that multiple seizure types, including tonic seizures and fast EEG rhythms, in addition to SSWs, are necessary criteria, the clinical presentation of LGS remains heterogeneous, and the limits of the syndrome are not easy to define precisely. Furthermore, LGS is a syndrome of multiple causes, and a diagnosis of the cause is important for prognosis and sometimes for therapeutic purposes.

Neuroimaging is essential for the etiologic diagnosis, but it does not contribute to the syndromic diagnosis. In most patients, no significant abnormalities are found, although various types of lesion can be present in symptomatic patients. Positron emission tomography (PET) studies have also given variable results that confirm the etiologic heterogeneity of LGS. Chugani et al. (1987) and Theodore et al. (1987b) found in 5 and 10 cases, respectively, that focal areas of hypometabolism were present in some and that multiple abnormal areas or diffuse hypometabolism was evident in others. These results suggest that both focal lesions with secondary bisynchronous diffusion of the discharge and multifocal damage can be responsible.

The clinical and etiologic heterogeneity of LGS probably accounts for the many clinical patterns that variably overlap with both one another and other syndromes that can be encountered, depending on the individual combination of seizure types and EEG abnormalities. Beaumanoir and Dravet (1988) found that 65 (63%) of 103 patients presented with a typical picture, including tonic seizures, 10-Hz EEG bursts, and episodes of status, whereas 38 (37%) exhibited only some of the classic features but also had other seizure types, including focal seizures or, rarely, generalized tonic-clonic seizures or even absences suggestive of primary generalized epilepsy.

Other investigators have also proposed separating some clinical presentations, variably regarded as subtypes of LGS or as differential diagnoses, from typical LGS. Gastaut et al. (1987b) suggested that cases characterized by a predominance of atonic drop attacks that were commonly associated with focal seizures and focal EEG anomalies should be separated from LGS and regarded as cases of *secondary bilateral synchrony* due to diffusion from focal epileptogenic lesions, similar to the cases of "partial epilepsy with a turn for the worse" reported by Pazzaglia et al. (1985). They thought that such cases differ from "true" LGS because the latter is classified as a generalized epilepsy. However, a distinction based on supposed pathophysiologic mechanisms is not warranted in the present stage of knowledge as long as the clinical and EEG criteria for the syndrome are fulfilled. It is possible that a significant proportion or even most cases of LGS are secondary to focal brain

lesions. Asymmetries of the EEG and focal neurologic signs, including hemiparesis, have been reported in typical cases of LGS (Gastaut et al., 1987b).

Cases of *posttraumatic epilepsy* with diffuse SSW complexes, such as those reported by Niedermeyer (1972b), can also be included in LGS if seizures typical of LGS are present.

The so-called "intermediate petit mal" described by Lugaresi et al. (1973) also fulfills the criteria for the diagnosis of LGS. According to these authors, these cases differ from LGS by the presence of relatively typical absence seizures during the initial course that are associated with or precede more characteristic LGS seizures and by the high proportion of fast (3-Hz) spike-waves in addition to the SSWs of LGS. Such differences do not suffice to exclude the diagnosis of LGS, and no single feature or combination of features clinically permits them to be separated from typical LGS. Moreover, the concept of an "intermediate petit mal" between absence epilepsy and LGS is no longer accepted.

A *myoclonic variant of LGS* has been reported (Giovannardi-Rossi et al., 1988a; Dravet et al., 1982; Aicardi and Chevrie, 1971). It features prominent myoclonic or myoclonic astatic seizures and, less commonly, tonic seizures that are usually of late onset, which are almost exclusively nocturnal and which are often grouped at the end of the night, and episodes of absence status, often with marked erratic myoclonus. The onset is later than that seen in the average LGS, and the outcome is less unfavorable. The EEG variably features fast spike-wave and SSW complexes. The cases reported as LGS occurring in the course of myoclonic astatic epilepsy (Hoffmann-Riem et al., 2000) seem to belong to the same category. The children reported by these authors initially presented with myoclonic jerks and myoclonic astatic seizures, as well as episodes of nonconvulsive status. In a second phase, they developed tonic seizures and a picture that fulfilled the major criteria for LGS. The duration and repetition of the episodes of absence status seemed causally related to the development of cognitive deterioration and tonic attacks (Hoffmann-Riem et al., 2000; Kaminska et al., 1999; Doose and Völzke, 1979). Although tonic seizures are usually considered an uncommon and a late feature only of myoclonic astatic epilepsy, Kaminska et al. (1999), Oguni et al. (2001), and Dravet et al., 2002 found them in a high proportion of their patients, thus emphasizing the potential diagnostic difficulty.

Aicardi and Gomes (1988, 1992) studied ten patients with a *possible mild variant* of the syndrome. All had normal neurologic examination results, a relatively late onset (43 months), and a predominance of absence attacks over tonic seizures. They had relatively normal background EEG tracings and a positive response to hyperventilation; typical 3-Hz absences were sometimes observed early in their course. These patients had some of the features attributed to the so-called "intermediate petit mal" (Lugaresi et al., 1973, 1974). However, complete separation as a subgroup was not possible because all of the patients fulfilled the criteria for the diagnosis of LGS, and several patients with typical LGS had exhibited similar features.

Other epilepsy syndromes clearly differ from LGS in terms of their course, prognosis, and therapy. Typical absences may be impossible to separate clinically from atypical absences. However, the EEG correlates are completely different, and, when associated seizures are present, they enable the recognition of these syndromes. Epilepsies with repeated falls pose a more difficult problem, and these should be clearly separated from LGS, even though they are often misdiagnosed as such. Epileptic falls can result from several mechanisms, and they are observed in several syndromes with different prognostic and therapeutic significance.

Severe myoclonic epilepsy of infants or Dravet syndrome (Dravet et al., 1992a; Dalla Bernardina et al., 1982, 1983a) (see Chapter 5), also termed *polymorphous epilepsy of infants* (Aicardi et al., 1972), also features brief seizures with falls and cognitive deterioration. However, the early history of these affected children is quite different; the onset is virtually always in the first year of life, in which repeated and often long-lasting convulsive seizures are commonly precipitated by mild fevers. At this stage, the differential diagnosis lies more with febrile convulsions than with LGS. The EEG never features SSWs, and no or only a few and late tonic seizures are seen (see Chapter 5).

The less severe types in the *spectrum of the myoclonic epilepsies* (including benign myoclonic epilepsy) and the other imperfectly classified types do not feature tonic attacks or SSWs, except in rare cases (Aicardi, 1994; Guerrini et al., 1994; Dravet et al., 1992b). Myoclonic astatic epilepsy and transitional forms between the myoclonic epilepsies and LGS are discussed later in this book (see Chapter XX).

Atypical partial benign epilepsy (Aicardi, 2000; Aicardi and Chevrie, 1982), also termed "pseudo–Lennox syndrome " (Hahn, 2001; Doose and Baier, 1989), can pose a more difficult diagnostic problem because of the multiple falls associated with gross EEG abnormalities in the form of diffuse SSWs on sleep records. It is characterized by rare, focal, and often nocturnal seizures and by periods, usually of a few weeks in duration, in which intense clinical and EEG epileptic activity is evident. During these periods, the seizures are characteristically atonic attacks that can be focal or generalized and that can result in multiple daily falls. The EEG abnormalities include brief discharges of spike-waves associated with the falls and "continuous spike-waves of slow sleep" or "electrical status epilepticus of sleep" during slow sleep. The active periods are separated by intervals that can reach several months, and, usually, only a few (two to five episodes) occur before complete recovery (Aicardi and Gomes, 1992; Aicardi, 1986a; Deonna et al., 1986a). The cognitive and behavioral outcome of this syndrome may be favorable, although no detailed neuropsychologic follow-up study is available; but deterioration may also occur, especially when multiple and long bouts of seizures occur. Atypical partial benign epilepsy probably represents an intermittent form of the syndrome of continuous spike-waves of sleep, and the poor cognitive outcome of some patients may be related to the duration of the paroxysmal activity.

Patients with only tonic seizures do not meet the criteria of LGS. However, some have a course quite similar to that of complete cases, and these can probably be regarded as variants of LGS, whereas others may have different syndromes. Vigilance-dependent tonic seizures (Rajna et al., 1983) and other sleep-related tonic seizures (Vigevano and Fusco, 1993) rarely pose serious diagnostic difficulties. Such cases probably represent focal seizures of frontal lobe origin.

In general terms, a diagnosis of LGS should not rely solely on the demonstration of diffuse SSW discharges on EEG (Roger et al., 1989), because this is not a specific pattern and other features, such as rapid rhythms during slow sleep, are also important but not constant. The latter pattern is not entirely specific, so the diagnosis relies on a conjunction of abnormalities.

MANAGEMENT

LGS is notoriously resistant to therapy, and it thus constitutes a common type of intractable epilepsy (Brett, 1988). Although complete control of all seizures is obtained only rarely, drug treatment can decrease the frequency of seizures in a significant proportion of patients. Because many cases are highly resistant to many drugs, the tendency is often to use multiple drugs in high doses. Care should be taken, however, to limit the use of multiple-drug combinations, especially of sedative drugs, because this may depress the level of consciousness and result in a paradoxical increase in seizure frequency. Some patients clearly improve with a decrease in polypharmacy, even though this does not result in complete control (Viani et al., 1977).

Because of the frequency of falls and attending injuries, the protection of these children is a major but difficult problem. Often inevitably, the child must wear a helmet, although most models do not afford protection of the chin and nose and few are cosmetically acceptable. The great refractoriness and often the poor prognosis constitute a heavy handicap, and these children require much attention and support, in addition to drug therapy. The special educational, medical, and social needs of the patients should be given great consideration, and every effort should be made to meet them. Cooperation between doctors, psychologists, social workers, and specialized agencies is imperative. The children and their families require considerable sympathy and support.

Drug Therapy

Most antiepileptic drugs are ineffective (Arzimanoglou, 2002b; Brett, 1988; Aicardi and Chevrie, 1986; Erba and Browne, 1983). In addition, because the syndrome consists of several seizure types, single-drug therapy rarely permits control, so combinations of drugs are often required.

Many drugs are being used in multiple combinations that are mostly guided by anecdotal evidence, common wisdom, or personal experience. Only a few controlled studies are available (Glauser and Morita, 2001).

Tonic seizures may respond to phenytoin (Erba and Browne, 1983), but the chronic use of this agent is associated with unpleasant side effects. Carbamazepine is deemed satisfactory by some clinicians for tonic seizures, but it has no effect—or it may perhaps even aggravate—on other types. Phenobarbital can be efficacious, but it may produce sedation and drowsiness, which may exacerbate the seizures. Sodium valproate and the benzodiazepines are regarded as first-line therapies by many investigators (Wheless and Constantinou, 1997; Brett, 1988; Aicardi, 1986a; Aicardi and Chevrie, 1986), especially in cryptogenic LGS (Farrell, 1993), because of the broad spectrum and good tolerability of sodium valproate. Good results have been reported with their use (O'Donohoe, 1985; Jeavons et al., 1977). The following three benzodiazepines are commonly used: clonazepam, nitrazepam, and clobazam (Schmidt, 1985; Gastaut and Lowe, 1979). Clonazepam produces drowsiness; drooling; incoordination; and, in some cases, severe behavior disturbances that limit its usefulness. Nitrazepam has similar, if less marked, side effects (Schmidt, 1985). Clobazam is useful because its side effects are much less marked than those of the other benzodiazepines (Aicardi and Chevrie, 1986; Allen et al., 1983; Gastaut and Lowe, 1979), and its clinical effectiveness seems good. With all benzodiazepines, the development of tolerance is a major concern. Tolerance often develops within 4 to 8 weeks, but it may be delayed for as much as 10 to 12 months. The benzodiazepines should be used with caution in the treatment of absence status because they can transform into the more dangerous tonic status (Ohtsuka et al., 1982; Bittencourt and Richens, 1981; Tassinari et al., 1972a).

The association of valproate and a benzodiazepine (preferably clobazam) is considered a choice combination by several authors, but it has not been formally tested. The fear that this combination could induce a state of stupor (Jeavons and Clark, 1974) has not been substantiated.

Vigabatrin has been found effective in open-label studies (Maldonado et al., 1995; Feucht and Brantner-Inthaler, 1994). Although complete control of attacks was obtained in only a small proportion of cases, the overall result was considered gratifying. However, its retinal toxicity does not make it the drug of choice, and its long-term use is not recommended.

Favorable results in LGS and in other cases of "secondary generalized" seizures have been reported with the use of adrenocorticotropic hormone (ACTH) or steroids (Beaumanoir and Dravet, 1992; Brett, 1988; Aicardi, 1986a; Snead et al., 1983; Yamatogi et al., 1979). No controlled study is available, however; the side effects are potentially dangerous; and relapse seems common. The recent experience seems to be moving away from long-term therapy with these agents. The authors occasionally use these drugs to tide some patients over a particularly difficult period, rather than as long-term therapy.

The use of intravenous immune globulins in high doses has shown some encouraging results (Van Engelen et al., 1994). Controlled trials of immune globulins did not, however, confirm those results (van Rijkevorsel-Harmant et al., 1994; Illum et al., 1990).

Felbamate, lamotrigine, and topiramate are new agents that have been tried in controlled double-blind studies. Felbamate was the first drug shown to be effective for LGS in a controlled trial (Felbamate Study in Lennox-Gastaut Syndrome, 1993). With a dose of 45 mg per kg per day, a 50% decrease of seizure frequency was obtained in 57% of the felbamate-treated patients, compared with only 9% of controls. Unfortunately, hematologic and hepatic toxicity have limited the use of this agent. Because of its possible hematologic and hepatic toxicity, repeated blood counts and a determination of transaminase levels are recommended. However, the frequency of severe toxicity is low in children, in whom no case of aplastic anemia has been reported (Pellock, 1999). At the time of this writing, the concern about toxicity appears to have been excessive, and felbamate remains a useful drug despite the practical difficulties of its use.

Lamotrigine as an add-on drug has proven safe and effective against all types of major seizures in a double-blind, placebo-controlled study (Motte et al., 1997), and it is commonly used. The combination of lamotrigine and a benzodiazepine is often employed (Pisani et al., 1993). The drug may be particularly efficacious against atypical absences and falls.

Topiramate has also proven effective in placebo-controlled studies (Glauser and Morita, 2000; Sachdeo et al., 1999). No comparison among these three agents (felbamate, lamotrigine, and topiramate) is available. Currently, the authors still prefer lamotrigine, which is better tolerated and easier to use, but all three agents should be tried in cases of refractoriness or in those with only partial results. The combination of lamotrigine and valproate may prove useful.

Nonconventional agents have been used. Corticosteroids or ACTH may be indicated to tide the patient over a particularly difficult period (Aicardi, 1994), but their prolonged use is fraught with unavoidable side effects. The value of immunoglobulins has not been properly assessed, although some favorable results have been reported (van Engelen et al., 1994; Rapin et al., 1988). Some authors have used amantadine (Shields et al., 1985) or thyroid-stimulating hormone in small numbers of patients, but these trials have apparently been abandoned.

Nondrug Treatment

The *ketogenic diet* is clearly efficacious in a proportion of cases (Kinsman et al., 1992; Schwartz et al., 1983a, 1983b; O'Donohoe, 1985), and it currently is used extensively in several centers (Trevathan, 2002; Abram and Turk, 1997). However, no controlled study is available, and the use of the diet remains controversial, although the clinical opinion is generally favorable.

Vagus nerve stimulation may be an alternative. Most of the studies show a small average reduction in seizure frequency (3 [17%] of 16 children studied by Parker et al., 1999; 4 [21%] of the 19 children reported by Aldenkamp et al., 2002). However, a worthwhile reduction is occasionally seen.

Resective surgery has been used in a few cases in which a focal lesion, especially cortical dysplasia

(Palmini et al., 1991c, 1991d), was thought to be responsible for the syndrome. In most case, the only surgical possibility is an anterior partial or total *callosotomy*. This operation has proven useful in selected cases (Oguni et al., 1991b; Pinard, 1991), especially as a treatment for seizures with falls, which represent the most incapacitating type of seizure. Recurrences have been observed, however, but gratifying results are sometimes obtained in apparently desperate cases.

SUMMARY

LGS is one of the most severe forms of childhood epilepsy. It is defined by the occurrence of multiple seizure types, the most characteristic of which are tonic and atonic seizures, atypical absences, myoclonic or myoclonic astatic seizures, and episodes of nonconvulsive status epilepticus. From the EEG standpoint, SSW complexes (less than 2.5 Hz), and bursts of rapid (10 to 20 Hz) rhythms during slow sleep, often corresponding to minimal or subclinical seizures, are important for the diagnosis. The syndrome may be cryptogenic in 25% to 30% of cases, or it may be symptomatic of congenital or acquired brain anomalies. The outcome of the syndrome is gloomy, as more than 90% of patients are left with mental retardation or behavioral disturbances. Cases following infantile spasms have an especially poor prognosis, whereas those resulting from focal lesions with bilateral synchrony may have a slightly better outlook; this also applies to cases with a prominent myoclonic component, which are sometimes distinguished as the myoclonic variant of LGS.

The mechanism of mental deterioration in "primary" cases remains in doubt, but it may be related to the interference of the prolonged paroxysmal epileptic activity, as indicated by the EEG, on brain function. This places LGS among the group of the epileptic encephalopathies as they are defined by the new proposal for classification of epilepsies of the ILAE (Engel, 2001).

The treatment of LGS is difficult, and even the new antiepileptic agents are not satisfactory. Palliative or rarely resective surgery is helpful only on occasion.

LGS shares some of the features of myoclonic astatic epilepsy, and an overlap is seen between these two syndromes, although important differences do exist.

Despite the common absence of obvious brain damage, genetic factors play only a minor role, which suggests that undetectable lesions may be a cause. Frontal lobe abnormalities with secondary generalization may be an important factor.

5

Dravet Syndrome

Severe Myoclonic Epilepsy or Severe Polymorphic Epilepsy of Infants

Severe myoclonic epilepsy (SME) initially was mistakenly considered a form of the Lennox-Gastaut syndrome because of the occurrence of repeated falls. However, its clinical and electroencephalographic (EEG) features and its treatment clearly differ, and it should thus be distinguished from the other syndromes that can be associated with myoclonic seizures.

Dravet syndrome was initially described as *SME of infants* (Dravet et al., 1982). Although it does often feature myoclonic phenomena (see Chapter 6 for description), only uncommonly are these the first manifestation of the syndrome, and they are usually overshadowed by other types of seizures (generalized, unilateral, or partial) often precipitated by fever, which suggests the diagnosis of febrile seizures. Moreover, myoclonic phenomena observed in Dravet syndrome are of the following two different types: (a) massive myoclonus with concomitant EEG paroxysmal transients and (b) erratic myoclonus that is usually fragmentary and is often unassociated with EEG paroxysms. The pathophysiologic mechanisms of these two types may well differ, and only one type of myoclonus may be present in a proportion of the cases. Not uncommonly, the myoclonic activity is mild and it may be intermittent, and cases with quite similar features but without myoclonus have been known to occur (Oguni et al., 1994; Kanazawa and Kawai, 1992; Fujiwara et al., 1990; Watanabe et al., 1989a, 1989b). Whether they belong to the syndrome has been disputed (Doose et al., 1998). Recently, however, a consensus that cases with and without myoclonus do not differ in any essential aspect except for the absence of myoclonus (and of other brief seizures in some cases) has been reached (Dravet et al., 2002; Kanazawa, 2001; Oguni et al., 2001). For these reasons, the term *SME* may be inadequate, and the use of the term *Dravet syndrome* may seem more appropriate because the first description of the syndrome (Dravet et al., 1982) was given by this investigator. Considering *Dravet syndrome* as one member of the group of the *epileptic encephalopathies* of infancy and childhood with West syndrome and Lennox-Gastaut syndrome may also be appropriate because it almost invariably features cognitive arrest or deterioration and, sometimes, neurologic abnormalities in addition to intractable seizures. A progressive course is also consistently observed.

ETIOLOGY

The *frequency* of Dravet syndrome is not known. Hurst (1990) placed the incidence between 1 in 20,000 and 1 in 40,000, but that figure may vary with the diagnostic criteria used and the populations studied. A significant number of cases likely remain undiagnosed. In tertiary centers, Dravet syndrome is a fairly common problem (Dravet et al., 1992a). In several studies, a variable excess of boys was present (Doose et al., 1998; Dravet et al., 1992a).

Antecedents of prenatal and/or perinatal abnormal events or risk factors, such as toxemia of pregnancy, severe emesis, low birth weight, or twin delivery, were found in 22% of the patients in the study conducted by Dravet et al. (1992a) and in 20% of those studied by Doose et al. (1998), but the significance of this finding is not clear. No metabolic abnormality has been detected in any case thus far (Dravet et al., 1992a). Repeated imaging studies have not demonstrated detectable brain abnormalities, even though a mild degree of atrophy has been demonstrated in some late-onset cases (Dravet et al., 1992a), and lesional factors are not thought to play an important role. In a biopsy specimen, Renier and Renkawek (1990) found typical images of microdysgenesias similar to those described by Meencke (1985) and Meencke and Janz (1984) in cases of idiopathic generalized epilepsy. The significance of this finding is not clear, and most investigators consider the cause of Dravet syndrome not to be structural brain abnormalities.

Genetic factors seem to play an important role. A family history of epilepsy or convulsions has often been noted, varying from 25% (Dravet et al., 1992a; Sugama et al., 1987; Dalla Bernardina et al., 1984) to 57% (Hurst, 1987b) and 64.4% (Ogino et al., 1986), with an average of about 50% (Scheffer, 2003). Affected monozygotic pairs of twins (Dravet et al., 2002; Doose et al., 1998; Fujiwara et al., 1990), and the occurrence of a similar syndrome in siblings (Doose et al., 1998) have been reported. Doose et al. (1998) studied the EEG in detail in siblings and parents of children with SME and related cases and found a high frequency of abnormalities, including generalized spike-waves, generalized monomorphic alpha rhythm, and photosensitivity. Recently, Claes et al. (2001) found several *de novo* mutations in the genes for α_1 subunit of the sodium channel SCN1A on chromosome 2q in seven children. Some investigators have suggested that Dravet syndrome represents the most severe end of the spectrum of the syndrome of generalized epilepsy with febrile seizures plus (GEFS+) (see Chapter 14) (Singh et al., 2001; Veggiotti et al., 2001). Indeed, missense *de novo* mutations in the same gene have been reported in families with the GEFS+ syndrome (Escayg et al., 2001). Interestingly, Veggiotti et al. (2001) found cases of Dravet syndrome in two siblings belonging to a family with a history of GEFS+ syndrome. The frequency of the mutation of this SCN1A channel in cases of SME is not yet clear because the figures vary in different series. Japanese groups found a mutation rate of 77% to 82% (Fujiwara et al., 2003; Ohmori et al., 2002; Sugarawa et al., 2000), whereas other groups found significantly lower rates of around 35%. Truncating mutations are the most common, but missense mutations have also been reported. Fujiwara et al. (2003) found 25 nonsense mutations, two frameshift mutations, and 12 missense mutations in a series of 33 patients with SME. Whether such *de novo* mutations are present in all patients with Dravet syndrome and are the only mutations found or whether similar, but genetically inherited, mutations can also be responsible for Dravet syndrome remains to be explored.

The possible role of immunizations, especially those against pertussis, has been hotly debated (Menkes and Kinsbourne, 1990). Doose et al. (1998) found that 6 of 33 infants with onset in the first 6 months of life experienced their first seizure within 48 hours of pertussis immunization with a whole-cell vaccine. Given the average age at occurrence, that this is a coincidence seems probable (Robillard et al., 1983).

CLINICAL AND ELECTROENCEPHALOGRAPHIC FEATURES

The following description is based on the classic description by Dravet et al. (1982, 1992a). However, the clinical and EEG features of cases without myoclonus, which present as severe generalized or unilateral convulsive seizures ("hemi–grand mal") with or without associated partial seizures, are also reviewed because drawing a clear delineation between the latter cases and SME seems difficult. This issue is further discussed.

Clinical Features

The clinical physiognomy and course of Dravet syndrome are highly suggestive, with an early appearance of convulsive seizures that are often prolonged and lateralized in a child with normal development. The onset of seizures occurs between 2 and 12 months of age (Dravet et al., 1992a; Giovanardi Rossi et al., 1991; Dalla Bernardina et al., 1982). The seizures are initially generalized, or they are often unilateral clonic seizures and less commonly tonic-clonic attacks. They are often long lasting (10 to 90 minutes). In the series by Doose et al. (1998), 67% of the attacks lasted more than 15 minutes, and 75% had localized symptoms. In more than three-fourths of infants, the lateralization of the attacks changed from one seizure to the next or even within the same attack. The seizures were related to fever in two-thirds to three-fourths of patients, although the level of fever was often modest, being either at or lower than 38°C. Even when the convulsions were nonfebrile, they were often triggered by minor infections. The precipitating effect of Japanese-style hot baths has been mentioned by Japanese investigators (Fujiwara et al., 1990; Sugama et al., 1987; Ogino et al., 1986), and it is common in the authors' experience.

The seizures tend to recur even without fever, and, in all cases, afebrile attacks appear. In one-third of infants, afebrile seizures are the presenting symptom (Doose et al., 1998). A rapid recurrence of febrile seizures within 2 months of the first attack is common, and this should make the clinician suspicious of the possibility of this form of epilepsy, especially if further recurrences follow.

In much less common cases, the mode of onset may be myoclonic seizures that usually occur in the hours preceding the first convulsion; rarely, however, they may supervene days or weeks before (Dravet et al., 1992a, 2002).

During the second or third year of life, the convulsions persist; they are repeated very frequently, but they do tend to become less long and less severe. This period is marked by the emergence of brief attacks that include myoclonic and partial seizures, and atypical absences.

Myoclonic seizures may be of the following two types: massive and segmental (or erratic). *Massive myoclonias* involve predominantly the axial muscles. They may be violent, and they can produce falls; but they can also be barely discernible, producing small forward or backward movements of the head, shoulders, or trunk. Myoclonias can be isolated, or they can be grouped in brief bursts consisting of two to three jerks. They tend to predominate on awakening, and they disappear during slow sleep. They can occur quite frequently, but they are often seen only in the minutes preceding a convulsion. They may be precipitated by variations in ambient light intensity (Dravet et al., 1992a, 2002), and about one-fourth of patients demonstrate self-stimulation by waving a hand in front of their eyes while looking at a source of light or

by looking intently at patterns such as grids and checkered fabric (Dravet et al., 1992a; Aicardi, 1991a; Aicardi and Gomes, 1988; Dalla Bernardina et al., 1987; Hurst, 1987b). On the EEG, massive myoclonias are associated with bursts of irregular spike-waves or polyspike-waves. In the series of Dravet et al. (1992a), they were present in a vast majority of the patients but were seen in only 47% of those in the study by Doose et al. (1998) and in only a part of those in other series (Dravet et al., 2002; Oguni et al., 1994; Kanazawa, 1992; Fujiwara et al., 1990; Watanabe et al., 1989a, 1989b; Ogino et al., 1986). *Segmental or erratic myoclonias* consist of mostly mild muscle jerks involving predominantly the limbs in a narrowly limited, mainly distal territory or the face (Fig. 5.1). They are present at rest, but they are enhanced by movement. They are seldom intense, and they may be more palpable than visible; they do, however, cause unsteadiness and disturbances of fine coordination. They are particularly common during periods of severe and frequent convulsions. Erratic myoclonias are *not* associated with EEG paroxysms.

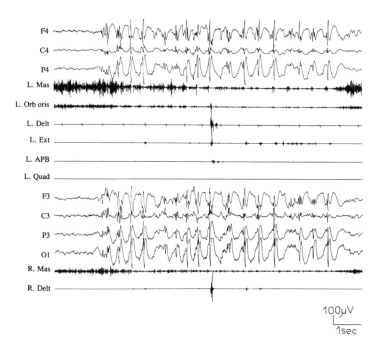

FIG. 5.1. A polygraphic recording of a 14-year-old boy with severe myoclonic epilepsy. A discharge of bilateral and synchronous quasi-rhythmic multiple spikes and waves and spike-wave complexes is accompanied by a series of myoclonic potentials, which are time locked with the spikes, most of which are visible only on the left masseter; one jerk is generalized. Such focal jerks, which were not reported by the patient, would have gone unrecognized if multiple muscles had not been sampled.

Erratic myoclonus were present in 36.5% of the patients studied by Dravet et al. (Dravet et al., 1982), in 31% of those studied by Doose et al. (1998), and in 38% of those studied Oguni et al. (2001). Both types can occur in the same patient, but each may also occur in isolation. This was the case for 21% of the patients studied by Dravet et al. (1992a).

The *atypical absences* noted in 40% (Dravet et al., 1992a) and 75% to 93% (Sugama et al., 1987, Ogino et al., 1986) of patients are brief episodes of decreased awareness that are sometimes associated with the fall of the head, a complete fall, or a myoclonic jerk of the upper limbs. These are associated with brief discharges or irregular spike-waves on EEG. They may be grouped in episodes of *nonconvulsive status epilepticus* lasting several hours or even days, usually with erratic myoclonus (Dravet et al., 1992a, 2002) that is often associated with unsteadiness, dribbling, or frank ataxia that may wrongly suggest the presence of a degenerative disease. Obtundation of variable, often fluctuating degree is a major feature.

Focal seizures occur in one-half to three-fourths of cases. Complex partial seizures with adversive movements and autonomic phenomena predominate, but simple partial seizures do occur (Doose et al., 1998). These may become generalized, or they may remain unilateral.

Doose et al. (1998) found *tonic seizures* in 36 (36%) of their 101 cases. This figure is much higher than that found by other investigators (Dravet et al., 2002; Oguni et al., 2001; Dravet et al., 1992a; Dulac and Arthuis, 1982), who have emphasized the rarity of this type of seizure in Dravet syndrome. This discrepancy might be due to the difference in selection criteria but also to the realization that tonic seizures were a late event (average onset at 6 years of age) that required prolonged and repeated EEG surveillance. All of the investigators have agreed that tonic seizures are only nocturnal and brief, and that they are not frequently repeated.

Initially, the affected children develop normally despite the frequent seizures. During the second or third year of life, however, their progress slows down and comes to a standstill, making the cognitive deficit increasingly evident.

Usually, the slowing of development coincides with the onset of "minor" seizures. The infants begin to walk alone at the normal age, but their gait remains unsteady. Their first few words are uttered normally, but their language progresses very slowly and many patients can never produce elementary sentences. Their unsteadiness increases progressively, and their behavior often deteriorates.

In one series of 50 patients (Aicardi, 1991a), only 2 eventually reached a borderline normal to mildly retarded level. The rest were severely or moderately retarded, and none could follow a regular school course. Only one child could read. Behavioral disturbances were often present in the form of attention-deficit hyperactivity disorder. Psychotic features are less common than they are in Lennox-Gastaut syndrome, and they may be of a milder degree.

Most patients develop fluctuating ataxia and erratic myoclonus between 3 and 14 years of age, and mild pyramidal signs that do not progress are seen in some patients. Ataxia and pyramidal signs were noted in 59% and 22%, respectively, of the patients studied by Dravet et al. (1992a, 2002).

In the long run, the myoclonic attacks have a tendency to subside and to disappear in most patients after 4 to 7 years, but the seizures persist in virtually all patients in the form of generalized tonic-clonic seizures, clonic seizures alternating from side to side, or complex partial seizures (Dravet et al., 1992a; Aicardi and Gomes, 1989; Giovanardi Rossi et al., 1988). Convulsive seizures are usually of shorter duration than the initial attacks, and they tend to occur in clusters, often with a nocturnal preponderance. However, episodes of nonconvulsive status epilepticus are common, and these may play a role in increasing the degree of cognitive and behavioral deterioration.

Electroencephalographic Features

The interictal EEG recordings are generally normal during the first months of the disease despite the frequent seizures. From the second year of life, generalized discharges of fast spike-wave or polyspike-wave complexes appear in bursts or in isolation, sometimes with a unilateral predominance. Focal or multifocal spikes are often observed. Photic stimulation is positive in 40% of patients, sometimes as early as the first year of life (4 months in one of the authors' patients), and the presence of a photoconvulsive response in patients younger than 12 to 18 months of age is suggestive of the diagnosis. A sensitivity to light may also be observed with continuous, rather than intermittent, stimulation (Oguni et al., 2001). Multifocal spikes or sharp wave discharges tend to become more common over the years, and background tracings become slower, especially during seizure clusters. A theta rhythm of 5 to 6 Hz in the central and vertex regions is usually present from the onset (Dravet et al., 1992a; Hurst, 1987b), and it was found in 95% of the patients studied by Doose et al. (1998). No slow spike-waves like those seen in the Lennox-Gastaut syndrome are found. Paroxysmal abnormalities tend to increase with slow sleep. Later, epileptiform discharges tend to occur less frequently, and the theta rhythm tends to disappear; it is replaced by diffuse polymorphic or rhythmic slowing.

LONG-TERM OUTCOME

The ultimate outcome of Dravet syndrome is poor (Kanazawa, 1992; Aicardi, 1991a; Giovanardi Rossi et al., 1991; Hurst, 1987b; Ogino et al., 1986). Dravet et al. (1992a) found that 10 (15.9%) of their 63 patients, followed to a mean age of 11 years, 4 months, had died. All 37 patients older than 10 years were dependent and institutionalized. Half had an intelligence quotient (IQ) of less than 50 (Dravet et al., 1992a), and two-thirds of those studied by Doose et al. (1998) were severely mentally impaired. Of the 101 patients in the study by Doose et al. (1998), 9 died by accident or of sudden death.

Virtually all patients (Dravet et al., 1992a; Aicardi, 1991a; Giovanardi Rossi et al., 1991; Dalla Bernardina et al., 1982) continued to have seizures at their last follow-up. The myoclonic seizures disappear before adolescence in most children. Short tonic-clonic seizures, especially those occurring in sleep, often with a focal component, are the most common seizure type at this age. The photosensitivity and pattern sensitivity often persist (Dravet et al., 1992a, 2002). The sensitivity of these children to fever and even to afebrile infections remains striking in late infancy and adolescence. Their neurologic signs tend to fluctuate with the frequency of the attacks, but they do not continue to progress, in contrast with that which is seen in neurodegenerative disorders. However, motor function remains poorly coordinated in adolescents and young adults, and a persistent tremor is common. Treatments usually have little effectiveness, and SME remains one of the most intractable forms of childhood epilepsy.

DIFFERENTIAL DIAGNOSIS AND NOSOLOGIC ISSUES

The differential diagnosis varies with the stage of the disorder. Dravet syndrome may raise difficult diagnostic problems. During the initial phase, the diagnosis of febrile convulsions is difficult to avoid. Indeed, the initial attacks are febrile convulsions. Some clinical nuances may, however, attract attention, such as the low degree of fever (often below 38°C), the prolonged duration of the seizures beyond 15 or 30 minutes, and a unilateral localization (Dravet et al., 1992a; Aicardi, 1986a, 1991a; Dalla Bernardina et al., 1987). The most suspicious features are the rapid and frequent recurrences of the attacks, usually within 2 months of the first episode, and the occurrence of nonfebrile seizures.

The diagnosis of encephalopathy due to whooping cough immunization is often suspected because the seizures are often prolonged in convulsive status epilepticus and because the modal age of the first seizure falls within the period when immunization is performed, making a temporal coincidence common (Menkes and Kinsbourne, 1990).

The diagnosis usually becomes obvious during the second year of life, with the appearance of brief seizures of multiple types. At this stage, recognizing the syndrome of polymorphic epilepsy of infants is easy, even though many children are still referred with a diagnosis of Lennox-Gastaut syndrome because of their repeated falls. More difficult may be differentiation from progressive degenerative disease, especially during periods of nonconvulsive status epilepticus when ataxia and regression become evident (Bennett et al., 1982; Aicardi and Chevrie, 1971; Roger et al., 1960). In a few patients with this syndrome, mild neurologic abnormalities such as increased reflexes or even a Babinski response may be present, but these are not progressive.

Other forms of myoclonic epilepsy do not usually pose major diagnostic problems because myoclonic attacks are clearly at the forefront of the clinical picture and the initial phase of long-lasting repeated, mildly febrile convulsions is not present (see Chapter 6). The EEG abnormalities are bilateral and symmetric. Falls resulting from atonic seizures are more characteristic of myoclonic astatic epilepsies than they are of Dravet syndrome, but they can occur in the latter. Some cases of myoclonic astatic epilepsy with episodes of nonconvulsive status epilepticus, which are sometimes associated with erratic myoclonus, may be difficult to classify properly, and, indeed, intermediate forms may exist.

The most difficult diagnostic problem is raised by a group of cases that are quite similar, clinically and electrically, to Dravet syndrome but that do not exhibit obvious myoclonic seizures. Such cases have been reported from Japan (Kanazawa, 1992, 2001; Fujiwara et al., 1990; Ogino et al., 1989; Watanabe et al., 1989a, 1989b) and from the Western world (Steinhoff and Kruse, 1992; Yakoub et al., 1992; Aicardi, 1991a; Ernst et al., 1988). Doose et al. (1998) collected a large series of 101 of these cases, which they termed *severe idiopathic generalized epilepsy of in-*

fancy with generalized tonic-clonic seizures; 56 of these also had massive myoclonic seizures. Their cases were selected based on the following criteria: (a) onset of an epilepsy with febrile, often prolonged and unilateral febrile, or afebrile convulsive seizures in the first 5 years of life; (b) absence of known progressive brain disease; (c) severe course with frequent intractability and developmental retardation; and (d) no response or only poor response to treatment. Cases with "minor" seizures (myoclonic, partial, or absence seizures) were not excluded.

Such cases may be more of a nosologic than a diagnostic problem. Their similarities with cases of "classic" Dravet syndrome featuring massive myoclonic seizures are striking in all other respects, and, clearly, a large overlap is seen between cases with and without myoclonic seizures in age at onset, types of seizures, EEG abnormalities, the absence of structural lesions, and the presence of strong genetic factors. Some of the differences, such as a relatively later onset in a few nonmyoclonic cases, a less severe outcome in some, and the more frequent occurrence of tonic seizures, may be due to slightly different selection criteria. The higher incidence of tonic seizures and EEG discharges of fast rhythms in the cases of Doose et al. (1998) is perhaps explained by the close surveillance of the EEG over prolonged periods, as these were observed only late (in patients older than 6 years) and they occurred only infrequently and only during sleep.

Although some of the differences between cases with and without massive myoclonias might represent true nosologic heterogeneity, the similarities are such that the conclusion that most cases in both groups belong to the same syndrome seems safe. Indeed, 13 of the 56 patients of Dravet et al. (1992a) did not have massive myoclonic seizures but only erratic myoclonus, and they therefore appear identical to those of Doose et al. (1998). Erratic myoclonus was present in about the same proportions (37% and 31%, respectively) in both series. The possible relationship between SME and the GEFS+ syndrome has already been mentioned, and the two conditions may well be part of an extended spectrum (Singh et al., 2001; Veggiotti et al., 2001).

Cases with "minor" seizures, including massive myoclonias, atypical absences, and partial attacks, tended to have a more unfavorable outcome (Doose et al., 1998), which Doose et al. thought might have resulted from the presence of modifying genes. More recently, the "atypical" cases were also shown to be associated with mutations in the same gene as the "classic" cases. However, cases manifesting exclusively with tonic-clonic seizures appear to be selectively associated with missense mutations (Fujiwara et al., 2003; Oguni et al., 2001; Kanazawa, 2001).

THERAPY

Therapy for Dravet syndrome is disappointing. The prevention and vigorous treatment of febrile diseases is recommended, but this measure is of uncertain value. The use of vaccines that can produce fever is not contraindicated, but temporary increases in anticonvulsive treatment (e.g., the administration of benzodiazepines) may be useful. Hot baths should be avoided.

Barbiturates and valproate are of limited efficacy (Steinhoff and Kruse, 1992; Tanaka et al., 1990; Woody, 1990). However, Hurst (1987a, 1987b) reported favorable results with valproate in a small series of patients. Unfortunately, these results have not been replicated in larger series. Benzodiazepines, especially clonazepam, may be useful. Carbamazepine might increase seizure frequency (Ernst et al., 1988), and the same might be true of phenytoin. Recent research has suggested that lamotrigine could also have a paradoxical effect and that its use is not indicated (Genton and McMenamin, 1998; Guerrini et al., 1998c). German and Japanese investigators have had more favorable results with bromides (Oguni et al., 1994; Steinhoff and Kruse, 1992; Tanaka et al., 1990; Woody, 1990). To obtain a blood level of 1,400 to 1,900 mg per L, the dosage for infants and young children is 60 to 70 mg per kg per day and, for older children and adolescents, is 40 to 50 mg per kg per day.

Some preliminary results with stiripentol are encouraging (Chiron et al., 2001; Perez et al., 1999); stiripentol is usually administered in combination with other agents, especially benzodiazepines and valproate. Recent work by Chiron et al. (2000) reported complete control of seizures in 9 of 21 treated children and a reduction of seizure frequency by 50% or more in 71%, as opposed to only one case of complete control in the placebo group. Anecdotal reports suggest that topiramate may also be of some help.

Uncontrolled trials of steroids or adrenocorticotropic hormone have been performed, but, even though several investigators have observed a reduced seizure frequency, the overall course of the disease does not seem to be modified. Immunoglobulins have also been tried, especially because the association of seizures with intercurrent infections is so striking (Dravet et al., 1992a; Aicardi, 1991a). However, determining whether cases of polymorphic epilepsy of infants were included in the short series of children with epilepsy treated with immunoglobulins is usually impossible, and, consequently, specific results cannot be ascertained.

The management of these children clearly should include, in addition to drugs, practical measures, such as wearing a helmet, and considerable psychosocial support.

SUMMARY

So-called SME does not present primarily as a myoclonic syndrome but rather as febrile convulsions of long duration and frequent occurrence in the first year of life. Myoclonic seizures are not the initial type of attacks, and, often, they are not even a prominent manifestation, as they are overshadowed by convulsive generalized or unilateral seizures and/or by other brief seizures, such as complex partial fits or atypical absences. The myoclonic seizures may be absent altogether in children with identical histories and clinical and EEG findings. Therefore, the term SME is not really appropriate. The term *polymorphic epilepsy of infants* better defines the phenomenology of this group. Other terms, such as *grand mal* or *hemi–grand mal* (Kanazawa, 1992) or *severe idiopathic generalized epilepsy of infancy* (Doose et al., 1998), have also been proposed. The term *Dravet syndrome* is now preferred, it is historically correct, and it is now advised by the Commission of Classification of the International League Against Epilepsy. Recent progress in molecular genetics has confirmed that Dravet syndrome, together with the related forms mentioned earlier in this chapter, is part of a continuum of severe epilepsies of infancy that may or may not feature additional partial seizures, atypical absences, and myoclonias. This continuum may have a close relationship with the GEFS+ syndrome, which may be associated with mutations in the same gene. However, the genetics of Dravet syndrome continue to raise questions, such as why a family history of epilepsy is so common, whereas the vast majority of mutations associated with SME are nonhereditary truncating mutations.

The diagnostic problems raised by this group are mainly those of tonic-clonic seizures, especially febrile convulsions. The prognosis for these children is extremely poor with regard to both seizure outcome and cognitive development, in which eventual severe or moderate mental retardation follows an initial normal period. No effective treatment is available, although new agents such as stiripentol may be promising.

6

Epilepsies with Predominantly
Myoclonic Seizures

Myoclonic seizures are a common feature of many types of epilepsy at all ages, and they are, therefore, a nonspecific manifestation. Epilepsies characterized by "true" myoclonic seizures can occur at any age. Those syndromes in which myoclonic attacks are the exclusive or predominant type of seizure are considered in this chapter, and they differ in outlook and therapy from the Lennox-Gastaut syndrome (LGS). Therefore, properly classifying the different types of seizures is important; this involves not only careful questioning of parents and caregivers but also the use of polygraphy and/or video-electroencephalograms (video-EEGs) when they are available. Video and neurophysiologic monitoring often reveals that different seizure types that are often referred to as *myoclonic* in the clinical histories because they involved a brisk movement are in fact brief tonic or atonic attacks. The precise determination of the other seizure types that often accompany myoclonic attacks is also important because the associated seizures are critical for classifying the myoclonic epilepsies.

In this chapter, after discussing the nosology and pathophysiology of myoclonic seizures, the authors review the nosologic and semantic problem of the myoclonic epilepsies and define the features common to all forms of myoclonic epilepsy, as well as the features of the different members of this heterogeneous group.

GENERAL NOTIONS ON THE MYOCLONIC EPILEPSIES

Definitions

The term *myoclonus* encompasses a group of neurophysiologically diverse phenomena of heterogeneous etiology whose common semiologic characteristic is represented by involuntary jerky movements that most commonly involve antagonist muscles (Patel and Jankovic, 1988). Myoclonus can be classified as "epileptic" and "nonepileptic" according to its physiology. Some authors define *epileptic myoclonus* as that occurring within the setting of epilepsy (Patel

and Jankovic, 1988), while others define the term as those forms in which the underlying neurophysiologic substrate is thought to be a paroxysmal depolarization shift, regardless of which population of neurons (cortical or subcortical) is primarily involved (Hallett, 1985). Guerrini et al. (2002b) suggested that epileptic myoclonus can be comprehensively defined as an elementary electroclinical manifestation of epilepsy involving descending neurons whose spatial (spread) or temporal (self-sustained repetition) amplification can trigger overt epileptic activity. According to its distribution, myoclonus can be classified as focal, multifocal, or generalized (Hallett, 1985).

The electroencephalographic (EEG) correlate of generalized epileptic myoclonus is a generalized spike-wave discharge, in which the spike corresponds to the myoclonic jerk (Fig. 6.1) and the following slow wave to a postmyoclonic muscular silent period. The EEG correlate of focal epileptic myoclonus is a focal spike in the contralateral sensorimotor cortex. Sometimes, such a correlate can be detected only by the use of jerk-locked (EEG or magnetoencephalogram) averaging. The duration of the "positive' myoclonic muscular burst ranges between 10 and 100 milliseconds. Antagonist muscles are involved simultaneously. The postmyoclonic silent period (200 to 300 milliseconds) is usually proportional to that of the myoclonic jerk. Epileptic myoclonus can either be spontaneous, or it can be evoked by sensorial stimulation such as tapping, muscle stretching, or photic stimulation.

Epileptic myoclonus can also be classified as "negative" (Guerrini et al., 1993b) when the jerking is mainly related to brief pauses of ongoing electromyographic (EMG) activity that lasts 50 to 400 ms. These silent periods are time locked to a contralateral spike-wave complex that is usually central or frontocentral (Tassinari et al., 1995; Guerrini et al., 1993b). Negative myoclonus is characterized by a brief involuntary lapse of posture, followed by a jerk that results from the individual's voluntary attempt to resume his or her original position (Fig. 6.2). Positive and negative myoclonus can be focal or generalized. However, generalized purely "negative" epileptic myoclonus is rare.

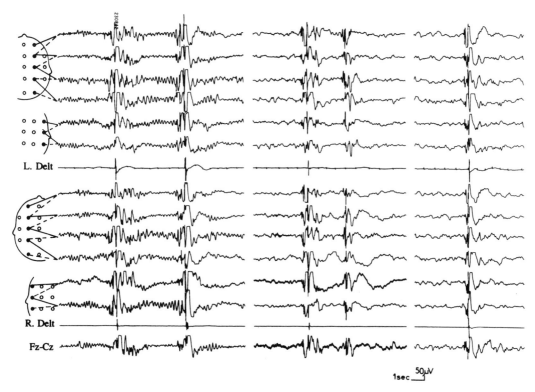

FIG. 6.1. A 4-year-old girl with childhood-onset myoclonic epilepsy having the characteristics of benign myoclonic epilepsy. Isolated generalized jerks are recorded while the patient is drowsy **(left)** and asleep **(middle and right)**. The jerks are accompanied by generalized spike-wave discharges, but they are clinically indistinguishable from sleep myoclonus. This patient is now 17 years of age, and she has been seizure free since the myoclonic jerks were identified at 4 years of age and were treated with valproate until the age of 7 years.

Epileptic myoclonus should not be confused with other forms of nonepileptic myoclonus. Spinal or segmental myoclonus involves muscle groups supplied by contiguous segments of the spinal cord or brainstem. The EMG burst duration is longer (more than 100 ms); the jerks usually have a rhythmic appearance (frequency of 1 to 3 Hz), and they constantly involve the same segments. Rhythmic distal myoclonus should be differentiated from tremor, which usually presents with an alternating EMG pattern between antagonist muscles and which is not associated with scalp potentials on back-averaged EEG. Fasciculations present as twitches involving a muscle fascicle, and they are usually well differentiated from myoclonic jerks. They are prominent if the motor unit is enlarged, as occurs in motor neuron diseases in which they usually involve different body segments. Myo-kymia can be confused with focal myoclonic jerks, but it presents as an undulating, irregular movement involving the facial muscles.

Nosologic Problems

The term *myoclonic epilepsies* has often been used as a collective designation for a large group of epilepsies characterized by repeated brief seizures that are often responsible for multiple falls, by a severe course that is often resistant to antiepileptic drugs, and by their usual association with mental retardation (Aicardi, 1982a, 1991a). As a result, confusion has arisen because this wide group clearly includes several syndromes with different seizure types that are only superficially similar (Arzimanoglou, 2001).

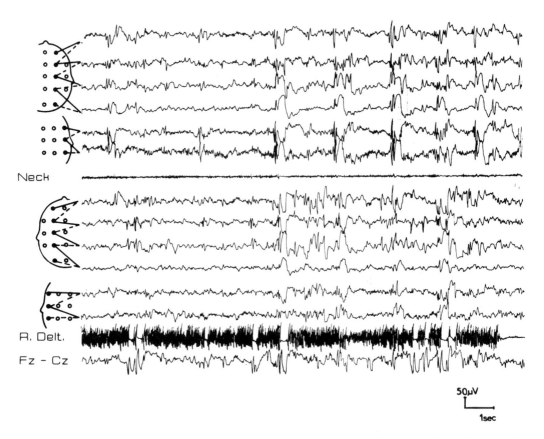

Neck

R. Delt.

Fz - Cz

50µV

1sec

FIG. 6.2. Polygraphic electroencephalographic–electromyographic recording of a 4-year-old boy with staggering gait and continuous postural lapses due to epileptic-negative myoclonus. Electromyographic silent periods lasting up to 300 ms appear irregularly, interrupting the ongoing interferential activity recorded from the right deltoid (*R. Delt*). Silent periods are time locked with sharp waves or spike-wave complexes recorded from the contralateral central area and from the vertex.

Part of the difficulty arises because several types of brief seizures are manifested by sudden, brief jerks. Although these seizures are superficially similar and, as a consequence, are often loosely termed *myoclonic*, they have different neurophysiologic mechanisms. Precise analysis of the ictal manifestations by combined clinical, EEG, EMG, and video monitoring permits the distinction of three different types of seizures. "True" *myoclonic seizures* are manifested on the EMG by biphasic or polyphasic potentials of 20 to 150 ms in duration that may be followed by a tonic contraction of the affected muscles or a transient suppression of normal tonic activity that lasts up to 400 ms; they may therefore be termed *myoatonic seizures* (Niedermeyer et al., 1979b; Gastaut and Tassinari, 1975a). On EEG tracings, myoclonic seizures are associated with generalized bursts of polyspike-waves or spike-waves. During *atonic*

seizures, the patient may fall to the ground suddenly or may slump in a rhythmic step-by-step fashion (Erba and Browne, 1983) or he or she may display only brief nodding of the head or sagging of the body. Atonic seizures are accompanied by slow spike-waves on EEG recordings (Lombroso and Erba, 1982; Gastaut et al., 1966a, 1974a), 3-Hz spike-waves (Aicardi and Chevrie, 1971), polyspike-waves (Chayasirisobhon and Rodin, 1981; Gastaut et al., 1974a), or fast recruiting rhythms (Chayasirisobhon and Rodin, 1981; Fariello et al., 1974). The EMG demonstrates the suppression of normal tonic activity in the involved muscles (Gastaut et al., 1974a; Gastaut and Regis, 1961). *Tonic seizures* involve the tonic contraction of certain muscle groups without a progression to a clonic phase (Erba and Browne, 1983; Gastaut and Broughton, 1972). They can also cause the patient to fall to the ground when the lower limbs are forcibly flexed or the patient is thrown out of balance, especially if the tonic contraction is asymmetric. Patients who fall in a rigid posture like a statue are having a tonic seizure; those patients who fall by collapsing may be having either an atonic seizure or a global tonic seizure with triple flexion of the lower extremities (Erba and Browne, 1983). During a tonic seizure, the EMG shows an interferential muscle discharge that is similar to that seen with a voluntary contraction. The EEG may show a simple flattening of all activity throughout the attack, a very fast activity (20 ± 5 Hz) of increasing amplitude, or a discharge of a 10-Hz rhythm with a high amplitude from the onset that otherwise is similar to the "epileptic recruiting rhythm" (Brenner and Atkinson, 1982; Fariello et al., 1974; Gastaut et al., 1963, 1974a) (Fig. 4.2). *Spasms* that, in fact, are quite similar to brief tonic seizures can also occur, and they are an important cause of sudden falls (Egli et al., 1985).

Conversely, myoclonic phenomena, whether massive, bilaterally symmetric, or fragmentary, can occur with different types of epilepsy at different ages (Aicardi, 1986a), and these do not define a single epileptic syndrome. Several types may occur in the same patient and even within the same attack.

The interictal EEG patterns associated with the seizure types described earlier comprise the following two main types: (a) the diffuse slow (1 to 2.5 Hz) spike-wave pattern (see "Clinical and Electroencephalographic Features Common to the 'True' Myoclonic Epilepsies") and (b) the fast (2.5 to 3.5 Hz) irregular spike-wave pattern. Only one of these patterns may be present, or they may be combined and variably distributed. Other EEG abnormalities may also be present. In some patients, especially those with fast spike-wave ictal pattern, the interictal tracings may be normal.

Atonic and tonic seizures are especially common in the epilepsies with brief repeated seizures beginning in children younger than 5 to 6 years. They are much less common in older children, in whom true myoclonic seizures are more common. Thus, separating study of the seizures by the various age-groups is justified.

In infants and children in whom the onset of epilepsy occurs at less than 5 to 6 years of age, several types of seizures, including tonic or atonic types, are usually present in the same patient, and the epileptic syndromes that are encountered are often associated with structural brain damage. The best-known subgroup in this category is LGS.

In older patients, true myoclonic seizures are the predominant form of attack. Organic brain damage is

seldom found; genetic factors are often of etiologic significance; and the prognosis is better, especially for cognitive development. These "true myoclonic epilepsies" are the subject of this chapter.

Even with this approach, some disagreement still exists over the degree of subdivision that is desirable and the limits of accepted syndromes; furthermore, a fair proportion of cases resist precise classification because they display features that are common to different subsyndromes. Therefore, a complete separation of the various syndromes is not possible in all children (Fig. 6.3).

Clinical and Electroencephalographic Features Common to the "True" Myoclonic Epilepsies

The abrupt brief myoclonic seizures usually are repeated many times a day. Like atonic seizures, with which they may sometimes be associated, they can produce only a slight head nodding, often with abduction of the arms, or they may be responsible for falls when the lower limbs are also involved either in the jerk or by the atonic phenomenon that immediately follows the jerk (Tassinari et al., 1992b; Erba and Browne, 1983). A diagnostically useful feature of myoclonic jerks is their short duration (less than 100 ms) and frequent saccadic character, with a rate of repetition at 2 to 3 Hz, which contrasts with the more sustained muscle contraction of most tonic seizures, however brief, and with the slumping of pure atonic attacks. Myoclonic seizures may affect the external ocular muscles and/or the eyelids or facial, especially perioral, muscles in a significant proportion of patients, but the axial type is the most common (57% and 89%, respectively, of 90 patients) (Aicardi and Chevrie, 1971).

Most myoclonic seizures are spontaneous, and they tend to occur at specific times of the day relative to the level of arousal. They occur predominantly on awakening in juvenile myoclonic epilepsy (JME) or while the child is drowsy in benign myoclonic epilepsy (BME). Some jerks may be precipitated by photic stimulation, most commonly in the EEG laboratory, but this may also be seen with natural stimuli (see Chapter 17). Tapping or sudden acoustic stimuli may also cause generalized epileptic myoclonic jerks in infants (Ricci et al., 1995). At times, myoclonic seizures supervene in prolonged series. In some cases, myoclonic status is observed, usually with partial preservation of consciousness (Doose, 1992; Dravet et al., 1992a; Giovanardi Rossi et al., 1991).

The spike-wave activity is usually fast (more than 2.5 Hz). However, occasional myoclonic jerks are

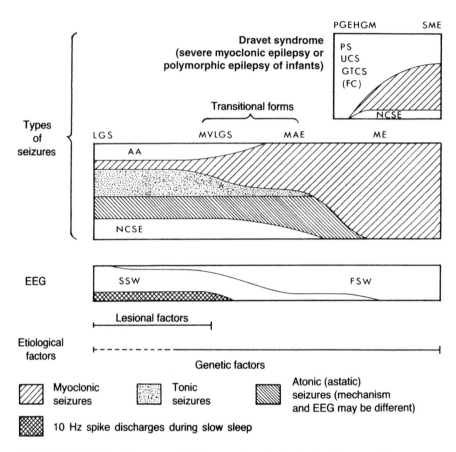

FSW: fast (>2.5 Hz) spike-waves; GTCS: generalized tonic-clonic seizures; LGS: Lennox-Gastaut syndrome; MAE: myoclonic astatic epilepsy; ME: myoclonic epilepsies; MVLGS: myoclonic variant of LGS; NCSE: non-convulsive status epilepticus; PGEHGM: primary generalized epilepsy with hemi Grand Mal; PS: partial seizures; SSW: slow (<2.5 Hz) spike-waves; UCS: unilateral clonic seizures.

FIG. 6.3. Nosologic concept of the myoclonic epilepsies and Lennox-Gastaut syndrome (LGS). LGS and benign myoclonic epilepsy (BME) are the ends of a clinical spectrum that also includes the myoclonic variant of the LGS (MVLGS), as described by Chevrie and Aicardi (1971); myoclonic-astatic epilepsy (MAE), as defined by Dravet et al. (1982); and other unclassified types of myoclonic epilepsy. **Doose's concept** of MAE is based on its supposed genetic etiology. It includes both the severe and the benign idiopathic myoclonic epilepsies. **Dravet syndrome** (previously termed severe myoclonic epilepsy [SME] or polymorphic epilepsy of infants) belongs to a clinically different spectrum. It begins in the first 2 years of life with convulsive seizures (often febrile), usually followed later by myoclonic and partial seizures. Myoclonic seizures may not be prominent in some closely related cases that feature generalized and/or unilateral tonic-clonic seizures, sometimes with partial attacks. The term *primary generalized epilepsy with hemi grand mal* has been used for such cases (Doose, 1985). Tonic and atonic seizures and atypical absences in association with interictal diffuse slow spike wave discharges predominate in LGS, while mostly myoclonic discharges associated with fast (>2.5 Hz) spike wave activity characterize the other end. Lesional damage may be predominant in cases of LGS, whereas genetic factors are most important in the myoclonic epilepsies.

associated with slower (2 to 2.5 Hz) discharges. The interictal tracings may be entirely normal or abnormally slow or asymmetric, or they may display focal abnormalities, depending on whether the myoclonic attacks occur as an idiopathic or a symptomatic phenomenon (Aicardi, 1980b). Interictal bursts of irregular polyspike-waves of short duration (less than three per second) often occur spontaneously, or they are induced by photic stimulation (Aicardi and Chevrie, 1971; Dalla Bernardina et al., 1982, 1992b; Dravet et al., 1992a). During non–rapid eye movement (REM) sleep, an increase in the frequency of discharges that generally feature multiple spikes and waves is often seen (Dravet and Bureau, 2002; Dravet et al., 1992a; Aicardi, 1980a; Aicardi and Chevrie, 1971).

Myoclonic attacks are the only type of seizure in a minority of patients (Dravet et al., 1992b; Aicardi, 1980a). More commonly, they are associated with other seizure types. Generalized tonic-clonic seizures (GTCSs) are most common (Erba and Browne, 1983; Aicardi and Chevrie, 1971), but generalized purely clonic seizures, unilateral clonic attacks, atypical absences, and especially *atonic seizures* are also observed (Dravet et al., 1992a; Dalla Bernardina et al., 1987). *Tonic seizures* are not usually seen in predominantly myoclonic epilepsies, but isolated tonic or short tonic-clonic attacks during sleep are not rare in children within the subgroup defined as *myoclonic astatic epilepsy* (MAE) (Oguni et al., 2002; Guerrini et al., 2002f) (see "Myoclonic Astatic Epilepsy").

Etiology of the Myoclonic Epilepsies

Symptomatic cases of myoclonic epilepsy are rather uncommon; most often, they are the result of prenatal or perinatal hypoxic-ischemic encephalopathies. Patients with brain damage start having myoclonic seizures between a few months and 2 to 3 years of age (Guerrini et al., 2002b; Elia et al.1998; Dalla Bernardina et al., 1992b; Aicardi, 1980a, 1980b, 1982a). They have developmental delay and clinical and/or imaging evidence of diffuse brain damage. Other seizure types are usually associated with the myoclonias. Myoclonic status may be prominent (Dalla Bernardina et al., 1992b, 2002; Guerrini et al., 1996b; Lombroso and Erba, 1982). The latter authors emphasized the occurrence of continuous mild rhythmic jerks that are hardly detectable without polygraphic recordings and the common association with dystonic movements during wakefulness. Most of their patients were later diagnosed as having Angelman syndrome. The mental outcome was generally poor, even though the myoclonus could sometimes be controlled.

A vast majority of cases are idiopathic or cryptogenic, and genetic factors play an important role in their origins, as indicated by the frequency of a family history of epilepsy in individual forms. The recent observation of mutations of the *SCN1A*, *SCN1B*, and *GABRG2* genes in some patients with a phenotype said to be consistent with MAE who belong to families with the "generalized epilepsy with febrile seizures plus" (GEFS+) spectrum (Meisler et al., 2001), and of the *GABRA1* gene in a family with JME (Cossette et al., 2002) suggests ion channel disorders may comprise the pathophysiologic substrate for many cases of myoclonic epilepsy.

However, simple inheritance is limited to a few families, and more complex mechanisms, possibly appearing in combination with other factors, are likely in most. The overall incidence of convulsions or epilepsy in first-degree and second-degree relatives of propositi with myoclonic epilepsy has been found to vary from 26% to 38% (Dravet et al., 1992a; Aicardi, 1991a; Giovanardi Rossi et al., 1991), an incidence that is higher than that seen in most other forms of early onset epilepsy and is similar to that in patients with febrile convulsions. A number of authors (Doose, 1992; Doose and Baier, 1987; Doose et al., 1984) have found a positive family history in 37% (16% in siblings) of their cases of "MAE," which probably includes most cases of cryptogenic myoclonic epilepsy.

Little information, however, is available regarding the pathologic substrate, if any, of the myoclonic epilepsies. Renier and Renkawek (1990) found typical images of microdysgenesis in a biopsy specimen that were similar to those described by Meencke and Janz (1984, 1985) in cases of idiopathic generalized epilepsy (IGE). The significance of such subtle abnormalities has been disputed (Lyon and Gastaut, 1985), and microdysgenetic changes were not observed in a recent study of the brains of five patients with IGE (Opeskin et al., 2000).

SYNDROMES OF MYOCLONIC EPILEPSY IN INFANCY AND EARLY CHILDHOOD

The clinical and EEG features, the etiologic factors, the developmental profile, and the type of seizures that are associated with the myoclonic attacks permit the delineation of some major syndromic groups. In a scheme that has been accepted by several investigators and that was incorporated into the International Classification of Epilepsies, Dravet et al. (1982) recognized the following three major syndromes: BME, severe myoclonic epilepsy (see Chapter 5), and MAE.

Other classifications have been proposed (Lombroso, 1990; Aicardi and Gomez, 1989; Giovanardi Rossi et al., 1988a). Giovanardi Rossi et al. (1988a) proposed the development of an "intermediate" form between the idiopathic and symptomatic epilepsies. Lombroso (1990) held that no firm basis exists for individualizing these two forms and that intermediate types that form a continuum of myoclonic epilepsies, which is somewhat arbitrarily dichotomized, do exist. However, recent findings challenge the view that all forms of myoclonic epilepsy belong to a single large category. Moreover, the recognition of the main syndromic groups does not imply that all cases of myoclonic epilepsies within the same age range must be forcefully classified.

Other investigators (Aicardi and Gomes, 1989) proposed classifying the myoclonic epilepsies simply according to the presence or absence of and the types of associated seizures.

No scheme is really satisfactory, and the differences among the "true" myoclonic syndromes are likely due to the difficulties, or perhaps the impossibility, in assigning precise criteria and limits to the different syndromes proposed.

Benign Myoclonic Epilepsy

The subgroup designated as BME includes cases presenting exclusively or primarily with myoclonic seizures that usually are repeated many times daily. The myoclonic attacks may have been preceded by febrile convulsions. The jerks are preponderantly axial or are generalized; they are usually symmetric. They may result in nodding; staggering; or, only rarely, in falls. Myoclonic seizures in infants, either alone or in combination with subsequent GTCSs do not define, *per se*, a homogeneous subgroup because idiopathic, cryptogenic, or symptomatic cases may present with similar features (Guerrini et al., 1994a) and these had been classified for many years under the confusing heading *myoclonic epilepsies* (Jeavons, 1977; Loiseau et al.; 1974; Harper, 1968).

Dravet et al. (1992a) and Dravet and Bureau (1981) initially classified as having BME only those children who had an age at onset of younger than 2 years and who had no other seizure types, except, eventually, febrile seizures. BME was understood to be an early and minor expression of IGE. Similar cases were subsequently recognized by other groups (Ohtsuka et al., 1993; Todt and Muller, 1992; Salas-Puig et al., 1990a; Dalla Bernardina et al., 1983a); a special subgroup, represented by cases of touch myoclonic epilepsy in infants (see Chapter 17) in whom myoclonic jerks are triggered by tactile or sudden acoustic stimuli, was also

recognized and may or may not be associated with spontaneous jerking (Ricci et al., 1995; Deonna and Despland, 1989; Revol et al., 1989). The total number of cases described initially remained low, and about half of the patients described by Dravet et al. (1992b) were mildly retarded or behaviorally disturbed at follow-up, casting some doubts on the benign outcome of the syndrome (Aicardi, 1994). Aicardi and Gomes (1988), studying a series of infants and young children presenting with only myoclonic seizures and occasional GTCSs, observed a relatively favorable outcome. However, about half their patients exhibited behavioral and/or learning problems at school age. Therefore, when cases with only myoclonic seizures of early onset were not identified retrospectively, they could apparently have a variable prognosis.

In a recent review of the 103 cases reported thus far under the heading "BME," Dravet and Bureau (2002) updated their description of the syndrome and slightly modified the initial concepts. They acknowledged that the age at onset may be as late as 5 years (Giovanardi Rossi et al., 1997; Guerreri et al., 1994a), that the term *benign* is questionable according to the most recent International League Against Epilepsy (ILAE) definitions (Engel, 2001), and that the difference from the milder cases of MAE may not be entirely clear.

For the sake of simplicity, in this section, the authors will continue to use the accepted term *BME*, bearing in mind the aforementioned uncertainty about its appropriateness.

Etiologic and Epidemiologic Data

BME is rare. Dravet and Bureau (2002) reported that children with such a syndrome represented less than 1% of the epilepsy population in their specialized center and 2% of all IGEs. Other authors observed BME in 1.3% to 1.7% of the children with seizure onset in the first year of life (Sarisjulis et al., 2000; Caraballo et al., 1997) and in 2% of those with onset in the first 3 years. The syndrome is almost twice as common in boys than in girls (Dravet and Bureau, 2002).

A family history of epilepsy or febrile seizures is observed in almost 40% of children with BME (Dravet and Bureau, 2002; Aicardi and Gomes, 1988). However, familial cases have not been described. Occurrence of MAE in the brother of an affected child has been reported (Arzimanoglou et al., 1996).

Clinical and Electroencephalographic Presentation

With very few exceptions, the child's development is normal before the first myoclonic seizures appear. The age at onset ranges from 5 months to 5 years. The initial jerks tend to be mild and rare, and they are often overlooked or misinterpreted as spasms or tics. They are usually manifested as head drops or upward eyeball rolling that is accompanied by a brisk abduction of the upper limbs (Dravet and Bureau, 2002). Myoclonic jerks occur several times daily, sometimes clustering within a short time, and they may vary in intensity in the same child. Stronger jerking that is accompanied by projection of objects or falling are rare, and it tends to appear later in the course, if at all. Rhythmic or quasi-rhythmic repetition of a short series of jerks within 5 to 10 seconds is another feature usually seen in older children.

If falling occurs, it characteristically is followed by the immediate resumption of the previous posture and ongoing activities, usually without injury. This behavior is extremely different from falling that is linked to an epileptic spasm (i.e., an atonic seizure), which clearly interferes with ongoing activity as the children appear confused and often cry because they are frightened or they have suffered injuries. Mild myoclonic jerks cause little displacement of the limbs, and their expression is influenced by the child's posture. An occasional myoclonic seizure may be asymmetric or even unilateral. Whether impairment of consciousness occurs is difficult to appreciate because the jerks are too brief and, in general, no detectable interruption of ongoing activities occurs; however, repeated jerks might be accompanied by a mild impairment of contact. Drowsiness appears to facilitate the jerks. Episodes of myoclonic status are extremely rare (Aicardi and Gomes, 1988).

A subset of children presents with generalized myoclonic jerks that are triggered by sudden tapping or acoustic stimuli, and these may or may not be associated with spontaneous attacks of an identical type (Ricci et al., 1995; Deonna and Despland, 1989; Revol et al., 1989). The electroclinical characteristics of this form are similar to those seen in children with only spontaneous jerks, and its evolution might be even more "benign" (Dravet and Bureau, 2002). The onset of reflex jerks may be as early as 4 months of age (Ricci et al., 1995). These jerks can be provoked while the child is awake or during sleep.

The EEG shows normal background activity in almost all children with BME (Dravet and Bureau, 2002; Guerrini et al., 1994a; Aicardi and Gomes, 1988). Interictal EEG, especially while the child is awake, may be normal because spike-wave discharges very rarely occur without concomitant myoclonic jerks. Focal EEG abnormalities have been reported occasionally (Dravet and Bureau, 2002; Lin et al., 1998; Giovanardi Rossi et al., 1997), but, in most patients, they disappeared in follow-up recordings.

Sleep recordings provide higher chances of capturing ictal discharges, which are represented by bursts of generalized fast spike-waves or polyspike-waves without rhythmicity, and of brief duration (less than 3 seconds). Most jerks are isolated and time locked with the spike component of the spike-wave complex (Guerrini et al., 2002b). In the reflex variety of BME, a refractory period lasting up to 2 minutes may be observed after a reflex-induced jerk (Ricci et al., 1995). In about 10% of all affected children, myoclonic jerks are also triggered by light stimuli, especially intermittent photic stimulation (IPS) in the EEG laboratory (Dravet and Bureau, 2002; Guerrini et al., 1994a; Aicardi and Gomes, 1988).

Course and Outcome

The course of BME is said to be benign, an opinion largely based on retrospective studies that mainly included children selected because of their favorable outcomes. In some series (Dravet and Bureau, 2002), one of the proposed criteria for diagnosis was a rapid response to valproate monotherapy, which is clearly also a strong criterion of benignity. However, some children did have cognitive or behavioral sequelae, indicating that, even with these strict criteria, a benign outcome could not be guaranteed.

The epilepsy outcome is said to be favorable. Myoclonic jerks were reported to have disappeared in all the children who were followed for a long period (Dravet and Bureau, 2002). Dravet and Bureau (2002) estimated that myoclonic seizures had been present for less than 1 year in most of the 52 published cases for whom this information was available. However, the mean delay for initiating an effective treatment was not known. In general, treatment had been withdrawn in most patients older than 6 years at follow-up. A minority of patients were reported to have experienced rare GTCSs when they were 9 to 16 years of age (Dravet and Bureau, 2002; Giovanardi Rossi et al., 1997; Dravet et al., 1992b). In some, these seizures occurred during valproate withdrawal, and they were subsequently controlled by the reinstitution of treatment (Dravet and Bureau, 2002). No detailed information is available for the remaining patients. The main cause for continuing treatment after that age was photosensitivity that had either persisted or had emerged after the spontaneous myoclonic jerks disappeared (Dravet and Bureau, 2002; Lin et al., 1998; Giovanardi Rossi et al., 1997).

Some children with BME did not receive any drug treatment (Dravet and Bureau, 2002). Although no additional seizure types were seen, the myoclonic jerks had persisted. These cases were thought to have an increased risk of impaired psychomotor development and behavioral disturbances, but evidence for this was unconvincing.

A critical review of the published information on treatment indicated that most children were well controlled with valproate monotherapy and that they were seizure free by school age (Dravet and Bureau, 2002). Other drugs, including phenobarbitone or nitrazepam monotherapy or combinations of valproate or phenobarbitone with clonazepam, clobazam (Giovanardi Rossi et al., 1997), or ethosuximide (Todt and Muller, 1992), have been used, especially in the past.

The cognitive and behavioral outcome is favorable (Dravet and Bureau, 2002). Only a minority (17%) of affected children experienced mild cognitive difficulties. Clearly, the good outcome of BME fulfilling the criteria of Dravet and Bureau (2002) might be due to the additional requirements for criteria of benignity, such as a rapid response to therapy, rather than to an intrinsic difference in the severity of the condition. Similar remarks could apply to those cases classified as "MAE" with a favorable outcome (Oguni et al., 2002; Kaminska et al., 1999). Thus, BME does not always have a benign outcome, nor is it the only relatively benign syndrome among the myoclonic epilepsies.

Diagnostic and Nosologic Aspects

Cases of early onset BME are sometimes mistaken for cryptogenic infantile spasms. However, infantile spasms are characterized by a more sustained muscle contraction, and they occur in periodic series differing from the brisk and often isolated myoclonic jerks of BME. In doubtful cases, polygraphic EEG–EMG recordings easily clarify the picture.

The so-called *benign nonepileptic myoclonus of early infancy* (Dravet et al., 1986; Lombroso and Fejerman, 1977) is a possible diagnosis in children who have normal development and present with clusters of jerky movements of the limbs, nodding, or axial shudder (Pachatz et al., 2002) but who have normal interictal and ictal EEGs. In such cases, polygraphic recordings show a short tonic, rather than myoclonic, contraction lasting 0.5 to 3 seconds (Pachatz et al., 2002).

The separation of BME, especially if it is of late onset, and the milder cases of MAE may be difficult. A complete distinction between these two conditions may even be improper because they might represent two extremes of a same syndromic spectrum. However, the statement that using the criteria of BME, perhaps because they are criteria of benignity, is usually more predictive of a good outcome is fair.

In summary, a reasonably favorable prognosis can be given when *all* the criteria, including those of benignity, are present (Dravet and Bureau, 2002). A later onset would not modify the good prognosis if these typical characteristics are present (Guerrini et al., 1994a). Those children who present with reflex myoclonic jerks, either as the only type of attacks or in addition to spontaneous ones, may have an even more favorable outcome, although the evidence for this is rather meager.

As Dravet and Bureau (2002) recently discussed, the denomination of the syndrome as "benign" might no longer be appropriate because the most recent definitions of a "benign" epilepsy syndrome require that it remit without sequelae (Engel, 2001).

Myoclonic Astatic Epilepsy

Doose et al. (1970) first proposed the use of the term *myoclonic astatic petit mal*, which was later changed to *MAE*, to designate the primary generalized epilepsies of childhood whose main clinical manifestations are myoclonic and/or astatic seizures. The latter seizures were characterized by falls attributed to lapses of muscle tone. However, myoclonic attacks involving axial muscles can also result in falls that may be impossible to separate from atonic seizures in the absence of polygraphic EEG–EMG recordings, so some doubt still exists about the mechanism of the falls in the cases described by Doose et al. These authors also stressed the value of biparietal theta activity in the EEG; the importance of genetic factors in the etiology; the absence of organic brain damage; and the preponderance of fast spike-wave or polyspike-wave complexes, as opposed to the slow spike-wave complexes and symptomatic nature of LGS. Doose (1992) considered MAE a form of primary generalized epilepsy and clearly indicated that his intent was not to describe a "rigidly defined syndrome" but rather a large group of early cases of epilepsies with myoclonic and atonic manifestations of idiopathic origin, with emphasis on "the wide variability of the IGEs of early childhood as a result of a multifactorial background responsible for electroclinical differences in presentation." His concept of MAE apparently embraced all forms of primary (or idiopathic) myoclonic epilepsies, including both severe and benign myoclonic epilepsies as later described in the ILAE classification (Commission on Classification and Terminology of the International League Against Epilepsy, 1989). Such classification included "Doose syndrome" in the list of myoclonic epilepsy syndromes on the same level as, and in addition to, severe myoclonic epilepsy and BME on the basis of the description of the clinical and EEG features of the seizures, without realizing that Doose's classification was based largely on etiology. Moreover, "Doose syndrome" was listed under the heading "cryptogenic and symptomatic epilepsy syndromes," in contradistinction to the statements of Doose, who had insisted on its primary or idiopathic nature.

Such inconsistencies explain why large differences in the concept of the myoclonic astatic epilepsies exist among different investigators.

The recent proposal of the Task Force of the ILAE for a new classification scheme (Engel, 2001) lists "epilepsy with myoclonic astatic seizures" with benign (BME) and severe myoclonic epilepsy (Dravet syndrome) and myoclonic absences among the recognized myoclonic syndromes. However, if severe myoclonic epilepsy is a well-defined syndrome that clearly differs from the other "myoclonic" epilepsies, the frontiers that separate BME from MAE are less clear cut, and these two forms can also be regarded as belonging to a single spectrum.

Moreover, a consensus on the necessary criteria for the diagnosis of MAE does not appear to have been reached. For example, whether falls were considered a necessary criterion for inclusion in MAE in several series, which apparently included patients with purely myoclonic seizures, is not clear (Oguni et al., 2002; Kaminska et al., 1999), and the contrast between the favorable course of BME and that of MAE is not always obvious. In the series by Kaminska et al. (1999), half the cases of MAE had an excellent outcome, and, in that by Oguni et al. (2002), who studied 81 patients, the spontaneous remission of seizures was observed in 26% of the children, 89% were free of myoclonic astatic attacks within 3 years, and approximately 60% eventually had a normal intelligence quotient (IQ). In practical terms, however, falls are of major importance because of their severe negative impact on the quality of life of the affected children. They may also have some unfavorable prognostic significance, although this is not true in all cases (see "Cause and Outcome"), because they seem to indicate a higher risk of occurrence of other seizure types (GTCSs, absences, nonconvulsive status epilepticus) and a greater likelihood of an unfavorable cognitive and behavioral outcome. However, no reliable predictors of the long-term course are currently known (Guerrini et al., 2002f; Kaminska et al., 1999), and an overall description of MAE, regardless of the ultimate course, is given in this section.

The relationship of MAE and LGS is discussed in Chapter 4. No clear differentiation is always possible, and the "myoclonic" variant of LGS is probably an evolutive aspect of MAE.

Etiologic and Epidemiologic Data

MAE is a relatively uncommon type of epilepsy. However, the variable systems of classification used by different authors make quantitative estimates unreliable. Series that include several dozens of patients have been published (Oguni et al., 2002; Kaminska et al., 1999; Aicardi and Gomes, 1988).

Although the 1989 ILAE classification regarded MAE as "symptomatic or cryptogenic," acquired factors appear infrequently as a cause. Neuroimaging mostly provides normal results. In contrast, genetic factors are often present. They were found in 32% of Doose's patients, who probably suffered from various syndromes of myoclonic epilepsy and who were classified on the basis of their idiopathic ("primary") etiology, and in 17% to 26% of cases selected on clinical and EEG criteria similar to those of the ILAE. In the studies of Doose and Baier (1987), the frequency of EEG markers such as photosensitivity, parietal theta rhythms, and spike-waves was distinctly increased in the siblings and parents of the affected children. These authors favor a multifactorial type of inheritance. Personal antecedents of febrile convulsions or other epileptic seizures were found in a substantial proportion of patients. The recent finding that the GEFS+ spectrum includes children with missense mutations of the *SCN1A* and *GABRG2* genes and a phenotype that might be consistent with MAE (Meisler et al., 2001) suggests febrile seizures and MAE may possibly have a common genetic background in some cases. However, the genetics of MAE is likely to be complex in most patients, and whether children with a good outcome differ genetically from those with an unfavorable outcome is not known.

A remarkable predominance of boys exists in most series. In the mixed series of Doose (1992), which also included other myoclonic syndromes, 74% were boys; more than 75% were boys in that of Kaminska et al. (1999), and 79% were boys in the series of Aicardi and Gomes (1988). The proportion of boys was also high (68%) in the studies of BME (Dravet and Bureau, 2002).

Clinical and Electroencephalographic Presentation

The onset is usually between 7 months and 8 years of age with a peak incidence between 2 and 6 years of age. Some cases have an early onset, which occasionally can be as early as 1 month of age (Kaminska et al., 1999). Most patients have normal development before the first seizures occur.

The generalized jerks or astatic falls are typically repeated several dozen times daily. In a recent series of 81 cases (Oguni et al., 2002), 29 were studied polygraphically. The seizures were myoclonic in 17 children, atonic with or without a preceding minor myoclonus in 11, and myoclonic atonic in 3. In the remaining 48 patients of this series who were not examined by polygraphy, in 39, the seizures were judged to be atonic from the history, and, in 18, they were thought to be myoclonic. Overall, 52 children (64%) had drop attacks resulting in falls. In a previous study, the same authors (Oguni et al., 1993) used video and EEG–EMG monitoring to record 36 drop attacks in five children with MAE. They found that 26 seizures were purely atonic, whereas 9 were purely myoclonic with a predominant involvement of the flexor muscles; only 2 were myoatonic. However, a change in facial expression and/or a brief twitch of the extremities might have preceded the atonic resolution, probably indicating the presence of a brief positive phenomenon that was visible only in a few muscles. Because only a few muscles can be sampled, limited myoclonic activity may escape recognition.

Myoclonic atonic seizures consist of brief massive or axial symmetric jerking involving the neck, shoulders, arms, and legs, often resulting in head nodding, abduction of arms, and flexion of the legs at the knees. Stronger jerks can precipitate a fall. The jerk is immediately followed by an abrupt loss of muscle tone that seems to be the most common cause of the fall (Tassinari et al., 1998). Falls in MAE can also result from purely myoclonic seizures (Dravet et al., 1997; Yaqub, 1993; Dravet and Roger, 1988). A violent myoclonus that is followed by an abrupt fall to the ground or on the table may result in severe injuries, especially to the nose, teeth, and face. The duration of such episodes is less than 2 to 3 seconds. The jerks may be isolated, or they may occur in short series at a rhythm of about 3 Hz, resulting in saccadic flexion of the head and/or abduction of the arms.

The EEG of myoclonic atonic seizures shows bursts of spike-wave complexes or polyspike-waves at 2 to 4 Hz (Fig. 6.4). The EMG shows that the muscle contraction responsible for the myoclonic jerk is usually followed by a brief period of EMG silence during which muscle activity disappears for up to 500 ms. The silent period sometimes occurs without a preceding jerk, although excluding the possibility of mild contractions in muscles that are not being sampled is difficult.

Neurophysiologic study of the myoclonic jerks in MAE has shown bilateral synchronous EEG dis-

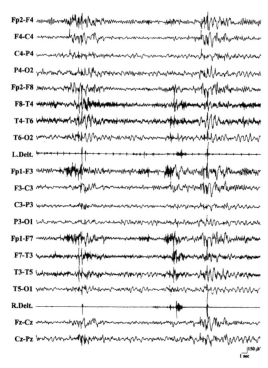

FIG. 6.4. A 6-year-old boy with myoclonic astatic epilepsy. Generalized myoclonic jerks causing brisk abduction of the arms and flexion of the head and knees are visible as high-amplitude myoclonic potentials on the electromyographic (EMG) channels (*L. Delt* and *R. Delt*). Myoclonic potentials are accompanied by a diffuse discharge of irregular spike-wave complexes. A clear time-locked correlation is observed between the electroencephalographic spikes and the myoclonic EMG potentials.

charges and bilateral synchronous jerks in muscles from both sides of the body, which indicates that myoclonic attacks were primary generalized. This differs from the observations in LGS, in which interhemispheric latency and side-to-side delay in the activation of muscles indicates that the jerks probably represent the secondary generalization of focal myoclonic activity (Bonanni et al., 2002; Guerrini et al., 2002b).

Other types of seizures, including generalized tonic-clonic attacks, atypical absences, and nonconvulsive status, are common. Episodes of nonconvulsive status are mentioned by all authors. They are marked by a variable blurring of consciousness (somnolence, stupor, apathy, or milder obtundation with drooling) that is often associated with erratic perioral and distal muscle twitching and by brief head nods that are due to the repeated lapses of axial muscle tone and/or jerking of the neck muscles. Sometimes, increased muscle tone may be seen, the child may have a fixed, rigid posture like a statue, and he or she may display mild vibratory movements (Guerrini et al., 1994a). These episodes can begin insidiously and then develop progressively, and they may last from minutes to hours, days, or even weeks, often with fluctuations. They can be repeated, and they have been considered indicators of a poor cognitive outcome when they are severe, frequent, and long lasting (Kaminska et al., 1999; Doose and Völzke, 1979). The EEG correlate of such episodes is often represented by long runs of slow waves and spike-wave complexes that are sometimes associated with sequences of slow spike-waves. More often, the EEG shows irregular polymorphous paroxysmal abnormalities that may be so severely disorganized that they simulate a hypsarrhythmic pattern (Genton et al., 2000c; Guerrini et al., 1994a) (Fig. 6.5). During such episodes, neurologic symptoms and signs may appear, especially ataxia and pseudocerebellar signs that can suggest the presence of a degen-

erative condition; they, however, fluctuate and eventually disappear (Bennett et al., 1982; Aicardi and Chevrie, 1971).

Tonic seizures have been considered to be absent by some authors (Oguni et al., 2002; Giovanardi Rossi et al., 1988a), but others have found them to be common. On the EEG, they are marked by the same fast rhythms as in LGS (Guerrini et al., 1994a, 2002f; Kaminska et al., 1999) (see Chapter 4). Kaminska et al. (1999) observed such seizures in up to 38% of patients, even those who had a favorable course, although they were distinctly less frequent and shorter in these latter cases. These authors stressed the occurrence of vibratory tonic seizures, which were also mentioned by Oguni et al. (2002). Tonic seizures are considered by some investigators to be an indication of a transition from MAE to LGS after a variable course that is marked mostly by myoclonic attacks (Hoffmann-Riem et al., 2000).

The interictal EEG of MAE may be normal at onset (Genton et al., 2002c). Bursts of 3-Hz spike-waves may occur without apparent clinical manifestations, and these may be activated by sleep. Slow-wave activity may be observed during bad periods. The most suggestive finding is the presence of 4-Hz to 7-Hz theta rhythms with parietal accentuation and occipital 4-Hz rhythms that are constantly blocked by eye opening (Oguni et al., 2002; Doose, 1992). Variable lateralization of paroxysmal bursts is possible; a consistently localized focus is, however, distinctly unusual (Bonanni et al., 2002). A considerable subset of these patients are photosensitive.

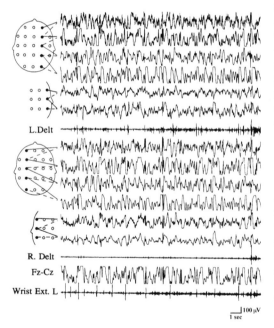

FIG. 6.5. An electroencephalographic (EEG) polygraphic recording in a 3-year, 5-month-old boy during an episode of myoclonic status. The child was vacant and unresponsive, and he presented with increased muscle tone; drooling; and tiny, arrhythmic, and erratic jerky movements of the face and hands. Irregular high-amplitude spike-wave EEG activity and the frequent multifocal myoclonic jerks are observed. (Abbreviations: Delt., deltoids; Ext., extensors; L., left; R, right.)

Course and Outcome

The course of MAE is unpredictable. In some children, despite the occurrence of frequent attacks of multiple types, the disorder seems self-limited, and the seizures abate after a few years. This occurred in about half of the patients studied by Kaminska et al. (1999), 54% of those of Doose (1992), and up to 89% of those of Oguni et al. (2002). The mean duration of the active phase was less than 3 years in this group, in which the cognitive and behavioral outcomes were satisfactory. Some of the children did have mild cognitive and behavioral problems, especially hyperactivity, as Kaminska et al. (1999) also mentioned. Oguni et al. (2002) found that 58% of their patients had a normal IQ, 20% had a borderline IQ or "mild mental retardation," and 21% had more severe retardation at the end of follow-up.

Other children have a more severe course because their epilepsy remains intractable. In most, cognitive and behavioral impairment becomes evident, and mental retardation of variable degree is present after a few years, even though the seizures may eventually disappear (Neubauer et al., 2002). Factors responsible for these different outcomes are not well understood. Doose et al. (1989, 1992) emphasized the association between a poor mental outcome with dementia and the repetition of prolonged episodes of nonconvulsive status. The hope that prompt effective treatment of these episodes can improve the cognitive outcome is reasonable, but this assumption has not been proven. Other factors thought to be associated with an unfavorable outcome include the occurrence of atypical absences, repeated GTCSs, and repeated falls. The occurrence of nocturnal tonic seizures is classically regarded as being indicative of a turn for the worse. However, some investigators have found that they are common, even in the "benign" cases, so they may not be incompatible with a favorable outcome (Guerrini et al., 1994a, 2002f; Hoffmann-Riem et al., 2000; Kaminska et al., 1999). According to Gundel et al. (1981), the persistence of rhythmic EEG slowing until adolescence, without the development of a stable alpha rhythm, may be an indicator of an unfavorable course.

Children with a poor outcome and those with a more favorable course cannot be separated on the basis of age, antecedents, or clinical presentation at onset or for the first year of the disorder (Kaminska et al., 1999; Aicardi, 1994a). The cognitive deterioration may perhaps be regarded as a form of "epileptic encephalopathy," a condition in which the epileptic activity itself plays an important role in the loss of the individual's mental abilities (Engel, 2001).

Diagnostic and Nosologic Aspects

Because of the lack of agreed criteria and the multiple classifications used, separating MAE from the other childhood epilepsies featuring prominent myoclonic seizures may still be difficult in clinical practice (Arzimanoglou, 2001).

Some of the conditions discussed in the differential diagnosis of LGS may also pose diagnostic problems with MAE, including atypical benign rolandic epilepsy in which negative motor phenomena may cause astatic postural lapses or full-blown falls mimicking myoatonic seizures (see Chapter 10).

The progressive myoclonic epilepsies (see Chapter 7), such as myoclonic encephalopathy with ragged-red fibers, Unverricht-Lundborg disease, or late infantile ceroid lipofuscinosis, can be clinically impossible to distinguish from MAE at their onset, but the later emergence of neurologic signs and continuous erratic myoclonus establishes the diagnosis. One difficulty can result from the appearance of neurologic signs, especially ataxia, erratic myoclonus, and apparent cognitive deterioration, during episodes of nonconvulsive status in the course of MAE when the disturbance of consciousness is slight and progressive and when such episodes are long lasting (Bennett et al., 1982; Aicardi and Chevrie, 1971). In these cases, the grossly abnormal EEG tracings and the fluctuating course are diagnostic.

Late-onset cryptogenic epileptic spasms (Bednarek et al., 1998) may be clinically similar to myoclonic astatic seizures. These children come to medical attention because of multiple daily episodes of violent falls. Although the individual attacks may seemingly have a similar semiology, the spasms appear in series with typical periodicity, and the EEG recording shows different ictal and usually interictal characteristics.

Nonepileptic myoclonus is rarely an important diagnostic consideration. However, erratic myoclonus such as that observed in some degenerative disorders, even without epilepsy, may rarely raise a suspicion of a diagnosis of MAE.

The distinction among LGS, Dravet syndrome, and MAE is often misunderstood because of the association of multiple seizure types in all three entities, so these three syndromes are often confused with one another. However, making a distinction is feasible in most cases with accurate history taking and the support of appropriate EEG (including sleep recordings) and simultaneous EMG investigations that, ideally, are accompanied by video recording for off-line analysis (see Chapters 4 and 5). The differential diagnosis is of considerable prognostic therapeutic and genetic importance because at least 50% of children with MAE have a good prognosis; MAE may be exacerbated by drugs used for the treatment of LGS, such as vigabatrin (Guerrini et al., 1998c); and the familial recurrence risk is higher in both MAE and Dravet syndrome than in LGS. Furthermore, Dravet syndrome has its onset earlier, in the first year of life, with febrile convulsions that are often prolonged, and myoclonus seldom appears before the second or third year of life. At this stage, multiple seizure types, including myoclonic jerks and episodes of nonconvulsive status, can wrongly suggest MAE, but the overall history is distinctive and it is dominated by the repeated and prolonged convulsive seizures, which are not seen in MAE.

Differentiation of MAE from LGS is usually straightforward (Dravet, 1996), as the main types of seizures in LGS are tonic attacks and atypical absences associated with atonic seizures in some patients. The EEG mostly features slow spike-waves and high-frequency ictal discharges (fast rhythms) that are extremely frequent during sleep. However, myoclonic seizures are present in some cases of LGS. The occurrence of tonic and atonic attacks and often of slow spike-wave complexes, although these are more consistent with the diagnosis of LGS, is not incompatible with MAE, thus emphasizing the limitations of classification based solely on clinical and EEG features.

Other epilepsies of childhood with predominant myoclonic attacks remain difficult to classify; in some cases, they may well belong to the spectrum of MAE. Dravet et al. (1982) left 34 of their 142 cases of myoclonic epilepsy without further classification. Other investigators (Giovanardi Rossi et al., 1988a) also encountered similar problems.

One cause of these classification difficulties is the absence of universally accepted criteria for the delineation of the syndromes. For example, some cases reported as MAE apparently did not have falls. Likewise, the proportion of tonic seizures that rules out a diagnosis of MAE is nowhere clarified, and the proportion of myoclonic attacks that are incompatible with a diagnosis of LGS is also not clarified. Those patients classified as having "type 1" MAE by Kaminska et al. (1999) (i.e., those patients who had a relatively short course of their epilepsy [less than 3 years] and a good cognitive outcome) frequently had several types of seizures, including nocturnal tonic attacks and brief episodes of nonconvulsive status epilepticus.

Given these difficulties, accepting that the epilepsies that feature prominent myoclonic activity, including BME, MAE, and other unclassifiable cases but excluding severe myoclonic epilepsy and LGS, which clearly belong to separate categories, are part of a continuum with different degrees of severity might be more realistic. One should also realize, however, that these probably are closely related in terms of their clinical presentation and idiopathic etiology and possibly in their genetics.

In summary, MAE is a relatively uncommon form of early onset, probably idiopathic epilepsy whose criteria have not yet been definitively established. No unanimous agreement has been reached on the definition and criteria of this syndrome, which seems closely related to other reported syndromes of idiopathic myoclonic epilepsy, especially BME, from which it may be impossible to differentiate. Intermediate forms between the different syndromes may exist, and the idiopathic myoclonic epilepsies might constitute a spectrum of related cases rather than a collection of distinct syndromes.

As the heterogeneous character of MAE may lead one to expect, the prognosis of the condition is variable. So far, only a few indicators of prognosis are known.

Available treatments are effective in roughly half the cases. Considerable therapeutic difficulties are encountered in the remaining patients.

Principles of Management of the Myoclonic Epilepsies in Infancy and Childhood

Because the myoclonic epilepsies are relatively rare, no controlled trials supporting the following suggestions exist; clinical experience from large series is the only available resource (Dravet and Bureau, 2002; Kaminska et al., 1999; Aicardi, 1994).

Treatment of prominent myoclonic seizures in infancy and childhood is primarily with sodium valproate, ethosuximide, and the benzodiazepines. Lamotrigine does not seem effective against myoclonic seizures, but it may be useful for treating the associated generalized seizures. However, in general, it should be used with caution in the epilepsies featuring myoclonic seizures because aggravations of the condition have been reported (Biraben et al., 2000; Guerrini et al., 1998e).

Avoiding the use of carbamazepine and vigabatrin is advised in most myoclonic epilepsies of infancy and childhood because these drugs may increase seizure frequency and can trigger episodes of myoclonic status (Guerrini et al., 2002b; Kaminska et al., 1999; Lortie et al., 1993), priming a vicious circle of heavy treatment, whereby the original disorder is no longer recognizable and transformed in an epileptic encephalopathy (Guerrini et al., 2002a).

Some patients with only myoclonic seizures respond dramatically to either valproate or ethosuximide in regular doses. Oguni et al. (2002) found ethosuximide to be the most effective, with a "good response rate" in 64% of patients. In other patients, higher doses of valproate may be necessary (Lin et al., 1998). The use of a combination of valproate and ethosuximide is sometimes effective when either drug has failed. Clonazepam may also be highly effective in such cases, but, unfortunately, its behavioral side effects may be intolerable in children. Second-line drugs include topiramate, levetiracetam, acetazolamide (Tennison et al., 1991; Green et al., 1974), methsuximide, and sulthiame. Topiramate and levetiracetam are currently being tested, and their use, although promising, does not have the benefit of validation from controlled trials or the consolidated experience of clinicians.

The optimum duration of treatment may vary from a few years to several years. Photosensitivity has been the main reason for restarting or maintaining treatment in some children with BME (Dravet and Bureau, 2002). One-third of the patients with prominent myoclonic seizures associated with other generalized seizure types were successfully discontinued after a 5-year period in one study (Aicardi and Gomes, 1988).

The main practical problem is represented by those children who present with resistant myoclonic astatic seizures causing disabling falls, whether or not they can be classified within a syndromic subgroup. Uncontrolled trials of steroids or adrenocorticotropic hormone have been performed, but, even though a reduced seizure frequency has been observed by several investigators, the overall course of the disease does not seem to be modified. The management of these children clearly should include practical measures (e.g., wearing a helmet) and considerable psychosocial support in addition to drug therapy. The ketogenic diet may be helpful, and it has proven particularly effective in MAE in the series by Oguni et al. (2002), in which 58% of those on the diet had "excellent results." However, maintaining the diet for long periods is difficult. Surgery, even in the form of callosotomy, is not indicated in the myoclonic epilepsies.

In summary, the myoclonic epilepsies are observed in a large fraction of those infants and young children with frequent brief seizures that are different from those in LGS. Myoclonic seizures are exclusive or predominant, and these occur in association with fast (3 Hz) spike-wave complexes.

Two main subgroups can be delineated among the myoclonic epilepsies according to whether the myoclonic seizures are isolated or they are associated with other forms of seizures, including GTCSs, tonic seizures, or other brief fits. Children with isolated myoclonic attacks or those that are associated only with an occasional tonic-clonic seizure have a relatively favorable outlook, and they generally respond well to treatment with valproate, ethosuximide, or benzodiazepines. This subgroup corresponds with the recently reappraised definition of BME by Dravet and Bureau (2002).

Those epilepsies usually beginning after the age of 3 years with myoatonic seizures with other brief attacks and that are often associated with tonic-clonic seizures and episodes of nonconvulsive status are now included under the heading "MAE." The outcome in these individuals is unpredictable because cases with similar characteristics have roughly the same chances of experiencing complete remission and normal cognitive and behavioral development as they do of evolving into epileptic encephalopathies. Recurrence of episodes of nonconvulsive status is the

only factor that might predict an unfavorable outcome.

These two main subgroups might represent extremes of the same spectrum. Many children cannot be classified in either group. In general, isolated myoclonic jerks, especially if they respond quickly to drug therapy, have a favorable significance.

All forms of myoclonic epilepsy have strong genetic determinants. However, the mechanisms responsible for the attacks and especially for the cognitive impairment (or possibly the deterioration) in some patients remain obscure.

SYNDROMES OF MYOCLONIC EPILEPSY IN LATE CHILDHOOD AND ADOLESCENCE

In some epilepsies of late childhood and adolescence, myoclonias constitute the exclusive type of seizure or a predominant proportion of the seizures. Myoclonic attacks are the typical generalized epileptic myoclonic jerks, as the first section of this chapter describes, although great differences in the severity of the attacks are seen. A phenomenon that is more typical of older children and adolescents is a succession of myoclonic jerks that may culminate in a GTCS, the so-called *clonic-tonic-clonic seizure* (Delgado-Escueta et al., 1982b; Delgado-Escueta, 1979). The epilepsies characterized by marked myoclonic phenomena in this age range are, in most cases, idiopathic in origin, and they are not associated with any evidence of organic brain damage. A strong genetic predisposition to convulsive disorders is extremely common, as the high incidence of a family history of epilepsy illustrates. The cognitive development of those affected is usually normal (Lombroso and Erba, 1982).

The following four main groups of epilepsy syndromes with prominent myoclonus are considered in this section: (a) those in which the seizures associated with the myoclonus are mainly absence attacks and have their onset in childhood; (b) those in which myoclonic attacks, whether isolated or associated with other types of seizures, are induced electively by intermittent photic stimulation; (c) those with onset in adolescence, in which grand mal attacks are the main type of associated seizure but which also may feature absence attacks; and (d) those with onset in a wide age range spanning from late childhood to well into adulthood, with prominent rhythmic distal myoclonus, as well as generalized jerks, GTCSs, and focal seizures in some patients (Guerrini et al., 2001; Okuma et al., 1998; Okino, 1997; Kuwano et al., 1996). This latter group is mostly familial.

A particular subgroup too small to deserve a specific section, but worth mentioning here, is composed of those adolescents who present with intractable myoclonic jerks and GTCSs of variable severity. Some of these patients are probably included among the "resistant" cases of JME in some series (Thomas et al., 2002; Gelisse et al., 2001), but they might, in fact, represent a distinct category. An important concept is that, since considerable overlap of seizure manifestations is seen from one syndromic group to another, a comprehensive definition of *IGE with variable phenotypes* (Engel, 2001) might be more suitable for including all those cases that do not fit any specific syndrome.

Myoclonic Attacks Alternating With or Preceding the Appearance of Absences

Not uncommonly, myoclonic attacks are observed in the course of absence epilepsies (see Chapter 8). Myoclonus may precede the absence attacks, it may occur at the same time, or it may appear after the absences. Myoclonus may be an integral component of certain types of absence seizures, including the myoclonic or clonic absences and eyelid myoclonia with absence of stimulus-sensitive epilepsies (see Chapter 17). In other more frequent cases, myoclonic attacks precede or do not alternate with typical absences that feature marked myoclonic components.

Myoclonic jerks of the axial or massive type may occur in young children before the advent of absences, with the latter type of seizure then replacing the myoclonic attacks. Myoclonic attacks may also be observed between absences in patients with otherwise typical absence attacks. In such patients, the myoclonic jerks involve the limbs only rarely, and they are strong enough to provoke falls. More commonly, the jerks involve mainly the head, neck, and the proximal muscles of the upper limbs, resulting in a saccadic flexion of the head with abduction of the arms. The EEG correlates of such attacks are bursts of irregular spike-wave complexes at a rhythm of 3 Hz or more that are mostly of short duration (less than 3 seconds). The associated absences may be both clinically and electrically typical (see Chapter 8). They often tend to be brief (about 5 seconds in duration), and are accompanied by bursts of irregular spike-wave complexes at 3 Hz. During the same burst, the complexes may vary in both duration and amplitude. Aicardi (1980a) reported 21 such patients (11 boys and 10 girls). The mean age at onset was 4.5 years. These absences could be induced by hyperventilation, which also facilitated the occurrence of spike-wave bursts but not of myoclonic attacks. GTCSs were observed in 29% of these patients. The outlook was less favorable than that seen in cases of pure absence epilepsy, but it was better than that for patients with only myoclonic seizures without absences. Forty-four percent had normal mentation, and neurologic deficits were rare. In several of these patients, the myoclonic jerks tended to disappear with time, although the absences did become more typical. The exact nosologic place of these cases relative to the absence epilepsies and the early myoclonic epilepsies remains unsettled. Genetic factors were present in 33% of affected children. The familial occurrence of myoclonic seizures and typical absence attacks in different siblings suggest that both are closely related epileptic manifestations (Italian League Against Epilepsy Genetic Collaborative Group, 1993).

Myoclonic (or Clonic) Absences

Myoclonic and clonic absences are described in greater detail in Chapter 8. Patients with myoclonic absences differ from those already described in that the myoclonic jerks are an integral part of the absences. The age at onset varies within a wide range (1 to 12 years) (Bureau and Tassinari, 2002), but it tends to peak around age 7 years. There is a remarkable male preponderance (70%), which is the reverse of what is usually seen in absence epilepsies. A family history of epilepsy is found in about 20% of patients, a rate lower than that usually seen in other epilepsies featuring absence or myoclonic seizures. The jerks occur at a rhythm of 3 Hz, and they are temporally correlated with the spike component of the spike-wave complex (Bureau and Tassinari, 2002; Tassinari et al., 1971). The EEG discharge during myoclonic absences is indistinguishable from the discharges accompanying simple typical absences (Tassinari et al., 1992b). About 66% of these cases demonstrate additional seizure types, especially GTCSs with variable severity (Bureau and Tassinari, 2002). Myoclonic absences are resistant to drug therapy, or they evolve into other seizure types in about 60% of the cases. Cognitive impairment is already obvious before the onset of myoclonic absences in about 50% of children, and its severity tends to worsen, especially, but not exclusively, in those children who also experience frequent GTCSs (Bureau and Tassinari, 2002). The prognosis of this disorder is therefore guarded.

Eyelid Myoclonia With and Without Absences

Eyelid myoclonia (see Chapter 8) with absences is a type of photosensitive epilepsy that is characterized by prominent jerking of the eyelids with upward deviation of the eyes occurring in association with what appears to be a typical absence from both the clinical and EEG points of view (Chapter 17). Jeavons (1982) and Jeavons and Harding (1975) emphasized the severity of the eyelid jerking in these patients, compared with the slight flicker of the eyelids that is common in typical absences. Isolated episodes of eyelid jerking that sometimes resemble eyelid flutter are also seen in children with different types of epilepsies, often in association with mental retardation and visual sensitivity. The phenomenon may be so short (1 to 2 seconds) that discovering whether a concomitant lapse of consciousness occurs may be impossible. The intensity of the jerking justifies the inclusion of these seizures in the group of myoclonic epilepsies, especially because the myoclonic phenomena are difficult to control and they persist into adulthood, whereas the absences are relatively easily controlled. The marked photosensitivity and the frequent autostimulation are also features that eyelid myoclonia, with and without absences, shares with the other myoclonic epilepsies of infancy and childhood.

Myoclonic Seizures Induced by Photic Stimuli

Myoclonic attacks can be induced by photic stimuli. Jeavons and Harding (1975) found that only 1.5% of pure photosensitive epilepsies (i.e., epilepsies induced exclusively by exposure to visual stimuli without any spontaneous attacks) were myoclonic in nature. Other investigators have suggested higher figures (Tassinari et al., 1989a, 1989b, 1990; Newmarck, 1983; Newmark and Penry, 1979). Very commonly, myoclonic jerks are provoked in the EEG laboratory by exposure to intermittent photic stimulation. They can also be observed in patients who have never experienced visually induced myoclonic seizures in daily life and even in those who are being investigated for reasons other than epilepsy.

Visually induced generalized myoclonic jerks are usually symmetric, and they occur predominately in the upper limbs. In most cases, they are mild, producing only head nodding and slight arm abduction. More generalized jerks involving the face, trunk, and legs occasionally may cause the patient to fall. The relationship of myoclonic jerks to the stimulus is complex. Sometimes, no definite time relationship is observed. On other occasions, the jerks may be repeated rhythmically at the same frequency as the stimulus or at that of one of its subharmonics (Kasteleijn-Nolst-Trenité et al., 2001). Isolated myoclonic jerks occur without any impairment of consciousness. However, when the generalized jerks are repeated, especially if the stimulus continues, the individual's consciousness may be impaired, and a GTCS may follow.

In the EEG recording, the jerks are associated with the photoparoxysmal response, which consists of a bilateral polyspike or a polyspike-wave discharge that, at times, is terminated by one or several diffuse slow waves (Kasteleijn-Nolst-Trenité et al., 2001; Gastaut and Broughton, 1972).

Spontaneous seizures are said to occur mainly, but not exclusively, when the polyspike-wave discharge persists after the discontinuation of the stimulation, which is known as the "prolonged photoconvulsive response" (Kasteleijn-Nolst-Trenité et al., 2001; Reilly and Peters, 1973). Myoclonic attacks can be provoked by television watching, especially when the patients are close to the screen, and by video game playing (see Chapter 17). Some patients, especially but not only those who are mentally retarded, induce their own myoclonic attacks by waving a hand between their eyes and a light source, flickering their eyelids in front of a light source, staring at patterned surfaces, or other similar maneuvers (Binnie and Jeavons, 1992; Tassinari et al., 1990; Binnie et al., 1980; Jeavons and Harding, 1975). Such self-stimulation is often observed in children with Dravet syndrome (Dravet et al., 1992a).

Seino and Fujihara, (cited in Dreifuss, 1985), reported a group of 27 patients with *photosensitive myoclonic epilepsy* who experienced "combined seizures of myoclonic absence, myoclonic jerks, and generalized tonic-clonic convulsions." These researchers considered photosensitive myoclonic epilepsy a tentative epileptic syndrome that was always associated with mental retardation and an obvious tendency toward resistance to drug therapy. Forty-four percent of their patients had neurologic antecedents, and the onset of epileptic seizures was before the age of 3 years in 82% of these patients. Their EEGs were characterized by a slow background activity and short bursts of irregular spike-wave complexes that were mostly faster than 3 Hz. Self-provocation of the seizures was common. The outcome for these patients was not indicated, but it was probably unfavorable.

Juvenile Myoclonic Epilepsy

The occurrence of myoclonic attacks in adolescent patients with no progressive central nervous system disorder has long been recognized (Janz, 1991; Loiseau, 1971). Janz (1962, 1969) and, later, a number of authors (Asconapé and Penry, 1984; Jeavons,

1977; Aicardi and Chevrie, 1971) studied such patients and delineated their EEG and clinical pictures. The term *impulsiv petit mal* was initially used in the German literature (Janz, 1991), but, subsequently, the terms *myoclonic epilepsy of adolescence* (Janz, 1991), *benign myoclonic juvenile epilepsy* (Asconapé and Penry, 1984), Janz syndrome (Delgado-Escueta, 1979), or the more descriptive JME (Janz, 1969, 1973, 1991) were proposed to avoid the use of the equivocal phrase *petit mal*. The term *benign* was also discarded when relapses were found to be common following treatment withdrawal, even late in life. The myoclonic attacks of JME are unrecognized more often than they are misdiagnosed (Panayiotopoulos, et al., 1991). Their most constant manifestation, the morning jerks, is very rarely mentioned by the patients, and it only emerges from the history after careful questioning. This often occurs retrospectively when the first grand mal attack finally brings the patient to a physician.

Epidemiologic and Etiologic Data

The frequency of JME among epilepsy patients seeking medical attention varies from 3.1% (Bamberger and Matthes, 1959) to 11.9% (Thomas et al., 2002; Janz, 1991). Among those patients with IGEs, 20% to 27% are diagnosed with JME (Thomas et al., 2002; Genton et al., 2000a).

The etiology of JME is dominated by genetic factors. Therefore, neuroradiologic or other investigations are not required when the diagnosis is clear. Some neuropathologic studies have suggested that the genetic predisposition to primary generalized epilepsies may be associated with morphologic cortical abnormalities (Meencke, 1985; Meencke and Janz, 1984) and an isolated report indicated the presence of abnormal cortical organization on quantitative MRI in JME (Woermann et al., 1999). However, these findings remain of controversial significance (Lyon and Gastaut, 1985; Meencke and Janz, 1985), and have not been confirmed in a recent study (Opeskin et al., 2000).

A family study of 319 patients by Tsuboi and Christian (1973) found a 27.3% incidence of relatives with various types of epilepsy, compared with a 9.9% incidence in a control epilepsy population. Fifteen percent of the affected relatives had myoclonic attacks; 17%, "awakening grand mal;" and 14%, absence seizures. Several studies (Janz, 1991; Panayiotopoulos and Obeid, 1989; Tsuboi and Christian, 1973) showed that the incidence of epilepsy in relatives varied between 13% and 50%. Close rela-

tives were affected in 4.1% of the patients of Tsuboi and Christian (1973) and in 5.8% of those of Janz et al. (1992). In the latter series, the following details on the epileptic syndrome encountered in affected relatives were given: about 31% had JME, 34% had absence epilepsies, and 28% epilepsies with GTCSs. The relatives of male patients were less commonly affected than were those of females, and identical twins were always affected by the same form (Berkovic et al., 1991b). The risk for children of affected parents was variably found to be 5.1% (Tsuboi and Christian, 1973) and 7.1% (Janz, 1991), with girls having a greater risk than boys.

The mode of transmission does not appear to be uniform. The rates of family members with epilepsy that are reported are consistent with those of complex inheritance in most cases. In addition, females have a greater heritability and a lower threshold (Tsuboi and Christian, 1973), which accounts for the 2-to-1 female-to-male proportion reported in some series (Wolf, 1992c; Tsuboi, 1977b; Tsuboi and Christian, 1973). Other investigators (Panayiotopoulos and Obeid, 1989) have favored inheritance by a monogenic recessive mode, but their results were obtained in a highly inbred population, making assessment difficult. A monogenic dominant inheritance that was affected by one or more modifying genes was initially hypothesized (Hodge et al., 1989; Greenberg et al., 1988a, 1988b). Recently, Cossette et al. (2002) reported a large French Canadian family in which four generations of affected members had typical JME and harbored a mutation of the *GABRA1* gene. In contrast with the usual finding of large kindreds affected with different types of IGE (Italian League Against Epilepsy Genetic Collaborative Group, 1993), the features were homogeneous in all of the affected members. However, this single gene might account for only a very small minority of cases. Digenic inheritance has also been hypothesized (Greenberg et al., 1988b). Linkage studies have provided discrepant information. A close linkage between a major gene for susceptibility to JME and the HLA-BF locus on the short arm of chromosome 6 was initially reported in three studies (Durner et al., 1991; Weissbecker et al., 1991; Greenberg et al., 1988a, 1988b), although recessive or dominant models were used. Subsequent linkage studies further refined the initial candidate region (*EMJ1*) (Sander et al., 1997; Serratosa et al., 1996; Liu et al., 1995) and identified an additional locus in the short arm of chromosome 6 (Delgado-Escueta et al., 2000). However, linkage to this region was not confirmed in studies of north European families (Elmslie et al., 1996; Whitehouse et al., 1993), which instead identified a susceptibility locus on chromosome 15q (Bate et al., 2000). At present, polygenic inheritance is favored, which might account for the partially contradictory results that linkage studies with monogenic inheritance models have provided in most series. The same genes might be responsible for susceptibility to other forms of IGE (Janz et al., 1992), and one or more specific genes might determine the expression of JME or another form of IGE (Sander et al., 2000).

Clinical and Electroencephalographic Presentation

The patients have no history of neurologic disorders, except possibly febrile seizures. Females are more commonly affected than males (61% and 57%, respectively) (Thomas et al., 2002).

Virtually always, the onset is between 6 and 22 years of age; in 78% of cases, it is between 12 and 18 years and in 50%, between 13 and 16 years of age. More than 75% of patients experience their initial seizures between 12 and 18 years of age (Obeid and Panayiotopoulos, 1988). The myoclonic jerks appear between 12 and 16 years of age, and GTCSs tend to peak at roughly 16 years of age (Thomas et al., 2002), but the latter most often are what brings these patients to medical attention.

The myoclonic jerks are sudden and lightning-like. They occur spontaneously, affecting mainly the shoulders and arms in a symmetric fashion, but, occasionally, they may also affect the lower extremities or the entire body, thus resulting in a fall on rare occasions. In rare cases, the jerks may be asymmetric or even unilateral, which may be a cause of misdiagnosis of focal epilepsy (Thomas et al., 2002). No apparent alteration of consciousness is observed during the jerks. These may occur singly at irregular intervals or in brief series that are usually arrhythmic. Although massive jerks are easily discernible, the mild jerks may be less apparent, and they may mimic postawakening clumsiness with dropping of objects. The patients may describe these jerks as a sort of electric shock. Most jerks occur in the morning within 20 to 30 minutes after awakening. In some patients, the jerks may also supervene with tiredness at the end of the day or, occasionally, at other times (Wolf, 1992c), usually when the individual is in a relaxing situation but not falling asleep. Sleep deprivation is the most effective precipitant of the jerks, and it is usually present when these occur repeatedly in status. A severe increase in the frequency of jerks may herald episodes of myoclonic status epilepticus, which were relatively common in the past (Asconapé and Penry,

1984) but which have become rarer (7.3% of patients in the series of Salas-Puig et al., 1990b) with improved syndrome recognition. Indeed, drug withdrawal and inappropriate drug choice are among the main factors that may precipitate status (Thomas et al., 2002). *Myoclonic status* lasts from a few minutes to several hours, and it is characterized by myoclonic jerks that recur every few seconds. Often, the intensity of the jerks may be so mild that only the patient can perceive them. Consciousness is preserved in most cases, but the patients are incapacitated by the involuntary movements, which may cause the patient to throw away or to knock objects in his or her hand or in the immediate vicinity. Facial or lingual and perioral jerks, which are usually isolated, may, in some patients, be precipitated by talking (Wolf and Mayer, 2000), a phenomenon analogous to the jerking that is observed in patients with primary reading epilepsy.

GTCSs occur in about 85% of patients (Genton et al., 2000a; Wolf, 1992c; Janz, 1991; Delgado-Escueta, 1979). Generally, they are infrequent, although they often are the reason for consultation. This suggests that pure cases of JME are probably more common than is clinically apparent (Janz, 1991). Because the jerks almost always precede the GTCSs by months or years (Janz, 1991; Asconapé and Penry, 1984), any young patient with grand mal attacks should be specifically asked about whether they have occurred (Asconapé and Penry, 1984). Many grand mal seizures in patients with JME are ushered in by salvoes of myoclonic jerks that crescendo in frequency and severity and then culminate in a generalized tonic-clonic episode (Delgado-Escueta, 1979). The circadian distribution and the facilitating factors of the GTCSs are the same as those for myoclonic jerks. The first GTCSs are often precipitated by one or more factors, among which sleep deprivation is most important (84% in the series of Pedersen and Petersen, 1998), followed by stress (70%) and alcohol intake (51%). Although the average number of these seizures is not higher than two per year (Thomas et al., 2002), those patients with an irregular lifestyle or who are noncompliant may experience numerous episodes. Some authors have reported that mental activities implying planning of manual praxis or decision making play a triggering role (Matsuoka et al., 2000; Inoue et al., 1994), a report that has been confirmed in up to one-third of patients who are specifically questioned about this (Wolf and Mayer, 2000).

Absence attacks occur independently of the jerks in a subset of patients. Older estimates had indicated their presence in about 15% of patients (Wolf, 1992c; Janz, 1991; Panayiotopoulos et al., 1989a), but more recent studies using intensive video-EEG monitoring have suggested that up to 33% to 38% of patients may suffer absences (Genton et al., 2000a). These absences are often very brief (2 to 4 seconds), and they may be difficult to recognize clinically because the impairment of consciousness can be extremely slight (Panayiotopoulos et al., 1989a, 1989b, 1991). They occur predominately on awakening, they may be associated with spike-wave complexes at 3.5 to 5 Hz that are initiated by a double or multiple spike (Wolf, 1992c; Janz and Christian, 1957), and they may be irregular in amplitude and rhythm (Panayiotopoulos et al., 1989a). Because of this mild expression, the patients or their caregivers may not be aware of the absences, which may be uncovered during an EEG recording (Thomas et al., 2002). Typical "pyknoleptic" absences are rare (6% in the series by Janz [1991]), and episodes of absence status are exceptional (Agathonikou et al., 1998; Kimura and Kobayashi, 1996).

The most common association of seizure types includes myoclonic jerks and GTCSs; absence seizures coexist with these two seizure types in about one-third of patients (Janz and Durner, 1998). The association of myoclonic and absence seizures without corresponding GTCSs is extremely uncommon (Thomas et al., 2002).

About 5% of patients suffer from clinical photosensitivity (Genton et al., 1994). In these individuals, the myoclonic jerks or GTCSs that may occur spontaneously can also be triggered by environmental stimuli, especially television, video games, or flashing lights in a dance club.

The ictal EEG of myoclonic jerks (Fig. 6.6) typically consists of a generalized, almost always symmetric, cluster of spikes of high frequency (10 to 16 per second), followed by several slow waves, which may, in rare instances, be absent (Janz, 1991; Simonsen et al., 1976a). The onset and maximum voltage are in the frontocentral areas with spread to the parietal, temporal, and occipital regions. Although similar complexes are often observed without any clinical manifestation, a correlation seems to exist between the number of spikes within a complex and the intensity of the time-locked jerk (Thomas et al., 2002), so those discharges with a low number of spikes are usually interictal. Such typical ictal EEG abnormalities are found in 85% to 95% of the patients by some au-

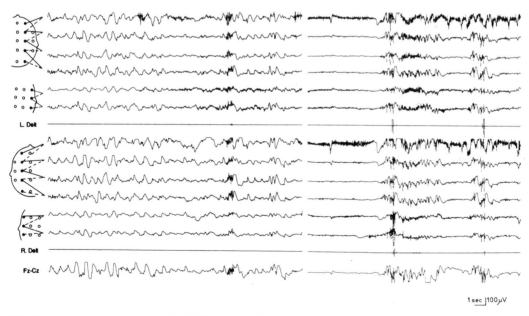

1 sec ⌐100µV

FIG. 6.6. An electroencephalographic (EEG) polygraphic recording of a 20-year-old man with juvenile myoclonic epilepsy, who had suffered two generalized tonic-clonic seizures since 16 years of age, and who reported "electric-like jerks" after awakening. **Left:** Provoked awakening is accompanied by the cessation of slow-wave activity of sleep (phase IV) and the immediate appearance of generalized multi–spike-wave complexes. **Right:** In the minutes that follow the awakening, two episodes of blinking are accompanied by generalized myoclonic jerks (myoclonic potentials are visible over the right and left deltoid) and a series of multiple spike-wave complexes.

thors (Wolf, 1992c; Janz, 1991), but they were observed much less frequently by others (Asconapé and Penry, 1984; Tsuboi, 1977b) and they are often followed by bursts of fast (3 to 5 Hz) irregular spike-wave complexes. Focal abnormalities, such as focal slow waves or asymmetric interictal discharges that do not show a consistent lateralization, are reported in 15% to 55% of patients (Thomas et al., 2002; Aliberti et al., 1994; Genton et al., 1994). The background EEG activity is consistently normal. The resting tracings are often within normal limits, so activating procedures are important. Recording of even a brief period of sleep and the subsequent awakening is usually sufficient to uncover the typical profile of activation of discharges that accompanies the arousal (Fittipaldi et al., 2001).

Classic spike-wave complexes (3 Hz) and fast spike-wave complexes (4 to 6 Hz) are each present in about half the patients (Wolf, 1992c; Janz, 1991), and they are rarely observed in the absence of polyspike-wave complexes (Janz, 1973). Approximately 30% to 40% of the patients will have a photoparoxysmal response (Janz, 1991; Wolf and Goosses, 1986) that is often accompanied by myoclonic jerks. However, in most such patients, the abnormal response in the EEG laboratory does not translate into clinical photosensitivity in everyday life. Girls are twice as likely to show a photoparoxysmal response than boys. Discharges of polyspike-wave complexes occur on eye closure in up to 21% of patients (Wolf, 1992c), but the occurrence of myoclonic jerks at that time is highly unusual (Baykan-Kurt et al., 1999). Sleep does not induce the jerks; however, the rate of discharges may be increased during stage 1 sleep, and it is particularly high when patients are awakening (Touchon, 1982). To the same extent that a sudden provoked awakening facilitates the appearance of myoclonic jerks or, more rarely, of other seizure types, such an awakening appears particularly effective in activating the discharges. For this reason, a sleep EEG recording including the awakening and the following 20 minutes, even after a short nap, is of great diagnostic yield, especially after sleep deprivation.

The neurologic status and the intelligence of the affected persons are normal. Peculiar psychologic traits, such as unsteadiness, hedonism, and indifference to the disorder, have been found by some, but not all, authors (Janz, 1991). The onset of JME very seldom occurs at younger than 8 years or older than 22 years. More than 80% of the patients in the Janz series had an onset of their jerks between 12 and 19 years of age (Janz, 1991), and the mean age at onset in the patients of Asconapé and Penry (1984) was 14.75 years. Unusual ages of onset of as early as 3

years or as late as 80 years have been rarely recorded (Gram et al., 1988). However, patients with an unusual age at onset may have other types of IGEs with partially overlapping phenotypes (Engel, 2001).

Course and Outcome

Response to treatment is excellent or good, achieving complete control in approximately 80% to 90% of patients (Thomas et al., 2002; Jeavons et al., 1977; Lennox-Buchtal, 1973) (see "Treatment"), but spontaneous remission is said to be extremely rare. Seizure relapse after the discontinuation of medication is, on the other hand, common, even after many years of seizure control (Baruzzi et al., 1988; Delgado-Escueta, 1979), but it can be delayed for several years in some patients (Penry et al., 1989). About 15% of patients resist treatment and continue to suffer seizures, and those with all three seizure types appear to have a higher risk of a resistant course (Thomas et al., 2002). The risk of sudden, unexplained death is not negligible in patients who continue to have GTCSs (Genton and Gelisse, 2001).

Diagnostic and Nosologic Aspects

Physiologic myoclonus, particularly sudden body jerks on falling asleep or sleep myoclonus (Hallett, 1985), rarely pose serious problems. They are not associated with other paroxysmal manifestations, and the EEG shows no abnormalities.

Distinguishing true myoclonic jerks from brief atonic or tonic seizures is often difficult, and EEG polygraphic and video recordings are required for so doing. However, the ages at occurrence and the accompanying manifestations are different, but transitional cases may be difficult or even impossible to classify. The myoclonic attacks of JME should be differentiated from myoclonic or clonic absences, which may have a more severe prognosis. In JME, consciousness is preserved, and the clonic jerks are arrhythmic. The differentiation of the primary types of myoclonic epilepsy from the progressive myoclonus epilepsies rests on the presence of mental deterioration; the occurrence of other types of myoclonus in addition to the massive myoclonic jerks, particularly erratic and/or intention myoclonus; and other clinical and EEG characteristics in the latter.

Among the progressive myoclonus epilepsies with an onset of symptoms at around adolescence, Lafora disease and some cases of Unverricht-Lundborg disease may initially be mistaken for JME. Subsequent worsening of the myoclonic syndrome, the appearance of slow background EEG activity, and cognitive deterioration suggest the possibility of a progressive disorder.

Nothing indicates that any of the myoclonic epilepsies of infancy and childhood (i.e., BME and MAE) subsequently evolve into JME. A possible source of confusion may arise from cases of MAE of late onset (5 to 7 years of age), but the characteristic association of myoclonic astatic seizures, nocturnal brief GTCSs, or tonic seizures and episodes of absence status clearly differ from the myoclonic jerks that occur alone or in association with very brief absences, which characterize JME at onset. Some cases of typical absences can, however, evolve to JME (see Chapter 8).

JME has no obvious link with febrile seizures, which were found in only 1.7% of the close relatives of affected individuals (Janz, 1991). The observation that the JME phenotype is not usually seen in families with a history of GEFS+ is consistent with the lack of significant association with febrile seizures. However, patients with GEFS+ do present with generalized seizures, and considerable clinical overlap exists among JME, awakening grand mal, and adolescent absence epilepsy (i.e., the syndromes featuring all three seizure types of IGE). These three syndromes quite commonly occur in association with one another in the same family (Italian League Against Epilepsy Genetic Collaborative Group, 1993), and, in the case of JME and adolescent absence epilepsy, they may have the same types of seizures, although in different proportions. Indeed, a precise diagnosis of either syndrome may be difficult in a number of patients. Some have thus suggested that these should be grouped into a single broad category of *IGE of adolescence*, which may feature any or all of them.

Treatment

The use of sodium valproate alone controls both the jerks and the other types of attacks in about 85% of patients (Genton et al., 2000a; Penry et al., 1989). Methsuximide has also been used with success as an alternative monotherapy (Hurst, 1996). The use of phenobarbital or primidone, which was originally recommended by Janz, is more effective against grand mal than myoclonic jerks. Uncommonly, a second drug is needed, especially for control of absence attacks (Wolf, 1992c). In resistant cases, the addition of small doses of a benzodiazepine (clonazepam or clobazam) may be effective (Obeid and Panayiotopoulos, 1988). Lamotrigine has been used in JME, either as an alternative to, or in addition to, valproate (Biraben et al., 2000; Wallace, 1998; Buchanan,

1996). However, in some patients, the withdrawal of valproate acid was associated with the recrudescence of both myoclonic seizures and GTCSs (Buchanan, 1996). Biraben et al. (2000) hypothesized that a specific pharmacodynamic action of lamotrigine caused clinical worsening in a small number of patients. Preliminary data suggest that topiramate might be an interesting alternative in some patients with difficult-to-treat JME (Kellett et al., 1999). A trial of primidone may also be worthwhile. Acetazolamide may also be effective (Resor and Resor, 1990). A particular profile of the pharmacologic sensitivity of JME, which is similar to that of other IGEs, has been delineated by Thomas et al. (2002), who stressed the potential for seizure aggravation that may be observed with the use of phenobarbital and especially of carbamazepine, which could even precipitate myoclonic status (Genton et al., 2000b).

An extremely important factor is preventing seizures that are precipitated by sleep deprivation by the elimination of those factors that may hinder physiologic sleep.

In summary, JME is among the most well-characterized epilepsy syndromes. In spite of its denomination, the myoclonic jerks may not be particularly disabling; and, although they are present in all affected individuals, they are often unrecognized by patients and clinicians alike. Considerable clinical and possibly genetic overlapping exists with other IGEs with onset in adolescence and complex inheritance. Recent data indicate that, rarely, JME can become segregated as an autosomal dominant trait. If JME is correctly diagnosed, it can be successfully treated with valproate in almost all patients, who, however, require lifelong treatment.

Epilepsies with Prominent Rhythmic Distal Myoclonus

Several families of mostly Japanese origin with a dominant disorder characterized by a peculiar form of rhythmic distal cortical myoclonus (generalized myoclonic jerks, also defined as *cortical tremor*), and GTCSs, have been described (Labauge et al., 2002; Okuma et al., 1998; Terada et al., 1997; Kuwano et al., 1996; Okino, 1997). This disorder is currently known as *familial adult myoclonic epilepsy*. The affected patients present with a great homogeneity of the following characteristics: (a) autosomal dominant transmission; (b) adult onset (mean age of 38 years; range of 19 to 73 years); (c) a nonprogressive course; (d) distal, fairly rhythmic myoclonus that is enhanced during movement; (e) rare, apparently generalized seizures that are often preceded by a worsening of distal myoclonus and appearance of generalized jerks; (f) the absence of other neurologic signs; (g) generalized interictal spike-wave discharges; (h) photoparoxysmal response; (i) giant somatosensory evoked potentials; (j) hyperexcitability of the C-reflex; and (k) cortical EEG potential that is time locked to the jerks. In two different studies, linkage analysis in five of the Japanese kindreds led to the localization of the disease gene to chromosome 8q23.3-q24.1 (Mikami et al., 1999; Plaster et al., 1999). The only European family with a similar disorder did not link to the same locus (Labauge et al., 2002).

Childhood onset of a comparable form of epilepsy was reported in an Italian family (mean age of 9 years), whose affected members had moderate mental retardation (Elia et al., 1998). Another family with 11 affected individuals over five generations but with an onset between 12 and 59 years of age of focal seizures and generalized seizures of variable severity has also been reported (Guerrini et al., 2001). Sporadic cases with similar characteristics have also been observed (Guerrini et al., 2002b). This form of distal and generalized myoclonus is associated with different types of epilepsy and probably is actually underdiagnosed rather than extremely rare.

SUMMARY

True myoclonic attacks constitute a common phenomenon in many types of epilepsy, and they therefore are not characteristic of any syndrome. They can occur at any age, but their diagnostic and prognostic significance is quite different with age.

In infancy and early childhood, myoclonic seizures are often associated with other types of brief seizures, as well as with cognitive and behavioral abnormalities even when no obvious brain lesion is present to account for it, and their prognosis is often guarded. In this age-group, they should be distinguished from other syndromes with frequent brief attacks and repeated falls that result from the tonic and atonic

seizures mostly observed in LGS. This differentiation may be difficult, and neurophysiologic studies may be required. The EEG features of myoclonic and tonic-atonic seizures are usually distinct.

In late childhood and adolescence, myoclonic attacks are mainly seen within the spectrum of the IGEs, in which genetic factors play a prominent role. Myoclonic attacks may be the predominant or the only type of seizure in a minority of patients, but, in general, they are associated with other types of attacks, mainly typical absences and/or GTCSs. Myoclonic attacks are often precipitated by photic stimulation, and, rarely, they may be self-induced using a visual trigger.

Myoclonic attacks are associated with absence seizures in some children. However, the association of myoclonic attacks with absences does not constitute a single, well-defined syndrome. Rather, myoclonic jerks are observed with several types of absence epilepsy, and the significance, course, and outlook of such cases remain unclear.

Myoclonic attacks in adolescents constitute a clearly defined epilepsy syndrome (JME). They are usually associated with GTCSs and, less commonly, with absences. In many patients, these three types of seizures appear in various associations, and they can be grouped in the broader entity IGE of adolescents and young adults.

The effectiveness of therapy for the myoclonic epilepsies varies with the syndrome causing them. The overall outcome is much more favorable in cases with onset in late childhood and adolescence because cognitive functions are not usually affected, whereas, in infancy and early childhood, cognitive problems are common and often severe.

The seizure outcome is more favorable in young children, in whom many cases remit after a few years. However, highly resistant cases are not rare. In older children and especially in adolescents, although pharmacological control is possible in most cases, the persistence of active epilepsy over very long periods is common.

7

Myoclonic Epilepsies Associated with Progressive Degenerative Disorders: Progressive Myoclonic Epilepsies

The progressive myoclonic epilepsies (PMEs) have received considerable attention in the neurologic literature (Genton et al, 2000; Roger et al., 1992; Berkovic et al., 1986; Diebold, 1973) even though, numerically, they represent only a small fraction of the myoclonic epilepsies. Aicardi and Chevrie (1971) found only nine patients with PMEs in a study of 90 children and adolescents with myoclonic seizures. Aicardi (1980b) extended this series to 145 patients, and found only 11 who had a progressive encephalopathy. Because these figures come from a specialized referral center, they certainly overestimate the proportion of severe and unusual cases, so the true figures would be even lower. The interest aroused by PME, however, is justified by the genetic origin of these disorders, the severity of their prognosis, and the insight that inborn errors of metabolism can provide into the normal functioning of the neuronal chemical machinery.

Following the early descriptions by Unverricht in 1881 and Lundborg from 1903 to 1913, the concept of PMEs as a single individualized and recognizable syndrome became firmly established. The PME syndrome is characterized by the following four main elements: (a) *myoclonic jerks*, which are segmental, fragmentary, and usually erratic in topography; (b) *epileptic seizures*, mainly generalized tonic-clonic or clonic-tonic-clonic seizures and massive myoclonic seizures; (c) *progressive mental deterioration*; and (d) variable neurologic signs and symptoms, mainly cerebellar, extrapyramidal, and action myoclonus (Fig. 7.1). Diebold (1973) separated the myoclonic epileptic syndromes with dementia into two groups. In the first group, the myoclonic epileptic syndrome is a constant and central characteristic of the causal disorders (e.g., Lafora bodies disease). In the second group, the myoclonic epileptic syndrome is a manifestation of the causal disorder only occasionally (e.g., in Huntington chorea).

More recently, the value of the concept of PME has been increasingly questioned. The PME syndrome clearly is comprised of a heterogeneous collection of unrelated disorders that are only superficially similar. The mechanism of the myoclonus itself varies with the causes, and neurophysiologic studies permit the separation of the several mechanisms responsible for the jerks. The remaining usefulness of the concept of PMEs is to offer a broad framework that permits temporary accommodation of some as yet unclassified conditions featuring epileptic seizures, myoclonus, and neurologic degeneration.

Most disorders responsible for PME with or without dementia have relatively characteristic clinical, electroencephalographic (EEG), and other features that permit individual recognition (Aicardi, 1982b), and enzymatic assays, linkage and/or deoxyribonucleic acid (DNA) studies, and/or peripheral tissue biopsies are available to confirm the diagnosis.

This chapter therefore describes the major conditions that are responsible for PMEs in infancy, childhood, and adolescence. Cases in young adults that pose the same problems as those in adolescence are included. However, most disorders that produce myoclonus in infancy and early childhood are quite different from the traditional picture of the PME syndrome in older children and adolescents, and they raise completely different diagnostic problems. These are dealt with only briefly, and the interested reader is referred to their descriptions in specialized articles (Genton et al., 2002; Livet et al., 2002; Delgado-Escueta et al., 2001; Berkovic et al., 1986, 1993). The late infantile type of ceroid lipofuscinosis is one such case, because differentiating it from the early myoclonic epilepsies and Lennox-Gastaut syndrome (LGS) is difficult, thus exposing this problem, especially since it has no real resemblance to the traditional PME syndrome (Harden and Pampiglione, 1982). Similarly, the late type of ceroid lipofuscinosis may pose difficult diagnostic dilemmas with some disorders of vision and/or hysteria, not with the PMEs, because the myoclonus is usually a late manifestation.

The main conditions that give rise to PMEs are listed in Table 7.1. In this table, the disorders have been di-

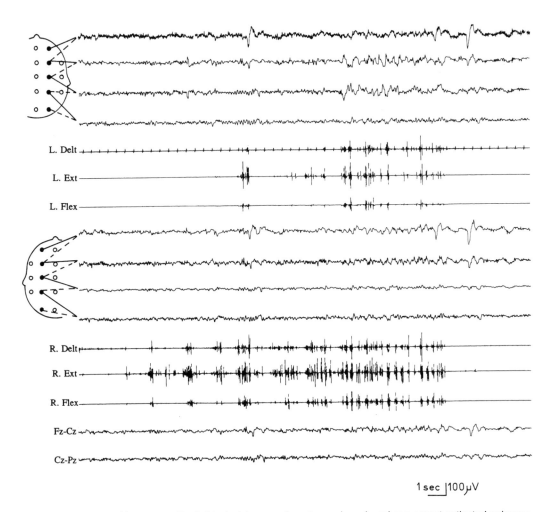

1 sec |100μV

FIG. 7.1. A 27-year-old woman with sialidosis (cherry-red spot myoclonus) and movement-activated seizures. When the patient raises her right arm to seize a hammer, a typical "cascade" of myoclonic potentials that are initially arrhythmic and that involve all of the sampled muscles on the right (right deltoid and wrist extensors and flexors) occurs; these then become more rhythmic, spreading to the contralateral muscles. This pattern of spread of myoclonic activity is typical of action myoclonus.

vided into three groups. The first group includes those disorders that produce a relatively typical PME syndrome, as described earlier in this chapter. The second group includes the diseases that give rise to myoclonic epilepsies that clearly differ from those in the first group in their associated signs. The third group comprises a variety of disorders that are associated with myoclonic jerks and other epileptic manifestations but that differ considerably from the classic PME syndrome in age at onset and clinical and EEG manifestations. A complete description of the conditions listed in Table 7.1 is, however, beyond the scope of this book.

Most of the conditions listed are genetic diseases that are mostly inherited as autosomal recessive traits. Their geographic and ethnic distribution varies. For example, Unverricht-Lundborg disease is common in Finland (Norio and Koskiniemi, 1979) and relatively common in northern European populations, whereas Lafora disease is most prevalent in the Mediterranean Basin and several Middle and Far East countries. However, extensive overlap does exist (Delgado-Escueta et al., 2001).

In some PMEs (e.g., Gaucher disease, several types of ceroid lipofuscinosis), the metabolic error respon-

TABLE 7.1. *Diseases that may cause progressive myoclonic epilepsy*

Group I: *typical or relatively typical progressive myoclonic epilepsy syndrome*
  Lafora disease
  Unverricht-Lundborg disease
  Juvenile neuronopathic Gaucher disease
  Galactosialidosis
  Dentatorubral-pallidoluysian atrophy
  Juvenile neuroaxonal dystrophy
Group II: *atypical progressive myoclonic epilepsy syndrome*
  Ceroid lipofuscinoses (see Table 7.2)
  Nonspecific poliodystrophy with lactic acidosis (Alpers disease)
  Huntington chorea (Aicardi, 1992a)
  Wilson disease
Group III: *very atypical progressive myoclonic epilepsy syndrome*
  Hyperglycinemia nonketotic (Seppäläinen and Similä, 1971)
  D-Glyceric aciduria (Brandt et al., 1974)
  Infantile hexosaminidase deficiency (Rapin, 1986)
  Biopterin deficiency (Smith et al., 1975)

sible for the disease is known, permitting both a confirmation of the diagnosis and reliable prenatal diagnosis. Linkage studies have defined 12 loci of the PME syndromes. More recently, DNA studies have led to the discovery of the mutated genes of several PMEs, including Lafora disease, Unverricht-Lundborg disease, dentatorubral-pallidoluysian atrophy (DRPLA), myoclonic encephalopathy with ragged-red fibers (MERRF), and five of the ceroid lipofuscinoses (Table 7.2).

In this chapter, only the salient features of the most important disorders, especially those in the first group, are reviewed.

LAFORA BODY DISEASE

Lafora body disease (Genton et al., 2000; Roger et al., 1992; Tassinari et al., 1978) is an autosomal recessive condition that usually begins between 10 and 18 years of age. The onset is almost always marked by generalized tonic-clonic seizures, with the myoclonic jerks appearing later. The jerks occur spontaneously, but they are increased by many stimuli, including sudden noises, flashing lights, touch, or movement. They are often of small amplitude, and they produce only limited movement of the limb or segment of the limb that is affected. The muscle twitches may be visible even if they do not induce any movement. The jerks are multiple, asynchronous, and arrhythmic. Massive myoclonic seizures may be associated with the jerks. Partial seizures are not uncommon. Tassinari et al. (1978) reported visual ictal phenomena in approximately 50% of their patients, and others have

TABLE 7.2. *The ceroid lipofuscinoses*

Type	Age	Epi-lepsy	Myo-clonus	Cognitive Deterior-ation	Visual Involve-ment	Cyto-somes	Mapping	Gene Product
Early infantile (Santavuori-Hagberg)	6–18 mo	+	++	++ (early)	+	GRODs	CLN1 (1p32)	PPT
Late infantile (Jansky-Bielschovsky)	2–4 yr	+++	++	++	+ (late)	CVL	CLN2 (11p15)	TPP1
Juvenile (Spielmeyer-Vogt)	4–10 yr	+	±	+	++	FPP	CLN3 (16p12)	Novel membrane protein
Late infantile variant (Finnish)	5–7 yr	++	±	++	++	FPP/CVL	CLN5 (13q21 −q32)	Novel membrane protein
Late infantile variant	2–6 yr	++	?	++	+ (early)	FPP/CVL	CLN6 (15q21 −23)	?
Late infantile (Turkish)	2–4 yr	+	?	++	±	FPP/CVL	CLN7 (?)	—
Juvenile variant with GRODs	2–8 yr	+	?	+	+	GROD ± CVL or FPP	CLN1 (1p32)	PPT

Abbreviations: CLN, ceroid lipofuscinosis; CVL, curvilinear inclusions; FPP, fingerprint profile; GROD, granular osmiophilic inclusions; PPT, palmitoyl-protein thioesterase; TPP, tripeptidyl peptidase.

recorded visual seizures in the EEG (Tinuper et al., 1983b). Mental deterioration is rapidly progressive once it appears, but, at onset, the disorder may appear quite similar to primary generalized epilepsy (i.e., juvenile myoclonic epilepsy), especially since the EEG demonstrates a photoconvulsive response and spontaneous polyspike-wave paroxysms on a relatively normal background rhythm. Later in the course of the disorder, cerebellar and/or extrapyramidal and pyramidal signs appear while the EEG rhythms slow down and become disorganized (Roger et al., 1992). The total duration of the disease varies between 5 and 10 years.

Lafora bodies, which are formed of abnormal glycogen with excessively long linear peripheral chains (polyglucosans), form Lafora cytoplasmic inclusion bodies and accumulate in the brain, striated muscle, liver, and skin. An axillary skin biopsy is the diagnostic procedure of choice (Tinuper et al., 1983b). Eighty percent of cases are due to a large variety of mutations in the *EPM2A* gene on chromosome 6q23-25, which codes for *laforin* (Minassian et al., 1998b, 2001; Serratosa et al., 1995, 1999), a protein tyrosine phosphatase that may also be involved in the regulation and folding of ubiquitin (Ganesh et al., 2000). Antiepileptic treatment may improve seizure control, but it is otherwise ineffective.

More recently, cases of earlier onset have been reported that are marked by slow cognitive decline, sometimes with partial seizures, and that precede by several years the completion of the PME syndrome (Delgado-Escueta et al., 2002). These may be associated with different mutations in the laforin gene.

Even though all of the known mutations can now be tested, the molecular diagnosis is difficult, even in those cases that involve the laforin gene, because a large number of mutations, none of which are clearly predominate, are known (Minassian, 2001). Therefore, axillary skin biopsy remains the best diagnostic test.

UNVERRICHT-LUNDBORG DISEASE

Unverricht-Lundborg disease, also known as *degenerative myoclonic epilepsy* (Shibazaki et al., 1978; Koskiniemi et al., 1974), Baltic myoclonus (Berkovic et al., 1986; Eldridge et al., 1983), Mediterranean myoclonus (Ellison et al., 1986), and EPM1, is the least uncommon of the PMEs. Previously, the condition was also reported as Ramsay Hunt syndrome (Roger et al., 1992), a term that should be abandoned because it has been applied to several conditions. Recent research has shown that both the Finnish and the Mediterranean types are due to the same mutation in the cystatin B gene and that they therefore represent a single entity (Lalioti et al., 1997).

The clinical picture conforms to that of classic PME. Onset with stimulus-sensitive erratic myoclonus is between 6 and 18 years of age. The precipitation of jerks by movement and intention is particularly disturbing, and the myoclonias progressively increase to the point of rendering all voluntary action almost impossible. Generalized tonic-clonic seizures occur later. They are mostly uncommon, and they are often associated with massive myoclonic jerks reminiscent of those in juvenile myoclonic epilepsy (see Chapter 6). The EEG picture is similar to that of Janz syndrome as well (Roger et al., 1992; Kyllerman et al., 1991). Photosensitivity is present in more than 90% of patients. The ataxia and myoclonus progressively increase at a variable, but generally slow, pace. These patients maintain normal cognitive functions for a long period of time, and moderate deterioration may take from 10 to 20 years. Treatment with phenytoin has been shown to be responsible for some of the cognitive decline and EEG slowing reported in Finnish patients (Koskiniemi, 1974). Differentiating this condition from juvenile myoclonic epilepsy may initially be difficult. However, the precipitation of myoclonus by stimuli is a suggestive feature. Furthermore, the demonstration of membrane-bound vacuoles in eccrine sweat glands on an axillary skin biopsy has been reported. However, the diagnosis can now be confirmed by the finding of an increased number of dodecamer repeats (Lalioti et al., 1997) in the promoter region of the *EPM1* gene on chromosome 21q22.3 that codes for cystatin B (Pennachio et al., 1996; Lehesjoki et al., 1991, 1993). DNA diagnosis is reliable because the condition is genetically homogeneous, and demonstration of the expansion is relatively easy. Homozygous point mutations in the cystatin gene have rarely been reported (Lalioti et al., 1997). Apparently, the *EPM1* expansion leads to a low expression of cystatin B, which probably has a role in the prevention of apoptosis, although the mechanisms are not fully understood. Interestingly, the age at onset and the severity of the disease are not related to the length of the repeats.

Although no cure is available, the myoclonus and seizures can be improved by the administration of valproate and clobazam and, in some cases, of topiramate or lamotrigine. Piracetam in extremely large doses may be highly effective (Koskiniemi et al., 1998; Brown et al., 1993), but it may also result in digestive difficulties. Levetiracetam may also prove efficacious while having fewer side effects (Genton and Gelisse, 2000; Genton and Van Vleymen, 2000).

MYOCLONIC ENCEPHALOPATHY WITH RAGGED-RED FIBERS

MERRF has a variable age at onset, ranging from 3 years to late adulthood (Fukuyama, 1991; Garcia Silva et al., 1987). It is characterized by myoclonus; generalized tonic-clonic seizures; sometimes atypical absences; ataxia; and the presence of subsarcolemmal aggregates of mitochondria, the so-called *ragged-red fibers* (Berkovic et al., 1986). Deafness is a common feature that should suggest the diagnosis. Additional features may include short stature, optic atrophy, neuropathy, migraine, fatigue, and diabetes. The inheritance is consistent with mitochondrial (maternal) transmission, and the course is highly variable. The EEG often shows paroxysmal features, and giant visual potentials can be elicited in all patients.

The disorder is associated with an A-to-G substitution at nucleotide 8344 in the transfer ribonucleic acid (tRNA) Lys in the mitochondrial DNA (Shoffner et al., 1990). At least two other mutations (T8356C and G8363A) in the same gene can cause a similar picture. In addition, forms that "overlap" with the Leigh and MELAS (mitochondrial myopathy, encephalopathy, lactic acidosis, and strokelike episodes) syndromes may occur (Canafoglia et al., 2001). The condition, since it is caused by mutations in the mitochondrial DNA, is inherited dominantly from the mother.

Some rare forms of myoclonic epilepsy, such as Ekbom syndrome (myoclonic epilepsy with lipomas) and May-White syndrome (myoclonic epilepsy with deafness), likely are related mitochondrial diseases (Berkovic et al., 1986).

Mitochondrial dysfunction may also be the cause of PME in infancy and early childhood. Harbord et al. (1991) reported eight such cases. Three of those patients had abnormalities in complex I of the respiratory chain with elevated serum lactate levels.

OTHER DISORDERS CAUSING TYPICAL PROGRESSIVE MYOCLONIC EPILEPSY

Juvenile Neuronopathic Gaucher Disease

Juvenile neuronopathic Gaucher disease (type III) is a rare disease that may be responsible for a typical picture of PME (Aicardi, 1998a). The associated signs are variable. The most common is supranuclear palsy of horizontal, and sometimes vertical, gaze.

Cerebellar and pyramidal or dystonic syndromes and cognitive difficulties may be present. Splenomegaly is often found. The EEG abnormalities may precede their clinical manifestations. Diffuse or multifocal paroxysmal discharges, a paroxysmal response to photic stimulation, and a progressive slowing of background rhythms may be observed (Aicardi, 1994a). Enzyme replacement therapy is highly effective in the treatment of type I. However, in type III, only limited improvement may be observed in a few patients.

Sialidosis, Type I

Sialidosis type I, or the cherry-red spot myoclonus syndrome, which is caused by a deficit of the enzyme neuraminidase, also produces a typical syndrome. Facial myoclonus and intention myoclonus may point to the diagnosis (Rapin, 1986), which can be made by the highly suggestive funduscopic examination, its slow progression, and the absence of mental deterioration. The EEG shows spike-wave discharges or polyspike-waves associated with clinical jerks, which are not provoked by photic stimulation. The somesthetic evoked potentials are abnormally large (Engel et al., 1977).

Galactosialidosis

Galactosialidosis results from a combined deficiency of neuraminidase and β-galactosidase, and its features are similar to those of sialidosis type I, with action and intention myoclonus. The course may be more rapid, however, and it is marked by the slow appearance of dysmorphic features reminiscent of Hurler disease (Aicardi, 1998a).

Dentatorubral-Pallidoluysian Atrophy

DRPLA is an autosomal dominant disorder caused by an unstable expansion of a CAG repeat in a gene at chromosome 12p13.31 (Yasawa et al., 1995). Most cases have occurred in Japan, although some cases are observed in persons of other ethnic origins (Norrenmolle et al., 1995; Burke et al., 1994; Warner et al., 1994). The disease can present as a movement disorder. In children and in young patients, it is expressed by a PME syndrome. This presentation is due to an expansion of a CAG trinucleotide repeat on chromosome 12. Early-onset forms are associated with longer repeats (anticipation) and they are usually severe. The repeat encodes a polyglutamine tract that induces cell death.

Juvenile Neuroaxonal Dystrophy

Juvenile neuroaxonal dystrophy is an exceptional cause of action and intention myoclonus. It is associated with a pigmentary retinopathy (Scheithauer et al., 1978).

CEROID LIPOFUSCINOSES

Among the disorders listed in Table 7.1 as group II, the ceroid lipofuscinoses, which are sometimes collectively referred to as *Batten disease*, are responsible for myoclonus with an almost universal regularity, in contrast to Huntington chorea, in which it is inconsistent, and Wilson disease or Hallervorden-Spatz syndrome, in which they are only occasionally seen. Myoclonus is seen in five forms of neuronal ceroid lipofuscinosis (CLN). It is an early manifestation in the early and late infantile types, but, in these, it presents mainly as massive myoclonic or myoclonic astatic seizures, rather than as erratic fragmentary jerks. As a result, the diagnostic problems in these cases differ from those posed by the "classic" PME syndromes, and these diseases must be distinguished from LGS and the severe types of non-PME (see Chapters 4 and 6). In the juvenile form of CLN, the myoclonus is more typical of the PME syndrome (Lake and Cavanagh, 1978). However, it is always preceded for months or years by visual disturbances and psychiatric manifestations. In all of the cases of ceroid lipofuscinosis, alterations or extinction of the electroretinogram are found early in the course (Harden and Pampiglione, 1982; Zeman et al., 1970).

The *late infantile form* (CLN, type 2) is the least uncommon form of ceroid lipofuscinosis, except in Scandinavia, where CLN, type 3, is the prevalent type. This autosomal recessive disease starts between 2 and 4 years of age and has a fatal course. The disease, which is also termed *Jansky-Bielschowsky disease*, was mapped to chromosome 11p15 (Sharp et al., 1997), on which the gene encoding tripeptidyl peptidase-1 (TPP-1) has several mutations (Sleat et al. 1997, 1999) that compromise the removal of tripeptides from the degrading proteins in lysosomes.

The following two variants of infantile or early juvenile CLN are known: the Finnish variant, or CLN, type 5, maps to chromosome 13q21-q32, a gene whose function is unknown; and CLN, type 6, which may also cause myoclonus, maps to 15q21-23.

Autosomal recessive juvenile ceroid lipofuscinosis (Batten or Spielmeyer-Vogt disease) (CLN, type 3) is responsible for resistant epilepsy that often has a myoclonic component. The disorder is prevalent in Sweden. The disease (Gardiner et al., 1990; Eiberg et al., 1989) maps to a gene on chromosome 16p that encodes a novel protein of unknown function. A large number of mutations have been reported.

The diagnosis of the ceroid lipofuscinosis is usually made by the demonstration of the cytosomes found by peripheral biopsies (skin or conjunctivae), which are characteristic of, although not entirely specific for, the diverse forms. It can now be made by molecular genetic means or by enzymatic determination for CLN-1, CLN-2, and CLN-3. After an index case, prenatal diagnosis is possible using similar methods.

At least eight different ceroid lipofuscinoses with variable presentations are known. Their main features are shown in Table 7.2. A recent review of the phenotypic-to-genotypic relationships is available (Wisniewski, 2001).

DIFFERENTIAL DIAGNOSIS

The diagnosis of any of the diseases studied in this chapter entails a poor prognosis, so less severe conditions should be absolutely excluded before the diagnosis of PME is accepted.

Essential (familial) myoclonus (Korten et al., 1974) does not feature other types of seizures, and it is a nonprogressive condition that is not associated with paroxysmal EEG abnormalities. Other forms of benign myoclonic epilepsies with prominent myoclonic phenomena include rare familial forms in both adults (Okino, 1997) and children (Zara et al., 2000) and infants (de Falco et al., 2001).

PMEs, especially Unverricht-Lundborg disease, may closely resemble primary generalized epilepsy at onset (Roger et al., 1992), and the diagnosis may be impossible for variable periods unless the family history is positive for similar cases. The differentiation of PME from nonprogressive epilepsies with myoclonic phenomena is not always easy. The frequent occurrence of cerebellar signs in the epilepsies presenting with prominent myoclonic phenomena is well established. Hodskins and Yakovlev (1930) found that 30 (10%) of 300 chronic epileptic patients showed signs of poor cerebellar function. Conversely, cerebellar abnormalities were present in one-third of their patients with myoclonic attacks, compared with one-tenth of unselected epileptic persons. These authors did not separate the transient signs from the chronic or progressive cerebellar syndromes. Roger et al. (1960) found that 20% of the patients with massive myoclonic jerks had cerebellar signs, versus 0.5% of unselected epileptics. Aicardi and Chevrie (1971) encountered cerebellar signs in 24 (27%) of 90 children with various types of myoclonic epilepsy. The cerebellar signs were permanent or progressive in only one-fourth of the cases and were transient in the remaining three-fourths. These latter were often recurrent. When such transient cerebellar signs are associated with both partial erratic myoclonus and a temporary lowering of the level of mental functioning as often occurs with myoclonic status epilepticus or in the so-called *absence status* often observed in patients with LGS, the diagnosis of a progressive disease is often wrongly made. The mechanism of this pseudoataxia (Bennett et al., 1982) is unclear. Although drug toxicity may play a part, the role of the subclinical status is probably essential. The so-called *minor epileptic status* (Brett, 1966) is also significantly associated with ataxia.

SUMMARY

The PMEs, or myoclonus epilepsies, include a heterogeneous collection of disorders, most of which are genetically determined. They all run a severe course that is always debilitating and often fatal.

Although a PME syndrome is traditionally described as being characterized by erratic myoclonus, massive myoclonic jerks, progressive mental deterioration, and evolving neurologic signs, the clinical picture observed with the various causes often departs from this scheme. Indeed, most disorders that produce PME give rise to specific or highly suggestive symptoms and signs. The myoclonus itself differs in its clinical manifestations and circumstances of occurrence depending on the causal disease. Nevertheless, the term *PME* has been maintained in the new guidelines for classification of seizures and syndromes (Engel, 2001).

The concept of a definite syndrome of PME has become obsolete, even though a few cases continue to remain unclassified. Several forms of epilepsy with myoclonic jerks that are not the result of progressive degenerative conditions can be complicated by transient episodes of ataxia and/or mental regression. This is especially true in the case of some types of myoclonic or myoclonic astatic epilepsy, as well as LGS, whose course may be marked by episodes of nonconvulsive status epilepticus often associated with erratic positive or negative myoclonus that may last days or even weeks and with temporary cognitive deterioration. Such episodes should not be misdiagnosed as progressive myoclonic encephalopathies because they have a much better prognosis and they are not genetic conditions.

8

Epilepsies with Typical Absence Seizures

Absences are generalized nonconvulsive epileptic seizures; in other words, they are seizures without local onset, expressed predominantly by disturbances of consciousness, with no or relatively little motor activity. The 1981 revision of the International Classification of Epileptic Seizures recognizes the following two types of absence seizures depending on their ictal electroencephalographic (EEG) pattern and clinical characteristics: (a) typical absence seizures characterized by an abrupt onset and offset and an EEG discharge of symmetric, synchronous spike-wave complexes recurring regularly at a rhythm of about 3 Hz and (b) atypical absences with a more progressive onset and offset that are often associated with different EEG patterns, including bursts of spike-wave patterns that are often irregular at a rhythm of less than 2.5 Hz and, at times, fast rhythms of small-amplitude or high-voltage 10-Hz activity (Erba and Browne, 1983; Commission on Classification and Terminology of the International League Against Epilepsy, 1981). In actuality, these distinctions are somewhat artificial, and some investigators consider typical absences to be those that occur in idiopathic epilepsy and atypical absences to be those associated with cryptogenic or symptomatic epilepsies, especially the Lennox-Gastaut syndrome (LGS) (Roger and Genton, 1995). However, typical absences may occasionally occur in symptomatic epilepsies (Ferrie et al., 1995).

Typical absence attacks can be classified as "simple" when only impairment of consciousness is present, possibly with simple and limited motor activity, such as eyelid fluttering or jerking or slight elevation of the eyeballs, and as "complex" when automatisms or prominent motor components (myoclonic, tonic, or atonic) are present (Gastaut et al., 1974b). This chapter deals with childhood epilepsies manifested exclusively or predominantly by typical absences, whether simple or complex. Atypical absences are considered elsewhere (see Chapter 4). The term *petit mal epilepsy* is often used synonymously with *typical absence epilepsy* (Lennox and Lennox, 1960; Livingston, 1960). However, the former term has been used loosely to designate a number of different epilepsy syndromes with relatively minor symptoms,

regardless of the precise description of the seizures and the associated EEG abnormalities. The term has also been variously used in a number of countries (Doose et al., 1970; Kruse, 1968). Thus, the use of the term *typical absence epilepsy* is preferable, as it avoids the ambiguities associated with the term *petit mal*.

Typical absence epilepsy does not designate a single type of epilepsy but rather a broad group of epilepsy syndromes with onset at different ages and varying associated seizures, courses, and outcomes. This chapter describes the clinical and EEG manifestations of typical absences and then reviews the several syndromes featuring typical absence attacks. These include the following:

1. A relatively pure form of typical absence epilepsy of childhood in which very frequent seizures occur in isolation, generally between the ages of 4 and 10 years (also called *pyknolepsy*) (Janz, 1969).

2. Typical absence epilepsy of adolescence in which absences occur less frequently than in the childhood type and they are more often associated with tonic-clonic seizures and other forms of attack. Panayiotopoulos et al. (1989a, 1989b) separated the absences observed with juvenile myoclonic epilepsy (JME) from the typical absences of adolescence on the basis of a mild decrease in consciousness and different EEG findings. However, the term *absence* may not be adequate if no alteration of awareness is observed.

3. Myoclonic absences, which are also known as *clonic absences*.

In addition to these syndromes, which are recognized by the International League Against Epilepsy (ILAE) classification, other syndromes with absences have been described (Panayiotopoulos, 1998a; Duncan and Panayiotopoulos, 1995b). These include the following: absences occurring in association with adversion (adversive absences) (Janz, 1969); absences occurring in association with focal features (Dalby, 1969; Bancaud et al., 1965); absences with evidence of a brain lesion, whether fixed or evolving (Sato et al., 1976; Loiseau and Cohadon, 1970; Dalby, 1969;

Lennox and Lennox, 1960); absences induced by intermittent light stimulation, television, and/or eye closure (Jeavons, 1982); absences preceded by generalized tonic-clonic seizures (GTCSs) other than febrile convulsions (Dieterich et al., 1985b). Such cases are not included in the ILAE classification (Commission on Classification and Terminology of the International League Against Epilepsy, 1985, 1989).

EPIDEMIOLOGY AND ETIOLOGY

The *epidemiology* of typical absences is not well known because of problems with case ascertainment, case definition, and patient-selection bias (Sander, 1995). Typical absences affect predominantly children and adolescents, and females are usually affected more than males. The incidence of typical absences ranges from 0.7 to 4.6 per 100,000 in children and adolescents up to 15 years of age. Granieri et al. (1983) estimated an average incidence of 1.9 per 100,000 in Italy, and Hauser et al. (1991) noted an annual rate of 1.3 per 100,000 population in Rochester, Minnesota. Higher figures (6 per 100,000) were found in children younger than 16 years, compared with 1.4 per 100,000 in the general population in France (Loiseau et al., 1990). The prevalence rate is quite low, but it may be underestimated in epidemiologic studies.

The proportion of patients with typical absences among those with epilepsy is often given as 3% in community-based or hospital-based studies (Sander, 1995).

The *etiologic factors* of typical absence epilepsy probably vary with the syndrome observed. Girls are more commonly affected than boys, with a ratio of 60% to 40% (Roger, 1974; Dalby, 1969; Gibberd, 1966). Typical absence seizures are mainly a disorder of children and adolescents, although adults are not immune (Loiseau and Cohadon, 1970). Holowach et al. (1962) indicated that 80% of their patients were between 2.5 and 9 years of age at the onset of typical absence. Livingston et al. (1965) found 2.6% of their patients to be younger than 2 years, 55% were between 4 and 8 years, and 93.1% were younger than 13 years. In the series by Dalby (1969), 17% were younger than 4 years, 64% were between 5 and 9 years, 17% were between 10 and 14 years, and only 2% were older than 15 years. The mean age at onset for the patients with typical absence seizures in the study by Oller-Daurella and Sanchez (1981) was 7 years. However, in the series by Lugaresi et al. (1974), 30% of patients had an age at onset of younger than 4 years, and 22.6% had an onset after 10

years of age. This series contained a very high proportion of patients with cerebral lesions, and, thus, it may be biased in favor of the more severe cases. Rare cases in the first year of life have also been reported (Aicardi, 1995; Cavazzuti et al., 1989).

Genetic factors are thought to be of major importance in the causation of typical absence seizures. Family studies indicate that the incidence of seizures or EEG paroxysmal abnormalities in first-degree relatives ranges from 15% to 44% (Degen et al., 1990; Rocca et al., 1987a; Sato et al., 1976; Lugaresi et al., 1973; Currier et al., 1963; Holowach et al., 1962). The occurrence of two cases of typical absence epilepsy in siblings, parents, and offspring is not uncommon (Loiseau and Cohadon, 1970; Lennox and Lennox, 1960). However, the occurrence of other forms of epilepsy in relatives of patients with typical absence seizures is more common than is that of the same typical absence type. Twin studies (Lennox and Lennox, 1960) found a concordance of 75% for typical absence seizures and of 84% for EEG abnormalities in monozygotic twins, whereas no dizygotic pair was concordant. Several investigators (Metrakos and Metrakos, 1970) favored a dominant mode of inheritance, but polygenic transmission appears more likely (Doose and Baier, 1987, 1988; Doose et al., 1973, 1984; Aicardi, 1973). Although a genetic relationship between typical absence epilepsy and other epilepsy syndromes, such as awakening grand mal, has long been known, this relation is, to a large extent, dependent on the syndrome, as the study of pedigrees with several affected members shows (Bianchi and the Italian League Against Epilepsy Collaborative Group, 1995). Juvenile absence epilepsy (JAE) is not usually found in relatives of patients with childhood absences, whereas absences associated with myoclonic phenomena are not encountered in families with pure absence attacks but they may be related to those with JME. Absences are preceded by febrile seizures in approximately 15% to 30% of patients (Wallace, 1991; Olsson, 1990; Hashimoto et al., 1989; Doose et al., 1973). Rare cases of such may be an expression of the spectrum of generalized epilepsy with febrile seizures plus (GEFS+), which can manifest with typical absences (see Chapters 5 and 9).

Linkage of typical absences to several loci has been found in some cases, including 8q24, 15q14, and 6p. In one family, the dominant transmission of absences and other seizure types following febrile seizures in early life was observed within the framework of GEFS+ (Wallace et al., 2001) and was associated with a mutation of the γ-aminobutyric acid (GABA) receptor (see Chapter 20). However, the responsible genes have not been cloned, and no linkage was found in a large number of cases.

Acquired factors may also play a role. Typical absence epilepsy may appear in children with brain lesions, and, at least in some, it is a result of the brain lesions (Ferrie et al., 1995). Perinatal difficulties, infections, or focal damage of undetermined origin are quoted as causes of typical absence epilepsy, but these are rarely proved. Cases of typical absence seizures apparently resulting from progressive brain lesions (Olsson and Hedström, 1991; Broughton et al., 1973), such as brain tumors (Farwell and Stuntz, 1984; Madsen and Bray, 1966) or neuronal lipidosis (Olsson and Hedström, 1991) are on record. Lesions in the mesial or orbital frontal cortex seem especially likely to produce absence seizures (Loiseau and Cohadon, 1970). Bancaud et al. (1974) showed that 3-Hz electrical stimulation of the mesial aspects of the frontal lobes can produce typical absence seizures in epileptic patients. The frequency of acquired brain damage in patients with typical absence attacks is poorly known, and it depends largely on the criteria that are used to define a lesion. Figures of up to 39% have been reported in some series (Bamberger and Matthes, 1959). Dalby (1969) found evidence of brain damage (as judged from the presence of neurologic antecedents, a low intelligence quotient [IQ], or interictal neurologic or pneumoencephalographic abnormalities) in 21% of patients with "pure petit mal," in 37% of those with absences associated with automatisms, and in 58% of those with "focal petit mal." Determining the exact significance of such abnormalities relative to strictly defined typical absence seizures is difficult, but they are rare in practice. However, localized brain damage undoubtedly may be a factor at the origin of typical absence. Olsson and Hedström (1991) found that 12 (10%) of 119 unselected children with typical absences had mental retardation and/or neurologic signs.

Typical absence epilepsy (*petit mal* in the restricted sense of the term) is regarded as the prototype of the primary or idiopathic generalized epilepsies in children (O'Donohoe, 1985; Gastaut et al., 1974b). The use of the term *primary* implies the absence of underlying brain damage as a cause of seizures (Gastaut, 1973). As was stated already, this absence is not constant.

The origin of the bilaterally synchronous 3-Hz discharge of typical absence epilepsy has received considerable attention (Coulter, 1995; Avoli and Gloor, 1994; Coulter et al., 1990; Gloor et al., 1990; Browne and Mirsky, 1983). A thalamocortical oscillatory system that includes neocortical neurons, the thalamic

relay neurons, and neurons of the nucleus reticularis thalami seems to play a major role. GABAergic mechanisms are essential for the maintenance of the oscillations underlying the spike-wave discharges. The thalamic oscillation is dependent on the deactivation of a low calcium $(Ca)^{2+}$ current that occurs when the membrane of the thalamic relay neurons is hyperpolarized (Gloor, 1995; Steriade et al., 1993). In addition to the mild hyperexcitability of the cortex, the excessively strong inhibition of the thalamic relay nuclei by the GABAergic reticular neurons results in the switching of the spindle-generating mechanism to the spike-wave mode (Gloor, 1995). The therapeutic role of ethosuximide is probably due to its decreasing effect on the low Ca T-current (Drinkenburg et al., 1991; Coulter et al., 1990).

Whatever the mechanisms of typical absence attacks, the study of which is beyond the scope of this book, one may consider the paroxysmal instability (in the corticoreticular system or any equivalent circuit) to be genetically determined or to be the result of diffuse pathologic processes involving the cortex or the deep structures implicated in the generation of typical absences.

CLINICAL AND ELECTROENCEPHALOGRAPHIC CHARACTERISTICS OF ABSENCE SEIZURES

Clinical Aspects

The most common and most typical symptomatology of absence epilepsy is that observed in childhood absence epilepsy (CAE), which can, therefore, be used as a paradigm for other syndromes. However, significant differences from this classic type may occur with other syndromes and ages at onset, and a variable course may be seen.

Simple Typical Absence

Simple absences in their most characteristic form in CAE are marked by a profound disturbance but not necessarily complete abolition of awareness, perception, responsiveness, memory, and recollection. Marked variability in the expression of absences may be observed even in the same child, and some patients may remember what they were told during the latter part of an absence. In most children, the impairment of consciousness is profound. When the absence is induced by hyperventilation with the eyes shut, eye opening occurs within the first 3 seconds of the absence (Panayiotopoulos, 1998a; Duncan and Panayiotopoulos, 1995a). According to Lennox and Lennox (1960), 90% of simple typical absences last between 5 and 15 seconds, and absences lasting more than 30 seconds are rare, occurring in only 3% of patients with typical absence epilepsy. In 14% of patients, both brief and long absences may occur (Loiseau and Cohadon, 1970). Absences lasting less than 5 seconds may be difficult to detect. The onset of an attack is sudden, and the child's ongoing activity is abruptly interrupted, with the child remaining motionless with a vacant stare. The eyes may drift upward, and slight beating of the eyelids at a rhythm of 3 Hz is common. The end of the attack is as sudden as its onset, and the patient returns to whatever activity he or she was engaged in at the onset of the seizure. Occasionally, a smile with a slightly dazed state is observed for 2 to 3 seconds, possibly indicating a very brief postictal phase (Gastaut and Broughton, 1972). This, however, is uncommon or hardly noticeable, and the lack of definite postictal confusion or fatigue is an essential clue for differentiating typical absences from complex partial seizures of limited expression (Holmes et al., 1987; Penry et al., 1975). The abruptness of both onset and termination is also important for distinguishing typical absences from atypical absences (Erba and Browne, 1983; Gastaut et al., 1974b).

In some typical absence attacks, the impairment of awareness is less profound, and the patient may be directly conscious of the time elapsed after the seizure, without external clues. Some responsiveness may be maintained, and, rarely, only confusion or mental clouding occurs with some memory of events (Browne and Mirsky, 1983; Mirsky and Van Buren, 1965). Only rarely in CAE is the degree of confusion so slight that it goes unnoticed by observers or even by the patient in the absence of specific tests. This occurs only in specific syndromes mostly seen in adults.

Typical absence seizures are of variable frequency. They are repeated several or dozens of times daily in a vast majority of children, but they may occur less frequently in other syndromes. Browne et al. (1983c), using telemetric EEG recording, recorded an average of about 100 seizures per day in 20 patients. In fact, attacks that do not recur daily rarely prove to be typical absences, and these should be accepted as such only with caution. The frequent occurrence of extremely brief "microabsences," during which the state of consciousness may be almost impossible to assess, makes any precise evaluation of the number of attacks difficult.

Typical absences in children are almost always easily precipitated by hyperpnea, which is one of the most powerful means of confirming the diagnosis without danger.

Photic stimulation is said to induce typical absences in some patients (Roger and Genton, 1995; Loiseau and Cohadon, 1970; Dalby, 1969). The frequency and significance of photic sensitivity is quite variable among the various syndromes with absences (see "Electroencephalographic Aspects"). Photic stimulation, especially watching television at very close range, may be used for self-induction of absences in some patients (mostly adolescents or adults) (Harding and Jeavons, 1994).

A number of factors can facilitate or reduce the occurrence of typical absences. Spike-wave discharges and absences decrease in number when the child focuses his or her attention on a particular task, especially if it is pleasant (Guey et al., 1965, 1969; Lennox and Lennox, 1960). Playful activities have a similar effect, whereas more demanding tasks may increase the frequency of typical absences. Occasionally, typical absences appear selectively in specific activities, whether physical or intellectual (Senanayake, 1989), thus showing that not only the degree of attention but also more complex psychologic factors play a role in the provocation or inhibition of attacks (see Chapter 17).

Simple typical absences seem relatively uncommon. Penry et al. (1975) observed that only 34 (10%) of the 347 typical absence seizures they monitored belonged to that type. This was a referral series, however, so atypical cases were likely overrepresented.

Complex Typical Absence

In complex typical absence seizures, the impairment of consciousness is associated with other phenomena, motor or otherwise. These phenomena are often relatively minor and inconspicuous, so the disturbance of consciousness remains the essential feature. *Motor components* (Janz, 1969) are part of many absence attacks. An increase in muscle tone, especially in the posterior neck muscles, may occur. This may lead to retropulsion of the head and trunk. Some asymmetry is possible, with resultant gaze deviation and head rotation to one side (versive absences) (Janz, 1969). In typical absences, phasic muscle contractions are limited to clonic jerks of the eyelids that are occasionally accompanied by mild clonias of the deltoid muscles. Diminution of the muscle tone in muscles subserving posture is a common phenomenon during typical absence (Loiseau, 1992; Gastaut et al., 1974b), but its degree is usually mild, producing only a slight slump or causing patients to lose objects they had in their hands. Hypotonia may result in intermittent or saccadic lowering of the head or arms that sometimes alternates with myoclonic jerks. Tonic loss rarely involves the lower limbs, with resultant falls or a mere sagging of the knees. However, 17% of the patients in the study by Dalby (1969) had atonic phenomena that, in 9%, were severe enough to cause the patient to fall.

Automatisms occur in a high proportion of typical absence seizures. *De novo* automatisms were present in 60% of the patients in the study by Penry et al. (1975) and in 55% of those in the study by Dalby (1969). Persistence of an action that has already been initiated is common, but the act is usually carried out imperfectly. Oral automatisms (e.g., licking, smacking, and swallowing) are extremely common, and simple gestural automatisms, such as crumbling or scratching movements, crossing the legs, carrying hands to the face, trying to take off the EEG electrodes, or fumbling with clothes, are also common. The patient may also mumble, sing, or utter incoherent words. The probability of automatisms occurring during an absence increases with the duration of the absence (Penry et al., 1975). Automatisms occur only when the loss of consciousness is severe, and they are not observed in patients with only mild impairment of awareness. Though automatisms are highly common in typical absence attacks, they are usually relatively minor in expression and different in character from those in complex partial seizures. Moreover, they stop abruptly at the same time as the EEG discharge, and they do not progressively merge with postictal automatisms and confusion, a frequent occurrence in partial attacks. *Autonomic phenomena* include changes in respiratory rhythms or apnea, pallor, heart rate modification, and mydriasis (Lennox and Lennox, 1960). Micturition occurs in 5% to 17% of patients (Loiseau and Cohadon, 1970; Janz, 1969; Holowach et al., 1962).

Complex absences are more common than the simple variety (Porter, 1992). However, very complex ictal phenomena are rarely observed; when they are, they are seen only in long-lasting absences and in absence status (see Chapter 16).

Electroencephalographic Aspects

The *EEG features of typical absence attacks* are the same whether the absence is simple or complex. The absence discharge essentially consists of generalized, symmetric, and synchronous complexes that feature a negative slow wave preceded by one (occasionally two or more) negative spike or sharp wave and that recur

at a rhythm of about 3 Hz (Fig. 8.1) in regularly organized bursts that last as long as the clinical absence does (generally 5 to 15 seconds). More detailed descriptions (Browne and Mirsky, 1983; Gastaut et al., 1974b; Gastaut and Broughton, 1972) indicate that the spike of the spike-wave complex consists of the following several components: (a) an initial low-voltage, negative deflection notching the descending limb of the preceding slow wave; (b) a positive transient turn; and (c) the final classic negative spike of 70-ms to 80-ms duration. The frequency of repetition of the complexes may vary somewhat but remains close to the basic frequency of 3 Hz. The first 1 or 2 seconds of the absence discharge may be at a faster rhythm and less regular than the rest. Very often, progressive and regular slowing of the discharge from about 3.5 to 2.5 Hz is observed. The onset and termination of the discharge are abrupt. The tracing resumes its interictal appearance without displaying depression or postictal slowing. Occasionally, a few postictal slow waves may be seen in the frontal areas (Gastaut et al., 1974b). In addition to being bilateral and symmetric with simultaneous onset in all leads, the spike-wave discharge of typical absence also exhibits (with a few possible variations [Lockman et al., 1979; Loiseau and Cohadon, 1970; Livingston et al., 1965]) a relatively stereotypic spatial distribution with a maximum amplitude over the frontorolandic regions, to which it, at times, is limited (Lennox and Lennox, 1960). Automatic frequency analysis indicates a more complex picture—several frequencies are mixed with a predominance of 3-Hz and 10-Hz rhythms. With regard to their synchronism and distribution of field potentials, these two rhythms behave independently (Gastaut et al., 1974b). In some cases (Lagae et al., 2001), a frontal onset and/or predominance has been thought to be associated with greater treatment resistance.

The spike corresponds to positive (excitatory) phenomena, particularly myoclonic jerks of eyelids or limbs, whereas the slow wave appears to be inhibitory in nature (Tassinari et al., 1971).

The ictal discharges differ from one patient to another. During slow sleep, they become fragmented and irregular, and they may be replaced by isolated generalized polyspike-wave or polyspike discharges. The discharges also become atypical with therapy and increasing age. Their amplitude frequently diminishes, and they tend to be less regular. In adolescents and adults, the spike-wave complexes may be repeated at a faster rhythm of 4 to 4.5 Hz (Gastaut and Tassinari, 1975a).

Sudden variations in the shape and rhythm of the discharge can occur, especially towards the end of a

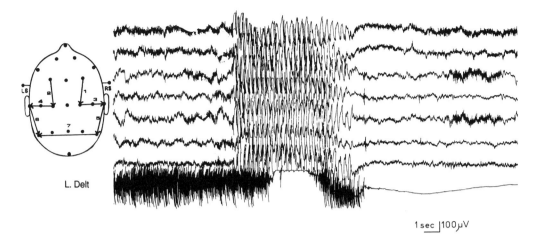

FIG. 8.1. Typical absence seizure in a 9-year, 5-month-old girl. This simple polygraphic recording with seven electroencephalographic channels and just one electromyographic (EMG) channel (L. Delt, left deltoid) is sufficient to show the phenomenology of a short absence seizure. The girl is asked to keep her arms raised and extended; this maneuver produces continuous interferential EMG activity on the muscle sampled. A discharge of generalized spike-wave complexes at 3 Hz that lasts about 7 seconds is accompanied by cessation of the task (the girl puts her arms down) in its central part (for about 3 seconds) and is followed by the resumption of the requested posture before its end. Soon afterwards, the girl drops her arms again and looks around puzzled.

discharge when slow spike-waves or slow and irregular waves may replace the 3-Hz complexes (Loiseau and Cohadon, 1970). According to Loiseau and Cohadon (1970), such changes have no prognostic significance. However, Panayiotopoulos (1994b) has stated that they are not observed in patients with CAE. The discharges may be asymmetric in up to 9% of patients at the onset of a seizure, but they rarely remain so throughout the attack (Gastaut et al., 1986a; Lockman et al., 1979). In a few cases, only rhythmic delta activity is detectable on standard EEG records, and the spike is invisible (Lee and Kirby, 1988). The significance of this discharge does not seem to differ from that of classic paroxysms. However, such rhythmic slow discharges during hyperventilation are not uncommon, and they should be distinguished from true absence discharges (Epstein et al., 1994).

Photosensitivity is present in 10% to 20% of patients (Smith, 1995). In a minority, photic stimulation precipitates absences. In a majority, it is a purely EEG phenomenon. All authors acknowledge that it usually heralds more severe syndromes with a greater likelihood of myoclonias and GTCSs (Panayiotopoulos, 1998; Roger and Genton, 1995).

The *interictal EEG records* are most often normal. Occasionally, the background rhythm is slower than

normal, of high amplitude, and poorly reactive (Sato et al., 1976). Brief irregular bursts of spike-waves are seen in 30% of patients. Whether such bursts are truly interictal has been disputed; some authors consider generalized spike-wave activity to be accompanied by impaired performance in all cases, while postulating that interseizure discharges probably do not occur in absence seizures (Browne and Mirsky, 1983; Browne et al., 1974). Posterior, rhythmic slow-wave activity at a frequency of 3 Hz is observed in 13% to 20% of patients with typical absences. This activity is often symmetric, it may occur in bursts, and it is blocked by eye opening (Fig. 8.2). Not uncommonly, ictal spike-wave discharges appear to surge from such trains of slow waves (Gastaut and Tassinari, 1975a; Loiseau and Cohadon, 1970).

Localized or focal interictal paroxysms are uncommon. Gibbs and Gibbs (1952) found them in 15 of 137 cases of typical absence attacks; Ricci and Vizzioli (1964), in 3 of 200 patients; and Niedermeyer (1972a), in 8% of his cases. Olsson (1990) found a higher proportion of focal anomalies (24%), especially in those children who later developed GTCSs (28%). Foci of paroxysmal activity are sometimes associated with 3-Hz generalized discharges. Dalby (1969) found such foci in 24 of the 161 patients with

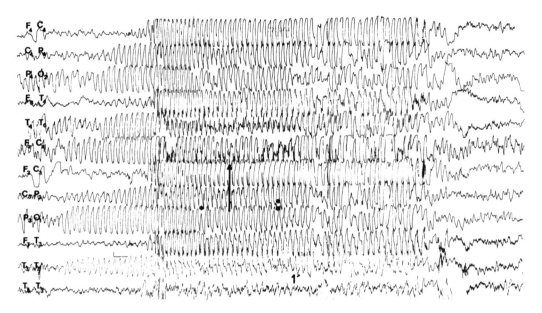

FIG. 8.2. Typical absence seizure preceded by a discharge of 3-Hz rhythmic waves over the posterior region of both hemispheres. The absence occurred after 1 minute of hyperventilation. The patient's eyes open (*arrow*); the patient does not answer (*first asterisk*); and the patient is responsive (*second asterisk*) (calibration: 1 sec, 50 μV).

typical absences that he studied. In most patients, the onset was later than in the other forms of typical absence attacks, with 45% having an onset after 10 years of age. In addition to typical absences, 20% of the patients had other types of seizures. Evidence of cerebral damage was found in 58% of patients with what Dalby termed "petit mal with focal component," but in only 21% of those with classic typical absences and 37% of those with an automatic component to their attacks. Not unexpectedly, the prognosis was unfavorable, with stabilization being observed in only 35% of these patients. At least some of the cases of petit mal with focal components as described by Dalby were likely cases of frontal lesions associated with typical absences. Several such cases are on record (Gordon, 1979; Marcus and Watson, 1966; Niedermeyer and Khalifeh, 1965), and the existence of secondary bilateral synchrony (i.e., the occurrence of bilateral bursts of rhythmic spike-wave complexes in patients with frontal brain damage) (Ohtahara and Yamatogi, 1990; O'Brien et al., 1959) has long been known (Penfield and Jasper, 1954).

The association of ictal 3-Hz discharges with a "functional" focus of rolandic spikes seems to be present in only 3% of patients (Genton, 1995a).

The correlations between clinical ictal phenomena and EEG events in typical absence epilepsy are complex. Although a strong relationship exists between changes in consciousness and the occurrence of ictal 3-Hz discharges, the depth of the loss of awareness does not seem to correlate directly with EEG characteristics, such as amplitude and diffusion of the discharge (Lennox and Lennox, 1960). Indeed, completely normal responsiveness has occasionally been noted during typical discharges (Loiseau and Cohadon, 1970), and all of the intermediary states between complete unconsciousness and normal awareness may be noted with EEG discharges of various morphology, amplitude, and rhythmicity.

Subclinical changes in awareness and/or responsiveness are known to occur with brief spike-wave discharges or with some discharges that are limited to the anterior part of the scalp and/or are of low amplitude. Various authors (Browne and Mirsky, 1983; Gastaut et al., 1974b; Goode et al., 1970; Guey et al., 1969; Mirsky and Van Buren, 1965) have demonstrated that some tests of the effects of epileptiform activity are more sensitive than others. Simple motor tasks (e.g., reaction time, rhythmic tapping) are less affected than short-term memory tasks, signal detection, or discriminative tasks. The use of such continuous tests for sufficiently long periods permits the detection of transient cognitive impairment that occurs in association with brief spike-wave bursts. Such events can be regarded as real, although minimal, epileptic seizures, and they may be of practical significance (Browne and Mirsky, 1983). However, only some of the spike-wave bursts in absence seizures are associated with evidence of cognitive impairment. Aarts et al. (1984) found that about half were not related to any clinical phenomenon. Careful testing of patients with repeated paroxysmal bursts has shown that the loss of awareness that accompanies them may appear before the onset of an EEG discharge and that it is generally maximal at the beginning of an absence and becomes less marked toward the end of the discharge (Gastaut et al., 1974b). Such minimal or "subclinical" absences have been described only in adults, most of whom have specific syndromes (see "Epilepsy with 3-Hz Rhythmic Spike-Wave Discharges without Clinically Evident Absences [Phantom Absences]").

Associated Seizures

Associated seizures occur in 40% to 50% of patients (Browne and Mirsky, 1983; Loiseau et al., 1983a; Livingston et al., 1965). GTCSs are most common, whereas focal seizures are rare. Myoclonic seizures are also commonly associated with absences. As is discussed later, the frequency of associated seizures varies greatly with the absence syndrome. GTCSs are rare in CAE but more common with juvenile absence epilepsy. They can precede; accompany; or, more often, follow the absences. Their occurrence is a cause for concern because they tend to persist into adolescence and adulthood. Myoclonic attacks are clearly associated with specific syndromes, and they rarely, if ever, occur in CAE (Panayiotopoulos, 1998). They are common in patients with JME (Janz and Waltz, 1995), occurring in 15% to 25% or more of such cases. In these cases, they do not occur simultaneously with the absences. Other syndromes are characterized by the prominence of the myoclonic attacks, in which the jerks occur simultaneously with the absences. In some of these syndromes, the myoclonic component is much more obvious than the absences, which may be brief and/or inconspicuous (e.g., in the proposed syndrome of eyelid myoclonia with absences), so such cases may be better classified among the myoclonic epilepsies. However, myoclonic jerks synchronous with the spike component of the spike-wave complexes can occur with typical childhood absence seizures that have a good outcome. They involve mainly the eyelids and the face, and they usually are relatively mild (Capovilla et al., 2001b).

Myoclonias may be limited to a single jerk, or they may be repetitive. They involve mostly the face, especially the eyelids and sometimes the eyeballs, but they may also affect the shoulders and, in a few patients, the peribuccal and masticatory muscles. They can be mild or intense and generalized, as occurs in myoclonic absences (Tassinari et al., 1995). The myoclonic phenomena are often closely correlated with EEG photosensitivity. Their presence is of prognostic significance because they often herald difficulties with achieving lasting control of seizures.

Mental and Neurologic Status

The *mental and neurologic status* of patients presenting with typical absence attacks is variable. Classically, typical absence epilepsy was considered to occur in patients of normal or even superior intelligence (Lennox and Lennox, 1960). More recent studies indicate that some mental defect is present in 10% to 42% of patients (Loiseau, 1992; Olsson, 1988; Sato et al., 1983; Holowach et al., 1962). Such differences are probably explained by the varying definitions of absence epilepsy by various investigators and by referral bias because the highest figures seem in excess of the true incidence. Olsson and Hedström (1991), however, reported two cases of progressive encephalopathy, one of myoclonic epilepsy with ragged-red fibers and one of Unverricht-Lundborg disease, in a series of 12 patients with absence and associated encephalopathy, an event already reported in a case of juvenile lipidosis and in one of subacute panencephalitis (Broughton et al., 1973; Andermann, 1967). A low IQ is significantly correlated with the following three factors: (a) resistance to treatment, (b) early onset before the age of 4 years, or (c) late onset after 9 years of age (Roger, 1974). The mental deficit, when it is present, does not appear to be progressive nor is it apparently related to the duration of the epilepsy. *Neurologic signs*, which are found in 2% to 6% of patients, are rare (Chevrie and Aicardi, 1978; Lennox and Lennox, 1960).

DIAGNOSIS

The diagnosis of typical absence attacks can be readily made in most cases by a careful clinical history, and it can be confirmed by EEG. The provocation of an attack by hyperventilation while the child is being watched is a highly useful test when an attack is produced. However, hyperventilation can induce other types of attack, especially brief complex partial seizures, and distinguishing these from typical absences is not always easy. Thus, an EEG recording of 3-Hz spike-wave bursts should be required in all cases. In some cases (Niedermeyer and Khalifeh, 1965), ambulatory EEG monitoring is useful, although it is seldom more effective than hyperventilation (Adams and Lüders, 1981). It permits correlating the occurrence of seizures with the patient's ongoing activity under natural conditions.

On one hand, the diagnosis of absence is often overlooked, especially when the absences are brief and mild. A long history of absences is commonly elicited on the occasion of a first tonic-clonic seizure. On the other hand, the diagnosis of absences is often made wrongly (Fish, 1995; Loiseau, 1992). One common error is confusing simple daydreaming at school or in front of the television screen for a typical absence seizure. Tics or other stereotyped movements (e.g.,, the head thrusts observed with oculomotor apraxia) also are mistaken for typical absences surprisingly often. Careful questioning about the abruptness of onset, the circumstances of occurrence, repetition, the appearance of the eyes, and the movement of the eyelids usually permits easy differentiation. A negative trial of hyperventilation in an untreated child makes the diagnosis unlikely. A normal EEG in a young child with a recent appearance of suspected absences is extremely unusual, and it almost rules out typical absences if adequate hyperventilation was performed. In adolescents, however, both a normal EEG and a negative response to hyperpnea are less exceptional (Loiseau and Cohadon, 1970). The occurrence of pseudo-absences has been reported in patients with hyperventilation syndrome (North et al., 1990).

The differential diagnosis of typical absence attacks and complex partial seizures is usually not difficult if proper attention is given to the following distinguishing features: typical absences have an instantaneous onset and lack any aura; their termination is abrupt without any postictal phase; and their duration is brief, lasting less than 30 seconds almost always and in 90% of patients, less than 10 seconds (Penry and So, 1981). However, complex partial seizures are still wrongly diagnosed as petit mal, on the basis of their relatively short duration and minor manifestations only.

Conversely, although less commonly, absences with automatisms may be wrongly interpreted as complex partial attacks because the frequent existence of automatic activity during typical absences is not widely recognized. Only in long-lasting typical absences, however, will the distinction between typical absences and complex partial seizures raise problems. In brief typical absences, the automatisms are much simpler and less prominent than in complex partial attacks. Brief myoclonic and/or atonic seizures may accompany typical absences, although they are more common with LGS. The differential diagnosis of typical absences and atypical absences is discussed in Chapter 4. The differences in EEG tracing and the distinctive clinical context generally permit an easy differentiation. The diagnosis of the different absence *syndromes* is important because their outcome may be quite variable.

COURSE AND PROGNOSIS

Widely discrepant views have been expressed regarding the outcome of patients with typical absence seizures. These discrepancies have resulted from the differing diagnostic criteria used by various investigators; the differences in origin and composition of the series studied; the variable duration of follow-up; and the heterogeneity of the epilepsies featuring typical absence seizures, with the consequent differences in the definition of what constitutes petit mal or typical absence epilepsy. In general, however, the outcome of typical absence seizures has been considered less favorable in recent series, and the commonly accepted tenet that, in most cases, typical absence epilepsy remits before adulthood is no longer accepted (Lugaresi et al., 1973; Barnhart et al., 1969; Pazzaglia et al., 1969). Control of absences before the age of 20 years was reported in 82 (70%) of 117 patients by Livingston et al. (1965) but in only 47% of patients by Gibberd (1966). Loiseau et al. (1983b) found that, after a 5-year follow-up, the absences were controlled in 32 (46%) of 69 patients with typical absence seizures and that the incidence of absences continued to decline over the following years. Gibberd (1966) also reported that the incidence of absences declined steeply during adolescence, a trend that then continued slowly but steadily until 50 years of age. Gastaut et al. (1986b) have reported on the prolonged persistence of absences in adults.

On the other hand, the incidence of other seizures increases with age (Oller-Daurella and Sanchez, 1981). Fifty-four percent of the patients of Livingston et al. (1965) experienced major seizures later in life; and only 52% of the patients of Loiseau et al. (1983b) had no major fits after a 10-year follow-up, even though only 18% still had absences. Even higher proportions of uncontrolled epilepsy have been reported

(Oller-Daurella and Sanchez, 1981), but, in some series, bias may have been introduced since well-controlled patients may not have reported for follow-up. The mere figures of incidence of uncontrolled epilepsy may be partly misleading because the overall handicap for patients depends also on the severity and frequency of fits. The major motor seizures that follow typical absence attacks are seemingly often relatively mild and infrequent, thus limiting the social and individual handicaps. Status epilepticus appears to be quite rare in such patients (Dieterich et al., 1985a; Roger, 1974).

Several researchers have attempted to evaluate the outcome, not only in the control of epilepsy but also in a more comprehensive manner that includes assessments of intelligence and social and psychiatric adjustment. Loiseau et al. (1983b) found that 29% of their patients with simple or automatic absences and 37% of those with clonic or atonic absences had psychiatric problems and that less than half were socially well adjusted. Lugaresi et al. (1973) had a large proportion (42%) of patients with a low IQ; this, however, was probably existent before the onset of typical absence attacks. They found no evidence of mental deterioration. Overall, they regarded the condition of 120 (48%) of their 249 patients as relatively benign, whereas, in 129 (52%), the outcome was considered unfavorable because of the persistence of seizures (10%), mental retardation (30%), or both (12%). Clearly, the conclusions that may be drawn from these figures, as well as others (Sato et al., 1983; Roger, 1974; Gibberd, 1966; Currier et al., 1963), are far from indisputable because many of them originate from specialized centers, which likely treat the most severe cases.

Olsson and Campenhausen (1993) studied an unselected population of 126 children and adolescents younger than 18 years with absence epilepsy diagnosed from 1973 to 1982 according to strict EEG and clinical criteria. Sixty-nine (55%) of these had active epilepsy, which was defined as either persisting seizures or regular medication, when they were 18 years of age.

At a mean age of 22.5 years, the remaining patients did not differ from a control group in family status and rate of employment. However, the patients had significantly more jobs requiring shorter training, and they were overqualified for their jobs. These patients were also significantly more socially isolated when they were compared to the reference group. Most thought that their everyday life had been influenced by their epilepsy, and they reported difficulties in school achievement, a limited choice of job, and difficulties in concentration and memorization.

The overall studies of absence epilepsy that do not take into account the variable outcome of different absence syndromes provide only a very rough estimate of the prognosis because considerable differences in the outcome and the management are seen among the various subgroups, depending on the age at occurrence and the electroclinical features. The outcome of specific absence epilepsy syndrome is discussed later in this chapter.

The prognosis for typical absence epilepsy depends on several factors, in addition to the absence syndrome causing the absences, which is, by far, the most important factor in the prognosis. General factors may be of interest, especially when syndromic diagnosis is difficult.

An age at onset between 4 and 9 years, the occurrence of typical absences as the only seizure type, and a normal intelligence were found to be associated with a favorable prognosis by Roger et al. (1974). The absence of other types of seizures (with the probable exception of febrile convulsions) and the lack of tonic and atonic components to the absences were regarded as favorable by Loiseau et al. (1983b). In their series, grand mal was more likely to occur (60% versus 35%) in patients in whom the onset of typical absences occurred after 8 years of age and, obviously, in those children in whom convulsive seizures had preceded the typical absences. The occurrence of automatisms during the absence had no prognostic value. The presence of rhythmic posterior delta waves is associated with a lower frequency of later grand mal (Oller-Daurella and Sanchez, 1981; Dalby, 1969). The precipitation of the absence by photic stimulation and the presence of marked myoclonic jerks are other unfavorable factors (Loiseau and Cohadon, 1970). Furthermore, evidence of brain damage and a low IQ are associated with a poor prognosis (Sato et al., 1983; Dalby, 1969). Likewise, absence of more than 30 seconds and a poor or delayed response to therapy indicate the likelihood of difficulties in both seizure control and social adjustment (Roger, 1974).

Sato et al. (1983) using a multivariate analysis with 24 variables in 83 patients to confirm that a normal IQ, no hyperventilation-induced spikes and waves, male gender, and normal neurologic examination results were significant favorable prognostic factors associated with cessation of all types of seizures. The presence of three or more significant factors correctly predicted arrest of the seizures in more than 90% of their patients. The presence of grand mal seizures or a family history of seizures was associated with an unfavorable outcome in univariate analyses, but this factor lost significance in the multivariate analysis. Overall, the rate of cessation of all types of seizures was 48%.

Olsson (1990) divided her 97 patients into those with absences only (n = 56); those with initial absences followed by GTCSs (n = 31), which were subdivided into 21 with GTCS before start of treatment and 10 with GTCSs after the start of treatment; and those with typical absences preceded by GTCS (n = 10). The remission rate after 3.5 years differed significantly among the subgroups. Children with absences only and those with initial absences followed by GTCSs before the start of treatment had an equally high remission rate of 91%. Those children who developed GTCSs after the start of treatment had a significantly lower remission rate of 50%.

In this study, the occurrence of GTCSs was low (11%) in patients with an onset of absences at 6 to 7 years of age, whereas all patients whose absences started at or after 12 years of age had GTCSs. A good response to therapy strongly predicted the absence of GTCSs.

EPILEPSY SYNDROMES FEATURING TYPICAL ABSENCE ATTACKS

The various types of typical absence attacks already described may occur in patients of different ages and neurologic status. They may display different clinical presentations, the absences may occur in association with other types of seizures, and they may run different courses. Certain clinical presentations are selectively encountered. Most researchers recognize at least the following three relatively well-individualized syndromes featuring typical absence attacks: (a) pure typical absence epilepsy or pure petit mal of childhood, which currently is termed *CAE* and is also called *pyknolepsy*; (b) typical absence epilepsy of adolescence; and (c) clonic or myoclonic absences. Other more recently described or less generally recognized syndromes involving absences are also considered.

Childhood Absence Epilepsy

CAE is commonly defined as a syndrome occurring in children of school age that is more common in girls than in boys; it is characterized by very frequent absences, explaining the use of the term *pyknolepsy*. However, some investigators (Duncan and Panayiotopoulos, 1995a; Panayiotopoulos et al., 1989b; Ross et

al., 1980) have proposed additional criteria to separate CAE from other syndromes with absences.

CAE, probably the most common absence syndrome, may represent 2% to 10% of cases of childhood epilepsy (Loiseau, 1992). It is an idiopathic generalized epilepsy in which genetic factors play a major role in its cause.

The age at onset is usually between 4 and 8 years, with a peak at 6 to 7 years. The absences have not been preceded by nor are they associated with other types of seizures, although the occurrence of febrile convulsions in the first years of life does not exclude the diagnosis. The typical absences are repeated many times (usually several dozen) daily. They consist essentially of a transient loss of consciousness without marked motor components, although both simple and complex absences with automatisms are common. The attacks usually last only a few seconds (10 to 15 seconds in most patients). The loss of consciousness appears to be rather profound in most children, and they usually have no direct perception of having the absence, of which they may become aware only by changes in their environment. When the absence occurs with eyes closed, the eyes usually open in the first 2 to 3 seconds of the discharge (Panayiotopoulos et al., 1989b). The absences are easily precipitated by hyperventilation.

The EEG background is normal in these children, and the ictal bursts consist of regular, well-aligned spike-wave complexes at 3 Hz with neither polyspike-waves nor photosensitivity. Some, but not all, authors consider the presence of photosensitivity to rule out the diagnosis of CAE (Duncan and Panayiotopoulos, 1995a, 1998a; Roger and Genton, 1995). The mental and neurologic status of the affected children is normal.

The outlook is usually favorable, with typical absences disappearing before adulthood in approximately 80% of patients. When they do persist into adulthood, associated GTCSs are usually observed. The GTCSs may develop after the absences, usually in adolescence but sometimes as much as several years later (Browne and Mirsky, 1983; Loiseau et al., 1982). The frequency of this occurrence is disputed. Loiseau et al. (1983b) found that 32% of their patients with typical absences beginning before 8 years of age developed grand mal seizures after a mean follow-up of 6.5 years, even though myotonic or atonic absences had been excluded. This figure compares favorably with that of 65% in typical absences of later onset. Grand mal seizures may appear as late as 20 to 30 years of age, but a majority arise between 10 and 15 years of age. The convulsive seizures, as a rule, occur infrequently, and they are often precipitated by factors such as sleep deprivation. Status epilepticus is not observed. Panayiotopoulos (1994b, 1998a) thinks that, with strict definition criteria, no more than 3% of children with CAE develop infrequent GTCSs in adult life. He maintains that the higher figures result from the admixture of cases that do not fulfill his criteria of inclusion and exclusion and that they probably represent other absence syndromes of less favorable outcome. Although the exclusion of absences with myoclonic features, photosensitivity, and atypical EEGs (especially polyspike-waves) probably results in an improved prognosis, some cases of classic absences undoubtedly evolve toward other syndromes, especially JME. Panayiotopoulos considers these cases as belonging to JME from their onset. However, separating such cases from CAE either clinically or by EEG sometimes appears impossible because the absences may be frequent and severe, they begin in the same age range, and the EEG may show typical spike-wave complexes.

Typical Absence Epilepsy of Adolescence

Juvenile Absence Epilepsy

Typical absence attacks in adolescence differ from those in childhood in a number of clinical and, at times, in their EEG features. The age frontier between the two types is not sharply demarcated because cases of CAE may have their onset at up to 12 years of age (Janz et al., 1994). JAE is also largely determined by genetic factors. Relatives of probands with JAE mainly have GTCSs, rather than CAE (Bianchi and the Italian League Against Epilepsy Collaborative Group, 1995). In JAE, absences are usually reported much less frequently than in CAE (a few daily), and those that do occur tend to cluster, especially in the hour following awakening. However, some patients have extremely frequent attacks. The onset ranges from 4 to 30 years of age (Janz et al., 1994), with an average of 13 years.

The absences show a variable, but usually rather severe, impairment of consciousness, although it is less severe than in childhood absences and it may vary considerably in the same patient. Not uncommonly, the patients may retain some awareness and responsiveness during some attacks, and they may be able to remember imperfectly what they were told during the absence and even to execute simple orders, especially when these are given in the late part of the attack. Eye opening is not constant, and it may occur later than in CAE (Panayiotopoulos, 1998a;

Panayiotopoulos et al., 1989b). Absences of JME are easily induced by hyperventilation, and the precipitation of absences by photostimulation has been reported (Harding and Jeavons, 1994; Binnie and Jeavons, 1992; Tassinari et al., 1989). Some adolescents and adults can induce absences by peering at a television screen closely, towards which they feel attracted. Whether such rare cases belong to the JAE syndrome is not entirely clear. The absences of JAE may last longer than in children.

The interictal EEG results may be normal, but, in about 20%, photosensitivity (Wolf and Gooses, 1986) and brief interictal discharges may be seen. The ictal discharges are rhythmic and regular. Their rhythm may be the classic 3 Hz. In a proportion of cases, the spike-wave complexes may recur at a rhythm of 4 Hz (Fig. 8.3) or even 5 Hz (Janz, 1969). Polyspike-wave formations and discharge fragmentation may occur.

The absences seldom remain the only type of seizure. In 80% of cases, they are associated with GTCSs that usually follow the onset of absences. Myoclonic jerks that are usually infrequent occur in 15% to 25% of patients (Wolf, 1995a; Janz et al., 1994; Panayiotopoulos, 1994b). All three types of seizure can occur in the same patient, thus suggesting that they are genetically related, although genetic differences do un-

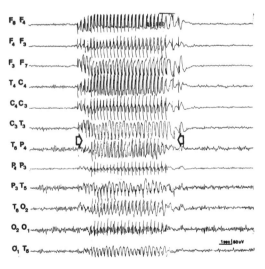

FIG. 8.3. Absence seizure in a 15-year-old boy. Note that the rhythm of occurrence of spike-wave complexes is 4 Hz, which is faster than in younger patients. Clinically, this patient's absences were infrequent, occurring mainly within 1 hour of awakening. This boy had three generalized tonic-clonic seizures, two of which occurred after sleep deprivation (*arrows* indicate apparent loss and recovery of consciousness).

doubtedly exist (Bianchi and the Italian League Against Epilepsy Collaborative Group, 1995).

The outcome of JAE is reasonably good for the absences that can be controlled in 70% to 80% of cases. Generalized convulsive seizures tend to persist, however, although, in general, they occur infrequently and they are often precipitated by lack of sleep, fatigue, and/or alcohol consumption.

Absences in Juvenile Myoclonic Epilepsy

The frequency of absences in JME is not known because their detection occurs as a result of special attention (Janz and Waltz, 1995). As a rule, the absences of JME are simple and brief. They often go unnoticed by others, and the patients experience them as brief disruptions of concentration that often go unreported or that may not even be perceived by them (Canevini et al., 1992; Janz, 1991). These absences are usually simple without automatisms. The age at onset is in the same range as that of JAE.

Ictal EEG shows rhythmic spike-wave discharges at 3 to 4 Hz. Some are regularly rhythmic, but the discharges tend to be less regular and, sometimes, they are frankly arrhythmic. Polyspike-wave discharges are common (Panayiotopoulos and Obeid, 1989; Panayiotopoulos et al., 1989a, 1989b), but the tracings do not need to differ from those in JAE (Janz and Waltz, 1995). Photosensitivity is present in 42% of patients, a higher figure than that of JAE (29%).

As was mentioned in "Childhood Absence Epilepsy" in this chapter, absences in JME may be the first manifestation of epilepsy (2 of 18 patients of Canevini et al. [1992], 11 of 51 patients of Janz and Waltz [1995]). When such cases have an early onset (i.e., within the age range of CAE), the absences tend to occur many times daily and to be profound. Whether they differ from CAE and represent a different syndrome may be a somewhat immaterial question because, in many cases, clinical differentiation is not possible. In such cases, the diagnosis of JME awaits the appearance of more characteristic manifestations.

GTCSs in most patients with JME occur with similar characteristics to those in patients with JAE. By definition, myoclonic jerks are present, and they usually occur after awakening or in the evening during a period of relaxation. JME is a lifelong disorder, but its response to therapy is often gratifying.

Myoclonic Absences or Clonic Absences

Clinically, clonic absences are distinctive because of the intensity of the myoclonic jerks, even though their EEG picture is indistinguishable from that of the usual type of typical absence seizure (Tassinari et al., 1969). They are characterized by rhythmic jerks that occur approximately three times per second and that are much more violent and diffuse than those seen in the usual forms of typical absences. The jerking may predominate in the upper limbs, but it also involves the lower limbs and often produces loss of posture. Usually, the jerks predominate on the proximal limb muscles (Lugaresi et al., 1973, 1974). Clonic or myoclonic absences should be separated from those typical absences that include eyelid or facial myoclonus, although the intensity and extent of myoclonus that are necessary to define clonic absences are difficult to quantify. A tonic contraction that is predominant in the proximal and axial muscles often accompanies the severe clonic jerking; it is often apparent on electromyographic (EMG) traces on polygraphic recording. As a result, the head may be tilted backward as the patient raises his or her arms (Tassinari et al., 1992b). According to Lugaresi et al. (1973) and Tassinari et al. (1992b), myoclonic or clonic absences not only constitute a special type of typical absence attack, but they also define a syndrome with a guarded prognosis. Lugaresi et al. (1974) studied 14 patients in whom clonic absences had their onset between 2 and 17 years of age. In three patients, the seizures were precipitated by watching television; in addition, paroxysms in the EEG recording were induced by photic stimulation in three patients and by hyperventilation in eight. The interictal EEG recording was normal in seven patients and was slowed in eight, and it displayed interictal bursts of spike-waves in 11. The course was unfavorable, and very frequently repeated absences were resistant to vigorous therapy in eight of 14 children. Mental development was impaired in 12 patients at the time of observation, two of whom had an IQ of less than 50. Two patients subsequently developed tonic seizures and atypical absences similar to those in LGS. In a study of 49 patients, Tassinari et al. (1992b, 1995) also reported that mental retardation was present before the onset of seizures in 45% and that deterioration occurred in an additional 25% of patients. Seizures were still present at a mean age of 10.7 years in 19 patients (53%). Associated seizures, most of which were GTCSs, were present in two-thirds of the patients, and they usually indicated a rather poor outcome. Five of their patients developed characteristic features of LGS. These authors emphasized the fact that prominent myoclonus during attacks was in itself of grave prognostic significance, whereas all of the other clinical manifestations observed during complex absences (automatisms and the like) did not appear to influence the prognosis.

The syndrome may not be homogeneous. Some patients respond well to antiepileptic drugs, especially to a combination of valproate and ethosuximide (Tassinari et al., 1995). The association of valproate or ethosaximide to lamotrigine also may have a favorable effect (Manonmani and Wallace, 1994). In half of the patients followed by these investigators, the disease remitted 5.5 years after onset, and, in the remaining half, seizures persisted at the end of follow-up, which, in some cases, was up to 29 years. Patients with refractory seizures had a high incidence of associated seizures (85%), mainly generalized tonic-clonic attacks. Patients with remitting absences had a lower (50%) incidence of associated seizures, most of which were of the absence type. Tassinari et al. (1995) believe that early vigorous treatment might prevent an unfavorable evolution and that a prolonged duration of uncontrolled seizures may be associated with a poor prognosis. However, no prospective study of this is available. In a recent review of the syndrome's characteristics (Bureau and Tassinari, 2000), the long-term evolution of the 40 patients followed at the Centre Saint Paul was reported. Myoclonic absences disappeared in 38% of the cases, while they persisted or the epilepsy manifestations changed in the remaining 25 patients. Adequate treatment from onset apparently did not influence the final outcome.

Myoclonic absences are considered a 'cryptogenic' type of epilepsy in the 1989 ILAE classification.

However, no lesion is usually found, and a significant proportion of patients have favorable outcome like those with other childhood absence syndromes.

Other Possible Syndromes with Typical Absence Seizures

A number of cases of epilepsy involving absence attacks do not fit into any of the categories described in this chapter. Some are described in this section, which is concerned with syndromes that are not generally recognized but that have been mentioned in one or more reports.

Typical Absences in Patients with Brain Damage

Typical absence seizures are sometimes seen in patients with neurologic evidence of diffuse brain damage from various causes. Figure 8.4 shows an attack in a 6-year-old child with a history of neonatal ventricular hemorrhage with subsequent shunted hydrocephalus. In such patients, the clinical features of the absences tend to be atypical, with atonic manifestations or focal symptoms such as head deviation. The EEG bursts may be asymmetric.

Several investigators have found widely differing prevalences of brain damage, ranging from 0% to 38%, in relatively old series (Ferrie et al., 1995). Some of these series were heterogeneous, and they included var-

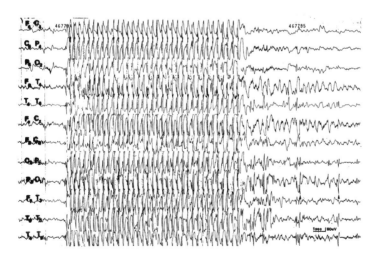

FIG. 8.4. Absence seizure in a 6-year-old boy who had ventricular hemorrhage at birth that was followed by the development of progressive hydrocephalus. A shunt had been inserted in the posterior part of the right ventricle, and neuromental development was only mildly retarded. At 3 years of age, he started to have generalized tonic-clonic seizures and multiple daily absences, some of which were accompanied by a loss of muscle tone that caused falls. The spike-wave burst was almost symmetric, but it was followed by interictal sharp waves (*arrowheads*) located over the left posterior temporal area. It was accompanied by a clinical absence.

ious types of absence with imperfectly defined EEG abnormalities. According to Ferrie et al. (1995), 5% to 14% of patients with typical absences may have central nervous system pathology. However, no distinction is usually made between cases in which brain damage is coincidental and those in which a causal role is likely.

Olsson and Hedström (1991) found that their 12 patients with absence and diffuse encephalopathy had "typical absences with 3-Hz spike-wave bursts on EEG during the course of a more severe type of epilepsy with myoclonic seizures, atypical absences, and GTCSs." The incidence of such cases is unknown, but the prognosis is obviously poor when frank neurologic signs such as a bilateral pyramidal syndrome exist and the mental defect is marked.

Focal pathology, including brain tumors, can also rarely be associated with 3-Hz spike-wave patterns (Farwell and Stuntz, 1984).

Cases of typical absence with focal brain damage, especially that which is frontal, may be interpreted as phenocopies of classic typical absence epilepsy if this is considered mainly a genetic type of epilepsy, or they can be interpreted as being due to the interaction of genetic and organic factors as conceptualized by Berkovic et al. (1987). Cases of absence epilepsy with encephalopathy are related to the following two other possible epilepsy syndromes: typical absences in patients with initial grand mal seizures and "intermediate petit mal" (see "Concept of 'Intermediate Petit Mal'").

Typical Absences in Patients with Initial Grand Mal Seizures

Afebrile GTCSs may precede the onset of absence attacks. In such cases, the prognosis is more guarded than that seen in pure absence epilepsy. In 39 of 83 patients studied by Dieterich et al. (1985a), the seizures persisted or secondarily recurred, and the social integration of these patients was more difficult than that seen in cases of pure absence epilepsy.

Doose et al. (1965) separated a subgroup of 33 patients from 149 patients with absence epilepsy; this subgroup was mainly composed of boys whose epilepsy started with grand mal before 5 years of age. These children often also had atonic or myoclonic attacks, and many were mentally retarded. The EEG recordings were often atypical, with irregularly rhythmic discharges.

Recently, Guerrini et al. (2002e) reported six patients in whom abnormal movements of various types developed following typical absence seizures of early onset in the first year of life. However, the type of

movement disorder was variable, and two children had only a tonic upgaze syndrome.

Epilepsy with 3-Hz Rhythmic Spike-Wave Discharges without Clinically Evident Absences (Phantom Absences)

Some patients (mostly adults) may have typical 3-Hz spike-wave discharges that are not associated with obvious clinical manifestations (Genton, 1995b). Video-EEG recording and close observation can demonstrate minimal function impairment, such as errors or arrest of counting during hyperventilation, that is sometimes associated with eyelid blinking or brief episodes of blank staring. The patient is often unaware of the dysfunction. Such phenomena have been termed *subclinical* or *larval absences* (Aarts et al., 1984) or, more recently, *phantom absences*. The frequency of such phenomena is not known, but they seem common in many idiopathic epilepsies.

Panayiotopoulos (1998a, 2001) has proposed that such episodes may be part of a syndrome that also features GTCSs and, in about half of the cases, absence status epilepticus. Given that "phantom" absences in and of themselves may not lead to medical investigation that results in their discovery, many "incomplete forms" of the syndrome may occur; the validity of this concept remains unconfirmed.

Eyelid Myoclonia with Absences

Eyelid myoclonia with absences was first described by Jeavons who regarded it as an unusual but clearly differentiated type of epilepsy (Jeavons, 1977; Jeavons and Harding, 1975). It consists of severe myoclonic jerking of the eyelids that is much more intense than the fluttering or mild twitching of the eyelids that is commonly seen with simple typical absences. The jerking is accompanied by upward deviation of the eyes, and marked photosensitivity is almost always present. The myoclonias are inconsistently associated with a brief absence that is often difficult to detect. The EEG pattern differs from the classic, regularly rhythmic 3-Hz spike-waves of typical absences. The discharges are brief, usually lasting 2 to 4 seconds, and they are often triggered by photostimulation. The eye closure that often precedes the jerking differs from the slow closure with forced elevation of the eyeballs that is used by some photosensitive patients for the self-induction of seizures (Binnie and Jeavons, 1992). In a few cases, arrest of foveal fixation—so-called *fixation-off epilepsy* (Panayiotopoulos, 1987)—has been the trigger of the attacks.

Eyelid myoclonia with absences is usually associated with other types of seizures, mainly GTCSs. Both the myoclonia and the grand mal attacks tend to persist into adulthood. Eyelid myoclonia with or without absences is regarded as a definite syndrome by several epileptologists (Panayiotopoulos et al., 1998; Appleton, 1995b; Appleton et al., 1993). However, the phenomenon of eyelid myoclonia is fairly common in photosensitive patients, and the other features of the proposed syndrome, especially GTCSs, may not be highly distinctive. In any case, eyelid myoclonia belongs more to the myoclonic epilepsies than to the absence group because the absences are not constant and they do not have the electroclinical characteristics of typical absence seizures.

Other Proposed Syndromes

Other syndromes with myoclonias associated with absences have been proposed. *Perioral myoclonia with absences* (Panayiotopoulos et al., 1995) can occur in children or in adolescents, and it is characterized by frequent seizures and ictal rhythmic localized myoclonus of the perioral muscles. The absences are usually brief, but absence status may also occur. Most patients develop GTCSs. Whether these features are sufficient to characterize a syndrome is a matter of debate (Hirsch et al., 1994). A proposed syndrome of *absences with single myoclonic jerks* (Panayiotopoulos, 1998) also has insufficient documentation.

Concept of "Intermediate Petit Mal"

The term *intermediate petit mal* was coined by the Bologna School to designate a group of cases with features of both classic petit mal (or typical absence attacks) and the LGS (Lugaresi et al., 1973, 1974). In individual patients, the seizures may present predominantly as typical absence attacks or as the tonic-atonic seizures of LGS. This concept has now been largely abandoned, and most cases that were reported under this name belong to the various absence syndromes reviewed earlier in this chapter or to some forms of myoclonic epilepsy (myoclonic atonic). They may also represent the least severe end of the spectrum of the LGS.

TREATMENT OF ABSENCE EPILEPSIES

The aim of treatment of patients with typical absences is complete seizure control without drug-re-

lated side effects. An important consideration is that, in many absence epilepsy syndromes, the occurrence of GTCS is common, and their treatment differs from that of absences.

Typical absence attacks do not respond to several antiepileptic drugs. In particular, drugs that are conventionally used for the treatment of generalized convulsive attacks or for partial seizures, such as phenytoin, phenobarbital, and carbamazepine, are essentially ineffective against typical absences. The diones, especially trimethadione and paramethadione, were the first compounds that proved effective. Their use now has been largely abandoned because of their high toxicity and the introduction of less dangerous drugs.

In 1958, ethosuximide superseded the diones, and it is still widely used today. The drug can be employed as monotherapy in most children presenting with absences without a history of GTCSs (Sherwin, 1983) (see Chapter 24 for dosing information). Caution is recommended for patients with tonic-clonic attacks because the drug may exacerbate the grand mal seizures (Todorov et al., 1978; Livingston, 1972), although the evidence for this is far from complete (Duncan, 1995). Ethosuximide remains the drug of choice for children with major side effects from valproate.

Sodium valproate or valproic acid now is generally regarded as the drug of first choice because it permits complete control in 80% of children with typical absence seizures (Sherwin, 1983; Covanis et al., 1982). It may be slightly more effective than ethosuximide, although this has not been demonstrated (Sato et al., 1982), and it has fewer minor adverse effects (Sherwin, 1983). Valproate is also efficacious against GTCSs, thus making monotherapy easier. In cases of failure of either one of these drugs, the patient should be gradually switched to the other compound. If seizure control is not attained with any one drug, a combination of both may be efficacious, so it should be tried (Rowan et al., 1983). According to Tassinari et al. (1995), the combination is particularly effective against myoclonic absences and other syndromes with myoclonias.

Lamotrigine is extremely effective against most absences, and its use is advised when valproate and ethosuximide have failed (Gram, 1995; Schlumberger et al., 1992a; Sander et al., 1991a).

A combination of lamotrigine and valproate may be effective when neither drug in isolation controls absences (Arzimanoglou, 2000b; Panayiotopoulos et al., 1993). This effect does not appear to be mediated simply through lamotrigine's slowing effect on valproate metabolism. Slow titration of lamotrigine is recommended.

Clonazepam and nitrazepam are effective in controlling absence attacks, but their side effects make them the third-choice agents (Sherwin, 1983). The development of tolerance is a problem with these drugs and with clobazam as well. Tolerance usually develops after 1 to 2 months and occasionally after 6 to 12 months (Schmidt, 1985; Allen et al., 1983). For difficult cases, clonazepam can be combined with valproate because the risk of absence status seems minimal (Jeavons and Clark, 1974). Acetazolamide used in association with major drugs has been advised for resistant cases (Lombroso and Erba, 1982). However, tolerance often develops rapidly as a result of the induction of new enzyme synthesis in glial cells; therefore, the drug should be used only on a short-term basis.

Other antiepileptic drugs generally are not effective. Indeed, some agents, especially those that act through a supposed GABAergic mechanisms, such as vigabatrin and especially carbamazepine (Snead and Hosey, 1985), may increase the frequency of absences or may facilitate the occurrence of myoclonias and GTCSs.

Monotherapy should always be used both at the onset of treatment and for maintenance, except in the unusual patient. The use of a second antiepileptic drug to prevent the development of tonic-clonic seizures has been advocated (Livingston et al., 1965), but its value has not been proven. Multiple drug treatment is required in a small minority of cases (Henriksen, 1980).

Clinical control is rapidly obtained in most patients, and it can be easily verified by having the child hyperventilate. The disappearance of the rhythmic ictal spike-wave bursts is necessary to confirm the effectiveness of therapy (Sherwin, 1983). Browne et al. (1974) advised that "therapy should be aimed at suppressing all spike-wave paroxysms." However, this view could only be accepted if "subclinical discharges" were established to be a significant handicap for the patients or to represent a significant risk. Although a decrease in responsiveness on some tests during such discharges has been well documented, its practical importance remains to be established.

Those syndromes that are known to be often or regularly associated with GTCSs or with a prominent myoclonic component need more prolonged, often lifelong treatment than CAE. In the latter syndrome, the discontinuation of treatment may be considered after a remission of 18 to 24 months.

SUMMARY

Typical absence attacks are characterized by the brief and sudden abolition or marked depression of awareness, responsiveness, and amnesic registration that lasts from 5 to 30 seconds. The disturbance of consciousness may be isolated (simple typical absences), or it may be associated with clonic, tonic, or automatic motor components (complex typical absences). Whether the absence is simple or complex, it is accompanied by a remarkable EEG discharge of spike-wave complexes at a regular rhythm of 3 Hz. The complexes are generalized and symmetric, and they start and stop suddenly, as do the clinical attacks.

Atypical absences have a different ictal EEG pattern, and they belong to other syndromes, especially LGS. Typical absence attacks should be differentiated not only from atypical absences but also from nonepileptic phenomena such as daydreaming or tics and from brief complex partial seizures. Typical absences are briefer, they are not preceded by an "aura," and they are not followed by postictal fatigue, confusion, or sleepiness. Complex partial seizures are not associated with the characteristic EEG discharge of typical absence. The course of typical absence epilepsy differs with the various absence syndromes. The most frequent absence syndromes include CAE, whose prognosis is most favorable; JAE; and JME with absences; in the last two, the development of generalized convulsive seizures is the rule. Rarer syndromes include myoclonic absences and some miscellaneous types with a variable, though more serious, prognosis.

Control of the typical absence attacks themselves is eventually attained in 80% to 90% of patients. However, other seizure types, especially GTCSs, appear in a variable proportion of patients. In general, onset during early childhood, the absence of any other seizure antedating the typical absences, and a normal intellectual and neurologic development are indicators of a favorable prognosis. Onset after 8 years of age, the occurrence of grand mal seizures before the onset of absences or while on therapy, and prominent myoclonic phenomena are predictors of a less favorable outcome.

Therapy for typical absences differs from that for other forms of seizures, a point of great interest that suggests the presence of different mechanisms. However, genetic relationships with other forms of generalized epilepsy and possibly with some partial nonlesional epilepsies have been found. Valproate and/or ethosuximide are the drugs of choice, and, whenever possible, they should be used as monotherapy. Lamotrigine is also an effective agent.

9

Epilepsies with Tonic-Clonic Seizures

Generalized tonic-clonic seizures (GTCSs), also known as *grand mal seizures*, represent the prototypical epileptic seizures. However, GTCSs do not constitute a homogeneous group, and they occur in a variety of clinical circumstances. Occasional seizures, especially febrile convulsions, are usually GTCSs (see Chapter 14). When GTCSs are a manifestation of a chronic seizure disorder, they are often associated with other forms of attacks of either a generalized or a focal nature. For example, GTCSs may precede, accompany, or follow typical absences in early childhood or adolescence, and they are often associated with myoclonias. In other patients, they alternate with partial seizures. In many patients, however, GTCSs are the only type of seizure, although the exact frequency of such an occurrence is poorly known; it probably varies with the origin of the patients and the investigations performed.

Large epidemiologic studies (Ross and Peckham, 1983; Ross et al., 1980) have indicated a high frequency of grand mal epilepsy. However, the classification of seizures in such studies is often debatable because of the manner in which data are collected. O'Donohoe (1985) states that 70% of all seizures in childhood are GTCSs that occur either as the sole type of attack or in association with partial seizures or other fits. On the other hand, the incidence of GTCSs that occurs in isolation and has no association with clinical and/or electroencephalographic (EEG) evidence of a local lesion seems much lower. Gastaut et al. (1973b) reported that GTCSs comprise 9.5% of the classifiable epilepsies of childhood. Oller-Daurella and Oller (1992) found only 80 cases that were characterized solely by GTCSs among the 392 children with generalized seizures in the 1,847 cases of childhood epilepsy that they studied, for an incidence of 5.4%. These figures may, however, be too low as they emanate from specialized centers to which patients with "ordinary" seizures often are not referred. The incidence also depends on age; GTCSs are uncommon before 3 years of age, although they do occur (Aicardi and Chevrie, 1982b). In this age-group, atypical seizures that are often difficult to classify are much more common than grand mal attacks (Chevrie and Aicardi, 1977).

From a pathophysiologic viewpoint, GTCSs can be divided into the following three subgroups:

1. GTCSs may be apparently generalized from the start. Such primarily GTCSs are often a manifestation of idiopathic epilepsy. Myoclonic jerks that immediately precede the seizure are common in this form.

2. GTCSs may represent the secondary generalization of a partial seizure; this is more common with a simple partial seizure than with a complex partial one. Such secondarily generalized seizures can be of two varieties. In some cases, the initial partial seizure is manifested clinically by localized motor, sensory, or other phenomena. This initial partial seizure traditionally was referred to as the "aura" of the GTCSs. In other cases, the seizure appears generalized from the outset, but EEG recordings demonstrate that an initial focal discharge occurs that remains clinically inapparent either because it involves a "silent" area of the brain or because the memory of any subjective manifestation experienced by the patient is erased by retrograde ictal amnesia. When no ictal records are available, those seizures that occur in patients who have a stable interictal EEG focus are commonly considered to be secondarily generalized. Such focal paroxysmal activity is found in the EEG recordings of 20% to 40% of patients with tonic-clonic seizures (Kreindler et al., 1969). Secondarily generalized attacks may alternate with partial attacks, or they may represent the only ictal manifestation. Only seizures that are not associated with clinical partial seizures are discussed in this chapter. Patients in whom both partial and generalized seizures occur are discussed in Chapter 10.

3. Finally, GTCSs may be the expression of an epilepsy with multiple independent foci. In this case, they are almost always associated with other seizure types such as absences, tonic seizures, or partial seizures; they also are often atypical with a less regular course and less regular EEG recordings (Chapter 10).

The epilepsies characterized by GTCSs have different etiologies, courses, and prognoses. They have only one type of seizure in common; this type is described before the various syndromes featuring GTCSs are considered.

SEIZURE PHENOMENA

Clinical Manifestations

The core of the attack consists of a stereotyped series of motor and autonomic manifestations that are associated with an immediate loss of consciousness (Gastaut and Broughton, 1972). The tonic phase comprises a sharp, sustained contraction of muscles that produces a fall to the ground that is often injurious when the patient is standing or sitting. The patient lies rigidly in an extensor posture that is often preceded by a transient stage of flexion. Opisthotonus is unusual. The tonic contractions of the diaphragm and intercostal muscles inhibit respiration, and cyanosis occurs. After 10 to 30 seconds, the tonic phase gives way to clonic jerks, which often follow a brief intermediate period of vibratory tremor (Gastaut et al., 1974a). The jerks are bilateral and symmetric. The jerks progressively slow as the seizure proceeds, while, at the same time, becoming increasingly violent. The jerks may be accompanied by brief expiratory grunts, as diaphragmatic contractions force air against the closed glottis. Froth appears at the mouth, and the tongue may be bitten during this stage. After 30 to 60 seconds, muscular relaxation occurs. Careful observation, however, reveals that a second tonic contraction, lasting only a few seconds in most cases, usually takes place before relaxation. During this second tonic phase, the muscle tone is preferentially increased in the cephalic muscles, and tongue biting is common (Gastaut and Broughton, 1972). The patient remains unconscious for variable durations. Respiration is stertorous, and pallor replaces cyanosis. Urinary incontinence occurs in one-third of these patients, but fecal incontinence is uncommon (Browne, 1983b; Gastaut et al., 1974a). The autonomic phenomena may include tachycardia, increased blood pressure, flushing, salivation, miosis, and increased bronchial secretions (Gastaut and Broughton, 1972). Some GTCSs are immediately preceded by a series of myoclonic jerks that, at times, are so prominent that the term *clonic-tonic-clonic seizure* has been proposed for such cases (Delgado-Escueta et al., 1983a), and an initial cry is common.

Atypical GTCSs are extremely common in children. The tonic phase may be much longer than the clonic stage, which may be limited to a few jerks. Both the tonic contraction and the clonic stage may

be asymmetric. In addition, asynchrony of up to several seconds between the two sides of the body is not unusual (Gastaut et al., 1974a), but clinical detection may be difficult. These seizures are usually much less violent in young children than they are in adults, and those injuries that are caused by muscular contractions during an attack, such as compression fractures of vertebrae, are generally not observed before late adolescence.

Electroencephalographic Manifestations

The tonic phase of a GTCS is characterized by a rhythm of 10 Hz that increases rapidly in amplitude; it has also been called the *epileptic recruiting rhythm* (Gastaut and Tassinari, 1975a; Gastaut and Broughton, 1972). Toward the end of the tonic phase, this rhythm tends to become discontinuous. During the clonic phase, bursts of 10-Hz rhythms become separated by intervals of inactive tracing or by slow waves. The bursts are synchronous with the jerks, which may be regarded as an interrupted tonus (Gastaut and Broughton, 1972). The bursts of fast rhythm become further apart and more brief. At the end of a seizure, single spikes are common, and they may be followed by a slow wave, forming atypical spike-wave formations. A phase of inactive flat tracing, the phase of cortical exhaustion, follows the clonic stage. Although the ictal phenomena are generally bilateral and synchronous, a significant degree of asymmetry is not uncommon in GTCSs in children.

The physiologic basis of GTCSs has been studied in animal models. Only pentylenetetrazol (Metrazol) and megimide (Browne, 1983b; Gastaut and Broughton, 1972) produce a sequence of events comparable to that observed in human primary tonic-clonic seizures. Studies in animals have demonstrated that subcortical structures, especially the midbrain reticular formation, play a key role in the initiation of megimide-induced seizures. High-voltage fast activity that is recorded in the midbrain reticular formation is synchronous with the myoclonic jerks, and it is continuous throughout the tonic phase. The origin of GTCSs in humans, however, remains controversial. Most investigators postulate a diffuse thalamocortical hyperirritability (Gloor et al., 1990; Gloor, 1983). Bancaud et al. (1974) showed that the stimulation of the mesial orbitofrontal cortex in epileptic persons could induce either GTCSs or generalized spike-wave activity similar to that recorded in typical absences, depending on the frequency of stimulation. A cortical origin of GTCSs is therefore possible, even though the subcortical structures undoubtedly play an important role in the elaboration of the discharge (Gloor, 1979).

DIFFERENTIAL DIAGNOSIS

The differential diagnosis of GTCSs is discussed in Chapter 21. The most common diagnostic problem is that of *syncopal attacks.* This is especially true for children in whom the tonic phase of GTCSs often predominates over the clonic phase. Seizures in syncope are mainly tonic fits, although, not uncommonly, a few jerks may follow the tonic phase. Opisthotonus is much more common in syncopal attacks than in grand mal seizures. Downward deviation of gaze is another important feature (Stephenson, 1990). Provocation of the fits by emotional stimuli (e.g., pain, anger), no matter how the fits are described, is a strong argument for syncope. Urination can occur during syncopes, and the tip of the tongue may be bitten as a result of the patient's fall. Lateral tongue biting or biting of the inner cheek, however, is also characteristic of GTCSs.

Hysterical attacks or pseudoseizures are uncommon in young children, but they do occur relatively frequently in adolescents (Chapter 21). Distinguishing other varieties of epileptic seizures from GTCSs may be difficult. In general, the label "GTCSs" tends to be applied loosely to a wide variety of epileptic seizures of different significance. For example, a number of partial seizures have generalized autonomic and some bilateral motor manifestations that are all too often regarded as sufficient evidence for GTCSs, resulting in misdiagnoses. Distinguishing tonic seizures (see Chapter 4) from grand mal attacks may also be difficult. However, the overall clinical picture and the association with other types of fits should permit diagnosis. Clearly, the management and prognosis of such cases differ from those in GTCSs.

SYNDROMES FEATURING GENERALIZED TONIC-CLONIC SEIZURES AS THE PREDOMINANT TYPE OF ATTACK

GTCSs are a common manifestation of epilepsy in children older than 2 to 4 years and in adolescents. They may be the only or the predominant type of seizures in some epilepsy syndromes in this age-group, although, in many patients, they are not the most characteristic type; they are, however, of relatively little value in the diagnosis of an epilepsy syndrome, which depends more on the characterization of the associated seizures. This section successively

considers the syndrome of idiopathic generalized epilepsy (IGE) with GTCSs in adolescents, the less well-defined spectrum of generalized convulsive epilepsy in childhood, and the syndrome of generalized epilepsy with febrile seizures plus (GEFS+) and then briefly reviews the significance of secondarily generalized seizures.

Idiopathic, or Primary, Generalized Epilepsy of Adolescents with Generalized Tonic-Clonic Seizures

Epilepsy syndromes that feature prominent GTCSs are also expressed with additional seizures in many patients (Fig. 9.1). The most common are those with myoclonic attacks and typical absences. The syndromes that include these types of attacks are studied in Chapters 6 (juvenile myoclonic epilepsy [JME]) and 8 (juvenile absences).

Epilepsies with exclusive or predominant GTCSs have also been classified into the following three categories according to their relationship to the sleep-waking cycle (Wolf, 1992a; Janz, 1974): awakening grand mal; grand mal of sleep; and diffuse grand mal,

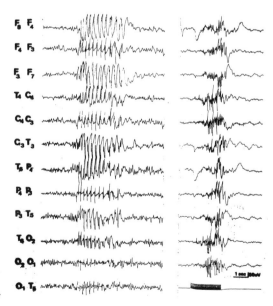

FIG. 9.1. An electroencephalographic recording of a 14-year-old girl with primary generalized epilepsy, showing 3-Hz spike-wave complexes preceded by several spikes (**left**), as well as a burst of polyspike-waves induced by photic stimulation (**right**). The patient had infrequent nocturnal seizures, jerks of the upper limbs on awakening, and brief absences.

which occurs in both sleep and wakefulness. In this type of classification, the only relatively well-defined syndrome (see discussion below) is that of awakening grand mal (Wolf, 1992a).

The syndrome may have its onset as early as 8 or 9 years of age, but, most commonly, it appears during the teens. More than two-thirds of patients have their first attack before 19 years of age, and the peak frequency of onset is between 14 and 16 years. Gastaut et al. (1973b) found that the affected females outnumbered affected males (54% vs. 46%) and that, in one-third of the female patients, the onset of seizures coincided temporally with the first menstruation.

The seizures typically are of the primary generalized type, and they occur most often in the half hour following awakening. The term *awakening grand mal stricto sensu* applies only to cases in which all of the seizures occur with this schedule. According to Janz (1969), the diagnosis depends on the occurrence of five GTCSs on awakening without other types or schedules of attacks. However, the occurrence of some seizures during sleep (Wolf, 1992a; Janz, 1991; Tsuboi, 1977b) or in the evening when the patient is relaxing (Janz, 1991; Touchon, 1982) is possible. The provocation of the seizures by sleep deprivation is common (Touchon, 1982; Gastaut et al., 1973b). The precipitating role of alcohol ingestion has also been stressed, but separating its role from that of sleep deprivation is difficult because both are strongly interrelated. The latter factor is, however, considered more important. Another precipitating factor is "naturally" occurring intermittent photic stimulation, which, in Gastaut's experience, induced seizures in 13% of patients, which is much lower than the EEG paroxysms induced by flickering light in 29% of the patients in the EEG laboratory. Natural photic stimulation may include such stimuli as riding a car along a road lined with trees or the reflection of the sun on water. Television watching, electronic games, and the flashing lights of dance clubs are much more common precipitants (see Chapter 17). The interictal EEG recording is normal in most patients (Wolf, 1992a). GTCSs are generally infrequent in primary generalized epilepsy, with 37% to 70% of patients having less than one seizure a year. Seizures that occur more often than once a week are unusual (12% of Gastaut's patients).

In many patients, the seizures of IGE include, in addition to GTCSs, typical absences, massive myoclonic jerks, or both (see Chapters 6 and 8). Completely separating the different syndromes is often difficult and perhaps artificial. The syndromes share, in addition to the seizures, a number of EEG features; similar triggering factors, especially sleep deprivation

and awakening; and the same drug sensitivity. In some adolescent girls, the seizures have a definite relationship to the menstrual cycle, generally occurring during the 3 to 4 days preceding menstruation. In some patients (catamenial epilepsy), the effect of the menstrual cycle is so marked that a trial of hormonal therapy is justified (Mattson et al., 1981; Newmark and Penry, 1980).

The three syndromes of awakening grand mal, JME, and juvenile absences with associated grand mal are now regarded as variants of a broader epilepsy syndrome termed *primary generalized epilepsy* (Andermann and Berkovic, 2001). This syndrome seems to be due mostly or exclusively to genetic causes. However, Meencke and Janz (1984, 1985) found cortical microdysgenesis in the brains of eight patients who died after a long history of primary generalized epilepsy, and they suggested that these abnormalities might play a role in the enhanced excitability of the cortex. The significance of this finding, however, remains disputed (Lyon and Gastaut, 1985). Recent magnetic resonance studies have suggested that the cortex of patients with IGE may be abnormal (Sisodiya et al., 1995), but no pathologic confirmation of this is available.

Several loci have been suggested as causative. These include a locus in the human leukocyte antigen (HLA) region on chromosome 6 (Durner et al., 1991; Greenberg et al., 1988a, 1990), another locus on chromosome 6 that is outside the HLA region, a locus on chromosome 15 (Sander et al., 1999; Elmslie et al., 1997), and one on chromosome 8 (Durner et al., 2001). The origin is likely multifactorial, and the variable expression could result from the varying combinations of known, and perhaps unknown, genes (Durner et al., 2001; Greenberg et al., 1995).

The seizures of primary generalized epilepsy supervene in persons without neurologic or mental disturbances. Janz (1974) suggested that patients with impulsive petit mal or awakening grand mal had certain psychologic characteristics, such as hedonism or passivity and a tendency to a less than orderly style of life. They are often inclined to go to bed late and to rise late, and they may thus be especially sensitive to precipitation of seizures by premature awakening. However, this finding remains an item of dispute.

Minor EEG differences can be found among the three types of primary generalized epilepsy. Patients with absences are often responsive to hyperventilation, whereas photosensitivity is present in 31% of cases of JME, in 18% of cases of juvenile absences, and in only 13% of those with awakening grand mal. Rapid spike-wave bursts at a rhythm of 4 to 6 Hz

(Janz, 1991) are present in 25% to 50% of patients. This type of fast discharge is almost pathognomic of the primary generalized epilepsy syndromes (Wolf, 1992a; Gastaut et al., 1973b). According to Tsuboi (1977b), the 3.5-Hz to 6.0-Hz pattern is present in 9.5% of patients with "awakening grand mal," and polyspike-waves are observed in 16%, a proportion that is lower than that observed in cases of JME, in which the corresponding figures are 22% and 26%.

The course of primary generalized epilepsy of adolescents is relatively favorable (Wolf, 1992a; Janz, 1991). Generalized tonic-clonic status is exceptional, although rare cases of myoclonic status have been recorded (Asconapé and Penry, 1984). Mental or neurologic deterioration never occurs. Anticonvulsant drugs given in moderate dosages control the seizures in 50% to 70% of patients (Gastaut et al., 1973b) and significantly reduce their frequency in an additional 10%. Patients who are followed for more than 10 years tend to have fewer seizures or to go into complete remission. The treatment should be maintained for at least 10 to 15 years and perhaps indefinitely because recurrences after 5 to 10 years of stabilization are common (Janz, 1991). The best results are obtained with valproate, especially when associated myoclonic jerks are present. Primidone, carbamazepine, and phenobarbital are also effective against the GTCSs (Browne, 1983b; Gastaut et al., 1973b), even though they are less effective for the control of myoclonic jerks. Lamotrigine, topiramate, and probably levetiracetam are also indicated (Arzimanoglou, 2002b).

Epilepsies with Generalized Tonic-Clonic Seizures in Childhood

Although most workers consider grand mal epilepsies the most common type of chronic seizure disorder in childhood (O'Donohoe, 1985), a paucity of reports on this topic exists in the literature (Gastaut et al., 1973b). The epilepsies of childhood that are characterized exclusively or predominantly by GTCSs are much more heterogeneous than the corresponding epilepsies of adolescence, and they do not represent a single syndrome but rather a collection of various seizure disorders with different causes and courses.

Gastaut et al. (1973b) published a report on a group of 295 patients with what they termed *primary generalized epilepsy of childhood*. These 295 patients represented 9.5% of 3,000 unselected epileptic patients younger than 15 years who had been referred to a specialized center. Criteria for inclusion in the group were (a) the exclusive occurrence of GTCSs

that were, at times, associated with bilateral myoclonus and (b) the presence of bilateral paroxysmal EEG abnormalities that excluded any focal paroxysm. This group had a definite male preponderance, as only 36% of the patients were girls. The age at onset of the seizures was between 2 and 14 years of age. All patients had GTCSs that were usually rather uncommon, and 36% also had bilateral massive myoclonic jerks. The interictal clinical examination was normal. In all patients, the interictal EEG tracings displayed irregular spike-wave or polyspike-wave complexes at a rhythm of 2.5 to 3.5 Hz. Faster complexes of 4 to 6 Hz, similar to those occurring in primary generalized epilepsy of adolescents, were never found. The precipitating factors of the seizures included natural intermittent photic stimulation in 17% of patients. Sleep favored the emergence of seizures in 44% of children. Gastaut et al. (1973b) found that the course was mostly favorable. Treatment was able to stop the attacks in 61% of patients, and it produced marked improvement in an additional 27%. No brain lesions were found. Antecedents in the form of febrile convulsions were present in relatives of 21% of the patients and of "true" epilepsy, in the relatives of 12%. However, a prediction of the outcome for such children is difficult. Ehrhardt and Forsythe (1989) found that 22 of 187 seizure-free patients had relapsed even on continuing treatment for some.

The isolation of such a distinct syndrome of primary generalized epilepsy in childhood is debatable. In the series of Gastaut et al. (1973b), 51% of the patients were between 9 and 14 years of age at the onset of seizures, and justifying their separation from those with primary generalized epilepsy of adolescence is difficult. The high proportion of massive myoclonic jerks in this series is in contradistinction to the experience of other authors, including those of this text, who do not mention myoclonic jerks as a common accompaniment of GTCSs in children (O'Donohoe, 1985). Some of the cases reported by Gastaut et al. (1973b) perhaps fit better into the various groups of myoclonic epilepsies (see Chapter 6) in which GTCSs frequently occur. Cases of JME with an abnormally early onset of 3 years of age have been reported (Gram et al., 1988).

The Syndrome of Generalized Epilepsy with Febrile Seizures Plus

Although GEFS+ is named after the occurrence of febrile seizures and GTCSs, these are not the only type of attack observed in the syndrome. Indeed, in some individual cases, GTCSs may be absent altogether. More often, they are associated with other seizure types (Sugawara et al., 2001; Scheffer and Berkovic, 1997). The very term *syndrome* may not be an appropriate designation for the condition because it is *not* characterized by the nonfortuitous association of signs and symptoms but rather by its genetic nature, which is indicated by the familial occurrence, and, in some cases, by the demonstration of the same genes in affected persons of GEFS+ families. The concept of a genetic syndrome has been introduced as a result of the description of GEFS+, but the meaning differs from that of the International League Against Epilepsy classification because the phenotypic manifestations often are quite variable and they do not occur together nonfortuitously. Instead of representing a syndrome, GEFS+, in fact, introduces a new concept.

The delineation of the "syndrome" of GEFS+ was based on the recognition that, in one large Anglo-Australian extended family, febrile seizures that were often of unusual duration or severity and afebrile generalized seizures of various types appeared to be transmitted as a dominant trait (Scheffer and Berkovic, 1997). In this family, the linkage of the condition to chromosome 19q was demonstrated (Wallace et al., 1998). Other similar pedigrees were later reported (Moulard et al., 1999; Singh et al., 1992a), and linkage to chromosome 2q could be demonstrated in some (Baulac et al., 1999). Eventually, mutations in the α subunit of the sodium channel SCN1A gene were evidenced in some families (Escayg et al., 2001; Wallace et al., 2001). The latter cases were termed GEFS+2, while those linked to chromosome 19 were termed GEFS+1.

The phenotype of this familial syndrome is variable. Simple febrile seizures constitute the most common manifestation (Scheffer and Berkovic, 1997). However, these often tend to occur beyond the usual upper limit of 4 to 5 years of age, and they may be unusually severe. Afebrile seizures, which mainly include generalized tonic-clonic ones but which, in some cases, can include myoclonic attacks, myoclonic astatic epilepsy, or even episodes of status epilepticus, occur in some pedigree members. The first family described by Scheffer and Berkovic (1997) included 25 affected persons over four generations, 23 of whom a history of often prolonged febrile convulsions. Nine later had afebrile seizures of variable severity, repetition rate, and duration that started at a median age of 2.2 years and remitted by 11.7 years of age (range of 6 to 25 years). All had normal intellect, and their EEG recordings were normal at last examination. One had myoclonic astatic epilepsy, four had infrequent absence seizures in ad-

dition to febrile seizures plus, and one man had atonic attacks that were mostly in the form of head falls. Overall, the phenotype of GEFS+ tends to be mild. The most common presentation is that of febrile convulsions, followed by infrequent generalized tonic seizures that often experience definitive remission by 9 to 12 years of age.

The latter subgroup of patients had previously been recognized on the basis of their clinical symptoms and course, and they were considered to belong to a possible syndrome of childhood epilepsy with GTCSs (Aicardi, 1994). Studies of febrile seizures had indicated that roughly 40% of children who developed afebrile attacks following febrile convulsions (2% to 6% of patients) had only a few GTCSs (Nelson and Ellenberg, 1976). Oller-Daurella and Oller (1992) had also noted that isolated grand mal in childhood often started with febrile convulsions and then was usually limited to a few seizures. Lennox-Buchtal (1971) reported that GTCSs following febrile convulsions were often nocturnal and that they were uncommon. The relative benignity and the spontaneous remission of grand mal following febrile seizures had also been noted. Nelson and Ellenberg (1978) found that 18 (1%) of their patients with afebrile seizures after febrile convulsions had only one or a few seizures, with remission occurring before 48 months of age. This incidence was one-third that of chronic epilepsy in the same study. This *clinical* syndrome of rare and benign GTCSs following febrile convulsions can perhaps now be included within the *concept* of GEFS+, of which it may represent a common, mild form. However, much more work is required to determine the actual frequency with which GEFS+ may be responsible for such a clinical presentation, as well as how often it is due to other genetic or nongenetic factors. That such cases may represent only a part of the spectrum of the GEFS+, which is clearly broader (Singh et al., 2001), is now apparent. In addition to the types of afebrile seizures mentioned, at least some cases of severe myoclonic epilepsy (Dravet syndrome) are likely closely related to GEFS+. Veggiotti et al. (2001) reported the cases of two brothers with severe myoclonic epilepsy who belonged to a family with a history of GEFS+. Singh et al. (2001) found a high incidence of a family history of febrile seizures in the families of 12 patients with Dravet syndrome. Like Veggiotti et al. (2002), they suggested that severe myoclonic epilepsy might be the most severe end of GEFS+ (see Chapter 5).

Several mutations in a gene coding for the α_1 subunit of the SCNA1 canal have been found in cases of GEFS+2 (Escayg et al., 2001; Wallace et al., 2001).

Recently, Claes et al. (2001) found different mutations of this gene in seven children with severe myoclonic epilepsy. These were sporadic cases of *de novo* mutations. Other mutations of the same gene may possibly be transmitted, and they thus may be responsible for cases of GEFS+ with other types of seizures (Singh et al., 2001), in which the variable picture results from the different types of mutations or from the influences of other genes.

GAB RG2 mutations in the gene for the GABA receptor were recently shown to be a possible cause of a variant GEFS+ (GEFS+3) (Baulac et al., 2001; Wallace et al., 2001) (see Chapter 20).

Epilepsies with Secondarily Generalized Seizures

Whether the localized onset is manifest clinically or is expressed only on the EEG recordings (i.e., secondarily generalized seizures), epilepsies characterized by generalized seizures with a partial onset have received little attention, although they are probably quite common. This is understandable because such cases are better defined by their focal features, which are more characteristic and more important from a therapeutic point of view than are the generalized attacks, and because the diagnosis of secondarily generalized seizures may be difficult to make in the absence of ictal EEG recordings. For practical purposes, patients with GTCSs whose interictal EEG recordings contain a fixed focus of abnormality are regarded as having secondarily generalized seizures. Epilepsies related to the presence of a localized brain lesion also are considered in this section. However, a small proportion of the epilepsies related to localized brain damage can manifest themselves exclusively as GTCSs, without an apparently localized onset on ictal EEG recordings (Bancaud et al., 1973). Such cases cannot be considered secondarily generalized seizures, but this rare possibility should be kept in mind. Brain tumors may even be expressed only by apparently primary GTCSs (Spencer et al., 1984a; Bancaud and Talairach, 1975; Aicardi et al., 1970), and this possibility should be considered when epilepsy characterized by these seizures is refractory to treatment (see Chapter 23).

Some studies (Okuma and Kumashiro, 1981; Gastaut et al., 1973b) have shown that secondarily generalized seizures differ in both their outcome and prognosis from epilepsies with partial seizures (or with a mixture of partial and generalized seizures) and primary generalized epilepsies. As a result, the recognition of secondarily generalized seizures may have practical prognostic implications.

Epilepsies with secondarily generalized seizures are slightly more predominant in males than in females (53% versus 47%, respectively). Their incidence is approximately equal to that of primary generalized epilepsy (Gastaut et al., 1973b). The onset occurred before 9 years of age in 20% of the patients in the series by Gastaut et al. (1973b). The etiologic factors do not differ from those associated with partial epilepsy. The seizures are, by definition, typical GTCSs. They are seldom associated with generalized myoclonic jerks, and they never have a clonic-tonic-clonic pattern of attack. The attacks may occur during sleep, but this is less common than in primary generalized cases; the respective proportions for secondarily generalized versus primarily generalized cases in the series by Gastaut et al. (1973b) were 24% and 57.5%. They do not occur on awakening, and they are not induced by photic stimulation. Interictal clinical signs are present in approximately one-fourth to one-third of patients (Pazzaglia et al., 1982). The clinical features may include intellectual deficits and/or focalized neurologic signs. Interictal EEG recordings show focal paroxysmal abnormalities, such as spikes or sharp waves, in 51% to 75% of patients and multifocal or diffuse abnormalities in 6% to 20%. Pazzaglia et al. (1982) found an abnormally slow and/or irregular EEG background rhythm in about 10% of their patients. These EEG paroxysms are located mainly over the frontal and parietal regions. Photic stimulation does not enhance the focal paroxysms, but it may induce bursts of bilateral spike-waves, which may also occur spontaneously. At times, they are asymmetric, and a lower amplitude is occasionally found over the abnormal hemisphere (Gastaut and Tassinari, 1975a).

The course of secondarily generalized seizures is less favorable than that of primary generalized epilepsy; Gastaut et al. (1973b) reported complete control of seizures in 41% of his patients, compared with 68% in primary grand mal, and "satisfactory" control in 32%, versus 22% in grand mal. Pazzaglia et al. (1982) found that secondarily generalized seizures could be controlled in 60% of their patients (both adults and children), whereas control was obtained in only 31.6% of their patients with simple partial seizures and in only 37.5% of those with complex partial attacks, a statistically significant difference between primary and secondary grand mal ($p=0.05$). These authors concluded that secondarily generalized seizures differ from partial seizures by their lesser initial severity and their better response to therapy; in those respects, they are similar to primary grand mal. Other authors (Knudsen and Vestermark, 1978), however, have found the remission rate for secondarily generalized seizures (39%) to be much lower than that for primary generalized epilepsy (69%), and Callaghan et al. (1988) reported that the remission of epilepsies featuring complex or simple partial seizures with generalization was much lower than that in seizures that did not generalize. The experience of Sofijanov (1982), which was also in children, differed—the remission rate achieved in patients with partial attacks was the same as that in those with secondarily generalized seizures. Different criteria for the classification of patients likely are responsible for the discrepancies seen among the various studies. Further studies are necessary before a definitive conclusion can be reached. If secondarily generalized seizures do indeed prove to have an outcome between the favorable one of primary generalized epilepsy and the severe course of the epilepsies characterized by partial seizures, their delineation as a distinct subgroup of GTCSs would be justified.

TREATMENT OF EPILEPSIES FEATURING GENERALIZED TONIC-CLONIC SEIZURES

Phenytoin, phenobarbital, carbamazepine, and primidone are the drugs most commonly employed to treat GTCSs. Most new antiepileptic agents are also effective (see Chapter 24 for detailed results and indications). Phenytoin (Reynolds and Shorvon, 1981; Wilder and Bruni, 1981) and phenobarbital (Strandjord, 1984; Gastaut et al., 1973b) have been considered the standard treatment for GTCSs occurring alone or in association with other seizure types. Carbamazepine, however, is also effective in controlling the GTCSs (Leppik, 1990; Shorvon et al., 1978). However, this drug may aggravate some types of idiopathic epilepsy, whether generalized or partial (Genton et al., 2000b). Valproate is the most effective drug for the treatment of idiopathic epilepsy. It is also effective in many cases of nonidiopathic forms (Tan and Urich, 1984; Wilder et al., 1983). Clonazepam or clobazam may also be effective as second-choice drugs. Most studies have found no evidence indicating that the rate of control differs significantly depending on whether the seizures are generalized or partial (see Chapter 24). Valproate appears to give similar results in the same groups of patients. Wilder et al. (1983) achieved control of seizures in 72 (83%) of their 87 patients. Turnbull et al. (1982) did not find a significant difference between phenytoin and valproate in adults. Comparative studies in children (Hosking, 1989) and adults (Mattson, 1992; Mattson et al., 1985, 1992) also show no major difference in the efficacy of four major antiepileptic agents—carbamazepine, phenytoin, phenobarbital, and valproate—but they do indicate that carbamazepine and valproate tend to be better tolerated.

Ernst et al. (1988) has proposed that bromides might be effective in the treatment of early onset intractable epilepsy with unilateral and tonic-clonic seizures.

In general, the authors of this text tend to use valproate as the first-choice treatment for GTCSs that belong to the primary generalized epilepsies of childhood or adolescence. This applies particularly to GTCSs associated with myoclonic phenomena, for which valproate is more effective than the other drugs. The new antiepileptic agents can be useful when conventional drugs have failed. Unfortunately, controlled trials in young children are lacking, and any comparison would be arbitrary. The prevention of known or potential precipitating factors, especially disciplined sleep habits and the avoidance of alcohol, is an essential part of treatment.

Surgical treatment (see Chapter 25) can be extremely effective when a focal lesion or a well-defined epileptogenic area can be identified in cases of secondarily generalized seizures.

SUMMARY

GTCSs (grand mal seizures) occur in a variety of circumstances. They are the usual type of attack in patients with occasional seizures. They often occur in association with other seizure types in chronic seizure disorders. Because seizures other than GTCSs have more specificity than grand mal attacks, the epilepsies featuring both GTCSs *and* other types of seizures are considered in the chapters corresponding to the most specific seizure types. The epilepsies that feature GTCSs exclusively (at times in association with myoclonic jerks) form a heterogeneous group. In adolescent patients, GTCSs that frequently occur on awakening or in sleep; that are unassociated with any neurologic or mental abnormality; and that feature generalized spike-wave paroxysms, especially those with a frequency of 4 Hz to 6 Hz, on the EEG, with a normal background tracing, constitute a well-defined syndrome. This syndrome is often associated with myoclonic jerks (benign JME) and less commonly with typical absences, thus constituting the common generalized epilepsy of adolescence. In most cases of young children, GTCSs are less stereotyped in their clinical presentation and association with other seizure types.

GTCSs are the most common type of seizure following febrile convulsions. The occurrence of a few grand mal attacks in children with previous febrile seizures may represent a benign, self-limited form of generalized epilepsy in this age-group. They may belong to the spectrum of GEFS+, but this remains to be proven.

GTCSs are often of the secondarily generalized type. In such cases, the seizures may constitute a manifestation of a local brain lesion, and their prognosis is less favorable than that fo the primary generalized types. Some inconclusive evidence indicates, however, that the epilepsies characterized exclusively by secondary generalized seizures may be of an intermediate severity between the primary generalized epilepsies and the epilepsies with partial seizures.

Epilepsies Characterized by Partial Seizures

Focal seizure is the term proposed by the Task Force of the International League Against Epilepsy (ILAE) to designate seizures in which the first clinical symptoms indicate the paroxysmal activation of an anatomofunctional system of neurons limited to part of a single hemisphere, with a correspondingly localized electroencephalographic (EEG) discharge (Engel, 2001). The terms *localization-related epileptic seizures* or *focal seizures* designate the same type of seizures. Focal seizures are often associated with generalized seizures in the same patient. In such patients, the epilepsy is usually considered to be focal because, in these patients, generalization is considered to be secondary to an initial focal seizure of partial seizures. Epilepsies with partial seizures are the most common form of epilepsy (Zarrelli et al., 1999).

Epilepsies with focal seizures were divided into the following two groups by the ILAE seizure classification of 1989: those with elementary (simple partial seizures) and those with complex (complex partial seizures) symptomatology (Commission on Classification and Terminology of the International League Against Epilepsy, 1981). Impairment of consciousness is defined operationally by the responsiveness and awareness of the patient during the seizure. It is preserved in simple partial seizures and is decreased or abolished in complex focal seizures, and it was the criterion for separating the two types. This criterion has been disputed, and the proposal for a new classification (Engel, 2001) does not include these terms.

This chapter describes the symptomatology of focal seizures without specific referencing to the dichotomy previously used. It is divided into three parts. The *first part* gives a description of the multiple types of focal *seizures* according to the nature of their clinical ictal manifestations; it successively considers motor, sensory, autonomic, and cognitive symptoms and impairment of consciousness, with or without associated cognitive or affective features. This section describes the topographic grouping of seizure symptoms according to the cortical areas involved in the discharges. The reader should keep in mind that the *areas involved by the first clinical and/or EEG manifestations are not necessarily those in which the discharge actually originates*; they can

be secondarily involved by its propagation. The *second part* is concerned with the description of the various recognizable topographic *epilepsy syndromes* that feature focal seizures with or without impairment of consciousness. The *third part* is concerned with the syndromes that are predominantly manifested by focal seizures.

SEIZURE SYMPTOMATOLOGY

FOCAL MOTOR SEIZURES

Motor seizures are characterized by motor symptoms as their main clinical manifestation. The ictal symptomatology may be either simple (a jerk) or complex (complex organized movements). Focal clonic and myoclonic muscle activity typically arises from seizure discharges in the primary motor cortex. Tonic muscular activity is typically produced by the activation of the premotor areas (Rasmussen, 1974) or the supplementary sensorimotor cortex (Penfield and Jasper, 1954). The epileptic discharges responsible for partial motor seizures may remain localized to a relatively small cortical area, which, in childhood, is often the lowermost part of the motor strip, but they may also spread slowly from their area of origin to involve the neighboring areas. When spread occurs within the motor or sensory strips, a progressive and regular extension of the territory involved in the convulsive activity or the paresthesias results. This *jacksonian march* often stops before affecting the whole motor or sensory area. A typical jacksonian march is uncommon. More commonly, the extension of a localized discharge is irregular. For example, a discharge that starts in the primary motor cortex may involve subcortical structures that, in turn, activate other cortical areas that may be relatively distant from the site of origin (Fig. 10.1). This type of propagation explains the common saltatory expression of many simple partial seizures, with their sequences of jacksonian march alternating with "jumps" of the paroxysmal activity to other parts of the body. Although distinctive patterns of motor activation of the primary motor cortex, premotor areas, and supplementary

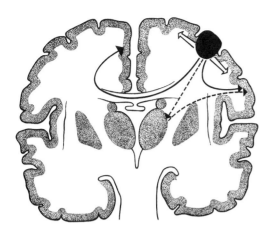

FIG. 10.1. Schematic concept of the various types of propagation of partial motor seizures. From its area of origin (epileptogenic zone) in the motor strip, the discharge may spread slowly along the motor strip (*open arrows*), but it may also move rapidly through normal anatomic pathways or through abnormally facilitated pathways to distant areas on the same or opposite side (*solid arrows*). This long-distance propagation explains the frequently irregular "saltatory" course of partial motor seizures and the occurrence of contralateral symptoms, particularly, ipsiversion of the head and eyes. A third unproved pathway (*dotted arrows*) may exist with activation of the corresponding area in the thalamus, which, in turn, would activate other cortical areas. (Adapted from Bancaud and Talairach, 1975.)

sensorimotor cortex may be observed, overlapping clinical manifestations also exist due to highly developed interconnectivity of the different cortical motor areas.

Ictal Manifestations

Somatomotor Seizures with Simple Clonic and Tonic Phenomena

Somatomotor seizures with simple clonic and tonic phenomena are characterized by localized convulsive movements that are often clonic from the start or that become clonic after an initial brief tonic contraction. Clonic seizure activity is characterized by rhythmic jerking or twitching of usually contiguous body segments due to short (50-ms to 200-ms) muscle contractions that alternate with postjerk silent periods.

However, purely tonic focal motor seizures do occur (O'Neil et al., 1991). Any part of one side of the body can be affected. Because of the respective sizes

of the cortical representation of movement, the seizures tend to involve the thumb, fingers, lips, eyelids, and great toe preferentially. In children, the involvement of the muscles of the face, tongue, pharynx, and larynx, with consequent salivation and dysarthria, is especially common. Facial buccolingual tonic-clonic contractures with aphemia point to the involvement of the lowermost part of the motor strip in the upper bank of the sylvian fissure (Loiseau and Beaussart, 1973; Lombroso, 1967). In some seizures, the convulsions remain narrowly localized (e.g., to one segment or limb). In *jacksonian attacks*, the symptoms travel slowly from one territory to another, following the order of their somatotopic representation, usually from the extremity to a proximal part. A *jacksonian* march or very narrowly localized clonic or tonic motor phenomenon is evidence favoring the primary involvement of the rolandic strip. *Jacksonian* seizures represent the only ictal symptom, thus allowing a seizure type to be assigned to a precise cortical area on the strength of clinical observation only (Chauvel et al., 1992b).

Partial motor seizures may vary from a few seconds to several hours in duration. When they are prolonged, they are usually clonic. *Postictal hemiplegia*, or a more restricted motor deficit (*Todd paralysis*), is common following long seizures, and it may last from minutes to several days. It may also be observed after brief seizures or even partial seizures without motor manifestations (Mauguière and Courjon, 1978; Gastaut and Broughton, 1972). The presence of Todd palsy indicates the focal character and location of the causal seizure when a precise history is lacking. When Todd paralysis lasts only minutes, it is probably caused by postictal inhibition. When it is more prolonged, it probably reflects the metabolic exhaustion of the cortical area involved in seizure activity or the existence of transient changes in local blood flow and/or the blood–brain barrier. Localized edema has been demonstrated in such cases (Sammaritano et al., 1985; Dillon et al., 1984).

Clonic seizures are often preceded by somatosensory auras (Mauguière and Courjon, 1978) that, however, are rarely reported in smaller children. Of 14 patients with clonic seizures, 7 were reported to harbor a structural lesion in the primary motor cortex (Geier et al., 1977). A total of 10 of 22 children with frontal lobe epilepsy studied with ictal single photon emission computed tomography (SPECT) by Harvey et al., (1993b) had clonic seizures that had been preceded by other symptoms, including a tonic phase in most. On the whole, clonic seizure onset appears to be more common with dorsolateral seizure onset than with mesial frontal or orbitofrontal origin (Noachtar and Arnold, 2000). Clonic seizures, which were often preceded by a somatosensory aura, were observed in up to 57% of patients with parietal lobe seizure onset that was posterior to the postcentral sulcus (Salanova et al., 1995b). Clonic movements following tonic posturing also occur during seizures originating in the supplementary sensorimotor cortex (Morris et al., 1988). Clonic seizure activity, which is usually preceded by subjective symptoms and automatisms, has also been reported in about one-fourth to one-third of patients with temporal lobe seizure onset (Noachtar and Arnold, 2000).

Unilateral Clonic Seizures

Unilateral clonic seizures (Gastaut et al., 1974c), which are common in childhood, are characterized by synchronous rhythmic jerking of most or all of the muscles of one-half of the body. The distribution of the jerks can be stable or variable, migrating on the affected side (Dravet, 1992a). The jerks may sometimes be very mild, only affecting the eyeballs or the orbicularis oris; they may sometimes cease on one side, subsequently starting contralaterally. Unresponsiveness is common, but this is not always observed; it can be either initial or gradual. Seizure onset is usually represented by lateral clonic turning of the eyes or the head and eyes, often with vomiting. Autonomic phenomena, including pallor, perspiration, or hypersalivation, are common. The child may recover consciousness quickly as seizure activity ceases while postictal hemiparesis is still present (Dravet, 1992a). The severity and duration of postictal hemiparesis are related to the duration of the seizure. Very prolonged unilateral seizures may be followed by permanent hemiparesis (Guerrini and Dravet, 1997; Gastaut et al., 1974b).

Seizures with Asymmetric Tonic Motor Phenomena

Seizures with asymmetric tonic motor phenomena include differing manifestations. The term *versive* seizure was proposed by Gastaut and Broughton (1972) to designate ictal turning of the head and eyes. This is a common type of motor attack involving conjugate, unnatural deviation of the head and eyes to one side (Wyllie et al., 1986a, 1986b), with tonic or clonic components. The ictal version must be differentiated from head and eye turning that occurs in some partial seizures but is not due to direct involvement of the motor system by the discharge but to such factors as external stimuli, or a visual hallucination

moving across his or her visual field, or ictal dysfunction of the attention mechanisms within the ipsilateral hemisphere (Chee, 2000). The deviation is most often away from the discharging hemisphere (contraversive seizures), but it may be toward the side of ictal EEG activity (ipsiversive seizures) (Ochs et al., 1984). Version is subserved by different reciprocally interconnected, discrete anatomic areas, including the frontal eye field, supplementary eye field, parietal eye field, calcarine cortex, and subcortical structures (Chee, 2000) that, when stimulated, produce similar clinical manifestations (Chee 2000; Fish et al., 1993). As a result, the localizing and lateralizing value of head and eye deviation is limited *per se* (Ochs et al., 1984; Robillard et al., 1983). However, a forceful tonic version that usually is accompanied by preservation of awareness seems to be preferentially associated with contralateral frontal origin in the dorsolateral cortex (area 8), and it may even be clonic (Jayakar et al., 1992; Wyllie et al., 1986a, 1986b). Clonic head version immediately preceding secondary generalization lateralizes the ictal onset to the hemisphere contralateral to the side of head turning (Wyllie et al., 1986a).

Conscious slow and saccadic deviation of the head and eyes that is followed by clonic eye movements is seen with purely occipital onset seizures (Williamson et al., 1992b; Bancaud et al., 1965) that can be either contralateral or, more rarely, ipsilateral (Bancaud, 1969). More complex attacks may comprise abrupt asymmetric tonic postural changes. These can be either a tonic flexion of the forearm, with abduction at the shoulder of the arm toward which the face is rotated and the assumption of an attitude reminiscent of the asymmetric tonic neck reflex, or, at times, repetitive vocalization. The lower limbs may also show abnormal posturing, with abduction at the hips and extension or semiflexion of the knees. This seizure pattern, which is also known as the *M2e posture*, has long been related to discharges involving the contralateral supplementary motor area on the internal aspect of the frontal lobe (Quesney et al., 1990; Ojemann and Ward, 1975; Ajmone-Marsan and Abraham, 1960; Ajmone-Marsan and Ralston, 1957), which, more recently, was defined as the supplementary sensorimotor area through electrical stimulation studies (Lim et al., 1994). Bilateral abduction of the upper limbs can also be observed (Morris et al., 1988). In some patients, extension of one upper limb with hyperextension of the arm and contralateral head rotation occur. Gyration of the whole body may be associated with head and eye deviation. Repetitive vocalization or loud moaning may be observed, and some patients may try to speak during the attacks or may be able to respond as soon as the tonic contraction relaxes (Bleasel and Lüders, 2000; Remillard et al., 1974). However, speech arrest is more common. Because of the predominantly axial involvement and the preserved consciousness, the children may still demonstrate spontaneous activity, which, with modifications in the intensity and distribution of muscle contraction, may lead to slow writhing, dystonic movements (Bleasel and Lüders, 2000). Focal clonic activity indicates seizure spread to the primary motor cortex and makes lateralization obvious (Chauvel et al., 1992b). A sensation of tension or heaviness in a limb or a more general body or cephalic sensation is reported by some patients before the tonic contraction becomes apparent (Morris et al., 1988; Penfield and Jasper, 1954). The characteristics of such subjective symptoms are in keeping with the sensory representation of the supplementary sensorimotor area (Lim et al., 1994).

Consciousness is most often preserved during attacks; the patient may, however, become unresponsive or a secondary generalization may follow. Supplementary motor seizures may be accompanied by unilateral tonic activity (Morris et al., 1988). The rapid spread of epileptic activity to the contralateral supplementary sensorimotor area is common (Baumgartner et al., 1996; Chauvel et al., 1992b; Morris et al., 1988), and this may account for some of the bilateral symptoms in some patients.

The seizure duration is brief, usually lasting between 10 and 40 seconds, and postictal confusion is rarely observed (Bleasel and Lüders, 2000). Childhood-onset seizures with bilateral asymmetric tonic activity and posturing are mainly seen in partial epilepsies of frontal lobe origin of either genetic or idiopathic or symptomatic origin (Scheffer et al., 1995a; Bleasel et al., 1993; Vigevano and Fusco, 1993).

Complex Motor Seizures with Hyperkinetic Automatisms: Complex Partial Seizures of Frontal Lobe Origin and Hypermotor Seizures

Some seizures feature prominent bilateral postural movements involving primarily the trunk, pelvis, and proximal extremities; they resemble natural movements and therefore differ from the tonic, clonic, or dystonic movements occurring during bilateral asymmetric motor phenomena. Numerous studies have tried to characterize such hyperkinetic postural phenomena and automatisms and their sequences. Different terms, such as *extreme motor restlessness* (Tharp, 1972), *complex motor automatisms*, *agitation* (Geier

et al., 1977; Williamson et al., 1985; Manford et al., 1996a), or many others (Chauvel et al., 1995; Munari and Bancaud, 1992; Fusco et al., 1990; Delgado-Escueta et al., 1987; Waterman et al., 1987), have been used to define them. The resulting motor sequences may vary from seemingly natural movements with mild postural changes to large-amplitude, explosive movements involving different body segments. Even the more bizarre motor sequences tend to have a stereotypic pattern in the same patient (Lüders et al., 2000; Williamson et al., 1985). The characteristic patterns of repetitive movements and automatic activities include kicking, cycling, thrashing, crossing and uncrossing the legs, rocking, genital manipulations, a peculiar repetitive vocalization, echolalia, screaming, kneading of objects, crumbling, gripping something or somebody, rubbing, and rhythmic fine finger movements. Sometimes, movements suggest defensive or sexual behavior (Tinuper et al., 2001). Asymmetric tonic or dystonic limb posturing is common. Phonatory phenomena in the form of continuous or repetitive vocalization may be present (Bancaud et al., 1973). In children, *aphemia* without a disturbance in the understanding of language is more common than vocalization. Ictal autonomic changes, such as tachycardia or tachypnea, are common (Tinuper et al., 2001). Staring or a facial expression of surprise or fear is often noted. The degree of concomitant consciousness impairment varies greatly, ranging from full awareness to complete unresponsiveness (Holthausen and Hoppe, 2000; Chauvel et al., 1995; Williamson et al., 1985). The individual's postictal recovery is rapid. Most studies have correlated these prominent motor manifestations with frontal lobe seizure activity involving the anterior cingulate and the orbitofrontal and frontopolar cortices (Chauvel et al., 1995; Bancaud and Talairach, 1992; Williamson et al., 1985).

Hypermotor seizures are characterized by "complex, organized movements that affect mainly the proximal portion of the limbs and lead to a marked increase in motor activity" (Lüders et al., 1993a, 1998). The term *hypermotor* is used in antithesis to *hypomotor*, which designates seizures characterized by a significant decrease in motor activity when ascertaining whether a concomitant alteration of consciousness (AC) has occurred is not possible (Lüders et al., 1998).

Purely "hypermotor" seizures occur in a minority of patients. In the great majority, the seizures include tonic phenomena that may be either mild or prominent (Holthausen and Hoppe, 2000). The order of the progression of motor manifestations is variable; the hypermotor behavior may precede or follow the tonic movements (Holthausen and Hoppe, 2000; Chauvel et al., 1995; Geier et al., 1977). Subjective symptoms that precede the hypermotor seizures are reported in 50% to 90% of patients, and they mainly consist of a somatosensory aura in the form of abdominal aura or ictal fear (Biraben et al., 2001b; Tinuper et al., 2001; Holthausen and Hoppe, 2000; Harvey et al., 1993a; Williamson et al., 1985; Geier et al., 1977). "Hypermotor seizures" often have their onset in childhood (Provini et al., 1999; Vigevano and Fusco, 1993), with one series reporting such an onset in up to 90% (Holthausen and Hoppe, 2000). Onset in the first year of life has been reported with seizures characterized by an initial tonic type of posturing that occasionally is followed by hypermotor behavior (Vigevano and Fusco, 1993). When ictal fear is present, such episodes can be mistaken for *pavor nocturnus* (Chapter 21).

The seizures tend to appear much more often during non–rapid eye movement (REM) sleep than during wakefulness (Tinuper et al., 2001; Holthausen and Hoppe, 2000; Fusco et al., 1990; Waterman et al., 1987). An arousal is often the first ictal manifestation during sleep (Fusco et al., 1990).

The motor activity usually lasts less than 1 minute (Provini et al., 1999; Tinuper et al., 2001), and, if no alteration of consciousness has occurred, the individual's recovery is rapid. Secondary generalization is rare.

Paroxysmal Arousals and Epileptic Nocturnal Wandering

Paroxysmal arousals are short-lasting seizures (duration of 2 to 20 seconds) that occur during sleep and are characterized by a sudden brief arousal (Montagna et al., 1990). Opening of the eyes is often followed by sitting up in the bed with a frightened expression, with or without concomitant tonic or dystonic asymmetric posturing of the limbs.

Epileptic nocturnal wanderings (Plazzi et al., 1995; Pedley and Guilleminault, 1977) designate the presence of longer attacks (duration of 2 to 3 minutes) that appear during sleep and are characterized by an initial arousal, followed by semi-purposeful ambulatory behavior during which patients, who usually show a frightened expression and are particularly agitated, scream and may attempt to escape.

Aphemic Seizures

Aphemic seizures feature the incapacity to speak, to produce words, or to vocalize. They are related to speech arrest accompanying supplementary motor seizures, and they must be distinguished from ictal

anarthria due to ictal activity in the *pes* of the third frontal gyrus and from pharyngeal constriction due to opercular involvement.

Focal Myoclonic Seizures

According to its distribution, myoclonus can be classified as focal, multifocal, or generalized (Hallet, 1985) (see also Chapter 6). Focal epileptic myoclonus (FEM) is usually restricted to a distal group of muscles; it is the result of an epileptic discharge involving the motor cortex (Chauvel et al., 1992b; Hallett, 1985). The focal jerks can be either spontaneous, or they may be evoked by sensory stimulation, such as tapping, muscle stretching, or electric shocks. In some patients, the jerks can rhythmically recur, producing a sort of tremor (Guerrini et al., 2001). Spontaneous or reflex intermittent focal myoclonus may be associated with focal motor seizures (Chauvel et al., 1978; Sutton and Mayer, 1974). Each jerk represents the discharge of a small group of cortical motoneurons that is somatotopically connected to a group of contiguous muscles. Frequently, the EEG correlate of FEM can be detected only by using jerk-locked (EEG or magnetoencephalogram [MEG]) averaging. FEM can also be classified as positive or negative (Guerrini et al., 1993b).

Focal Epileptic Negative Myoclonus

Epileptic negative myoclonus (ENM) is defined as a brief, jerky, involuntary movement due to muscular silent periods lasting less than 400 ms that is time-locked to paroxysmal EEG activity (usually a spike-wave [SW] discharge) in the contralateral sensorimotor cortex. The atonic phenomenon may not be preceded by a myoclonic jerk (Tassinari et al., 1998; Guerrini et al., 1993b). Focal ENM is usually manifested as jerky movements of the outstretched arm(s) or leg(s). In small children, the involvement of axial segments may produce an ataxic-like picture. The affected children should be tested during the maintenance of a tonic contraction, because the SW discharges are not associated with clinical manifestations in the relaxed muscle.

In some children, severe negative myoclonus may reduce the motor initiative in the affected body part, resulting in a sort of motor neglect. The ENM can also be multifocal (Guerrini et al., 1993b; Kanazawa and Kawai, 1990) or generalized.

Inhibitory Seizures

Focal inhibitory seizures, or partial atonic seizures (PASs), represent a rare seizure type (Guerrini et al.,

2002d; Hanson and Chodos, 1978; Gastaut and Broughton, 1972) characterized by ictal paresis or paralysis of one body segment that is sometimes preceded or accompanied by numbness. Gastaut and Broughton (1972) identified the following two types of PASs: *unilateral atonic seizures* involving one hemibody and *somatic inhibitory seizures* with focal distribution. The associated manifestations include deviation of the eyes or head toward the side of the paralyzed limb (Thomas et al., 1998; Globus et al., 1982; Waltregny et al., 1969), clonic jerks in a different body part (So, 1995; Penfield and Jasper, 1954), or dysphasia and/or aphasia (Globus et al., 1982; Fisher, 1978). PAS can be difficult to differentiate from ictal or postictal paresis (Hanson and Chodos, 1978). The duration of PAS ranges from a few seconds to hours. Both children and adults have been reported to present with prolonged seizures (i.e., lasting more than 30 minutes) that can be considered "nonconvulsive epileptic status."

Subdural recordings have shown that the seizure activity involves the mesial frontal or the primary sensorimotor cortex (Matsumoto et al., 2000; Noachtar and Lüders, 1999; Hanson and Chodos, 1978). Electrical stimulation studies suggest that "negative motor areas" in the inferior frontal gyrus (primary negative motor area) and anterior to the mesial portion of the superior frontal gyrus (supplementary negative motor area) (Lim et al., 1994) inhibit voluntary movement as long as they are activated (Lüders et al., 1995). Epileptic activity involving these areas can lead to apraxia and motor inhibition that is manifested as PAS (Lüders et al., 1995). However, epileptic discharges in the primary sensorimotor cortex could also produce negative motor phenomena via the direct inhibition of the spinal motoneuron (Matsumoto et al., 2000).

Most paroxysmal attacks of paralysis in childhood are *not* of epileptic origin, and the diagnosis of "inhibitory seizure" can be accepted only when strong EEG evidence is available.

Drop Attack Seizures in Focal Epilepsy

Drop attack seizures may be the sole or main ictal manifestation in some patients. They may apparently be indistinguishable from generalized tonic or atonic seizures (Dravet et al., 1997; Tassinari et al., 1997) or from epileptic spasms. Two main types of drop attacks occur in focal seizures (Rubboli et al., 1997). One type is characterized by an initial stiffening or tonic posturing and is thought to result either from the involvement of the frontal or supplementary motor areas (Broglin et al., 1992; Waterman and Wada, 1990; Del-

gado-Escueta et al., 1987; Geier et al., 1977) or from a pathologic startle response in children with startle-induced epileptic seizures. Versive phenomena and vocalization may also be present. Although ictal involvement of the frontal cortex appears to be essential in producing the changes in muscle tone and posture causing this type of drop attack, posterior seizure onset that often is bilateral, followed by anterior propagation, is not uncommon (Biraben and Chauvel, 1997). A second type of epileptic drop attack is characterized by a sudden, possibly atonic, fall without preceding motor phenomena (Pazzaglia et al., 1985; Gambardella et al., 1994), followed by confusion and reduced responsiveness for about 2 to 3 minutes. Such attacks are often associated with temporal lobe phenomena, and they have also been termed *temporal lobe syncopes*. Depth electrode studies in one patient showed ictal onset in the amygdala and hippocampus, with subsequent rapid spread to the contralateral hippocampus and frontoorbital areas bilaterally (Gambardella et al., 1994). Accurate characterization of the focal origin of the epileptic drop attacks may be important when surgery is contemplated.

SENSORY SEIZURES

Somatosensory Seizures

Somatosensory seizures can originate from any of the following three sensory areas of the parietal lobe: the primary sensory area on the postcentral gyrus (Brodmann areas 1, 2, 3a, and 3b), the second sensory area on the superior border of the sylvian fissure, and the supplementary sensorimotor cortex in the mesial superior frontal cortex (Bleasel and Morris, 1996; Lüders et al., 1985; Martin, 1985). Clinical symptoms resulting from ictal activity in these brain areas are usually referred to the contralateral half of the body, but bilateral involvement is possible. The somatosensory symptoms can spread during the seizure, often in a jacksonian way, starting from the face or an extremity, but they rarely affect the whole half body (Mauguière and Courjon, 1978). Concomitant motor activity occurs in about 50% of sensory seizures with jacksonian march (Sveinbjornsdottir and Duncan, 1993).

Elementary paresthesias (i.e., prickling or tingling sensations, pins and needles, a sensation of something crawling under the skin, or numbness) are the most frequent ictal symptoms (Mauguière and Courjon, 1978; Ajmone Marsan and Goldhammer, 1973). The duration of sensory symptoms is brief, usually lasting less than 1 or 2 minutes (Mauguière and Courjon, 1978). Most somatosensory seizures are related to the involvement of the postrolandic primary sensory area (Mauguière and Courjon, 1978). Paresthesias and numbness originating in this area usually have a somatotopic distribution and spread that is consistent with a somatotopic representation (Critchley, 1966). The sensation is contralateral, usually involving the hands and the face, and it has a good localizing and lateralizing value (Mauguière and Courjon, 1978). Involvement of the supplementary sensorimotor area is usually characterized by imprecise paresthetic, often bilateral, sensations involving large proximal body regions. Patients often report a general body aura or nonspecific sensations of the trunk (Tuxhorn and Kerdar, 2000). The second sensory area can produce bilateral sensory seizures with the involvement of more than one body region (Penfield and Rasmussen, 1951).

The incidence of somatosensory seizures is low in children. In large series, somatosensory symptoms were reported in 8.5% to 25% of patients experiencing auras (Penfield and Kristiansen, 1951). A much lower incidence was reported by Mauguière and Courjon (1978), who diagnosed somatosensory epilepsy in 1,034 (1.4%) of 9,938 patients with epilepsy. Tuxhorn and Kerdar (2000) observed somatosensory auras in 72 (12%) of 600 consecutive patients undergoing presurgical evaluation. The age range in this subgroup varied from 6 to 61 years, and the mean age at epilepsy onset was 8.8 years.

Painful Seizures and Thermal Sensations

Painful seizures and thermal sensations are much rarer than paresthetic attacks. Ictal pain is often described as severe; it is cramplike in the extremities, and throbbing or stabbing in the head and face. The hands, face, and head are most commonly involved. Headache-like symptoms or abdominal pain are also possible (Young and Blume, 1983). Unilateral painful seizures have been linked with parietal epileptic activity (Young and Blume, 1983; Talairach et al., 1960; Whitty, 1953; Penfield and Rasmussen, 1951). Ictal pain is rare in children, and it should not be considered of psychogenic origin (Trevathan and Cascino, 1988). Sensations purely of cold or heat are exceptional. Bilateral sensations and thermal sensations may be related to the involvement of the secondary sensory area in the parietal operculum (Russell and Whitty, 1953; Penfield and Jasper, 1954).

Sexual sensations in the course of seizures are exceptional, and they never occur before puberty. *Body image disturbances* are rare (Mauguière and Courjon,

1978; Arseni et al., 1966); they are demonstrable only in older children and adolescents, who variably describe kinesthetic illusions of movement or displacement of a motionless limb (Penfield and Gage, 1933); a feeling of floating, twisting or torsion of a body limb (Epstein, 1967); and illusions of swelling or shrinking of a body part. Unilateral asomatognosia with a sensation of absence of a body part has also been reported. Their presence points to the involvement of the inferior parietal lobe posterior to the primary sensory area (Mauguière and Courjon, 1978; Penfield and Jasper, 1954), most often on the nondominant hemisphere (Hecaen and de Ajuriaguerra, 1952).

Ictal Vertiginous Sensations

Ictal vertiginous sensations are not uncommon, and they are often related to disturbances in body image (Smith, 1960; Lennox and Cobb, 1933). Ictal epileptic vertigo can be isolated, or it can precede loss of consciousness. It is usually brief, and it is never accompanied by nystagmus (Karbowsky, 1982). Smith (1960) noticed a strong association with visuospatial illusions and somatosensory sensations.

VISUAL SEIZURES

Visual Hallucinations

Visual hallucinations are the most frequent symptoms; these include bright, colorful, multicolored or occasionally dark rings or spots or simple geometric forms that are continuous or flashing. They are usually, but not necessarily, in the periphery of the visual field contralateral to the ictal discharge and rotate or move slowly to the opposite side (Guerrini et al., 1994, 1995; Williamson et al., 1992b; Bancaud, 1969; Penfield and Jasper, 1954; Russell and Whitty, 1953). Ictal amaurosis, blindness, or severe blurring of vision that is limited to one hemifield or quadrant or involves the entire visual field may follow the visual hallucinations; occasionally, however, it may be the first symptom (Salanova et al., 1992; Williamson et al., 1992b; Bauer et al., 1991; Huott et al., 1974). Hemianopia and quadrantanopia have high localizing value. Testing visual avoidance is important when the clinician witnesses a patient experiencing visual symptoms, both ictal and postictal.

More complex visual hallucinations include scenes often related to past experiences. They may be accompanied by macropsia, micropsia, or perception of scenes of people or animals described as static, moving horizontally, approaching, or moving away

(Sveinbjornsdottir and Duncan, 1993; Williamson et al., 1992b; Blume, 1991). Hallucinations may also include letters or numerals (Sowa and Pituck, 1989; Gastaut and Zifkin, 1984). Older children are usually aware of the hallucinatory nature of the perception. Ictal activity producing complex hallucinations involves the occipital association cortex and the posterolateral temporal cortex.

Visual Illusions

Visual illusions involving part or the whole of the visual field may be experienced during occipital lobe seizures (Sveinbjornsdottir and Duncan, 1993). They may consist of alterations in the size, shape, or motion of objects or a change in color quality with monochrome vision or lack of color (achromatopsia). More complex illusions may result in altered perception of objects in space. Ictal palinopsia, or the persistence or recurrence of visual images once the real object of perception is no longer present, has been reported (Critchley, 1951; Lefebre and Koelmel, 1989).

Head and Eye Deviation

Visual phenomena are often accompanied or followed by "conscious" tonic or, in rare instances, clonic eye or eye and head deviation that is usually, but not always, toward the side of the initial visual symptoms (contralateral to the side of seizure origin) (Guerrini et al., 2000d; Williamson et al., 1992b; Furman and Crumrine, 1990; Kanazawa et al., 1989; Munari et al., 1984; Bancaud, 1969). Determining whether eye and head turning is part of the seizure or if it is related to the patient's attempts to follow the images and hallucinatory figures may be impossible. However, ictal eye deviation of occipital origin has an initial tonic phase that is followed by a clonic phase with eye jerks. Oculoclonic movements were defined by Gastaut and Roger (1955) as *epileptic nystagmus*.

Ictal Manifestation Resulting from Extraoccipital Seizure Propagation

The patients' ability to recall the visual symptoms points to the initial localization of the ictal discharge near the calcarine fissure, followed by a slow propagation to adjacent areas. When the discharge is occipitotemporal from the onset, the visual phenomena usually cannot be recalled (Munari et al., 1993).

Infrasylvian propagation to the mesiotemporal limbic structures is common (Olivier et al., 1982; Ajmone-Marsan and Ralston, 1957); it is accompanied by automatisms typical of temporal lobe epilepsy (Salanova et al., 1992; Williamson et al., 1992b; Takeda et al., 1969; Bancaud et al., 1961). Some children experience vomiting in the course of prolonged visual seizures (Guerrini et al., 1994, 1995). Propagation to the lateral occipital cortex and temporal neocortex is responsible for complex visual and auditory hallucinations (Munari et al., 1993; Geier et al., 1973; Penfield and Perot, 1963). Suprasylvian propagation to the primary motor cortex is accompanied by focal motor or hemiclonic activity and propagation to the supplementary sensorimotor cortex, by asymmetric tonic posturing (Williamson and Spencer, 1986; Babb et al., 1981; Takeda et al., 1969). Secondary generalization is common when suprasylvian spread occurs.

Ajmone Marsan and Ralston (1957) observed that infrasylvian spread occurs more often when the seizure origin is below the calcarine fissure, whereas suprasylvian spread is most often related to supracalcarine onset. This pattern was not confirmed in another study (Aykut-Bingol et al. 1998). One-third of all patients have more than one seizure type, which indicates multiple possible spread patterns (Aykut-Bingol et al., 1998; Salanova et al., 1992; Williamson et al., 1992b; Bancaud et al., 1965). The manifestations of seizure spread are often the most prominent clinical feature, and these tend to overshadow the visual symptoms (Williamson et al., 1997).

AUDITORY SEIZURES

Auditory seizures or auras originate from the primary and association auditory cortices. Detailed clinical studies on auditory seizures are rare, and no study has specifically addressed their clinical characteristics in children.

Clinical manifestations include elementary and complex hearing symptoms (Foldvary et al., 2000). The elementary symptoms usually include ringing, buzzing, chirping, or humming noises. Complex auditory symptomatology include illusions, with alterations in perception of distance or loudness or temporal characteristics and hallucinations of voices, music, or meaningful sounds that may be referred to a specific source or that may be more vaguely identified (Gloor, 1990; Hurst and Lee Soo, 1986; Wieser, 1983b). The symptoms are referred to one or both ears. When they are unilateral, they most often are referred to the ear contralateral to the discharging hemisphere (Hurst and Lee Soo, 1986; Penfield and Perot, 1963; Penfield and Jasper, 1954).

The incidence of initial or isolated auditory symptoms in patients with focal epilepsy varies, ranging from 1.7% and 7% (Lennox and Cobb, 1933). More recent series, especially those including patients with temporal lobe epilepsy, have reported auditory auras in 1.7% to 16% of patients (Foldvary et al., 2000).

GUSTATORY AND OLFACTORY SEIZURES

Recent studies indicate that about 7.1% of adult patients with partial epilepsy (Manford et al., 1996a) and about 10% of those having sensory auras (Ebner and Kerdar, 2000) experience gustatory and olfactory sensations. In a large series of 222 adults diagnosed with temporal lobe epilepsy, 6.3% had olfactory and gustatory auras (Ebner and Kerdar, 2000). No studies on their prevalence and ictal characteristics in children are available.

Gustatory Seizures

Gustatory seizures are rarely an isolated symptom. Most patients experience hallucinations of taste that are associated with a sensation of smell. Abnormal taste sensations are bitter, acidic, or sweet and usually are disgusting (Sveinbjornsdottir and Duncan, 1993).

Gustatory hallucinations are considered an expression of either parietal-opercular or anterior temporal seizure activity, without lateralizing value.

Olfactory Auras

Olfactory auras are most often a symptom of a mesial temporal origin (Ebner and Kerdar, 2000). However, posterior orbitofrontal origin has also been demonstrated with depth electrodes (Roper and Gilmore, 1995; Bancaud and Talairach, 1992). The quality of the sensation is generally described as disagreeable (Ebner and Kerdar, 2000).

ICTAL AUTONOMIC PHENOMENA

Autonomic symptoms may be predominant in some children (Afifi et al., 1990; Coulter, 1984; Marshall et al., 1983); they may include respiratory (Southall et al., 1987; Davis et al., 1986), cardiovascular (Davis et al., 1986), pupillary (Wieser, 1987), gastrointestinal (Jacome and Fitzgerald, 1982), sudomotor, pilomotor, and salivatory manifestations. They may occur as isolated symptoms in a fully aware child, or, more often, they may be part of a more complex seizure symptomatology in an unconscious child. They may sometimes be prominent during the motor seizures that are typical of childhood, especially unilateral clonic seizures (Dravet, 1992a). Some autonomic auras represent the subjective awareness of a change in the activity of the autonomic nervous system (So, 1993). Others consist of objective changes in autonomic function (O'Donovan et al., 2000). Often, autonomic manifestations are reported by the parents of children with epilepsy, who describe seizures with alteration of consciousness and "dilated pupils," "pallor, or flushing around the mouth." Some degree of hemispheric lateralization of autonomic functions does exist, with the right hemisphere having a predominant effect (O'Donovan et al., 2000), but the localizing and lateralizing value, if any, is limited. In addition, autonomic changes during a seizure may result from the child's anxiety reaction to experiential symptoms (Ledoux, 1992; Gloor et al., 1982b).

Cardiovascular symptoms include tachycardia and bradycardia, arrhythmias, hypertension, flushing, or pallor. Bradycardia and arrhythmogenic seizures are rare (Zelnik et al., 1990; Davis et al., 1986; Gilchrist, 1985); they may sometimes be of a dramatic character that may be a cause of the sudden infant death syndrome (Smaje et al., 1987; Kiok et al., 1986; Southall et al., 1985). Both limbic and extratemporal areas, including the cingulate, orbitofrontal cortex, and amygdala, may be involved (O'Donovan et al., 2000; Anand and Dua, 1956). According to Stodieck and Wieser (1986), the slowing of the heart rate correlates with discharges from the amygdala.

Respiratory symptoms may present as short respiratory arrest, deep inspiration at seizure onset, or apnea or hyperpnea (Monod et al., 1988; Coulter, 1984) accompanying partial seizures (Wieser et al., 2000). Stimulation studies indicate that the mesiobasal limbic structures are involved in causing ictal apnea (Wieser, 1983b; Nelson and Ray, 1968).

Pupillary manifestations with mydriasis or myosis are a common symptom accompanying the arrest reaction (Wieser et al., 2000). The mydriasis can be asymmetric (Wieser, 1987).

Gastrointestinal symptoms include the classic epigastric aura or *rising epigastric sensation* of mesial temporal lobe epilepsy, eructation, borborygmus, nausea, and vomiting. The so-called *abdominal epilepsy* is one possible manifestation of limbic involvement. It features abdominal discomfort or pain that may be periumbilical, epigastric, or poorly localized, and it is often accompanied by disturbances in gastrointestinal motility and/or vomiting (Mitchell et al., 1983). Abdominal manifestations rarely occur in complete isolation without a subsequent loss of consciousness or automatisms. The authors have seen children suffering from abdominal seizures, with or without loss of awareness, due to temporal ganglioglioma, who were treated for several years in gastroenterology units for gastroesophageal reflux. Isolated vomiting or ictus emetica (Thomas and Zifkin, 1999; Devinsky et al., 1995; Guerrini et al., 1994; Panayiotopoulos, 1988; Fiol et al., 1988; Kramer et al., 1988; Jacome and Fitzgerald, 1982) is rare. The link between abdominal aura and mesial temporal lobe epilepsy represents the most reliable association of an autonomic aura with the area of seizure onset.

Ictal *pilomotor and sudomotor manifestations* are very rare. Sudomotor manifestations, especially if they are accompanied by tachycardia and fear, are a common symptom of panic attacks (Guerrini et al., 1998b).

Genitourinary or sexual sensations are exceptional in children. Feindel and Penfield (1954) noted that 8% of their patients with temporal lobe epilepsy reported a "desire to void" as their initial ictal symptom.

COGNITIVE SEIZURES

Paroxysmal disturbances of cognitive functions are a common feature of a number of focal epilepsies, and they are further considered (see "Focal Seizures Characterized by Prominent Disturbances of Consciousness with or without Automatisms and Cognitive and Affective Manifestations"). In such cases, the cognitive disturbances may constitute the "aura" of a more complex seizure event. In less common cases, cognitive dysfunction constitutes the whole seizure, and the term *cognitive seizures* is more specifically applied to such cases. This section considers all cases in which cognitive disturbances are a *prominent component* of the seizures, irrespective of their association with other ictal events, such as disturbances of consciousness, automatisms, or other motor or autonomic phenomena. Isolated impairment of consciousness is not included. Paroxysmal affective changes often accompany cognitive phenomena, and they contribute to both their clinical presentation and the subjective experience of the patients. They are indeed often impossible to analyze separately from the cognitive manifestations, and the previously proposed term *affective-psychic seizures* is probably justified (Aicardi, 1994a).

Dreamy State

The *dreamy state* first described by Hughlings Jackson is the most classic form of cognitive seizure. It involves a disruption in the perception of reality that affects both time and memory processes. The ictal state interferes with ongoing cognition, producing what Jackson called "double consciousness." The dreamy state is associated with *dysmnesic symptoms*, which consist of illusions of recall that the patient cannot separate from his or her current experience. Best known is the *"déjà vu"* feeling in which the patient believes that he or she is recognizing and living again a previous experience; the converse sensation of unfamiliarity and strangeness may, however, also occur (*jamais vu* feeling). Hallucinations that include vivid reminiscences of past experiences, the *experiential hallucinations* of Penfield and Jasper (1954) and Penfield and Perot (1963) are often part of the dreamy state. During these episodes of abnormal mental state, a considerable degree of awareness may be preserved, and the patient may be able to perform complex acts requiring the use of normal faculties (Jackson quoted by Aicardi, 2001a), although these acts have not been memorized. The dreamy state seems to require temporal lobe involvement (especially of the right) in the discharge.

Forced Thinking

Forced thinking is a rare ictal manifestation in which a thought unrelated to the current situation imposes itself on the patient's mind (Reinikainen, 1987; Broglin et al., 1992); it seems to be observed with frontal lobe discharges. Multiple other cognitive dysfunctions are also present. They are described in the section on disturbances of consciousness, with which they are often associated.

Other Manifestations

One interesting manifestation of cognitive seizures is the transient and isolated disturbance of selective mental processes, resulting in errors or slowness in the execution of specific mental tasks thought to affect localized cortical areas involved by the epileptic discharge (e.g., visuospatial tasks with discharges in the right parietooccipital area and verbal tasks with those affecting the left frontotemporal hemisphere). Such paroxysmal dysfunctions may be very brief, and they may go undetected. Recognizing these may require EEG recording during the performance of continuous tasks (Kasteleijn-Nolst Trenité et al., 1988, 1990; Shewmon and Erwin, 1988; Tsuchiya et al., 1978). These so-called *transient cognitive impairments (TCI)* are often ignored by the patient, but they can, in some circumstances, significantly disturb their life. This can also be the case with discharges in areas involved in amnesic recall, as in the patient reported by Aarts et al. (1984), who could not retrieve the information required by his profession of librarian, demonstrates. Interestingly, this occurred only when he was under stress, and the EEG at rest was normal; it did show SW activity only when he was challenged. The possible role of SW activity unassociated with clinical seizures has been proposed as an explanation for deterioration in some epilepsy syndromes, such as Landau-Kleffner and continuous spike-waves of slow sleep (CSWS) (Aicardi, 1999a; Deonna, 1996) (see Chapter 11).

Aphasic seizures are rare in children. The most common aphasia associated with epilepsy is Landau-Kleffner syndrome (Chapter 11). Ictal aphasia has been well described in adults (Wells et al., 1992). In children, however, isolated ictal aphasia has not been reported. Speech arrest and especially aphemia are common with seizure discharges involving the operculum in rolandic epilepsy (RE), but this is rarely isolated. Ictal aphasia should be distinguished from the more common confusion and postictal aphasia that may follow temporal lobe seizures.

FOCAL SEIZURES CHARACTERIZED BY PROMINENT DISTURBANCES OF CONSCIOUSNESS, WITH OR WITHOUT AUTOMATISMS OR COGNITIVE AND AFFECTIVE MANIFESTATIONS

This section deals with focal epileptic seizures that feature alterations or abolition of consciousness in the absence of generalization of the attack. This section first considers the general characteristics and pathophysiology of these seizures and then the effect of age, their different clinical expressions, and their diagnosis.

Alteration of Consciousness

Historical Note and Definitions

Disturbances of consciousness during partial seizures have long attracted the interest of neurologists, and their association with cognitive or affective manifestations has been known for a very long time.

In 1937, Gibbs et al. (1937) used the term *psychomotor* to encompass all the psychic and motor manifestations encountered in partial seizures in which alteration of consciousness was a prominent feature, but the same term was subsequently applied to automatisms as a specific ictal manifestation (Penry, 1975). The discovery that many of the seizures presenting with such phenomena originated in the temporal lobe, especially its limbic part (Lennox and Lennox, 1960; Penfield and Jasper, 1954), and that they were often associated with anterior temporal

spike foci (Gibbs et al., 1937) led to the introduction of the term *temporal lobe seizures* to designate the same type of attacks, even though a possible origin from other sites was quickly recognized (Penfield and Jasper, 1954; Ajmone-Marsan and Abraham, 1960). The terms *psychomotor seizures*, *temporal lobe seizures*, and *limbic seizures* have often been used synonymously regardless of the fact that they refer to different conceptual categories (topographic, descriptive, EEG), thereby producing increasing confusion. The term *complex partial seizures* was introduced by the International Classification of Epileptic Seizures in 1970 (see Chapter 2), which hoped to end the confusion by selecting the clinical and EEG manifestations as the main basis for classifying the seizures. The 1970 classification, however, used the term *complex partial seizures* synonymously with *temporal lobe seizures*. Subsequent studies addressing the anatomic substrate(s) of clinical seizure semiology, which were mainly derived from studies for epilepsy surgery, have clarified that both temporal and extratemporal seizures may be associated with alteration of consciousness. The 1981 revision of the International Classification of Epileptic Seizures, while retaining the distinction between simple and complex partial seizures based on the presence of alteration of consciousness, did not assign alteration of consciousness to any specific anatomic substrate. Additional evidence gathered during the last 20 years has led to the belief that the designation of partial seizures as "simple" or "complex" has lost meaningful precision for classifying seizures in terms of topography; pathophysiology; and, at times, clinical semiology (Engel, 2001). Consequently, the distinction "simple" versus "complex" is no longer recommended.

Because of the close, although not necessary, association between automatisms and alteration of consciousness, this section also includes some discussion of the automatic motor activities and subjective symptoms more commonly associated with and essential to the understanding of the phenomenology of seizures with alteration of consciousness. More details about clinical semiology of automatisms and affective psychic phenomena are provided in specific subsequent sections of this chapter.

Isolated impairment of consciousness was recognized as a distinct type of partial seizure by the 1989 international classification. Such attacks consist of a brief episode of confusion for which the patient is subsequently partially or entirely amnesic (Daly, 1982). In most of these seizures, a few inconspicuous automatisms likely occur. Such seizures differ from absences by their longer duration (30 to 90 seconds);

their more gradual termination; and the presence of some postictal tiredness and sleepiness, which is a major distinctive characteristic in children (Penry et al., 1975). From a purely semiologic perspective, the term *dialeptic* seizures (Lüders et al., 2000; Noachtar et al., 2000) has been suggested to define the ictal alteration of consciousness that is accompanied by staring and a loss or minimal persistence of motor activity, regardless of its pathophysiology (i.e., focal versus generalized).

In the same semiologic classification (Lüders et al., 2000), the term *hypomotor seizures* was suggested for seizures with a significant reduction in or arrest of behavioral motor activity occurring in small children or severely mentally retarded individuals in whom an appreciation of the level of consciousness during an attack is impossible (Acharya et al., 2000; Wyllie, 1995). The term *akinetic* was suggested for seizures in which a patient is unable to follow a simple motor command but retains full recall of the event (Noachtar and Lüders, 2000). An advantage of this proposal is that the level of "consciousness," which is so difficult to assess in young patients, need not be defined.

Other seizures that often alter "consciousness" are characterized by the predominance of motor activity, and different terms can be used according to the specific type of activity (e.g., "automotor" in the presence of automatisms, "clonic" when rhythmic jerks occur). In the present chapter, the authors do not use these terms because they are not generally accepted.

Automatisms (see "Automatisms") are behavioral sequences reproducing normal body movements that unfold without voluntary control and that, in a majority, occur with a loss or impairment of awareness. They occur with different types of seizures, whether generalized or partial, or as postictal manifestations (Talairach et al., 1974). Simple automatisms, especially of those of an oral alimentary type, can occur without impairment of consciousness (Munari et al., 1980a). Seizures in which distal automatisms are prominent are also described as "automotor" seizures (Kotagal, 2000), and these are considered highly characteristic of mesial temporal lobe epilepsy. Automatisms also occur in seizures arising from the frontal, parietal, and occipital lobes (Salanova et al., 1995b; Munari et al., 1980a; Geier et al., 1976).

Affective-psychic ictal phenomena are considered simple partial seizures in the 1981 classification because consciousness is often not impaired, even though the ictal events are highly complex. The state of consciousness during such seizures is often modified in a subtle way that is not necessarily part of the operational definition given. Affective-psychic phenomena often evolve into loss of consciousness.

In *summary*, focal epilepsies with alterations of consciousness have long been regarded as a relatively homogeneous disorder. However, they clearly constitute a heterogeneous group with different sites of origin of the discharges (Wieser, 1983b; Talairach and Bancaud, 1974). Two major categories are represented by seizures originating in the limbic system, especially its temporobasal part, which includes the hippocampus, amygdala, and adjacent temporofrontal cortex, and those originating from the neocortex, whether in the temporal lobe or outside it, especially the frontal lobe. These two groups have different clinical manifestations (Engel, 1987, 1992; Quesney, 1987; Wieser, 1987) and different courses, and they pose different therapeutic problems.

Pathophysiology of Alteration of Consciousness in Focal Seizures

Alteration of consciousness in focal seizures can be produced by at least the following four mechanisms: (a) widespread diffusion of the ictal discharge to the cortex, which consequently is diffusely inactivated (Bancaud and Talairach, 1992); (b) spreading of the discharge to the upper brainstem (Noachtar et al., 2000); (c) inactivation of the hippocampal formation bilaterally, with a consequent inability to store memories (Lüders et al., 2000); and (d) involvement of one or more of the language areas (Broca, Wernicke, or basal temporal area), leading to global aphasia (Lüders et al., 1987a, 2000; Lesser et al., 1986). These mechanisms may operate independently, or they may be combined in various proportions.

A fundamental concept is that alteration of consciousness is indicative of extensive seizure diffusion to the limbic or neocortical temporal and extratemporal areas and that it therefore reflects the amount of cortex involved but does not indicate *per se* any specific area of seizure origin or topographic distribution (Munari et al., 1980a). Therefore, alteration of consciousness is not particularly important for seizure localization, but it is a factor of major importance when assessing the level of seizure-related disability.

Neurophysiologic analyses of alteration of consciousness in focal seizures have been conducted mainly in patients with frontal and mesial temporal epilepsies. Electrical stimulation of the mesial frontal lobe can elicit "frontal absences" and generalized SW discharges on scalp EEG (Bancaud et al., 1974). Spontaneous ictal activity in the mesial frontal lobe may be responsible for a blank staring ictal symptomatology (Wieser, 1987). Electrical stimulation studies of the frontal lobes have also identified areas that can produce motor arrest (Lüders, 1992). Close connections linking the prefrontal cortex with nonspecific and intralaminar thalamic nuclei of the midline region might facilitate rapid ictal spread from the anterior frontal lobes to the reticular formation, causing alteration of consciousness and generalization (Noachtar et al., 2000).

Most focal seizures with loss of consciousness appear to originate in the temporal lobe(s), especially the limbic formation and various areas of the neocortex within the temporal lobe(s); the frontal lobe(s); or other areas. The limbic structures consist of the following three major interconnected neuronal constellations, each of which is centered around a particular group of nuclei: (a) the frontotemporal limbic cortex and the amygdala, through which impulses come from and go to the brainstem; (b) the hippocampal and parahippocampal cortex and the septal nuclei; and (c) the cingulate cortex and the anterior thalamus (Koella, 1987; Pandya and Yeterian, 1987). From animal experiments, these structures are thought to subserve autonomic and behavioral functions related to individual and species preservation, although the evidence in humans is far from complete (Koella, 1987). They are involved in the elaboration of behavioral responses to external stimuli, as well as corresponding affects and internal sensation, and integrate at the highest level most autonomic functions.

The temporal neocortical part of this system plays an essential role in integrating the sensory inputs from primary receiving areas in order to elaborate perceptions, then to match them with previous experience, and finally to evaluate whether they are motivationally meaningful for the individual (Gloor et al., 1982b). The mesial temporal structures also play an essential role in the mechanisms of memory. Disruption of this system by an epileptic discharge results in a distortion of perceptions, inappropriate associated affects, and inability to match ongoing perceptions to previous experience, thus disturbing the evaluation of a perception as novel or strange. Automatic motor activity, which may accompany alteration of consciousness, may result from the involvement of certain motor nuclei (e.g., the amygdaloid complex in oral alimentary automatisms), or it may be a release phenomenon caused by bilateral diffusion of the discharge (Wieser and Kausel, 1987) or a postictal phenomenon.

Seizures with alteration of consciousness are a dynamic process. Depth electrode studies during seizures have shown paroxysmal activity in several limbic system areas (cingulate gyrus, amygdala, hippocampus) and extralimbic sites (selected thalamic nuclei and various neocortical areas in or outside of the temporal lobes) (Wieser and Elger, 1987; Engel et al., 1981; Spencer, 1981; Bancaud et al., 1973). Determination of the actual site of origin of the discharge necessitates the convergence and compatibility of several of the following types of data: clinical manifestations; surface electrode and intracranial electrode findings; electrical stimulation studies; neuroradiologic evidence; positron emission tomographic (PET) scans; and SPECT scan studies, if they are available (Krakow et al., 1999; Engel, 1982, 1992; Theodore et al., 1983a, 1984a, 1988, 1990; Bancaud et al., 1973). The discharge migrates from its site of origin to neighboring or distant homolateral and contralateral structures. Preferential pathways of propagation can then be recognized (Wieser et al., 1993; Wieser and Elger, 1987; Wieser and Müller, 1987; Talairach and Bancaud, 1974). For example, Wieser and Kausel (1987) found that most limbic seizures have a focal or regional unilateral mesiobasal onset that usually involves both the hippocampus and the amygdala with spread to the contralateral hippocampal formation. Conversely, some seizures that originate in other brain areas such as the posterior, temporal, parietal, occipital, or frontal lobes often spread to the ipsilateral mesiobasal-limbic structures, which can then act as secondary "pacemaker zones" (Wieser and Müller, 1987), further distributing and maintaining the ictal event. The sequence of the symptoms and of EEG phenomena should therefore be carefully analyzed when surgery is contemplated.

Clinical Manifestations of Focal Seizures with Ictal Alteration of Consciousness as the Main Characteristic

Seizures with alteration of consciousness can manifest with a variety of associated symptoms that may differ considerably with the site of origin and propagation of the ictal activity, the age of the patient, and the nature and extent of the causative lesions. The clinical features of focal seizures with alteration of consciousness have been well defined in adults (Kotagal, 2001; Engel, 1992; Van der Wens and Binnie, 1987; Wieser and Kausel, 1987; Munari et al., 1982b; Bancaud, 1973), but information about their characteristics in children is less abundant (Mohamed et al., 2001; Acharya et al., 2000; Hamer et al., 1999; Wyllie et al., 1989; Wyllie and Lüders, 1989; Duchowny, 1987; Dinner et al., 1984; Holmes, 1984; Holowach et al., 1961).

Peculiarities of Seizures with Alterations of Consciousness in Infants and Young Children

The level of consciousness during seizures in infants and small children or in individuals with mental retardation is difficult to assess. Duchowny (1987) acknowledged that alteration of consciousness is difficult to demonstrate and that it often is assumed only on the basis of unsuccessful attempts to draw attention during an episode (Acharya et al., 1996). Therefore, using the objective term *hypomotor* to designate seizures, both focal and generalized, with a prominent reduction of behavioral motor activity might seem preferable. These authors studied seizure semiology in 23 children from 2 to 24 months of age who had focal epilepsy. Retrospective video-EEG assessment of the level of AC, as tested by the ictal assessment of reactivity to external stimuli, proved unreliable in most patients. A subgroup of children presented with a homogeneous ictal pattern consisting of arrest or a marked reduction of behavioral motor activity lasting a few minutes, followed by the resumption of preictal activity or an increase of activity. None of the children presented with fine motor or complex automatisms, but some did have oral alimentary activity. However, the "hypomotor" ictal behavior may be the consequence of the limited clinical repertoire that is typical of infants, more than it is an expression of bland "complex partial seizures" (Hamer et al., 1999; Nordli et al., 1997). Hamer et al. (1999) reviewed 296 videotaped seizures from 76 children younger than 3 years of age. A total of 81% of the attacks could be classified within four main categories, with 20% being hypomotor seizures. Hypomotor seizures were associated with focal (14 [70%] of 20) or generalized (6 [30%] of 20) ictal EEG activity. Nordli et al. (1997) proposed the term *behavioral seizures* to designate the abrupt change in behavior that is seen in infants without additional features and that sometimes include the sudden cessation of movement. Recently, Folgarasi et al. (2002) showed that brain maturation significantly affects the seizure semiology. Motor phenomena of multiple types, including spasms and tonic or hypotonic seizures, are more common in infants than are the typical features of temporal lobe origin.

A common sequence in children is the initiation with an aura of abdominal discomfort that often wells up from the belly and tightens the throat or with vague feelings referred to the alimentary tract (e.g., "fear in my stomach"); it continues with a vacant stare and loss of contact, followed by a period of confusion. In small children, behavioral arrest with unresponsiveness and a change in facial expression may represent the whole seizure.

Associated autonomic features are often present. Pallor of the face with cyanosis around the lips and dark circles around the eyes are often observed. Facial flushing is less common. Blume (1989) underlined the predominance of gastrointestinal symptoms, abdominal sensations, and/or fear, which he found in 11 of 22 patients. Initial staring, which has no localizing value, is commonly observed during alteration of consciousness (Wieser and Kausel, 1987). An abrupt loss of consciousness without automatisms is a well-recognized manifestation of some focal epilepsies, mainly in those with a mesial frontal and frontoorbital seizure origin (Chauvel et al., 1995; Chauvel and Bancaud, 1994; Bancaud and Talairach, 1992), and this may be difficult to distinguish from absence seizures of generalized epilepsy. However, seizure characteristics may point to a specific topographic origin (e.g., arrest of speech and movement, simple automatisms, conjugate eye and head deviation, and quick recovery). An abrupt lapse of consciousness and an arrest of movement without automatisms are also seen in patients with temporal lobe seizure onset (Noachtar et al., 2000; Delgado-Escueta and Walsh, 1983). A cluster analysis of ictal symptoms in patients with frontal and temporal lobe seizure origin indicated that ictal alteration of consciousness with minor or no motor activity occurred in both groups and that it could not be differentiated clinically (Manford et al., 1996a). In a study of 34 patients with focal epilepsy in whom arrest of activity and alteration of consciousness ("dialeptic seizures"), documented by video-EEG recordings, were the predominant ictal features, epilepsy was classified as having a temporal lobe origin in 11 patients, a frontal origin in 6, and a parietooccipital origin in 2, but the origin could only be lateralized and not defined further topographically in a large subgroup of 15 patients (Noachtar et al., 2000).

Subjective Symptoms

Auras, which are observed in most adult patients (Kanemoto and Janz, 1989; Taylor and Lochery, 1987; Gupta et al., 1983), are identified in less than one-third of children (Holmes, 1984). The simple partial seizure termed *aura* is probably present in more patients, but infants and young children cannot describe their feelings; they are, however, suggested by the fact that, before losing consciousness, the child may look panicked or otherwise "abnormal" for a few seconds.

Simple partial onset, the pathophysiologic substrate for subjective symptomatology, can be manifested with a wide range of symptoms.

Psychosensory Symptoms

Psychosensory symptoms include hallucinations (i.e., a perception in the absence of the appropriate stimulus) and illusions (i.e., disturbed perceptions of ongoing stimuli). Depending on the cortical areas involved, hallucinations and illusions can be visual and formed, with figures and scenes; unformed; auditory; vertiginous; olfactory; gustatory; somatosensory; or multimodal. The elaborateness of visual and auditory hallucinations is variable (Daly, 1982; Gastaut and Broughton, 1972). Multimodal hallucinations (Daly, 1982) consist of complex scenes with combined visual and auditory sensations, that often occur in association with affective changes, especially fear.

Cognitive Symptoms or Auras

Cognitive symptoms or auras, or "experiential phenomena," designate abnormal experiences resulting from dysmnesic (e.g., *déjà vu*) and cognitive (e.g., dreamy state, distortion of time sense) seizures (Commission on Classification and Terminology of the International League Against Epilepsy, 1981). During electrical stimulation of the "memory cortex, things [that are] seen or heard may seem strangely familiar, or they may seem strange, absurd, terrifying. They may seem suddenly more distant or nearer" (Penfield and Jasper, 1954). The resulting experience, which is usually retrieved from the patient's personal past, may be even more vivid than when it was experienced in normal life, with a combination of perception, memory, and affect (Gloor, 1990).

Affective Symptoms

Affective symptoms include mainly unpleasant feelings, the most common of which is fear, that are often referred to the epigastric region. The *fear* is often intense, and it occurs either in isolation (Biraben et al., 2001) or in combination with autonomic or psychosensory symptoms, particularly with hallucinations that may motivate the affect. A frightened expression associated with an epigastric sensation, pallor, or perioral cyanosis is often observed before the child becomes unresponsive. On some occasions, the child may scream loudly with a terrified expression and then run to hug the parents in a state of confusion. Depth-electrode recordings in patients with ictal fear, anguish, or a combination of the two have proved that the epileptic discharge spreads to involve the amygdala and hippocampus, the frontoorbital region, and the anterior cingulate gyrus (Bancaud and Talairach, 1992). Panic attacks of epileptic origin, which are not easily distinguishable from the more common ictal

fear, have been associated with right parietal ictal activity (Alemayehu et al., 1995). Depressive feelings or pleasurable sensations are unusual (Holden et al., 1982), and anger is rare, especially in children. Crying or laughing inappropriately may occur (Offen et al., 1976; Gascon and Lombroso, 1971; Loiseau et al., 1971). Both manifestations in children may be more common with diencephalic lesions (see "Symptoms of Lesional Epilepsy of Subcortical Origin").

Autonomic Symptoms

Autonomic symptoms have been dealt with in a separate section in this chapter. Here, only the abdominal aura, an ictal manifestation often preceding alteration of consciousness, is considered. *Abdominal or epigastric auras* are the most commonly identifiable subjective symptoms (Kramer and Bracht, 2000). About 30% of patients with seizure onset in the temporal lobe who were able to report an aura described an abdominal sensation (Kotagal, 1991). Abdominal aura is reliably associated with mesiotemporal epilepsy. However, in few patients, an abdominal sensation may be the expression of mesial prefrontal onset.

Automatisms

Automatisms are involuntary, more or less coordinated motor activities that often, but not necessarily, are associated with the impairment of consciousness. Ictal activity confined to the amygdala and anterior hippocampus can cause oral alimentary automatisms without impairment of consciousness (Munari et al., 1981, 1982b). Automatisms may apparently arise without preceding symptoms, or they may represent the extension of an episode with prominent sensory or affective-psychic manifestations. They may also follow simple partial motor seizures, especially with attacks of frontal origin. Most automatisms are relatively simple, and they affect mainly the oral alimentary domain (Theodore, 1983b; Daly, 1982; Ajmone-Marsan and Ralston, 1957). Chewing, smacking, swallowing, lip pursing, and hissing are particularly common in children (Holowach et al., 1961; Glaser and Dixon, 1956). More complex automatisms include looking around, searching, grimacing, fumbling with clothes or sheets, and scratching movements. Verbal automatisms (e.g., humming noises, repetition of phrases or more often of senseless words) may also occur. The most complex automatisms, such as coordinated gestures or ambulation toward some goal, are usually influenced more or less by environmental events. Some automatisms feature violent motor activity, shouting, and emission of profanities, and these are more common with a seizure of orbitofrontal origin. A large majority of automatisms are simple, primitive, and undirected (Theodore et al., 1984b; Theodore, 1983b). Automatisms during which some interaction is seen between the patient's activity and the outside world have been termed *reactive*, whereas those without interaction have been called *released* or *unreactive* (Penry, 1975). Gastaut and Broughton (1972) have classified automatisms into the following types: alimentary, mimetic, gestural, ambulatory, and verbal.

Ictal automatisms must be distinguished from *postictal automatic behavior*, which can arise in a state of confusion or which can be the expression of residual localized ictal activity (Devinsky et al., 1994). The postictal state may often not be readily apparent, and postictal automatic behaviors are usually of a different nature; thcy consist of getting up, walking, or running (Kotagal, 2000).

Ictal automatisms result from the activation of specific brain structures or represent release phenomena (Jasper, 1964). Stereotypic oral alimentary and hand automatisms only occur ictally, supporting the hypothesis that at least some automatic activities are the expression of direct epileptic activation of codified behavioral sequences. Stimulation studies have shown that masticatory (oral alimentary) activity, which may be accompanied by nausea or sickness and confusion, results from the direct stimulation of the amygdala and periamygdaloid region but not of the hippocampus (Feindel and Penfield, 1954).

Approximately 40% to 80% of patients with temporal lobe epilepsy have stereotypic automatisms of the mouth and hands, as well as other complex motor manifestations (Kotagal, 2000). In infants and children, oral alimentary activities are predominant, and the automatisms have less purposefulness (Brockhaus and Elger, 1995; Bye and Foo, 1994; Jayakar and Duchowny, 1990; Yamamoto et al., 1987b). More complex manual and gestural automatisms, such as fumbling or picking at clothes, are uncommon, and these tend to occur after 5 years of age (Wyllie et al., 1993). Automatisms were seen in 78% of children 3 to 13 years of age (Yamamoto et al., 1987b) and 87% of those who were 5 to 19 years of age (Holmes, 1984). In newborns and infants up to 2 years of age, the frequency varies from 57% (Holmes, 1984) to 80% (Yamamoto et al., 1987b). In the same age-group, Yamamoto et al., (1987b) observed that, although the location of initial ictal EEG changes was variable, the clinical manifestations were stereotypic, with the most common sequence being represented by motionlessness or simple automatisms, followed by convulsive movements and oral automatisms. Duchowny (1987) observed that the most common

automatism in 14 infants younger than 2 years was behavioral arrest with forced head turning and asymmetric tonic posturing that were inconsistently accompanied by sucking, mouthing, and blinking. Holmes (1984) studied 69 complex partial seizures in 24 children. He classified the seizures into the following three basic types: those that began with a motionless stare followed by automatisms (type I); those that began with automatisms (type II); and those (in only one patient) that started with a sudden loss of body tone, followed by confusion, amnesia, automatisms, and gradual recomposure (type III). As in adults (Delgado-Escueta and Walsh, 1985), the type I seizures were usually associated with lateralized ictal discharges, whereas type II and type III seizures were generally associated with bilateral ictal EEG abnormalities. Two additional studies of "complex partial seizures" in children with temporal lobe epilepsy, which was defined by the good seizure outcome after temporal lobectomy (Wyllie et al., 1993) or by EEG and MRI findings (Brockhaus and Elger, 1995), concluded that older children had seizure symptomatology analogous to that of adults but that smaller children had no (retrievable) auras and complex automatisms.

Adolescents and older children can exhibit the full range of automatic activities expressed in adult patients and reviewed in many papers (Lüders et al., 2000; Bancaud, 1987; Munari et al., 1982b; Delgado-Escueta et al., 1977; Ajmone-Marsan and Abraham, 1960). A retrospective cluster analysis of 91 seizures in 31 patients who had EEG monitoring before surgery and were subsequently rendered seizure free after temporal lobectomy showed that oral alimentary and repetitive hand automatisms occurred in 63% of the seizures and that these were correlated with each other and with loss of consciousness and looking around. Auras occurred in 29% of the seizures, an initial behavioral arrest in 36%, and staring in 10% (Kotagal et al., 1995b). Motor phenomena that involved bilaterally the trunk (e.g., flexion, lateral incurvation, rotation) may also occur. *Dystonic posturing* of one upper limb or of both upper and lower limbs on one side during alteration of consciousness points to a temporal lobe origin in the hemisphere opposite the side involved (Kotagal, 1991; Kotagal et al., 1989). The close temporal relationship between oral alimentary and manual automatisms and dystonic posturing could be due to the involvement of the basal ganglia, as demonstrated on invasive EEG recordings and ictal SPECT studies (Newton et al., 1992; Kotagal et al., 1989). Automatic activity in seizures of temporal lobe origin tends to be predominant or to be limited to the limbs ipsilateral to the involved hemisphere.

The combination of ipsilateral automatisms and contralateral dystonic posturing is highly characteristic of temporal lobe seizures (Kotagal, 1999; Wieser et al., 1993), and it has a good lateralizing value. Unilateral automatisms do not have a lateralizing value on their own (Kotagal, 2000; Bleasel et al., 1997).

Secondary generalization of complex partial seizures may occur; this is more common in seizures of frontal origin than in those originating in the temporal lobe, but estimates have indicated that it occurs in up to 60% of temporal lobe seizures (Kotagal, 2000). Automatisms can occur during or following generalized seizures with similar characteristics to those seen during focal seizures.

Diagnosis of Focal Seizures with Alteration of Consciousness

Difficulties in diagnosis are apt to arise in cases in which only sensory phenomena or automatisms occur because these may be difficult to distinguish from nonepileptic behavioral aberrations, especially in small children who are unable to report subjective symptoms. In the authors' experience, focal seizures with alteration of consciousness in children are of brief duration, and they feature stereotypic and usually relatively simple manifestations. They may be overlooked, but they are rarely mistaken for nonepileptic phenomena. More complex psychic and affective manifestations are less common, and many of them are not epileptic in nature, even though they often arouse a suspicion of limbic seizures.

The following three problems of diagnosis should be considered: (a) nonepileptic, nonictal manifestations; (b) nonepileptic, ictal manifestations; and (c) other epileptic manifestations. The first category includes such phenomena as episodes of depersonalization; derealization; feelings of déjà vu or strangeness; hallucinations or illusions; or amnesic phenomena, such as flashbacks. Although all may be part of a focal seizure, they may be seen in patients who are not suffering from epilepsy (especially in adolescents) as a result of the use of certain drugs, such as cannabis derivatives or hallucinogenic agents. Similar symptoms are a hallmark of psychosis, and these may be difficult to distinguish from true epileptic events, with which they may occasionally be associated. More often, similar but vaguely described symptoms are reported by children or adolescents to attract the attention of adults or their peers. In all such patients, the duration of the events is longer than in epileptic seizures, and overt phenomena such as alimentary or simple motor automatisms are lacking, which should arouse suspicion. The common fugue of adolescents is rarely interpreted

erroneously as epileptic. Occasional cases of "hysterical" fugue with amnesia have been recorded, and they very seldom raise a diagnostic problem with "complex partial" status (Gastaut et al., 1956).

A number of *ictal nonepileptic events* are often mistaken for epileptic seizures (see Chapter 21). Migrainous attacks, especially those accompanied by visual illusions, often raise such a problem. This is particularly the case with micropsia, often occurring in association with somatosensory illusions, which is much more commonly a manifestation of migraine than of epilepsy (the "Alice in Wonderland syndrome") (Breningstall, 1985). In addition, confusional states occurring with migraine are at times interpreted as seizures with alteration of consciousness, although their duration is much longer (Gascon and Barlow, 1970). Recurrent abdominal pain with or without vomiting is seldom the only manifestation of focal seizures. However, ictal vomiting, with prolonged alteration of consciousness and often version, is a common feature of the early onset idiopathic childhood epilepsy with occipital paroxysms (Ferrie et al., 1997; Guerrini et al., 1994, 1997a; Panayiotopoulos, 1989b).

Pseudoepileptic seizures may present with manifestations suggestive of seizures with alteration of consciousness in 20% to 40% of patients. The sequence of events is often stereotypic, but rarely does it closely resemble that classic clustering of manifestations seen during focal epileptic seizures with alteration of consciousness, if careful analysis is able to be conducted. (The diagnosis of pseudoseizures is discussed fully in Chapter 21.)

Focal epilepsies featuring seizures with alteration of consciousness should be distinguished from *other types of seizure disorders*. Absences may resemble episodes of motionless staring with a brief lapse of consciousness, which may be seen during focal seizures, especially when the latter are followed by a few simple automatisms. However, important differences permitting a relatively easy clinical diagnosis do exist. First, focal seizures are usually longer. Absences almost never last more than 30 seconds, and only 15% last more than 10 seconds (Penry et al., 1975), whereas the mean duration of focal seizures with alteration of consciousness is approximately 90 to 110 seconds (Penry et al., 1975). Furthermore, the onset of absences is sudden, and they are never preceded by an aura, whereas an aura precedes alteration of consciousness in 23% to 83% of patients with focal epilepsy (Theodore et al., 1994; Ajmone-Marsan and Ralston, 1957). More important, focal seizures with alteration of consciousness are followed by a period of confusion and/or tiredness that may be extremely brief and inconspicuous but that rarely is altogether absent; this is not missed if the patients and their families are specifically questioned on that point (O'Donohoe, 1985; So et al., 1984). Finally, absences are easily triggered by hyperventilation, which provoke focal seizures much more rarely. Automatisms may be present in both seizure types, and, although these differ in character in focal seizures and during absences, they are not a very good discriminative symptom. A correct diagnosis between absences and focal seizures with alteration of consciousness is clearly essential because the treatment of these two conditions is different.

The differential diagnosis between focal seizures with alteration of consciousness and sylvian seizures of benign epilepsy with centrotemporal (or centrorolandic) spikes (BECTS and BECRS, respectively) is easy, although the two conditions have sometimes been confused. Diagnosing these correctly is important because the prognosis is much better in rolandic epilepsy. The confusion may stem from the prominent oropharyngeal phenomena that are the hallmark of sylvian seizures; these can be erroneously interpreted as rudimentary oral alimentary automatisms. The presence in BECTS of a midtemporal spike focus may be another confusing finding. However, the midtemporal spike focus is distinct in both location and morphology from the anterior temporal focus of temporal lobe epilepsy, and it originates from the lowermost part of the rolandic area, not from the temporal lobe (Gregory and Wong, 1992; Lombroso, 1967). Some of the favorable outcomes reported in series of patients with "temporal lobe epilepsy" (Lindsay et al., 1979a) or in some antiepileptic drug trial of "partial epilepsy" are likely the result of the inadvertent inclusion of cases of RE.

TOPOGRAPHIC SYNDROMES: ICTAL, CLINICAL, AND ELECTROENCEPHALOGRAPHIC MANIFESTATIONS ASSOCIATED WITH SEIZURE ACTIVITY ORIGINATING FROM SPECIFIC CORTICAL AREAS

Accurate description of the semiology of focal seizures is important for a correct clinical diagnosis and for attempting a *topographic diagnosis*, especially when surgical treatment can be an option. The characteristics of the clinical manifestations and the ictal and interictal EEG features can help localize the origin of a seizure to a particular cortical area (Rasmussen, 1974; Penfield and Jasper, 1954). However, definitive localization of an epileptogenic area for surgical purposes demands that the topography suggested by clinical and EEG data be confirmed by other means, including CT and MRI scans; neuropsychologic studies; and, in some patients, subdural strips or grids, depth electrodes, interictal PET scan, and ictal and interictal SPECT scan, so that grave errors are avoided (Juhász et al., 2000a, 2001b; Krakow et al., 1999; Cross et al., 1997; Devinsky et al., 1989; Duchowny, 1989; Wieser and Elger, 1987; Engel et al., 1981, 1982b; Talairach and Bancaud, 1974).

Some elements of localization, as summarized by the Commission on Classification and Terminology of the International League Against Epilepsy (1989) and subsequently refined in several reviews (Williamson et al., 1997; Wieser and Williamson, 1993; Engel, 1989), are tentatively indicated in the following section. The reader should keep in mind that the involvement of a cortical area does not mean that the origin of the discharge is located within that area. An epileptic seizure is a dynamic process that does not remain stationary but rather propagates to neighboring and distant areas by both normal and abnormal (facilitated) pathways, and the area of origin does not necessarily produce the symptoms that often originate from a larger zone, the symptom-producing area. Similarly, the relationship between the location of a lesion and that of the resulting epileptic discharge is complex, and no absolute concordance exists between them. With these reservations in mind, some elements of localization are tentatively indicated.

FRONTAL AND CENTRAL SEIZURES: CLINICAL AND ELECTROENCEPHALOGRAPHIC FEATURES

Clinical Features

Seizures originating in the *frontal lobe* may or may not be accompanied by alteration of consciousness, and they tend to have prominent motor manifestations. The initial subjective symptoms are brief and difficult to describe. When alteration of consciousness predominates, the seizures are brief (so called "frontal absences"), and they may be accompanied by forced thinking and urinary incontinence (Wieser and Williamson, 1993) and followed by short postictal confusion. Asymmetric posturing (fencing posture) or focal tonic activity with vocalization or speech arrest, usually with preserved consciousness, is suggestive of the involvement of the *supplementary motor area*. Olfactory hallucinations and illusions that are followed by early motor signs and "hyperkinetic," repetitive gestural automatisms (or "hypermotor seizures") may originate in the orbitofrontal cortex (Lüders et al.,

2000; Bancaud and Talairach, 1992). Changes in mood and affect accompanied by vegetative signs and early elaborate gestural automatisms suggest the involvement of the cingulate cortex (Williamson et al., 1997; Engel, 1989). Tonic or clonic motor activity and lateral head and eye deviation (version) indicate dorsolateral frontal involvement. Drop attack seizures may occur. With the exception of the subjective symptoms, most of the features indicated are already apparent in late infancy and childhood. Small children tend to demonstrate postictal sleepiness, even after short attacks.

Seizures involving the *central region*, which includes the portion of the cortex surrounding the rolandic sulcus corresponding to the primary sensorimotor cortex, feature a *jacksonian march* or very narrowly localized clonic or tonic motor phenomena, which are evidence favoring the primary involvement of the rolandic strip. Concomitant sensations of tingling, a feeling of electricity, or loss of muscle tone are common. *Reflex activation* of simple motor seizures by sudden contact or the contraction of specific muscles is observed in some patients. Facial buccolingual, tonic-clonic contractures with aphemia, swallowing, salivation, and masticatory movements that are often accompanied by sensory symptoms, including tongue sensations of crawling, stiffness or coldness, gustatory hallucinations, and/or laryngeal symptoms, point to the involvement of the lowermost part of the perirolandic strip in the upper bank of the sylvian fissure (Wieser and Williamson, 1993; Loiseau and Beaussart, 1973; Lombroso, 1967). More extensive insular involvement is accompanied by vegetative symptoms, which may be digestive, urogenital, cardiovascular, and respiratory. These manifestations are easily misinterpreted as being of temporal lobe origin. Adversion of the head associated with a posture reminiscent of the asymmetric tonic neck reflex and, at times, with repetitive vocalization suggests the involvement of the supplementary sensorimotor area on the internal aspect of the frontal lobe. In such cases, the ictal EEG usually displays diffuse flattening that may be followed by fast low-amplitude rhythms (Bancaud and Talairach, 1992; Chauvel et al., 1992a; Rasmussen, 1983c). Secondary generalization is common.

Electroencephalogram of Frontal Seizures

Interictal Electroencephalogram

Capturing interictal EEG abnormalities in epilepsies arising from the frontal lobe(s), especially from mesial and orbitobasal areas, may be particularly difficult. The interictal EEG is often normal, or it shows midline spikes or sharp waves (Pedley et al., 1981). When such abnormalities appear only during sleep, they may be difficult to differentiate from vertex sharp waves, especially in children (Pedley et al., 1981), in whom such physiologic transients have a large amplitude. Even ictal recordings may fail to show focal seizure activity in such areas (see later discussion). In a study of 100 consecutive cases of nocturnal frontal lobe epilepsy (Provini et al., 1999), roughly half the patients showed interictal abnormalities during EEG recordings performed while both awake and asleep. The use of both sphenoidal and zygomatic electrodes were essential for documenting EEG discharges in some patients. The ictal EEG failed to reveal clear-cut epileptiform changes in approximately half of the patients. Normal recordings were obtained in 20% to 40% of patients in series reporting frontal lobe epilepsy at large (Laskowitz et al., 1995; Salanova et al., 1993). Spikes consistent with the side of seizure onset were observed in only about 25% of patients (Laskowitz et al., 1995), and bilateral or "generalized" discharges were common.

When a main spike focus can be identified, it reliably localizes the epileptogenic zone with greater precision in patients with alteration of consciousness than in those with supplementary motor or focal motor seizures (Manford et al., 1996a; Salanova et al., 1993, 1995b). Studies of pediatric series have reported a higher yield of EEG investigations, both ictally and interictally, than in adults, especially during sleep (Vigevano and Fusco, 1993). The ictal and interictal EEG characteristics of rolandic epilepsy and Rasmussen syndrome are covered in a later section in this chapter.

Ictal Electroencephalogram

According to the distribution of ictal motor phenomena, scalp EEG recordings may be contaminated by various degrees of muscle artifacts resulting from the contraction of muscles in the scalp and face, often obscuring EEG activities. *Clonic seizures* are the expression of direct activation of the motor cortex. Although single focal myoclonic jerks may occur without a recognizable spike on conventional scalp EEG (see later discussion), sustained clonic jerking is usually accompanied by a contralateral discharge (Fig. 10.2) that may be independent of the frequency of jerks or time locked

FIG. 10.2. Partial motor (tonic-clonic) seizure in a 15-month-old girl. The onset of seizure occurs in the left frontocentral region with progressive slowing of the discharge. At the end of the discharge, paroxysmal complexes appear over the opposite hemisphere.

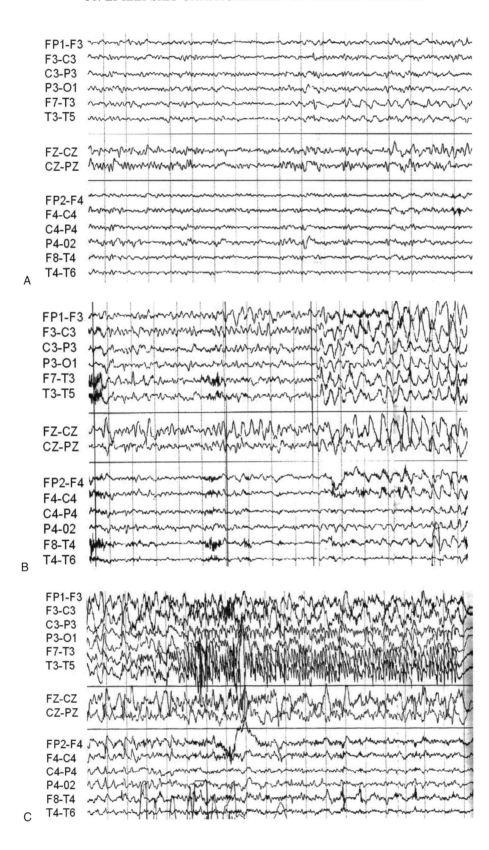

with them. Unilateral clonic jerking affecting one hemibody, which is typical of infants and small children, is almost always accompanied by rhythmic SW activity, which may be contralateral or bilateral, with predominating amplitude over the contralateral hemisphere (Guerrini and Dravet, 1997). Usually, the frequency of SW discharges is the same as that of clonic jerks (Gastaut et al., 1974b). However, the correlation between the extent of the discharge on the scalp and the amount of body segments involved is far from good because bilateral asymmetric discharges may sometimes be accompanied by discrete clonic movements involving, for example, only one hand or the eyes (Dravet, 1992a).

Asymmetric tonic motor seizures may be accompanied by a range of ictal EEG changes according to the nature of the phenomenon and its area of origin. In most cases, the lateralizing value of the ictal EEG is poor. Diffuse flattening that may be followed by bilateral frontocentral or diffuse fast low-amplitude rhythms (Bancaud and Talairach, 1992; Chauvel et al., 1992a; Rasmussen, 1983c) is more common with a seizure origin in the supplementary sensorimotor area. Although electromyographic (EMG) activity may obscure ictal EEG changes, these may still be recognizable at the vertex, where muscle artifacts are less prominent and electrical activity originating from the mesial hemispheric surface is better recorded. A seemingly normal ictal EEG recording is not uncommon. An estimated one-third of seizures are either obscured by artifacts or they show no ictal changes; one-third are accompanied by early bilateral changes (Fig. 10.3); and one third demonstrate lateralized changes that are often inconsistent with the side of seizure origin as determined by other techniques (Laskowitz et al., 1995). Versive phenomena caused by seizure origin in the dorsolateral frontal cortex may be accompanied by contralateral EEG changes, but bilateral frontal slowing is also possible. Contraversive or ipsiversive seizures can also originate in the occipital lobe; however, an occipital origin is more often accompanied by a contralateral ictal EEG

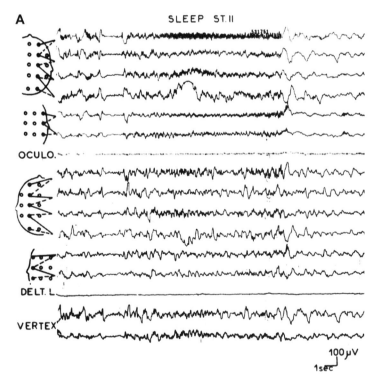

FIG. 10.3. An 8-year-old boy. **A:** The electroencephalogram shows a subclinical seizure appearing during sleep stage II. The seizure activity starts with an electrodecremental event lasting about 2 seconds that is bilateral but maximal on the right hemisphere, followed by rhythmic fast activity over the right frontal region during the following 13 seconds.

discharge involving the occipital and posterior temporal electrodes (Ochs et al., 1984) (see "Occipital Lobe Seizures"). Therefore, not only may those seizures arising in the frontal lobe, especially its mesial and orbital surface, lack a clear EEG correlation, but, even in the 30% to 50% of "positive" ictal recordings, the reliability of the data for the purpose of lateralization and localization is often questionable (Risinger, 2000; Provini et al., 1999).

Pure *inhibitory motor seizures* are accompanied by focal ictal EEG changes usually involving the contralateral frontocentral area (So, 1995).

Polygraphic recording of EEG and EMG represents the basic investigation in patients with *focal myoclonic jerks*. EEG should be recorded from at least frontal, central, and parietal derivations of the international 10-20 system. EMG activity from antagonist muscles (i.e., wrist flexors and extensors) should be recorded simultaneously. Digital recordings allow the off-line averaging of EEG segments centered on the onset of the EMG burst. The neurophysiologic features required for a diagnosis of focal myoclonus of cortical origin include a time-locked EEG transient on raw or back-averaged EEG and an EMG burst du-

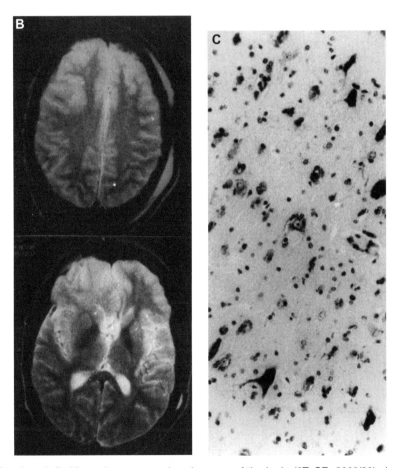

FIG. 10.3. *Continued.* B: Magnetic resonance imaging scan of the brain (2T, SE, 2000/90) shows abnormal thickening of the cortex of the base of the right frontal lobe that extends as far back as the striatum. The subjacent white matter is diminished in volume and is distorted. The morphologic anomalies extend to the insular cortex posteriorly and to the middle aspect of the lateral surface of the frontal lobe superiorly, up to the superior frontal sulcus. C: The neuropathologic study after a right frontal lobectomy showed focal cortical dysplasia with a loss of horizontal lamination, the scattering of large often hyperchromatic neurons throughout the cortex, and the proliferation of glial cells arranged in small groups. Cresyl violet stain; magnification ×80.

ration shorter than 100 ms for FEM or a silent period of 50 to 400 ms for focal ENM. Somatosensory evoked potentials, which are associated with C-reflex recording, are useful for determining the reflex nature of myoclonic jerks. Usually, a close correlation exists between muscular silent periods of ENM and contralateral sharp waves or SWs in the centroparietotemporal regions (Shibasaki et al., 1994; Guerrini et al., 1993; Oguni et al., 1992c; Cirignotta and Lugaresi, 1991; Kanazawa and Kawai, 1990).

PARIETAL LOBE SEIZURES: CLINICAL AND ELECTROENCEPHALOGRAPHIC FEATURES

Clinical Features

Symptoms produced by ictal involvement of the parietal lobe may be difficult to diagnose (Salanova et al., 1995a), especially in children, because they are mostly subjective. Furthermore, they may be shadowed by symptoms produced by the contiguous central, temporal, and occipital cortices. Focal seizures arising from the parietal lobe are characterized by positive or negative somatosensory symptoms (rarely pain) or by nausea or an intraabdominal sensation, illusions of movement or loss of awareness of a part of the body (asomatognosia, especially with nondominant hemisphere involvement), vertigo, or disorientation in space. Receptive or conductive language impairment with dominant hemisphere involvement and postural or rotatory movements may also be seen, and visual symptoms may appear with the involvement of the parietotemporooccipital junction. Inferior parietal involvement may be accompanied by contralateral or ipsilateral rotatory movements with posturing of the limbs contralateral to the involved hemisphere. Visual illusions, such as macropsia, micropsia, or metamorphopsia, suggest the involvement of the posterior parietal cortex or parietotemporooccipital junction.

Electroencephalogram of Parietal Seizures

Interictal Scalp Electroencephalographic Recordings

Interictal scalp EEG recordings are often unrevealing in patients with focal seizures of presumed parietal origin (Williamson et al., 1992a; Mauguière and Courjon, 1978; Ajmone-Marsan and Ralston, 1957). About 20% of patients show no abnormalities (Williamson et al., 1992a), and the discharges are often widespread or they are localized to the midtem-

poral regions or the frontal and contralateral parietal regions (Williamson et al., 1992a; Swartz et al., 1990; Mauguière and Courjon, 1978). Painful seizures have been associated with interictal centroparietal, parietooccipital, or parietotemporal spikes (Trevathan and Cascino, 1988; Young and Blume, 1983). Disturbances of body image have been associated with interictal temporal, temporoparietal, or temporooccipital spikes (Kawai and Fujii, 1979).

Ictal Electroencephalogram of Parietal Seizures

The surface EEG is often normal during a simple somatosensory seizure (Cascino et al., 1993b; Williamson et al., 1992a; Devinsky et al., 1988), or it may show diffuse suppression or widespread abnormalities without a clear focal onset (Williamson et al., 1992a). However, parietal sharp waves may follow a nonlocalizing onset. A clearly lateralized ictal discharge can be observed in less than one-third of patients, and it is confined to the parietal lobe in only about 10% (Risinger, 2000).

OCCIPITAL LOBE SEIZURES: CLINICAL AND ELECTROENCEPHALOGRAPHIC FEATURES

Clinical Features

Symptoms of occipital lobe involvement are mainly subjective, and they may be shadowed by manifestations resulting from the spread to the contiguous cortex. Epileptic discharges affecting the *primary visual cortex* are characterized by elementary visual phenomena, which may be either positive (e.g., flashes, phosphenes, rotating colors) or, less commonly, negative (e.g., scotomas, hemianopsia, amaurosis). The location is in the visual hemifield contralateral to the lobe involved. With discharges that are located more anteriorly, the conjugate deviation of the head and eyes (version) is common. Version is, however, not necessarily contralateral. The deviation of the eyes may periodically be interrupted by brief jerks that return the eyes to the primary position, the so-called *epileptic nystagmus* (Thurston et al., 1985; Beun et al., 1984; White, 1971). Additional manifestations include eyelid flutter or forced closure of the eyelids and a sensation of eye pulling (Williamson et al., 1992b; Bancaud, 1969). Occipital discharges originating below the calcarine fissure tend to propagate to the temporal lobe, producing secondary alteration of consciousness, whereas supracalcarine discharges propagate to the parietal lobe and rolandic areas (Williamson et al., 1992b; Bancaud et al., 1973). Rapid spread of ictal activity to the frontal region and bilateral diffusion may cause drop attacks, consequently producing an impression of frontally originated seizures. Secondary generalization is occasionally observed (Wieser and Williamson, 1993).

Electroencephalographic Features of Occipital Seizures

Interictal Electroencephalogram

EEG recordings in children with visual seizures or clinical suspicion of an occipital lobe seizure origin should always be performed with a median occipital electrode, as well as with the conventional 10-20 system electrodes (Guerrini et al., 1995). In addition to improving the detection rate of abnormalities originating from the calcarine cortex, which is mesially located, such electrode positioning facilitates the evaluation of the background activity and the many physiologic activities whose maximum expression occurs in the occipital lobes (rhythm, posterior slowing in children).

Interictal paroxysmal EEG activity is commonly seen in patients with visual seizures. Only in a minority is such activity localized in the occipital lobe(s) on scalp EEG recordings (Aykut-Bingol et al., 1998; Munari et al., 1993; Salanova et al., 1992; Williamson et al., 1992b; Paillas et al., 1959). In most patients, spike or sharp waves are recorded over the temporal lobes; they are bilaterally independent in about one-fourth and bilaterally synchronous in more than one-third (Guerrini et al., 2000; Salanova et al., 1992). In no more than 10% of patients are the interictal spikes confined to the occipital lobe. An increase in posterior discharges upon eye closure is a common phenomenon in occipital epilepsies, whether lesional or idiopathic. Intermittent photic stimulation may produce asymmetric photic driving that is usually, but not necessarily, depressed on the side of the structural abnormality. A photoparoxysmal EEG response may be observed in about one-third of patients (Guerrini et al., 1997a; Ludwig and Ajmone-Marsan, 1975).

Ictal Electroencephalogram

Scalp EEG findings are of little avail for occipital lobe localization, and ictal recordings may be electrically silent (Bancaud, 1969). About 50% of cases show regional discharges involving the occipital and posterior temporal areas (Munari et al., 1993;

Salanova et al., 1993; Williamson et al., 1992b; Bancaud, 1969). In one series (Blume et al., 1991), seizures recorded with scalp EEG permitted the identification of the abnormal occipital lobe in 63% of cases. The latter value is relatively high, when one considers that occipital seizure onset is often of a multilobar origin and that a pure occipital seizure onset, as determined by depth electrodes, might be relatively rare (Kennett, 2000; Munari et al., 1993).

Extraoccipital spread may be rapid or remarkably slow, and it can occur after many minutes of discharge that is limited to the occipital area (Guerrini et al., 2000; Naquet et al., 1960; Jasper, 1954). With spread, the visual symptoms are often overshadowed by the most prominent manifestations resulting from extraoccipital involvement. Version, with slow turning of the head and eyes toward the side contralateral to the discharge, is particularly common when seizure activity involves the occipital convexity.

Invasive EEG studies are often necessary to clarify seizure origin and spread (Munari et al., 1994). Depth-electrode studies confirm that, even when the clinical semiology is strongly indicative of occipital origin, ictal discharges can involve the mesial temporal structures or the parietal cortex immediately (Munari et al., 1993; Williamson et al., 1992a). The origin of the occipital discharge is more commonly pericalcarine, but simultaneous involvement of the lateral occipital cortex may also occur (Munari et al., 1993). A location of the discharge in the calcarine cortex in the mesial occipital surface explains why ictal electrographic changes during visual seizures may be difficult to recognize on surface recordings.

TEMPORAL LOBE SEIZURES: CLINICAL AND ELECTROENCEPHALOGRAPHIC FEATURES

Clinical Features

Seizures originating in the temporal lobe are thought to account for a large majority of cases of seizures with alteration of consciousness (Wieser and Kausel, 1987; Wieser and Metes, 1980). However, extratemporal seizures may be even more common, especially in children (Williamson et al., 1993; Chauvel et al., 1992a; Fusco et al., 1990). Seizures with and without alteration of consciousness often coexist in the same patient. The attacks are usually prolonged, lasting 1 to 2 minutes. Autonomic manifestations and psychic and sensory symptoms can represent the whole of a more complex episode evolving into alteration of consciousness or only its onset (aura) (Bancaud, 1987).

Hippocampal-amygdala (mesiobasal-limbic [Wieser, 1986]), *primary rhinencephalic* (Munari et al., 1979; Bancaud and Talairach, 1975), or *mesial temporal seizure origin* (Wieser et al., 1993) is characterized by an initial sensation of rising epigastric discomfort or nausea, often accompanied by fear, panic, and intense autonomic phenomena (pallor or flushing of the face are especially prominent in children). According to Wieser (1987), 65% of such seizures have their onset in both the hippocampus and the amygdala, 26% in the hippocampus only, 6% in the amygdala only, and 4% in other limbic formations. The seizures preferentially propagate along certain pathways, although a wide variability may be seen among patients and even within a single patient (Wieser, 1987). The propagation of seizures with mesiobasal onset is rapid, and it mainly occurs to the contralateral hippocampus; however, some attacks spread to the cingulate gyrus or to the orbital and lateral frontal cortex (Lieb et al., 1976, 1981).

Lateral (or neocortical) temporal origin is often characterized by auditory or complex perceptual visual hallucinations, illusions, a dreamy state, or vertiginous symptoms (Commission on the Classification and Terminology of the ILAE, 1989). The impairment of consciousness may begin with motor arrest or staring, followed by oral alimentary automatisms. However, the automatisms may appear while the patient is still responsive or when his or her consciousness is fluctuating. Amnesia for the ictal event is generally seen after alteration of consciousness, but this may be present even when the patient has apparently retained consciousness. Postictal confusion and, in small children, postictal sleep are common.

Temporal lobe seizures of neocortical origin are less common than limbic attacks (Avanzini et al., 2001). Such seizures often spread to the ipsilateral mesiobasal-limbic stations, which can act as secondary "pacemaker areas," permitting maintenance and further propagation of the ictal events that are thus relayed (Wieser and Kausel, 1987). This is the rationale for "palliative amygdalohippocampectomy" as treatment for seizures originating in surgically inaccessible areas (Wieser, 1988; Wieser and Yasargil, 1987).

Neocortical and rhinencephalic epilepsy can combine. The generation of a dreamy state requires simultaneous involvement of both the temporal neocortex and the mesial limbic structures (Bancaud et al., 1994; Munari and Bancaud, 1985; Munari et al., 1979). A dual pathology, with dysplastic or tumoral lesions of the neocortex and associated hippocampal sclerosis, is not rare (Raymond et al., 1994a; Levesque et al., 1991).

Language impairment indicates the involvement of the dominant hemisphere. The typical manifestations of complex partial seizures of temporal lobe origin are fully expressed in children beginning at a preschool age; motionless staring with minor or no automatisms (also defined as "hypomotor seizures") (Lüders et al., 2000) predominate in infants and small children (Hamer et al., 1999; Brockhaus and Elger, 1995; Wyllie, 1995).

Electroencephalographic Features of Temporal Lobe Seizures

Interictal Electroencephalogram

The most common interictal EEG pattern associated with focal seizures of temporal lobe origin are spikes or sharp waves over the anterior temporal area (Gibbs and Gibbs, 1952). These may be unilateral, but, even in such cases, in only 84 (63%) of 133 patients was the interictal surface paroxysmal activity in good agreement with the side of seizure activity recorded through depth electrodes, whereas partial disagreement was seen in 27% and total discrepancy in 10% (Wieser, 1983b). Some patients may have an additional spike focus at the midtemporal or posterior temporal area (Kanner et al., 1993). Anterior temporal delta activity is seen in some patients with mesial temporal sclerosis who have seizures with alteration of consciousness (Gambardella et al., 1995a). In some patients, a specific theta-wave rhythm is present in the temporal area (Gastaut et al., 1985). The determination of the dipolar source of the paroxysmal abnormalities indicates that anterior temporal lobe epilepsy is associated with a dipole of characteristic orientation (Ebersole, 1992; Ebersole and Wade, 1990, 1991). However, anterior temporal foci may also be observed in patients with frontal (Quesney, 1992) or occipital (Williamson et al., 1992b, 1993) epileptogenic areas.

Bilateral discharges are present in one-fourth to one-third of patients (Gibbs and Gibbs, 1952), even when unilateral hippocampal atrophy is proven to exist (Gambardella et al., 1995b). The bilateral foci were independent in 23% (Daly and Pedley, 1990) to 80% (Gastaut et al., 1953) of patients. Some have suggested that a more than 90% side predominance of bilateral interictal spikes indicates lateralization for the purpose of epilepsy surgery (Chung et al., 1991). This view is not universally accepted, however (Spencer et al., 1982).

Extratemporal foci are seen in 15% to 20% of patients experiencing focal seizures with alteration of consciousness (Quesney, 1986, 1992). Bilateral spike or SW discharges are less common. They may be triggered by "buried foci" in the temporal or frontal cortex (Sadler and Blume, 1989; Gastaut et al., 1953). Exceedingly diverse ictal symptoms may occur in patients with alteration of consciousness whose interictal EEG discharges are indistinguishable with regard to appearance and location (Daly and Pedley, 1990). Fish et al. (1991) studied 20 adult patients with small, indolent extratemporal lesions who showed secondary involvement of the hippocampus, as indicated by ictal and interictal EEG and clinical features. Seven of these had hippocampal sclerosis, gliosis, or cell loss in the hippocampus. Conversely, clinically significant epileptiform potentials may be seen over other parts of the temporal lobe (Daly and Pedley, 1990) or outside its anatomic limits, especially in the frontal region (Quesney, 1987). Ictal fear was more common in patients with unilateral temporal spikes, than in those with bilateral temporal spikes. Automatic behavior was seen in 95% of patients with temporal spiking, compared with 53% of patients with frontocentral foci and 61% of those with central paroxysms (Gastaut et al., 1953).

Nonparoxysmal tracings are common in children with alteration of consciousness (Holmes, 1986; Yamamoto et al., 1987b). A normal interictal EEG was found in roughly 20% to 40% of patients of all ages with "complex partial seizures" (Gibbs and Gibbs, 1952). This figure is reduced to approximately 10% when sleep records, activation procedures, and additional electrodes are used (Degen and Degen, 1984).

Acharya et al. (1997) observed that unifocal interictal spikes were uncommon in infants and small children with "hypomotor seizures" who tended to have either no spikes or multiregional spikes. Other authors had previously stressed that interictal spikes are rarely observed in infants with "complex partial seizures" (Yamamoto et al., 1987b; Holmes, 1986). However, when interictal spikes are present, they correspond with the ictal onset area (Acharya et al., 1997; Blume, 1989). Interictal EEG seems, therefore, to have a low sensitivity but a high specificity for identifying the seizure focus in infants and young children with alteration of consciousness.

Ictal Electroencephalogram

Focal seizures with alteration of consciousness have been extensively studied from an EEG point of view (Morris et al., 1987; Lindsay et al., 1984; Engel et al., 1982b; Spencer, 1981; Wieser and Metes, 1980; Lieb et al., 1976; Bancaud et al., 1973; Ludwig et al., 1962; Gastaut and Roger, 1955), and a detailed description is

beyond the scope of this book. Gastaut and Broughton (1972) indicated that the complete absence of any recognizable EEG discharge during "complex partial seizures" is rare and that this is present in only 5% when consciousness is lost (versus 30% to 40% when it is intact). However, brief seizures with alteration of consciousness of frontal or parietal origin tend to occur without concomitant changes on the surface EEG (Risinger, 2000; Williamson et al., 1985, 1992b).

Because consciousness becomes impaired only when the seizure activity has propagated to a sufficiently large area of the brain, extracranial EEG recordings almost always show discernible changes during alteration of consciousness (Risinger, 2000). Widespread or asymmetric, rhythmic or arrhythmic changes represent the most common EEG correlate of alteration of consciousness. A progression can be identified in most patients in the surface EEG (Risinger, 2000), which consists of a sustained rhythmic or nearly rhythmic discharge with a variable degree of regional predominance, if any, evolving with more diffuse, higher-amplitude, slower frequencies. A less commonly observed ictal pattern is represented by focal or lateralized SW discharges, which are apparent from the onset of the seizure (Risinger, 2000; Engel, 1987).

More characteristic ictal EEG changes relative to seizure origin in specific brain areas may sometimes be encountered. In approximately 70% to 80% of patients in whom alteration of consciousness occurs during seizures of mesial temporal lobe origin, a "prototypic" EEG pattern is observed (Gastaut and Tassinari, 1975a). It includes rhythmic, 4-Hz to 7-Hz activity, which becomes progressively slower, possibly reaching 2 Hz. The discharge may be unilateral at onset, generally predominating over one temporal or temporofrontal region (Blume et al., 1984; Geiger and Hanrer, 1978); it then tends to diffuse bilaterally as the seizure proceeds while still remaining asymmetric in most cases (Fig. 10.4). The use of additional surface electrodes reveals that this characteristic "temporal" rhythm predominates in the anterior and inferior temporal regions (Risinger, 2000). This rhythmic pattern may either appear as the initial ictal EEG change, or it may follow a diffuse attenuation of EEG activities. The first scalp EEG changes may occur after clinical onset in about 90% of patients (Williamson et al., 1993). Less commonly, a positive rhythm located at the vertex or parasagittal convexity has been observed either in isolation or in association with the more typical rhythmic anterior temporal discharge (Pacia and Ebersole, 1997).

Discharges confined to the hippocampus do not usually produce recognizable scalp abnormalities (Pacia

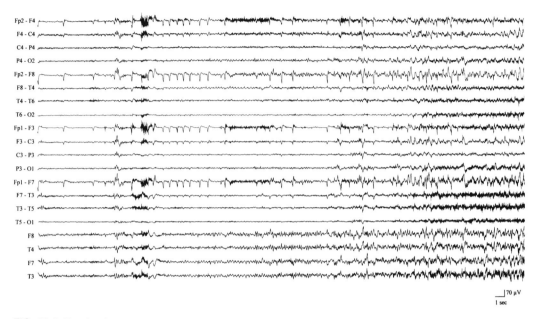

FIG. 10.4. Focal seizure recorded in a 14-year-old girl with right hippocampal sclerosis and intractable partial epilepsy since the second year of life. At the age of 2 years, she suffered a right unilateral clonic febrile status. Electrographic seizure onset is characterized by a generalized burst of sharp waves with frontotemporal emphasis, followed by a buildup of rhythmic theta activity that clearly is predominant over the anterior temporal and centrotemporal area (F8–T4). The rhythmic ictal activity remains focal for about 30 seconds to become subsequently more diffuse. During the first 15 seconds of the seizure, the girl complains of an epigastric sensation but remains calm; she then initially looks frightened; subsequently appears terrified; screams meaningless sentences, becoming unresponsive; and starts oral alimentary automatisms. The whole episode lasts about 1 minute, and it is followed by slow recovery. A right temporal lobectomy at the age of 15 years rendered the patient seizure free.

and Ebersole, 1997), and, in general, temporal lobe seizures without alteration of consciousness are accompanied by surface ictal abnormalities in only about 40% of patients (Sirven et al., 1996; Bare et al., 1994).

Postictal abnormalities, especially slow waves but also the attenuation of background activity or the activation of spikes, are often present in the area of the seizure's origin (Kaibara and Blume, 1988). The "prototypic" ictal EEG pattern described earlier is not specific to mesial temporal seizure onset, as it may sometimes be observed even with temporal neocortical seizures, which probably have rapidly propagated to the mesial structures (Risinger, 2000). Therefore, considerable overlap is seen between cases of mesial and lateral onset in both the mechanisms and the patterns underlying the EEG expression of such seizure types (Ebersole and Pacia, 1996).

Other types of discharges occur in 20% to 30% of patients with temporal lobe seizure origin. The absence of spikes or sharp waves and the diffusion of the discharges that are usually recorded over the relatively large scalp areas even at onset appear to be due to the fact that seizure generators are remote from the recording electrodes; therefore, they represent projected activity from the deep limbic structures. The localizing and lateralizing value of this type of EEG abnormality is consequently limited (Sammaritano et al., 1987, 1991).

An electrodecremental event (flattening of the EEG traces) occurs in two-thirds of the seizures just before or at the time of onset, but it generally is of brief duration. Flattening is not restricted to seizures of temporal origin. In those, however, it occurs without any recognizable initial paroxysmal complex, whereas an initial SW is often observed with frontal seizures (Wieser, 1983b). Low-voltage, very fast (18 to 30 Hz) activity that is either localized or bitemporally located is relatively common (Feldman, 1983b). Several patterns may occur in succession during the same seizure, or they may alternate in different attacks (Blume et al., 1984; Anziska and Cracco, 1977).

Typical 3-Hz SW complexes have been described in children with "complex partial seizures." Many of these discharges probably are examples of the so-called SW stupor or absence status (Doose, 1992), rather than complex partial seizures. However, little doubt exists that temporal or especially frontal foci can trigger generalized SW complexes (Bancaud et al., 1974).

Ictal scalp EEG recordings in infants and young children with "hypomotor" seizures (Acharya et al., 1997) has shown seizure onset in the posterior temporal, temporoparietal, and temporooccipital areas of one or both hemispheres independently in most. An anteromesial temporal seizure onset was seen in none of these. A similar posteriorly predominant seizure onset was also stressed by Duchowny et al. (1994) in children with temporal lobe epilepsy.

SYNDROMES WITH PREDOMINANTLY FOCAL SEIZURES

This section is devoted to those epilepsies that are characterized predominantly or exclusively by focal seizures, even though other types of seizures, especially generalized tonic-clonic ones, commonly are associated with them. As Chapter 2 indicates, in the 1981 revision of the International Classification of Epileptic Seizures, focal seizures are defined as seizures with a local onset in one cerebral hemisphere (Aird et al., 1989; Parsonage, 1983; Commission on Classification and Terminology of the ILAE, 1981).

The symptoms of focal seizures may be of many different kinds, including motor, sensory, cognitive, or affective. In a significant proportion of the patients, the clinical manifestations include disturbances of consciousness with alteration of awareness or responsiveness. Such cases were termed *complex partial seizures* in the ILAE classification of 1989, and those seizures in which consciousness remained intact were termed *simple partial seizures*.

This dichotomy based on the level of consciousness is no longer advised in the proposal for a new classification from the Task Force of the ILAE (Engel, 2001). Instead, this scheme prefers the term *focal* to *partial* or *localization-related* seizures and the criterion of alteration of consciousness because the presence or absence of a decrease in or the loss of awareness or responsiveness seems too difficult to assess accurately. In addition, the occurrence of seizures with and without alteration of consciousness, as it was previously defined, in the same patient is common, and the presence of such changes simply indicates a wider propagation of the epileptic discharge, which does not fundamentally change the localizing significance of the seizures. Any localized discharge can propagate to other structures, especially to limbic ones, with a resulting secondary "complex partial" seizure. Finally, the generalization of a partial seizure is not uncommon. This may take place following the complete sequence of a "simple partial seizure" followed first by involvement of half the body or suddenly at any moment in a "simple partial seizure" sequence. Generalization of a simple partial seizure can be so rapid that the initial focal features of the seizure may not be apparent to the observer, even though the patient may experience a brief sensory or autonomic sensation. Alternatively, a partial discharge can occur in a clinically "silent" cortical area so that even the patient is not aware of any focal feature. Such rapid generalization is especially common with discharges originating in the frontal lobe. These seizures, which are termed *secondarily generalized seizures*, are often misclassified as primary generalized ones unless they occur at the time of EEG recording or they are regularly associated with a localized spike focus. Sleep studies may help differentiate seizures with secondary generalization from seizures that are generalized from onset. In the first group, sleep often activates an EEG focus that is imperceptible in waking records, whereas, in the second group, the EEG records only bilateral synchronous paroxysms. Likewise, a focus may sometimes be evidenced by the suppression of the associated generalized abnormalities that were masking it (e.g., by injection of diazepam) (Blume and Pillay, 1985) or by techniques of activation (e.g., the use of methohexital) (Erba and Browne, 1983).

Although focal seizures had been widely thought to be due primarily to the presence of a brain lesion, which, therefore, implied the need for performing multiple investigations to determine the nature and plan management, the recognition of the common occurrence of focal seizures that are unassociated with any detectable structural brain abnormality has represented a major progress in the understanding and management of focal seizures. The first such syndrome was benign rolandic or centrotemporal epilepsy, which was followed by the recognition of several other types, leading to the concept of idiopathic focal epilepsy syndromes. This concept is important from both the theoretical and practical points of view. A complete neuroradiologic evaluation of all patients with partial seizures is not warranted if many suffer from epilepsies unassociated with structural brain damage. In addition, such epilepsies are usually less severe than those caused by structural lesions, and some disappear quite predictably, thus leading to the concept of "benign" partial epilepsies (see Chapter 22).

In this chapter, the main epilepsy syndromes with predominantly focal seizures are classified into the following two subgroups: (a) *b*enign *e*pilepsy with *c*entro*r*olandic *s*pikes (BECRS) or *b*enign *e*pilepsy with *c*entro*t*emporal *s*pikes (BECTS) and related syndromes, including occipital and parietal epilepsies, as well as other less well-defined types without evidence of a lesion; and (b) the lesional epilepsies of childhood with partial seizures with or without AC.

These various syndromes are variably defined, and they have differing significances. Some, like BECRS, have been extensively studied, and, thus, they are extremely well defined, whereas others are only tentatively isolated or poorly delineated.

IDIOPATHIC FOCAL (OR PARTIAL) EPILEPSIES

Idiopathic focal epilepsies comprise a large group of syndromes characterized by seizures of focal origin in which no structural brain abnormality is detectable and for which a functional mechanism for the epilepsy and EEG features is generally accepted (Panayiotopoulos, 1999; Dalla Bernardina et al., 1992c; Loiseau, 1992; Roger et al., 1990). This group includes several syndromes, including benign rolandic epilepsy; benign epilepsy with occipital paroxysms with an early onset and those types with a late-onset; idiopathic photosensitive occipital lobe epilepsy; and some less well-defined syndromes, such as benign epilepsy with evoked parietal spikes and benign epilepsy with affective symptoms. These syndromes share common clinical and EEG features (Dalla Bernardina et al., 1992c). The seizures occur infrequently, and they are often related to sleep. They remit spontaneously after a few years, and they are not associated with neurologic disturbances or mental retardation (except in some special cases, see "Relatively Benign Epilepsies" in Chapter 22). Some mild neuropsychologic anomalies are possible, but they usually do not outlast the period of active seizures. Certain types of manifestations, such as automatisms, and predominating disturbances of consciousness are not observed. The EEG abnormalities feature mainly high-amplitude sharp waves that often appear in clusters. They are exaggerated in sleep, during which time polyspike-waves are not seen and they appear on an essentially normal background.

These features, which vary with the degree of brain maturation and with specific syndromes, have been interpreted as representing different aspects of a "syndrome of benign childhood seizure susceptibility" (Panayiotopoulos, 1999, 2002; Ferrie et al., 1997) that is closely age (and maturation) related and that virtually always remits before adolescence.

Although this favorable course is the rule, rare cases with more severe outcome are possible and the term *benign* may not apply to certain forms, such as CSWS and Landau-Kleffner syndrome (see Chapter 11), which seem to have a close relationship with the benign idiopathic epilepsies. Moreover, milder cognitive and behavioral disturbances may be present, although their practical significance has not been fully assessed.

In the past few years, several other epilepsy syndromes, including the following, have been added to the group of idiopathic partial epilepsies: frontal lobe nocturnal epilepsy, familial temporal lobe epilepsy with or without auditory symptoms, idiopathic epilepsy with multiple foci, and RE with bulbar symptoms and anticipation. Although some of the reported cases of these proposed syndromes clearly belong to the idiopathic group, as the demonstration of their genetic origin proves (Hirose et al., 2002; Picard et al., 2000), the nosologic situation of many of these cases is not yet entirely clear, especially in those cases in which a monogenic origin has not yet been demonstrated. Moreover, the determination of the topographic origin is often uncertain, because a clear EEG localization of the origin of the seizures and even of their involvement by the discharge has often not been proved. These syndromes are, therefore, described separately because of the uncertainties about their origin and mechanisms.

Rolandic Epilepsy, Benign Epilepsy with Centrorolandic or Centrotemporal Spikes

BECRS is also known as *benign partial epilepsy of childhood* (Aicardi, 1983b), sylvian epilepsy (Lombroso, 1967), lingual syndrome, and BECT (Heijbel et al., 1975a). It is the most common and most characteristic form of "idiopathic" partial epilepsy. The term implies the absence of a brain lesion and a genetic propensity to seizures (Commission on the Classification and Terminology of the ILAE, 1989). Both have been demonstrated in BECRS, but it is possible that the presence of localized brain damage may act as a triggering and localizing factor in genetically predisposed children or that, in rare cases, it may even be the sole cause of seizures mimicking BECRS (Ambrosetto, 1992; Lüders et al., 1987b). In a vast majority of patients, a genetically determined cortical excitability is sufficient to produce the characteristic EEG abnormalities, which, in a few patients, are accompanied by clinical seizures. Lüders (1987b) estimated that only 8.8% of children with rolandic spikes have seizures, which indicates the low epileptogenicity of this type of neurophysiologic dysfunction. The localized character of the EEG abnormalities and seizures might be explained by local variations in cortical excitability as a function of brain maturation, with epileptogenicity disappearing when a particular cortical area has reached full maturation (Roger et al., 1990; Lüders et al., 1987b).

The syndrome is characterized by (a) the onset of the seizures between 2 and 14 years of age (usually between 3 and 10 years), (b) simple partial motor seizures as an exclusive or dominant type of seizure in the vast majority of cases, (c) characteristic EEG foci occurring on a normal background tracing in the lower rolandic (sylvian or "midtemporal") area, and (d) the absence of neurologic or intellectual abnormalities before and during the period of seizure activity.

BECRS, the most common type of partial motor epilepsy in childhood, accounts for 16% of the epilepsies beginning before 15 years of age (Cavazzuti, 1980; Heijbel et al., 1975a) and 24% of those with onset between 5 and 14 years of age (Beaussart, 1972). In specialized centers for epilepsy, BECRS accounts for 62% to 67% of idiopathic partial epilepsies (Roger et al., 1990). Deonna et al. (1986b) found a much higher figure (36%) for the incidence of BECTS in a presumably less biased series. The peak frequency of onset is at 5 to 8 years, and 83% of cases begin between 4 and 10 years of age (Beaumanoir et al., 1974); virtually all patients have an onset by 13 years of age. A smaller peak may exist around 3 years of age (Dalla Bernardina et al., 1992c).

Some investigators (Blume, 1989; Dravet et al., 1989; Maekawa et al., 1980) have discussed the possibility of early cases in the first 2 years of age. However, the recent description of a number of cases of idiopathic partial epilepsies of infancy (the genetic cases are reviewed in Picard et al., 2000) (see Chapter 13) that may belong to several syndromes casts doubt on the existence of early cases of RE because most cases appear to have different clinical and EEG features and they seem to be genetically unrelated to RE, even when small spikes were recorded (Bureau et al., 2002; Capovilla et al., 2000) (see Chapter 13).

The Seizures

Partial seizures comprise 70% to 80% of the fits (Loiseau and Beaussart, 1973). These may be the only type of attack, or they may alternate with generalized fits, which occur in 24% to 80% of patients. Most partial seizures are mainly motor in type, but sensory phenomena occur in 7% to 100% of patients (Roger et al., 1990; Lüders et al., 1987b). The discrepancy is probably due to underreporting by children and to difficulties in differentiating between sensory and motor phenomena.

Remarkably, partial seizures involve one side of the face preferentially (37%); the oropharyngeal muscles (53%); and, to a lesser extent, the upper limb (20%). The lower limb is affected in only 8% of seizures (Loiseau and Beaussart, 1973). Facial seizures consist of a tonic contraction of one side of the face and/or clonic jerks of the cheek and eyelids. Oropharyngeal signs comprise one or several of the following: guttural sounds, often described by parents in nocturnal seizures as "sounds from the throat, gurgling noise" or "as if the child were about to vomit;" movements of the mouth (e.g., "my mouth moved, my teeth chattered, my tongue trembled"); the contraction of the jaws, which feel tight or deviate to one side; a feeling of suffocation; and profuse salivation. The sensory symptoms most often involve the corner of the mouth, the inside of one cheek, the tongue and gums, or teeth, and a narrowly localized sensation inside or about the mouth that may be described as "a dry throat" or "my tongue prickled" may be present. Buccal paresthesias are a common feature, and the child should systematically be questioned about these because they may represent the most characteristic sign of some seizures that can be difficult to recognize.

The profuse salivation is often particularly striking even in the absence of marked motor oropharyngeal phenomena. Arrest of speech with preservation of comprehension occurs in more than 40% of seizures (Loiseau and Beaussart, 1973).

Such seizures have been sometimes referred to as *rulandic seizures* after the sixteenth century author Martinus Rulandus, who gave their first precise description in a 10-year-old boy with such seizures (Van Huffelen, 1989). Indeed, such attacks are highly suggestive of the diagnosis. Consciousness is retained throughout the seizure in most attacks and, less often, only in their initial phase. An inability to speak is common (39%), although the children know what they want to say and they may utter inarticulate sounds. When the arm is involved, it mostly consists of clonic jerks; a jacksonian march is, however, rare.

Strictly localized seizures are extremely brief, lasting from a few seconds to 1 or 2 minutes; they occur more often in children older than 5 years of age; and they are often diurnal, especially in the early morning (Roger et al., 1990; Beaussart, 1972). In younger children, the seizures tend to be less localized, and they may involve a complete half of the body. Such seizures tend to be nocturnal, and they are often longer than the more localized attacks, lasting several minutes or even half an hour. Long attacks are followed at times by a Todd hemiplegia, although this is uncommon (Dalla Bernardina et al., 1982). Some impairment of consciousness is the rule with prolonged fits. The incidence of these long-lasting seizures has been variably estimated from 12% (Loiseau and Beaussart, 1973), 14% (Beaussart, 1972), to up to 22% (Dalla Bernardina et al., 1985b, 1992c).

Generalized seizures may be the only ictal manifestation of BECRS. However, such generalized fits are mainly nocturnal; therefore, a focal onset may easily go unrecognized, particularly because diffusion of a paroxysmal discharge occurs much faster in slow sleep than in the waking state. Indeed, in several cases (Panayiotopoulos, 1999; Ambrosetto and Gobbi, 1975; Dalla Bernardina and Tassinari, 1975), the sequence of a focal onset that is rapidly followed by generalization has been recorded on sleep tracings.

The relationship of the seizures of BECRS with sleep is striking (Dalla Bernardina et al., 1985b). Only 5% to 25% of them occur exclusively during wakefulness. In more than 50% of patients, the attacks occur only during sleep; in the remaining children, they occur in both states. Approximately 25% of the nocturnal fits take place during the middle part of the night; 20% appear upon falling asleep, and 35% occur upon awakening or in the 2 hours that precede awakening. Diurnal seizures often are observed when the children are inactive or bored (e.g., during automobile journeys), and these are probably at least partially related to episodes of dozing off. Nonetheless, some seizures do occur when the child is fully alert; these are almost always of the localized facial type.

Other types of seizure are rare. Febrile convulsions can precede the seizures of BECRS in 10% to 20% of patients (Bouma et al., 1997). Absences with typical EEG abnormalities were often found by Beaumanoir et al. (1974), but, since then, these have been rarely mentioned (Panayiotopoulos, 1999).

The frequency of seizures in BECRS is usually low. Approximately one-fourth of the patients have only one attack (Beaussart and Faou, 1978), and, in such cases, using the term *epilepsy* seems disputable, although the clinical and EEG characteristics are the same as those in patients with repeated fits. Approximately half of the patients have fewer than 5 fits, and only 8% have 20 seizures or more (Loiseau and Beaussart, 1973). When the seizures do occur frequently, they are generally seen in clusters that are separated by long intervals (up to several months). The total duration of seizure activity tends to be brief. It is less than 1 year in 21%, 1 to 2 years in 18%, 2 to

5 years in 20%, and 3 to 8 years in only 7% (Beaussart and Faou, 1978). The clinical expression often varies during the course; for example, diurnal fits may replace nocturnal attacks without apparent reason, or focal seizures may follow generalized ones.

The absence of frank interictal neurologic or mental impairment is one of the criteria of BECRS. A variety of minor disturbances in behavior and in fine motor control have, however, been reported in association with rolandic spike foci with or without seizures (Massa et al., 2001; Van der Meij et al., 1992a, 1992b, 1992c; Dalla Bernardina and Beghini, 1976; Loiseau et al., 1962).

The reported disturbances have included a possible effect on language lateralization on the side opposite the focus (Piccirilli, 1988); small differences in cognitive performance, mainly on tests of attention and visuomotor skills between patients and controls (Croona et al., 1999; d'Alessandro et al., 1990); intellectual and behavioral deficits on a battery of neuropsychologic tests (Weglage et al., 1997); and language dysfunction on some tests (Staden et al., 1998). The significance of these abnormalities is not easy to assess. Loiseau et al. (1983b) found that the achievements of children with RE were within the limits of the general population and that they were clearly superior as a group to those of children with absence seizures. The social insertion of children with RE was also satisfactory, and it was better than that in the absence group. Hommet et al. (2001) studied 33 adolescents and young adults who recovered from RE, comparing them with 33 controls without history of neurologic problem. They found no significant difference with respect to memory, language, and executive function. They found some differences on one task of language lateralization and speculated that these could result from the interference of paroxysmal abnormalities with the development of cortical specialization. Overall, these minor dysfunctions do not seem to outlast the active epilepsy period or to interfere with cognition and behavior in later life. They may, however, have a practical importance by temporarily disturbing learning processes and school achievement (Deonna et al., 2000).

A possible association of RE with migraine has been suggested (Dalla Bernardina and Beghini, 1976; Vassella et al., 1973; Loiseau et al., 1962), but the frequency of migraine does not seem to be increased over that in the general population and no well-controlled study is available.

Interictal Electroencephalographic Abnormalities

Interictal EEG abnormalities are, on the other hand, an essential part of the syndrome. The typical pattern of benign focal epileptiform discharges (Van der Meij et al., 1992b; Lüders et al., 1987b) is characterized not only by its location, which may indeed be variable, but also mostly by its waveform, field of distribution, and activation by sleep.

The waveform consists of a negative sharp wave (average duration of 88 ms) with a relatively blunted peak, followed by a prominent positive wave whose amplitude may be up to 50% of that of the preceding sharp wave (Lüders et al., 1987b) and only inconsistently by a smaller negative wave. The sharp waves are usually of high amplitude (mostly more than 100 µV), and they tend to be remarkably stereotypic in form and distribution. They do not form polyspikes, but they do tend to occur often and they are often grouped in short bursts of 1.5 to 3 Hz (Van der Meij et al., 1992b; Blume et al., 1984). No relationship is found between the frequency or extent of the sharp waves and the seizure frequency or duration. The discharges usually appear on a normal background rhythm. In the rare patients in which repeated seizures occur, some slowing may be observed in the same location (Fig. 10.5).

Drury and Beydoun (1991) have suggested that, in some cases, monomorphic sharp waves replace the classic sharp waves and that they have the same significance.

The benign epileptiform discharges are mainly localized to the centrotemporal region of the hemisphere contralateral to the clinical seizures. However, they may be located more posteriorly, especially in children younger than 5 years (Lüders et al., 1987b).

Some investigators think that foci can "migrate" from the occipital to the centrorolandic area but not in the reverse direction (Andermann and Oguni, 1990). Others believe that the succession of foci first in the occipital area and then in the rolandic area is the result of an age-dependent shift in cortical excitability, rather than a real migration (Panayiotopoulos, 1999). In one-third of patients, sharp waves occur bilaterally in either a synchronous or an asynchronous manner. The topography of the paroxysms may change, and bilateral and unilateral foci may be found on different tracings in the same patient. Legarda et al. (1994) found two subgroups among their 33 patients; 23 had a classic focus at the lower part of the central region,

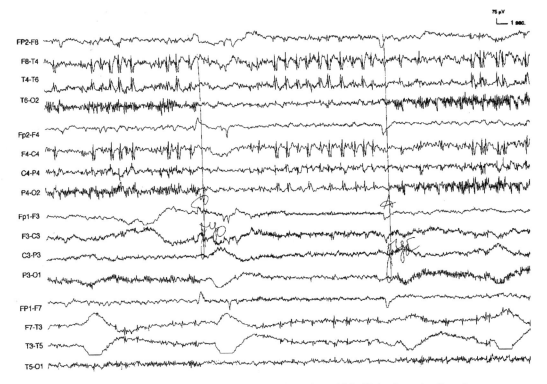

FIG. 10.5. Front left centrotemporal sharp wave focus in a child with benign rolandic epilepsy.

and 10 had a focus in the high central region. The clinical symptomatology varied in accordance with the topography; low foci were associated with orofacial ictal features, and high foci were seen with seizures that often involved the hand. Multifocal independent foci may be found in a few patients (Loiseau and Cohadon, 1981). The topography and frequency of the sharp waves is not correlated with the frequency or severity of the seizures (Van der Meij et al., 1992c).

Most investigators think that the morphology of the sharp waves in BECRS is characteristic and that the sharp waves associated with epilepsies caused by brain damage are of briefer duration and sharper configuration (Lüders et al., 1987b; Blume, 1982; Beaussart, 1972). However, quantitative analysis (Van der Meij et al., 1992a, 1992c) has shown that differentiating the rolandic sharp waves in BECRS from those in

patients without seizures and those in cases of cerebral palsy or other organic brain lesions may not be possible. Topographic analysis with brain-mapping techniques of the ascending phase of the rolandic spike, rather than the peak, seems to differentiate patients with epilepsy from those without (Van der Meij et al., 1992b).

The field of distribution is characteristic. The main negative spike component of the rolandic spike can usually be modeled by a single and stable tangential dipolar source, with the negative pole at the centrotemporal region and the positive pole at the frontal regions (Gregory and Wong, 1992). This tangential dipole has been confirmed by MEG (Baumgartner et al., 1995). Quantitative topographic study of the rolandic spikes has shown a unipolar rather than a bipolar field with a negative potential in the centrotemporal region in some children (Van der Meij et al., 1992b), and a

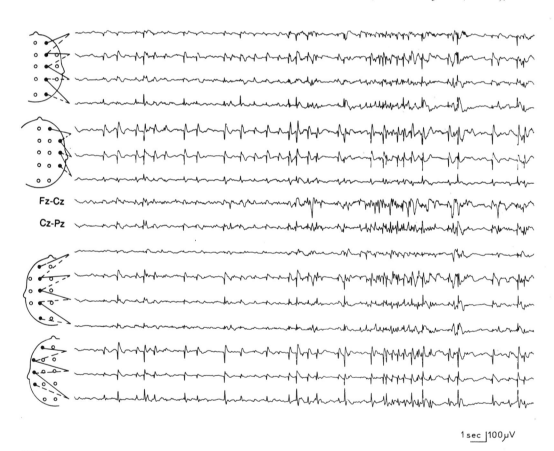

1 sec |100μV

FIG. 10.6. An 11-year, 6-month-old boy with benign rolandic epilepsy. Upon falling asleep, an important activation of typical rolandic sharp waves that are bilateral and synchronous occurs. Such discharges are intermingled with sleep transients, such as vertex spikes and spindles (right side of the figure, especially over the Fz-Cz and Cz-Pz channels), giving the false impression of multiple spike activity. Such an activation of discharges upon falling asleep is not unusual in rolandic epilepsy but it tends to be less pronounced during deeper sleep.

similar field distribution could also be observed in patients with organic brain damage. Van der Meij et al. (1992c) found using dipole source analysis that the estimated source could be ascribed to the depth of the lowermost point of the precentral cortex, which is in very good agreement with the cortical representation of the oropharyngeal region, so the term *midtemporal spikes* is inaccurate. The EEG paroxysms vary with time. They may disappear or reappear suddenly, or they may switch from one side to the other, an observation that argues against the presence of a structural lesion (Roger et al., 1990). They significantly increase in frequency during drowsiness and all the stages of sleep (Dalla Bernardina and Beghini, 1976). The amplitude of the paroxysms increases during slow sleep but decreases during REM sleep. During slow sleep, they tend to diffuse to the ipsilateral and sometimes the contralateral hemisphere. The absence of paroxysms on one or even several tracings cannot be taken as definite evidence against the diagnosis of BECRS. However, their consistent absence on repeated EEGs, *including sleep records*, is very rare, and, in such patients, the diagnosis should be accepted only with great reservation.

The frequency of bursts of generalized SW activity is diversely appreciated. Figures ranging from 13% to 40% have been reported (Dalla Bernardina et al., 1992c; Beaumanoir et al., 1974; Beaussart, 1972), whereas Lüders (Lüders et al., 1987b), who asserts that true SW discharges are very rare, believes that many reported SWs may have been physiologic elements, such as hypnagogic discharges.

The usual activating procedures (hyperventilation and intermittent photic stimulation) do not provoke the occurrence of paroxysms. Sleep consistently and considerably increases both the frequency and the diffusion of interictal abnormalities (Dalla Bernardina et al., 1978b, 1985b; Blom and Heijbel, 1975). Both slow sleep and REM sleep enhance the spike activity (Dalla Bernardina and Beghini, 1976), whereas, in patients with rolandic spikes but without seizures, only slow sleep is said to activate the EEG (Fig. 10.6).

Ictal Electroencephalograms

A few ictal EEGs in cases of RE have been recorded (Fig. 10.7). Focal seizures begin with fast rhythms and spikes in the rolandic area that is contralateral to the seizure, with a progressive increase in amplitude and admixture of slow waves that can produce SW or polyspike-wave figures. The generalized seizures that have been recorded had a similar focal onset with secondary generalization (Panayiotopou-

los 1999; Gutierrez et al., 1990; Ambrosetto and Gobbi, 1975; Dalla Bernardina and Tassinari, 1975; Lerman and Kivity, 1975). The reversal of the dipole during seizures (i.e., positive ictal spikes at the lower rolandic electrode in the late part of a seizure) has been considered a diagnostically significant feature (Gutierrez et al., 1990).

Course and Prognosis

The course of *BECRS* is remarkable in that the epilepsy consistently remits before 16 years of age, usually around the age of 9 to 12 years (Loiseau et al., 1988, 1992; Beaussart, 1972; Blom et al., 1972). In the series of Beaussart and Faou (1978), 98% of the patients were seizure free by 12 years of age, and all of them were by 17 years of age. Similarly, Blom and Heijbel (1982) found that 36 of 37 patients who were followed for 14 to 23 years were seizure free, with 32 being off antiepileptic drugs for more than 5 years. Lerman and Kivity (1975) observed no recurrence in patients older than 15 years of age. The mean duration of the period of seizure activity was 2.4 years, varying from 0 (a single attack) to 11 years. In a metaanalysis of 20 reports comprising 794 patients, Bouma et al. (1997) found the mean duration of the active disorder to be less than 3 years. Remission occurred in 50% of patients by 6 years of age, in 92% by 12 years of age, and in 99.8% by age 18 years, with a marked peak of remission by 13 years.

Remission occurs regardless of initial resistance to treatment, which may be present in up to 20% of patients (Loiseau et al., 1988), and even in patients with more severe seizures, such as attacks followed by Todd paralysis (Dalla Bernardina et al., 1982) or status epilepticus (Colamaria et al., 1991; Boulloche et al., 1990; Roulet et al., 1989; Fejerman and Di Blasi, 1987). The latter may be unilateral, or, rarely, they may simulate a cortical pseudobulbar opercular syndrome (Colamaria et al., 1991; Boulloche et al., 1990; Roulet et al., 1989).

The normalization of the EEG tracings occurs usually later than clinical remission, with the average interval being 2 years in a personal series (Aicardi, 1979). The remission of BECRS at adolescence has been shown to be long lasting. Beaussart and Faou (1978) followed 159 patients for 1 to 11 years after the discontinuation of therapy. Sixty-nine of their patients had been off treatment for more than 6 years, and, in only one of these, did a seizure occur in the form of a tonic-clonic generalized convulsion. Beaussart (1981) reported the occurrence of generalized tonic-clonic seizures in 5 patients at 3 to 10 years af-

L. Delt.

R. Delt.

Fz-Cz

R. Ext.

A

1 sec ⌐100 μV

B

C

ter remission of BECRS. The seizures were isolated episodes, and some were precipitated by extraneous factors, especially alcohol. The later presentation of occasional patients with BECRS with other common types of epileptic seizures is not unexpected. This is a rare event, however, and the favorable prognosis attached to BECRS is not substantially modified by this finding nor by a single report of persistence of BECRS into adulthood (Ambrosetto et al., 1985).

The global prognosis, particularly regarding social outcome, school achievement, and later professional activity, appears to be as good as the prognosis for the seizures. The achievements of patients with BECRS as a group do not differ from those of a normal population (Loiseau et al., 1983b; Heijbel and Bohman, 1975). These favorable results are obtained no matter what treatment is used, even in those patients in whom seizures persist despite treatment. In the remaining children, treatment rapidly and completely controls the fits.

The effect of drug therapy on the EEG abnormality has not been assessed. Clinical experience indicates that the EEG is often relatively unchanged, even with effective treatment. Similarly, fluctuations in the location, activity, and number of EEG paroxysms are not related to the frequency of seizures, and extreme discrepancies between the rarity of seizures and the activity of the EEG foci are not uncommon (Aicardi, 1979; Beaussart, 1972). BECRS generally has a limited impact on the life of affected children because of the time of occurrence of the fits; their infrequency; and, in most cases, their good response to therapy. However, unfavorable consequences in the form of emotional disturbances may result from anguish, overprotection, or rejection if the epilepsy is not recognized as benign and the good prognosis is not adequately explained to parents. Overtreatment to suppress EEG abnormalities or in those cases that do not respond to anticonvulsant drugs is a definite hazard that should be avoided by the proper diagnosis of the syndrome.

Diagnosis

The *diagnosis of BECRS* is easy when the existence of the condition is known. Because of the presence of orofacial phenomena and of the "midtemporal" location of the spike focus, the condition has for many years been confused with temporal lobe epilepsy, and cases of BECRS likely account for some of the reported cases of complex partial seizures with a favorable course (Lindsay et al., 1979a). In fact, the buccopharyngeal manifestations of BECRS clearly differ from the oral alimentary automatisms seen in complex partial seizures (Daly, 1982; Morikawa et al., 1979). The complete persistence of consciousness and memory, as well as the purely motor nature of speech difficulties, during the seizures of BECRS help to distinguish the two types. Patients with repeatedly normal EEG tracings should have sleep tracings made because the diagnosis, in the authors' opinion, requires the presence of the characteristic paroxysms. Very seldom, a brain lesion involving the lower rolandic area can produce an identical clinical picture with very different consequences. The EEG signs in such cases are usually distinct, with changes in the background rhythms occurring in association with the spikes. However, Gobbi et al. (1989) showed that symptomatic partial epilepsy can share all the clinical and EEG characteristics of BECRS, at least for short periods; and Van der Meij et al. (1992c), using quantitative analysis, could not separate "organic" from "functional" spikes, either by their morphology or by their field distribution. In some patients, the seizures may have atypical features, such as visual phenomena, generalized body sensation, or lateral torsion of the body (Loiseau and Beaussart, 1973).

The presence of rolandic spikes is not sufficient to make the diagnosis of RE. Spikes or sharp waves identical to those in RE can be encountered in pa-

---

FIG. 10.7. Rolandic seizure in a 4-year-old boy; 15 minutes after sleep onset, an electrographic seizure appears that initially is subclinical but that is followed about 25 seconds after the onset by rhythmic clonic jerks of the left side of the face lasting around 1 minute. The child was not awakened by the seizure. At seizure onset, the electroencephalogram showed bilateral right predominant increments of spikes, followed 5 seconds later by a buildup of rhythmic theta activity intermingled with faster rhythms and frequent spikes. Ill-defined spike-wave complexes disrupted the rhythmic activity for 15 seconds; some complexes were clearly related to the facial jerks, as the muscular artifacts on left temporal and frontal electrodes show. A short train of 8-Hz right centrotemporal rhythmic ictal activity then appeared; it was accompanied by 8-Hz rhythmic jerks. The seizure end was marked by the reappearance of spike-wave complexes and inconsistently related slower clonic jerks, and it was followed by attenuation of background activity on the right hemisphere. The episode lasted 1 minute, 30 seconds.

tients with fragile X syndrome, in those with Rett syndrome, or in patients with structural abnormalities. A relatively large proportion of children in the general population also have similar spikes in EEGs recorded for various reasons or in systematic studies.

In a significant proportion of patients with only generalized seizures, the diagnosis of RE rests mainly on the finding of a rolandic focus (Van der Meij et al., 1992b). In such cases, an EEG is essential to separate BECRS from generalized epilepsies, thus allowing a favorable prognosis to be given to the individual and his or her parents.

In some patients, the paroxysms may be abnormally located, especially over the parietal region, or they have unusual shapes (e.g., very-high-amplitude sharp-wave and slow-wave complexes with a duration of up to 1 second). Such minor deviations should probably be accepted if the rest of the picture is typical (Wirrel et al., 1995; Lüders et al., 1987b; Aicardi, 1979). On the other hand, a diagnosis of BECRS should never be made solely on the basis of an EEG focus. Similar foci have been found by systematic studies (Cavazzuti et al., 1980; Eeg-Olofsson et al., 1971) in 1.9% to 2.4% of normal school-age children, an incidence that is several times greater than that of all types of epilepsy in the same age-group. Such foci are also common in children with cerebral palsy, especially those with spastic diplegia or hemiplegia (Lüders et al., 1987b). In the latter case, they are usually located on the side opposite the paralysis, thus suggesting a causal relationship with the brain lesion. Therefore, one must not make a diagnosis of epilepsy purely on the basis of the EEG because most patients with rolandic spikes do not suffer seizures.

In its typical form, BECRS is not caused by organic brain pathology, and all of the neuroradiologic investigations that have been performed in many early cases have given normal results, except for incidental findings. Therefore, such investigations should not be performed when the clinical and EEG picture is typical. However, typical cases of BECRS have been reported in association with focal brain lesions (Lerman and Kivity, 1986; Santanelli et al., 1989; Ambrosetto, 1992), but these are exceptions too rare to modify this general recommendation.

Etiology of Benign Epilepsy with Centrorolandic Spikes

Genetic factors play an important role in the etiology of RE and the rolandic spikes. The temporocentral EEG abnormalities seemingly are the major features of a genetic trait that is only relatively rarely associated with rolandic seizures. However, the mode of transmission of this trait has not yet been clarified, and the factors determining the occurrence of clinical seizures have not been clarified.

In some families, RE was found in several members of the same pedigree in the same or successive generations (Heijbel, 1980), and it has been reported in identical twins (Kajitani et al., 1980). Bray and Wiser (1964) showed that, in cases of "temporocentral" epilepsy, which is probably the same as BECRS, identical paroxysms could be found in 31% of first-degree relatives, especially those between 6 and 10 years of age. Seizures in relatives may be of the same type as those in the propositus (Bray and Wiser, 1964), or they may take other forms (e.g., febrile convulsions or primary generalized epilepsy). However, only few subjects with EEG foci had seizures. Bray and Wiser (1964) suggested that the EEG trait may be transmitted dominantly, with reduced clinical penetrance and age limitation of the expression. Heijbel (1980) and Heijbel et al. (1975b) also favored an irregularly dominant inheritance with age dependency, with a maximum susceptibility between 5 and 15 years of age. Degen and Degen (1990) also prefer a dominant inheritance. Doose et al. (1984) and Doose and Gerken (1973) think that a multifactorial inheritance is more likely, with the sharp waves representing the major genetic marker of not only RE but also a series of disorders that comprise various types of seizures but also nonepileptic disturbances (cognitive and behavioral) that these researchers include with various types of seizures in a wide concept of "hereditary impairment of brain maturation" (Doose and Baier, 1989).

Kajitani et al. (1981) stressed the frequent succession of febrile seizures in patients with RE and their association with febrile convulsions in first-degree and second-degree relatives, which has been frequently reported (Roger et al., 1990; Lüders et al., 1987b; Heijbel, 1980; Heijbel et al., 1975b). One item of note is that no case of RE in twin pairs was found in the study of Berkovic et al. (1994a).

Recently, Neubauer et al. (1998) found a linkage to chromosome 15q14 in 22 families with 54 members with rolandic spikes (11 without seizures). No specific gene, however, could be ascribed to this region and this linkage more likely represents an etiologic factor of RE, rather than accounts for the whole genetic problem.

Treatment

In all patients, the treatment of RE should be limited to a single antiepileptic drug, preferably one with few side effects and low toxicity. Because of the benign nature of the condition, any form of overtreatment should be absolutely avoided. Many physicians prefer not to give anticonvulsants because BECRS interferes little with the normal activities of the patients, it is not hazardous, nor is it socially unacceptable as a result of the timing of the fits. Ambrosetto et al. (1987) have proposed not giving antiepileptic drugs until after the second seizure because many patients have only one or two attacks. Moreover, they think that no treatment is indicated even after two fits if these occurred more than 6 months apart or if they were generalized, because the frequency of seizures seems low in such patients. This attitude appears eminently reasonable (Freeman et al., 1987).

Carbamazepine (CBZ) has been the most commonly used agent because of its efficacy for partial seizures. It is generally effective and well tolerated (Lerman and Kivity, 1975). However, a possible aggravating effect has been reported, with an increase in the frequency and diffusion of the spikes that leads in some cases to status epilepticus or to the full syndrome of CSWS (Colamaria et al., 1991; Lerman, 1986). The same effect of phenytoin has also been mentioned (Guerrini et al., 1998c). The actual frequency of aggravation of RE by antiepileptic agents remains poorly known. Corda et al. (2001) studied 82 patients treated with various drugs retrospectively and found only one case of electroclinical aggravation among 40 patients exposed to CBZ (5 in polytherapy) and one of marked increase of EEG anomalies without worsening of seizures among 14 children receiving phenobarbital and CBZ, and they concluded that the risk was minor. Sulthiame has been shown to be effective in the treatment of RE (Rating et al., 2000; Gross-Selbeck, 1995). Rating et al. (2000) found the drug to be significantly superior to a placebo in a double-blind controlled study. Some investigators use valproate rather than CBZ to avoid the risk of aggravation with the latter agent.

Probable Phenotypic Variants of Benign Rolandic Epilepsy

Epilepsy with Evoked Parietal Spikes

De Marco and Tassinari (1981) and Tassinari et al. (1988) have described 12 children between 2 and 10 years of age who presented with focal, often adversive attacks without loss of consciousness or with generalized seizures. The EEG displayed foci of sharp waves or SWs in one or the other parietal parasagittal region. These patients exhibited or had exhibited before their seizures the curious EEG phenomenon of unilateral parietal spikes that were elicited by tapping the sole of the contralateral foot. None showed any evidence of brain damage. A systematic EEG study showed that a vast majority of the subjects who exhibited evoked parietal spikes on tapping of the sole did not develop clinical attacks (De Marco and Tassinari, 1981). Tassinari and De Marco believe that those who do develop attacks have a special form of benign epilepsy of childhood and early adolescence that follows a four-stage course. First, only evoked parietal parasagittal spikes are seen in an otherwise normal EEG. In a second stage, a spike focus with the same topographic and morphologic characteristics as the evoked spikes appears in sleep. In the third stage, the focus is seen in the awake stage. The fourth stage is marked by the appearance of clinical fits. The seizures are usually only transient, and they are said to disappear in less than 2 years. They are unprovoked, thus differing from the startle epilepsies (see Chapter 17). These interesting cases deserve further study before a *bona fide* syndrome of parietal epilepsy of a benign type can be recognized.

However, similar "extreme somatosensory evoked potentials" that were elicited by tapping the fingers instead of the toes have been found in cases of RE (Panayiotopoulos, 1999; Manganotti et al., 1998), and this EEG feature is probably not specific of a separate syndrome.

Alleged Syndrome of Benign Epilepsy of Childhood with Affective Seizures

Dalla Bernardina et al. (1985) described 20 patients with epileptic seizures in which affective manifestations, especially fear, were the exclusive or predominant ictal manifestations. According to this report, the seizures were brief, uncommonly contained motor symptoms, and they did not feature a loss of consciousness. They occurred frequently (up to several times daily) in both the waking and the sleeping state without a change in symptomatology. In a typical seizure, the child would turn pale or red, cry out for his or her parents, and run toward them. A look of terror or a terrified stare would follow. Autonomic symptoms, such as abdominal pain or simple oral alimentary automatisms, were common. Occasionally, eyelid jerking or head turning was observed. Additional important features included the onset of the fits from between 15 months or 2 years to 10 to 12.5 years of age; the stereotypic character of the fits in the same patient, although the symptoms could vary in different children; and the absence of neurologic signs or abnormal antecedents. Except for occasional febrile seizures before the onset of the "affective" fits, no other type of seizure was observed in any of these patients.

The interictal EEG recordings consistently showed a normal background activity. Slow spikes with a diphasic or triphasic shape were recorded over the temporal or rolandic areas in some of the patients. Bursts of generalized SW complexes were occasionally present. Ictal records showed rhythmic theta waves or spikes that were either localized over the temporocentral area or were diffusing to one hemisphere, to the same area of the contralateral hemisphere or diffusely. The seizures responded favorably and rapidly to medical treatment, and the outcome seemed favorable in those patients who were followed more than a few months. No mention of mental or behavioral disturbances was made.

Such cases now appear to be only a variant of RE, and Dalla Bernardina et al. (1992a) admitted that this syndrome is difficult to delineate and that it can be easily confounded with lesional cases.

A syndrome of *benign childhood frontal seizures* that was initially described by Beaumanoir and Nahory (1983) is discussed in "Focal (Partial) Epilepsies Caused by Brain Lesions: Nonidiopathic Focal Epilepsies and Syndromes" in this chapter.

Atypical Forms of Idiopathic Epilepsies Related to Rolandic Epilepsy

Some patients present with epilepsies that manifest some of the features of BECRS, especially nocturnal partial seizures and focal EEG paroxysms, but that also display other types of attacks and unusual EEG abnormalities not observed in RE (Stephani, 2000). Although, in most cases, these atypical forms are not associated with structural brain abnormalities, their idiopathic origin has not been proven in all cases, and cortical abnormalities may be present in some.

This group comprises the following three presentations: atypical partial benign epilepsy (Doose et al., 2001; Hahn et al., 2001; Fejerman et al., 2000a; Morikawa, 2000; Doose and Baier, 1989; Deonna et al., 1986a; Aicardi and Chevrie, 1982a) orofacial status epilepticus with or without opercular syndrome; and CSWS, which is also known as "electrical status epilepticus of slow sleep (ESES)." The last of these is mentioned only briefly as a full description is given in Chapter 11.

Atypical Benign Partial Epilepsy of Childhood

The term *atypical benign partial epilepsy* (APBE) was proposed by Aicardi and Chevrie (1982a), who used it to contrast this type of epilepsy with the Lennox-Gastaut syndrome, for which it was often mistaken because of the repeated atonic falls, absences, and diffuse slow SW activity on drowsiness and sleep records. However, during the active periods, some degree of mental slowing or behavioral disturbance, although it is often subtle, is usually present, so the benignity of this syndrome is only by contrast with more severe epilepsy types. The abnormalities do disappear during seizure-free periods. Doose and Baier (1989), Doose et al. (2001), and Hahn et al. (2001) have termed the condition *pseudo–Lennox syndrome.* However, the definition they use includes cases with more severe mental retardation and without the intermittent occurrence of CSWS, so some degree of confusion still persists in the classification of such cases. The criteria of Doose et al. (2001) and Hahn et al. (2001) include the occurrence of "generalized minor seizures as previously described for APBE and the detection of focal sharp waves indistinguishable from those of RE with generalization during slow sleep." His report included 43 cases with an onset of seizures between 2 and 5 years of age; these included atonic astatic seizures; atypical absences; and, less often, myoclonic seizures in 67% and status of minor seizures in 40%. Multifocal sharp waves were present in 88% of patients; these were activated to electrical status during sleep in 56%. No tonic seizures or fast 10-Hz discharges were recorded. At the last follow-up, 84% of the patients and all of those older than 15 years were seizure free. Retarded mental development was seen in 26 (60%) of their patients before the onset seizures and in 24 (56%) at the end of follow-up.

Fejerman et al. (2000) described 11 cases with onset between 2 and 7 years of age. All of these children showed periods of frequent inhibitory seizures, five with pseudoataxia caused by negative myoclonus of the lower limbs. Five children had learning difficulties, but all attended normal school. Nine patients also had atypical absences, and eight had partial seizures. Six showed interictal CSWS. These authors felt that these cases followed an initial period of typical RE, which, on average, lasted 18 months.

In the authors' series of 12 patients (Aicardi and Gomes, 1988, 1991), the onset was between 2 and 6 years of age in children with a normal development and neurologic examination. All patients had at least two different seizure types at some time. The initial seizures were often partial nocturnal, reminiscent of those of BECRS, and they were usually infrequent. Some patients had tonic-clonic seizures, and one had focal sensory motor attacks. Atonic attacks, the most characteristic seizure type, occurred in periods of 1 to several weeks' duration that were usually separated by free intervals of several weeks or months. The atonic attacks may involve the whole axial musculature and/or both lower limbs and may then result in multiple daily falls that can produce severe injuries, or they may be localized, generating repeated episodes of atonia in the head or one limb that lasts only 1 to 2 seconds. These latter can be demonstrated by having the patient maintain his or her arms extended. Such atonic attacks are associated with the slow-wave component of the SW complexes, and the location of the EEG discharges corresponds to that of the atonic episodes (Dalla Bernardina et al., 1990; Cirignotta and Lugaresi, 1991; Kanazawa and Kawai, 1990; Wang et al., 1984). Other types of seizure, including generalized tonic-clonic attacks, brief absences, and partial motor seizures, may also be present, but the predominance of atonic seizures is characteristic.

The EEG recording is highly abnormal during slow sleep or even in drowsiness, showing an intense, diffuse, slow SW activity that is similar or identical to that of the so-called ESES, which have been renamed CSWS. This activity seems to be present only during the periods when atonic seizures occur and to disappear between the clusters of attacks (Aicardi and Gomes, 1991; Aicardi, 1986a) (Fig. 10.8), even though this temporal correlation may not be absolute. Usually focal spiking involving one central region, often with considerable contralateral diffusion, is observed. Bursts of diffuse 3-Hz SWs are usually demonstrable during seizure periods both with and without concomitant clinical seizures.

The course of the 15 patients studied so far by the authors has been self-limited with apparently complete remission that has been maintained for up to 15 years in the 11 children followed after 9 years of age. None of them has experienced gross cognitive-behavioral sequelae, although no detailed psychologic study has been performed, and all have remained in normal classes. This favorable course sharply contrasts with the gloomy outlook of Lennox-Gastaut syndrome and justifies the separation of this group of cases to avoid errors in prognosis and treatment escalation. Indeed, antiepileptic drugs have seemed ineffective against these seizures, and they have not modified the EEG paroxysms. Neither adrenocorticotropic hormone nor steroids have been effective in a few cases.

In some children, the electroclinical picture may be slightly different. Deonna et al. (1986a) noted patients in whom no focal seizure or focal EEG paroxysms were present, and they questioned the relationship of such cases to benign partial epilepsy. Likewise, the occurrence of the full-fledged syndrome of CSWS may be preceded by many types of seizures and only uncommonly by BECRS (Roger et al., 1990). At the time of this writing, it seems that CSWS and atypical benign partial epilepsy are probably related, but they do differ in that the paroxysmal activity in sleep is continuous in one and is interrupted in the other, with differing effects on learning and behavior. The continuous paroxysmal activity seemingly interferes gravely with higher functions.

Both conditions also appear to be etiologically heterogeneous. A clinical and EEG picture of partial epilepsy, with considerable diffusion of the EEG paroxysms from the focus during sleep and even during wakefulness in the form of bursts of bilateral SWs with brief minor clinical attacks at certain periods, can occur with either localized organic brain lesions or purely functional foci without detectable brain pathology (Montagna et al., 1990; Morikawa et al., 1985). The prognosis probably varies accordingly.

The authors have observed several patients with a type of epilepsy reminiscent of atypical benign partial epilepsy (e.g., with diffusion of the EEG abnormalities and atonic seizures) that were due to demonstrable central lesions. In these patients, atonic seizures of very brief duration (usually less than 1 second) affected either the axial muscles (neck, trunk, and lower limbs), with consequent falls or head nods, or the upper limbs resulting in "negative myoclonus." During the active periods, the EEG recording displayed continuous SW activity in slow sleep and, occasionally, in the awake state. The paroxysmal activity often predominated over the side of the brain lesion, but it was always diffuse. The attacks were grouped in episodes of nonconvulsive status epilepticus that usually lasted several days.

All patients had hemiparesis and variable degrees of mental retardation. Despite the presence of a lesion, the seizures eventually remitted in the three patients followed for 3 years or more. Similar cases have been observed by other investigators (Caraballo et al., 1999; Guerrini et al., 1996d). These investigators have described the occurrence of a relatively "benign" epilepsy with a few focal seizures reminiscent of those of BECRS and of CSWS that persisted for extended periods in patients with a mild congenital hemiplegia; these were caused by polymicrogyria involving a whole hemisphere or at least extensive cortical areas unilaterally. The electrical continuous activity eventually subsided with the complete disappearance of seizures before adolescence. However, the learning and cognitive sequelae can persist.

Retrospectively, the six patients described by Aicardi (1994) likely were examples of this syndrome, as a reevaluation of CT scans, which, in one

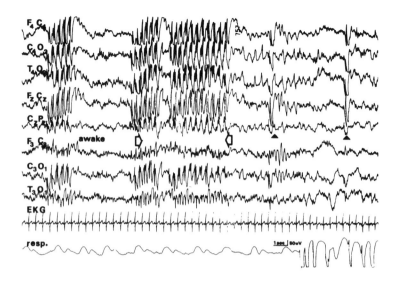

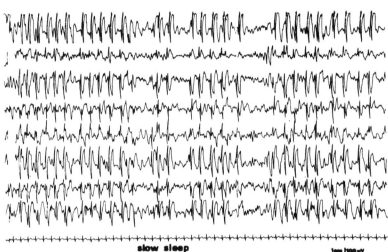

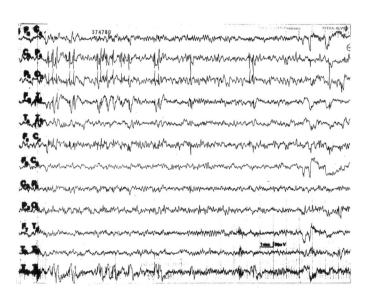

case, also were demonstrated by MRI, confirmed the presence of an extensive unilateral malformation.

The reader may therefore consider atypical partial benign epilepsy to be only the most benign end of a continuum of epilepsies of partial (or focal) origin, whether due to structural or "functional" causes, with considerable diffusion from the focus at certain periods, especially during sleep. Such a diffusion may originate from an area of a structural lesion (e.g., microgyric cortex) or functional disturbance. Several authors have suggested that a similar picture may result from the use of CBZ in patients with focal seizures (Colamaria et al., 1991; Caraballo et al., 1989; Lerman, 1986). However, none of the authors' patients had received CBZ.

Continuous Spike-Waves in Slow Sleep or Electrical Status Epilepticus in Slow Sleep

The phenomenon of CSWS clearly is closely related to that of atypical partial benign epilepsy, and the latter may well be part of the ESES syndrome; it at least overlaps with it. CSWS describes an EEG phenomenon, the presence of continuous, generalized slow spikes and waves of high amplitude, and a special morphology that persists through a major part of slow sleep (Tassinari et al., 1992a) (see Chapter 11). It also applies to a syndrome that is characterized by the regular presence both of this EEG abnormality and of seizures, which include partial seizures closely resembling those of BECRS but which, in addition, comprise atonic and atypical absence attacks, negative myoclonus, and cognitive and/or behavioral deterioration that is only partly reversible after the cessation of the paroxysmal EEG abnormalities. CSWS are also a feature of most cases of Landau-Kleffner syndrome (Hirsch et al., 1995; Beaumanoir et al., 1995; Beaumanoir, 1992; Paquier et al., 1992; Deonna et al., 1977).

Status Epilepticus of Benign Partial Epilepsy in Children

Continuous, repetitive localized jerks affecting the face unilaterally or bilaterally that occur in association with almost continuous rolandic or generalized spiking during wakefulness, sleep, or both have been reported as episodes of status epilepticus in a few patients with RE (Colamaria et al., 1991; Boulloche et al., 1990; Roulet et al., 1989; Fejerman and Di Blasi, 1987). They are often associated with drooling, swallowing difficulties, and other features of the cortical opercular syndrome, which may be the most striking manifestation, and with only minimal jerking (Boulloche et al., 1990). These may only respond to corticosteroid treatment (Fejerman and Di Blasi, 1987). De Saint Martin et al. (1999) reported such a case, but they interpreted the facial weakness and oral motor problems as inhibitory phenomena and the twitches as being due to negative myoclonus. They preferred the term *paraictal phenomena* instead of *status epilepticus*. Such episodes may recur with periods of normality in between.

Landau-Kleffner Syndrome of Acquired Epileptic Aphasia

Landau-Kleffner Syndrome of acquired epileptic aphasia is described in Chapter 11. Although this syndrome is probably heterogeneous, a large proportion of cases appear to be closely linked to atypical rolandic epilepsies. The sleep EEG recording of these patients often shows CSWS (Beaumanoir et al., 1995; Hirsch et al., 1995; Deonna et al., 1977), and the language disturbances have been hypothesized to result from the epileptic activity itself (see Chapter 11).

The four conditions described in this section ("Atypical Forms of Idiopathic Epilepsies Related to Rolandic Epilepsies," including "Atypical Benign Partial Epilepsy," "Continuous Spike-Waves in Slow Sleep," "Status Epilepticus of Benign Partial Epilepsy," and "Landau-Kleffner Syndrome of Acquired Epileptic Aphasia") clearly overlap, and they may be different aspects of a same process. Some discussion exists about whether they are a complication or a special evolution of RE (Fejermann et al., 2000) or if they instead represent distinct, although overlapping, conditions. However, the former view seems more likely.

FIG. 10.8. Atypical partial benign epilepsy in a girl who started having seizures at 19 months of age. The seizures were of the following three types: absences with eyelid jerking and often a fall; left partial motor seizures that were mainly nocturnal; and an occasional generalized tonic-clonic seizure. Absences and falls occurred many times daily for periods of 3 to 12 weeks, separated by free intervals lasting weeks or months. Neuromental development was normal, and the computed tomographic scan showed no abnormality. At the age of 6 years, the seizures have become infrequent. **A:** Age of 39 months and awake: absence with eyelid jerks. The *arrows* indicate the onset and termination of absences. **B:** During slow sleep continuous slow spike-wave activity (so-called *electrical status epilepticus of slow sleep*). **C:** Age of 5 years and awake: right posterior spike focus reminiscent of tracings observed in benign rolandic epilepsy.

Autosomal Recessive Rolandic Epilepsy with Paroxysmal-Induced Dystonia and Writer's Cramp

This syndrome was reported by Guerrini et al. (1999) in one pedigree, and it was found to map to chromosome 16p, on which other genes for paroxysmal movement disorders have been localized. The autosomal recessive inheritance is unusual because all other similar syndromes are dominantly inherited.

Benign Partial Epilepsy with Occipital Spikes

The realization that epilepsies with centrotemporal spikes do not comprise all cases of benign or relatively benign epilepsies of childhood and that benign epilepsies with occipital paroxysms also occur came only several years after RE had been thoroughly studied (Panayiotopoulos, 1999). The common presence of occipital spikes in young patients had been long recognized in infants and children with various types of seizures but also in some without clinical manifestations of epilepsy (Gibbs and Gibbs, 1952).

Continuous, more or less rhythmic, high-voltage sharp-wave and slow-wave activity over one or both occipital areas that is completely or significantly suppressed by eye opening is a relatively uncommon abnormality in children (Aicardi and Newton, 1987). This abnormality has been described in association with overlapping syndromes, such as benign occipital epilepsy (Gastaut, 1992) and basilar migraine with severe epileptic EEG abnormalities (Camfield et al., 1978).

The following two different syndromes of childhood epilepsy with occipital spikes have been described: a "late-onset" form (Gastaut, 1992; Gastaut and Zifkin, 1987) with prominent visual manifestations and an early onset form (Panayiotopoulos, 1989a, 1999, 2002) that is characterized mainly by ictal vomiting; head and eye deviation; and, sometimes, prolonged loss of awareness. This second type is by far the most common, with its frequency being perhaps as high as one-third of that of RE, although no epidemiologic study is available.

Late-Onset Benign Occipital Epilepsy or Gastaut Type

According to Gastaut (1992) and Gastaut and Zifkin (1987), *benign occipital epilepsy* is an epilepsy syndrome that is as clearly defined as BECRS. The mean age at onset of the syndrome in 36 patients was 6 years. Of these patients, 17 (47%) had a family history of

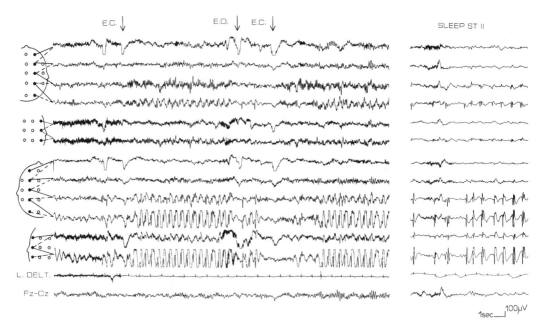

FIG. 10.9. A 9-year-old boy with spontaneous visual seizures in the context of idiopathic childhood epilepsy with occipital paroxysms (Gastaut type). Interictal electroencephalogram shows left predominant continuous occipito-posterior temporal spike-wave activity upon closing of the eyes that is promptly stopped upon opening the eyes. During sleep stage II, bilateral left predominant almost continuous discharges occur over the same regions.

epilepsy, and seven (19%) had a family history of migraine. The seizures were mainly partial, generally beginning with visual symptoms that could remain isolated or that were followed by hemisensory, motor, or psychomotor phenomena. The visual symptoms included transient amaurosis in 65% of the patients; elementary visual hallucinations in the form of phosphenes, colored or luminous discs, or formed visual hallucinations in 23%; and visual illusions in 12%. Nonvisual seizures often followed the visual onset, but they occasionally occurred in isolation. In addition, 41% of the patients had hemiclonic seizures, 19% had complex partial seizures, and 8% had generalized tonic-clonic attacks. One-third of these patients had a severe postictal long-lasting headache, which was sometimes accompanied by nausea and/or vomiting, with definite migrainous features.

The ictal EEG showed a localized sustained discharge over one occipital lobe (Gastaut, 1992; Fois et al., 1988a), even when the interictal SWs were bilateral. The interictal EEG recording displayed a normal background activity and very peculiar localized paroxysms. These were high-amplitude (200 to 300 μV) SW complexes occurring only when the eyes were closed, and they recurred more or less rhythmically at roughly 2 to 3 Hz over the occipital or occipitoparietotemporal region of one or both hemispheres (Fig. 10.9). When the paroxysms were bilateral, they could be synchronous or asynchronous and symmetric or asymmetrical. Intermittent photic stimulation and sleep did not facilitate the occurrence of the paroxysms, but hyperpnea often activated them (Newton and Aicardi, 1983). In some patients, the paroxysms were arrhythmic and/or of different morphology (e.g., mainly spikes without associated slow waves). Suppression of the SWs by eye opening was at times incomplete.

Visual fixation was shown to be responsible for the suppression of the paroxysms, as these persisted in bright light when lenses prevented fixation (Lugaresi et al., 1984) but disappeared, even in darkness, when the patients fixed on red spots of low luminance (Panayiotopoulos, 1979). The term *scotoepilepsy,* meaning that darkness is the trigger of the phenomenon, is therefore inappropriate as absence or arrest of fixation is the real cause (Lugaresi et al., 1984).

In Gastaut's patients, the course of the syndrome was said to be benign. "Full remission" of the seizures occurred in 92% by the age of 19 years. Drug treatment was successful in preventing attacks in half of the patients, but the duration of follow-up was not indicated. Eighteen similar cases have been reported by Beaumanoir (1983), but only eight had visual phenomena as part of their seizures. A few such isolated

cases were on record (Deonna et al., 1984; Panayiotopoulos, 1979, 1980). Similar cases have since been reported (Cooper and Lee, 1991; Kuzniecky and Rosenblatt, 1987; Terasaki et al., 1987), confirming the existence of a benign epileptic syndrome with well-defined features, as described by Gastaut.

Early Onset Benign Occipital Epilepsy: Panayiotopoulos Type of Benign Occipital Epilepsy or Panayiotopoulos Syndrome

In this syndrome, the onset is between 1 and 14 years of age with the average age being 4 to 5 years. The seizures are relatively rare, and up to 30% of children have a single episode.

The seizures are nocturnal in approximately two-thirds of patients, and, in the whole course, their mean number is three. They usually begin with a feeling of sickness and nausea that evolves into vomiting, which may be protracted. Deviation of the eyes to one side is present in most patients, and it is usually slow and pursuit-like.

The phase of eye deviation, vomiting, or both often evolves into loss of consciousness or obtundation of variable degree. A progression to a unilateral clonic convulsion occurs in about 30% of seizures. The duration of seizures varies between a few minutes and several hours (Panayiotopoulos, 1999, 2002). Such long-lasting seizures with loss of consciousness can suggest severe neurologic disorders (Panayiotopoulos, 1999, 2002; Ferrie et al., 1997; Kivity and Lerman; 1992; Panayiotopoulos and Igoe, 1992). However, except in the immediate postictal period, the neurodevelopment of these children is unaffected.

The interictal EEG is usually characterized by occipital spike complexes with a morphology similar to the centrotemporal spikes of RE. These can occur singly or in brief clusters; more characteristically, however, they present as continuous rhythmic repetitive paroxysms at 1 to 3 Hz, and they may last as long as the eyes remain closed. They are often of high amplitude (up to 300 μV), but a high degree of variability exists. The spikes are increased in sleep. Characteristically, they are arrested by eye opening (fixation-off phenomenon) (Panayiotopoulos, 1987). The EEG abnormalities tend to persist for several years after the disappearance of seizures (Panayiotopoulos, 1999, 2002). Ictal EEGs have only rarely been recorded. They show a mixture of repetitive slow waves and spikes contralateral to eye deviation (Panayiotopoulos, 2002).

The course of early onset benign occipital epilepsy seems to be regularly favorable with both the disappearance of seizures and normal development being observed in these patients. In a few cases, a typical picture of RE occurs following the syndrome, and rolandic spikes are seen in up to 10% of the patients followed (Ferrie et al., 1997).

The electroclinical picture of early onset benign occipital epilepsy syndrome may not be as stereotyped as was initially proposed. Some seizures may consist purely of vomiting (ictus emeticus). According to Panayiotopoulos (2002), in about 20% of patients, syncope is the major paroxysmal manifestation, and this may not be associated with convulsions. Infrequently, visual symptoms may occur, but their absence may be difficult to assess in young children. Symptoms suggestive of RE, such as a speech arrest and oropharyngeal manifestations, may be present. Hemiconvulsions are present in one-third of patients, and these may be the only manifestation of seizures that are not directly observed. They could account for a significant proportion of the cases of prolonged afebrile epileptic seizures in children 3 to 5 years or age (Aicardi, 1976). The EEG is quite variable because many patients have no occipital seizures, and an anterior distribution of the spikes is not rare (Panayiotopoulos, 2002). The paroxysms may be delayed in appearance (Guerrini et al., 1997), or they may even be repeatedly absent in some patients.

The precise limits of the syndrome are, therefore, not entirely clear from both the clinical and the EEG points of view. Undoubtedly, however, a sizable group of children with early onset seizures characterized by prominent autonomic ictal phenomena, multifocal spikes, and a tendency to prolonged seizures with vomiting and coma does exist; these may be frightening, but they are in fact benign. Such patients share several features with the syndrome of RE, and grouping the two subgroups into a syndrome of childhood seizure susceptibility that is age limited and that tends to disappear spontaneously with brain maturation appears seems legitimate.

Idiopathic Photosensitive Occipital Lobe Epilepsy

Idiopathic photosensitive occipital lobe epilepsy (Guerrini et al., 1994, 1995), in which focal occipital lobe seizures are induced by photic stimulation, represents a third syndrome of occipital epilepsy. This uncommon syndrome features seizures with visual hallucinations that are often brightly colored, blurring of vision, or blindness. The seizures may last up to 2 hours, although they are often shorter (a few minutes). Headache commonly accompanies them, and sensitivity to flickering light may be obvious, or it may have to be looked for carefully, which, in some

cases, requires prolonged exposure. Such seizures may be induced by television viewing or video-game playing (Ferrie et al., 1994). The outlook is favorable. Treatment should include the avoidance of precipitating factors and possibly drug administration, most commonly valproate.

Diagnosis of Idiopathic Occipital Epilepsies

An important diagnostic problem is posed by the long-lasting severe seizures of early onset occipital epilepsy. They must be differentiated from severe neurologic conditions, such as encephalitis or complications of head injury, and from nonneurologic emergencies, especially abdominal ones, because of their vomiting and autonomic phenomena.

Migraine is a common diagnostic issue because all types of occipital epilepsy syndromes can feature prominent headache that is often migraine like and some also feature visual hallucinations. The syndrome of *basilar migraine with epileptiform EEG abnormalities* (Panayiotopoulos, 1980; Camfield et al., 1978) is clinically characterized by typical migrainous headaches that usually have a throbbing character, are associated with nausea and/or vomiting, and are heralded by visual symptoms of an elementary type, with infrequent epileptic seizures. The EEG demonstrates the abnormality described earlier. This syndrome is part of the migraine epilepsy syndrome, but not all cases are associated with the EEG abnormality (Aicardi and Newton, 1987). However, basilar migraine with continuous SWs appears to be only a manifestation of occipital epilepsy rather than a distinct syndrome (Panayiotopoulos, 1980) as migraine-like headache is commonly observed in patients with occipital epilepsy (Wallace, 1977).

Benign occipital epilepsy syndromes can be difficult to separate from other epileptic phenomena with less favorable prognoses. The mere presence of continuous SW activity is not a guarantee of benignity because a similar pattern may occur with structural lesions.

Newton and Aicardi (1983) studied 21 children with typical EEG abnormalities and found that the range of clinical manifestations and the course were more variable than that indicated by Gastaut. Visual symptoms were lacking in 12 of their patients, who exhibited a wide spectrum of epileptic seizures. Migrainous features were noted in 10 of the children. The prognosis in such patients was not as good as that seen in other series. The epilepsy was difficult to control in 14 patients, and 13 had educational problems. The differences between reported series probably reflect differences in the types of patients referred, indicating that occipital epilepsy is not a homogeneous syndrome. Some cases, at least, appear to be the result of organic brain damage, even though their clinical and EEG presentations are similar. Therefore, this electroclinical syndrome does not necessarily indicate a benign prognosis (Fois et al., 1988a; Aicardi and Newton, 1987; Aso et al., 1987; Newton and Aicardi, 1983).

Seizures of occipital origin are also a feature of the syndrome of *epilepsy with occipital calcifications* that was initially reported by Gobbi et al. (1988, 1991, 1992) and has since been observed by several other investigators (Maggauda, 1991; Giroud et al., 1990).

Two types seem to exist. In the severe form, at onset, the epilepsy features the same clinical and EEG characteristics seen in cases of "benign" occipital epilepsy. However, sleep tracings may then show the presence of polyspike bursts, which are not observed in idiopathic cases. At a later stage (usually after several years), the patient has a turn for the worse with the appearance of atonic or tonic seizures and diffuse EEG abnormalities similar to those observed in secondary generalized epilepsies. Mental slowing and severe learning difficulties are also present. In less severe cases, the picture remains similar to that of "benign" occipital epilepsy; this evolution seems common.

The CT scan shows the presence of calcifications that are reminiscent of those seen with methotrexate encephalopathy. These are bilateral, and they predominate in the occipital regions but extend to the temporal, parietal, and occasionally frontal areas as well. They are not associated with cortical atrophy (Maggauda, 1991), which is an important feature for differentiating them from Sturge-Weber syndrome. Indeed, some cases that were reported as bilateral Sturge-Weber syndrome without facial angioma may well belong to this entity (Ambrosetto et al., 1983). In one patient, the gadolinium-enhanced MRI scans were normal, which appears to be of great value for the exclusion of a pial angioma (Lipski et al., 1990; Sperner et al., 1990). The origin of these calcifications is obscure. In one familial case (Tateno et al., 1985), a cortical angioma was demonstrated pathologically, but this probably represented a different problem.

In most, if not all, patients with apparently idiopathic epilepsy with occipital calcifications, the presence of celiac disease has been demonstrated by clinical signs or, more commonly, only by jejunal mucosal biopsy (Gobbi et al., 1991). However, the latter may be negative in rare cases in whom antigliadin antibodies have been demonstrated. The relationship between celiac disease and this syndrome is not understood. A deficit in folates as a result of malabsorption has been shown in some cases,

but this is not consistently present and it probably does not play a causal role (De Marco and Lorenzin, 1990). Immunologic factors probably have a major role in the etiology. The apparent frequency of the syndrome in Italy may be related to the high incidence of celiac disease in this population.

Treatment of Idiopathic Occipital Epilepsy

The *treatment* of idiopathic occipital epilepsies follows the same guidelines as that of BECRS. In particular, the mere presence of the EEG abnormality is not a sufficient indication for treatment because this may exist without causing epileptic seizures. Likewise, the persistence of occipital SWs does not necessarily indicate that therapy should be continued.

Newly Recognized Syndromes of Probable Idiopathic Focal Epilepsy Whose Nosology Is Not Yet Completely Clarified

In the past few years, several new syndromes predominantly characterized by focal seizures that apparently are not associated with brain lesions have been reported. Some of these are genetically transmitted (Picard et al., 2000), mostly in a dominant manner, and the responsible genes have been identified in a few cases. In a majority, however, evidence of a genetic transmission rests on pedigree studies, and, indeed, a genetic origin has not been convincingly demonstrated in many cases. This section successively considers frontal epilepsy (Scheffer et al., 1995a), epilepsy with multiple foci (Scheffer et al., 1998), familial temporal lobe epilepsy with (Ottman et al., 1995) and without (Berkovic et al., 1994, 1996) auditory symptoms, and autosomal dominant RE with speech dyspraxia (Scheffer et al., 1995b).

Idiopathic Frontal Lobe Epilepsy

Although a few cases of benign frontal lobe epilepsy had been described by Beaumanoir and Nahory (1983), their characterization was not precise, and their differentiation from other frontal lobe epilepsies was not easily accomplished.

Scheffer et al. (1995a) described 47 affected persons in five families. They termed the syndrome *autosomal dominant nocturnal frontal lobe epilepsy* (ADNFLE). Their description has since been confirmed by several investigators.

ADNFLE is characterized by clusters of brief nocturnal motor seizures with hyperkinetic or tonic manifestations. The patients often experience an aura (fear, forced thinking), and they usually remain conscious throughout the events. The seizures are brief (generally less than 1 minute), and often recur in clusters in which several attacks occur in one night, especially on dozing or shortly before awakening. The epilepsy can begin at any age, but the onset is usually in childhood. It seems to last throughout adulthood, with considerable variations in severity. Interictal EEG studies may be unhelpful. In some cases, focal theta or delta rhythms or sharp waves are recorded in the frontal area. EEG abnormalities are sometimes present in clinically unaffected members of families with this syndrome; some family members may also have focal EEG anomalies that are localized outside of the frontal lobes (Picard et al., 2000). The ictal EEG may also be uncharacteristic, or it may be blurred by movement artifacts. A frontal onset has been demonstrated in some patients (Hayman et al., 1997). Most patients respond to CBZ, but up to 30% of cases may be pharmacoresistant. Neuroimaging shows no abnormalities.

The disorder has an autosomal dominant inheritance with a high penetrance. Mutations of the gene for the α_4 subunit of the neuronal acetylcholine receptor located on chromosome 20q13 have been discovered in a few families; this is now termed ADNFLE type 2. Subsequently, a second locus on chromosome 15q24 was found involving a gene for the α_2 subunit (nicotine acetylcholine receptor subtype B [CHRNB] 2, type 3) (Phillips et al., 1998), and a third locus has been mapped to chromosome type 1 (Gambardella et al., 2000). A systematic search for these loci has been negative in most cases, which suggests further heterogeneity. Sporadic cases may occur, and a *de novo* mutation has been reported in a sporadic case (Phillips et al., 2000).

In several families, several types of seizures are observed in different members, although, in some families, all of the affected members suffer similar attacks (Picard et al., 2000).

The diagnosis may be difficult with some types of parasomnias and with pseudoseizures. The dystonic attacks are probably identical to those described as nocturnal dystonia by Lugaresi et al. (1984). Most, if not all, cases of this condition are now considered a manifestation of frontal seizures (Tinuper et al., 1990).

Cases of ADNFLE share common features with the 10 children reported by Vigevano et al. (1993); these cases were characterized by hypnogenic tonic or tonic-automatic seizures that frequently were repeated and that had a benign outcome. Both the interictal and ictal EEGs of these patients indicated frontal lobe involvement; they could, however, be normal. An interesting form of familial RE that is associated with exercise-induced dystonia and writer's cramp has been reported by Guerrini et al. (1999). It is transmitted as an autosomal recessive trait that was mapped to chromosome 16. Recently, Kinton et al. (2002) reported a syndrome of autosomal dominant epilepsy with pericentral spikes that featured various types of seizures, including complex partial and unilateral motor attacks with linkage to chromosome 4p15.

The nosologic situation of ADNFLE and related cases remains partly unsettled. Demonstration of a genetic origin has not yet been brought about for many cases, and sporadic cases and/or phenocopies are possible. Small areas of dysplasia that escape diagnosis by MRI may produce a similar picture, and the presence of such lesions remains plausible in some cases. The localization of the epileptogenic area has often not been confirmed, and, although a frontal location is probable, various areas within and outside the frontal lobe can be the origin for similar seizures. Finally, the course is rather variable, and achieving seizure control may be difficult in some patients.

Autosomal Dominant Epilepsy with Variable Foci

Autosomal dominant epilepsy with variable foci concerns only a small number of patients (Picard et al., 2000; Oldani et al., 1996, 1998; Thomas et al., 1998; Scheffer et al., 1998). It involves children with different seizure types, some of which closely resemble those of ADNFLE.

Individualization of this "syndrome" is based mainly on molecular genetic data. Linkage to chromosome 2 was reported by Scheffer et al. (1998) and to chromosome 22 by Xiong et al. (1999). Therapy with CBZ seems effective.

Familial Temporal Lobe Epilepsy

Berkovic et al. (1994b,c, 1996b) drew attention to the fact that temporal lobe epilepsy, a common type of epilepsy that was generally believed to be of lesional origin, could occur as a familial genetic trait that was transmitted in a dominant fashion. They reported patients with "complex partial" seizures associated with a temporal focus. Similar cases have since been reported (Picard et al., 2000). The condition seems fairly common. The "syndrome" has its onset in adulthood or adolescence. The clinical and EEG features do not differ from those of the lesional temporal epilepsies. Most patients have altered awareness, and autonomic and/or psychic auras are common. Disturbances of language and oral alimentary automatisms have been reported (Picard et al., 2000).

Berkovic et al. (1994b) emphasized the good response to antiepileptic agents, especially CBZ. That this "syndrome" is entirely defined by genetic data must be emphasized because the clinical and EEG features do not seem to differ significantly from those of the more common temporal lobe epilepsies.

Even though the initial cases (Berkovic et al., 1994b) were reported as having a benign course, Cendes et al. (1998) challenged this view by reporting cases of familial temporal lobe epilepsy that were difficult to control. The exact frequency of familial temporal lobe epilepsy and its significance in terms of prognosis need more thorough definition.

However, even though questions still persist, the realization that not all cases of temporal lobe epilepsy are due to brain damage or are likely to be intractable is clearly of great significance in terms of the prognosis and investigations.

A second type of familial temporal lobe epilepsy with dominant inheritance is characterized by the presence of auditory ictal symptoms (Ottman et al., 1995). At the time of this writing, six such families have been reported (Boneschi et al., 2002; Poza et al., 1999), and linkage to chromosome 10q24 has been determined (see Chapter 20). Other symptoms of involvement of the lateral aspect of the temporal lobe have been associated with the auditory features.

Autosomal Dominant Rolandic Epilepsy with Speech Dyspraxia

Autosomal dominant rolandic epilepsy with speech dyspraxia comprises a rare syndrome described by Scheffer et al. (1995b). They reported a family with nine affected children in three generations that had nocturnal oral faciobrachial focal seizures and centrotemporal epileptiform discharges associated with oral and speech dyspraxia and cognitive impairment. The electroclinical features resembled those of benign RE, except for the orolingual dyspraxia. The syndrome was dominantly inherited with anticipation, which suggested the possibility of the expansion of an unstable triplet repeat.

The recent discovery of epilepsy syndromes that are transmitted as monogenic mendelian traits (Hirose et al., 2002; Berkovic and Scheffer, 1997) has significant implications for the understanding of epilepsy mechanisms. The diagnosis of these "syndromes" rests on the genetic history because none has clinical and EEG features that are sufficiently characteristic to permit a diagnosis in isolated cases, in whom the presence of a hidden lesion is difficult to exclude. Although the major types appear to be well established, a number of cases have common clinical and EEG features, and actual proof of their area of origin in the brain is not always given.

A Syndrome of Benign Focal Seizures in Adolescents

A benign syndrome of partial seizures in adolescents has been recognized. Loiseau and Orgogozo (1978) and Loiseau (1983a) have pointed out that simple partial seizures that do not exhibit the features of BECRS are frequent in adolescents. Many such seizures are not due to brain lesions, and they remain isolated or occur as a single episode with two or more seizures that cluster in a period of 24 or 48 hours. In their series of adolescents with partial seizures (purely motor and mixed motor and sensory seizures, with or without autonomic symptoms), 67% and 76% were seizure free and off drug therapy after a 5-year and a 10-year respective follow-up. However, this high remission rate was entirely due to the frequency of isolated seizures, and patients with repeated fits (i.e., those not grouped in a single episode) had a prognosis similar to that of adults with partial seizures. Although such epileptic seizures do not represent epilepsy because repetition of the seizures is required in the definition of epilepsy, separating them from true epilepsy at the time of their occurrence is impossible.

Predictors of a favorable prognosis include, in addition to the age at occurrence and the absence of central nervous system abnormality, a normal EEG recording. If no seizure occurs in the year following the initial attack(s) and the EEG recording then remains normal, the likelihood of a favorable course is extremely high. Loiseau et al. (1983a) believe that isolated partial seizures in adolescents represent a separate benign convulsive, if not epileptic, syndrome. This syndrome is important to recognize to avoid giving a poor prognosis to adolescents at their first partial seizure.

This syndrome has been recently confirmed by King et al. (1999) in eight patients and by Capovilla et al. (2001a) in 37 adolescents (see Chapter 14). In the series of Loiseau and Orgogozo (1978), 100% of adolescents with *isolated* simple focal seizures were seizure free after 3 years. Those with seizures that were associated with loss of consciousness or generalization had a less favorable outcome, but they still remained seizure free in 68% and 89% of cases at 5 and 10 years, respectively (Loiseau et al., 1983a), if they had no recurrence in the year following the initial episode.

FOCAL (PARTIAL) EPILEPSIES CAUSED BY BRAIN LESIONS: NONIDIOPATHIC FOCAL EPILEPSIES AND SYNDROMES

Focal lesional epilepsies represent one of the major problems among childhood epilepsies because of their frequency and the difficult therapeutic problems they pose. This group is highly heterogeneous with respect to etiology, pathology, and clinical presentations. Thus, establishing precise semiologic and prognostic criteria is much more difficult than in the idiopathic focal epilepsies.

Only a few reasonably well-defined syndromes can be individualized among the epilepsies of lesional origin. *Most of the proposed syndromes of nonidiopathic epilepsy are defined mainly by the characteristics of the seizures rather than by the non-random association of several symptoms,* which is part of the definition of syndromes. This is the case for the topographic syndromes reflecting the involvement of, although not necessarily an origin in, various regions of the brain that have been proposed by the ILAE classification of 1989 (Commission on the Classification and Terminology of the ILAE, 1989). They are essentially based on a description of the *seizures*. As a result, the causes and the prognosis often have to be determined on the basis of an *individual* combination of signs and symptoms, as well as on the results of multiple investigations, in which neuroimaging holds a prominent place (discussed in Chapter 19). In a high proportion of cases, some symptoms and signs, although not defining a syndrome, suggest the lesional origin of an epilepsy.

This section discusses the etiology of lesional epilepsies and briefly describes the associated pathology; it then discusses the general clinical and EEG features that suggest, more or less strongly, the presence of a brain lesion that is responsible for the seizures in those cases that do not belong to a recognizable syndrome. Finally, the few well-delineated syndromes of symptomatic focal epilepsy are described.

Etiology and Pathology

The frequency of lesion-associated focal epilepsy is high even in childhood and adolescence. Of the patients of Currie et al. (1971), 26% developed "complex" partial seizures before 15 years of age. A total of 59% of the surgical patients of Mathieson (1975), 46% of those of Falconer et al. (1964), and 42% of those of Aird et al. (1984) developed their habitual seizures in the first decade. The mean age at the first temporal attack in the series of Ounsted et al. (1966)

varied from 3 years 10 months to 7 years 6 months, depending on the cause. Cavazzuti (1980) indicated that 18% of the epilepsies of school-aged children included complex partial seizures, and Glaser (1967) proposed a figure of 20%. Other investigators have noted a figure of at least 40% of children younger than 15 years (Viani et al., 1988; Cavazzuti, 1980; Gastaut et al., 1975).

Any lesion involving the cerebral cortex can be responsible for epilepsy. This section discusses only the most important types of lesions, most of which are described in more detail in Chapter 19, which deals with epileptogenic tumors, cortical dysplasia, hippocampal sclerosis, Sturge-Weber syndrome, and other vascular abnormalities (traumatic epilepsy is discussed in Chapter 18). The known causes of lesional seizures do not essentially differ, whether or not the seizures feature altered consciousness. Indeed, seizures with and without alteration of consciousness often coexist, and disturbances of consciousness depend on the diffusion of the discharge much more than on its location. However, some differences with the anatomic site of origin of seizures do exist. Most of the initially published works dealt with temporal lobe epilepsy; the temporal lobe, especially the hippocampus, appears particularly susceptible to insult. However, extratemporal lesions are clearly common, especially in children, in whom they may outnumber temporal lesions.

In infants and children, congenital lesions, especially cortical malformations, outnumber destructive ones. Destructive lesions of prenatal, perinatal, or postnatal origin, however, and/or cortical scars are a significant cause of epilepsy. Residual damage following infections (e.g., meningitides or meningoencephalitides) often gives rise to severe focal epilepsy (Trinka et al., 2000; Lancman and Morris, 1996; Marks et al., 1992). In some of these patients, the temporal lobe is involved on one or both sides. Imaging abnormalities are present in up to 78% of patients (Trinka et al., 2000). The onset may be long delayed, and most cases remain medically intractable.

The high incidence of perinatal insults reported in some adult series is not duplicated in children. Only 7 of 100 patients of Ounsted (1966) had an uncertain history of birth trauma, and no difference in birth weight was evident between his patients and the general population. *Isolated* complex partial seizures rarely, if ever, follow a mechanically difficult birth. The relationship between status epilepticus and epilepsy, especially of temporal lobe origin, is discussed with febrile convulsions and hippocampal sclerosis. Some evidence indicates that hippocampal sclerosis is sometimes observed *de novo* following status (see Chapters 14 and 19). The partial or secondarily generalized seizures that occur in patients with shunted hydrocephalus remain a subject of debate. In 117 such cases, Hosking (1974) found an incidence of epilepsy of approximately 30%. A few patients had fits that were related to an episode of shunt dysfunction. Other researchers have reported an incidence of epilepsy of up to 40% following shunt placement (Ines and Markand, 1977), and the location of the EEG foci has been found to correspond to the location of the ventricular catheter (Dan and Wade, 1986; Copeland et al., 1982). In a study of 171 patients, Di Rocco et al. (1985) found that 34 had seizures after shunting, compared with only 25 before surgery, but the cause of the hydrocephalus was thought to be responsible for the seizures. The correspondence of EEG foci with the position of the catheter has not been confirmed by all authors. Bourgeois et al. (1999a) has conducted a review the literature that discusses the possible causes.

The role of genetic factors seems to be secondary in the etiology of partial seizure epilepsies (Ottman, 1989; Treiman, 1989; Rocca et al., 1987c; Andermann, 1982; Andermann and Straszak, 1982). Ounsted et al. (1966) reported that the frequency of any type of convulsive disorder, mostly febrile convulsions, among the siblings of children with temporal lobe epilepsy varied with the etiology. In their series, 30% of the siblings were affected by the temporal lobe epilepsies that followed status epilepticus in infancy, 9% by epilepsies of unknown cause, and only 1.9% by temporal lobe seizures attributable to cerebral insults of known etiology. These researchers thought "a number of subpopulations in respect of genetic influence within the overall group of temporal lobe epilepsies" existed. In a majority, the genetic factor was merely a predisposition to febrile convulsions. When these chanced to be severe and prolonged, a resulting lesion could then produce partial seizures (Ounsted et al., 1987). In a few patients, such as those with tuberous sclerosis, simple mendelian inheritance could be responsible. Aird et al. (1984) and Andermann (1982) believe that genetic factors are implicated in the origin of partial epilepsies as a part of a multifactorial causation, with the genetic factors facilitating the expression of brain lesions that otherwise would not become epileptogenic.

In many cases of epilepsy with partial seizures, the causes remain obscure. This was the case, for example, for 32 of the 100 patients of Ounsted et al. (1966) and for 14 of 36 patients with intractable complex partial seizures reported by Schmidt (1982). In the large series of Pazzaglia et al. (1982), in which half of the cases had their onset before the age of 15 years, no brain pathology was found in 134 (37.3%) of 332 patients with complex partial seizures compared with 292 (49%) of 596 patients with simple partial seizures.

General Features Suggestive of a Lesional Origin

All types of partial seizures can be manifestations of symptomatic epilepsy, which is not the case for idiopathic focal epilepsies. However, some features are more characteristic of lesional cases. Moreover, symptomatic epilepsies may also have suggestive interictal features that may be even more important for diagnosis than are the seizures themselves.

Ictal Clinical Features Suggestive of Lesion-Related Epilepsies

Focal seizures with AC, which formerly were known as *complex partial seizures*, are only rarely a manifestation of idiopathic epilepsies (see earlier discussion). Seizures with epigastric aura, automatisms, loss of awareness, postictal amnesia, and/or sleep are, therefore, suggestive of a symptomatic nature, but other features can also be observed (e.g., "hypermotor" and hypomotor seizures). The association of several types of seizures may also be suggestive of brain damage.

An age at onset of younger than 15 to 24 months also makes a diagnosis of idiopathic epilepsy unlikely (Dulac et al., 1989). However, the description of benign infantile partial epilepsy challenges this statement.

Even when no alteration of consciousness is present, a number of features are of some value. These include the common occurrence of global motor semiology with a diffusion of motor phenomena to a large territory, in contrast with the more discrete contractions seen in idiopathic seizures, the frequency of motor symptoms that involve the entire half of the body, the progressive development during an attack of new symptoms over a relatively long duration, and the frequency and duration of any postictal paralysis (Revol, 1992). Bilateral motor phenomena, pedaling movements of the lower limbs, and forced eye and head deviation are also suggestive of brain lesions, but these may occur in certain frontal idiopathic seizures. Atypical absences with progressive onset and termination and with additional motor phenomena favor a symptomatic origin.

Clearly, however, the symptoms are strongly dependent on the localization of the epileptogenic area, as was previously indicated.

Interictal Clinical Features Suggestive of Lesional Epilepsies

Epilepsies of lesional origin are frequently associated with a high incidence of intellectual, emotional, and psychiatric abnormalities. Many of these have been regarded as being particularly related to temporal lobe seizures (Lindsay et al., 1980a, 1980b; Geshwind, 1979). However, a precise origin has not been established in most series, and complex partial seizures of frontal origin may also be associated with behavioral and cognitive difficulties (Jambaqué and Dulac, 1989; Boone et al., 1988).

Neurologic signs are lacking in many patients. Extensive brain damage may be manifested by hemiparesis or other evidence of cerebral palsy. *Intellectual disturbance* has been fairly common in pediatric series of partial seizures. Holowach et al. (1961) indicated that one-fourth of their 120 children with temporal lobe seizures were mentally deficient. Glaser and Dixon (1956) described disturbances in attention, concentration, memory, abstraction, and language in 30 of 67 children with limbic seizures. They also mentioned a tendency to concrete thinking and distortions of body image. These abnormalities were more marked in those patients with the longest histories of most severe seizures who were receiving the highest dosages of medication. More subtle neuropsychologic involvement has been described, especially differences between the verbal and performance intelligence quotient (IQ) (Fedio and Mirsky, 1969).

Involvement of memory and language is common in older patients with complex partial seizures, especially those of temporal lobe origin (McMillan et al., 1987; Mayeux et al., 1980).

Emotional disturbances have been reported in most child and adult series (Gates and Gumnit, 1990; Trimble, 1990b; Ounsted et al., 1966; Holowach et al., 1961; Glaser and Dixon, 1956). The main problems in childhood have been hyperactivity, impulsivity, distractibility, destructiveness, and outbursts of rage (Dongier, 1977; Taylor, 1972). Ounsted et al. (1966) found outbursts of rage in 36 of 100 patients with temporal lobe seizures and in 26 children with the hyperkinetic syndrome. The latter syndrome was especially common in males with cerebral insults (14 of 35 patients) and in patients with complex partial seizures following early status epilepticus (9 of 32 patients). It was significantly associated with mental retardation, with the mean IQ of hyperkinetic patients being 59. Outbursts of rage also were much more common in patients with cerebral insults or early status, but their presence was not related to a low intellectual level. According to Taylor (1972), aggressiveness is the result of a defect in learning more than of an interference with mechanisms specifically controlling aggressive behavior.

A relationship of psychosis with complex partial seizures has been repeatedly reported (Shepherd and Stephenson, 1992; Tondi et al., 1987; Sindrup and Kristensen, 1980; Jensen and Larsen, 1979; Dongier, 1959), and the association seems too common to be coincidental (Stevens, 1975, 1983). Temporal lobe lesions of early onset are especially prone to an association with psychoses (Shepherd and Stephenson, 1992; Pritchard et al., 1980; Taylor, 1975) that are not manifested before adolescence. Psychoses can result from several mechanisms, including prolonged ictal discharges, some of which may not be recordable from the scalp (Wieser, 1983a, 1991; Wieser et al., 1985) the so-called *forced normalization* (Pakalnis et al., 1991; Trimble, 1991), in which the suppression of clinical seizures and paroxysmal EEG activity is associated with psychosis; and the noxious action of some antiepileptic drugs such as vigabatrin, especially in patients with a personal or family history of mental disorder. In adults, psychosis has occasionally been observed to follow complex partial seizures (Fagan and Lee, 1990; Savard et al., 1987), and the authors have observed similar cases in two children following serial seizures. This phenomenon has been linked to Todd paralysis following motor seizures.

Considerable controversy still exists regarding psychologic peculiarities in patients with complex partial seizures, especially those of temporal lobe origin. Some investigators think specific behaviors, such as excessive religiosity and hypergraphia (Trimble, 1990b), are common, but this is not universally accepted (Gates and Gumnit, 1990). Sexual problems, especially hyposexuality and sexual indifference, are common in adults with complex partial seizures of early onset (Lindsay et al., 1979b).

The high incidence of psychopathology in patients with complex partial seizures has been questioned by several researchers (Ounsted et al., 1987; Feldman, 1983b; Ounsted, 1969; Tizard, 1962). Several large studies (Currie et al., 1971) have failed to find a close relationship between complex partial seizures and aggressiveness or other emotional disturbances when the individual's mental level was considered. Lindsay et al. (1980c) prospectively followed into adulthood the 100 patients studied as children by Ounsted et al. (1966). They found that 75% of them had no psychiatric disorder in later life, even though 85% of them had psychologic problems as children. Although the problem is not easy to solve, some specificity of the epilepsies with complex partial seizures relative to certain psychiatric disorders has been reasonably demonstrated (Stevens, 1983). Conversely, the incidence of mental retardation in patients with complex partial seizures may not differ from that of other types of partial epilepsy of probable lesional origin (Sofijanov, 1982). The differences observed are probably the result of different types of referral, different ages of the patients at time of study, and the type of investigation performed. They reflect the obvious heterogeneity of the epilepsies with complex partial seizures in childhood.

Electroencephalographic Features Suggestive of Lesional Epilepsy

Interictal EEG patterns associated with symptomatic epilepsy vary with the localization of the epileptogenic zone. With temporal lobe lesions, the most characteristic finding is the presence of spikes or sharp waves over the anterior temporal area (Gibbs and Gibbs, 1952). These may be unilateral, but, even in such cases, in only 84 (63%) of 133 patients was the interictal surface paroxysmal activity in good agreement with the site of recording of ictal activity through depth electrodes; partial disagreement was observed in 36 (27%), and total contradiction in 13 (10%) (Wieser, 1983b).

Bilateral discharges are present in one-fourth to one-third of patients (Gibbs and Gibbs, 1952). The bilateral foci are independent in 23% (Daly and Pedley, 1990) to 80% (Gastaut et al., 1953) of patients. Anterior temporal foci are usually associated with a temporal origin of discharges, but they may also be observed in patients with frontal (Quesney, 1992; Lindsay et al., 1984) or occipital (Williamson et al., 1992b, 1993) epileptogenic areas. In some patients, a specific theta-wave rhythm is present in the temporal area (Gastaut et al., 1985).

Extratemporal foci that can involve any area are common in children. Frontal foci are relatively uncommon despite the frequency of frontal lobe seizures. This explains the mechanism for how many lesions remain silent—they are located in areas remote from scalp electrodes, such as the mesial and orbital aspects of the lobe, which accounts for the frequency of normal nonparoxysmal tracings in such cases. Furthermore, EEG paroxysms of spikes or SWs tend to diffuse bilaterally quite rapidly, producing bilateral and apparently synchronous SW paroxysms, the so-called *secondary bilateral synchrony* (Blume and Pillay, 1985; Penfield and Jasper, 1954).

SW bursts may be at 3 Hz or often slower, so some cases of Lennox-Gastaut syndrome could be caused by focal unilateral lesions (Gastaut and Zifkin, 1988).

EEG paroxysms in lesional epilepsies are not strongly as activated by sleep as are those of idiopathic cases (Revol, 1992). Repetitive paroxysms are observed over the site of the focus or, more commonly, on the contralateral hemisphere (Gobbi et al., 1989).

Multiple independent foci are not necessarily related to the lesional epilepsies, and they have been reported in idiopathic RE (Loiseau and Cohadon, 1981) and idiopathic "occipital" epilepsy (Panayiotopoulos, 2002). They have also been found often in severe lesional epilepsies with bilateral lesions and mental and neurologic deficits (Blau and Wiles, 1983; Noriega-Sanchez and Markand, 1976). This pattern may also evolve following Lennox-Gastaut syndrome or infantile spasms (Ohtahara and Yamatogi, 1990; Ohtsuka et al., 1990).

Alteration of background tracings, focal or diffuse areas of low-amplitude EEG rhythm, and polymorphic slow waves are classic features of brain lesions (Gobbi et al., 1989). Rapid low-amplitude rhythm or runs of repetitive spikes usually indicate the presence of dysplastic cortical lesions (Palmini et al., 1991b, 1991c) (see Chapter 19).

Course and Prognosis of Epilepsies Caused by Brain Lesions

Epilepsies caused by brain damage carry a poor prognosis, whether or not the seizures are associated with alterations of consciousness. Cases of known etiology have a poorer prognosis than do idiopathic cases, while epilepsies termed "cryptogenic" in the ILAE classification probably have an intermediate outcome.

Classically, partial epilepsies with alteration of consciousness during seizures (complex partial seizures) have had a particularly poor outcome. Only 12 (7%) of 167 untreated patients with complex partial seizures reported by Janz (1969) were seizure free over a 20-year period. The belief that complex partial seizures are less often controlled by drug treatment has been challenged. In a large series of patients with temporal lobe epilepsy, Currie et al. (1971) found that 40% had been seizure free for 4 years or more, 33% exhibited a marked reduction in seizure frequency, and only 22% were unchanged. Juul-Jensen (1963) found that 88 (40%) of 222 patients with temporal lobe epilepsy were uncontrollable, 80 (36%) became seizure free with drug therapy, and 54 (24%) had only mild epilepsy. Pazzaglia et al. (1982) reported a control rate of 125 (38%) in 332 patients (mainly adults) with complex partial seizures, compared with 32 (32%) of 102 patients with epilepsies with mainly seizures of partial elementary symptomatology. Similarly, Okuma and Kumashiro (1981) found identical remission rates for the epilepsies with "complex partial seizures" and those with simple partial seizures (60% vs. 61%), and this was also the experience of Hauser and Kurland (1975). Studies specifically dedicated to "complex partial seizures" in children have conflicting results (Currie et al., 1971; Holowach et al., 1961). In 100 patients, Lindsay et al. (1979a) reported a control rate of 33%. However, Roger et al. (1991) found that seizures without alteration of awareness outnumbered complex partial seizures when the most severe cases were considered.

Prognostic factors for lesional epilepsies are the same regardless of the clinical types. The association of generalized tonic-clonic seizures with partial ones is unfavorable (Schmidt et al., 1985; Juul-Jensen, 1963), although this has not been the universal experience (Currie et al., 1971; Janz, 1969). The prognosis for intellectual accomplishments is variable, depending on the nature and extent of the lesion, as well as on the course of the epilepsy. In reviews by Lindsay et al. (1979a, 1979b, 1980a, 1980b, 1980c) and Ounsted et al. (1987), 33 of their 100 patients who were followed for 25 years were seizure free without taking drugs, and they were leading fully independent lives. Another 32 were independent, but they still took medication and some had fits. Thirty who were dependent were either living with their families or in institutions, and five had died. An unfavorable course was more common when two or more of eight adverse factors were present. Those factors included (a) an IQ of less than 90, (b) an onset before the age of 2 years 4 months, (c) the occurrence of five or more generalized tonic-clonic attacks, (d) the occurrence of more than one "complex partial seizure" per day, (e) a left-sided EEG focus, (f) the presence of catastrophic rage, (g) the hyperkinetic syndrome, and (h) the need for special schooling. Conversely, a history of seizure disorders in first-degree relatives had a favorable prognostic significance for the long-term outcome of temporal lobe epilepsy in childhood, even when some of the adverse factors were present. Not unexpectedly, the worst prognosis was found in patients with organic brain insults or a history of early status epilepticus. The 33 patients with complex partial seizures of unknown cause did well, as only 2 became dependent. Although this series may have included some patients with benign partial epilepsy, a proportion of patients with focal seizures with alteration of consciousness undoubtedly run a favorable course.

The response to treatment of partial epilepsy associated with brain lesions is often poor, and resistance to antiepileptic drugs is especially common with extensive brain damage. However, even lesional epilepsy can remit but often only after a protracted period (see Chapter 19), and some patients may respond satisfactorily to medical therapy. Epilepsies associated with neurologic signs and mental subnormality are often intractable (Aicardi, 1988a; Holowach-Thurston et al., 1982; Emerson et al., 1981). Surgical treatment probably should be considered in such patients. The therapeutic problems are basically the same as those in the epilepsies with focal seizures associated with disturbances of consciousness.

Syndromes Featuring Focal Epilepsies Caused by Brain Lesions

Mesial Temporal Lobe Syndrome

The mesial temporal lobe syndrome is defined not only on a topographic criterion— the involvement of the hippocampus and other mesial temporal structures—but also on the clinical, EEG, and evolutive features. In addition, imaging evidence of hippocampal sclerosis is often present.

The syndrome often occurs in patients with a history of complex febrile convulsions in infancy, especially those with long-lasting attacks. Such a history is found in at least 40% of patients, and it is sometimes considered the first phase of the syndrome. It is followed by a second phase of latency of variable duration. Focal seizures mark the third phase of chronic epilepsy, which often appears during the second half of the first decade of life; however, an earlier onset is not unusual with focal epilepsy starting within a few years after the initial febrile seizures (Harvey et al., 1995; Abou-Khalil et al., 1993). Seizures are typical of involvement of the mesial aspect of the temporal lobe. An epigastric, often rising sensation that is frequently associated with fear is usual, and it is rapidly followed by the occurrence of oral alimentary automatisms (see "Temporal Lobe Seizures"). Ipsilateral automatisms of the hand or upper limb may then become apparent, whereas a dystonic posture of the contralateral upper limb with internal rotation of the arm and flexion at the wrist is probably indicative of involvement of the basal ganglia. Head turning, which is of little localizing value because it may be ipsilateral or contralateral and not forceful, may or may not be present. Some seizures may be limited to the aura, and loss of awareness is not constant, even in some patients with oral alimentary automatisms (Munari et al., 1980a, 1996). Fear is quite common, although it is difficult to describe precisely. More complex psychic or cognitive subjective phenomena, including a dreamy state in some older children, indicate the probable associated involvement of at least the external aspect of the temporal lobe.

Interictal EEGs show slow (1 to 2Hz), rhythmic sharp waves or sharp slow-wave complexes that are either isolated or in brief runs, occurring unilaterally or bilaterally. An anterior temporal location is usually unilateral or at least predominantly unilateral. Ictal EEGs typically show a buildup of a lateralized sharp theta recruiting rhythm, often following an attenuation of EEG activity. However, different types of discharge can be recorded by invasive monitoring. Interestingly, even in the same patient, the discharges can variably originate from different limbic structures, indicating the involvement of neuronal networks rather than punctual structures. Recent work suggests that mesial temporal seizures may originate from the amygdala or the parahippocampal gyrus more often than from the hippocampus proper (Wennberg et al., 2002).

Memory disturbances are common, especially with left-sided involvement. This picture is mainly associated with hippocampal sclerosis, which may be well demonstrated by MRI showing a shrunken hippocampus on one side with a loss of its internal structures on T1-weighted sequences and an abnormally intense signal on T2-weighted sequences, probably indicating the presence of hippocampal gliosis. Often, other limbic structures, especially the entorhinal cortex, are also atrophic.

Confirmatory evidence can be obtained by noninvasive investigations in most cases. PET shows temporal hypometabolism that often extends beyond the pathologic limits of the lesions (Harvey et al., 1993a, 1993b; Silver et al., 1991). Interictal SPECT may also show an area of relatively low blood flow; ictal SPECT is of more value as it shows increased blood flow involving mostly the internal aspect of the temporal lobe (Engel, 1984, 1992b; Engel et al., 1982a, 1982b, 1990). A PET scan using flumazenil, a ligand of GABAergic receptors, may allow a more precise delimitation of the epileptogenic area, which usually has a more limited extension than the zone of abnormal blood flow (Duncan and Koepp, 2000). When doubt exists about the localization or extent of the lesions, invasive investigations are in order (Lüders et al., 1993b; Engel, 1992b; Wieser et al., 1987, 1993). Some investigators use foramen ovale electrodes (Wieser and Morris, 1997).

Epilepsy of the mesial temporal syndrome is resistant to drug therapy in most cases (Semah et al., 1996), so this is an excellent indication for anterior temporal lobectomy, amygdalohippocampectomy, or tailored temporal cortectomy, which give good results in 60% to 95% of cases (Lüders et al., 1993b). Thus, surgery should probably not be delayed after antiepileptic agents have failed for more than 2 or 3 years.

Hemiconvulsion–Hemiplegia–Epilepsy Syndrome

The hemiconvulsion–hemiplegia–epilepsy (HHE) syndrome, as described by Gastaut et al. in 1960, comprises an initial phase of unilateral or predominantly unilateral convulsive seizures that are usually of long duration (hemiconvulsions); a second phase of hemiplegia (usually permanent), immediately following the hemiconvulsions; and a third stage that is characterized by the appearance of partial epileptic seizures (epilepsy).

The first two stages constitute a particular form of status epilepticus (see Chapter 16), rather than a distinct syndrome. The third phase of partial epilepsy represents, in conjunction with the history of the temporal sequence of hemiconvulsions and hemiplegia, a characteristic epilepsy syndrome (Chauvel et al., 1992b).

The hemiplegia immediately follows the convulsions. It is initially flaccid and fairly massive, but it tends to become spastic and less marked as time passes. The minimum duration of the hemiplegia is arbitrarily set at more than 7 days to separate it from the more common postictal or Todd paralysis. In 20% of the cases recorded by Gastaut et al. (1960), the hemiplegia was not permanent, and it disappeared within 1 to 12 months. In the authors' experience (Arzimanoglou and Dravet, 2001; Aicardi et al., 1969), some degree of spasticity, increased deep tendon reflexes, and pyramidal tract signs persist, even after the paralysis clears. The hemiplegia is usually predominant in the arm, but the face is consistently involved, an important sign differentiating an acquired hemiplegia from a congenital one in cases of early onset. Hemiconvulsion–hemiplegia syndrome has its peak incidence during the first 2 years of life; 60% to 85% of the cases occur between 5 months and 2 years of age, with only few patients who are 4 years or older (Aicardi and Chevrie, 1976; Roger et al., 1974). In approximately three-fourths of patients, hemiconvulsion–hemiplegia syndrome evolve to the secondary appearance of partial seizures that are clearly different from the initial hemiclonic attack

(Gastaut et al., 1974c). In a proportion of the patients, partial seizures may appear even after the hemiplegia has completely cleared. The average interval from initial convulsions to chronic epilepsy was 1 to 2 years, with 85% of the epilepsies having started within 3 years of the initial hemiconvulsion in one study (Aicardi et al., 1969). However, this series was biased in favor of the early onset of complex partial seizures, and these often occur 5 to 10 years after the initial episode.

Approximately two-thirds of the late seizures are partial seizures with alteration of consciousness (Roger et al., 1974; Aicardi et al., 1969). Other types of seizures are commonly associated with the complex partial seizures. Simple partial seizures occur in approximately one-third of the patients, secondarily generalized seizures in 20%, and repeat status in approximately 10% (Roger et al., 1974). The emergence of seizures is usually preceded or accompanied by the appearance of paroxysmal EEG abnormalities, especially in the temporal area. Multifocal paroxysms are not uncommon. Bursts of bilateral SWs are less common. They may be asymmetric with a paradoxically higher amplitude over the hemisphere ipsilateral to the hemiplegia, especially when the amplitude of the background tracing is diminished over the opposite hemisphere (Gastaut et al., 1974c). The lateralization of the late seizures of HHE syndrome is closely related to that of the inaugural convulsion (Aicardi and Chevrie, 1983).

Late epilepsies of HHE syndrome run an unpredictable course, but most are severe and difficult or impossible to control.

The incidence of the syndrome has considerably declined over the past 20 years (Roger et al., 1982) in industrialized countries, but cases are still common in third-world countries (Arzimanoglou and Dravet, 2001).

The causes of the initial convulsions in HHE syndrome are multiple. Meningitis, subdural effusions, and trauma have been recorded. In many patients (Aicardi and Chevrie, 1983), no cause is obvious. Such cases may be the result of the epileptic activity itself, as has been observed in febrile status epilepticus (Soffer et al., 1986; Aicardi et al., 1969; Norman, 1964). Alternatively, a small, asymptomatic hemispheric lesion of perinatal or prenatal origin could be responsible for the initiation or localization of the seizure, which then produces epileptic brain damage with a resultant increase in the extent of the original lesion and the appearance of new clinical and radiologic signs. The likelihood of such a mechanism in many cases is suggested by the frequency of an-

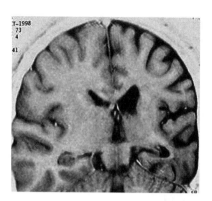

FIG. 10.10. Magnetic resonance imaging (MRI) scan of a patient with hemiconvulsion–hemiplegia syndrome. The left hemisphere is uniformly atrophic with ventricular dilatation and cortical atrophy. The MRI picture corresponds to the neuropathologic aspect known as *hemiatrophia cerebri*. It differs from the localized atrophy observed in congenital hemiplegias resulting from arterial occlusion, and it is seen only with acquired postconvulsive hemiplegia.

tecedent abnormalities in the history of patients with prolonged unilateral infantile convulsions (Chevrie, and Aicardi, 1975; Wallace, 1972, 1976b). Roger (1974) thought that, in 33 of 92 cases, the hemiplegia had the same cause as the hemiconvulsions, whereas, in 59 patients, it was the consequence of the status itself. Neuroradiologic studies at the time of the initial convulsive status and a few weeks or months later (Kataoka et al., 1988; Aicardi and Baraton, 1971; Gastaut et al., 1960) have demonstrated that an acquired atrophy can appear very rapidly following status epilepticus. Atrophy often is preceded by swelling and edema of the hemisphere involved in the epileptic discharge (Soffer et al., 1986). Eventually, when the hemiplegia persists, generalized atrophy of the hemisphere sets in (Figs. 10.10 and 10.11), producing the so-called *hemiatrophia cerebri* (Tan and Urich, 1984), which is highly suggestive of postepileptic atrophy. This lesion differs from the more limited atrophies observed with ischemic lesions of vascular origin. Indeed, postconvulsive hemiplegia is rarely associated with vascular obstruction (Aicardi et al., 1969; Norman, 1962).

Syndrome of Cystic Dilation of the Occipital Horn with Epilepsy

Remillard et al. (1974) have reported cases of partial seizures with alteration of consciousness associated with cystic dilation of the posterior part of one lateral ventricle. Similar cases have since been re-

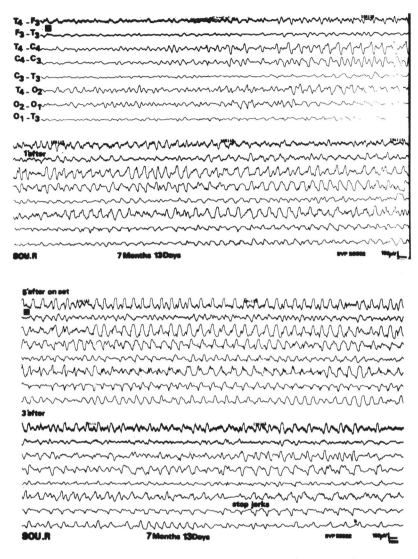

FIG. 10.11. Hemiplegia–hemiconvulsion syndrome. **Top:** Onset of seizure over the right central region. **Bottom:** Continuation of the seizure with spike-wave activity over the right hemisphere and diffusion to the opposite side.

ported (Deonna and Prod'hom, 1980; Roger et al., 1977). Like HHE syndrome, this syndrome includes two sets of events that usually occur several years apart. The initial events generally occur during the neonatal period. Compression or thrombosis of one posterior cerebral artery is responsible for the development of a large temporooccipital ischemic lesion, which is later responsible for the seizures. The compression is probably the result of herniation of one temporal lobe into the incisura tentorii. In the series of Remillard et al. (1974), 5 of 8 patients had difficult

neonatal periods, with convulsive seizures, drowsiness, and vomiting. The process of birth itself had been traumatic, and/or the neonatal period had been abnormal in several patients of Roger et al. (1977). In a few cases, symptoms and signs pointing to temporal lobe herniation with compression of the third nerve have been described (Deonna and Prod'hom, 1980). Herniation might result from an acute subdural hematoma or massive hemispheral edema. However, the initial phase of the syndrome does not need to be symptomatic or, even necessarily, to take place during the neonatal period. In a personal case, the syndrome was apparently the result of a subdural effusion that occurred at 9 months of age.

The seizures associated with this syndrome are probably of occipital origin, but they may spread to the anterior temporal lobe. They occur frequently, and they are difficult to control (Remillard et al., 1974). Definitive diagnosis rests on neuroimaging, which reveals atrophy of the temporooccipital cortex with dilatation and outpouching of one occipital horn. In one series (Roger et al., 1977), 2.2% of all epileptic patients submitted to CT scan and 5% of those younger than 20 years had the characteristic lesion.

Partial Continuous Epilepsy (Epilepsia Partialis Continua, Kojewnikow Syndrome) and Rasmussen Syndrome

Epilepsia partialis continua is defined as the occurrence of continuous myoclonic jerks that are localized to a limited area on one side of the body. The jerks are of brief duration, and they typically affect the agonist and antagonist muscles, persist in sleep, are worsened by action or stress, and continue relentlessly over time. The jerks are sometimes associated with jacksonian seizures starting in the same area and occasionally with other seizure types (Bancaud, 1985; Bancaud et al., 1970). The twitches often involve only a few muscles. They are usually arrhythmic, but the individual jerks usually occur no more than 10 seconds apart (Thomas et al., 1977). The hand and foot and the face are affected more often than the proximal segments of the limbs. Typically, one thumb or the great toe jerks continuously. The jerks may increase spontaneously, with attempts at voluntary movements and maintenance of postures or with sensory stimuli. From time to time, they may extend toward the proximal part of the limb with a jacksonian march and may involve the whole side of the body; rarely, they become generalized.

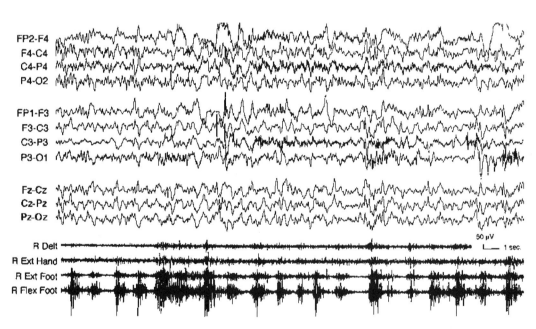

FIG. 10.12. *Epilepsia partialis continua* in a 12-year-old girl with left-sided Rasmussen encephalitis. The child also presented with numerous somatomotor and somatosensitive (intense pain) seizures of the right arm and leg. Complete control of her epilepsy was achieved following hemispherotomy at the price of a right hemiplegia and aphasia. The polygraphic recording, including right extensor and flexor of the foot, corresponds to subcontinuous myoclonic jerks of the right leg that often diffused ipsilaterally to the right arm. The electroencephalogram shows diffuse abnormalities with asymmetry of background activity that were slower and less well organized over the left derivations. A high-voltage angular delta activity is registered, with slow spikes over the left frontocentral regions and the vertex. This activity is organized in pseudorhythmic subcontinuous discharges, some of which were concomitant to the myoclonic jerks. (Courtesy of Dr. Pierre Thomas, Nice, France.)

The EEG may show very little paroxysmal abnormality, and the background rhythm may be normal (Bancaud, 1985; Watanabe et al., 1984; Dulac et al., 1983b). In such cases, time-locked EEG events can be detected by back-averaging. In other cases, the EEG displays occasional spikes, either localized or in clusters, which may remain localized even during a jacksonian march. In more severe cases, unilateral or bilateral runs of abnormal rhythms may occur (Fig. 10.12). Rarely, periodic lateralized discharges that are time locked to the jerks are observed (PeBenito and Cracco, 1979). A neurologic examination may produce normal results, or it may show monoplegia or hemiplegia, which may be fixed or which may fluctuate with the frequency and intensity of the attacks.

This rare type of somatomotor seizure is almost always the result of brain lesions of variable extent (Drinkenburg et al., 1991), and it regularly involves the *rolandic cortex* (Chauvel et al., 1992b; Bancaud, 1985; Bancaud et al., 1970, 1982). Rare cases of epilepsia partialis continua of extracortical origin have been reported, but these do not conform to the current definition of epilepsia partialis continua (Cock and Shorvon, 2002).

The following two major forms of epilepsia partialis continua are recognized: cases due to a fixed circumscribed cortical lesion and those associated with a progressive course with evolutive brain atrophy (Dulac et al., 1983b; Bancaud et al., 1970).

In the first group, the disease is not progressive. Some degree of weakness may be associated with seizures in the same localization. This rare type of somatomotor status is due to cortical lesions of variable extent (Drinkenburg et al., 1991). Most cases are caused by static brain damage. Atrophic, and especially dysplastic, lesions are much more common in children than are tumors or vascular disturbances (Palmini et al., 1991b; Kuzniecky et al., 1988; Dulac et al., 1983b). The epilepsia partialis continua may persist for hours to months or years. It may stop suddenly, only to reappear after variable periods, but the reasons for the appearance or disappearance of epilepsia partialis continua in patients with old lesions are unknown.

Partial continuous epilepsy also occurs as the main component of a progressive syndrome (*Rasmussen syndrome*) that includes other types of seizures, especially partial complex attacks, and evolving neurologic deficits, such as hemiplegia, abnormal movements, aphasia, and mental deterioration. Neuroimaging in such patients shows a progressive atrophy that may involve the frontotemporal region or a whole hemisphere but that rarely affects the contralateral hemisphere.

The onset is usually between 18 months and 14 years of age, with a mean of 7 years, and the child's development is usually normal before the onset of epilepsy. In about half the patients, a history of infectious or inflammatory episodes in the weeks preceding onset can be elicited, and these may play an etiologic role. Seizure of multiple types, especially focal seizures, can occur. In a series of 47 patients, 20 had generalized tonic-clonic attacks, 37 had "simple partial seizures," and 15 had "complex partial seizures." Twenty-seven patients had partial continuous epilepsy. The syndrome evolves in three phases (Bien et al., 2002; Oguni et al., 1991a). (a) A first prodromal phase is characterized by a relatively low seizure frequency and, only rarely, by a mild degree of hemiparesis; this lasts an average of 7 months, but it may be longer in adolescents. (b) The second acute phase features an abrupt increase of seizures with partial continuous epilepsy in 50% to 60% of patients, and the development of hemiplegia in almost all cases (Oguni et al., 1991a; Zupanc et al., 1990; Rasmussen and Andermann, 1989). Its median duration was 8 months in a recent study (Bien et al., 2002), Most of the atrophy develops during this phase. (c) The third stage follows with a permanent and usually stable hemiparesis. Unfortunately, cognitive decline is an almost constant feature of the disease.

Unilateral hemispheric atrophy involving predominantly the frontotemporal region is apparent on CT scans. MRI better defines the lesion, showing an abnormal T2 signal involving the white matter and the cortex of the frontal and temporal lobes around the sylvian fissure (Bien et al., 2002; So and Andermann, 1998; Yacubian et al., 1997). Interestingly, involvement of the caudate nucleus on the side of the lesion is usually present, accompanied by marked atrophy and consequent widening of the frontal horn. Atrophy of the caudate may be an early and even the first imaging abnormality in some patients (Koehn and Zupanc, 1999). This relatively neglected finding is even more interesting because cases of Ramussen syndrome that begin with unilateral choreic movements mimicking Sydenham chorea have been reported (Oguni et al., 1991a) and these have been responsible for diagnostic errors (Lascelles et al., 2002).

The lesions are progressive with increases in both the intensity and extent of the atrophy, which eventually may involve the whole hemisphere.

The EEG also shows progressive deterioration of the background activity, which is virtually constant and often bilateral, although it is asymmetric. Abnormal slow-wave activity is constant, usually with asymmetric polymorphic delta activity and sometimes with runs of monomorphic slow waves. Interictal paroxysmal discharges of multiple independent foci lateralized over one hemisphere are seen in about half the cases. Bilateral discharges are common, and they are usually asymmetric but they do not indicate bilateral pathology (So and Andermann, 1998). Such cases are also termed *Rasmussen encephalitis*, and they were originally reported by Rasmussen and Andermann (1989). Neuropathologic studies of resected (Honavar et al., 1992; Robitaille, 1991) or postmortem (Gray et al., 1987) specimens have shown definite inflammatory signs with glial nodules and perivascular infiltrates containing plasmocytes and lymphocytes, as well as microglial cells (Honavar et al., 1992). The lesions generally predominate in the posterior frontal and anterior temporal regions. Remarkably, they are limited to one side, and they do not cross to the opposite hemisphere.

Attempts at demonstrating a conventional virus or unconventional agents have mostly failed. Reports on the presence of cytomegalovirus or Epstein-Barr virus deoxyribonucleic acid in the brain (Power et al., 1990) have an uncertain significance (Atkins et al., 1995); the presence of herpes simplex virus type 2 in a case of smoldering encephalitis with temporal lobe epilepsy presenting similarities to Rasmussen syndrome is difficult to interpret (Cornford and McCormick 1997). Oligoclonal bands in the cerebrospinal fluid were present in several cases (Iivanainen et al., 1981; Dulac et al., 1983b).

Current opinion favors the presence of immunologic allergic mechanisms (So and Andermann, 1998; Larner and Anderson, 1995; Rogers et al., 1994). The presence of antibodies against the glutamate R_3 receptor has been demonstrated in some, but not all, cases (Rogers et al., 1994). These have been shown to stimulate the receptors, and they might thus play a role in the origin of seizures.

Rasmussen syndrome has a severe course. Neurologic signs, especially hemiplegia and mental deterioration, develop in almost all cases, but the disease rarely progresses to death (Rasmussen and Andermann, 1989; Oguni et al., 1991a). In most patients, the disease burns out after several years, leaving severe residua. A fluctuating course is common, and it may last for several years (Rasmussen and Andermann, 1989). Stabilization at a limited level of disability is possible (Oguni et al., 1991a), and the prospect that some cases of partial epilepsy without special EEG or imaging features are "formes frustes" of Rasmussen syndrome has been entertained.

Antiepileptic drug treatment is ineffective in almost all cases of Rasmussen syndrome. Therapy with corticosteroids in large doses (Dulac et al., 1991b) or with immunosuppressant agents and immunoglobulins has been proposed, but these have not been properly tested.

Treatment with corticosteroids in large doses may be temporarily effective (Hart et al., 1994; Dulac et al., 1991b), but it does not seem to alter the ultimate outcome. Immunosuppressors also may have some immediate effects. Immunoglobulins given intravenously have gained some measure of success (Wise et al., 1996; Hart et al., 1994). The same applies to plasmapheresis (Palcoux et al., 1997; Andrews et al., 1996), which has been associated with improvement, although this, unfortunately, has only been transient (Gordon, 1997b). Surgical treatment seems to be efficacious in many cases, but only large resections and especially hemispherectomy seem to help (Vining et al., 1993, 1997; Andermann et al., 1992; Villemure et al., 1991; Polkey, 1989). The expected sequelae limit the indications for surgery to patients who are already hemiplegic, even though some investigators (Rasmussen and Villemure, 1989) have proposed hemispherectomy even in the face of mild hemiplegia because they think that the course is relentlessly progressive. However, an occasional patient may stabilize with very mild hemiparesis, making an early surgical decision extremely difficult.

Epilepsia partialis continua is known to occur with demonstrated viral infections as a manifestation of acute or subacute viral encephalitides. These include Russian spring-summer encephalitis in which continuous jerking develops months after the acute phase; this was the cause of the cases reported by Kojewnikow (1992). Continuous partial epilepsy is also a major feature of the subacute type of delayed measles encephalitis, a syndrome that is usually observed in immunosuppressed children (Aicardi et al., 1983). In two such cases, the partial continuous hemiplegia was attributed to subcortical lesions (Colamaria et al., 1988). Epilepsia partialis continua may also result from mitochondrial disorders, especially the myoclonic epilepsy with ragged-red fibers (MERRF) and the mitochondrial myopathy, encephalopathy, lactic acidosis, and strokelike episodes (MELAS) syndromes (see Chapters 7 and 15), and as a manifestation of nonketotic hyperglycemia.

Other Possible Syndromes of Lesional Focal Epilepsy

Most cases of seizures originating outside the temporal lobe are not part of clusters of symptoms and signs that are not randomly linked, and, therefore, they do not qualify for categorization as syndromes, even though frontal and occipital *seizures* have characteristic features. However, the clinical context and course of such cases are often variable, and they do not conform to the definition of epilepsy syndromes.

However, some patients with frontal lobe seizures share, in addition to their characteristic ictal manifestations, certain characteristics, such as predominant emergence during sleep; frequent repetition of clusters of seizures; rapid bilateralization; and frequent generalization that confers to them a certain similarity, albeit with important differences. In rare cases, a behavioral syndrome resembling the classic frontal syndrome of adults has been described (Jambaqué and Dulac, 1989). Such cases partially satisfy the criteria for epilepsy syndromes, even though they are rather loosely defined ones.

Occipital seizures are also characteristic as such, but, like frontal seizures, they occur in multiple contexts and they are due to multiple causes, lesional or genetic. In addition, they can be part of several syndromes with a variable outcome. As this chapter discussed in "Occipital Lobe Seizures," cases of benign (probably genetic) occipital epilepsies have been classified into several subsyndromes, but lesional cases do not lend themselves to this categorization because of their multiple clinical presentations, courses, and etiologic contexts.

Syndromes of Lesional Epilepsy of Subcortical Origin

Hypothalamic Hamartoma

Hypothalamic hamartomas are ectopic masses of neuronal and glial tissue that may be sessile or pedunculated; they vary from small masses that are sometimes difficult to evidence by imaging to large masses (Fig. 10.13). They arise from the region of the tuber cinereum or mamillary bodies and develop into the interpeduncular cistern or within the third ventricle; they are due to multiple causes, either lesional or genetic; and they can be part of several syndromes with variable outcomes. Their histologic structure resembles that of gray matter, with varying proportions of neurons, glia, and fiber bundles. They do not behave as true tumors. Rather, they grow at about the same rate as the rest of the brain, and they do *not* produce signs of nerve tissue compression.

Hamartomas present most often with epilepsy, although they may also produce precocious puberty. The *epilepsy syndrome* of hamartomas has an early onset between birth to 2 years of age, and it is characterized by frequent, repeated attacks of unnatural, mirthless laughter (gelastic seizures) or, more rarely, by crying (dacrycystic seizures) (Tassinari et al., 1997). After several years, the seizures often become secondarily generalized with tonic or atonic features

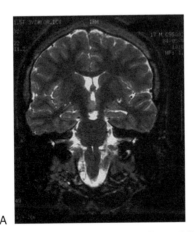
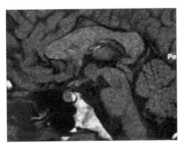

A   B

FIG. 10.13. A, B: Hypothalamic hamartoma. Coronal **(A)** and sagittal **(B)** magnetic resonance imaging scan of a small hypothalamic hamartoma impinging on the right side of the third ventricle. The onset of epilepsy occurred at the age of 7 years with gelastic seizures and partial seizures characterized by deviation of head to the right, facial contraction, and clonic jerks of the right arm. The epilepsy was intractable to all antiepileptic drugs in several combinations. When the patient was 17 years old (October, 2001), the patient was submitted to gamma-knife surgery. A classic surgical approach was not feasible because the patient also suffered from familial angioneurotic edema. Following an initial amelioration, the seizures relapsed. In some patients, remission is observed only 12 to 18 months after radiosurgery.

that are often uncontrollable (Berkovic et al., 1986). Interictal EEG may show only bilateral paroxysmal discharges (Berkovic et al., 1986). However, focal paroxysms of spikes or sharp waves are often recorded from the temporal lobe. Temporal resection, however, has proven ineffective (Dubeau et al., 1995). Evidence that the seizures originate from the hamartoma itself has been shown by ictal SPECT, which shows increased blood flow in the hamartoma (Kuzniecky et al., 1997), and by direct recording from intralesional electrodes (Munari et al., 1995, 1999a; Kahane et al., 1997). Surgical excision or disconnection of the lesion can give excellent results, and it may prevent the secondary cognitive and behavioral deterioration (Berkovic et al., 2003), which is usually associated with generalization of the seizures, itself associated with the diffusion of EEG paroxysms of spikes and SWs (Berkovic et al., 1986).

Cerebellar Congenital Neuroglial Tumors

Several reports (Al Shawan et al., 1996; Arzimanoglou et al., 1999) of a syndrome of frequent, repeated brief attacks of tonic facial contractions of early onset that resemble the facial hemispasm observed in adults have been published. The attacks may occur in both wakefulness and sleep, and they may consist of short, mostly unilateral, contractions around the mouth and eye without loss of awareness.

Harvey et al. (1996) showed that these attacks were associated with a typical EEG discharge that was closely related to the lesion. In all reported cases, the lesion was an apparently static mass localized in the cerebellar peduncle that was impinging on the brainstem and the fourth ventricle. The tumor was regarded as a hamartoma by some (Arzimanoglou et al., 1999) or as a ganglioglioma by others (Harvey et al., 1996). Removal of the mass with subsequent control of the seizures is possible. Such cases may be thought of a subcortical epilepsy.

SUMMARY

Focal (or partial) seizures are a most important category of seizures. Although they are commonly thought to be due to focal brain damage, this actually applies only to part of such seizures. In the past few decades, the importance of nonlesional (or idiopathic) focal seizures, in which genetic factors play a prominent etiologic role, has been recognized, and these form a significant category of partial epilepsies with usually favorable outcomes.

Focal seizures can present with a variety of clinical manifestations. Depending on their area of origin, they can feature motor, sensory, visual, auditory, cognitive, autonomic, or behavioral manifestations.

The traditional dichotomy between simple or complex partial seizures based on the state of consciousness during attacks is no longer universally accepted. Disturbances of consciousness are often difficult to recognize, especially in children, and both "simple" and "complex" types of partial seizures can occur in the same child, depending mostly on the diffusion of the discharge. Seizures that remain localized to their area of origin usually do not disturb consciousness; disturbances result with a larger diffusion of the epileptic discharge.

Partial seizures of symptomatic origin can be due to a wide variety of brain lesions. The extent and nature of damage are largely responsible for the outcome.

A significant proportion of cases do respond to antiepileptic drug treatment. However, focal epileptic seizures caused by brain lesions are often difficult to control or are medically intractable. For such patients, surgical therapy is promising for many cases. However, not all focal intractable seizures are amenable to surgery, and a careful study of each case is mandatory. The investigation of possible surgical cases is best performed in specialized centers that use modern techniques of anatomic and, if necessary, functional imaging, as well as the most recent surgical techniques. With careful preoperative localization, the results can be rewarding.

Focal epilepsies are related to the activation of localized cortical areas. They can result from brain damage of multiple causes or they can be unassociated with any detectable cortical lesion. In this latter case, the seizure discharges appear to result from a purely functional disturbance that for reasons that are still obscure is limited to a restricted cortical zone. In such cases, the localization of the abnormally excitable area can move from one place to another, either in the same hemisphere or contralaterally, or it can become "generalized." Epilepsies that are due to this mechanism are termed "idiopathic" epilepsies. Genetic factors are probably a determinant cause of such cases, even though the exact mode of inheritance remains unsettled in most patients. Idiopathic focal epilepsies are often benign, in terms of both seizure control and cognitive and behavioral development. The major syndromes in this group include rolandic epilepsy, which represents about 15% of epilepsies in the 3-year-old to 16-year-old age group; occipital epilepsies; and a few rarer types.

Recently, rarer idiopathic syndromes with a established mode of inheritance (usually autosomal dominant) and, in a few cases, with an identified gene have been recognized. In spite of their authenticated genetic origin, they may not all be benign. The identified genes code either for protein constituents of ionic channels or for subunits of receptors for neurotransmitters. Despite their rarity, these monogenic idiopathic epilepsies are important for the understanding of epileptic mechanisms.

A large heterogeneous group of epilepsies is associated with the presence of brain lesions that involve essentially the cerebral cortex. All types of lesions may be a cause of seizures, and the clinical picture is highly variable, depending on the location, extent, and nature of the lesion(s). Collectively, such lesional epilepsies tend to be more difficult to control with antiepileptic agents than idiopathic cases are, to be more polymorphic in their clinical expression, and to be associated more often with cognitive behavioral or psychiatric problems. However, not all epilepsies of lesional nature necessarily have poor prognosis. Because of their variability of expression, lesional epilepsies often do not present as well-defined syndromes. However, some clinical subgroups, such as mesial temporal epilepsies, Rasmussen syndrome, and a few other presentations, constitute relatively well-delineated syndromes that are clinically recognizable and that have different prognostic and, sometimes, etiologic significances.

11

Landau-Kleffner Syndrome and Syndrome of Continuous Spike-Waves of Slow Sleep

SYNDROME OF EPILEPTIC APHASIA WITH SEIZURE DISORDER

Since Landau and Kleffner (1957) described six children who developed aphasia after apparently normal acquisition of language, the association of unusual types of aphasia with electroencephalographic (EEG) abnormalities and, often, a seizure disorder has been recognized as a specific syndrome.

The Landau-Kleffner syndrome (LKS) is currently defined as an acquired childhood aphasia with mainly bitemporal paroxysmal EEG abnormalities, a seizure disorder without demonstrable focal brain lesions, and a regression or stabilization of the disease after a variable time (Tassinari et al., 2002). Even though cases with paroxysmal EEG recordings but no seizures are not epilepsy in the strictest sense, they are covered in this chapter because they do not differ in any other way from the most common cases with clinical attacks. The EEG abnormalities are often very marked, and they tend to increase during slow sleep, often producing continuous spike-waves of slow sleep (CSWS), also termed *electrical status epilepticus of sleep* (ESES), thus suggesting a close relationship between LKS and the "syndrome of CSWS." (In this chapter, for the sake of clarity, the terms CSWS and ESES are used to designate the EEG abnormalities, and CSWS syndrome refers to the electroclinical picture.)

Before onset, the affected children have normal motor and intellectual development, and their language is at a normal level for their age. The language disturbances develop over a relatively brief period. The loss of acquired language is usually total or profound, but nonverbal skills are generally completely or at least relatively preserved. Behavioral disturbances of various types can be observed in up to two-thirds of patients (Tassinari et al., 2002; Deonna, 1991; Sawhney et al., 1988; Dugas et al., 1982), and persistance of the aphasia is not rare (Beaumanoir, 1992; Paquier et al., 1992; Deonna, 1991; Dulac et al., 1983a). The epilepsy tends to remit before adulthood. All patients consistently display paroxysmal

EEG abnormalities that commonly are bilateral and that often have a predominantly temporal or posterior location. Clinical seizures are experienced by 75% to 85% of patients at some time, although they do not necessarily appear at the very beginning of the disorder. The course is initially progressive, but fluctuations, stabilization, or improvement of speech may occur over the years, although long follow-up is available for only a few cases.

Cases of temporary aphasia following unilateral status epilepticus, as well as postical aphasia occurring in association with certain types of transient attacks, particularly brief complex partial seizures, probably belong to different epilepsy syndromes, so these are not considered here (see Chapters 10 and 16).

At least 248 publications on this topic have appeared in the last 32 years (Panayiotopoulos, 1999), and the syndrome is diagnosed increasingly often (Beaumanoir, 1992; Paquier et al., 1992). Not all patients with acquired aphasia associated with seizure disorder display the same clinical, EEG, and evolutive features, which suggests the possibility of subgroups within the syndrome and raises the question of the criteria used to define the syndrome.

Etiologic Data

Reported cases of the syndrome of acquired epileptic aphasia indicate that its onset occurs between 18 months (Uldall et al., 2000) and 13 years of age. In most, the onset is between 4 and 7 years of age, with three-fourths of the cases appearing before the age of 7 years. Late-onset cases have been reported, however (Dugas et al., 1995).

Among affected patients, males are more preponderant than females. Beaumanoir (1992) found 98 boys and only 59 girls. Most patients appeared normal before the onset of the syndrome. Extensive studies have failed to detect an identifiable cause. By definition, no evidence of structural brain pathology is found. However, a few cases with similar presentations, including the same intense EEG anomalies, and a focal lesion have been recorded; these may, in fact, be due to the same epileptic mechanism, which, in these cases, is initiated by a lesion instead of being purely "functional" (Galanopoulou et al., 2000; Cole et al., 1988; Lou et al., 1977). Worster-Drought (1971) suspected an inflammatory cause, but no positive data are available to support this hypothesis. Lou et al. (1977) reported inflammatory infiltrates in a biopsy specimen of temporal lobe in a patient with Landau syndrome. Their findings, however, were not entirely convincing. No organic cause was demonstrated in another patient submitted to brain biopsy (McKinney and McGreal, 1974), and the computed tomographic (CT) and magnetic resonance scan results are almost always normal. Positron emission tomography (PET) studies have variably shown areas of hypometabolism or hypermetabolism (Maquet et al., 1990). Pascual-Castroviejo et al. (1992) found abnormal arteriograms in four patients, and they considered these individuals to have arteritis that was limited to the central nervous system. They claimed that they had obtained excellent results with the combined use of steroids and calcium-entry blockers. However, the significance of these findings has been disputed (Deonna, 1991). One case of neurocysticercosis associated with LKS has also been recorded (Otero et al., 1989).

Epilepsy Characteristics and Electroencephalographic Abnormalities

Seizures

Seizures are the first manifestation of the syndrome in about 60% of patients. In the remaining patients, aphasia is the first manifestation, and 17% to 25% of the patients with this syndrome do not have clinical attacks (Gordon, 1997c; Beaumanoir, 1992; Dulac et al., 1983a; Deonna et al., 1977). The frequency of seizures is quite variable; many patients have one or few fits, and others may have several attacks daily. The seizures do not represent a major problem, and episodes of status epilepticus seem unusual (Deonna et al., 1977). The attacks, which may be either diurnal or nocturnal, are often well controlled by drug treatment (Mantovani and Landau, 1980). A precise description of the seizures in 44 patients (Beaumanoir, 1992; Dulac et al., 1983a) indicated that 19 had partial motor seizures with or without generalization that, at times, was followed by Todd paralysis; 7 had complex partial seizures; 7 had atypical absences, often with atonia of head; and 17

had generalized motor attacks, which often were the first epileptic manifestation (Bureau et al., 1995a). Facial and ocular myoclonias have also been mentioned (Morrell et al., 1995; Dulac et al., 1983a), but tonic seizures have not been reported. In most patients, the seizures seem to remit before adulthood (Beaumanoir, 1992; Dulac et al., 1983a; Mantovani and Landau, 1980). In exceptional cases (Cole et al., 1988), the epilepsy persists into adult life and represents a major problem, at times necessitating surgery.

Neurophysiologic Abnormalities

EEG abnormalities, by definition, are present in all patients. The background rhythms are usually normal, but slow waves in the theta range are occasionally present in the same regions as the spikes. The repetitive spikes or sharp waves or spike-wave complexes of high amplitude are generally bilateral, but, frequently, they are prevalent over the temporal and parietal regions (Beaumanoir, 1992; Hirsch et al., 1990; Dulac et al., 1983a; Shoumaker et al., 1974; Gascon et al., 1973). They rarely, if ever, involve the anterior temporal areas (Deonna et al., 1977). Contrary to expectations, the paroxysms predominate over the right hemisphere as often as they do over the left, and, when they are unilateral, they may shift from side to side.

The paroxysmal activity is usually predominant over the temporal areas (Beaumanoir, 1992). A striking feature in most cases is the variability of the EEG abnormalities with regard to time and intensity. Nakano et al. (1989) used brain-mapping techniques to study the topographic features of the discharges. Using the methohexital-suppression test, Morrell et al. (1995) demonstrated that spikes on one side always anticipated those on the contralateral side by 20 to 40 ms, thus suggesting that one hemisphere has a leading role. Magnetoencephalography has confirmed that the spikes originate on the dorsal surface of the superior temporal gyrus (Paetau et al., 1999). Other investigators also showed that the spikes could interfere with the auditory evoked responses (Seri et al., 1998; Isnard et al., 1995), which strongly implicates the auditory cortex in the genesis of the epileptic activity.

Multifocal discharges are common, and the spike or sharp-wave foci may resemble those observed in benign partial epilepsy of childhood (Dulac et al., 1983a; Billard et al., 1981). In keeping with this, the frequency and intensity of discharges often are considerably augmented in slow sleep. Massa et al. (2000) compared the EEG features in seven children with LKS with those of seven other children with benign rolandic epilepsy and suggested that some patterns, including the presence of unilateral slow-wave foci, bilateral independent spike-waves discharges, and an increase of spike-wave discharges by more of 40% in the first sleep cycle, were predictors of the continuous paroxysms. In slow sleep, a prominent increase is often seen in the activity of spike foci that is accompanied by the disappearance of the landmarks of sleep (Billard et al., 1990; Kellerman, 1978), an aspect reminiscent of that of the so-called ESES or CSWS (Billard et al., 1981, 1990; Hirsch et al., 1990). However, some investigators (Giovanardi Rossi et al., 1999; Genton et al., 1990b; Tiberge et al., 1988) have noted that the paroxysmal activity may continue during rapid eye movement (REM) sleep in patients with the LKS, in contrast with its disappearance at this stage in cases of "electrical status epilepticus of slow sleep," and they have suggested that this might differentiate the two syndromes. The EEG abnormalities tend to subside with increasing age. Dulac et al. (1983a) noted that they had disappeared by the age of 15 years in 17 of 18 adolescents.

Characteristics of Language Disturbances

The typical language disturbance in epileptic aphasia is a marked deficit of auditory comprehension, which differs from the usual features of the more common aphasias of childhood. This may be so profound that many of the children are initially considered deaf. Indeed, a disturbed understanding of language is often the first manifestation, and the progressive disappearance of spoken language follows, apparently as a consequence of the receptive disturbance (Kaga, 1999; Paetau et al., 1991; Billard et al., 1990; Hrachovy et al., 1979). Kaga (1999) suggested that the language disorder evolves in a systematized manner, beginning with sensory aphasia, followed by auditory agnosia and finally by word deafness. The full deficit evolves over weeks or even months, although an abrupt onset or a sudden aggravation following the occurrence of a seizure has been reported in some cases (Dugas et al., 1982; Deonna et al., 1977; Shoumaker et al., 1974). In at least some patients, the disturbance in auditory gnosia appears to extend beyond the verbal field. These children are not able to recognize other sounds, such as the cries of animals or other familiar sounds. The tonal audiograms are, however, normal, indicating that the defect is an inability to decode sounds, which is a necessary step in language

understanding (Rapin et al., 1988). The affected children understand little or no spoken language, and, consequently, their verbal expression deteriorates. Their visual-verbal abilities, on the other hand, may be remarkably well preserved and they can be taught to lip read and write quite well. However, errors in reading and spelling are not uncommon. Auditory inattentiveness is present in some patients, who may have difficulties localizing the origin of a sound (Beaumanoir, 1983).

Some cases of fluent aphasia (Lerman et al., 1991; Rapin et al., 1977), as well as the use of jargon (Mantovani and Landau, 1980; Rapin et al., 1977; Landau and Kleffner, 1957), have been reported. Paraphasias, asyntaxia, and verbal stereotypies are common in those children who are not completely mute, and such abnormalities may lead to a misdiagnosis of autism or psychosis (Dugas et al., 1982). The difficulties may extend to written language, although this is affected less than verbal expression is. All patients, however, do not have the same type of language disturbance. Dugas et al. (1982) found that, in 6 of 77 patients, the aphasia was predominantly expressive, and Deonna et al. (1977, 1982) has emphasized the complexity of the problem and the likelihood of diverse mechanisms being at play in different cases.

The authors' personal experience also indicates great variability in the language disturbance. In some children, the expressive component of language is more affected than is auditory gnosia, which was also the case in two of the original patients of Landau and Kleffner. One of our patients (Chevrie-Muller et al., 1991) had very marked expressive and repetition difficulties, and her EEG abnormalities were also atypical, with continuous spike-waves in wakefulness and in sleep on some tracings that did not have a clear relationship to the phasic disturbances.

Behavioral Disturbances

Behavioral disturbances commonly accompany the syndrome, and they may be prominent. Most commonly, they consist of hyperkinesia and outbursts of rage with aggressiveness and opposition (Roulet et al., 1991; Dugas et al., 1982), and they may occur in reaction to a primary auditory defect. In some patients, anxiety, gestural stereotypies, the avoidance of interpersonal contact, or bizarre behavior may suggest the presence of a psychotic component (Rapin, 1995; Deonna, 1991; Sawhney et al., 1988; Papini et al., 1984; Dugas et al., 1982). Roulet et al. (1993) and De Negri (1993) suggest that the LKS and the behavioral disturbances observed in patients with "electrical status epilepticus of slow sleep" represent the two poles of a continuum, in which the latter is characterized by predominant psychiatric disturbances and the former, by predominant language difficulties. The individual's intellectual efficiency is usually relatively preserved, although a marked discrepancy between his or her nonverbal and verbal abilities is present (Dugas et al., 1982).

In some children, apraxic components may be evident (Hirsch et al., 1995), and motor disturbances, including abnormalities of tonus, abnormal movements, ataxia, and marked clumsiness, may be more common than researchers had suspected (Neville et al., 1998).

Course and Relationship between Epilepsy and Language Disturbances

The relationship between the activity of clinical epilepsy and/or the intensity of EEG disturbances and the degree of aphasia in the LKS probably differs from case to case. Indeed, continuous paroxysmal EEG activity may appear long before the language disturbances, and its intensity may fluctuate independently of the severity of language problems (Hirsch et al., 1990). In some cases, continuous spike-wave activity precedes aphasia by periods of as long as 1 year (Hirsch et al., 1990). Some investigators (Giovanardi Rossi et al., 1988b; Nanda et al., 1977) have found a relationship between predominantly temporal activity and language difficulties, although this may be difficult to ascertain by surface recording. Several authors have suggested that the evolution of aphasia may depend on the occurrence of continuous spike-wave activity during slow sleep (Giovanardi Rossi et al., 1999; Deonna, 1991; Paetau et al., 1991; Billard et al., 1990; Shinnar et al., 1990; Hankey and Gubbay, 1988) because the individual's language appears to deteriorate during periods of electrical status and to improve during periods when the sleep EEG is less abnormal. This correlation is far from being tight or consistent (Beaumanoir, 1992; Deonna et al., 1977), but, in all cases in which this could be documented, the disappearance of continuous spike-waves during slow sleep has preceded the clinical recovery.

The relationship of EEG paroxysms to clinical features is no doubt a complex one because not only the intensity but also the spatial distribution and the precise timing relative to the phases of sleep must be taken into account. Reliable cases without CSWS have been recorded (Beaumanoir, 1992; Papini et al., 1984), although one cannot be certain that CSWS were not present at some stage. In one of the authors'

patients, the correlation between spike-wave and clinical language disturbance could be studied in detail, and the temporal relationship of spike-waves to the course of the disease was not obvious (Chevrie-Muller et al., 1991). Giovanardi Rossi et al. (1999) emphasized that disturbances in language were correlated with the diffusion of the paroxysms beyond the temporal regions and with the duration of the period of continuous spike-waves as well. The latter was also true in the experience of Veggiotti et al. (2002). In some patients, the severity of aphasia clearly fluctuates with the frequency and/or severity of the clinical seizures, and these cases may represent one subgroup of the syndrome of epileptic aphasia.

In cases in which a dissociation between epilepsy and aphasia is present, the epilepsy tends to fluctuate in severity, whereas the aphasia is usually stable, at least for periods of months in a row. Beaumanoir (1992), in a review of 77 cases, found that the aphasia remained stable in 40 patients, whereas it was more or less variable in the remaining 37. Even in these cases, the periodicity of the fluctuations usually extended over several months. Sudden increases in the severity of the aphasia may even occur relatively late in the syndrome; they have been seen up to 7 years after onset (Dugas et al., 1982).

The ultimate outcome is still unclear (Hirsch et al., 1990; Mantovani and Landau, 1980). Some patients improve to the point of being able to lead completely normal lives. Even in these cases, however, a few residual aphasic phenomena, such as word-finding difficulties and occasional paraphasias, can be detected by systematic language examination (Curatolo et al., 1987). The proportion of such favorable cases varies in the literature from 40% to 60% of cases (Dugas et al., 1982) to a low of 18% (Giovanardi Rossi et al., 1999). Other patients do recover useful language but still experience substantial limitations (Deonna et al., 1989). A few patients are left with more severe residua, such as a reduction of oral expression, diminished comprehension, dysnystaxis, or other defects leading to a moderate or severe handicap. Among nine patients followed to adulthood by Mantovani and Landau (1980), one of whom was not tested, three had normal language, two had mild verbal difficulties, and three had significant persistent defects. Paquier et al. (1992) found that four of their six patients still had significant language problems.

The prognosis is quite unpredictable. It tends to be more favorable in patients with a relatively late onset, whereas onset before the age of 5 years is associated with a more severe outlook (Loonen and Van Dongen, 1990; Bishop, 1985; Dulac et al., 1983a; Dugas et al.,

1982). However, the frequency and types of seizures do not affect the outcome. The persistent localization of EEG anomalies to the speech cortex and the duration of CSWS activity are also associated with an unfavorable outcome (Tassinari et al., 2002).

The effect of the treatment of the epilepsy on the final outcome is impossible to assess because a variety of regimens have been used. Many anticonvulsants, including adrenocorticotropic hormone (ACTH) and steroids, have been used even in patients without clinical seizures. The consensus is that conventional antiepileptic drugs have little efficacy with regard to the language disorder. Most authors (Paquier et al., 1992; Deonna and Roulet, 1991; Lerman et al., 1991; Marescaux et al., 1990) recommend the use of high-dose ACTH or corticosteroids for prolonged periods of 2 to several months; encouraging results have been reported with the use of this regimen. No controlled trial is available, however, and the unpredictable fluctuations of the disorder make any assessment difficult. Some investigators (Beaumanoir, 1983; Mantovani and Landau, 1980) have found that ethosuximide alone or in combination with corticosteroids might have a beneficial effect. Benzodiazepines, particularly clobazam, are also used. Surgical treatment by subpial transection may shorten the active period and may lessen the sequelae (see "Treatment" in this chapter).

Differential Diagnosis

Children with epileptic aphasia are often initially considered to be affected with psychologic or psychiatric disturbances, especially because they often display abnormal behavior in association with the speech difficulties. In some patients, several months may elapse before the language problem is recognized (Deonna et al., 1977). Such errors can easily be avoided if the child's language is systematically studied, even on a clinical basis.

Distinguishing deafness from epileptic aphasia is more difficult. The language disturbances observed in acquired deafness, which produces the loss of oral expression through the failure of auditory feedback mechanisms, may closely resemble those in LKS. This confusion is often compounded by the fact that the auditory agnosia in LKS may not be limited to language sounds but may involve a wide variety of other sounds as well. Distinguishing between deafness and acquired epileptic aphasia may require the clinician to perform not only an audiogram, which is compulsory but not always easy to interpret in young children, but also more sophisticated electrophysio-

logic investigations, including an electrocochleogram and brainstem and cortical auditory evoked responses.

Other acquired aphasias in childhood, which mostly result from vascular occlusion or herpes simplex encephalitis, are relatively easy to distinguish from LKS because most of these are mainly characterized by a reduction in expressive language activity but with the relative preservation of understanding. However, paraphasias, jargon aphasia, and difficulties with language comprehension can occur in vascular or inflammatory aphasias (Loonen and Van Dongen, 1990).

Some of the acquired aphasias may occur in epileptic patients. For example, postictal aphasia, which is transient, or acquired aphasia, which accompanies postconvulsive acquired hemiplegia. Difficulties may be encountered in the occasional cases of epileptic aphasia with predominant involvement of expressive language. Differentiating acquired epileptic aphasia from "congenital" developmental dysphasia may be difficult in cases of early onset. Indeed, developmental dysphasia associated with intense paroxysmal EEG activity (Ebersole, 1992; Rapin et al., 1988; Maccario et al., 1982) may actually be an early variant of the LKS, although no definitive conclusion can be drawn at this time.

Possible Variants of Epileptic Aphasia

The nosologic situation of LKS is not entirely clear. In reality, acquired epileptic aphasia may not be a single entity. A very low number of cases may be the result of an acquired structural abnormality of one or both temporal lobes, which may perhaps be of an inflammatory nature (Lou et al., 1977). Most cases, however, seem to result from purely functional disturbances, but, even in such cases, different mechanisms may be at play. Deonna et al. (1977) proposed separating acquired epileptic aphasia into three different categories. The first subgroup contains cases of abrupt onset after severe focal seizures, followed by rapid regression or by marked fluctuations in severity that bear a direct relationship to the occurrence of seizures, especially right-sided attacks, that are likely to involve the cortical areas of speech. Such cases may represent extreme examples of postictal aphasia, with a mechanism similar to that of Todd paralysis and of abnormally long duration. In such patients, the recovery is too rapid to be explained by a shift in hemispheral dominance for speech. The origin of the epileptic focus could be congenital, especially in those cases in which language difficulties antedated the onset of the syndrome.

The second group proposed by Deonna includes those cases in which no recovery takes place following a severe seizure or repeated episodes of seizures. In such cases, the aphasia might result from acute or progressive damage to the speech cortical areas. An argument supporting this hypothesis was that, in one of Deonna's patients, the recovery occurred slowly and it was associated with an inversion of original manual laterality.

The third group comprises the most typical cases, with few clinical seizures and marked auditory agnosia that may precede the first seizure.

Even more variability in clinical manifestations and mechanisms may well exist. For example, the aphasia may be predominantly of an expressive type, and a linguistic analysis of the language disorder will probably, in that case, show that several different disturbances exist (Deonna et al., 1982).

Treatment

The treatment of epileptic aphasia is disappointing. A number of antiepileptic drugs have been used, but the results have almost uniformly been limited or entirely negative (Beaumanoir, 1992; Dugas et al., 1982). The interruption of paroxysmal EEG activity in those cases in which it occurs in the form of a so-called ESES has proved difficult, even though the administration of benzodiazepines, valproate, and ethosuccimide has obtained some measure of success in a few cases of electrical status epilepticus. Others have also had this limited experience (Marescaux et al., 1990). De Negri et al. (1995) found that cycles of diazepam three weeks apart were useful, but other investigators think that such an effect is transient.

Many investigators consider ACTH and/or corticosteroids to have a definite effect on EEG activity and language (Deonna, 1991; Lerman et al., 1991; Marescaux et al., 1990; Ounsted et al., 1966). Large doses over prolonged periods (e.g., 2 to 3 mg per kg of prednisolone for at least 3 months) are generally advised. Because the effects are often slow to appear, the possibility of EEG improvement being due to a coincidence of treatment timing cannot be dismissed, especially as the spontaneous course is often fluctuating. Some investigators use repeated injections of these agents several days apart to try to prevent major side effects. Pending further more definitive studies, ACTH or steroid treatment for at least 3 months is currently advised. Immunoglobulins have been found

useful by some investigators (Mikati and Saab, 2000; Lagae et al., 1998), and they are probably worth trying systematically.

Trials of surgical treatment using subpial transection (Polkey, 1989, 2003; Morrell et al., 1989) have been performed, but, despite some encouraging results, the value of this approach is difficult to evaluate (Morrell et al., 1989). Surgical treatment by multiple subpial transections (Morrell et al., 1989) has resulted in long-lasting improvement in several patients (Grote et al., 1999; Morrell et al., 1995; Polkey, 1989). Some authors have found that the effect on behavioral abnormalities is particularly gratifying (Robinson et al., 2001).

Remedial treatment of the language disorder is always indicated. Its efficacy was, however, fairly limited in the experience of Deonna et al. (1989), who found that teaching nonverbal communication paradoxically was of little help because patients did not tend to use it.

SYNDROME OF CONTINUOUS SPIKE-WAVES OF SLOW SLEEP

In children, the occurrence of behavioral disturbances that are temporally related to the presence of an intense, subcontinuous paroxysmal activity made of slow spike-wave complexes in the EEG was first reported by Patry et al. (1971). The term CSWS is used synonymously with that of ESES, although some investigators (Galanopoulou et al., 2000) have proposed that ESES should be used to designate the EEG abnormalities and CSWS syndrome, for the association of a neuropsychologic syndrome with the paroxysmal abnormalities.

Tassinari et al. (1977) defined ESES as diffuse, continuous 1-Hz to 3-Hz spike-waves appearing at the onset of sleep that persist during the entire slow sleep period, occupying at least 85% of the EEG slow sleep tracing. Subsequent studies have, however, shown that the neuropsychologic symptomatology may be present even when the proportion of paroxysms is less than 85% (Tassinari et al., 2002; Beaumanoir et al., 1995; Jayakar and Seshia, 1991). Therefore, accepting a direct relationship between the EEG abnormalities and the presence of neuropsychologic disturbances, even when the proportion of spikewaves is less than 85%, now seems reasonable when a dramatic aggravation of epileptiform activities occurs in slow-wave sleep, compared with wakefulness, and it is accompanied by a constellation of clinical symptoms of gradual cognitive and behavioral deterioration.

The present definition of the CSWS syndrome includes the presence of continuous diffuse spike-waves during slow-wave sleep that persist for months to years but eventually disappear either spontaneously or following therapy, although the benefit of treatment remains uncertain. From a clinical viewpoint, various seizure types are possible, including mainly partial or generalized seizures occurring during sleep and atypical absences when the individual is awake (Boel and Casaer, 1989). Neuropsychologic disturbances are regularly associated with the EEG abnormalities.

Clinical Features of the Continuous Spike-Waves of Slow Sleep Syndrome

The *syndrome of CSWS* may appear in extremely diverse clinical settings in either previously normal or delayed children (Tassinari et al., 1992a; Morikawa et al., 1989; Dalla Bernardina et al., 1978b). Morikawa et al. (1989) and Roulet et al. (1989) found that 20% to 30% of children with CSWS had identifiable brain pathology, whereas a positive family history of epilepsy or febrile seizures was relatively uncommon; 3% had a family history of epilepsy and 15%, a personal history of febrile convulsions. One pair of affected monozygous twins is on record (Bureau et al., 1995b). Galanopoulou et al. (2000) list congenital hemiparesis, psychomotor retardation, and neonatal convulsions among the antecedents of one-third of affected children. A shunted hydrocephalus has been found in 30% of patients (Veggiotti et al., 1998). Neuroradiologic abnormalities are found in 30% to 50% of patients. These include developmental lesions, especially polymicrogyria involving a whole hemisphere or large areas in the central region that may represent a definite syndrome (Guerrini et al., 1996d), and, less commonly, acquired damage, such as porencephaly (Tassinari et al., 1992a).

The *onset of the syndrome* is usually insidious. *Before recognition of the CSWS*, seizures are often present, most commonly around 3 to 5 years of age. They are usually nocturnal, focal, or unilateral, but generalized seizures have been reported as well. In many patients, the focal seizures resemble those of rolandic epilepsy, and they are often associated with interictal EEG features similar to those of idiopathic rolandic epilepsy; however, features of an organic etiology may be present. Multifocal spikes are frequent, and a considerable increase in the frequency of spikes or spikes and waves is obvious at the onset of slow sleep. An interictal focus, which usually is frontal, is often found.

The mental level of these individuals is normal in more than half the patients before the full-fledged syndrome, which contrasts with an intelligence quotient of between 45 and 78 at the end of follow-up in most cases.

The *onset of the CSWS period* is seldom sudden. Usually, the first symptoms are imprecise, and a change for the worse often becomes apparent several months or a year after the first seizures. During the period of ESES, 80% of the patients have seizures of variable severity. Some children continue to have rare partial nocturnal seizures, although most have frequent nocturnal and/or diurnal attacks. The presence of *atonic seizures* is highly suggestive of the syndrome, as these occur in approximately half the cases (Tassinari et al., 1992a) and they are not a feature of the LKS (Bureau et al., 1995). They were found to herald the appearance of CSWS in 23% of patients (Morikawa et al., 1989). A prominent atonic component is commonly associated with the emergence of CSWS (Tassinari et al., 1977, 1992a). It is often manifested by falls that may occur several dozen times daily; some may be limited to a head nod or a sagging at the knees without a complete fall. Absences are also common. These *absences* are usually associated with bursts of generalized spike-wave activity on the EEG; these burts also occur independently of clinical seizures in many patients. Some children may have myoclonic absences and generalized nonconvulsive seizures (Gaggero et al., 1995; Dulac et al., 1983a). Approximately 12% of patients have a single type of seizure (Bureau, 1995a). Tonic seizures are not a feature of CSWS, a major differentiating factor from Lennox-Gastaut syndrome.

The *major EEG feature* during the CSWS period is the presence of continuous, spatially diffuse spike-wave discharges at 1.5 to 2.5 Hz during slow-wave sleep that appear as soon as the patient falls asleep and then persist throughout all slow sleep stages (Fig. 11.1A–D). The paroxysms are particularly intense during the first sleep cycle (Genton et al., 1995a). Although an arbitrary decision was initially made to require a proportion of 85% of spike-waves for the diagnosis, a lower proportion of spike-waves is now accepted by several authors (Beaumanoir et al., 1995; Yashura et al., 1991; Billard et al., 1982). Some investigators have suggested that an index of less than 85% may be associated with less severe neuropsychologic impairment (Beaumanoir et al., 1995). Although the paroxysms were initially described as generalized, they may be asymmetric and they can shift from side to side in the same child, so a unilateral predominance does not rule out the diagnosis.

Some controversy exists with regard to REM sleep EEGs; in most cases, the paroxysmal activity tends to fragment and the records become similar to awake tracings (Tassinari et al., 2002). Some authors have emphasized that the disappearance of spike-waves during REM sleep distinguishes CSWS from LKS. In contrast, Genton et al. (1990b) and Giovanardi Rossi et al. (1999) have found that the spike-wave activity continues during REM sleep in LKS.

A more precise analysis of the tracings indicates that, in slow-wave sleep, the diffuse-appearing spike-wave discharges usually originate focally and then rapidly propagate within and between the hemispheres (Farnarier et al., 1995), suggesting secondary bilateral synchrony. Studies with single photon emission CT and PET also support a focal origin in some cases (Gaggero et al., 1995).

The most serious feature of CSWS is mental and/or behavioral deterioration, which is present to some degree in almost all patients (Tassinari et al., 2002; Morikawa et al., 1985, 1992; Jayakar and Seshia, 1991; Boel and Casaer, 1989). The onset of deterioration may be acute, but, more often, it is progressive; rarely is it the first manifestation. A constant and marked decrease in IQ is seen (Roulet-Perez et al., 1993). Attention deficits and hyperactivity are reported in roughly two-thirds of patients (Morikawa et al., 1995; Yashura et al., 1991). Language disturbances are noted in 40% to 60% of patients, and deciding whether these are of an aphasic nature or a consequence of the psychotic behavior may be difficult. A tendency toward expressive rather than receptive aphasia, in contrast to that seen in patients with LKS, has been noted (Rousselle and Revol, 1995).

Aggressiveness, a deficit of inhibition, and emotional lability are often prominent, and they may represent a major management problem. Autistic-like features have been reported (Kyllerman et al., 1996; Hirsch et al., 1995). Inattention, impulsivity, perseverations, and difficulties in abstract reasoning may be particularly common, suggesting frontal lobe dysfunction (Jayakar and Seshia, 1991), which is consistent with the location of the interictal foci and the predominance of bisynchronous frontal

spike-wave discharges. Roulet Perez et al. (1993) have suggested that LKS and CSWS with behavioral disorder might be the two extremes of a spectrum of conditions featuring variable proportions of either type of disturbance and that both syndromes are merely two aspects of a basically identical underlying disorder. The variable expression of the neuropsychologic disturbances could be due to the predominant location of the EEG paroxysms.

Some investigators have reported patients with CSWS who have never shown even transient mental impairment (Tassinari et al., 1992a; Billard et al., 1990).

The *long-term course of epilepsy* is always favorable, even in lesional cases (Guerrini et al., 1998f). The mean duration of epilepsy was 12 years in one series (Tassinari et al., 2002), and some authors include CSWS among the "benign" epilepsies solely on this basis (Roger et al., 1990). The disappearance of the seizures preceded that of CSWS in about half of the patients. However, focal abnormalities did persist in 12 of 25 patients. Abnormalities of sleep structure consistently disappeared. Unfortunately, variable degrees of mental deficit persisted permanently in most patients, and the mental level (IQ) of most patients was around 50 or less. In 50% of patients, the behavioral disturbances persisted, even though they tend to fade away with the disappearance of paroxysmal discharges. A long duration of the CSWS (2 years or more) appears to be the major factor for a poor outcome of cognitive and behavioral prognosis (Veggiotti et al., 2002; Giovanardi Rossi et al., 1999; Rousselle and Revol, 1995).

The epileptic syndrome described by Aicardi and Chevrie (Aicardi and Chevrie, 1982a) as "benign atypical partial epilepsy" now appears to bear a close relationship to CSWS, of which it may be a mild and intermittent form (see Chapter 10). In this syndrome, CSWS are observed during brief periods of a few days to a few weeks, separated by long intervals (months) of relatively normal sleep EEG recordings. During the active periods, behavioral changes commonly manifest with some decrease in intellectual efficiency. The brief duration of the episodes of electrical status and their separation by long intervals without seizures or major EEG anomalies may explain the more favorable outcome of these affected children. Overall, the effect on development is small or absent, although being sure that no mild decrease in intellectual potential occurs in at least in some cases is impossible because no detailed neuropsychologic study is available.

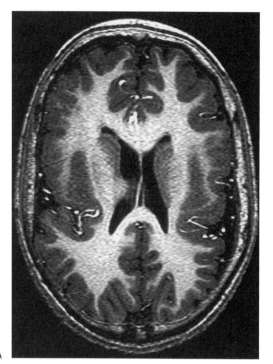

A

FIG. 11.1. A: Child with epilepsy with continuous spike-waves during sleep and asymmetric bilateral perisylvian polymicrogyria. FSPGR, axial section. The perisylvian cortex is thickened and irregular, and the left hemisphere is smaller than the right. **B:** At 7 years of age, an atypical absence seizure with a marked atonic component that caused head drop and saccadic falling to the ground was recorded; note that the seizure is accompanied by slow spike-wave activity. The rhythmic discharge accompanying the episode is both preceded and followed by nonrhythmic spike and slow-wave complexes that are not as generalized as the ictal discharge; they do, however, predominate on the left and they show phase reversal over the centrotemporal regions. **C:** During sleep stage II, the continuous spike-wave activity is abruptly interrupted by a short rolandic seizure (duration of about 20 seconds) that is clinically characterized by mild bilateral perioral facial twitching with arousal; its electrographic characteristics include a discharge of rhythmic spikes that predominate over the left central area and that are progressively intermingled with spike-wave activity. **D:** A sleep electroencephalogram shows that, when continuous spike-wave activity subsides, bilateral independent spikes become obvious over both temporal lobes, which suggests secondary bilateral synchrony.

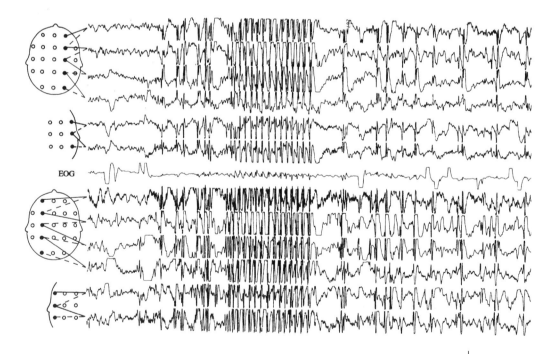

EOG

B

1 sec   ⌐   100 μV

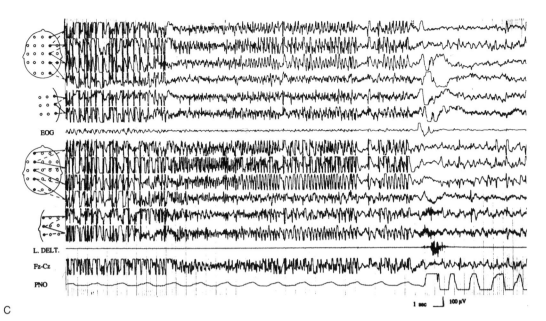

C

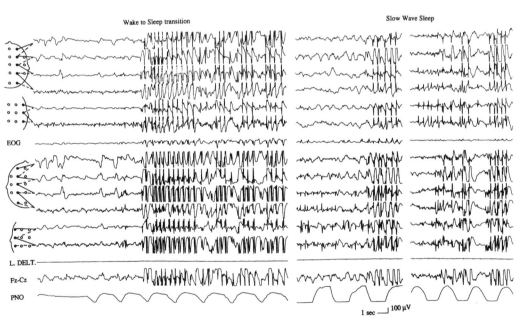

D

Treatment

The treatment of CSWS is perhaps even more difficult than that of LKS. The continuous paroxysmal activity is resistant to conventional antiepileptic agents. Prolonged therapy with ACTH and/or corticosteroids is probably indicated (Tassinari et al., 1992a; Yates et al., 1986), but their efficacy is far from established. Immunoglobulins have given some encouraging results (Mikati and Saab, 2000; Fayad et al., 1997). Ethosuximide may be of some value, and sulthiame is widely used by German authors (Gross-Selbeck, 1995).

POSSIBLE MECHANISMS OF ELECTRICAL STATUS EPILEPTICUS OF SLEEP, LANDAU-KLEFFNER SYNDROME, AND SYNDROME OF CONTINUOUS SPIKE-WAVES OF SLOW SLEEP

As was indicated earlier in this chapter, ESES or CSWS seems to be due to the diffusion of the EEG paroxysms from one or several cortical foci. The location and the type of focus, whether it is due to a structural lesion or of a purely functional nature, varies with the clinical syndrome. The primary focus is usually temporal, and it rarely, if ever, is of lesional nature in LKS, whereas it is more often frontal or central and it is associated with pathologic abnormalities in the CSWS syndrome. However, the two syndromes do exhibit differences in their EEG aspects. In LKS, CSWS are not consistently present during the whole duration of the active period (Giovanardi Rossi et al., 1999), and their topography is more posteriorly located than in the CSWS syndrome. Moreover, the persistence of the diffuse paroxysmal anomalies during REM sleep has been reported in LKS but not in the CSWS syndrome (Giovanardi Rossi, 1999; Genton et al., 1990b). Any generalization is, therefore, likely an oversimplification of a complex problem, and trying to determine mechanisms on the fragile basis of present-day knowledge is hazardous. However, one may accept that, in most patients, the bilateral cortical involvement is related to the paroxysmal EEG abnormalities responsible for the neuropsychologic disturbances, because auditory agnosia or cognitive deterioration is not explicable on the basis of unilateral brain dysfunction. A unilateral abnormality would hardly be compatible with the absence of complete recovery or at least the long duration of the neuropsychologic deficits. Because structural damage is absent in many patients, some functional but lasting disturbance must explain the syndrome.

In both syndromes, the most likely hypothesis is that the epileptic activity itself, even if it is not manifested clinically by seizures, produces functional exclusion of the cortical areas that are the seats of the repeated discharges, with resulting agnosia and secondary loss of speech in LKS (Lerman and Lerman-Sagie, 1995; Beaumanoir, 1983) and cognitive and behavioral deterioration in CSWS syndrome. The good correlation between the EEG paroxysmal activity and the neuropsychologic deficits supports the opinion that these are a direct result of the epileptic process, thus permitting the consideration that both LKS and the CSWS syndrome belong to the group *epileptic encephalopathies*. If this functional exclusion is sufficiently prolonged, and it occurs at a period that is critical for language and/or other cognitive acquisition, definitive sequelae will result. This is in keeping with the more unfavorable language outcome that is seen in cases of early onset (Bishop, 1985; Dulac et al., 1983a). If this hypothesis is accepted, the interruption of paroxysmal activity would be essential even in the absence of seizures, and vigorous treatment would be essential. Although this hypothesis remains unproved (Holmes et al., 1980), it should, from all appearances, be temporarily accepted as a pragmatic concept. However, a primary disturbance responsible for both the epilepsy and the language disorder is possible, but little proof of its nature or, indeed, of its existence has been found.

SUMMARY

Acquired aphasia in association with paroxysmal EEG activity and, usually, with a seizure disorder is a rare but puzzling condition. The language disorder primarily involves the decoding of language sounds, but difficulties with the decoding of other sounds are often associated. The epilepsy is often relatively mild, but paroxysmal EEG abnormalities may be extremely marked in some of the cases. The language disorder sets in progressively over a period of weeks or months, and it is usually long lasting or permanent. The epilepsy seems to remit spontaneously before adulthood in most patients. The ultimate prognosis for language is guarded, although significant improvement or even complete recovery may occur in a sizable proportion of patients followed over many years. The causes of epileptic aphasia are not known. Likely, all cases do not depend on the same causes and mechanisms, as a careful analysis of the symptoms and signs suggests that the syndrome is heterogeneous, with different types of language disorders and quite different patterns of epilepsy and course.

The syndrome of CSWS, or ESES, shares many of the features of LKS, especially the same type of EEG activity and probably many of the mechanisms. In this syndrome, behavioral and cognitive disturbances predominate over language difficulties, which are, however, present in many patients. Some cases of aphasia with convulsive disorders and CSWS may represent two aspects of a basically similar condition, and they may be part of the group *epileptic encephalopathies.*

The treatment of both conditions is currently based on ACTH and corticosteroids. These are thought by several authors to be effective in treatment of epileptic aphasia, but are considered less so in CSWS. Immunoglobulins are being tried. Surgical treatment by subpial transection has given some promising results.

12

Neonatal Seizures

The variable terminology used in the literature when neonatal paroxysmal events (e.g., convulsions, seizures, epileptic seizures, nonepileptic seizures, muscular twitching, and motor automatisms) are discussed reflects the difficulty with recognizing and interpreting motor phenomena and autonomic signs in the newborn. Such difficulties may result either in the overdiagnosis of epileptic seizures or in the delay of the diagnosis of true "epileptic" attacks because not all paroxysmal neonatal events are epileptic seizures. The electroencephalographic (EEG) and clinical phenomena that characterize neonatal seizures differ from the usual epileptic patterns of older age. Typical absences, jacksonian attacks, and generalized tonic-clonic convulsions are not observed in neonates, although some of the rapidly migrating movements that occur in multifocal clonic seizures or in bouts of shudders and tremors may mimic motor seizures. The commonly atypical manifestations and most types of bizarre or unusual transient events in the neonatal period may be epileptic seizures, especially if these are stereotyped, insensitive to stimuli or restraint, and periodically recurring.

The differences between epileptic attacks in newborn babies and those in older children probably reflect the incomplete neuroanatomic and neurophysiologic development of the neonatal brain. Although virtually all neurons are in place by the time of birth, their axonal and dendritic processes and synaptic connections are still incompletely developed in the neonatal human brain (Levene et al., 2001; Volpe, 2001), and myelination is limited to a few pathways, which do not include the main hemispheric commissures. Changes in the receptors for and roles of both excitatory (glutamate and aspartate) and inhibitory (γ-aminobutyric acid [GABA]) circuits play a major role in the modulation of cortical excitability, and their differential rate of maturation with age may explain the changing susceptibility to epilepsy at various ages (Holmes, 1997; Johnston, 1996; Moshé, 1987) and the variability in the clinical expression of seizures. In particular, $GABA_A$ receptors seem to play an excitatory role at this age as a result of differences in the concentration of intracellular chloride in the immature brain (Cherubini et al., 1991; Ben-Ari et

al., 1988). A detailed study of the mechanisms that are supposedly responsible for the generation and propagation of epileptic discharges in neonates is beyond the scope of this chapter. The absence of generalized tonic-clonic seizures (GTCSs) probably reflects both the lack of a sufficient degree of the cortical organization necessary to propagate and to sustain the electrical discharge and the failure of interhemispheric transmission resulting from commissural immaturity.

However, not all clinical phenomena in neonates have the same mechanisms (Mizrahi and Kellaway, 1998; Aicardi, 1991b; Camfield and Camfield, 1987; Kellaway and Mizrahi, 1987). Some are regularly associated with rhythmic EEG discharges that are clearly epileptic in nature, whereas others are unassociated or only inconsistently associated with paroxysmal EEG changes.

- In the first group of seizures, which consist mainly but not exclusively of clonic events, the origin of the ictal discharges appears to have a cortical focus, and these may often be correlated with discrete cortical insults. Morphologically, the discharges are quite reminiscent of the epileptic events observed in older patients, leaving little doubt about their epileptic nature.
- In the second group, which consists mainly of tonic and subtle seizures, the mechanism is uncertain; although some such seizures are associated with cortical epileptic discharges that are not picked up on the scalp, such an explanation is unlikely to apply in all cases. At least part of these are probably not epileptic; they may instead represent "release" phenomena caused by the liberation of the subcortical (especially brainstem) structures from cortical control, usually because of extensive cortical destruction or dysfunction (Kellaway and Mizrahi, 1990; Volpe, 1990; Camfield and Camfield, 1987).

Such an explanation for the second group is supported by the fact that "release" phenomena are often graded rather than being an all-or-none phenomena, and they can be elicited by stimulation and inhibited by restraint. In addition, they may demonstrate spatial and temporal summation, which is not observed in true epileptic seizures. Similar features have been demonstrated in animal models of reflex physiology, which supports the suggestion that these clinical phenomena may actually be nonepileptic in origin, representing exaggerated reflex behaviors (Mizrahi and Kellaway, 1998). Alfonso et al. (2001) reported two neonates who presented with clinically similar episodes of sustained tonic posture of the right upper limb, which, in one, were considered as brainstem release phenomena on the basis of EEG and clinical data and, in the other, as epileptic seizures. Ictal single photon emission computed tomography (SPECT) scans showed focal cerebral hemisphere hyperperfusion only in the second case. According to the authors, different perfusion characteristics of two similar clinical events suggest a different mechanism, refuting the theory that brainstem release phenomena are due to EEG seizures that are not detectable by scalp or nasopharyngeal EEG.

A growing body of information in neonates and older children (Arzimanoglou et al., 1999; Arzimanoglou, 1996; Harvey et al., 1996) suggests that epileptic phenomena can also be generated at subcortical levels. The studies of Scher et al. (1993) and Weiner et al. (1991) also support the possible role of subcortical structures because those groups with EEG accompaniments for the subtle seizures were clinically similar to those without EEG accompaniments and both had similar neurologic outcomes. Studies in rats support this hypothesis (McCown and Breese, 1992).

The problem is further compounded by the frequent occurrence of electrical discharges without clinical manifestations (Glauser and Clancy, 1992; Connell et al., 1989; Clancy et al., 1988; Bridgers et al., 1986; Hellstrom-Westas et al., 1985). These may be much more common than electroclinical seizures. Although they may precede, follow, or alternate with electroclinical attacks, they also occur in isolation. The converse phenomenon of typical clinical seizures without electrical concomitants has also been reported (Herranz Tanarro et al., 1984).

The distinction between epileptic and nonepileptic seizures may be of practical significance for therapy and prognosis (Volpe, 1989; Lombroso, 1992, 1996). However, clinical differentiation of these two types of seizures may be extremely difficult or even impossible. Indeed, clinically identical seizures in the same patient may only occasionally be associated with epileptic paroxysms, and seizures occurring late in long-lasting series are sometimes unaccompanied by EEG discharges (Delgado-Escueta and Enrile-Bacsal, 1984; Dreyfus-Brisac and Curzi-Dascalova, 1979). Scher et al. (1989) and Scher and Painter (1990)

found ictal paroxysms in only 8 of 18 newborn infants with clonic seizures, although most investigators have noted a closer correlation (Lombroso, 1992). This is even more likely in newborn infants whose brains may have been gravely injured and whose EEG background activities may be quite abnormal or diffusely depressed (Lombroso, 2002). EEG monitoring and, even better, video-EEG are desirable, even if they do not answer all the questions. Important clinical indications include the stereotypic nature of the events, as well as the absence of sensitivity to stimuli and to restraint, which are easily looked for and have considerable value (Mizrahi and Kellaway, 1998).

The etiologic context and global neurologic evaluation provide a solid and indispensable basis for decision making (Arzimanoglou and Aicardi, 2001). The issue of "epileptic" versus "nonepileptic" seizures has been debated extensively, and the interested reader can consult the pertinent articles mentioned earlier for the different views, as well as a recent review of the issue (Lombroso, 2002).

As a result of these diagnostic difficulties, the true *incidence of neonatal seizures* varies in different series from 0.15% to 1.4% (Aicardi, 1991b; Legido et al., 1988; Goldberg, 1983; Bergman et al., 1982). The reported incidence in the general population of neonates was 3.5 per 1,000 livebirths in a retrospective cohort study by Lanska et al. (1995) and 2.5 per 1,000 livebirths in the prospective study from Ronen and Penney (1995). The incidence probably varies with gestational age, with most cases being observed in full-term infants (Curtis et al., 1988; Bergman et al., 1983; Hopkins, 1972). However, preterm infants do appear in most series (Scher et al., 1988; Painter et al., 1986; Bergman et al., 1983; Radvanyi-Bouvet et al., 1981). Of 121 neonates with seizures that were reported by Dreyfus-Brisac et al. (1981), 40 were premature, with 19 being born before 33 weeks of gestation. The extremely high incidence rate (up to 23%) that Bergman et al. (1983) reported in premature infants is probably due in part to the frequency of nonepileptic events in this group (Mizrahi, 1987; Mizrahi and Kellaway, 1987). Stratification of data according to birth weight (Lanska et al., 1995) shows a much higher incidence of an estimated 57.5 cases per 1,000 livebirths in very-low-birth-weight (i.e., less than 1,500 g) infants. Scher et al. (1993) estimated that 2.3% of all infants cared for in an intensive care unit experienced seizures.

Intrauterine seizures have been suspected in several reports (Holmes, 1985; Bejsovec et al., 1967), and they have been directly observed by ultrasonography (Du Plessi et al., 1993; Landy et al., 1989). Movements that the mothers later recognize as probably being convulsive in nature mainly occur in the last days or weeks of gestation. Pyridoxine dependency is another possible cause of intrauterine convulsions (Bejsovec et al., 1967; Mikati et al., 1991), but other causes, especially brain dysplasia (Du Plessis et al., 1993), are possible.

This chapter first describes the clinical manifestations of neonatal seizures, including all stereotypic events in which no sensitivity to stimuli is present and which are not abolished by restraint. The relationship of the various clinical phenomena with EEG events is then considered, followed by a discussion of the diagnostic, etiologic, and treatment issues.

CLINICAL AND ELECTROENCEPHALOGRAPHIC FEATURES

The seizures of newborns require a different classification than those that are applied at other ages. Most authors recognize the following four main types of seizures: subtle (Volpe, 1989) or minimal, clonic, tonic, and myoclonic. Several seizure types often occur together in the same infant; subtle seizures are often associated with other types in severely ill neonates (Aicardi, 1991b). The possibility that some seizures may occur in the absence of simultaneous EEG seizure activity is widely accepted. The increasing use of EEG polygraphic video-monitoring techniques during the last decade has allowed a more precise description and classification of neonatal seizures and a better understanding of their pathophysiology.

Clonic Seizures

Clonic seizures consist of rhythmic muscle jerking that can involve any part of the body. The following two subtypes are recognized: *focal clonic* and *multifocal*. Unifocal seizures may affect one extremity or one side of the face; at times only a very limited territory may be influenced. Rarely, they can involve a whole side of the body. In some infants, the jerks remain confined to a limited muscle group or to the tongue, or they may involve the diaphragm or other axial muscles. In multifocal seizures, localized clonic movements shift, often quite rapidly, from the site of origin to another nonadjoining body part or to the opposite side in a disordered nonjacksonian fashion. Several segments can be involved simultaneously, but the jerking is not synchronous, even though the rapid

shifting may superficially simulate a generalized seizure (Lombroso, 2002). The terms *erratic* (Lombroso, 1992; Volpe, 1990) and *migratory* have been applied to such seizures (Legido et al., 1988; Aicardi, 1985b). Such multifocal seizures probably have the same significance as focal clonic seizures as far as prognosis is concerned, but they do not indicate the presence of a fixed focal lesion, as is often true with unifocal seizures (Aicardi, 1991b). In neonates, these can, however, can be due to metabolic disturbances, and all variations of the spectrum between frank multifocal seizures and subtle seizures with minimal jerking and poor organization may be seen.

Unifocal seizures usually have good correlation with EEG activity, but they do not necessarily imply a focal pathology. Multifocal discharges usually accompany multifocal seizures. Careful direct observation and manipulation maneuvers (restraint, repositioning, stimulation) allow the seizures to be distinguished from manifestations seen in nonseizure states (Mizrahi and Kellaway, 1998; Lombroso, 2002), such as jitteriness, tremor, shudders, hypnic jerks, and benign myoclonus of sleep.

Subtle Seizures

The term *subtle seizures* was used to describe various behavioral phenomena that may involve the limbs, the axial muscles, or the face and eyes. Lip smacking, sucking or swallowing movements, mouth puckering, grimacing, eye deviations (lateral or vertical), repetitive blinking, and staring can all be observed. Abnormal limb movements may include complex patterns such as pedaling, boxing, swimming, or stepping or the assumption of a tonic posture by one limb or a segment thereof (Aicardi, 1991b; Volpe, 1990; Mizrahi, 1984; Rose and Lombroso, 1970). Autonomic phenomena, such as vasomotor changes, salivation, or modification of heart rate, may occur in an isolated fashion, but they are more often associated with motor automatisms. Several abnormal events are usually associated (Dreyfus-Brisac and Monod, 1972, 1977), and abnormal eye movements, especially in the horizontal plane (Blume, 1978), have a high diagnostic value. Subtle paroxysmal phenomena mostly occur in newborns with central nervous system insults (Lombroso, 2002).

Some authors (Mizrahi and Kellaway, 1998) prefer the term *motor automatisms* to describe these phenomena, which they usually consider nonepileptic in nature. Although this may be true for a number of cases, the use of video-EEG suggests caution when interpreting such phenomena. These motor behaviors or automatisms may occur in premature or encephalopathic babies. When they are nonictal in nature, they are usually not accompanied by autonomic changes, they can be stopped by restraining or repositioning the child, or they can be triggered by stimulation. Drooling may, however, occur (Lombroso, 2002).

Apneic seizures are common, and they rarely occur as the sole manifestation (Navelet et al., 1989; Fenichel, 1985; Watanabe et al., 1982). More often, they are seen in association with ocular or autonomic signs. Fenichel et al. (1980a) found that apneic seizures were not accompanied by bradycardia, while this was seen in the much more common nonepileptic apneas of the premature infant when these last 20 seconds or more. Central nonictal apnea is usually accompanied by agitated asynchronous movements of the limbs, whereas mainly oral automatisms, nystagmus, or eye deviation is observed with apneic ictal manifestations. Some apneas may be iatrogenic (Lombroso, 2002). Further investigations are needed to understand more fully the paroxysmal tachycardia, hypertension, or tachypnea that can be the sole manifestations of paroxysmal brain activity.

Tonic Seizures

Tonic seizures most often are *generalized*, featuring tonic extension of all limbs or, occasionally, flexion of the upper limbs with extension of the legs. These symmetric tonic postures are rarely true seizures. They more commonly represent "release" phenomena, and they can be triggered by stimulation. The background activity is usually abnormal, but ictal paroxysmal activity is not observed. However, abrupt tonic limb extension and/or flexion with abduction may represent true epileptic spasms (see Chapter 3).

Focal tonic seizures consist of sustained asymmetric posturing of one limb with flexion of the trunk toward the involved side. Tonic eye deviation may be associated with these. Autonomic phenomena, such as apnea, flushing, or mild cyanosis, are usually present. They are not affected by restraints nor are they triggered by stimulation. Eye signs, such as opening or closing movements of the eyelids, staring, or gaze deviation, or the occurrence of a few clonic jerks may be a clue to the epileptic mechanism. Ictal discharges may be of the delta, alpha, or beta-like types.

Myoclonic Seizures

Myoclonic seizures are uncommon. When they do occur, they can be erratic or fragmentary. More often,

myoclonic jerks are generalized, and these may be associated with tonic spasms or multifocal clonic patterns. They often persist into infancy as more or less atypical infantile spasms (Lombroso, 1974, 1992). They may be provoked by stimulation, and, from a pathophysiologic point of view, they may or may not be epileptic. The overall neurologic context, which usually favors the presence of a severe neurologic insult, allows them to be distinguished quite easily from shudders or benign neonatal sleep myoclonus.

REPETITION OF SEIZURES

Isolated seizures are relatively uncommon in the neonatal period. The occurrence of at least a few attacks is the rule. In a significant proportion of the patients, the seizures continue for long periods.

Clancy and Legido (1987b) found that the average duration of 427 seizures in 42 newborns was 137 ± 11 seconds, with extremes of 10 seconds and 46 minutes. Most (97%) seizures lasted less than 9 minutes, and only 2 seizures lasted more than 30 minutes. Discharges occupied 22% of total recorded time. Presumably, the patients in this study were more severely affected than was the average infant with neonatal seizures, and patients with only a few seizures were underrepresented. The total duration of the seizure period varies from a few seizures up to several days or rarely weeks. However, neonatal seizures tend to be self-limited, and they generally last 24 to 96 hours (Camfield and Camfield, 1987; Bout et al., 1983; Cukier et al., 1976), another factor complicating the assessment of therapy.

The term *status epilepticus* in the neonatal period has been used by French investigators (Dreyfus-Brisac and Monod, 1972, 1977; Cukier et al., 1976; Monod et al., 1969) and Schulte (1966). Neonatal status epilepticus was defined by Dreyfus-Brisac and Monod (1977) and Monod et al. (1969) as the repetition of clinical and/or purely electrical seizures with the interictal persistence of an abnormal neurologic status. Using this definition, Dreyfus-Brisac et al. (1981) reported that, in one study, 79 of 121 newborns had status epilepticus rather than isolated convulsions. Cukier et al. (1976), redefining the term with greater precision, required the occurrence of electrical seizure discharges, each of which lasted for at least 10 seconds and was repeated for several hours in association with an abnormal neurologic state and unconsciousness. Clinical seizures may or may not be present. The latter definition does not include repeated clinical seizures without ictal EEG concomitants, as may occur in neonates who have been convulsing for many hours (Dreyfus-Brisac et al., 1981; Dreyfus-Brisac and Monod, 1977).

The use of the term *serial seizures* is perhaps preferable to that of *status epilepticus* in the neonatal period because it does not refer to an abnormal inter-ictal neurologic state, which may be impossible to assess reliably because of the interference of drug treatment. Whatever the repetition rate and duration of the seizure period, the occurrence of several seizure patterns in the same patient is the rule rather than the exception. With prolonged convulsive episodes, the individual seizures tend to progress from well-marked to poorly organized attacks both clinically and electrically (Dreyfus-Brisac and Monod, 1977).

ICTAL AND INTERICTAL ELECTROENCEPHALOGRAPHIC CORRELATES OF NEONATAL SEIZURES

The combination of both EEG and clinical criteria accurately diagnoses and classifies seizures in neonates. The interpretation must take into account the gestational age, medical history, and the results of clinical and laboratory examinations. The maturational aspects and the normal and abnormal features of neonatal EEG are beyond the scope of this chapter (Mizrahi and Kellaway, 1998; Hrachovy et al., 1990; Dreyfus-Brisac and Curzi-Dascalova, 1979).

Except for the more generalized activity associated with myoclonic jerks or infantile spasms, almost all paroxysmal electrical activity in the neonate begins focally. Ictal discharges in the full-term neonate are exceedingly variable in appearance, voltage, frequency, and polarity (Rowe et al., 1985; Estivill et al., 1983; Dreyfus-Brisac, et al., 1981). Changes occur between discharges in the same infant and even within the same discharge. The modification in rhythm and polarity may be either progressive, usually with slowing of the rhythm toward the end of a discharge, or quite sudden, with abrupt changes in the frequency, morphology, and amplitude of the paroxysmal complexes (Fig. 12.1). Any schematic presentation is therefore inaccurate.

The following two main elements constitute the EEG discharges in newborns: *abnormal paroxysmal rhythms* and *repetitive spikes* or *sharp waves*. Both are commonly encountered (Estivill et al., 1983; Dreyfus-Brisac and Curzi-Dascalova, 1979; Dreyfus-Brisac, 1979; Harris and Tizard, 1960).

- The abnormal ictal rhythms include alpha-like, theta-like, and delta-like rhythms (Fig. 12.1), with the last being most common (Willis and Gould, 1980; Dreyfus-Brisac, 1979). In a few patients, very fast (12 to 14 Hz) rhythms are recorded, especially at the on-

set of discharges. Fast rhythms, especially those in the beta range, may constitute the only abnormality in some seizures (Willis and Gould, 1980; Knauss et al., 1978). These are suggestive of a poor prognosis, and they are most often associated with other paroxysmal figures. Fast and slow rhythms are variably combined. They may occur in succession, with the fast rhythms usually coming first, or simultaneously, with the fast rhythms being superimposed on the delta rhythms. As a result of the combination of these various elements, the ictal EEG discharges in full-term babies are usually quite polymorphic (Tharp, 1981; Dreyfus-Brisac and Monod, 1977). The duration is quite variable. Most authors require a discharge to last at least 10 seconds to be considered ictal (Clancy et al., 1988; Radvanyi-Bouvet et al., 1985).

- The focal discharges of sharp waves may be relatively fast (2 to 4 Hz), or they may occur at a slow (about 1 Hz) rate, a pattern resembling the periodic lateralized electrical discharges (PLEDs) of older patients (Holmes, 1985; Lombroso, 1982). The spikes or sharp waves are more frequently observed in the late part of the paroxysm, although they may represent the only abnormality. They are focal or multifocal, and they tend to involve the rolandic regions preferentially (Estivill et al., 1983; Dreyfus-Brisac et al., 1981). More often, they are associated with abnormal ictal rhythms, and, in combination with these rhythms, they may produce indented or notched diphasic or triphasic repetitive complexes (Estivill et al., 1983).

In premature infants, the EEG findings tend to be more stereotypic. Spikes are uncommon. They were observed in only 5 of 12 premature infants by Radvanyi-Bouvet et al. (1981, 1985), whereas spikes were present in 13 of the 15 full-term babies they studied. The most typical discharge in preterm infants is a delta rhythm with a steeply ascending initial deflection. Focal low-frequency discharges and multifocal spikes or sharp-wave rhythmic discharges are also observed (Rowe et al., 1985). The ictal discharges tend to be more synchronous over one hemisphere in premature infants than they are in full-term neonates. The duration of ictal discharges is quite variable, ranging from a few seconds to several minutes. In most patients, their diffusion remains quite restricted.

Some ictal patterns occur in neonates with severe encephalopathies; *electrical seizures in the depressed brain* are typically low in voltage, long in duration, and narrowly localized. These are usually seen in EEG recordings whose background activity is depressed and undifferentiated (Mizrahi and Kellaway, 1998).

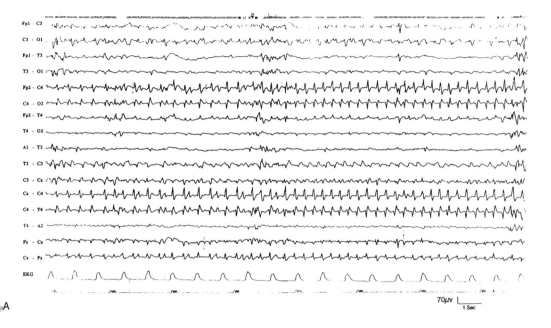

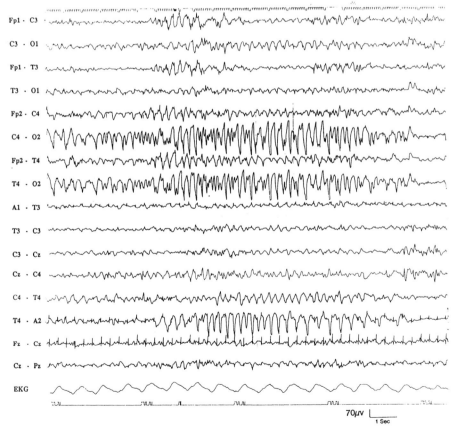

FIG. 12.1. Left frontocentral discharge **(A)** and right occipitotemporal seizure **(B)** in two newborn infants with seizures.

**RELATIONSHIP BETWEEN CLINICAL AND
ELECTROENCEPHALOGRAPHIC ICTAL
MANIFESTATION IN NEONATAL SEIZURES**

Not all clinical phenomena traditionally regarded as seizures are regularly associated with EEG seizure discharges temporally (Legido et al., 1988; Camfield and Camfield, 1987; Fenichel, 1985; Mizrahi, 1984). In a video-EEG study of 420 neonates from 28 to 44 weeks of gestational age, 100 of whom had either clinical seizures or electrographic seizures that were unaccompanied by clinical seizures, Kellaway and Mizrahi (1990) found that all patients with focal or multifocal clonic seizures, all those with focal tonic seizures, some of those with generalized myoclonic seizures and apneic seizures, and only a few of those with generalized tonic and subtle seizures had consistent ictal EEG activity. The experience of other investigators has been largely similar. Fenichel et al. (1980a) recorded 52 episodes of subtle seizures in 15 neonates, only one of whom had accompanying EEG discharges; and only 4 of 23 infants with such seizures recorded by Scher and Painter (1990) had concomitant EEG discharges. Radvanyi-Bouvet et al. (1981) recorded ictal discharges in 50 premature infants with mostly subtle seizures, but whether the association between the clinical and EEG events in these patients was consistent is unclear.

Concluding that most subtle and generalized tonic seizures are not accompanied by EEG seizure discharges and that at least some of these may well have a "nonepileptic" mechanism seems safe, but the possible occurrence of epileptic discharges in any clinical seizure precludes reaching definitive conclusions.

Clonic seizures are mostly associated with well-formed, repetitive spike and sharp-wave discharges (Kellaway and Mizrahi, 1990; Mizrahi, 1984; Lombroso, 1982; Fenichel et al., 1980b). Abnormal paroxysmal rhythms tend to be present in seizures with less conspicuous clinical manifestations, such as focal tonic seizures (Aicardi, 1991b; Fenichel et al., 1980b), apneic attacks (Kellaway and Mizrahi, 1990), and subtle seizures (Holmes, 1985; Rowe et al., 1985; Fenichel et al., 1980b).

EEG seizure discharges without detectable clinical manifestations are common in neonates, as the practice of long-duration EEG monitoring has shown. This is especially common in infants receiving antiepileptic drugs, particularly phenobarbital, which often produces "uncoupling" of the clinical and EEG seizure manifestations (Clancy et al., 1988; Shewmon, 1983). An undefined proportion of newborns may have such discharges without ever having behav-

ioral seizures. This was the case for 11 patients of Mizrahi and Kellaway (1987), and it has also been found in several other studies (Mizrahi, 1987; Kellaway and Hrachovy, 1983). Hellstrom-Westas et al. (1985) used a cerebral function monitor to detect seizure discharges in 87 neonates over several days in an intensive care unit. Fourteen infants had seizures that lasted an hour or more, and, of these, two never had detectable clinical seizures. Similar results were obtained by Eyre et al. (1983) and Bridgers et al. (1986) using cassette recording. In some of these patients, the absence of clinical manifestations was due to therapeutic paralysis, but the same results were then obtained in several nonparalyzed neonates. Connell et al. (1989) found EEG seizure activity in 55 (25%) of 275 full-term or preterm neonates, and clinical seizure manifestations were totally absent in 23 of these infants. Clancy et al. (1988) indicated that up to 79% of EEG discharges may not have clinical accompaniment. The frequency of silent seizures seemed especially high in infants who were receiving antiepileptic drugs.

Conversely, clinical seizures that are deemed to be epileptic but that have no typical EEG abnormalities are also encountered (Weiner et al., 1991; Dreyfus-Brisac and Monod, 1977; Chariton, 1975). Weiner et al. (1991) compared 33 newborns with both clinical and EEG seizures to 18 with only clinical seizure activity. They found that those without electrographic discharges had more interictal background EEG abnormalities and a higher frequency of subcortical lesions. Dreyfus-Brisac and Monod (1972, 1977) and Cukier et al. (1976) indicated that clinical seizures without EEG discharges were more common in cases in whom several seizures occurred after a long period of seizure activity (Clancy et al., 1986).

DIAGNOSIS OF NEONATAL SEIZURES

The most difficult issues in the diagnosis of neonatal seizures are deciding (a) which atypical ictal behavioral events can be regarded as epileptic seizures and (b) whether subclinical EEG seizures are occurring. For both purposes, EEG monitoring is essential, and this should occur over a prolonged period to answer the question regarding subclinical seizures (Lombroso, 1992; Scher and Painter, 1990; Scher and Beggarly, 1989; Legido et al., 1988).

The best methods of monitoring are still under discussion. Conventional multichannel EEG recording, cassette EEG monitors, cerebral function monitors, and compressed spectral array have all been used (Eaton et al., 1992). The essential point with the use of any neurophysiologic technique is that the technician and doctor in charge should be familiar with the EEG of the newborn, which is quite different from that of adults (Lombroso, 1992; Plouin, 1990; Tharp, 1981). The issue of whether behavioral seizures that are unaccompanied by EEG discharges should be regarded as different in nature from electroclinical seizures or whether they represent only a variant of the same basic epileptic phenomenon has been discussed earlier in this chapter.

A number of abnormal phenomena in the neonatal period generally are not epileptic seizures, or they are only on rare occasions. *Jitteriness*, which is characterized by tremulous movements of a periodic nature that have equal speed in the alternating phases of flexion and extension, is usually easy to distinguish from convulsive jerks, which have a fast active phase and a slower release component. Jittery tremor is usually generalized to all four limbs, but they may be observed in a single limb or in a particular position of that limb; this is not accompanied by abnormal eye movements (Fernandez-Alvarez and Aicardi, 2001; Brown and Minns, 1980; Brown, 1973). Almost one-half of normal full-term neonates exhibit jitteriness during the first days of life, when they are excited or crying (Parker et al., 1990), but the phenomenon can also occur in infants with hypoxic-ischemic encephalopathy (HIE), hypocalcemia, hypoglycemia, and drug withdrawal (Volpe, 2001). Jitteriness and seizures can occur coincidentally, and they can be difficult to differentiate.

Shuddering episodes can also be observed in the first months of life. They consist of brief (5 to 15 seconds) bursts of rapid tremor of the head and arms that are reminiscent of a shiver (Pachatz et al., 1999; Vanasse et al., 1976). Such cases might be associated with those of "benign myoclonus of infants" (Lombroso and Fejerman, 1977).

Benign neonatal sleep myoclonus (Resnick et al., 1986) is characterized by clonic movements of the limbs that occur only during slow sleep. The phenomenon is less common or is absent during rapid eye movement (REM) sleep (Di Capua et al., 1993), and waking the infant up always stops the jerks. In most patients, the jerks predominate in the upper limbs, especially distally, and they may be bilateral or localized, rhythmic and arrhythmic, and even migratory or multifocal (Fernandez-Alvarez and Aicardi, 2001). They may occur in salvoes, mimicking clonic seizures or even status epilepticus (Alfonso et al., 1995) when they occur repetitively for 20 to 30 minutes or even up to 90 minutes. No associated interictal or ictal EEG abnormality is present. Benign

neonatal sleep myoclonus fades spontaneously from the second month onward, and it usually disappears before the sixth month of life (Fernandez-Alvarez and Aicardi, 2001).

Motor automatisms (Mizrahi and Kellaway, 1998; Kellaway and Mizrahi, 1990; Fenichel, 1985) can include several types (see "Subtle Seizures" earlier in this chapter), and they are only rarely associated with EEG discharges. This is especially applicable to the pedaling and boxing movements observed in metabolic disorders, such as leucinosis or organic acidurias (Livet et al., 2002). The multifocal myoclonic jerks observed in nonketotic hyperglycinemia (Seppäinen and Similä, 1971) may or may not be associated with EEG bursts, and these are often accompanied by other more or less typical electroclinical seizures (Aicardi and Goutières, 1978). True convulsive seizures are late events in most neonatal metabolic disorders, except for in the neonatal hyperammonemias, in which they may be the presenting symptom (Livet et al., 2002).

Clinical recognition of nonepileptic phenomena in neonates is often possible. Important diagnostic clues include the ability to elicit the abnormal phenomena by stimulation, whether tactile or otherwise; the demonstration that spatial or temporal summation of stimuli is effective; and the ability to prevent or interrupt abnormal events by restraint. Epileptic seizures are not usually stimulus sensitive, and they persist despite restraint (Lombroso, 1992, 2002; Volpe, 2001; André et al., 1988). More importantly, the clinician must consider the neurologic context within which the paroxysmal phenomena are observed (Arzimanoglou and Aicardi, 2001).

The value of interictal EEG for the diagnosis of neonatal seizures is limited. Normal newborns often show sharp waves on EEG (Clancy, 1989; Tharp, 1981; Dreyfus-Brisac, 1979), especially in the central and/or frontal regions. Even though such transients are statistically more common in babies with seizures (Hughes et al., 1983; Chugani et al., 1988), the mere presence of such abnormalities in a neonate does not establish an epileptic origin of seizures. In contrast, the prognostic value of the EEG is considerable.

ETIOLOGY OF NEONATAL SEIZURE DISORDERS

During the last decade, the development of neonatology, emergency facilities, and more rapid access to sophisticated investigations and techniques has changed the relative importance of various etiologic factors. The survival rate of very sick neonates has significantly improved, creating a larger population of infants that is at risk of developing seizures. Table 12.1 lists the main etiologic factors of neonatal seizures.

Mizrahi and Kellaway (1998) discussed the changes in etiologic factors in four studies conducted at Texas Children's Hospital between 1962 and 1995. For example, hypocalcemia was reported in 31% of cases in 1971 and in only 4% in 1995, whereas the 23% of infants presenting with unknown etiology in 1971 was reduced to 9%. The percentage of those diagnosed with an infectious disease cause increased from 4% to 14%.

The probable diversity of the mechanisms responsible for neonatal paroxysmal events makes determining whether some types of seizures are specifically related to certain etiologic factors difficult. Moreover, several factors are often operative in the same patient, such as hypocalcemia, hypoxia, and infection (Lombroso, 1992), each of which requires prompt recognition so that specific therapies can be adopted when possible. Although HIE and metabolic disorders more often cause subtle seizures of "nonepileptic" nature, they can also produce typical epileptic events.

Hypoxic-Ischemic Encephalopathy

HIE remains a common cause of neonatal seizures (Arzimanoglou and Aicardi, 2001; Volpe, 1989; Legido et al., 1988; Minchon et al., 1987; Holden et al., 1982). However, the true incidence is not known. Considerable variability in the HIE diagnostic criteria and terminology renders any comparison between old and recently published series difficult. Mizrahi and Kellaway (1998) noted out that the incidence had diminished from more than 60% in the early studies (Craig, 1960; Harris and Tizard, 1960) to 20% to 30% in the late 1960s (Hopkins, 1972; Rose and Lombroso, 1970), followed by an gradual increase from 30% to the current level of 50% (Bergman et al., 1983).

The clinical signs and laboratory findings lack specificity, which makes long-term outcome predictions difficult (Aicardi, 1998b; Paneth, 1993; Nelson and Leviton, 1991). The exact mechanism is often uncertain, so investigators (Leviton and Nelson, 1992) now prefer the use of the more general term *newborn or neonatal encephalopathy*. The criteria for the diagnosis of "neonatal asphyxia" have been reassessed. The combination of profound metabolic or mixed acidemia, an Apgar score of 0 to 3 for longer than 5 minutes, neonatal neurologic manifestations, and multisystem organ dysfunction are required (Committee on Obstetric Practice and American Academy of Pediatrics, 1996). Special attention has been given to the Apgar score as an indicator of the degree of hypoxia in the brain. However, most children with Apgar scores of 3 or less even at 10 and 15 minutes do well. The occurrence of seizures following a low Apgar score, however, has an ominous significance (Nelson and Ellenberg, 1981a). Several authors agree that individual parameters in isolation do not consistently predict the outcome (Aicardi, 1998b; Mizrahi and Kellaway, 1998; Perlman, 1997; Vanucci, 1997). The diagnosis of HIE requires unequivocal evidence of fetal distress; depression at birth; and clinical manifestations of encephalopathy, including seizures. Prenatal or intrapartum difficulties are not a sufficient argument for making a diagnosis of HIE.

Many cases are probably of prenatal origin, as the frequency of prenatal placental damage shows (Scher, 2003; Burke and Tannenberg, 1995). The disorder is most common in full-term infants or in infants born af-

TABLE 12.1. *Main causes of neonatal seizures*

Hypoxic-ischemic encephalopathy—may produce both clearly epileptic attacks and seizures that are probably nonepileptic in nature
Intracranial hemorrhage
    Subarachnoid hemorrhage—clonic seizures in term infants who are 1–5 days of age
    Intraventricular hemorrhage—mainly tonic seizures and episodes of apnea without EEG correlates, occasionally typical EEG discharges
    Intracerebral hematoma—fixed localized clonic seizures
Intracranial infections
    Bacterial meningitis and/or abscess
    Viral meningoencephalitis
Cerebral malformations—Hemimegaloencephaly, abnormalities of cortical development
Metabolic causes
    Hypocalcemia—clonic, multifocal seizures
    Hypoglycemia
    Hyponatremia
    Inborn errors of amino acids or organic acids and NH_3 metabolism—often atypical, mostly unassociated with EEG discharges
    Molybdenum cofactor deficiency
    Bilirubin encephalopathy—atypical, no EEG discharges
    Pyridoxine dependency
    Biotinidase deficiency
    Carbohydrate-deficient glycoprotein syndrome
Toxic or withdrawal seizures—probably nonepileptic phenomena in most cases
Familial neonatal convulsions
"Benign" neonatal seizures of unknown origin

Abbreviation: EEG, electroencephalogram.

ter gestations longer than 41 weeks. This was the case in 28 of the patients in the series of Dreyfus-Brisac et al. (1981), 14 of whom had a gestation of more than 42 weeks. Postnatal respiratory insufficiency causes less than 10% of cases of hypoxic encephalopathy (Volpe, 2001). Ischemia is secondary to intrauterine asphyxia with cardiac insufficiency. Postnatal heart disease and cardiovascular collapse resulting from hemorrhage or sepsis are uncommon causes of neonatal cerebral ischemia (Levene et al., 2001).

Overdiagnosis is probably common, and this may have serious consequences. It may impede the recognition of potentially treatable causes (e.g., meningitis and pyridoxine dependency) or genetic disorders. As yet undescribed genetic conditions that are responsible for neonatal seizures (outside the benign familial cases) likely exist, and these will likely continue to be unrecognized if the convulsions are too readily attributed to anoxia. In addition, overdiagnosis may be responsible for a wrong prognosis, because anoxic seizures are difficult to control and their long-term outcome is often unfavorable.

Seizures in HIE occur between 4 and 24 hours after birth (Minchon et al., 1987; Fenichel, 1983; Hill and Volpe, 1981), and 60% of the patients with this condition have already had fits by 12 hours (Volpe, 2001). The seizures are often isolated at the start. They tend to become severe and serial within 12 to 24 hours of birth. A total of 75% to 85% of the cases of "neonatal status" have been attributed to hypoxic insult (Volpe, 2001). The seizures are often fragmentary or subtle (Lombroso, 1983b), but no relationship between the cause and seizure types was found in other studies (Holden et al., 1982). The convulsions are accompanied by other manifestations of the causal disorder, such as apathy, hypotonia, or hypertonia; absence of the Moro reflex; and bulbar palsy (Brown and Minns, 1980).

In severe cases, the interictal EEG is of the *tracé paroxystique*, or inactive tracing, type (Dreyfus-Brisac, 1979). A history of prenatal or perinatal adverse factors (e.g., toxemia, *abruptio placentae*, meconium staining, cord prolapse, slow or fixed fetal heart rate, type II dips on monitoring, prolonged labor, or prolonged failure to establish spontaneous respiration) is the only presumptive evidence that hypoxia is responsible for the convulsive state.

Localized Ischemic Events

Localized ischemic events resulting from obstruction of major arterial branches are increasingly being recognized in neonates (Clancy et al., 1985; Levy et al., 1985; Ment et al., 1984; Billard et al., 1982). In such patients, the seizures appear between a few hours to 4 to 5 days after birth. They are mostly focal clonic, and, in most patients, they remain localized to the same territory, even when they persist for hours. The neurologic status is fairly well preserved. The computed tomographic (CT) scan shows an area of hypodensity located in the territory of one major cerebral artery (Fig. 12.2). The course is variable (Sreenan et al., 2000). Some patients recover without sequelae even when residual cavitation is evident on later CT scans. In other cases, hemiplegia or other localized deficits eventually appear. This neonatal stroke syndrome accounted for the occurrence of seizures in 7 (14%) of 50 full-term neonates reported by Levy et al. (1985). Ultrasonography usually permits the diagnosis (Volpe, 2001), although some investigators think that a CT scan is the only reliable technique.

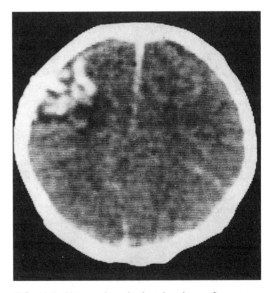

FIG. 12.2. Neonatal stroke in a boy born after an uneventful gestation and delivery. Left focal mainly clonic seizures started when he was 36 hours old and were repeated many times over the next 30 hours. Hemiparesis was noted between the seizures and for 48 hours after their arrest. At the age of 3 years, the child has no neurologic signs, and his neuromotor development is normal. Computed tomographic scans show an area of hypodensity with marked contrast enhancement in the cortical zone in the territory of the right sylvian artery.

Hemorrhage

Intracranial hemorrhages are a significant cause of neonatal convulsions. In two large series, they were found in 14% to 15% of affected newborns (Lombroso, 1983c; Bachman et al., 1976). Such figures should, however, be accepted with some caution because (a) intracranial bleeding is extremely common in the neonate so a coincidental occurrence is by no means unlikely and (b) some of the phenomena attributed to hemorrhage, especially tonic seizures with *intraventricular hemorrhages*, may well be "release" phenomena rather than true epileptic seizures. Intraventricular hemorrhage can, however, be associated with definite seizures that are confirmed by EEG recordings, especially when the hemorrhage spreads from its subependymal origin into the brain parenchyma or toward the ventricular system (Fenichel, 1985; Maynard and Garrel, 1983; Cukier et al., 1976). Dreyfus-Brisac (1979) and Dreyfus-Brisac and Curzi-Dascalova (1979) found intraventricular hemorrhage in 15 of 29 premature infants with neonatal seizures at autopsy but in only 2 of 13 full-term infants. Such seizures, especially in the premature infant, are associated with a very poor prognosis (Marret et al., 1997; Shinnar et al., 1992; Tharp et al., 1981). Their clinical features are generally limited to apneas or subtle motor manifestations (Volpe, 2001). Rolandic spikes in the EEG are common but not characteristic with intraventricular hemorrhages (Clancy and Tharp, 1984; Blume and Dreyfus-Brisac, 1982; Cukier et al., 1972).

Subarachnoid hemorrhage can be associated with seizures in the full-term infant, although, in most patients, it is of little clinical significance. The convulsions are often focal or multifocal clonic. In the interictal periods, the infant often appears remarkably well. The onset may be any time between 1 and 4 or 5 days after birth, most often on the second postnatal day. The cerebrospinal fluid is generally grossly bloody, but, after a few days, a marked white blood cell reaction may be seen that may mimic purulent meningitis. A similar picture is seen with *intracerebral hematomas*, which may be of traumatic origin but which most commonly are unassociated with any obvious trauma (Chaplin et al., 1979). Resorption of the hemorrhage leaves behind a residual cavity that may not be associated with any neurologic deficit.

Subdural hemorrhage is most commonly of traumatic origin and when accompanied by seizures is located on the convexity of the hemispheres. In one series, convulsive phenomena occurred in 50% of newborns with subdural hemorrhage and appeared in the first 48 hours of life (Lombroso, 1978).

Intracranial Infection

Intracranial infections account for 12% of neonatal seizures, according to Volpe (2001), and the relative incidence has remained constant. Bacterial meningitis is the major cause, so lumbar puncture must be performed for any seizure occurring in the neonatal period, especially after the first 2 or 3 days of life. In some patients, especially those with meningitis caused by *Proteus mirabilis* and *Citrobacter* organisms, seizures appear in infants without any obvious sign of infection; these are commonly associated with multiple intracerebral abscesses (Levy and Saunders, 1981). Nonbacterial infections can include encephalitides following toxoplasmosis, herpes simplex virus, rubella, coxsackie B, and cytomegalovirus (Lombroso, 1983c; Kairam and DeVivo, 1981).

Developmental Brain Defects

Developmental brain defects can be the cause of fits from the very first days of life. *Severe* dysgenesis produces early seizures. Clinically, the attacks commonly are myoclonic seizures or infantile spasms, but fixed focal clonic seizures or subtle attacks are also observed (Lombroso, 1983b). The EEG not uncommonly demonstrates a suppression-burst pattern (see Chapter 3). According to Lombroso (1982), in some patients with brain malformations, the tracings tend to exhibit ill-formed discharges of the alpha, theta, or delta types rather than spikes, but these patterns are by no means specific. Major or minor peripheral malformations may suggest the presence of brain dysgenesis. The relative incidence of congenital brain malformations or migration disorders will certainly increase with the broader use of high-resolution neuroimaging.

Metabolic Disturbances

Metabolic disturbances, especially those that affect the metabolism of glucose and electrolytes (e.g., calcium, magnesium, sodium), are now less commonly associated with neonatal seizures. Therefore, they cannot be accepted as an explanation for neonatal convulsions without a due consideration of the clinical history and the associated signs and symptoms.

Seizures from congenital enzymatic disorders usually have their onset in early infancy (Livet et al., 2002; Ogier and Aicardi, 1998). Some congenital aminoacidurias may cause dystonic posturing or characteristic repetitive athetoid movements that may be mistaken for convulsive episodes (Lombroso, 2002). Features like "pedaling" or "boxing" have been often described in maple syrup urine disease or organic acidemias. However, erratic myoclonus is particularly suggestive of nonketotic hyperglycinemia, although it may be observed with other disorders, including those of a metabolic nature.

Hypocalcemia

Hypocalcemia (calcium levels of 7 mg per dL or less) best exemplifies the various significances of the same metabolic abnormality in different contexts. *Early hypocalcemia* occurring during the first 2 or 3 days of life is a common finding in premature and low-birthweight infants; in infants of diabetic mothers; or in those who experienced neonatal distress from any cause, especially hypoxic injury (Lombroso, 1978, 1983b; Keen and Lee, 1973). Early hypocalcemia is thus associated with other potential etiologic factors that appear to play a major role at the origin of the convulsions. The role of hypocalcemia itself seems, at best, to be accessory, as both the almost universal failure of calcium therapy alone to stop the fits and the poor prognosis of children with early as opposed to late hypocalcemia demonstrate.

Late hypocalcemia manifests only by the end of the first week or the onset of the second week of life in full-term babies fed large quantities of formula with nonoptimal phosphorus-to-calcium and phosphorus-to-magnesium ratios. It probably results from functional hypoparathyroidism because of the inability of the immature kidney to excrete the excess phosphate load contained in such formulas. Associated *hypomagnesemia* is often seen in these patients, and, in few patients, it may even occur in isolation. The clinical picture is distinctive, with well-formed focal or multifocal seizures that repeatedly occur in a conscious, jittery, hyperactive infant who often also has a ravenous appetite (Brown, 1973). The seizures of late hypocalcemia are regularly controlled by the administration of calcium salts. The long-term prognosis is excellent, and sequelae have not been reported even following prolongation of the seizures for several days (Lombroso, 1983c). Late hypocalcemia is now rare. Its high incidence in Great Britain in the 1960s, which included more than half of the patients of Brown et al. (1972), was probably related both to feeding habits and to some subclinical vitamin D–deficiency state in the mothers (Purvis et al., 1973; Roberts et al., 1973). Today, the finding of hypocalcemia and hyperphosphatemia in a newborn should initiate investigations for latent maternal hyperparathyroidism or rare agenesis of the parathyroid glands (DiGeorge syndrome), or they may be associated with cardiac disease, which has a guarded prognosis (Lynch and Rust, 1994).

Hypoglycemia

Hypoglycemia raises problems similar to those posed by early hypocalcemia. The rare patient with persistent hypoglycemia, whether it is idiopathic or is related to abnormalities in glycogen metabolism or to a pancreatic lesion, convulses early and repeatedly; these infants fare poorly, with high mortality and morbidity. Such babies often present with episodes of apnea, tremors, and lethargy. Transient hypoglycemia is common in low-birth-weight infants and in those born of diabetic or prediabetic mothers. In addition to seizures, the neurologic symptoms include jitteriness, apneas, and hypotonia, which occur more commonly than the seizures. In the series of Cornblath and Schwartz (1967), 80% of small-for-gestational-age neonates with hypoglycemia had symptoms, and 50% exhibited seizures. The convulsions occurred early (mainly on the second day). Because hypoglycemic babies almost always have other possible causes for their seizures, the role of hypoglycemia *per se* is difficult to assess (Lombroso, 1983c). The hypoglycemia should nevertheless be corrected immediately, because some evidence does indicate that symptoms are related to the duration of the hypoglycemia (Kovisto et al., 1972). Seizures and neurologic symptoms are much less common in the infants of diabetic mothers, possibly because the duration of hypoglycemia is relatively brief in such neonates (Cornblath and Schwartz, 1967).

Pyridoxine Dependency

Pyridoxine dependency is a rare but curable condition, the presence of which should be systematically investigated. In a recent prospective study (Baxter, 1999), the point prevalence of definite (i.e., response to pyridoxine confirmed after formal withdrawal trial) and probable (i.e., a second successful trial after the recurrence of seizures or a first trial in children with an affected sibling) cases in children younger than 16 years of age was 1 per 687,000, and the birth incidence was 1 per 783,000. With the inclusion of possible cases (i.e., those defined earlier but without an attempt to withdraw pyridoxine), these become 1 per 441,000 and 1 per 313,000, respectively. When all forms of pyridoxine-responsive seizures were included, the prevalence becomes 1 per 317,000, and the birth incidence 1 per 157,000.

Pyridoxine dependency is classically marked by early (i.e., in the first few days of life or even in the days preceding birth) (Bejsovec et al., 1967) and intractable seizures that respond dramatically to the intravenous injection of pyridoxine and that recur within a few days if therapy is discontinued. Recent evidence indicates that the seizures may occur long after the neonatal period up to 12 or even 18 months of age, that they may respond temporarily to antiepileptic drugs, and that they may not recur for weeks or even months after the discontinuation of vitamin B_6 (Connolly et al., 1991; Haenggeli et al., 1991; Mikati et al., 1991; Goutières and Aicardi, 1985; Bankier et al., 1983; Krishnamoorthy, 1983). Atypical presentations are relatively common. The seizures vary in type, and infantile spasms have even been reported (Bankier et al., 1983). The most common presentation is that of episodes of generalized or unilateral status epilepticus. Intravenous pyridoxine (100 mg) should be given systematically for all cases of severe seizures of unknown origin occurring during the first 18 months of life.

Other Metabolic Disturbances

Other metabolic disturbances are uncommon in the newborn. *Hyponatremia* may occur as a result of inappropriate secretion of antidiuretic hormone (ADH) resulting from meningitis or intracranial hemorrhage. *Hypernatremia* is observed occasionally with dehydration or excessive bicarbonate administration. *Disturbances of amino acids and organic acids* (e.g., leucinosis, propionic acidemia, methylmalonic acidemia, and isovaleric acidemia) are characterized by the occurrence of neurologic symptoms after a symptom-free interval of a few hours or days. Abnormal movements of a nonepileptic nature are more common than true convulsions, which occur usually as a relatively late symptom (Lombroso, 2002). Hyperglycinemia is associated with fragmentary myoclonus and partial seizures with a suppression-burst EEG pattern.

Other rare metabolic causes include a familial spongiform encephalopathy with neonatal seizures and a low activity of the Na^+/K^+ adenosine triphosphatase pump in the brain (Goddard et al., 1969) and familial folinic acid–responsive seizures (Hyland et al., 1995).

Toxic Causes

Local-Anesthetic Intoxication

Local-anesthetic intoxication has been reported mainly in the United States. It results from local anesthetics being inadvertently injected into the infant's scalp at the time of placement of a paracervical, pudendal, or epidural block. The infants have a low Apgar score, hypotonia, bradycardia, and hypoventilation (Volpe, 2001; Kim et al., 1979). The pupils are fixed to light, and the vestibular (doll's head) reflex is abolished. Seizures occur within 6 hours of birth. The prognosis is excellent if vigorous supportive treatment is given.

Drug Withdrawal

Drug withdrawal rarely produces seizures, although it is becoming a common cause of neurologic symptoms. Maternal addiction with narcotic-analgesic drugs during pregnancy usually results in irritability and jitteriness during the first 24 hours of life, but seizures occur in only 1.2% to 3% of cases (Doberczak et al., 1988). A similar syndrome may occur in the neonate experiencing withdrawal from short-acting barbiturates (Desmond et al., 1972) or alcohol (Pierog et al., 1977). Delayed withdrawal seizures can occur as long as 4 weeks after birth in infants born to methadone-addicted mothers (Kandall and Gartner, 1974).

Idiopathic Neonatal Convulsions

No cause can be assigned to neonatal seizures in 10% (Volpe, 2001; Dennis, 1978) to 25% (Lombroso, 1983c) of patients. In a review of 2,042 cases that had been reported since 1959, 224 had no demonstrable cause (Plouin, 1990). The proportion of undiagnosed cases varies with the type of referral and the criteria required for the diagnosis of hypoxic encephalopathy and some metabolic disturbances. Cases without a recognizable cause often have a relatively benign outcome. However, the prolonged repetition of fits, resistance to therapy, or a rapid relapse after discontinuation of treatment indicates the probability of some basic defect in the newborn (Lombroso, 1983c). Two syndromes were identified as part of the idiopathic group in the International League Against Epilepsy (ILAE) classification (*familial and nonfamilial benign idiopathic neonatal convulsions*), and these are discussed in the following section. The main difference between these two syndromes is the presence or absence of a family history of neonatal convulsions of unknown etiology and a favorable outcome. In individual patients, the initial diagnosis may be difficult because the "benign evolution," which often is wrongly thought to be part of the definition of the syndrome, can only be suspected but not confirmed until an undetermined lapse of time has passed.

NEONATAL SEIZURES IN THEIR OVERALL CONTEXT: SYNDROMES IN NEWBORNS

Although some relationship does exist between the age at onset of seizures and the associated clinical manifestations, on the one hand, and etiology and prognosis, on the other, isolating well-defined "epileptic syndromes" during the neonatal period is difficult. Most groupings are rather loose, and only familial seizures and a few rare syndromes, such as neonatal myoclonic encephalopathy (NNME) (Schlumberger et al., 1992b; Aicardi and Chevrie, 1976), stand out clearly. Although the ILAE classification recognizes four syndromes for that age group, two are classified within the group "idiopathic epilepsies" (benign idiopathic familial and nonfamilial neonatal convulsions) and the remaining two within the group of symptomatic epilepsies (early myoclonic epileptic encephalopathy and early epileptic encephalopathy with suppression bursts). In clinical practice, the age at emergence and the neurologic examination results allow distinction into one of the following two groups: (a) early onset seizures in severely affected neonates and (b) early or late onset seizures in relatively well infants.

Early Onset Seizures with Marked Neurologic Involvement

Seizures that occur during the first 3 days of life are often fragmentary or subtle, and they tend to occur in long series or to constitute episodes of status epilepticus (Cukier et al., 1976; Monod et al., 1969; Schulte, 1966). The neurologic status of neonates with early fits is often poor, with many infants exhibiting hypotonia, disturbances of sucking, lack of reactivity, absent primary reflexes, or other serious signs (Brown et al., 1972). Hyperexcitability and tremors may occur in less severely affected babies. This is the group in which the more abnormal EEG patterns, such as flat records, *tracé paroxystique*, and inactive tracing, are often obtained (Marret et al., 1997; Tharp et al., 1981; Dreyfus-Brisac, 1979).

Many cases of early onset neonatal convulsions are the result of HIE (Minchon et al., 1987; Freeman, 1983), and the prognosis is, therefore, guarded (see "Hypoxic-Ischemic Encephalopathy"). Metabolic disturbances, especially hypoglycemia, hypocalcemia, or hypomagnesemia, are common, and these should be corrected. However, they play, at best, a secondary role. Intracranial hemorrhages, especially intraventricular hemorrhages in premature infants, are also a cause in this group. Positive rolandic sharp waves are common in this context, although they are not specific (Okumura et al., 1999; Tharp et al., 1981; Cukier et al., 1972) as a similar pattern can result from local-anesthetic intoxication. Because the prognosis is completely different, a careful inquiry into the obstetric history and a search for needle marks on the infant's scalp are mandatory.

Within this group, the following two syndromes have been more clearly delineated (Aicardi and Ohtahara, 2002) and included in the ILAE classification: *early myoclonic encephalopathy or NNME*, which was first described by Aicardi and Goutières (1978), and *early infantile epileptic encephalopathy* with suppression burst, which was described by Ohtahara et al. (1987, 1992) (see Chapter 3).

The neurologic status of infants with NNME is always poor, even at birth or as soon as the onset of the seizures occurs, with marked hypotonia of truncal muscles and progressive deterioration. More than half of these babies die before 1 year of age.

Seizures in Neurologically Well Babies

Early onset seizures, which most often begin on the second day of life, are relatively uncommon (Volpe, 2001). They may remain focalized to the same site or shift from one area to another, or they may be multifocal. In the interictal period, the infant is conscious, displaying no neurologic signs. The EEG recording is usually almost normal between the seizures, and this continues in the areas not involved by the paroxysmal discharges even during the seizures. This syndrome is characteristically associated with neonatal strokes caused by localized vascular obstruction resulting in brain softening (Mantovani and Gerger, 1984; Ment et al, 1984; Mannino and Trauner, 1983). It is also observed with primary subarachnoid hemorrhage (Volpe, 1989; Lombroso, 1983b) and localized intracerebral bleeding. In both stroke and hamartomas, the seizures usually remain localized to the same area throughout the course. Although localized deficits may follow intraparenchymal hemorrhage, the prognosis for this group is rather favorable.

Late-onset seizures, with an onset after the third day of life, uncommonly are associated with severe neurologic signs, except in the case of bacterial meningitis. Affected infants are well until the onset of the seizures, and most are full-term babies without abnormal antenatal or obstetric antecedents. Although the seizures, as a rule, tend to recur serially for many hours or even several days, no obvious compromise of the main vegetative functions is seen. The syndrome of late-onset seizures may be due to late hypocalcemia. In that case, the infants are jittery, and they have increased tendon reflexes in addition to their fits. More commonly now, no cause is found. Even in cases without a known cause, the prognosis is better than that in early onset seizures.

Two syndromes, benign familial neonatal convulsions (BFNCs) and the syndrome of "fifth-day fits," have received special attention. However, the only difference between the two is the presence or absence of a family history.

Benign Familial Neonatal Convulsions

BFNCs have their onset within 2 to 15 days of birth, most commonly on day 2 or 3, in most patients. The prevalence of the syndrome is unknown. Plouin (1994) reviewed data from the 334 cases of BFNC belonging to 38 families that had been reported since the initial description by Rett and Teubel (1964). The seizures, which are usually clonic, are often repeated up to several dozen times per day (Arts et al., 1991; Plouin, 1990; Pettit, 1987; Tibbles, 1980; Pynnönen et al., 1977; Bjerre and Corelius, 1968), but they stop spontaneously after a variable duration. Hirsch et al. (1993) reported video-EEG data on 14 seizures recorded in three children from two families who presented with BFNCs. All of the seizures occurred during sleep after a short arousal reaction. The seizures started with bilateral, symmetric flattening of the EEG for 5 to 19 seconds; apnea and tonic motor activity were simultaneously present. The EEG flattening was followed by a long (1 to 2 minute) bilateral discharge of spikes and sharp waves; vocalizations, chewing, and focal or generalized clonic activity occurred simultaneously. The prominence of EEG and motor abnormalities varied between the left and the right side from one seizure to the next in any given child.

The interictal status is either normal or not severe. The EEG confirms the epileptic nature of the fits (Camfield et al., 1991). Interictal EEG recording is normal, or it may show minimal focal or multifocal abnormalities or a pattern of "theta pointu alternant." Further psychomotor development is favorable. The overall rates of secondary epilepsy and febrile convulsions were 11% and 5%, respectively. The rate of febrile convulsions is comparable to that of the general population.

Despite the absence of a clearly focalized EEG discharge, the generalized nature of these seizures (Hirsch et al., 1993) has been debated. Some authors (Mizrahi and Kellaway, 1998) consider the clinical presentation suggestive of an age-dependent partial idiopathic epilepsy. The diagnosis rests entirely on the family history, which may be difficult to elicit because early seizures in family members may have been forgotten. The condition is transmitted in an autosomal dominant fashion with regular penetrance (Bate and Gardiner, 1999; Tibbles, 1980) but variable expression. The occasional occurrence of neonatal seizures in the siblings of unaffected parents in families in which previous generations have been unaffected (Goutières, 1977) may suggest that the trait is recessive in rare cases.

A linkage on chromosome 20 (EBN1) was demonstrated in 1989 by Leppert et al. (1989) and was confirmed by another study (Malafosse et al., 1990). Ryan and Wiznitzer (1990) and Ryan et al. (1991) presented data indicating that the syndrome is clinically and genetically heterogeneous. Other family pedigrees have been identified in which a linkage to chromosome 20 has been ruled out, and a second locus was found in chromosome 8 (EBN2) (Steinlein et al., 1995). A third family pedigree in which both chromosome 20q and 8q were ruled out by linkage studies has also been identified (Lewis et al., 1996). The gene for EBN1, also called *KCNQ2*, was identified by two teams in 1998 (Biervert et al., 1998; Singh et al., 1998) (for details, see Chapter 22).

Benign Idiopathic Neonatal Convulsions

Benign idiopathic neonatal convulsions were first described by Dehan et al. (1977) under the name *fifth-day fits*. The attacks are of the following two main types: clonic focal or multifocal convulsions and apneic spells (Dehan et al., 1977). They last on an average 20 hours. The interictal EEG recording shows preserved rhythms and a normal organization of sleep. Bursts of alternating theta rhythms, or *theta pointu alternant*, are observed in three-fourths of the patients. They are suggestive, although not characteristic, of the syndrome (Navelet et al., 1981).

Many authors have emphasized the benign nature of fifth-day fits when all the criteria of the syndrome are present (Pryor et al., 1981; Dehan et al., 1977). These include a full-term birth; a normal pregnancy and delivery; an Apgar score of more than 8 at birth; onset between days 4 to 6 (in 80% of patients); a normal neurologic status before and between seizures, at least in the beginning; clonic and/or apneic but not tonic seizures; normal laboratory investigations; the frequent presence of *theta pointu alternant* on the EEG recording and the absence of paroxysmal, inactive, or low-voltage records; and only brief seizures with no alpha-like pattern. However, mental retardation or later convulsions and epilepsy have been reported (Levy et al., 1985).

Plouin (1994) reviewed the literature on 299 cases and noted that no etiology was identifiable. The syndrome of fifth-day fits may be related to environmental factors, as the cases seem to cluster in certain places and periods. Pryor (1979) found that the incidence of the syndrome in Sydney reached a peak in

1973 and that thereafter it declined to low levels. A low concentration of zinc in the cerebrospinal fluid was found in 25 patients (Goldberg and Sheehy, 1982).

Identification of fifth-day fits as a separate syndrome remains questionable. The syndrome has no specific clinical or EEG features, and it may have a less than optimal outcome. That seizures occurring relatively late in the neonatal period, without a known cause and with a relatively normal or little altered clinical examination and EEG, have a generally benign course is perhaps not unexpected because the criteria for the syndrome are also factors for a favorable prognosis. Other causes of unknown etiology may have an unfavorable course when some of the criteria are lacking, so the individualization of the syndrome is dubious (Lombroso, 1992). This may explain the widely different incidences reported for the syndrome (Lombroso, 1992; Levy et al., 1985).

PROGNOSIS IN NEONATAL SEIZURES

The uncertainties regarding the true nature of neonatal seizures and the variability of causes and types explain why attempts at identifying the overall prognosis of neonatal seizures have been neither successful nor particularly helpful (Painter et al., 1986; Goldberg, 1983). Some have suggested that the prognosis of neonatal seizures has improved over the past decade. Volpe (2001) gathered a composite series of 1,000 cases from reports published before and after 1969 and found that mortality had decreased from 40% to 15%. Such studies, however, relied on seizure diagnosis by clinical criteria only. In one study including only neonates with EEG-proven seizures, the mortality rate was 32.5% (Clancy and Legido, 1987a).

The incidence of neurologic sequelae in survivors, however, has remained approximately the same (35%). In one series, Lombroso (1983c) found a mortality rate of 16%, and a 34% rate of long-term handicap. Bergman et al. (1982, 1983) found a mortality rate of 25%, moderate or severe abnormalities in 24%, and mild abnormalities in 5% of convulsing newborn infants, whereas 47% of them developed normally. As part of the United States National Collaborative Perinatal Project, Holden et al. (1980) and Mellits et al. (1981) studied 277 infants who were recognized to have neonatal seizures. This project was a prospective study of approximately 54,000 pregnancies, and it thus avoided the selection biases present in hospital series. However, some of the reported results must be interpreted with caution because they reflect the known etiologic factors and the level of recognition

of neonatal seizures in the period covered by the study (1959 to 1966). In this study, 35% of the infants who experienced seizures died, 29% of them during the first 36 hours. In addition, 19 of the 181 survivors had mental retardation with or without cerebral palsy, 2% had only cerebral palsy, and 9% had isolated epilepsy; 70% of the survivors had no sequelae. In the Dublin collaborative study, the mortality and severe sequelae were 18% and 25%, respectively (Curtis et al., 1988). Mental retardation and motor deficits are common sequelae. The possibility of later perceptual disabilities or of specific learning disabilities in children with neonatal convulsions is unknown.

The incidence of late recurring seizures varies among authors. Holden et al. (1982) indicated an incidence of 9%, and Bergamasco et al. (1984), 7.1%, whereas Schulte (1966), Lombroso (1978), and Dennis (1978) reported recurrence rates of 22%, 26%, and 20%, respectively. Following EEG-confirmed seizures, Clancy and Legido (1987a, 1991) and Legido et al. (1991) found that epilepsy developed in 15 of 27 survivors of a group of 40 patients, most of whom had HIE. The first postnatal seizure occurred at an average corrected age of 12.7 months despite ongoing anticonvulsant treatment in 9 of the 15. Predictors of recurrent seizures included the presence of coma at the time of the neonatal events, a duration of neonatal seizures of more than 10 hours, and an abnormal background EEG recording in 68% of patients. The age at onset of the neonatal seizures, Apgar score at birth, and gestational age were not indicative of the risk of later epilepsy. The late seizures were infantile spasms in 7 (47%) of 15, complex partial seizures in 4, and GTCSs in 4. Uncommonly, recurrent seizures are only an isolated sequela (Nelson and Ellenberg, 1982, 1986; Bergman et al., 1983). In most cases, the later seizures are associated with cerebral palsy and mental retardation. Infantile spasms associated with tetraplegia and microcephaly have been observed in a small proportion of infants with repeated neonatal convulsions of anoxic origin (Nelson and Ellenberg, 1981a).

The outcome of neonatal seizures depends mainly on their cause (Table 12.2). Other factors have a significant bearing on the prognosis, and attempts have been made to predict the development of epilepsy and other neurologic problems by combining the EEG, neurologic examination, etiology, duration and type of seizures, birth weight, and gestational age (Brod et al., 1988; Ellison et al., 1986).

Seizures in the *premature infant* have a gloomy outlook, with mortality rates of 89% to 100% (Watkins et

TABLE 12.2. *General outcome following neonatal seizures*

Study	Year	Number of Neonates	Mortality (%)	Incidence of Postneonatal Epilepsy (%)	Neurologic Impairment (%)	Normal (%)
National Collaborative Perinatal Project	1959–1966	277	35	20	30	35
Lombroso	1983c	117	16	56	35	48
Clancy and Legido	1991	40	33	17 (pre-term), 30 (full term)	38	30
Ortibus et al.	1996	81	29	28	49	22
Bye et al.	1997	32	25	21	31	38

al., 1988; Knauss and Marshall, 1977; Cukier et al., 1976). In a recent series (Bergman et al., 1983), the neonatal mortality associated with seizures was 17% for those born at term, 57% for those born at 32 to 36 weeks, and 84% in those born at 31 weeks or less. However, the rate of abnormalities in the survivors was not higher for the premature babies compared with that of full-term babies. The frequent repetition of seizures (status epilepticus) and the long duration of the individual attacks are also associated with a poor outcome. The mortality rate for infants with status epilepticus varied from 35% (Monod et al., 1969) to 87% (Dreyfus-Brisac et al., 1981) in full-term babies to up to 100% in premature babies (Cukier et al., 1976).

The early onset of seizures is a predictor of severe prognosis. In general, onset within 48 hours of birth is of grave significance, whereas seizures starting after the fourth day of life are often relatively harmless. Seizures occurring between 2 and 4 days of age are almost equally divided between favorable and unfavorable results (Ellison et al., 1986; Ziegler et al., 1976, 1981). Brown et al. (1972) found that, when seizures began on the first day, one-third of the infants died and 60% of the survivors were abnormal at 1 year. When seizures started between 2 and 6 days, 97% of the infants survived. Half of the infants whose seizures started on the second day, 70% of those whose seizures began on the third day, and 90% of those whose seizures began on the fourth day appeared normal at follow-up. The relationship between date at onset and outcome is mainly indirect because most early seizures are the result of hypoxic encephalopathy. Exceptions to the general rule do exist, especially in the case of local-anesthetic intoxication, in some cases of benign familial convulsions, and hemorrhage. In one old series (Dennis, 1978), the good prognosis associated with a late onset of the fits was entirely accounted for by the cases of late hypocalcemia. In other series, however, a favorable prognosis has also been associated with cases of unknown causation and late onset (Lombroso, 1983c; Dreyfus-Brisac et al., 1981).

Certain types of seizures, such as tonic spasms or massive myoclonus, have a very severe significance (Bergman et al., 1983; Brown, 1973). Subtle seizures are regarded as less favorable than well-formed clonic seizures by several authors (Volpe, 2001; Mizrahi, 1987; Goldberg, 1983), but this has not been a universal experience (Freeman, 1983). Purely electrical ictal discharges without clinical seizures are also of poor prognosis (Dreyfus-Brisac and Monod, 1977). McBride et al. (2000) recently reviewed the EEG and outcome data from 68 infants who met the at-risk criteria for neonatal seizures and underwent prolonged continuous EEG monitoring. Forty infants had electrographic seizures. The etiology of EEG seizures included asphyxia in 23 and stroke in 7. Ten infants with EEG-proven seizures and one without died from causes related to neurologic instability. The occurrence of EEG seizures was correlated with microcephaly, severe cerebral palsy, and failure to thrive. Conversely, Weiner et al. (1991) found that seizures without EEG concomitants had a severe outcome and that they were associated with EEG background interictal abnormalities more often than those with EEG ictal discharges.

Several investigators have found a good correlation between the results of the neurologic examination and the prognosis. Severe neurologic abnormalities are associated with an adverse outcome (Staudt et al., 1982; Brown and Minns, 1980; Zielinski, 1975; Keen and Lee, 1973), but exceptions to this are common, and several authors have emphasized the uncertainties of this approach, except in extreme cases (Freeman, 1983; Costeff and Avni, 1982). A low Apgar score at 5 minutes and the need for resuscitation after 5 minutes were predictors of death or sequelae, as was the presence of apneic episodes (Holden et al., 1980). Bergman et al. (1983), however, did not find a significant predictive role for the 5-minute Apgar score.

Interictal EEG data are of definite value, especially if several polygraphic recordings can be obtained during the first few days of life (Fisher and Clancy, 1987; Mizrahi and Tharp, 1982; Dreyfus-Brisac and Monod, 1972; Tibbles and Prichard, 1965; Ajmone-Marsan and Abraham, 1960).

Lombroso (1983c) showed that a normal EEG pattern with well-organized sleep stages in a newborn with convulsive attacks is associated with at least a 75% chance of the infant being normal by 5 years of age. Conversely, the presence of paroxysmal or low-voltage (flat) tracings or of a multifocal pattern (Tharp, 1981; Tharp et al., 1981) reduces the outlook for normality at 5 years to less than 10%, regardless of the clinical impression. Intermediate patterns have a less clear-cut value. In patients with such tracings, repeated EEG recordings are particularly important. If the background tracing and organization of sleep remain normal, the prognosis seems to be as good as that with a normal EEG, despite the presence of focal paroxysms (Clancy, 1983; Lombroso, 1982; Mizrahi and Tharp, 1982). The prognosis remains uncertain in 25% to 35% of full-term babies with borderline tracings or mild abnormalities (Lombroso, 1982, 1983c). Although the value of the EEG in premature infants has been questioned (Bergman et al., 1983), Rowe et al. (1985) recently confirmed the its value as a prognostic tool, even in premature infants. They found that low-voltage (less than 5 μV) tracings, inactive tracings, and the suppression-burst pattern were regularly associated with a poor outcome. Marret et al. (1997) reached similar conclusions in a prospective study of 417 neonates born before 33 weeks of gestation. The prognostic value of EEG findings relative to the motor and cognitive outcome was investigated in a group of preterm infants affected by different degrees of cystic periventricular leukomalacia (Biagioni et al., 2000). The study indicated that the EEG recording was a useful prognostic tool for preterm infants during the early postnatal period, whereas, at term age, the role of EEG tracings appeared secondary. The clinician should remember that a discontinuous EEG recording is normal in children of younger than 36 weeks of gestational age (Scher et al., 1988; Bachman et al., 1976).

The possible role of the seizures themselves in producing or aggravating brain damage is variably appreciated (Nehlig et al., 1999). Some investigators (Lombroso, 1992; Kellaway and Mizrahi, 1990) think that neonatal seizures are not likely to generate brain damage because they are usually focal and short lasting and they are without severe systemic accompaniment. However, other authors (Swartz et al., 1989;

Volpe, 1989; Lou and Friis-Hansen, 1979; Wasterlain, 1978) believe that the adverse effects of seizures on ventilatory function, circulation, and cerebral metabolism that have been observed in experimental animals also occur in humans, especially in those with repeated seizures. Furthermore, excitotoxic mechanisms related to excitatory amino acids might also produce brain damage. Although the question has not yet been settled, recent work (Holmes et al., 1999; Lombroso, 1996; Holmes, 1991a) has cast doubt on the importance of such effects in the human baby and has emphasized the great resistance of young animals (and probably of the human newborn) to seizure-induced damage. Clearly, a definite answer to this question is of considerable significance with regard to management. *In vivo* neonatal magnetic resonance spectroscopic measurement of cerebral high-energy phosphate compounds has shown minimal changes in adenosine triphosphate (ATP) content during seizures. ATP levels begin to decline only if prolonged exposure to intense hypoxia (30 mm Hg) exists and when the level of phosphocreatine has declined to less than half its normal value. Its recovery following seizures is rapid (Delgado-Escueta et al., 1996; Young et al., 1987; Younkin et al., 1986). These results suggest that seizure-induced damage may occur, but possibly only under special circumstances. On balance, the role of the seizures themselves should not be neglected, but it is minor in comparison to that of the causal disorder.

MANAGEMENT OF NEONATAL SEIZURES

The management of neonatal seizures should depend on the mechanism of the attacks. As was indicated earlier in this chapter, not all paroxysmal events have the same mechanisms, and the following guidelines apply to seizures of epileptic nature, not necessarily to those that are due to other mechanisms (e.g., release of brainstem tonigenic centers from cortical inhibition). Indeed, in such cases, antiepileptic drugs that may produce further cortical depression might be potentially dangerous (Kellaway and Mizrahi, 1990; Camfield and Camfield, 1987).

All authors agree that the most potent predictor of prognosis for infants with neonatal seizures is the cause of the convulsions. Therefore, establishing the etiologic factor or factors and treating them promptly are essential (Volpe, 2001; Aicardi, 1986a; Bergman et al., 1982). Pharmacologic treatment of the seizures is of lesser importance, although it is clearly required in all patients who experience more than an occasional attack. Because of the uncertainties regarding the effect of seizures on the brains of neonates, the degree of emergency in the treatment of neonatal convulsions and the best therapeutic techniques remain in dispute (Volpe, 1987; Aicardi, 1985b; Freeman, 1983). However, treating all recurring seizures early seems reasonable.

Continuous EEG recording is extremely useful because many neonatal seizures continue without clinical manifestations (McBride et al., 2000; Monod et al., 1969).

General Management

A newborn baby with convulsive seizures should be carefully observed. Monitoring of respiration and heart rate is essential. EEG recording is desirable, but obtaining an EEG recording should never delay treatment and it can be dispensed with if no *trained* electroencephalographer is available. A bedside ultrasound scan indicates if bleeding, infarction, or gross malformation is present in the central nervous system.

An intravenous line rapid correction of any metabolic derangement for the administration of glucose following blood glucose determination and rapid correction of any metabolic derangement. Maintaining blood glucose at a slightly supranormal level is advised by some (Lombroso, 1992) because glucose may help prevent the depletion of energy reserves (Dwyer and Wasterlain, 1985). However, in hypoxic injury, whether glucose administration may induce lactate production and acidosis is not known. Therefore, the optimum supply of glucose remains undetermined, especially because newborn babies may not produce lactate (Younkin et al., 1986).

Severely disturbed infants may require therapeutic respiratory muscle paralysis to facilitate assisted ventilation. This prevents the clinical manifestation of seizures, thus necessitating EEG monitoring (Eaton et al., 1992; Clancy et al., 1988).

The levels of electrolytes, pH, calcium, and magnesium should be obtained, and fluid administration should be restricted to 75% of the normally required amount to avoid dilutional hyponatremia. Proper ventilation and the maintenance of body temperature are essential, and a lumbar puncture is imperative. Treatment of "cerebral edema" with dexamethasone was considered essential by some (Brown and Minns, 1980), but the evidence in favor of such a treatment is limited because the edema is usually due to a cytotoxic mechanism that responds poorly to steroids (Lombroso, 1992; Hill and Volpe, 1981). Such treatment, however, may be indicated for the treatment of established edema due to the cause of seizures.

All children with early onset (younger than 3 years old) intractable seizures or status epilepticus should receive a trial of pyridoxine (usual dose is intravenous administration of 100 mg within 30 minutes) *before* that of any long half-life anticonvulsant and whatever the suspected cause so that cases of pyridoxine dependency, though rare, are not missed (Baxter, 1999; Goutières and Aicardi, 1985).

Specific Treatment

Specific treatment is immediately indicated whenever a treatable cause for the seizures is found (Aicardi, 1980c, 1991b). If hypoglycemia is present, 2 mL per kg of a 10% solution of glucose is given intravenously during the acute phase, followed by a dose of up to 8 mg per kg per minute as maintenance therapy. If hypocalcemia is found, 2 mL per kg of a slow (10 minutes) intravenous injection of 2.5% to 5% calcium gluconate is administered with electrocardiographic monitoring. After the restoration of normocalcemia, tapering the dosage may help in preventing rebound hypocalcemia (Mizrahi and Kellaway, 2001). Magnesium sulfate, 2 to 8 mL of a 2% to 3% solution intravenously or 0.2 mL per kg of a 50% solution intramuscularly, is added when associated hypomagnesemia is present. The serum levels of magnesium should be monitored to avoid its potential curare-like effect. Other metabolic derangements are uncommon, and, more often, they are responsible for nonepileptic abnormal movements than they are for true seizures.

Pyridoxine dependency should be systematically prevented. Biotinidase deficiency is only an exceptional cause of early seizures, but it responds dramatically to the intravenous administration of 10 mg of biotin.

Other specific therapies (e.g., for meningitis or hemorrhages) are applied according to usual techniques in appropriate cases.

ANTIEPILEPTIC THERAPY

Antiepileptic drug therapy is indicated for infants whose seizures do not have a specific treatment, as an adjunct to the treatment if it does not control the fits rapidly, or when the diagnosis makes it likely that the seizures will persist (e.g., malformations, infarcts, fetal infections) (Table 12.3). At the moment, no agreement exists on which seizures require antiepileptic drug treatment, the timing for starting them, or what drug should be used preferentially.

Those authors who think that neonatal seizures of whatever cause can harm the brain (Volpe, 1989) rec-

TABLE 12.3. *Main drugs for treatment of neonatal seizures*[a]

Drug	Loading Dose	Maintenance	Usual Range	Apparent Half-life
Phenobarbital	20 mg/kg i.v. (up to 40 mg/kg)	3–4 mg/kg/day in two doses	20–40 µg/mL	100 hr (declines rapidly after days 5–10)
Phenytoin	20 mg/kg i.v. (up to 35 mg/kg)	2–5 mg/kg/day in four doses	15–35 µg/mL	100 hr (40–200), declines as phenobarbital
Diazepam	0.25–1 mg/kg i.v. or rectal administration	May be repeated one to three times	200–800 µg/mL	31–84 hr
Lorazepam	0.05 mg/kg	May be repeated		17 hr
Paraldehyde	400 mg/kg i.v. (200 mg/kg/hr in 5% dextrose)	20–50 mg/hr	100–200 mg/mL	18 hr
Lidocaine	4 mg/kg/hr	Decrease loading dose by 1 mg/hr on days 2–5 then discontinue	—	3 hr
Clonazepam	0.1 mg/kg i.v. (infusion over 5 min)	—	28–117 mg/mL	—

Abbreviations: i.v., intravenous; —, no data available.

[a]Despite the considerable increase in the number of new antiepileptic drugs, no serious effort has been made by either the industry or the regulating authorities to develop drugs for use in neonates. However, everybody recognizes the need. See "Antiepileptic Therapy" for information about the occasional use of other drugs. No controlled studies to confirm the appropriate dose and range have been conducted.

ommend immediate therapy with large doses of long-acting anticonvulsants. The drug of first choice is usually *phenobarbital* (Aicardi, 1986a, 1991b; Painter, 1983, 1988; Fenichel, 1985; Dodson, 1983; Ouvrier and Goldsmith, 1982; Painter et al., 1981). Blood levels of at least 20 µg per mL are required in order to be therapeutic; to achieve this level promptly, a loading dose of 20 mg per kg is administered intravenously. Some advocate doses of up to 35 to 40 mg per kg so that levels of about 40 mg per mL are achieved (Gal et al., 1982). The maintenance doses are 3 to 4 mg per kg per day in two doses by intravenous or intramuscular routes, as the oral route is unreliable (Painter, 1988; Painter et al., 1986; Aicardi, 1985b; Fisher et al., 1981). Because the apparent half-life is very long (average is 100 hours after days 5 to 7) in the first 1 or 2 weeks of life and it rapidly shortens thereafter (Pitlick et al., 1978; Pippenger and Rosen, 1975), close monitoring of blood levels to permit rapid dosage adjustment is mandatory.

Phenytoin is usually the second drug used (Aicardi, 1985b; Painter et al., 1978, 1981), and it is often combined with phenobarbital because it is often used after failure of this agent. A recent study (Painter et al., 1999) compared the effectiveness of the acute administration of phenobarbital versus that of phenytoin in seizure control and found no significant difference between the two drugs. Phenytoin should be used par-

enterally to obtain plasma levels of 15 to 20 µg per mL (Painter et al., 1981). Some authors use even higher doses to obtain levels of 35 to 40 µg per mL (Fenichel, 1985). A loading dose of 15 to 20 mg per kg is usually effective, and it should be followed by a maintenance dose on the order of 3 to 5 mg per kg per day. The loading dose should be administered slowly at a rate not exceeding 50 mg per minute to avoid disturbances of cardiac rhythm.

Fosphenytoin, a prodrug of phenytoin, was administered in 11 neonates in a study that included 75 children and adolescents (Morton et al., 1998). The range of values for the conversion half-life of *fosphenytoin* and the resultant plasma total and free phenytoin concentration-time profiles following intravenous administration were greater in neonates, although, globally, these were similar to values in older children and adults. Kriel and Cifuentes (2001) have published a report on the use of fosphenytoin in two low-birth-weight infants.

Valproate has been used by some in neonatal seizures at doses of 50 mg per kg rectally or orally to achieve blood levels of 60 to 80 µg per mL (Lombroso, 1992; Gal et al., 1988), but the safety and efficacy of this drug have not been fully assessed. Alfonso et al. (2000) measured serum valproate concentrations in two neonates at 45 minutes and 3 hours after the initiation of the infusion. They found that each 1 mg per kg of intravenous valproate increases the 45-minute and 3-hour postinfusion serum valproic acid concentrations by approximately 4 µg per mL and 3 µg per mL, respectively.

Other agents that have been used include primidone (loading dosages between 15 and 12 mg per kg, followed by maintenance doses of 12 to 20 mg per kg per day) and carbamazepine (loading dose of 5 mg per kg every 12 hours), but few data are available for these agents (Sapin et al., 1988; Mackintosh et al., 1987; Powell et al., 1984; Painter, 1983). Lidocaine, which is administered by pump infusion at a rate of 4 mg per kg per hour the first day, 3 mg per kg per hour the second day, 2 mg per kg per hour the third day, and 1 mg per kg per hour the fourth day and is discontinued on the fifth day, has been proposed by some investigators (Radvanyi-Bouvet et al., 1990; Gamstorp and Sedin, 1982), but its effects are difficult to judge because concomitant therapy was generally present. Radvanyi-Bouvet et al. (1990) reported seizure control in 20 of 26 babies. Interestingly, the agent seems to produce discontinuous EEG activity without the ominous implications of this pattern. Paraldehyde has also been advocated (Koren et al., 1986; Brown and Minns, 1980).

Data are scarce concerning newer antiepileptic drugs. Reports on *vigabatrin* are anecdotal (Baxter et al., 1995). *Lamotrigine* was given to a 17-day-old neonate, after failure of several agents, at a single daily dose of 4.4 mg/kg per day for 3 days, followed by divided daily doses every 12 hours. Control of seizures could be obtained 75 minutes after the first dose was administered.

Those investigators who believe that only prolonged seizures are harmful tend to postpone the initiation of long-acting antiepileptic agents until the diagnosis is clarified, unless evidence of systemic effects is noted (Lombroso, 1992; Kellaway and Mizrahi, 1990). Lombroso (1992) favors the initial use of short-acting drugs, especially in cases in which seizures seem likely to be transient, such as mild HIE, sepsis, or cryptogenic seizures. *Diazepam* can be used intravenously or rectally at doses of 0.5 to 1 mg per kg, repeated at 4-hour to 6-hour intervals for 24 to 48 hours. Alternatively, continuous infusion at a rate of 0.7 to 2.7 mg per hour for up to 24 hours, followed by slow tapering, has given good results (Gamstorp and Sedin, 1982). *Lorazepam* is also rapidly effective, and it has the advantage of longer action and the absence of secondary release from brain and fat tissue (Maytal et al., 1991). The usual dose of 0.05 mg per kg can be repeated at 6-hour intervals. In dosages of 0.1 and 0.2 mg per kg, *clonazepam* has also been used

successfully in neonates (André et al., 1986). Recently, Sheth et al. (1996) reported the administration of *midazolam* (loading dose of 0.15 mg per kg, followed by maintenance doses from 0.1 to 0.4 mg per kg per hour given intravenously) to six neonates.

A number of neonates continue to have seizures despite the adequate use of drugs. Many of these have severe underlying brain damage and interictal EEG patterns of unfavorable significance. In such cases, increasing the antiepileptic dosage may do more harm than good (Lombroso, 1992), especially because at least some of these events are not epileptic seizures of cortical origin (Kellaway and Mizrahi, 1990; Camfield and Camfield, 1987).

Whether electrical discharges without clinical manifestations justify antiepileptic treatment has not been established (Volpe, 2001; Lombroso, 1992; Hakeen and Wallace, 1990). Such discharges may theoretically produce excitotoxic damage, even though no systemic consequences are noted. However, the newborn brain seems to be highly resistant to this form of insult. The suppression of electrical seizures may require high doses of antiepileptic agents with their attending dangers. Although dogmatic pronouncements are not possible, only moderate efforts at suppressing purely electrographic seizures appear to be justified.

The *optimum duration of therapy* for neonatal seizures has not been determined. No specific guidelines have been established (Mizrahi and Kellaway, 2001). The discontinuation of the antiepileptic drugs after a period of clinical seizure control should be individualized. Some investigators advise the discontinuation of drug treatment as soon as the seizures have stopped (Gal et al., 1984; Freeman, 1983; Gal and Boer, 1982; Gillam, 1982), whereas others advocate the continuation of therapy until all of the neurologic abnormalities have disappeared (Volpe, 2001). The intermediate approaches take into account the likelihood of recurring seizures after the discontinuation of treatment (Brod et al., 1988; Ellison et al., 1986), but this is difficult to predict (Camfield and Camfield, 1987), and recurrences may not be very common, even after major neurologic damage. For instance, Labrecque et al. (1984) found that only six infants developed epilepsy after major neonatal encephalopathy. Moreover, the continuation of treatment does not regularly prevent later epilepsy (Clancy and Legido, 1991; Watanabe et al., 1988) even though few data are available in this regard. The authors' opinion is that the continuation of antiepileptic treatment for more than a few weeks is justified only when the likelihood of recurrent seizures is high, specifically in cases of dysgenetic brain defect.

For acute conditions such as hemorrhages, mild or moderate HIE, and cryptogenic neonatal seizures, continued therapy is not needed. In cases of severe HIE or other forms of acquired brain damage, most authors advise maintenance therapy (Aicardi, 1985b, 1992a; Lombroso, 1992; Volpe, 1987), although the frequency of later epilepsy is poorly known (Clancy and Legido, 1991; Labrecque et al., 1984) and the feasibility of preventing later epilepsy is at best uncertain. A recent analysis of the published results of controlled clinical trials regarding the benefits and harm of the administration of anticonvulsants to infants following perinatal asphyxia with the primary aim of preventing death, subsequent neurodevelopmental disability, and/or seizures (Evans and Levene, 2000) concluded that no evidence supports immediate prophylactic treatment. Waiting for epilepsy to appear and thus avoiding the potential risks of chronic antiepileptic drug administration to developing infants (Farwell et al., 1990) is probably a safer alternative.

SUMMARY

Seizures in the neonatal period often result from serious neurologic disorders. As a consequence, their prognosis is often unfavorable, with a mortality rate of 15% to 30% and serious sequelae in approximately one-third of the survivors. However, approximately two-thirds of the infants who survive neonatal convulsions do well.

Not all paroxysmal events in the neonatal period are accompanied by epileptic EEG discharges. The nature of those events that are not associated with typical EEG abnormalities is uncertain. Some probably differ from true seizures, and they therefore may not require the same treatment.

One of the predominant causes of neonatal seizures is HIE. However, that diagnosis should not be accepted on the sole basis of abnormalities in the prenatal or perinatal periods if other conditions that, at times, are treatable are to be diagnosed. An onset of attacks before the infant is 24 hours of age and the presence of abnormal neurologic signs before and between the seizures are essential for substantiating the diagnosis of HIE. Many other processes (e.g., intracranial hemorrhage, infections, metabolic disorders, developmental brain defects) are responsible for a considerable proportion of cases, and the prognosis for these infants is not necessarily poor. Age at the onset of the fits is of considerable value as a guide to both their cause and their prognosis. Early onset attacks (in the first days of life) are mainly caused by anoxia and/or intracranial hemorrhage, and they generally have a poor outcome. Metabolic disturbances, although they are commonly encountered in this group, rarely have more than a secondary importance, and their correction does not modify the attacks. Late-onset seizures (from the fourth day onward) are mostly the result of metabolic disturbances or they are of unknown cause, and they have a much brighter outlook. In the latter group, the incidence of late hypocalcemia, which used to be a major etiologic factor, has steadily decreased over the past decade, whereas idiopathic seizures are more commonly recognized. These usually have the favorable prognosis that is attached to late hypocalcemia. Some may be genetically determined.

Convulsive phenomena take distinctive forms in the neonate because of the incomplete development of brain structures and connections. GTCSs do not occur, and most attacks remain localized or erratic.

The treatment of neonatal seizures is primarily directed at the causal condition when specific therapy is available, such as in late hypocalcemia, hypomagnesemia, pyridoxine dependency, or some cases of hypoglycemia. Anticonvulsant treatment is often the only therapeutic option available. The value of anticonvulsant treatment remains controversial because no clinical evidence conclusively indicates that neonatal seizures are a hazard to the brain. However, the clinician should keep in mind that no evidence indicates that neonatal seizures are innocuous, and common sense suggests that prompt and active treatment should be instituted. The various modalities of treatment are still being debated, but an awareness of the pharmacokinetic properties unique to the neonatal period permits a more rational use of anticonvulsant drugs.

13

Epilepsy in Infants

This chapter deals with convulsive disorders in the first 2 years of life, with the exception of those that occur in the neonatal period (first 28 days of age); occasional seizures, including febrile convulsions (see Chapter 14); and acute symptomatic seizures. Convulsive disorders in this period constitute a heterogeneous group, with some belonging to well-recognized syndromes, such as infantile spasms, Lennox-Gastaut syndrome (LGS), or various types of myoclonic epilepsy (see Chapter 6), while other epilepsies that have their onset in the first 2 years of life (even more so, in the first year) do not belong to the currently categorized epilepsy syndromes and have been relatively little studied (Abe et al., 2000; Watanabe and Okumara, 2000; Cavazzuti et al., 1984; Chevrie and Aicardi, 1977, 1978, 1979).

CHARACTERISTICS OF SEIZURES

The seizures observed in this age-group are difficult to classify because of their atypical features and, in particular, because the state of awareness and responsiveness often cannot be properly assessed (Watanabe et al., 2002; Kramer, 1999). They are often expressed by uncharacteristic features, which makes the distinction between focal and generalized seizures difficult.

Generalized tonic-clonic seizures are rare (Brunon et al., 1978; Sillanpää, 1973), and a detailed analysis of those attacks that are apparently generalized often reveals a lack of synchrony and symmetry of the motor phenomena that may predominate successively in different parts of the body, thus giving the impression that its components are more or less independent (Dalla Bernardina et al., 1978a). The generalized seizures also tend to be purely or predominantly tonic or clonic, rather than consisting of a regular tonic-clonic sequence. A unilateral predominance in the amplitude of the ictal electroencephalogram (EEG) discharge and irregularities in their rhythm are common, and their hemispheric synchronization is often imperfect (Gastaut et al., 1974c; Gastaut and Broughton, 1972).

Partial seizures are much more common (Cavazzuti et al., 1984; Aicardi and Chevrie, 1983; Dalla

Bernardina, 1978a), but, often, their expression is less clearly indicative of a localized discharge than that in older children. A relatively common type is marked by head and/or eye deviation toward one side and is accompanied by a predominantly tonic contraction involving only half the body or, more commonly, both sides symmetrically or asymmetrically (Watanabe and Okumara, 2000; Duchowny, 1987). These authors termed the attacks "complex partial seizures of infancy"; they were manifested by head turning; tonic, often lateralized motor phenomena; and apparent loss of contact. However, such features are often encountered in early seizures with or without alteration of consciousness, and many seizures are limited to hypertonia or hypotonia; mild convulsive movements; simple staring; and autonomic manifestations, such as flushing of the face, pallor, perioral cyanosis, or disturbances of respiratory or cardiac rhythms. Such seizures are classified as "hypomotor seizures" by some investigators (Hamer et al., 1999; Acharya et al., 1997) (see Chapter 10). Precise video-EEG study in 32 infants (Rathgeb et al., 1998) confirmed that the main features were motor phenomena that involved mostly the head, face, and trunk; arrest of activity; and autonomic symptoms. The degree of awareness is often impossible to determine. Such atypical seizures may alternate with or may evolve into more characteristic attacks as the infants grow older; in addition, lesions of the temporal lobe that initially are atypical in expression have been shown to develop later into typical temporal lobe seizures (Aicardi, 1970). Because of the difficulty in assessing the level of consciousness, the distinction between simple and complex partial seizures as defined by the International League Against Epilepsy (ILAE) classification of 1985 (Commission on Classification and Terminology of the ILAE, 1985) is not valid in this age group.

The EEG patterns associated with atypical partial seizures are quite variable (Aicardi, 1994a) in morphology and localization. In some patients, they may not be detectable on the scalp. Focal discharges have been recorded in infants with bilateral motor phenomena or diffuse autonomic manifestations (Aicardi and Chevrie, 1982b; Dalla Bernardina et al., 1978a), thereby indicating that partial seizures can easily be mistaken for generalized ones; differentiation may be impossible without simultaneous EEG recordings. Motor phenomena tend to be associated with anterior EEG discharges, and arrest and autonomic features with posterior discharges.

The relative lack of organization of the infantile seizures probably results from the incomplete development of the central nervous system (CNS), with the variable excitability being caused by changes in synaptic organization and the maturation of neurotransmitters, as well as by imperfect myelination and function of the interhemispheric connections (Holmes and Stafström, 1997; Moshé, 1987). However, the infant brain can occasionally produce massive epileptic myoclonus with bilateral, irregular spike-waves and, very rarely, even atypical absences (Aicardi, 1995).

ETIOLOGY

The etiology of infantile seizures is dominated by the presence of brain lesions (Aicardi and Chevrie, 1982b). The nature, localization, and extent of organic brain damage partly determine the ictal symptomatology. For example, tuberous sclerosis is not commonly responsible for seizure types other than infantile spasms in the first year of life (Pampiglione and Harden, 1973). Most of lesions responsible for early infantile epilepsy are prenatal in origin, and they are often quite extensive, even when they give rise to focal seizures (Chevrie and Aicardi, 1977). However, a close relationship exists between the lateralization of the lesions and that of seizures when both are unilateral or predominantly unilateral. The responsible lesions include brain damage of prenatal and perinatal origin, brain malformations, and diffuse or localized cortical dysplasias. Gross malformations were found in 57 patients in a large series in which 175 infants were thought to have acquired brain damage of prenatal or perinatal origin (Chevrie and Aicardi, 1977). The overall incidence of brain malformations would probably be higher with modern neuroimaging, which was not available in this series. Magnetic resonance imaging (MRI) has shown that cortical dysplasias and other developmental abnormalities are among the most common causes of infantile epilepsy (Guerrini et al., 1996c; Kuzniecky et al., 1992a; Palmini et al., 1991d; Andermann and Straszak, 1982) (see Chapter 19).

From a neuropathologic standpoint, the damage caused by prenatal and perinatal factors is mainly represented by ulegyrias and clastic lesions, such as the porencephalies. However, gyral abnormalities can be induced by prenatal factors such as anoxia and infections (e.g., cytomegalovirus).

The risk of early epilepsy is significantly increased following an abnormal birth. It is 7.2% even after low forceps delivery, and it reaches 11.3% following mid-cavity forceps. It is also increased by uterine dysfunction during labor and instances in which the lowest recorded fetal heart rate drops below 60 beats per minute. Conversely, the induction of labor, abnormalities of the cord, polyhydramnios, breech delivery, and abruptio placentae had no predictive value (Nelson and Ellenberg, 1986).

Metabolic causes of infantile seizures are uncommon. *Hypocalcemia* is unusual beyond the neonatal period (Oki et al., 1991), but this should be systematically investigated. *Pyridoxine dependency*, however, should always be kept in mind, even in those patients past the neonatal period. Recent reports (Baxter and Aicardi, 1999; Mikati et al., 1991; Goutières and Aicardi, 1985; Bankier et al., 1983; Stephenson and Byrne, 1983) have noted that the disorder may manifest at up to 18 to 24 and even 36 months of age with any type of seizures, including infantile spasms (Aicardi, 1999b). A test of the therapy for this condition (injection of 50 to 200 mg of pyridoxine) is the only way of establishing the diagnosis; therefore, this should be systematically performed.

Other metabolic causes include biotinidase deficiency, which can be easily diagnosed and treated by the administration of 10 to 20 mg of biotin, and neuroglycopenia resulting from a deficiency of the glucose transporter GLUT-1 (De Vivo et al., 1995), which is also treatable by the ketogenic diet. The latter justifies lumbar puncture to demonstrate low cerebrospinal fluid (CSF) sugar even when no cause is found for the seizures as the blood sugar level is normal.

In a large series by Chevrie and Aicardi (1977) and one by Cavazzuti et al. (1984), symptomatic cases were more common than cryptogenic (or idiopathic) ones. This was especially applicable to infantile spasms, in which 60% of cases were thought to be symptomatic and 40% were considered cryptogenic. However, the significance of these figures is open to discussion because the more severe symptomatic cases may be selectively included in such series, which originated from third-referral centers. On the other hand, they were collected at a time when modern neuroimaging was not available, and a number of CNS lesions could have been missed.

More recent work (Abe et al., 2000; Watanabe and Okumura, 2000; Vigevano et al., 1994) suggests that a significant proportion of infantile seizures may not be due to brain lesions and that, thus, they may have a more favorable prognosis. At least some such cases appear to be familial or at least to occur in patients with a strong family history of seizures of various types, thereby supporting the role of genetic factors in the origin of epileptic phenomena in the first 2 years of life. More than half the patients studied by Watanabe et al. (1990) had a family history of epilepsy or febrile convulsions, and "benign infantile convulsions" (Vigevano et al., 1992a, 1992b; Malafosse, 1990) appear to be dominantly inherited. Likewise, genetic factors are probably important in cases of epilepsy not manifested by infantile spasms. In one large series (Chevrie and Aicardi, 1977), a positive family history of seizures was present in 28% of infants with uncharacteristic seizures versus in 16% of those with infantile spasms, and the proportion of positive family history was higher in those with apparently generalized seizures than in those with partial seizures, especially when only nonsymptomatic cases were considered.

Thus, genetic factors likely are more important in the etiology of infantile seizures than was previously thought. Such factors may be of major importance in some syndromes of early epilepsy, some of which are apparently of monogenic origin (Hirose, 2002; Bate and Gardiner, 1999), or they may represent a significant factor in cases with multifactorial inheritance, in which several genes and environmental factors are involved.

SYNDROMES WITH INFANTILE SEIZURES

In several large series of infantile seizures published in the late 1970s and early 1980s (Cavazzuti et al., 1984; Chevrie and Aicardi, 1971, 1975, 1977), classification was limited to broad categories defined according to the dominant types of seizures. Only a limited number of epilepsy syndromes were recognized, especially West syndrome (or the presence of infantile spasms), with other cases being defined by the occurrence of uncharacteristic, (apparently) generalized or partial seizures.

In a study of 437 cases of chronic seizure disorders beginning before the age of 1 year, Chevrie and Aicardi (1977) classified 230 of them as "infantile spasms," whereas 207 could not be ascribed to specific syndromes. A few of the 207 cases were probably myoclonic epilepsies or an early form of LGS, but the vast majority could be divided only into partial (57 cases) and generalized (99 cases) seizures; 51 patients with seizures lasting 30 minutes or more were classified as "status epilepticus." Cavazzuti et al. (1984) similarly divided their patients into the fol-

lowing three groups: infantile spasms (183 cases), status epilepticus (66 cases), and "others" (138 cases). The last group included 51 infants with partial seizures and 87 with generalized seizures.

In a study of 504 children with epilepsy who had their first seizure between the ages of 28 days and 36 months, Dalla Bernardina et al. (1982) used a more complex classification. They ascribed 163 patients to the group "epileptic encephalopathies," which included West syndrome and LGS, with several subdivisions. They classified 189 as "partial epilepsies," also with various subgroups, and 80 as "generalized epilepsies," 43% of which were "myoclonic epilepsies." Only 72 cases remained unclassified. Only 37 (8%) of the patients in this series had a generalized epilepsy of a type other than myoclonic. Because the upper age limit was set at 3 years, more precise classification might have been possible than in the two preceding studies, which were limited to infants younger than 1 year. Clearly, a large proportion of the cases of LGS or myoclonic epilepsy cannot be diagnosed before 1 year of age, and this also applies to most of the subtypes of partial epilepsies reported by Dalla Bernardina et al. (1982). Though complex partial seizures are difficult to identify because of the problem of ascertaining the level of consciousness of infants ictally, these have been increasingly recognized (Watanabe et al., 1990; Duchowny et al., 1988; Dalla Bernardina et al., 1982). Most are probably associated with organic brain damage (Duchowny, 1992; Duchowny et al., 1988), and they have a poor prognosis that likely is related to the diffuse distribution of the lesions.

More recent studies have emphasized the existence of *recognizable epilepsy syndromes in infants younger than 2 years*. However, the definition of syndromes in this age group may be difficult because of the rapidly changing state of brain maturation, which is responsible for changes in seizure types and the associated features in the same patient. Thus, an epilepsy that, at 6 months, is expressed by infantile spasms can be expressed a few months later by atonic falls and/or atypical absences. More commonly, early epilepsies are initially manifested by atypical, abortive, or unclassifiable seizures that are later replaced by fits that are more specific for the accepted epilepsy syndromes, such as LGS. As a result, categorization of a syndrome is often impossible for a long period, consequently leading to prognostic uncertainties.

Some of the epilepsy syndromes that can occur in the first 2 years of life may be early forms (or the initial manifestations) of classic syndromes that also exist in older children, and these are described in other chapters of this book (see Chapters 3, 10, and 17). However, as the chapter indicated earlier, LGS often becomes characteristic only after 2 years of age and very seldom in the first year of life. The diagnosis of severe myoclonic epilepsy (Dravet syndrome) can be suspected in infants on the early occurrence of convulsions that are often prolonged and unilateral and that are triggered by mild fevers and then recur within a short period of time (usually less than 2 to 3 months). Confirmation of the diagnosis, however, has to await the appearance of myoclonias and/or other "minor" seizures in the second or third year of life. The diagnosis of "benign" myoclonic epilepsy rests, in principle, on the exclusive occurrence of brief isolated myoclonic jerks without other types of seizures, except febrile convulsions, but a definitive confirmation is possible only later with the appearance of no other types of paroxysms. A recessive form of infantile myoclonic epilepsy with seizures that may persist into adulthood has been reported in an Italian family and has been mapped to chromosome 16p13 (Zara et al., 2000).

Seizures associated with hypothalamic hamartomas can have very early onset, even within the neonatal period. Giggling seizures may occur (Pérez-Jiménez et al., 2003). In two personal cases, the authors have seen episodes of bizarre frantic agitation, with crying and grimaces that could last for hours and that were later followed by more typical gelastic attacks.

A rare type of early clinical paroxysmal seizures has been seen in infants, and it may start almost from birth. The attacks are exclusively motor, consisting of brief contractions of a hemiface without loss of consciousness and occurring repeatedly; these have sometimes been termed *hemifacial spasms*. These are associated with hamartomatous lesions in the middle cerebellar peduncle that impinge on the fourth ventricle (Arzimanoglou et al., 1999). Recording in the neighboring cerebellum has captured discharges similar to those of seizures, possibly justifying the use of the term *subcortical* or *cerebellar* epileptic seizures (Harvey et al., 1996).

Another early epilepsy syndrome of lesional origin was reported in 15 infants by Coppola et al. (1995). It features multifocal seizures with an onset in the first 3 months of life. The seizures are partial, with mostly motor manifestations; they occur with a high frequency in different localizations, generally involving both hemispheres alternately; and they often are of long duration. Controlling the attacks is quite difficult, and the rapid repetition of seizures is rapidly ac-

companied by severe neurologic and developmental deterioration, leading to death in a matter of months. Imaging is normal, and pathologic abnormalities are diffuse but not specific. A few similar cases since have been reported (Veneselli et al., 2001; Wilmhurst et al., 2000). The origin of such cases remains undetermined, but it does not seem to be genetic. Whether the clinical and EEG picture that has been described is characteristic of a unique syndrome has recently been debated by Ishii et al. (2002), who reported eight similar cases, five of which did not have a progressive course; these also had different etiologies, including two cases of mitochondrial disorder.

In contrast to these lesional and often severe convulsive disorders, other syndromes of apparently idiopathic epilepsy have been recently delineated, most of which feature partial seizures.

Syndromes with Partial Seizures of Idiopathic Origin

Vigevano et al. (1992a, 1992b) described a familial convulsive disorder that they termed *benign infantile convulsions* and distinguished from the previously described syndrome of benign familial neonatal convulsions. In their patients, the seizures first appeared in normal infants between 3 and 8 months of age. The affected infants had no history of prenatal or perinatal difficulties and no neurologic or imaging evidence of brain abnormality. This study included 31 infants from 17 families who had a family history of similar events at the same age in first-degree or second-degree relatives. The seizures often occurred in clusters, and they were marked by psychomotor arrest, cyanosis, head and eye deviation to one side, diffuse tonic contraction, and bilateral clonic jerks. Interestingly, the side of head deviation could change in the same patient. Ictal EEGs showed typical localized spike discharges arising from one or the other hemisphere, usually in the posterior region of the head (Vigevano, 1992a, 1992b, 1997). The seizures were short lived, as they disappeared in all patients within a few days, weeks, or months, and the later development of the affected children remained normal. A history of similar episodes in previous generations strongly suggested a dominant inheritance. A locus on chromosome 19q has been reported in some (Guipponi et al., 1997), but not all (Malafosse et al., 1990), such infants (see Chapter 19).

Somewhat similar cases have been described by Watanabe et al. (1987b, 1990) as *benign partial epilepsy of infancy*. These investigators initially reported nine patients with what they termed *complex partial seizures.* The age at onset was younger than 1 year in all but one case. The seizures occurred one to ten times daily in clusters for periods of 1 to 3 days, and they could recur in the same form within 1 to 8 weeks later. They were brief (30 to 217 seconds), and they appeared both in wakefulness (11 cases) and sleep (2 cases). They were marked by motion arrest; decreased responsiveness, thus satisfying the criteria for complex partial seizures; staring; simple automatisms involving the arms and leg movements or a change in facial expression; and mild convulsive movements. The latter variably included eye deviation or head rotation, mild clonic jerks of the face and limbs, and increased limb tone. The interictal EEG recordings were normal in all. The ictal EEG recordings disclosed focal discharges of repetitive sharp alpha or theta waves of increasing amplitude and decreasing frequency with gradual or rapid spread to other regions. The initial site of discharge was temporal in eight; central in two; and frontal, parietal, and occipital in the remainder of patients. The total duration of the disorder with antiepileptic treatment was short; treatment was discontinued in all infants after 1.5 to 5 years, and their later development was normal. The same group later reported on 7 (Watanabe et al., 1990) and then 11 (Watanabe et al., 1993) infants with a highly similar age at onset and comparable seizure manifestations that were followed, however, by generalized tonic-clonic convulsions of 40 to 120 seconds in duration that occurred in both asleep and awake patients as well. The EEG recordings in all showed a focal onset of the seizures (central in four, parietal in two, occipital in five, and posterior temporal in one), with secondary diffusion. Recurrences were limited to the first 1 to 5 months after onset. The response to antiepileptic agents was good, and the outcome was excellent. However, no history suggestive of a genetic origin was found in most families, even though a history of febrile convulsions was present in some. Similar cases have since been reported in Western countries (Capovilla et al., 1998; Berger et al., 1997; Camfield, 1987). Capovilla et al. (1998) described 12 cases with focal EEG ictal discharges arising from the occipital or temporal regions that also had a benign course.

Thus, one or several syndromes of benign partial seizures may exist in infancy. The ictal discharges may become generalized or remain focal, but this difference does not affect the clinical features or the outcome, and separating such cases may not be justified. Indeed, Watanabe et al. (1990, 1993) emphasized that differentiating between secondary generalized and partial seizures may be difficult because the ictal features of the latter may mimic generalized seizures or nonepileptic phenomena such as apneas (Symonds, 1959). In infants with complex partial seizures, the onset on EEG recordings may more often be temporal (Capovilla and Beccaria, 2000; Watanabe and Okumara, 2000; Watanabe et al., 1990), but such differences are subtle and their significance is uncertain. Further cases of this syndrome have been published in patients of European origin. The 12 Italian patients reported by Capovilla et al. (1998) had early onset seizures often marked by apnea, staring, motion arrest, cyanosis of the face, and loss of consciousness. Lateralizing signs were present in three of these infants. The attacks started between 13 months and 2.5 years of age, and they often occurred in clusters. All infants had a benign course, with the final attack being no later than 3 years, 7 months of age. Half the infants had a family history of epilepsy. The interictal EEG recordings were consistently normal both in sleep and in wakefulness. The ictal EEGs recorded paroxysmal discharges in the temporal or occipital areas. The same group (Capovilla and Vigevano, 2002; Capovilla and Beccaria, 2000) reported 12 cases of benign infantile convulsions associated with vertex spikes on interictal EEGs, a feature previously reported by Bureau et al. (1998), and proposed they represented a new syndrome, even though the presentation and course differed from the benign cases of Bureau et al. (1998), with a lower frequency of attacks and the absence of clusters.

The relationship between the syndromes described earlier has not yet been elucidated, but it appears to be close. A major difference is the evidence for dominant transmission in the cases of Vigevano (1992a, 1992b) and in the cases of this syndrome that have been reported since. This genetic transmission justifies the isolation of such cases as a separate group. The situation of other cases in whom genetic transmission is unknown is less clear. Whether the presence of small spikes, which are difficult to detect on routine EEG, and minor clinical differences are sufficient for separating other subgroups is also debatable. They seem to have many common features with other cases that have been reported, especially in the Japanese literature, as benign infantile convulsions (Fukuyama, 1963). Fukuyama (1963), followed by other several investigators, reported cases defined by the occurrence before 2 years of age of generalized symmetric tonic-clonic convulsions lasting 1 or 2 minutes, the absence of prenatal or perinatal antecedents, no recognized etiology, a normal interictal EEG, and a benign course. These infants did not have a history of familial epilepsy or febrile convulsions.

Although the clinical description was that of generalized seizures, no ictal EEG was reported, so some investigators suggested that a focal onset could have been missed (Watanabe and Okumara, 2000). Tsurui et al. (1989) observed that at least some seizures of this type that they witnessed and recorded had a partial onset and complex features. Therefore, whether these benign infantile convulsions are really distinct from the partial seizures described by other authors is uncertain. The most important difference seems to be the absence of a family history in the cases of Fukuyama (1963). However, very similar cases with a definite family history of convulsions were reported from Hong Kong by Lee et al. (1993). Interestingly, several of the infants in this series had a mild associated gastroenteritis at the time of the convulsive clusters. Similar cases from Japan have been reported by Abe et al. (2000); these occurred in association with gastroenteritis caused by infections with rotavirus and small round viruses, as well as in cases of undetermined cause. Whether these cases truly differ from those not associated with gastrointestinal disturbances remains undetermined.

However, the genetics among the cases seem to differ, as they are dominant in the cases of infantile convulsions (Vigevano et al., 1992a, 1992b) but they have a strong, but not specific, genetic component in those of Watanabe et al. (1987b, 1990, 1993). Genetic heterogeneity has been established as only some cases are linked to chromosome 19q.

At this writing, one or probably several syndromes of benign partial seizures clearly exist in infancy. However, their mode of inheritance seems to differ, and even the cases of typical benign infantile convulsions appear genetically heterogeneous because only some cases show linkage to chromosome 19q. In all these syndromes, however, the benign outcome seems well demonstrated.

This benignity, however, may be mitigated to some extent by the recent recognition that paroxysmal movement disorders may occur several years after the convulsive episodes in children who had recovered from infantile benign convulsions (Szepetowski et al., 1997). The movement disorder appears between 3 and 17 years of age and consists of paroxysmal kinesigenic choreoathetosis. A linkage to the centromeric region of chromosome 16 has been demonstrated (Szepetowski et al., 1997). Thirty cases have been reported in 17 French families, and other cases were later reported from other countries (Valente et al., 2000). The frequency of such an occurrence among cases of infantile convulsions is not known, and it may vary with the populations; a longer follow-up is needed to determine this. Some other cases of paroxysmal dyskinesias linked to the same region of chromosome 16 are not regularly associated with seizures or infantile convulsions (Valente et al., 2000). Similar cases with slightly different features (Lee et al., 1998) have been reported in different populations. Another syndrome featuring paroxysmal exercise-induced dyskinesia, writer's cramp, and rolandic epilepsy following infantile convulsions (Guerrini et al., 1999b) also maps to the same area of chromosome 16, but it is transmitted as an autosomal recessive disorder. Finally, another paroxysmal movement disorder, episodic ataxia type 1, which has been linked to chromosome 12p, may be expressed by seizures that are either associated with the movement disorder or occur even in isolation (Eunson et al., 2000); epilepsy may be ten times as common in this rare condition as it is in the general population (Zuberi et al., 1999).

Such an association of movement disorders and epilepsy is probably not fortuitous, and it suggests the importance of ionic channel dysfunctions in the mechanisms of several types of epilepsy.

Other Syndromes with Partial Seizures That May Manifest in Infancy

Other syndromes with partial seizures of genetic origin have been recently isolated (Picard et al., 2000). Although they can manifest clinically at any age, including in adulthood, they may have an early onset in the first 2 years of life. Several syndromes have been described, including familial frontal lobe nocturnal frontal epilepsy (Thomas et al., 1998; Oldani et al., 1996; Scheffer et al., 1995a), epilepsy with variable foci (Scheffer et al., 1998), and familial temporal lobe epilepsy (Berkovic et al., 1996a). The latter has, thus far, not been reported in infancy, and only two cases of epilepsy with variable foci have been reported (Poza et al., 1999; Ottman et al., 1995).

Frontal nocturnal epilepsy, the most common form, has repeatedly been observed in children younger than 2 years (Scheffer et al., 1995a), although it is more common in older children and adults. The clinical manifestations include tonic attacks that are often asymmetric with or without loss of consciousness (Vigevano and Fusco, 1993), nocturnal episodes of automatism, and sometimes violent and dystonic episodes (see Chapter 16). Usually, the child has a strong family history of seizures and/or "sleep disorders" that is retrospectively recognized as epileptic in nature. The outcome of these syndromes is not necessarily benign, and the seizures may persist into adulthood. In fact, quite similar seizures may also be symptomatic of various frontal lesions, so a benign outcome is not ensured (see Chapter 10).

PROGNOSIS

The prognosis of infantile seizures is often guarded (Matsumoto et al., 1983a, 1983b; Brunon et al., 1978; Harrison and Taylor, 1976; Hauser and Kurland, 1975). Precise information, however, is available for some syndromes, especially infantile spasms and some of the syndromes of benign infantile convulsions, whereas data concerning the epilepsies that are initially expressed by uncharacteristic fits or that are not part of recognized syndromes are extremely scant. Three hospital-based series (Cavazzuti et al., 1984; Dalla Bernardina et al., 1982; Chevrie and Aicardi, 1978) have reported broadly comparable results for such cases (Table 13.1). Overall, only 14% to 35% of the patients in these series had an intelligence quotient (IQ) of 81 or higher. The type of seizures experienced by the affected infants has a variable influence on the outcome (Table 13.2). Mortality and severe mental retardation tend to be more common in patients with infantile spasms than in those with other seizure types. Even in the series of Chevrie and Aicardi (1978), in which mental retardation was as common with other types of seizures as with infantile spasms, severe mental subnormality was more common in the latter. The different figures found in various series can probably be accounted for by varying referral patterns. As the reader may expect, the incidence of mental subnormality in all three series was much lower in patients with idiopathic or cryptogenic seizures than in those with symptomatic seizures. Similarly, the occurrence of epilepsy and neurologic abnormalities is much less common in cryptogenic cases.

The incidence of persisting epilepsy tends to be relatively lower in cases of infantile spasms than in the rest of the cases. Again, the higher figure found by Dalla Bernardina et al. (1982) is probably the re-

sult of different case referrals and a shorter duration of follow-up. The incidence of persistent epilepsy tends to decrease with increasing age (Chevrie and Aicardi, 1979). The type and severity of the persistent epilepsy varied widely according to the age and the initial expression of the seizure disorder. Many patients had several types of seizure, either in succession or simultaneously, and the general tendency was for the attacks to remain in conformity with their original type. The epilepsy that was the most serious and difficult to control generally occurred after infantile spasms or status epilepticus. Several disabilities (e.g., epilepsy, mental retardation, and cerebral palsy) were quite commonly encountered in these patients, so the total handicap was major.

In all three series, the factors associated with a poor prognosis included the symptomatic nature of the epilepsy and an early onset (before the age of 6 months), whereas a positive family history of epilepsy and/or febrile convulsions was associated with a less gloomy prognosis. Cavazzuti et al. (1984) also found that an epileptic pattern in the EEG had an unfavorable influence on the outcome. Some disagreement existed between two series about the significance of the type of seizure. According to Cavazzuti et al. (1984), whether the first seizures were generalized or partial did not seem to affect the subsequent development of epilepsy, whereas Chevrie and Aicardi (1979) found a higher incidence with partial attacks.

Some investigators (Dravet et al., 1992a) have stressed the unfavorable prognostic significance of myoclonic phenomena appearing during the second year of life (see Chapters 4 and 6) in association with other types of attacks.

In most series, however, the mental and neurologic development was noticeably better after generalized seizures. The less favorable outcome after partial seizures is probably the result of more extensive brain damage. A severely damaged brain may be unable to

TABLE 13.1. *Outcome of epilepsies starting in the first year of life*

Outcome	Chevrie and Aicardi (1978) (N = 293)	Cavazzuti et al. (1984) (N = 387)	Dalla Bernardina et al. (1982) (N = 319)
Mortality (%)	12	5	7
Neurologic abnormalities (%)	31	19	NA
Severe mental retardation (%)	55	43	NA
No mental retardation (%)	21	35	14
Persistent epilepsy (%)	59	50	72.5
	(at 5 yr)	(5–10 yr)	(≥2 yr)

Abbreviations: N, number of subjects; NA, not available.

TABLE 13.2. *Outcome of epilepsies of the first year in three series of infantile seizures according to type of seizure*

Outcome	Infantile Spasms (%) (N)	Status Epilepticus (%) (N)	Brief Seizures Other Than Infantile Spasms (%) (N)
Mortality			
Chevrie and Aicardi (1978)	8 (230)	22 (51)	14 (156)
Cavazzuti et al. (1984)	8 (183)	3 (66)	0.7 (138)
Dalla Bernardina et al. (1982)	12 (147)	—	3 (290)
Normal neuromental development			
Chevrie and Aicardi (1978)	20 (151)	25 (31)	20 (111)
Cavazzuti et al. (1984)	20 (168)	40 (64)	46 (137)
Dalla Bernardina et al. (1982)	6 (129)	—	20 (285)
Persistent epilepsy			
Chevrie and Aicardi (1978)	52 (151)	79 (31)	61 (111)
Cavazzuti et al. (1984)	34 (168)	74 (64)	70 (137)
Dalla Bernardina et al. (1982)[a]	80 (129)	—	30 (285)

Abbreviations: N, number of subjects; —, no data available.
[a]Followed 2 years or more.

produce relatively well-organized generalized seizures. Indeed, partial seizures were most common in patients with neurodevelopmental retardation antedating the first seizure or with demonstrated brain pathology (symptomatic group), whereas generalized seizures were more common in infants with cryptogenic seizures.

More recent studies (Datta and Wirrell, 2000; Czochauska et al., 1994) have generally confirmed the serious prognosis of early afebrile seizures. The mortality rate of seizures occurring in the first year life varies between 6% and 15% (Datta and Virrell, 2000; Czochauska et al., 1994; Matsumoto et al., 1983a, 1983b; Chevrie and Aicardi, 1978, 1979). In a recent series, 21 of 41 infants with seizures before 1 year of age had developmental delay, and they continued to have seizures at the end of follow-up. Infants with seizures that began when the child was younger than 3 months, those with infantile spasms, those with neurologic abnormalities, and those whose seizures were difficult to control and/or were associated with EEG discharges on the first recording had the worst outcome. The use of more than one antiepileptic agent was also a predictor of uncontrolled epilepsy (Datta and Wirrel, 2000).

The recent realization that some early seizures may have a favorable outcome tends to mitigate the classic severe prognosis of infantile seizures. Watanabe and Okumara (2000) recently suggested that the benign convulsive syndromes may represent up to 50% of all cases but that many are not recognized because they are not seen in tertiary referral centers and thus they are not reported. The relative frequencies of severe and benign cases are currently unknown. All investigators agree that the earlier onset is, the more severe the prognosis. In the prospective study of Ellenberg et al. (1984), in which 296 children who had at least two unprovoked afebrile seizures by the age of 28 days were followed, 27% had an IQ of 70 or less by age 7. The frequency of mental retardation was higher in children who had seizures between 7 and 24 months of age than in the rest of the series. The relatively low frequency of mental deficiency is probably due to the fact that this was a population-based, rather than a hospital-based, study, thus avoiding the selection bias toward the most severe cases. A contrary bias, however, may be operative in population-based studies. As Chapter 21 indicates, the overdiagnosis of various paroxysmal nonepileptic episodes as "epilepsy" is not uncommon, and it is probably more common in infants than in older children because atypical attacks are more common at an early age and because the differential diagnosis is consequently more difficult. Thus, Costeff and Avni (1982) reported that only 3 of 40 children with early afebrile seizures, excluding breath-holding spells, had become epileptic after a follow-up of 14 years. All three cases of epilepsy were observed in patients who had their early afebrile seizures after the age of 13 months, whereas none of those with an onset before 13 months of age developed a chronic seizure disorder. Presumably, the inclusion of such cases in a population-based study is difficult to avoid, particularly because of the large number of examiners involved, and they may falsely increase the proportion of apparently benign cases significantly. Although early onset epilepsies certainly have a less ominous prognosis than that reflected in studies originating from specialized centers, the conclusion that, even with seizures other than infantile spasms, they carry a higher risk of mental retardation and neurologic problems than do the epilepsies of later onset is difficult to avoid.

TREATMENT

The treatment of seizures and epilepsies of early onset, not including infantile spasms, is based mainly on the use of antiepileptic drugs. Most of the anticonvulsants used in older patients can be employed in infants. However, caution is required, especially in those younger than 6 months. This is especially the case with sodium valproate because most cases of severe hepatotoxicity have been reported in children younger than 2 or 3 years (Dreifuss et al., 1987). Dreifuss et al. (1987) reported that fatal hepatotoxicity occurred in as many as 1 in 500 patients younger than 2 years who were treated with these. This figure seems unduly high, and the later studies have seemed more optimistic. Most cases of fatal hepatotoxicity have been in infants with severe epilepsy and mental retardation. Likely, an unknown number of such patients have an underlying metabolic disorder, such as a urea cycle defect or organic aciduria (Coulter, 1991) that may be precipitated by the use of valproate but that is not due to the drug alone. Alpers disease can mimic valproate toxicity, and it may well be responsible for apparent hepatotoxicity (Bicknese et al., 1992).

Valproate has been successfully used, even in high doses, especially in infantile spasms (see Chapter 3), but its use should proceed with great caution and it is not generally advised. Among conventional agents, phenobarbital is still widely used in this age-group. Carbamazepine and the benzodiazepines have a more limited use. Phenytoin is an effective agent, but it is particularly difficult to handle in infants because of its erratic biodisponibility by the oral route and its nonlinear kinetics. Several new antiepileptic agents (e.g., lamotrigine, vigabatrin) can also be effective, but their use in infants is often not licensed and their undesirable side effects may not be fully known.

With all agents, careful monitoring of the treatment is mandatory because rapid changes take place after the neonatal period (Morselli, 1977). After the age of 2 to 4 weeks, the catabolic rate of many drugs is considerably accelerated, with a resulting decline in the previously high levels often obtained in the neonatal period when catabolism is slow (Wasterlain and Vert, 1990). Relatively high levels of the drug are often necessary, and fractionation of the daily dosage into multiple doses may be required. Moreover, side effects can easily go unrecognized in this age group (Dodson, 1987b), and a blood level determination is more useful than in older children.

Pyridoxine should always be given a trial in infantile epilepsy, especially when long-lasting seizures and/or episodes of status epilepticus occur (Goutières and Aicardi, 1985). Large doses (200 mg) of the drug should be given intravenously as early treatment for status before any long-lasting agent is administered. Resuscitation equipment should be available because severe apnea can occur after administration. An oral dose of 40 to 50 mg per day should be tried in refractory epilepsies with brief seizures. *Biotin* also should be given a trial, although biotin deficiency is rarely isolated (Wolf et al., 1983).

The ketogenic diet is relatively easier in infants than in older children. It is the only effective treatment of the uncommon condition of neuroglycopenia, and it can be maintained, with good results on seizures and development, for several years (De Vivo et al., 1991).

Surgical treatment is being increasingly used in infants, and its results may be satisfactory (see Chapters 3 and 25). It has been used in the treatment of both infantile spasms (Shields et al., 1985) and intractable partial epilepsies, which also are collectively termed *catastrophic epilepsies* (Wyllie, 1997; Shewmon et al., 1990). In such cases, the rationale for surgical therapy was not only the control of attacks but also the limitation of the possible effects on neurodevelopment and on cognitive functions (Deonna, 1996; Aicardi, 1994a), even though these have not been conclusively demonstrated. Surgery often necessitates large resections (multilobar or hemispherectomy and/or hemispherotomy). In several recent studies, the results of surgery in children younger than 3 years have not differed significantly from those in older patients (Sugimoto et al., 1999; Duchowny et al., 1998; Wyllie et al., 1996).

The ultimate degree of global impairment that can result from large resections is less than in older patients because of the greater plasticity of the infant brain. Thus, left hemispherectomy does not result in definitive aphasia even when transient disturbances of language are observed.

Several investigators are convinced that surgical control of seizures also results in better cognitive and behavioral development. However, Caplan et al.

(1992) noted that the rate of cognitive improvement following effective surgery for infantile spasms remained suboptimal, even though some improvement in the prognosis was seen in most infants. Anecdotal reports of marked cognitive or behavioral improvement are on record (Arzimanoglou et al., 2000b; Hoffman, 1997; Neville et al., 1997; Arzimanoglou and Aicardi, 1992; Shields et al., 1992a; Erba and Cavazzuti, 1990; Hoffman et al., 1979b). In any case, the control of seizures can considerably improve the quality of life for patients and families.

SUMMARY

Convulsive disorders that occur during the first 2 years of life include those that can be recognized as specific epilepsy syndromes, such as infantile spasms, early cases of LGS, and early cases of myoclonic epilepsies, and a large residuum of unclassifiable cases.

Nonspecific seizures of early infancy are not commonly generalized, and they almost never present as classic tonic-clonic seizures. Partial seizures are more common, but they often have an atypical expression and they may manifest as bilateral motor activity or by autonomic symptoms, so their focal origin often cannot be determined without concomitant EEG recordings.

The prognosis of seizures in early infancy should be guarded, even though the reports from specialized centers tend to give an excessively pessimistic impression. Nonspecific seizures have a less gloomy outlook than that of infantile spasms. The poor outcome is largely due to the frequency and extent of causal brain lesions. Infants with a previously normal development that experience generalized seizures starting after the first 6 months of life have a reasonable chance of a better outcome. Idiopathic epilepsy syndromes largely caused by genetic factors are increasingly being recognized, and these have a more satisfactory course for both seizures and development.

Infants with brief episodes of convulsions, often occurring in clusters without signs of brain damage and with a family history of convulsive disorders, tend to have a short-lived course and an excellent prognosis. The term *epilepsy* may not be entirely appropriate for such cases, but their recognition is obviously important, particularly because their real frequency is not yet accurately known but it may be significant.

The treatment of infantile seizures is often difficult because of the severity of lesional cases and the problems encountered in the handling of antiepileptic drugs. For intractable cases, surgery may be a possible option.

14

Febrile Convulsions

Febrile seizures are the prototype of occasional epileptic seizures (see Chapter 1). That young children have a high susceptibility to convulsions in a setting of acute fever has long been known. This vulnerability to seizures with fever is common, and it appears to cluster in families. The relationship of seizures induced by fever to epilepsy has been hotly debated (Addy, 1986; Hauser, 1981; Millichap, 1968). Undoubtedly, however, the natural history of febrile convulsions (FCs) is quite different from that of the epilepsies, and the population affected by FCs differs considerably from that affected by epilepsy, especially with regard to age and family history.

FCs can be defined as occasional seizures that occur in association with fever but without evidence of intracranial infection or other definable cause. Seizures with fever in children who have suffered a previous nonfebrile seizure are excluded. FCs must be distinguished from epilepsy, which is characterized by recurrent nonfebrile seizures (Consensus Development Panel, 1980).

This definition is rather imprecise. Not all paroxysmal events occurring with fever are FCs. The term applies only to those attacks that are of "epileptic" mechanism. The presence of a typical ictal electroencephalographic (EEG) discharge has been demonstrated in a few cases (Gastaut et al., 1962), and it is thought to be present in all cases of true FC, whereas it is not found in anoxic or syncopal attacks induced by fever (Stephenson, 1983; Gastaut, 1974), which may be difficult to separate clinically from FC.

FCs occur in childhood, and, although the age limits are not clearly defined, an upper limit of 5 years for a first seizure is often accepted. The degree of fever sufficient for a diagnosis of FC is not specified. In addition, the height of fever at the time of a convulsion is often unknown. Likewise, the absence of intracranial infection or of a recognized acute neurologic illness remains an unproved assumption in at least some children. Differentiation of an acute febrile encephalopathy from a severe FC (febrile status epilepticus) may be difficult if no specific signs are present and the cerebrospinal fluid (CSF) analysis is normal (Aicardi and Chevrie, 1970, 1983; Chevrie and Aicardi, 1975).

If all cases of prolonged FCs are considered to be due to some unrecognized causal disease, no case of febrile seizures will have sequelae. On the contrary, if all are regarded as FCs, an artificial increase in the frequency of sequelae due to FCs will result. Pneumonia (Nelson and Ellenberg, 1976), salmonellosis, or shigellosis (Lahat et al., 1990) can produce brain damage without an abnormal CSF analysis, though these are not true febrile seizures. For practical purposes, however, febrile status epilepticus, even if it is followed by permanent neurologic damage, should be included in the FC syndrome, as long as no cause or specific mechanism of brain insult is demonstrable.

Difficulties in precisely defining FCs are likely due to the variable mechanisms of seizures associated with fever, which clearly constitute a heterogeneous group of convulsive disorders. Three subgroups can be recognized. The first and largest subgroup consists of those children who have seizures in response to fever as a result of individual susceptibility, which usually is of genetic basis. In the second subgroup, which probably is small, the seizures are due to a brain insult that has resulted from the febrile illness. The third subgroup includes children with a previous latent epilepsy in whom fever acts merely as a trigger of the seizure. This heterogeneity would explain the different outcomes of some cases. The overwhelming majority of FC cases have an excellent outcome. The rare cases that do not could, however, belong to subsyndromes with a more severe outcome. Recent work has shown that such subsyndromes may feature abnormal prolongation of the FCs beyond the age of 5 or even 10 years or the occurrence of afebrile seizures of different types and severity following the onset of febrile seizures (Wallace et al., 1998; Scheffer and Berkovic, 1997). However, clinical recognition of such subsyndromes is difficult because the clinical features and durations of the seizures are not good predictors of outcome. Future progress in the study of FCs will probably permit reliable diagnostic criteria to be established and will determine more precisely the prognosis.

INCIDENCE OF FEBRILE SEIZURES

FCs are the single most common problem in pediatric neurology. Although the definitions and methods of case ascertainment have varied, that 2% to 5% of all children will experience at least one convulsion with febrile illness before 5 years of age is widely accepted (Fukuyama, 1991; Forsgren et al., 1990b; Annegers et al., 1987; Verity et al., 1985a; Leviton and Cowan, 1982; Lennox-Buchtal, 1973). Higher rates have been reported in some nonoccidental countries, including rates of 7% in Japan and of up to 14% in the Marianna Islands (Tsuboi, 1984, 1986; Mathai et al., 1968). These high rates may be explained by several factors. In developing countries, some common infections of childhood (e.g., measles) may occur earlier, on an average, than in industrialized countries, thus taking place during the period of maximum susceptibility to FCs; the number and/or severity of febrile diseases may therefore be greater.

Living conditions (e.g., the whole family living in a single room) may result in improved case identification. Other unknown factors, whether genetic or environmental, also may play a role. FCs are more common in males (Hauser, 1981; Lennox-Buchtal, 1973; Millichap, 1968), with the sex ratio varying between 1.4 to 1 and 1.2 to 1. This male excess may be the result of an excess of one-sex (male) sibships (Ounsted et al., 1966).

RISK FACTORS FOR FEBRILE CONVULSIONS

The main risk factors for FCs include age, fever, and genetic predisposition. Other factors of lesser importance may be a history of abnormal prenatal and perinatal events that may facilitate the occurrence of FCs or influence their clinical expression and outcome (Forsgren et al., 1991; Wallace, 1976a, 1976b Chevrie and Aicardi, 1975). In one study, heavy smoking during pregnancy was associated with a higher rate of febrile seizures in offspring (Nelson and Ellenberg, 1982, 1990) and was perhaps related to the increased frequency of respiratory illness in young children exposed to passive smoking, but this relationship was not found in another study (Forsgren et al., 1990b).

The *initial development* of the child has a definite impact on the expression and the outcome of febrile seizures. Wallace (1972, 1976b) considered FCs a possible indication of lifelong developmental defects of prenatal or perinatal origin.

The studies of Wallace (1972, 1976b) and those of Nelson and Ellenberg (1982, 1990) have found that previous developmental abnormalities were associated with complex febrile seizures and that these had a less favorable outlook. Nelson and Ellenberg (1981b) found an extraordinarily high incidence of suspect or abnormal development before the occurrence of FCs on at least one examination in the large National Collaborative Perinatal Project (NCPP). In

this study, 22% of their patients had such a history. However, the rate of abnormal development in nonconvulsive children is not stated, although that it was also quite high, possibly on the order of 12%, has been indicated by Nelson and Ellenberg (1976). Thus, the population of children with FCs likely was somewhat biased by the presence of children considered worrisome or abnormal on early examination when compared with a normal population, but the precision of the measurement limits the value of such evaluations.

Fever

Fever responsible for the occurrence of FCs is most often caused by upper respiratory tract infections, otitis media, pneumonia, influenza-like diseases, gastroenteritis, and urinary tract infections. Such infections are the cause of most febrile disorders of childhood. FCs usually supervene during the earliest hours of acute infectious illnesses and, in a vast majority, during the first 24 hours of fever. The term *initial* convulsions reflects this time distribution (Lennox-Buchtal, 1973) and emphasizes the fact that convulsions occurring later in the course of infectious disease, especially in exanthemas, are apt to be the expression of encephalitic complications. The seizure was the initial symptom of the illness recognized by the parents in 25% of the patients studied by Wolf et al. (1977). Further convulsions are uncommon even when temperature remains high. However, the seizures do not always occur at the time of highest fever, and they may even supervene at the time of defervescence (Lennox-Buchtal, 1973; Herlitz, 1941). Likewise, for a child who has had an FC to tolerate a higher fever later without a fit is not unusual (Nelson and Ellenberg, 1978).

The degree of temperature observed with FCs is variable. In one large series, 75% of children had a temperature of 39°C or higher at the time of the fit, and 25% had a temperature higher than 40°C (Herlitz, 1941). Children who convulse with relatively low levels of fever may have a greater risk of repeated seizures, and these should be observed with care (Offringa et al., 1992; Tsuboi et al., 1991; Tsuboi, 1986). The diagnosis of FCs should be regarded as tentative in such patients, especially when they are younger than 10 months of age (Dravet et al., 1982). The rate of increase in fever is deemed important in the causation of FCs by some workers (Millichap, 1968), but no definite evidence of its importance has been found (Michon and Wallace, 1984; Gastaut et al., 1962). Whether the cause of the fever has a role in the occurrence of FCs that is independent of the degree of fever remains debatable. The predominance of viral infections probably reflects their frequency rather than representing a specific factor (Lewis et al., 1979; Stokes et al., 1977). However, long focal convulsions may be more common with demonstrated viral diseases than with those in which no evidence of viral infection is found (Wallace and Zealley, 1970).

Seizures occurring with exanthem subitum (roseola infantum) or with febrile disorders with neutropenia have received special attention. Lennox-Buchtal (1973) thought that such diseases were associated with FCs in 14% to 20% of patients. Data (Nelson and Ellenberg, 1981b) have suggested that the risk of recurrence in cases of roseola infantum is no higher than that with other causes of fever. However, herpesviruses 6 and 7 may be responsible for encephalitic complications, in addition to triggering febrile seizures (Asano et al., 1992, 1994). Rotavirus infections have also been associated with encephalopathic manifestations (Keidan et al., 1992).

Bacterial infections less commonly cause FCs. However, the presence of occult bacteremia (McIntyre et al., 1983) and other bacterial disorders should always be considered. Specific infections have been reported to be associated with a higher than average rate of FCs or with unusually severe FCs. The high rate of seizures with shigellosis (Lahat et al., 1990) and salmonellosis may be related to a toxemic effect (Fischler, 1962). Lahat et al. (1990) found the incidence of febrile seizures with shigellosis to be 19.7%. However, only 2 of their 66 patients followed for an average of 9.7 years had recurrent FCs. This suggests that febrile seizures with shigellosis differ from the usual FCs.

Fever resulting from immunizations can provoke febrile seizures. Children who had fits after immunizations were almost always febrile, and, in one large study (Hirtz et al., 1983), more than half of the children who had seizures after immunization procedures had a personal history of other febrile seizures or a family history of FCs in a sibling or parent. The prognosis of such seizures seems favorable in most cases. Cases with severe convulsive encephalopathies probably result from a mechanism different from that of FCs. Seizures following immunizations are seen mainly with the pertussis (Hirtz et al., 1983; Fenichel, 1982) and measles vaccines. However, immunization against measles can produce FCs in 1.9% of recipients, compared with a rate of 7.7% in wild disease (Landrigan and Witte, 1973).

Age Dependence

FCs are strongly age dependent. In all series, the shape of the distribution curve by age is similar. Few infants have FCs before the age of 5 or 6 months; 80% have had their first seizure by the age of 4 years and 90% by the age of 5 years. The median age varies between 17 and 23 months, depending on gender and type of seizure. Unilateral and severe FCs occur earlier than those that are bilateral and brief (16 months versus 21 months). Occasional first FCs are seen late, with onset after 5 years up to 7 or 8 years of age. Persistence of FCs beyond the age of 5 or 6 years is not very rare (see "Course and Outcome"). Convulsions before 5 or 6 months are much more common with infections of the central nervous system (CNS) than they are with FCs. Purulent meningitis should be strongly suspected in this age group.

Genetic Factors

FCs occur with increased frequency among the family members of patients with FCs (Hauser and Anderson, 1986; Hauser et al., 1985; Annegers et al., 1982a, 1982b; Fukuyama et al., 1979; Tsuboi, 1977a; Van den Berg, 1974; Schiottz-Christensen, 1972). The estimates of this frequency vary. Annegers et al. (1976) found a level of risk to siblings that was two to three times higher than that expected in the local population. Tsuboi (1977a) found an incidence of FCs of 17% for parents and 22% for siblings of FC probands. Aicardi and Chevrie (1976) found an incidence of 31% in first-degree relatives. Verity et al. (1985a) reported a 26% incidence of a positive family history. The low figure of 7.3% of first-degree relatives found in the series by Nelson and Ellenberg (1978) may be explained by the difficulties inherent in a large-scale population study. Familial clustering of FCs suggests that genetic factors play an etiologic role. The frequent transmission from parent to offspring and the risk to siblings of less than 25% in most studies tend to rule out a recessive mode of inheritance. Most studies suggest a dominant mode of inheritance with reduced penetrance and variable expression (Degen et al., 1991; Fukuyama et al., 1979; Lennox-Buchtal, 1973; Frantzen et al., 1970) or a polygenic mode; the latter is currently preferred (Hauser and Anderson, 1986).

Anderson et al. (1990) and Rich et al. (1987) have proposed that a different mode of inheritance may apply to cases in which the proband has had three or more FCs. In such cases, dominant transmission seems likely, whereas a multifactorial model better fits the observed rates in patients who have had fewer than three seizures. Doose et al. (1983), Doose and Baier (1987), and Gundel and Doose (1986) have suggested that the risk of a child having FCs and/or another form of epilepsy is associated with the presence of one or several EEG characteristics that are inherited independently. The EEGs of children with FCs commonly show a monomorphous parietal theta rhythm in the awake state. In this concept, each inherited EEG characteristic could depend on a single gene, and the various combinations could account for the diverse types of genetic epilepsy of polygenic inheritance.

Several different loci on chromosome 8q (*FEB1*); 2q23–24 (*FEB2*); 19p (*FEB2*); and 5q14–15 (*FEB4*) have been mapped in multiple families with dominant inheritance of FCs. A possible third gene on chromosome 2q23-24 has been reported by Peiffer et al. (1999). However, this gene could be one of the genes for the syndrome of generalized epilepsy with febrile seizures plus (GEFS+), a syndrome that is related to but probably distinct from classic FCs (Scheffer and Berkovic, 1997), as discussed below (also see Chapter 20).

The more frequent involvement in boys may also be considered a genetic factor. However, it could also be due to the increased susceptibility of boys to febrile illnesses rather than being specifically due to FCs (Berg et al. 1995).

The empirical risk for a further offspring in a family with one affected child is approximately 10%. This risk is higher if one of the parents has had FCs, and it rises to almost 50% if one parent and one offspring have had febrile seizures. Some studies have reported a higher than expected rate of nonfebrile seizures among relatives of FC probands (Verity et al., 1985a; Van den Berg, 1974), whereas others have found no increased rate over the expectancy in the general population (Annegers et al., 1982a, 1982b; Frantzen et al., 1970).

CLINICAL MANIFESTATIONS OF FEBRILE SEIZURES

All febrile seizures are either tonic-clonic or possibly hypotonic (Gastaut et al., 1962). They never manifest as myoclonic seizures, spasms, or nonconvulsive attacks. The great majority are bilateral clonic or tonic-clonic attacks of short duration (less than 15 minutes). These are termed *simple FCs*. These seizures are followed by very brief postictal manifestations but no others; their virtual absence is of great diagnostic significance. *Complex febrile seizures* are those of long duration (15 minutes or more), those with focal features (most commonly unilateral), or those that recur two or more times within a single illness episode. Up to one-third of febrile seizures may have one or more of these complex features. Seizures

of long duration were noted in 18% of the children in the Gentofte series (Frantzen et al., 1968), in 16% in an old series by Herlitz (1941), and in 35% in studies by Wallace (1974, 1976a, 1988). In the large population study of Nelson and Ellenberg (1978), 4.3% of the FC attacks lasted longer than 30 minutes and 7.6% longer than 15 minutes; 4% had a focal onset. Some of the unilateral seizures may be followed by a Todd hemiplegia that usually lasts a few hours but that may persist for up to several days. The incidence of Todd hemiplegia is probably in the range of 0.4% of all cases of FC (Nelson and Ellenberg, 1978). Seizures lasting 30 minutes or more qualify as status epilepticus. Rarely, they can constitute the initial stage of the hemiconvulsion–hemiplegia syndrome or acquired postconvulsive hemiplegia (see Chapter 10). However, the outcome is favorable in most cases of febrile status (Shinnar et al., 1992; Maytal and Shinnar, 1990). Such patients need emergency treatment. Most long-lasting convulsions (approximately 75%) are the initial seizure (Nelson and Ellenberg, 1978; Aicardi and Chevrie, 1970, 1975), an important finding that indicates the impossibility of prevention.

The occurrence of more than one seizure in 24 hours during the same febrile episode is not uncommon; it amounted to 16% of the cases in the Collaborative Childhood Perinatal Project series (Nelson and Ellenberg, 1976). Repeated seizures are also seen in the initial attacks in 6% of cases. They are usually brief convulsions, and they generally occur within 2 to 4 hours after the onset of fever.

Complex seizures more commonly occur in children with previously abnormal development or neurologic findings than do simple seizures. Aicardi and Chevrie (1983) showed that children with unilateral FCs, most of which were also of long duration, had a lower incidence of a positive family history of FCs than did those with brief bilateral seizures (18% versus 35%) and a higher incidence of abnormal and perinatal antecedents, thus suggesting the possible role of acquired, possibly lesional factors in their determination. Their prognosis, however, is favorable, although they may carry a slightly increased risk of febrile recurrences (Offringa et al., 1994).

ELECTROENCEPHALOGRAPHIC FINDINGS WITH FEBRILE CONVULSIONS

Paroxysmal EEG abnormalities were found in 35% to 45% of patients for whom serial EEGs were obtained before the age of 5 years (Doose et al., 1983; Lennox-Buchtal, 1973). Sofijanov et al. (1992) found that the initial EEG of 676 children with FCs contained paroxysmal abnormalities in 22%. In all series, spike-waves at 3 Hz or more were most common, with focal spikes being second in frequency (about 10% of cases) (Lennox-Buchtal, 1973).

Generalized spike-waves should be distinguished from the so-called *hypnagogic bursts* that are a normal finding in children in the age bracket of FCs and that therefore are often found in these patients (Alvarez et al., 1983). The presence of paroxysmal EEG abnormalities is correlated with age. Paroxysmal anomalies are rare before the age of 1 year, but they are found in 51% of patients who had an initial EEG recording after 4 years of age (Sofijanov et al., 1992). Paroxysms are also significantly more common in children who had complex febrile seizures lasting more than 15 minutes, but they are related neither to the birthweight, gender, the nature of the febrile illness, the family history of convulsions, or epilepsy nor to the occurrence of multiple seizures in the same 24-hour episode. The number of previous febrile seizures is strongly related to the occurrence of EEG anomalies. These were found in 18% of children who had a single seizure and in 63% of those who had four or more seizures (Sofijanov et al., 1992). In the same study, EEG paroxysms were also more common in children with abnormal neurologic signs antecedent to the convulsions and with focal seizures, but the association was not as close as that of age and number of previous convulsions.

Most prospective studies have found no correlation between the presence of EEG paroxysms and the later emergence of nonfebrile seizures (Lennox-Buchtal, 1973; Frantzen et al., 1968). Millichap and Colliver (1991) did, however, find the incidence of paroxysmal EEG abnormalities to be five times greater in children who developed epilepsy than in those who did not. Even so, the EEG is of little, if any, practical value for the prediction of recurrences or epilepsy in the individual patient; paroxysms are found in a high proportion of the older patients who are least likely to develop severe or recurrent seizures of epilepsy, whereas they never appear on the EEGs of the young infants who are at maximum risk for recurrences, status epilepticus, and epilepsy. Biparietal theta rhythms were present during wakefulness in 54% of their patients, spike-wave activity in the resting record in 49%, and photosensitivity in 42%. The last two patterns were strongly age dependent.

DIAGNOSIS

The diagnosis of FCs is not always easy. Clearly, seizures associated with CNS infections, a topic dis-

cussed later in this chapter (see "Investigations in Children with Febrile Convulsions"), must not be diagnosed as FCs. Convulsions associated with fever may also be observed with toxic exposure, septic embolization, hemolytic-uremic syndrome, and other acute encephalopathies (Nelson and Ellenberg, 1983). Biotinidase deficiency may be responsible for both seizures and repeated infections (Aicardi, 1992a), and this condition is important to recognize because it is lethal condition if left untreated. Malaria and other parasitic diseases are important in many parts of the world, and these require specific therapy (Newton and Warrell, 1998). Severe FCs may raise the problem of the acute encephalopathies of obscure origin. Lyon et al. (1961) has suggested that some of the cases of acute encephalopathy in childhood are nothing more than severe and complicated cases of FCs. Whether such cases should be separated from FCs remains uncertain, as discussed in the introduction to this chapter.

Gastaut (1974) and Stephenson (1983, 1976, 1990) emphasized the fact that seizures occurring with fever were not necessarily of an epileptic nature. Syncopes, or reflex anoxic seizures, also can be triggered by fever, and the distinction between anoxic and epileptic seizures may be difficult (see Chapter 21). Stephenson (1976) divided 100 children who had fits with fever into the following three subgroups on the basis of the clinical description of attacks; 14 children were considered without doubt to have anoxic seizures, 35 had epileptic seizures, and the remaining 51 children could not be definitely classified. An exaggerated oculocardiac reflex was rare in the epileptic group, it was extremely common in the anoxic group, and it occurred with intermediate frequency in the undetermined group. However, an excessive oculocardiac reflex may be found in a child with authentic epileptic seizures, and the findings of Stephenson (1976) are difficult to interpret, even though they certainly suggest that febrile anoxic seizures may be common.

Other nonepileptic acute phenomena induced by fever include febrile delirium that, at times, is associated with marked agitation that can superficially resemble a seizure. Febrile shivering can be intense enough in some infants to be mistaken for FC. The confusion is favored by the autonomic phenomena associated with shivering, such as intense pallor and peribuccal cyanosis, which are often mistaken for autonomic seizure manifestations.

Severe myoclonic epilepsy (Dravet et al., 1992a) or polymorphic epilepsy of infants (Dravet syndrome) (Aicardi, 1991a) begins with febrile seizures that later evolve into a distinctive epileptic syndrome (see

Chapter 5). At onset, it cannot be differentiated from febrile seizures. However, the diagnosis can be suspected early when the evolution is characteristic. The best predictors of this syndrome include the long duration and often a localized (and alternating) character of the seizures and the recurrence of the attacks (usually multiple) within 2 months of the initial seizure (Dalla Bernardina et al, 1983a; Aicardi, 1991a). This syndrome has its onset between 4 and 10 months of age in most patients. Therefore, its occurrence has often coincided with the diphtheria-pertussis-tetanus (DPT) vaccine, to which it has been attributed by some (Menkes and Kinsbourne, 1990). A coincidental association is highly likely in such cases.

COURSE AND OUTCOME OF FEBRILE CONVULSIONS

The outcome of FCs has long been a subject of controversy. The reported frequency of residua has varied from 0% to 100% (Hauser, 1981). Such discrepancies were doubtless the result of different definitions of FCs, case selection, and the type and duration of follow-up. The dates and places of the studies are also possible influences on the incidence of residua. Evidence has indicated that severe sequelae, such as postconvulsive hemiplegias, have become much rarer in France over the past 15 years (Roger et al., 1982).

The consensus now is that FCs are benign events with an excellent prognosis (Roulet et al., 1991; Consensus Development Panel, 1980) and that residua, if any, are the result of the febrile disorder responsible for the convulsions or of previous abnormalities of development rather than being the consequences of the convulsions themselves. This conclusion has been reached as a result of prospective studies of cohorts of unselected children with FCs (Annegers et al., 1987; Nelson and Ellenberg, 1978), which demonstrated the rarity of unfavorable outcome with respect to both the later development of epilepsy and the intellectual and neurologic development.

However, the occurrence of apparent sequelae in children with febrile seizures has been repeatedly reported in retrospective studies (Aicardi and Chevrie, 1976; Ounsted et al., 1966), and the relationship of FCs to hippocampal sclerosis has been hotly discussed (Van Lierde and Mira, 2001; Holthausen, 1994). Clearly, retrospective studies cannot give any information on the frequency of such unfavorable outcomes, but they do prove their existence. However, the succession of events does not imply that they are causally related. On the other hand, prospective stud-

ies also have limitations, and their capacity to detect rare events (e.g., those occurring at a frequency of 1% or 2%) is limited because a large number of participants is required, usually in multicentric studies with their attendant problems. In addition, the incidence of sequelae may be underestimated if cases of severe febrile seizures followed by neurologic signs are regarded as being due to the causal disease because of their very existence. Moreover, epileptologists working with adult patients still identify cases of mesial temporal sclerosis that were due to prolonged febrile seizures in infancy (Wieser et al., 1993), thus raising the possibility of subtle sequelae that have a very late emergence.

Recurrence of Febrile Seizures

Recurrence of febrile seizures is by far the larger risk associated with FCs. Approximately 30% to 37% of patients with FCs experience at least one recurrence (Berg et al., 1990; Nelson and Ellenberg, 1978; Wallace, 1974; Frantzen et al., 1968). Annegers et al. (1990) found a recurrence rate of 25% in a cohort of 639 children that was prospectively followed. Half of the children who have one recurrence experience a further attack (Hauser, 1981). In most other cases, the number of recurrences is limited to two or three. Only 9% to 17% of patients experience more than three recurrences. Half of the recurrences take place within 6 months of the initial episode, and roughly three-fourths of all recurrences occur within 1 year (Nelson and Ellenberg, 1981b). Recurrences are more common when the first seizure occurs early. Infants who had their first FC before the age of 1 year have a 50% risk of recurrence, whereas the risk is only 28% for children whose first seizure occurs after the age of 1 year (Nelson and Ellenberg, 1981b). Multiple recurrences are also three times more common among younger babies. However, Offringa et al. (1994) found that the important factor was the age attained at the first recurrence, rather than age at the time of the first seizure. They found that the recurrence risk was highest for infants in the first year of life (48%) and lowest for those who were 4 years of age (15%).

Children whose seizures occur at a relatively low grade of fever (lower than 40°C and especially 39°C) are more likely to experience recurrences, which is consistent with the hypothesis of a threshold temperature for FCs.

A family history of febrile seizures in first-degree relatives seems to be associated with an increased recurrence rate that may be twice the usual figure (MacDonald et al., 1999; Offringa et al., 1992; Annegers et al., 1980). A family history of epilepsy does not seem to predict recurrent febrile seizures.

Complex FCs and the presence of neurodevelopmental abnormalities before the seizures may be associated with more frequent recurrences, although this effect is inconsistent and small.

The association of several factors (child younger than 1 year or 18 months, complex seizure, and a positive family history of FCs) seems to increase the recurrence rate from 15% in those with no risk factor to 30% when only one risk factor is present, to 40% in those with two risk factors, and up to 65% when all three factors are found (Al Eissa, 1995; Berg et al., 1992; Offringa et al., 1992; Annegers et al., 1980).

The risk of a severe febrile recurrence is relatively low. Most long-lasting seizures are the first episode (Chevrie and Aicardi, 1975). Nelson and Ellenberg (1978) found that a prolonged or another form of "complex" seizure followed an initial uncomplicated FC in 8% of children. In only 1.4% of their patients did the convulsion last longer than 30 minutes, in 0.7%, an hour or longer, and, by the age of 7 years, none of the children had experienced an afebrile seizure. Prolonged and/or unilateral seizures at the time of a febrile recurrence may also be related to the presence of a history of FCs and perinatal abnormalities in female children (Wallace, 1974).

Although the risk of recurrence is higher for patients with prolonged febrile seizures (Wilkins and Lindsay, 1985), the risk of recurrence of febrile status epilepticus is low when the initial development of the children has been normal. In addition, patients with previous neurologic abnormalities accounted for 88% of recurrences in 95 children with febrile status studied by Shinnar et al. (1992).

In summary, the results of recent prospective studies on the outcome of FCs are reassuring.

Mortality

Mortality from FCs is almost nonexistent. Only one death occurred in a quadriplegic retarded patient in the prospective study of Frantzen et al. (1968). In the NCPP study (Nelson and Ellenberg, 1976), no death was directly attributable to FCs among the 1,821 patients with FCs. Likewise, the mortality in 660 patients studied by Annegers et al. (1987) did not exceed the expected figures. Even status epilepticus now has a low mortality when it occurs in previously well infants (Maytal and Shinnar, 1990). The poor outcome of some patients of Viani et al. (1987) was probably due to the inclusion of symptomatic cases.

Mental and Neurologic Development

The mental and neurologic development of patients with FCs remains normal in most patients who have developed normally before the onset of FCs.

Wallace and Cull (1979) noted no apparent reduction of intelligence quotient (IQ) score in patients hospitalized for febrile seizure. Ross and Peckham (1983) found that academic achievement was unaffected by the occurrence of FCs. Two large studies have shown that FCs are not associated with significant intellectual deficits. Ellenberg et al. (1978) examined 431 children with febrile seizures who, during the course of the follow-up period, had not developed unprovoked seizures and for whom a sibling control was available. No difference in full-scale IQ scores was observed at 7 years of age between the index cases and their siblings in those children who were known to be neurologically normal before their initial FC. However, only full-scale IQ was examined, and no analysis of specific cognitive functions or educational and behavioral outcomes was performed. Verity et al. (1985b) compared 381 children who were developing normally before their first seizure with the rest of the population-based cohort with respect to 102 measures of intelligence, behavior, and academic performance. They found significant differences for only four tests, a finding consistent with chance occurrence. Schiottz-Christensen (1973) found subtle differences between 47 children with FC and their twin controls, but the significance of this finding is uncertain. Chang et al. (2001), however, found evidence of slightly better working memory function in children with antecedent febrile seizures than in the population-based controls.

Of interest is that children who developed afebrile seizures following FCs had a fivefold increase in the frequency of mental retardation, as defined as an IQ of less than 70 at the age of 7 years, regardless of whether their development before their FCs had been judged normal. Two-thirds of patients with later afebrile seizures came from the group of FC children with a low risk for later epilepsy (see "Nonfebrile Seizures Following Febrile Convulsions"). Thus, mental retardation cannot be easily predicted at the time of FCs, even though, in the FCs group as a whole, the subgroup of children who were not neurologically or developmentally normal before any seizure did score lower than their normal siblings. This result can be interpreted in various manners, such as positing the existence of lesions before the FCs. However, excluding the possibility that multiple sequelae tend to occur together and that both cognitive difficulties and epilepsy might be the result of FCs is not possible.

The relationship, if any, between the severity of febrile seizures and the occurrence of mental retardation is unclear. Nelson and Ellenberg (1978), Verity et al. (1985b), and Wallace (1991) found no correlation between intellectual dysfunction and the type and duration of FCs. This is in contradistinction to several studies that indicated an association among long and complicated attacks, mental retardation, and neurologic sequelae (Tsuboi and Endo, 1977). The effect on mental development of repeated FCs has been variably assessed. Ellenberg and Nelson (1978) and Verity et al. (1985b) found no difference in IQ scores between patients with single febrile seizures and those in whom they were recurrent. Smith and Wallace (1982) found a significant decrease in IQ in children with repeated febrile seizures. This lowering of IQ was greater in those children with three or more seizures than in those with two FCs. The treatment was not responsible for the decreasing IQ score. Thus, to say that FCs have no great effect on neurologic and mental development, except in uncommon cases, and that the best predictor of cognitive and behavioral difficulties is the status of the child before seizures is fair.

Hauser (1981) stated that no new permanent neurologic signs were reported in prospective studies. Such signs have, however, been well documented in several retrospective studies (Lindsay et al., 1984; Aicardi and Chevrie, 1976; Wallace, 1976b; Ounsted et al., 1966) and in a prospective study (Wallace, 1982). The sequelae most commonly reported are hemiplegias and, less often, more devastating residua such as diplegia, choreoathetosis, or decorticate rigidity. Obviously, retrospective studies cannot give a valid indication of the frequency of sequelae. However, such neurologic accidents do occur in the rare patient, and they are severe enough to merit consideration despite their rarity. Whether they are a consequence of seizures or of the causal disease has not been established.

Nonfebrile Seizures following Febrile Convulsions

Nonfebrile seizures following FCs occur in 2% to 7% of patients (Wallace, 1988; Annegers et al., 1987; Ross and Peckham, 1983; Nelson and Ellenberg, 1976; Frantzen et al., 1968), a rate that is two to ten times higher than that expected in the general population. The much higher incidence rates in some series result from case selection (Aicardi and Chevrie, 1976) or different definitions of FCs (Tsuboi et al., 1991). In population studies, a tendency to recurring unprovoked seizures follows febrile seizures in 2%

before the age of 5 to 7 years (Annegers et al., 1987; Nelson and Ellenberg, 1976), in 4.5% by the age of 10 years (Annegers et al., 1987), in 5.5% by the age of 11 to 15 years (Ross et al., 1980), and in 7% by 25 years of age (Annegers et al, 1987). Thus, they have lasting effects up to the third decade of life.

Nonfebrile seizures occur with an increased frequency in patients with developmental abnormalities antedating the first FC, in those with a first-degree relative with epilepsy, and in those with complex (or complicated) FCs. Verity and Golding (1991) found that 9.4% of children with complex febrile seizures developed epilepsy, compared with 2.3% of their whole series of 398 patients.

In the NCPP study (Nelson and Ellenberg, 1976), children with none of these risk factors had a 0.9% risk of developing afebrile seizures; in those with the three risk factors, epilepsy developed in 9.2%. Sixty percent of the patients with FCs had no risk factor. Despite the low risk for epilepsy in children with one or none risk factor, approximately three-fourths of the cases of epilepsy followed FCs occurring in this group, by the mere fact of the large number of low-risk cases, thus pointing out the limitations of predictive ability. Annegers et al. (1987) found a range for the development of later epilepsy to be 2.4% in children with no risk factor, 6% to 8% in those with a single complex feature (e.g., focal or prolonged seizures or repeated episodes of febrile convulsions within the same illness), and 49% in those with all three features. Most unprovoked seizures following FCs are brief generalized tonic-clonic seizures (Aicardi and Chevrie, 1976). Some children (Scheffer and Berkovic, 1997; Aicardi, 1994) experience only one or a few afebrile seizures with relatively rapid remission. The NCPP study included 18 such cases in which afebrile seizures remitted before the age of 48 months, compared with 52 cases of epilepsy (i.e., patients with afebrile seizures after the age of 4 years). Verity and Golding (1991) found that 2.7% of their 398 patients had recurrent nonfebrile seizures following FCs but that 3.4% developed nonfebrile seizures, so these were probably nonrecurrent in 0.7% of their cases. The distinction between such early remitting seizures and epilepsy may be somewhat fragile.

Generalized epilepsies following FCs are commonly benign, and they often remit after only a few seizures (see Chapter 9). The inclusion of early remitting afebrile seizures with the epilepsies does not substantially modify the prognosis of FCs, with the incidence of afebrile seizures remaining below 3% to 5%.

The risk of nonfebrile seizures after FCs is highest in the months soon after the first seizure (Nelson and

Ellenberg, 1978). However, in the Rochester study (Annegers et al., 1987), some increase in the risk of nonfebrile seizures was seen until middle life. This risk remained small (2.4% at 25 years of age) for persons who had simple seizures, but it was substantially higher for the small group with several risk factors. The types of afebrile seizures following FCs were not different for those in epilepsies not preceded by FCs in the NCPP study (Melchior, 1977), and their distribution was similar. The problem of lesional, especially temporal lobe, seizures and their relation to epilepsy is discussed later in this section.

The risk of epilepsy was found to increase with the number of febrile seizure recurrences in some (Annegers et al., 1987), but not all (Berg et al., 1996), studies. The magnitude of the increased risk is probably limited, and it may not apply to all subgroups of FCs.

A short interval between the onset of fever and the febrile seizure may also be associated with an increased risk of epilepsy (Berg et al., 1996).

The *relationship of FCs to later partial epilepsy*, especially that of the temporal lobe, has been a subject of controversy for decades (Lado et al., 2002; Holthausen, 1994). This issue has been approached from both the clinical point of view, as well as from that of the pathology often found in cases of temporal lobe seizures, the so-called *mesial temporal sclerosis* or *hippocampal sclerosis* (see also Chapter 19).

Falconer et al. (1964) found a history of early childhood convulsions, usually with fever, in 30% to 40% of patients in whom mesial temporal sclerosis was found at surgery in their two series of "temporal lobe epilepsy." This experience has since been replicated in several studies of surgical patients (Abou Khalil et al., 1993; Cendes et al., 1993a, 1993b, 1993c; Duncan and Sagar, 1987) in whom a history of FCs was recorded in about 30% to 50% of cases. Although some studies did not find an unusual number of cases of lesional partial epilepsy following complex FCs (Nelson and Ellenberg, 1976), others (Annegers et al., 1979, 1987) found that complex features of FCs strongly correlated with the development of partial but not generalized seizures. The same lesion was assumed to be the cause of the temporal epilepsy in the series of patients diagnosed clinically with temporal lobe epilepsy without pathologic confirmation who also had a history of severe febrile seizures (Wallace, 1976b; Roger et al., 1974; Ounsted et al., 1966; Gastaut et al., 1960). A long duration of the seizures was considered the most important factor (Maher and McLachlan, 1995). More recently, magnetic resonance imaging (MRI) studies have shown frequent evidence of hippocampal atrophy and sclerosis in patients with intractable temporal lobe epilepsy and a history of prolonged febrile seizures (Harvey et al., 1995; Abou-Khalil et al., 1993; Grattan-Smith et al., 1993; Kuks et al., 1993).

Although retrospective studies suggest a connection between febrile seizures and temporal lobe epilepsy, prospective population-based studies of FCs, even when they are prolonged in status epilepticus, have failed to find this association (Berg and Shinnar, 1997; Shinnar and Babb, 1997; Annegers et al., 1987; Lee et al., 1981). This discrepancy may be explained by the rarity of mesial temporal sclerosis and temporal epilepsy following FCs because such rare events are quite difficult to detect by prospective studies. Other factors may also be contributory, such as the late occurrence of temporal lobe epilepsy at an adult age that is beyond the age limits of the current prospective series.

Therefore, concluding that the sequence of febrile seizures followed by partial seizures, especially the temporal lobe seizure, is a real occurrence is fair. Its frequency is low, but the FCs may be of some significance in the etiology of temporal epilepsy. Clearly, this temporal sequence does not need to be regarded as causal, and three hypotheses can be envisioned. The first is that FCs cause mesial temporal sclerosis, which, in turn, is responsible for temporal lobe epilepsy. The second is that FCs and temporal epilepsy are both a consequence of a previous abnormality that may facilitate the prolongation and focalization of the FCs and that may then be responsible for the epilepsy. The third hypothesis is that no relationship exists between FCs and focal epilepsy, which appears less likely in view of the evidence from retrospective studies, even though these cannot give a true idea of the frequency of the event.

The hypothesis that prolonged FCs are the cause of mesial temporal sclerosis is mainly based on data from surgical series of patients who have undergone operation for intractable temporal lobe seizures, therefore representing a highly selected group of patients (Falconer, 1976; Falconer et al., 1964; Falconer and Cavanagh, 1959; Cavanagh and Meyer, 1956), and on the history of antecedents of FCs in patients with severe temporal epilepsy, which is also a selected group. Thus, if about one-third of the patients in pediatric series have such antecedents, this may not apply to all children with complex partial seizures because the figure is drawn from series from referral centers, which likely represent the most severe part of the spectrum. Moreover, the condition of the hippocampus before the FCs is unknown (Shinnar, 1998).

The hypothesis that a previous abnormality of the temporal lobe is the origin of the FCs or, at least, of their long duration and focalization may be supported by the frequent history of abnormal development in children with FCs, who often develop mental retardation or epilepsy (Nelson and Ellenberg, 1976). It has also received some support from the finding of minor malformations of the hippocampus in familial cases of FC followed by temporal epilepsy (Fernandez et al., 1998; Sloviter and Pedley, 1998).

Similar lesions have been experimentally associated with a greater susceptibility to FCs. Duplication of the granule layer of the dentate gyrus is found fairly frequently in temporal lobectomy specimens from patients with temporal lobe epilepsy and a history of FC. Whether this is a congenital or an acquired lesion is uncertain (Lado et al., 2002).

The role of malformations in the etiology of temporal lobe seizures following FCs may be considered either as explaining the whole sequence of the febrile seizures that are followed by unprovoked seizures or as a factor determining the localization and severity of FCs. The latter would then constitute a second insult in the full picture of hippocampal sclerosis.

The development of MRI, which clearly shows the hippocampus and its abnormalities, has enabled some progress in the controversy about the role of FCs. Van Landingham et al. (1998) obtained MRI scans in 27 infants shortly after their febrile seizure. In two children, bilateral hippocampal atrophy was found, indicating old damage that probably was of perinatal origin. In four children with long FCs, changes suggestive of acute edema with swelling and increased T2 signal intensity in the hippocampus in the hemisphere of seizure origin were present. In two of them, a subsequent MRI demonstrated acquired hippocampal atrophy. A similar sequence of events has also been shown to occur in cases of status epilepticus of other origins (see Chapter 16). Therefore, acquired atrophy of an apparently normal hippocampus can occur during or proximal to an acute febrile convulsive episode. The frequency and factors associated with these MRI changes must be studied in further cases.

Epilepsy Syndromes Related to Febrile Convulsions

Some specific epilepsy syndromes appear to have a relationship with febrile seizures (Wallace, 1991). *Absence epilepsy* (see Chapter 8) occurs in 15% to 25% of children who have a personal history of FCs (Hashimoto et al., 1989). A history of febrile seizures can also commonly be obtained from relatives.

Benign rolandic epilepsy, or benign epilepsy with centrotemporal spikes, is clearly linked to FCs, even though no case was reported in the NCPP study (Nelson and Ellenberg, 1976). The incidence of FC in patients with benign rolandic epilepsy in several series (Lerman and Kivity, 1975, 1986; Lüders et al., 1987b) ranged from 9% to 20%, which clearly is in excess of its incidence in the general population. Kajitani et al. (1981) found that focal epileptiform discharges were present in a subgroup of patients with febrile discharges and that both febrile seizures and benign partial epilepsy could occur together in both members of twin pairs (Kajitani et al., 1980), suggesting common genetic factors at the origin of these syndromes.

Other syndromes, including Lennox-Gastaut syndrome, benign myoclonic epilepsy, and myoclonic absences, have been observed to follow FCs, but the frequency of such an occurrence is poorly known (Wallace, 1991). Juvenile myoclonic epilepsy has been found to be often preceded by FCs in some studies (Wallace, 1991), but the large study of Janz (1991) concluded that a relationship between the two conditions is lacking.

Other possible mechanisms can also account for the sequential occurrence of FCs and unprovoked epileptic seizures, and a number of epilepsy syndromes that may begin with a febrile seizure may be impossible to distinguish from the FC syndrome initially. Scheffer and Berkovic (1997) reported a large multigenerational family with febrile seizures and generalized epilepsy, in which 25 individuals were affected over four generations in one branch of their pedigree. The most common phenotype was "febrile seizures plus" denoting FCs, usually with multiple recurrences, that continued after the age of 6 years and that were often associated with nonfebrile generalized seizures. Six family members had absences, myoclonic seizures, or atonic seizures, in addition to febrile seizures. The authors proposed that the affected family members carried a dominant gene with variable phenotypic expression, and they coined the term **GEFS+** to describe their cases. A gene for GEFS1 was mapped to chromosome 19q, and a mutation in the *SCN1B*, which encodes the β_1 subunit of a voltage-gated channel, was demonstrated (Wallace et al., 1998). Subsequently, other cases were reported (Singh et al., 1999a), and a second mutation in *SCN1A*, which encodes the α_1 subunit of the same sodium channel, was found in patients with a similar picture, which was termed GEFS2 (Escayg et al., 2000; Lopes-Cendes et al., 2000; Baulac et al., 1999; Moulard et al., 1999).

Recently, a mutation in a α-aminobutyric acid receptor gene (*GABRG2*) was found in one family. In addition to febrile seizures, some patients had multiple seizure types and resistant epilepsies. The proportion of children initially presenting with FCs that are then proved to belong to the GEFS+ spectrum is currently unknown, although some believe this may be common (Singh et al., 1999a). Recent work has suggested that severe myoclonic epilepsy (Dravet syndrome), which usually presents initially with long-lasting febrile seizures, may be related to the GEFS+ spectrum, of which it could represent the most severe form (Singh et al., 1999b, 2001). Families in which both severe myoclonic epilepsy and GEFS+ presented in different individuals have been reported (Veggiotti et al., 2001). Claes et al. (2001) found mutations (usually truncating ones) in seven children with polymorphic epilepsy who did not have any family history of FC. Now, the sodium channel mutation does not appear to be present in all such patients, and further work on this problem is warranted.

MANAGEMENT OF FEBRILE SEIZURES

Investigations in Children with Febrile Convulsions

The most important investigation in the acute stage is an examination of the CSF, and some authors advised it in all infants with a first febrile seizure (Ouelette, 1974). Most physicians perform a lumbar puncture only in selected cases, especially for patients who do not show rapid improvement and obviously for those with clinical signs of meningitis. Meningitis, however, may evolve without specific signs, and it may present as simple FCs, especially in young infants. Therefore, a lumbar puncture is imperative for infants younger than 6 months (Heijbel et al., 1980), and it is recommended in those younger than 18 months (Rutter et al., 1970). Even when a first lumbar puncture is negative, remaining vigilant is necessary because clear CSF at the first lumbar puncture does not exclude the possibility of later bacterial infection (Wallace, 1985; Rutter et al., 1970).

Routine blood sugar, calcium, and electrolyte determinations are costly and generally unhelpful (Millichap and Colliver, 1991; Nealis, 1981; Millichap, 1968), and plain skull radiographs are of no value (Millichap and Colliver, 1991; Heijbel et al., 1980; Hayes and Shopfner, 1973). Neuroimaging is not indicated unless neurologic abnormalities are present, and it is not urgent. An EEG is generally not indicated because it has little prognostic value, and it cannot be used as a means of selecting candidates for prophylactic therapy. Blood counts and other investigations, especially appropriate cultures, that are designed to elucidate the etiology of fever are indicated depending on the clinical situation.

Acute Treatment

The acute treatment of FCs is limited to elementary supportive measures in the most common case of brief seizures. If a convulsion is observed, the child should be placed in the semiprone lateral position to limit the danger of aspiration, and an adequate airway should be maintained. Prolonged FCs must be treated vigorously as this is the best way to avoid the preventable sequelae that can result from prolonged seizure activity. In practice, treatment should be started when the seizure lasts 5 to 10 minutes or more. Diazepam, the drug of first choice, should be administered by the intravenous or the intrarectal route (Milligan et al., 1982, 1984; Franzoni et al., 1983; Deonna et al., 1982) but not as suppositories (Knudsen, 1977). Alternative treatments can include lorazepam, clonazepam, or midazolam (see Chapter 24). The intracranial or sublingual routes of administration are probably satisfactory with these drugs. Prompt treatment is probably of more importance than the exact modalities of therapy, and sending the child to the hospital over a long distance, instead of starting emergency treatment, is inexcusable (O'Donohoe, 1985; Hoppu and Santavuori, 1981).

The importance of lowering body temperature has also been stressed (Bacon et al., 1979; Ouelette, 1974), but few data are available. Overheating of the child should absolutely be avoided, and blankets should be removed immediately. Reduction of temperature by sponging or tepid baths is usually advised (O'Donohoe, 1985), although no data regarding its effectiveness for stopping a fit or preventing rapid recurrences seem available. The use of antipyretics is more controversial. Camfield et al. (1980) reported that intermittent antipyretic treatment with aspirin was ineffective in the prevention of febrile seizures. Bethune et al. (1993) and Uhari et al. (1995) did not find acetaminophen effective in the prevention of recurrences. The recurrence of a seizure within the same febrile episode is common, but no precise regimen has been advised for this purpose. Recurrence within a few hours can possibly be prevented by the administration of diazepam as suppositories or via an oral route because sufficient blood levels can be obtained within the time available after the first convulsion, but whether this method is justifiable and efficacious remains undetermined.

Prophylactic Treatment against Recurrences

Given the relative infrequency of recurrences and their mostly benign nature, no treatment is necessary in most cases. Prophylaxis may be indicated in some cases, especially when the parents are excessively anxious. Although many physicians do not advise continuous antiepileptic drug treatment after a first simple seizure, they do consider it after complex, especially long-lasting seizures even though no clear evidence indicates its necessity (Shinnar et al., 1992; Maytal and Shinnar, 1990).

The following three types of prophylactic treatment exist: (a) intermittent prophylaxis given at the first sign of a febrile illness, (b) continuous prophylaxis with the daily administration of anticonvulsant drugs, and (c) the prevention of *prolonged* seizures only by the immediate administration of an anticonvulsant agent in the event of a seizure.

The last method employs the intrarectal administration of benzodiazepine solution by parents or guardians. The feasibility of this method has been tested by Ventura et al. (1982). These clinicians instructed the parents of 601 children who had a first febrile seizure to give the drug rectally only in the case of a recurrence. In 76 children, 109 recurrences were observed during the observation period. In 70 children, the drug was judged to have been correctly administered; in 26 of the 39 remaining cases, no drug was given because the seizure stopped spontaneously before it could be used. Only eight children had a long (longer than 15 minutes) seizure. Six of these had not been given diazepam, and two had expelled it. No adverse incident was noted, and the authors concluded that the method was safe and valuable. Further work along this line seems warranted, especially in areas in which medical or hospital facilities are not easily accessible.

Intermittent prophylaxis against recurrences of FCs, as opposed to early treatment of seizures, consists of giving medication only when the child is sick with fever. Intermittent prophylaxis is based on the assumptions that parents or guardians are able to recognize the onset of any febrile illness so that medication can be given early enough, that someone who recognizes the prodromes can give the medication effectively and quickly, and that the absorption of the drug that is given and its entry into the brain is relatively fast and invariant. Some doubt exists that the first assumption can be reliably satisfied. In addition, the need to recognize early symptoms of a febrile illness and to avoid too frequent, unnecessary treatment can generate considerable anxiety. Certainly, phenobarbital cannot be expected to satisfy the third assumption (see Chapter 24) because of its slow buildup in the blood and brain. Intermittent prophylaxis with phenobarbital, however, was found in one study to be partly effective in preventing recurrences. Failure of intermittent phenobarbital prophylaxis has been confirmed in the most recent studies (Wolf et al., 1977; Wolf, 1981). Intermittent prophylaxis with a benzodiazepine appears to be more satisfactory because of the rapid absorption and brain entry of the drug (Browne and Penry, 1973; Knudsen, 1979; Rosman et al., 1993). Diazepam given as suppositories at a dose of 5 mg every 8 hours appeared to be as effective as daily phenobarbital in one study (Knudsen, 1985b, 1988). However, no control (untreated) group was used, and the rate of failure of the phenobarbital prophylaxis was higher than that seen in other reports. Thorn (1975, 1981) gave intermittent diazepam to 207 children with FCs, of whom only 12 had a recurrence. The recurrence rate was 41% in untreated patients, and 20 of the 226 children to whom phenobarbital was prescribed had a recurrence; however, the compliance in this group was said to be poor. In addition, many patients with recurrences had not had diazepam before the seizure, and, in one-third, the fever was not noted before the fit. This study did not include a control group. More recently, Knudsen (1988, 1991) used a rectal solution of diazepam with a dose of 5 (younger than 3 years) to 7.5 mg (3 years or older) every 12 hours whenever the temperature was 38.5°C or higher; this intermittent prophylaxis was given alternating febrile patients in a group of 290 children. The recurrence rate, with the assumption that 25% of patients were lost to follow-up, was 12% in treated and 39% in untreated children. Similar results were reported with oral diazepam given at a dose of 0.5 mg per kg (Dianese, 1979), and some evidence also indicates that clonazepam, administered orally, can be effective. This may also apply to clobazam (Tondi et al., 1987).

Rosman et al. (1993) conducted a randomized, double-blind placebo-controlled trial among 406 children who had at least one febrile seizure. Oral diazepam (0.33 mg per kg of body weight) resulted in a reduction of 44% in the risk of febrile seizures in an intention-to-treat analysis. In only those children who actually received the medication, the risk of recurrence was reduced by 82%. The side effects seen in 39% of cases were mild to moderate. In a double-blind study, Autret et al. (1990) did not find a difference in the recurrence rate, but the treatment was not regularly given in the treatment group, so a firm conclusion is not possible. Other studies have confirmed the possibility of preventing some recurrences with intermittent therapy (Rosman, 1990; Vanasse et al., 1984). They also emphasize the difficulties associated with any type of intermittent prophylaxis. In addition to the problems raised by the early detection of fever, side effects such as ataxia, drowsiness, and hypotonia were frequently observed.

Continuous daily prophylaxis with anticonvulsant drugs avoids the drawbacks of intermittent prophylactic therapy, but it raises the difficult problems of compliance and exposure to the hazards of the long-term use of drugs. Several drugs have been more or less extensively tested for this purpose.

Phenobarbital at a dose of 4 to 5 mg per kg per day was shown to decrease the recurrence rate of FCs significantly in six prospective randomized studies with the use of concurrent controls and blood level monitoring (Mamelle et al., 1984; Bacon et al., 1981a; Camfield et al., 1980; Ngwane and Bower, 1980; Wallace and Smith, 1980; Wolf et al., 1977). A seventh study (McKinlay and Newton, 1989; Newton, 1988) showed an insignificant reduction in the frequency of recurrences, but the number of patients studied was too small to demonstrate a decrease in recurrence rate that would be of the magnitude observed in the positive studies. Other studies also indicate the effectiveness of phenobarbital, but these suffer various methodologic defects. These include the studies of Faero et al. (1972) and Thorn (1975), in which no concurrent controls were run; those of Wallace (1975) and Cavazzuti (1975), in which drug levels were not monitored; and those of Herranz et al. (1988) and Minagawa and Miura (1981), which were not randomized. In most phenobarbital studies, the recurrence rate varied between 4% and 13% (Wolf, 1981) compared with an average rate in controls of 20% to 30%. Wolf et al. (1977), who found a recurrence rate of 8% at 6 months for the treated children, compared with 24% in controls, also found no *severe* seizure in their treated patients, as opposed to the occurrence of severe seizures in 4.4% in the nontreatment group; however, the numbers were small. Newton and McKinlay (1988) mentioned the occurrence of prolonged febrile seizures in two patients, one of whom was receiving phenobarbital and the other, sodium valproate. Both were said to have "therapeutic levels" of the drugs.

Despite methodologic criticisms (Newton and McKinlay, 1988), phenobarbital appears to be mostly, but not completely, effective when blood levels of 16 mg per L are regularly maintained. The negative results of some randomized trials (McKinlay and Newton, 1989) based on an intention to treat are also subject to criticism, and they do not negate, in the authors' opinion, the results of previous studies (Wallace, 1988). Phenobarbital is equally effective against simple and severe FCs and in patients with or without abnormal antecedents of early life, such as complications of maternal pregnancy, low birth weight, prematurity, difficult birth resuscitation, abnormal neonatal period, delay in milestones, more than one seizure, a previous complex seizure, or abnormal neurologic examination results (Wolf, 1981).

Valproate reduces the recurrence rate about as much as (Cavanagh et al., 1974; Ngwane and Bower, 1980; Wallace and Smith, 1980) or more (Agbato et al., 1986) than phenobarbital. Wallace and Aldridge-Smith (1981) found a recurrence rate of 12.8% with valproate, 13% with phenobarbital, and 34% in untreated controls.

The experience with other drugs is rather limited and unsatisfactory. Phenytoin was considered ineffective by Frantzen et al. (1968), but the blood levels were very low in two-thirds of their patients. Melchior et al. (1971) found no decrease in the recurrence rate but no severe seizures in children given phenytoin prophylactically; however, the numbers were small, and the study suffered severe methodologic deficiencies. Primidone seemed about as effective as phenobarbital in two uncontrolled studies (Herranz et al., 1988; Minagawa et al., 1986). Wallace (1975) thought that primidone might be better tolerated than phenobarbital, and further study is desirable. Carbamazepine seems to be ineffective (Antony and Hawke, 1983).

The adverse effects associated with continuous prophylaxis are not negligible (Wolf et al., 1981; Wolf and Forsythe, 1978). Phenobarbital may be responsible for acute poisoning in the child or his or her siblings (Thorn, 1975). The abrupt discontinuation of phenobarbital treatment may itself provoke a seizure (Wolf, 1981). The interactions of the drug with other medications may occasionally raise problems, as in children treated chronically with steroids. The interference of phenobarbital with calcium-phosphorus metabolism is well known (Elwes et al., 1991; Christiansen et al., 1975), but the practical significance of this effect for the treatment of FCs is probably limited. The main side effect of phenobarbital is that on behavior. As many as 30% to 50% of the treated children display irritability, overactivity, temper tantrums, and aggressiveness (Wolf et al., 1981; Wolf and Forsythe, 1978). Fussing and sleep disturbances may be pronounced (Camfield and Camfield, 1981). These effects may be dose related, and they may be controlled by lowering the dose to obtain a blood level of 11 mg per L or less (Camfield and Camfield, 1981). However, some authors did not find that the adverse effects were influenced by dosage (Bäckman et al., 1987; Wolf et al., 1981). The behavioral side effects are bad enough to lead to the discontinuation of treatment in approximately 20% of patients (Wolf, 1981), and they are partly responsible for relatively low compliance. Even when great care was taken in instructing and encouraging the parents, the compliance rate did not exceed 60% to 65% (Camfield and Camfield, 1981; Wolf et al., 1981).

A widely publicized study (Farwell et al., 1990) found that, after 2 years, the mean IQ of the children assigned to phenobarbital was 7 points lower than that of children receiving placebo. Furthermore, no significant reduction in seizure frequency was found in the phenobarbital group. The latter result is difficult to assess, however, because the study was based on intention to treat, and limited compliance and crossing over between the study groups may have led to an underestimation of the effectiveness of phenobarbital in preventing recurrences. The effects on intelligence tests, however, are worrying.

A subtle effect on memory-related tasks of dubious significance has been noted (Camfield and Camfield, 1981; Hellström and Barlach-Christoffersen, 1980), so use of the smallest dose possible seems reasonable. Valproate seems much better tolerated (Wallace and Smith, 1980). However, refraining from its use in a benign condition like FCs seems wise because the risk of hepatotoxicity is difficult to justify in the treatment of a benign condition (Eadie and Tyrer, 1989; Hirtz et al., 1986; Lee et al., 1986b). The possibility of an adverse effect on testicular development, although this has not been documented in humans, is also of some concern.

The balance of risks, as currently evaluated, does not favor continuous prophylactic therapy for all patients following a first FC because the incidence of recurrences and complications is too small to justify treatment with potentially hazardous drugs in 3% or more of children.

Continuous prophylaxis for selected patients is favored by several investigators (Wallace, 1988; O'-Donohoe, 1985; Wolf, 1981), but this view has increasingly been challenged because of the realization that antiepileptic drugs may be more toxic than was previously thought. The common practice of starting prophylactic therapy after a second seizure has no obvious rationale. The use of selective prophylaxis after the first seizure rests on the assumption that the determination, from the time of a first seizure, of a population at risk of developing recurrent febrile seizures, later epilepsy, or both is possible. Such an assumption is untenable because more than 90% of cases of epilepsy come from the low-risk group (Nelson and Ellenberg, 1983).

Currently, the place of unselected continuous prophylaxis is, at best, very limited in patients in whom psychologic factors are paramount. The authors' current practice is to treat only patients younger than 12

months with continuous anticonvulsant therapy, but giving dogmatic advice is not possible.

The best technique under present circumstances is to concentrate efforts on establishing an effective *emergency treatment* of FCs and to make this treatment readily available to those who need it. The rapid administration of an agent that is capable of quickly arresting any lasting FC is the only possibility for preventing brain damage that could be incurred during a first seizure. This technique appears to be safe and effective (Camfield et al., 1989a). It obviates the need for any type of continuous therapy when medical help is at hand or if treatment can be administered by the parents themselves.

Possibilities of Prevention

Little can be done to prevent the occurrence, as opposed to the recurrences, of febrile seizures. Although some children, especially those with a family history of febrile seizures and possibly those with neurologic abnormalities, have a higher risk of having later FCs (Bethune et al., 1993; Berg et al., 1995), the magnitude of this effect is too small to justify specific measures.

On the other hand, anticonvulsant treatment may be advisable for those immunizations that are likely to induce fever. Immunization against measles is definitely indicated in patients with an increased risk of FCs. Febrile seizures were observed in 1.9% of recipients of measles vaccine, whereas the incidence of convulsions in wild disease is 7.7% (Landrigan and Witte, 1973). Immunization against whooping cough is contraindicated if an increased risk of convulsion, such as previous developmental or neurologic abnormalities, is present (Ross and Peckham, 1983), even though the objective evidence supporting this attitude is slim.

SUMMARY

Febrile seizures are the single most common neurologic problem in childhood. Most febrile seizures are brief, bilateral tonic-clonic convulsions that occur in children between the ages of 6 months and 4 years with a fever of 38°C or more and that are not caused by intracranial infections. However, long-lasting and unilateral or focal FCs may occur, and these may be associated with residual brain damage.

Genetic factors play an essential role in the genesis of FCs. A definite clustering of cases of FCs does occur in relatives of affected children. Acquired factors of prenatal, perinatal, or postnatal origin probably influence the severity of FCs, and they may determine the localization (or lateralization) of some seizures. The infections associated with FCs are mostly common infectious illnesses that are readily recognized. In younger patients and in the case of severe seizures, however, infections of the CNS may present as FCs, thus raising difficult diagnostic problems.

The long-term outcome of FCs is favorable in more than 95% of patients. The incidence rate of epilepsy following FCs has been between 2% and 5% in recent series, and neurologic and/or mental sequelae are rare. Long-lasting convulsions, however, deserve vigorous anticonvulsive treatment, and they should not go unchecked for more than 10 to 15 minutes. Recurrences of FCs occur in 30% to 35% of patients. They are usually benign as most severe FCs are initial seizures. Some recurrences are long lasting, and even short recurrences may increase the risk of later epilepsy. In most patients, only one or two recurrences are observed. Although individualization of subgroups within the general category of FCs is desirable for prognostic purposes, efforts to separate simple FCs with a consistently benign course from those cases associated with later epilepsy that, at times, are termed *epilepsy triggered by fever* or *atypical FCs* have been largely unsuccessful. The recent recognition of genetic syndromes with FC will, hopefully, help to improve the prognostic ability of clinicians. The risk of later epilepsy is higher when the child was developmentally abnormal before his or her first seizure; when the first seizure was long, lateralized, or repeated during a single febrile episode; and when familial antecedents of epilepsy were present in relatives. However, the vast majority of cases of epilepsy following FCs occur in patients who have had none of these features, and the terms *simple* and *complex* seizures are merely descriptive, giving relatively little indication about the prognosis.

The need for emergency treatment of the underlying illness if it is severe and of any prolonged seizure is generally agreed on. After an initial seizure, the parents should be thoroughly informed of the nature of the disorder, the attendant risks, and what they should do in the event of a recurrence.

Prophylaxis against recurrences by the intermittent use of fast-acting anticonvulsant drugs for every febrile disease is difficult to implement, and its results are limited. The long-term use of anticonvulsant medication is effective in preventing approximately two-thirds of recurrences. The hazards and inconvenience associated with continuous anticonvulsant prophylaxis are not negligible, so such treatment should be used only, if at all, for patients at special risk. Such patients are, in these authors' view, only those children younger than 1 year. The only rationale for giving prophylactic treatment is the prevention of febrile seizure recurrences, including those that might be severe enough to produce brain damage. No evidence indicates that prophylaxis has any effect on the incidence of later epilepsy, so this "should not be treated until it occurs" (Hauser, 1986).

15

Occasional Seizures Other Than Febrile Convulsions

Seizures precipitated by extracerebral factors, seizures resulting from acute brain insults, and single epileptic attacks, by definition, differ from epilepsy, which is a chronic condition characterized by the repetition of unprovoked seizures (see Chapter 1). This chapter successively deals with (a) occasional convulsions other than febrile convulsions and (b) the single or isolated epilepsy attack not related to any obvious precipitant.

Occasional seizures provoked by factors other than fever are also referred to as *reactive seizures*, *provoked seizures*, or *acute symptomatic seizures*. Acute symptomatic seizures are those that occur during a systemic disorder involving the central nervous system (CNS) or in close temporal association with a documented brain insult (Commission on Classification and Terminology of the International League Against Epilepsy [ILAE], 1985). They fall into the category of "situation-related seizures" in the 1989 classification of the ILAE. Acute symptomatic seizures differ from epilepsy in that they have a clearly identifiable proximate cause and they are not characterized by a tendency to recur spontaneously (Hauser and Annegers, 1998).

Occasional seizures are generally expressed as motor attacks (convulsions), most commonly of the bilateral tonic-clonic type. Focal or unilateral seizures, however, are not unusual with acute neurologic illnesses or even with disturbances of homeostasis, such as hypoglycemia or hypocalcemia (Tasker et al., 1991; Aicardi, 1980c). Seizures described as *absences* and *atonic attacks* have rarely been reported (Vohai and Barnett, 1989; Gastaut and Gastaut, 1958), and complex partial seizures may occur with metabolic disturbances such as hypoglycemia. Episodes of status epilepticus are not uncommon with certain causes, especially acute intoxications.

The frequency of acute symptomatic seizures is poorly known, in part because of the difficulties involved in their identification. Hauser and Annegers (1998) suggest they account for more than half of all newly occurring seizures.

Most occasional seizures occur before the age of 3 or 4 years because many of the responsible disorders, such as meningitis, trauma, or acute dehydration, take place predominantly in infancy and early childhood and because the brain may be more sensitive to certain stimuli, especially fever, during the period lasting from 6 months to 4 years of age. In one series (Ellenberg et al., 1984), only 12% of occasional seizures other than febrile convulsions supervened after the age of 48 months.

CAUSES OF OCCASIONAL SEIZURES

Occasional seizures other than febrile convulsions may be associated with fever as a consequence of the causal disorder. However, the definition of febrile convulsions excludes infections of the CNS (see Chapter 14). The main causes are listed in Table 15.1.

The most common causes of symptomatic seizures with fever are *meningitis and encephalitis*, which amounted to 82 (62%) of the 133 patients of Ellenberg et al. (1984). Seizures with bacterial meningitis are significantly associated with a young age, a delay in diagnosis, a low serum sodium level, and evidence of infarction and/or ventricular enlargement on a computed tomographic (CT) scan (Snyder, 1984). A small proportion of seizures associated with purulent meningitis may be caused by the fever itself (Ounsted et al., 1985), and patients with meningitis may certainly present with simple febrile convulsions (Wallace, 1985; Ratcliffe and Wolf, 1977) without meningeal signs, especially in children younger than 18 months. Therefore, a lumbar puncture should be systematically considered in infants with febrile convulsions at younger than 18 months. However, Green et al. (1993) found that children with meningitis were usually obtunded or comatose; only 8 of their 523 patients had a normal level of consciousness, and only 47 (1.7%) of the 2,780 patients they reviewed had no meningeal signs. Seizures with fever in infants younger than 6 months should always raise the suspicion of CNS infection (Heijbel et al., 1980; Aicardi and Chevrie, 1970; Van den Berg and

TABLE 15.1. *Main causes of occasional epileptic seizures*

Fever resulting from extracranial infections: febrile seizures, initial convulsions
Intracranial infections
 Bacterial: meningitis, brain abscess, subdural or extradural empyema
 Viral: primary encephalitis (mainly herpes simplex), postinfectious encephalitis, viral meningoencephalitis
 Fungal or parasitic
Acute encephalopathies of obscure origin, including Reye syndrome, acute encephalopathies associated with exanthemata or immunizations
Metabolic disturbances
 Hypocalcemia
 Hypoglycemia and hypomagnesemia
 Hyponatremia with water intoxication
 Hypernatremia—convulsions occur principally during correction of hypernatremic dehydration
 Inborn errors of metabolism
Intoxications
 Endogenous: uremia, hepatic encephalopathy, and others
 Exogenous: accidental or iatrogenic; lead encephalopathy, drugs
Head trauma, with or without intracranial hemorrhage
Hypertensive encephalopathy
Renal diseases: acute nephritis, hemolytic-uremic syndrome
Acute cerebral anoxia: cardiac arrest, drowning, acute vascular collapse caused by shock or dehydration
Cerebrovascular accidents
 Arterial thrombosis
 Venous thrombosis
 Hemorrhage from vascular malformations
Burn encephalopathy

Yerushalmi, 1969). In one series (Ellenberg et al., 1984), 25% of infants with symptomatic febrile seizures were younger than 6 months, whereas only 6.4% of those with true febrile convulsions were in that age group. The occurrence of seizures with bacterial meningitis has an unfavorable prognosis (Snyder, 1984), especially when the seizures are prolonged and focal. This is usually attributed to the complications responsible for the emergence of seizures. Some evidence, however, indicates that the convulsive activity itself may produce or favor brain damage (Ounsted et al., 1985). In the authors' opinion, systematic anticonvulsant treatment from the onset of the illness is justified in all children younger than 4 years with bacterial meningitis, because seizures supervene in 10% to 40% of patients. Early diagnosis and treatment, as well as careful attention to electrolyte balance, could possibly decrease the incidence of this major complication.

Viral meningitis is probably a fairly common cause of symptomatic convulsions with fever. Rutter and Smales (1977) found three cases of viral meningitis in a series of 328 children with febrile convulsions who were submitted to systematic lumbar puncture. Only 1 of the 328 children had purulent meningitis. All types of encephalitis and meningoencephalitis can be responsible for seizures. Herpes simplex is the most common cause of encephalitis in Western Europe and the United States. Early diagnosis is important because this is a treatable condition. Seizures are often the first symptom, and they are an indication for performing lumbar puncture. The seizures are localized and often prolonged, and they are associated with neurologic signs and depression of consciousness that does not clear rapidly after the arrest of convulsions. Other viruses, especially herpesvirus 6 (and 7), may also produce encephalitis, which usually is of a lesser severity (Barone et al., 1995; Jones et al., 1994; Asano et al., 1992).

Dehydration associated with acute diarrheal disease was responsible for 15% of the symptomatic convulsions with fever in the series by Ellenberg et al. (1984). The seizures are usually attributed to electrolyte imbalance, particularly to that resulting from the rapid correction of hypernatremia (Plouin et al., 1979; Swanson, 1977; Hogan et al., 1969). This mechanism is probably not exclusive, and convulsions may also result from vascular collapse, which, at times, is associated with intracranial venous thrombosis (Aicardi and Goutières, 1973); from the action of bacterial toxins, particularly with shigellosis (Lahat et al, 1990) and salmonellosis; and from the fever itself (Lennox-Buchtal, 1973). A good correlation between the degree of fever and the incidence of convulsions has been reported (Mélékian et al., 1962), and at least some of the seizures that occur with febrile dehydration are probably true febrile convulsions. The seizures often present as status epilepticus, but various types may be encountered (Andrew, 1991; Plouin et al., 1979). Recently, a number of reports of clusters of seizures in infants that usually occur without fever in association with a mild gastroenteritis have been reported in infants (see Chapter 13).

Malaria is a major cause of occasional seizures with fever in endemic areas. Convulsions may occur with any form of malaria, but they are an extremely common manifestation of cerebral malaria due to *Plasmodium falciparum* infestation, in which they are present in up to 80% of patients. In such patients, the seizures are associated with coma lasting more than 6 hours. Status epilepticus is present in 10% to 20% of patients. The mortality rate is high, and emergency treatment is essential. Simple febrile seizures without cerebral involvement are mainly associated with benign malaria (Phillips and Solomon, 1990; Molyneux et al., 1989).

Afebrile occasional seizures may have a number of causes (Table 15.1). In the series by Ellenberg et al. (1984), 34% of cases resulted from head trauma and 20% from toxic encephalopathy, mainly lead poisoning. The latter condition is now uncommon in its major convulsive form.

Accidental intoxications are common, with drug intoxication accounting for a significant proportion of cases. Seizures resulting from drug toxicity are usually fairly severe and prolonged attacks, and they are associated with disturbance in consciousness. The list of convulsant toxics is long, including such widely used drugs as tricyclic antidepressants, β-blockers, isoniazid, and local anesthetics. A review of 53 cases (children and adults) seen over a 10-year period has been published (Messing et al., 1984). Most seizures were described as generalized, but focal features were common. In two patients, the seizures were of the partial motor type.

In children, most cases of acute poisoning with convulsions are marked by severe, repeated seizures with coma. Intoxication must always be considered in children with seizures and coma or other disturbances of consciousness. Special mention should be made of theophylline toxicity because of its wide use in pediatrics; although cases have been reported following improper therapeutic use (Gal et al., 1980; Schwartz and Scott, 1974), they have also been seen, on occasion, with levels that were within the accepted therapeutic range (Yarnell and Chu, 1975). Seizures have also resulted from the use of theophylline for the treatment of apnea in the neonatal period or later during episodes of near-miss sudden death (Davis et al., 1986). In such cases, however, seizures might also result from hypoxia incurred during the episode, and status epilepticus has been attributed to such a mechanism (Constantinou et al., 1989; Aubourg et al., 1985). In older patients, anoxic and toxic metabolic seizures often present as status myoclonus (Celesia et al., 1988). Brief episodes of anoxia may induce an occasional epileptic seizure, as occurs in some children who present with a genuine epileptic attack immediately after an apneic episode, often a breath-holding attack (Stephenson, 1990). Such seizures are usually tonic-clonic ones, but they may occasionally present as absence status (Battaglia et al., 1989).

In acute cerebral anoxia, such as occurs after cardiac arrest, carbon monoxide poisoning, or drowning, the seizures are regularly associated with disturbed consciousness and often with characteristic electroencephalographic (EEG) patterns.

Other causes of severe seizures include phenylpropanolamine administration (Bale et al., 1984) and contrast myelography (Levey et al., 1988).

Seizures associated with head trauma may reveal the presence of a chronic subdural hematoma. Isolated afebrile seizures in infants should always raise the suspicion of a subdural effusion and the possibility of nonaccidental trauma (see Chapter 18).

Withdrawal seizures can occur with the discontinuation of any anticonvulsive agent. They may occur after the withdrawal of anticonvulsive agents, but they are more common after the withdrawal of phenobarbital (Rust, 2001) and the benzodiazepines, especially clonazepam (Farrell, 2001) but not phenytoin (Marks et al., 1991; Duncan et al., 1989, 1990; Bromfield et al., 1989; Theodore et al., 1987a; Marciani et al., 1985). Withdrawal can also follow the rapid discontinuation of some new antiepileptic agents, especially vigabatrin and gabapentin.

Burn encephalopathy is an uncommon cause of seizures. Its mechanism remains unclear, (Mohnot et al., 1982) but it probably has several etiologies. Partial seizures may occur (Mohnot et al., 1982).

Seizures associated with *acute nephritis* may not have obvious clinical signs, and even the urinary findings may be minimal. *Arterial hypertension* is not a common cause of convulsions in childhood. With headache, visual disturbances, and disturbances of consciousness, it is, however, a major manifestation of posterior leukoencephalopathy, which can also result from therapy with immunosuppressive agents, such as cyclosporine or tacrolimus (Hinchey et al., 1996; Schwartz et al., 1995), and sometimes with corticosteroids (Antunes, 2001). Status epilepticus is common, but atypical presentations are sometimes observed as well (Del Giudice and Aicardi, 1979).

The treatment of occasional seizures is essentially that of the causal disorder. Anticonvulsive drugs are indicated in long-lasting attacks and during the acute period of the causal disease (see Chapter 23). Because children with convulsions symptomatic of an acute neurologic or metabolic condition have no continuing liability to recurrent seizures, no prolonged treatment is needed after the acute episode.

THE SINGLE SEIZURE

All epilepsies begin with a first seizure, and, although unprovoked recurrence is common but, by no means, constant, isolated seizures, which have also been termed *single seizures*, can be defined as solitary seizure events that occur only once in a lifetime (Wolf, 1998). A seizure event may consist of one single seizure, a short series of seizures in the course of 24 hours, or an isolated episode of status epilepticus. Such a definition is obviously impractical, so the term *isolated seizure* applies also to those cases in which a very long seizure-free period without therapy follows the initial event (Wolf, 1998).

The frequency of single seizures can be determined only by studying the relapse rate after a first seizure, which is the inverse expression of the likelihood of its remaining isolated. This question has been studied only for generalized tonic-clonic seizures and partial seizures, as absences, drop attacks, and myoclonias virtually never occur as a single attack and they have a high frequency of repetition. Generalized tonic-clonic seizures are by far the most common types of single seizure, and these have been reported in 61% of cases. Simple partial seizures have been described in 27% and complex partial seizures in 10% (Hauser et al., 1990).

The magnitude of the risk of a subsequent seizure after a first unprovoked generalized or focal seizure is imperfectly known, particularly in children (see Chapter 22). Variable risks for recurrence ranging from 27% (Hauser et al., 1990; Hauser, 1986) to 67% (Hart et al., 1990) have been given in mixed series of adults and children and in those limited to adults. Studies exclusively concerned with children (Berg and Shinnar, 1991; Shinnar et al., 1990; Boulloche et al., 1989; Camfield et al., 1985a; Hirtz et al., 1984) have indicated similar or slightly higher figures, so a first generalized or focal seizure has a probability of remaining isolated in roughly one-third to half of children. Such overall figures are of relatively little practical value because the recurrence rate varies greatly with several factors. These include the cause of the seizure, in which the incidence is significantly higher in patients with remote symptomatic seizures than it is in those with cryptogenic or idiopathic seizures; the presence or absence of EEG abnormalities; and a family history of epilepsy (see Chapter 22). The occurrence of the seizure during sleep is also associated with a higher risk of recurrence (Shinnar et al., 1993). The type of seizure is also strongly indicative of the risk. Camfield et al. (1985a) found an overall recurrence rate of 52% after a 32-month follow-up in their study of 168 children with a first unprovoked seizure. In their series, 77% of the first recurrences occurred within 1 year of the first seizure. The risk of recurrence was highest for those patients with sylvian (rolandic) seizures (70% with a normal EEG and 97% with an abnormal EEG); next highest for patients with partial seizures, whether simple or complex (50% to 83% depending on type, EEG, and neuro-

logic examination results); and lowest for patients with generalized tonic-clonic seizures (30% without neurologic or EEG abnormalities and 63% with both neurologic and EEG abnormalities).

The age at occurrence of a first unprovoked seizure does not seem to influence the outcome in overall studies. However, the high incidence of isolated epileptic seizures, especially those of a partial motor or complex partial type, in adolescents has been emphasized (Capovilla et al., 2001a; King et al., 1999; Loiseau et al., 1983a); this is discussed in more depth in Chapter 10. When a single partial seizure or cluster of seizures occurs in an adolescent, the overall prognosis is favorable, with a likelihood of remaining seizure free of 52% after 1 year, of 67% after 5 years, and of 76% after 10 years (Loiseau et al., 1983a). If the patient had a simple partial seizure(s) with no associated grand mal, no etiologic factor, and normal EEG recordings, the prognosis was excellent (100% were seizure free at 3 years). The prognosis was less favorable for those with complex partial seizures, associated generalized tonic-clonic seizures, or an abnormal EEG recording or a combination of these factors. For patients with complex partial seizures, the prognosis cannot be made without a 1-year follow-up. If the seizure does not recur within 1 year, the prognosis is globally favorable; 68% of patients are likely to be controlled at 5 years and 89% at 10 years (Loiseau et al., 1983a). The favorable outcome of partial motor seizures in adolescents was recently confirmed in a group of 92 patients by King et al. (1999), who found rare recurrence in three of their patients, and by Capovilla et al. (2001a).

The presence of provoking factors, such as stress and lack of sleep, may be of importance because these might indicate a lesser risk of recurrence (Wolf, 1998). However, little firm evidence is available in this respect.

The long-term prognosis of an isolated seizure cannot be determined before time has elapsed. The duration of the seizure-free period that is necessary to consider the probability of a single seizure is difficult to determine. According to Wolf (1998), in most cases, the issue of whether a first seizure will remain isolated or whether it marks the onset of epilepsy is resolved within 1 or 2 years. This statement is probably applicable to epilepsy with relatively frequent attacks. Clearly, late recurrences are possible after several years. Usually, long seizure-free intervals indicate that the seizures, even if recurrent, will remain infrequent and that they thus may be considered "occasional." The common epidemiologic definition of epilepsy as two or more unprovoked seizures is arbitrary, and, for practical purposes, rare seizures have different consequences for the patient.

The *problem posed by a first seizure* is one of secondary prevention rather than one of therapy (Wolf, 1998). The decision to treat requires answers to several questions.

The first one is that of differential diagnosis. Nonepileptic attacks may be difficult to distinguish on the basis of limited, usually second-hand information, and the epileptic nature of the event has to be established before treatment is considered. If it remains in doubt, treatment is not likely indicated. Realizing that a first tonic-clonic seizure may not be the first epileptic event and that it may have been preceded, sometimes for months or years, by unrecognized seizures of limited clinical expression, such as absences, is important, as this completely changes the therapeutic problem.

The second question is whether an acute or progressive illness may be responsible for the seizure. The answer requires full clinical investigation, and additional studies, such as brain imaging, may be required because treatment must include the cause.

A third question is that of whether precipitants can be uncovered. What constitutes an unprovoked seizure is subject to debate. Hauser et al. (1990) considered seizures that occur in the context of precipitants of dubious significance, such as sleep deprivation or stress, are unprovoked. However, seizures that occur in the wake of an acute illness may be less likely to recur, but little information is available in this regard. Whether seizures occurring in a setting of emotional distress may be regarded as provoked is debatable. Some (O'Donohoe, 1985) believe that severe emotional upset and severe fatigue may combine to precipitate a single seizure, but this is not well documented and probably does not justify withholding therapy. However, Wolf (1995b) thinks that presence of provoking circumstances may alter the therapeutic decision in favor of nondrug prevention.

Even with the help of available statistical data, arriving at a decision regarding the individual patient is difficult. The problem should be discussed frankly with the parents and child. Some elect treatment because of personal preferences, because they are especially exposed to hazards from a fit as a result of their professional or sports activities, or because they think the occurrence of a fit might ruin their professional or personal life. Others are reluctant to take any long-term therapy; this often applies to adolescents. The risks of both positions should be fully explained, and a reasonable attitude should be encouraged. Treating the child following the first seizure is a simple method, but a substantial number of children who, even if left untreated, would never have had a repeated seizure, will be treated for 2 to 4 years. Most authors now think that such a policy is rarely justified. Another approach would be to make an individual decision according to whether factors indicative of a high risk of recurrence are present. The presence of paroxysmal abnormalities in the EEG, antecedent neurologic or mental abnormalities, and possibly a family history of seizures certainly favors starting treatment after the first seizure (Shinnar et al., 2000). Also, excessive parental anxiety about recurrence can impact the decision to start early treatment (Robinson, 1984). No completely rational justification can be made regarding the treatment of a first nonfebrile seizure, and further studies on the outcome of isolated seizures in children are needed before any firm recommendation can be made. The authors' attitude is to advise treatment of *proved* first epileptic seizures only in patients with risk factors and in those whose epilepsies are extremely likely to recur, such as those who experience complex partial seizures or myoclonic or absence attacks. Even in such patients, a decision to treat is rarely, if ever, urgent, and adopting a wait-and-see attitude may be defended. In children with a first generalized tonic-clonic attack, the decision not to treat seems wiser after the first seizure. Moreover, the efficacy of such a treatment is open to question (Camfield et al., 1985b). The final decision requires an acceptance of the treatment by the parents and adolescent patients.

If treatment is not started after the first epileptic attack, certain precautions should be taken. First, the patient should be brought back at once if he or she has a second seizure; treatment will almost certainly be recommended at that time. Second, dangerous activities (e.g., motorcycling and swimming) should be discouraged until the risk of a recurrence has fallen significantly (probably after 1 year).

SUMMARY

Occasional seizures other than febrile convulsions are mainly caused by meningitis or meningoencephalitis, head trauma, and acute or chronic intoxications. Seizures may be the first manifestation of bacterial meningitis, and they may present in young infants as simple febrile convulsions without meningeal signs. Before the age of 6 months, seizures with fever are more likely to be caused by meningitis than to represent true febrile convulsions. In that age group, afebrile convulsions may be the first and, at times, the only manifestation of subdural hematoma. In toddlers, severe convulsions with lasting disturbances of consciousness are a common manifestation of intoxication, especially of drug toxicity, and that cause should be investigated. A general examination is important at all ages, and urine examination and measurement of blood pressure should be included, because hypertension may provoke severe and repeated seizures.

A first epileptic attack can remain isolated. That is generally the case with generalized tonic-clonic seizures unassociated with neurologic or mental deficits. In such a situation and depending on individual preferences, lifestyle, and the circumstances of the occurrence of the attack, the treatment may be deferred until a second seizure has occurred. Treatment after the first seizure is rarely indicated in the absence of neurologic abnormalities, and it may not be indicated even in such cases. Seizures that are regularly recurrent, such as myoclonic or absence attacks, are virtually never seen as a first attack, and the most common form of partial seizures in childhood, rolandic epilepsy, may be left untreated until the second or third seizure, depending on the family's and child's preference.

16

Status Epilepticus

Status epilepticus (SE) is defined as "an epileptic seizure that is sufficiently prolonged or repeated at sufficiently brief intervals so as to produce an unvarying and enduring epileptic condition" (Gastaut, 1973). The duration necessary to diagnose SE has been variably estimated. Modern works generally accept duration of 30 minutes or more (Rothner and Erenberg, 1980; Chevrie and Aicardi, 1978) for continuous seizures. In other studies, a duration of 1 hour or more (Aicardi and Chevrie, 1970) was selected. The same durations apply to seizures repeated at brief intervals, without complete recovery of consciousness between individual attacks (Hauser, 1983). Some authors, however, consider that two seizures or more occurring without an intervening recovery of consciousness constitute SE (Janz, 1969).

The difficulties for a universally accepted definition based on duration are directly derived from the common clinical practice of treating all seizures lasting longer than 5 or 10 minutes and from data from clinical and fundamental research that suggests that prolonged seizures (longer than 30 minutes) are required to produce CNS metabolic disturbances. If a duration component should be included in the definition of status to be used for the evaluation of new drugs or for epidemiologic studies, this should be the minimum duration (10 minutes) after which medical care is usually applied. Care should be taken not to include the postictal period. Recently, Lowenstein et al. (1999) discussed the need for a revised, more operational definition (specifying a seizure duration of at least 5 minutes) of status. The studies by Theodore et al. (1994) evaluated the overall duration of the convulsive portion of a "typical" isolated seizure as lasting slightly more than 1 minute and rarely in excess of 2 minutes, supporting the operational definition proposed by Lowenstein et al. (1999).

SE is distinct from *serial seizures*, which are series of attacks in which consciousness is regained between episodes. Serial seizures not uncommonly evolve into SE, and they should, therefore, be treated energetically.

From a clinical point of view, SE can be classified into as many types as there are epileptic seizure categories (see Chapter 2). From a symptomatic point of view, the classifications of SE separate them into the following two major forms: (a) generalized status, which may be convulsive (with tonic-clonic, tonic, clonic, and myoclonic varieties) or nonconvulsive (absence or petit mal status), and (b) partial SE, which includes the simple partial forms (somatomotor and aphasic) and complex partial status (Gastaut, 1983).

From a practical viewpoint, however, considerable differences exist between the various types of status. Generalized tonic-clonic or clonic SE has a much more serious prognosis than does absence status and requires different treatment. On the other hand, a large proportion of cases of *convulsive* SE in infants and young children are localized or they predominate on one side of the body. Although such episodes of status should theoretically be classified as "partial convulsive SE," in practice, they share many features with generalized SE. In particular, they may produce the same type of sequelae as generalized status, even though the motor and epileptic sequelae are usually limited to the side affected by the convulsive activity (Aicardi et al., 1969a; Gastaut et al., 1960). They also share many causes with generalized convulsive status; for example, they may be caused by fever (Chevrie and Aicardi, 1975; Aicardi and Chevrie, 1970) or generalized metabolic disturbances, such as hypocalcemia or pyridoxine dependency (Baxter, 2002; Roger et al., 1974). In such cases, the limitation of the convulsive activity to one hemisphere is probably the result of incomplete maturity of the developing brain or of the unequal threshold between the two hemispheres because of lesional or other causes (Yakovlev, 1962). In this chapter, such episodes of unilateral status are described with generalized SE, even though at least some of them are accepted to be the result of localized hemisphere lesions. The episodes are clinically and prognostically quite distinct from those that remain strictly localized to a restricted part of one side of the body, which are described as "partial SE."

From an etiologic point of view, SE can be divided into several categories (Shinnar et al., 1992; Maytal and Shinnar, 1990; Hauser, 1983). *Acute symptomatic status* is due to acute brain insults, such as trauma, brain infections, or metabolic disturbances. The term *remote symptomatic status* has been used in various studies for status due to chronic encephalopathies (Phillips and Shanahan, 1989; Hauser, 1983), and this includes cases due to previous congenital or acquired epileptogenic brain damage. Some investigators (Shinnar et al., 1992) separate a category of progressive encephalopathies that others (Phillips and Shanahan, 1989; Aicardi and Chevrie, 1970) include with the remote symptomatic group. *Idiopathic status*, which sometimes is also termed *cryptogenic*, does not appear to be associated with any causal brain damage. It may be febrile, representing the extreme of the spectrum of febrile convulsions (Maytal and Shinnar, 1990), or afebrile.

In a recent extensive review of SE, Shorvon (1994) devised a new classification scheme based not on seizure type alone but on other features such as age of the subject, the pathophysiologic mechanisms, and clinical features (anatomy, electroencephalographic [EEG] findings, etiology, and clinical phenomenology). Shorvon (1994) considers his proposal provisional and incomplete. He underlines the fact that future modifications, based on advances in the knowledge of the mechanisms and etiologies involved, are desirable. The major subdivision of Shorvon's proposal is age (neonatal period, infancy and childhood, childhood and adult life, status confined to adult life).

This chapter successively considers (a) convulsive tonic-clonic or clonic SE, whether generalized, predominating on one side of the body, or limited to one side; these are the most common forms of status, and they raise the most difficult prognostic and therapeutic problems (Hauser, 1983; Aicardi and Chevrie, 1970); (b) other less common types of convulsive status, such as tonic and myoclonic status; (c) nonconvulsive generalized SE; and (d) nonconvulsive partial status (complex partial status). Neonatal status was discussed in Chapter 12, and the so-called electrical SE of slow sleep, more correctly termed *continuous spike-waves of slow sleep*, was considered in Chapter 11. For each category, etiologic factors, outcome, and consequences are discussed, with ictal clinical phenomena. Treatment of the various types of status are considered at the end of this chapter.

CONVULSIVE TONIC-CLONIC OR CLONIC STATUS EPILEPTICUS

Frequency and Etiology

Convulsive SE is the most common form of status, but its real frequency is difficult to document, precisely because the various types of status are not specified separately in most published series. The proportions quoted for convulsive status range from 1.3% to 16% of all patients with epilepsy (Hauser, 1983). Contrary to the situation that prevails in adults, status is often the first epileptic seizure in infants and children. This was the case for 184 (77%) of the 239 patients of Aicardi and Chevrie (1970). Similarly, 24% of all children with a first afebrile seizure before 10 years of age who were seen in Minneapolis (Hauser, 1983) presented with SE. Status is particularly common during the first 2 years of life, and approximately 75% to 85% of cases occur before the age of 5 years (Phillips and Shanahan, 1989; Aicardi and Chevrie, 1970). In children older than 3 years of age, the annual frequency remains stable at around 3% to 5% until the age of 15 years (Aicardi and Chevrie, 1970). The overall incidence of SE does not appear to have declined. A recent prospective population-based study (DeLorenzo et al., 1995) from Richmond, Virginia, evaluated the incidence of SE at 41 patients per year per 100,000 population. Total SE events and the incidence per 100,000 individuals per year showed a bimodal distribution, with the highest rates being observed during the first year of life and after 60 years of age (DeLorenzo et al., 1996).

However, the frequency of different causes of status appears to have changed during the past 30 years. In 1971, Aicardi and Chevrie noted 126 symptomatic cases and 113 cryptogenic ones, with half of these being associated with fever. They did not find any essential difference between the patients with febrile seizures and those with status, except for the duration of the attack. Thus, because of their frequency, febrile convulsions were probably a major cause of cryptogenic SE in children younger than 3 years of age. In this series, the proportion of cases due to changes in or interruption of treatment was not given. Although precise figures are not available, most investigators agree that drug withdrawal is a common cause of status in children with epilepsy (Delgado-Escueta et al., 1983b).

Symptomatic causes are more common in recent series, especially acute encephalopathies, whereas afebrile idiopathic cases and chronic encephalopathies appear less frequently; febrile cases remain the most common form. Lesional causes are particularly common in younger children (Chevrie and Aicardi, 1977). They were responsible for 69% of the cases in one series (Aubourg et al., 1985). Overall, approximately one-fourth of cases are afebrile idiopathic, one-fourth are febrile, and the rest are almost equally divided between chronic (remote symptomatic) and acute encephalopathies (Shinnar et al., 1992; Maytal and Shinnar, 1990; Dunn, 1988). Specific causes in

TABLE 16.1. *Causes of convulsive status epilepticus in various series*

	Aicardi and Chevrie (1970) (N = 239)	Phillips and Shanahan (1989) (N = 193)	Shinnar et al. (1992) (N = 95)	Aubourg et al. (1985) (N = 79)
Acute neurologic (acute symptomatic) or systemic insult	63 (26%)	84 (44%)	18 (19%)	37 (49%)
CNS infection	29	28		13
Electrolyte disorders	17	21		2
Toxic exogenous	9	6		2
Acute anoxic insult	5	7		2
Trauma	2	—		6
Metabolic disorder	1	2		2
Miscellaneous				6
Chronic CNS disorder (remote symptomatic)	50 (21%)	20 (11%)	18 (19%)	12[a] (19%)
Neonatal hypoxic-ischemic insult	11	2		2
				2
Nonprogressive encephalopathy of obscure origin	23 (23%)	7	24 (25%)	2
CNS malformation	6	8		2
Progressive encephalopathy	10	2	6 (6%)	2
Cryptogenic or idiopathic	126 (53%)	89 (46%)	55 (58%)	13 (21%)
Febrile	67	62	29 (30.5%)	—
Afebrile	59	27	26 (27%)	—

Abbreviations: CNS, central nervous system; N, number of subjects.
[a]Includes four cases of severe myoclonic epilepsy.

four large series are shown in Table 16.1. Brain tumors are the cause of status in children only on rare occasions. The preponderance of frontal lesions that are mentioned in most adult series is not evident in children. Toxic causes, especially theophylline toxicity, should always be considered (Dunn and Parekh, 1991). The recent study released by the Richmond group (DeLorenzo et al., 1996) highlights the marked differences in etiologies between the adult and pediatric populations. For example, SE related to remote etiologies was considered a cause in 27% of the pediatric patients and in only 16% of the adult patients. The percentages for noncompliance to antiepileptic drugs (AEDs) (15% in children and 22% in adults) and especially of infection (37% in children versus 5% of all etiologies in adults) also differed.

Precipitating factors in patients with previous epilepsy include intercurrent infections; sleep deprivation; and, especially, anticonvulsant drug withdrawal. In a Finnish study (Sillanpää and Shinnar, 2002), status occurred in 44% of patients with remote symptomatic epilepsy and in 20% of those with idiopathic epilepsy.

Clinical Features

Convulsive SE is sometimes *preceded* by serial seizures separated by intervals of recovery of consciousness, especially in patients with known epilepsy. During this period of serial seizures, prompt treatment can prevent the emergence of true status (Shorvon, 1994).

Convulsive status proper may present either as a series of generalized tonic-clonic seizures *without* intervening recovery or as a more or less continuous seizure, which usually is purely clonic in nature. The latter type is especially common in children, and it was noted in 40% and 80%, respectively, of the individuals studied in two pediatric series (Congdon and Forsythe, 1980; Aicardi and Chevrie, 1970). In the cases presenting as a series of convulsions, generalized tonic-clonic seizures last 1 to 3 minutes. They tend to become briefer as time elapses, and the clonic phase may disappear or become inconspicuous (Roger et al., 1974). Interictally, the patients are in a coma, with vegetative disturbances, such as salivation, bradypnea, cyanosis, and arterial hypotension. Circulatory collapse may be the cause of 20% of deaths. The EEG displays typical tonic-clonic seizures (Gastaut and Tassinari, 1975a, 1975b). Interictally, the tracings show slow arrhythmic delta waves or, less commonly, faster rhythms in the alpha or beta range (Roger et al., 1974). The interictal neurologic signs may include unilateral or bilateral Babinski responses. The possibility of cerebrospinal fluid (CSF) pleocytosis as a consequence of status has been mentioned in adults (Edwards et al.,

1983; Schmidley and Simon, 1981) and, more recently, in infants and children (Woody et al., 1988b; Aicardi and Chevrie, 1970).

Clonic seizures are often predominantly unilateral, or they may shift from side to side (seesaw seizures) (Roger et al., 1974). Approximately 75% of patients with unilateral clonic seizures are 3 years of age or younger (Chevrie and Aicardi, 1975). Clonic seizures tend to be continuous and long-lasting rather than to consist of repeated attacks. They may last hours or even days, waxing and waning in intensity. They may involve an entire half of the body, but, at some periods, they may be restricted to one limb or segment; at other times, they may involve part of the contralateral side or they may transiently become generalized. The rhythm of the jerks is variable. Frequently, the jerks are at different rhythms in the various segments affected (Gastaut et al., 1974c). A postictal hemiplegia that may be persistent is usually observed. The first manifestation of the hemiconvulsion–hemiplegia–epilepsy syndrome (see Chapter 10) is a sudden prolonged hemiconvulsion in the form of status (Arzimanoglou and Dravet, 2001). The individual's consciousness is variably affected, and it may be preserved during a part or the whole duration of an episode. The EEG during clonic status typically shows more or less rhythmic slow waves of higher amplitude over the hemisphere opposite the convulsing side that are associated with a predominantly posterior rapid rhythm at about 10 Hz (the epileptic recruiting rhythm). The elements of fast and slow rhythms can variously combine, and they may produce more or less typical spike-wave complexes (Gastaut et al., 1957, 1974c). Flattening of the tracing or arrhythmic slow waves are usual in the postictal phase (Gastaut et al., 1960). After prolonged convulsive activity, a suppression-burst tracing that has a serious prognostic significance may be observed.

Treiman et al. (1980) distinguished five successive phases in adults. After the establishment of continuous discharges (the first three phases), brief episodes of low-amplitude tracing appear, first sporadically and then more and more frequently, ending with periodic epileptic discharges on a "flat" background. Periodic epileptiform discharges (PEDs) are also observed in children. Autonomic involvement is generally less pronounced than with tonic-clonic seizures, but fever, respiratory embarrassment, and a decrease in blood pressure often occur with long-lasting status.

Outcome and Prognosis

The *outcome* of convulsive SE has improved considerably over the past three decades. The death rate ranges between 6.6% and 17% in most adult series (Hauser, 1983; Aminoff and Simon, 1980). The mortality rate of the Richmond study was 22% overall (DeLorenzo et al., 1996). However, the mortality rate in children is only 3% in some series, and most pediatric deaths occur between the ages of 1 and 4 years (Leszczyszyn and Pellock, 2001). Aicardi and Chevrie (1970) found a mortality rate of 11% in a series of 239 children younger than 15 years. In other series, the mortality has varied between 3.6% and 7% (Maytal and Shinnar, 1990; Phillips and Shanahan, 1989; Dunn, 1988; Vigevano, 1986), except in two series (Aubourg et al., 1985; Chevrie and Aicardi, 1977) of children younger than 1 year, in which it reached 25%. Most deaths are caused by the underlying disorder. Death during status is associated with respiratory or cardiac arrest (Hauser, 1983; Tassinari et al., 1983).

Long-term mortality after a first episode of afebrile status was recently evaluated in a population-based retrospective cohort study in the Rochester Epidemiology Project Records (Logroscino et al., 2002). Cases surviving the first 30 days (145 out of 184) were followed until death or study termination. In this study, 19 (13%) were younger than 1 year, and 35 (24%) were between the ages of 1 and 19 years old. At 10 years, the cumulative mortality among 30-day survivors was 43% (62 deaths), 76% for patients 65 years or older, but only 5% and 2% in patients younger than 1 year and in the age group of 1 to 19 year olds, respectively. Using generalized SE as the reference group, only those with myoclonic SE had a significantly higher mortality. Within etiologic subgroups, the highest mortality rate was seen in the acute symptomatic group (27 of 66 patients) and the lowest in the idiopathic or cryptogenic group (8 of 28 patients). The mortality rate was 50% in the group that experienced SE for more than 24 hours, compared with 28% for those in whom SE lasted for less than 2 hours. These observations extend the findings of an earlier report by the same group on short-term mortality (Logroscino et al., 1997), which showed that the highest mortality was for acute symptomatic SE; similar studies (Towne et al., 1994; Lhatoo et al., 2001) demonstrate that the prognosis and outcome are mainly determined by the nature of the acute or progressive neurologic or systemic disorders that precipitate the status.

Neurologic sequelae were found in 88 of 239 children and infants with convulsive status (Aicardi and Chevrie, 1970). In 47 patients, the sequelae apparently were acquired at the time of status (20%). The neurologic syndromes encountered included diplegia, extrapyramidal syndromes, cerebellar syndromes, and decorticate rigidity. Hemiplegia, which was found in 28 patients, was always acquired at the time of status, the so-called hemiconvulsion–hemiplegia syndrome (see Chapter 10). These figures are difficult to interpret because the sequelae may represent complications of the causal disease rather than of the status itself, or they may have antedated the convulsive episode. Of 59 patients with idiopathic status seen at the time of the initial episode and followed for at least 1 year, 12 (20%) had neurologic sequelae (Aicardi and Chevrie, 1983). In the same series, mental deficits were noted after the status in 114 (48%) of 239 patients; they apparently were acquired at the time of status in 79 (33%) of all patients and in 14 (24%) of those with cryptogenic status. Similarly, Fujiwara et al. (1979) found mental and/or neurologic sequelae in 40 of 79 children with status lasting 1 hour or more, 25 of whom had hemiplegia. Mental and neurologic deficits are often associated with each another and with the epilepsy. In the series of Aicardi and Chevrie (1970), epilepsy was present after the episode of status in 44% of patients, compared with an incidence of 23% with epilepsy before the status. Furthermore, seizures occurring after SE were mainly of a type that is usually associated with brain damage (Fujiwara et al., 1979; Aicardi and Chevrie, 1970).

The outcome in symptomatic cases is significantly poorer than that in cryptogenic cases (Aicardi and Chevrie, 1983). Other unfavorable factors include young age; long duration of status; and, possibly, female gender (Chevrie and Aicardi, 1978). Sequelae of cryptogenic status were found in 35% of children younger than 3 years and in only 9% of those older than 3 years. In infants younger than 1 year, Chevrie and Aicardi (1978) found neurologic abnormalities and severe mental retardation in 8 (40%) of 20 patients with symptomatic SE and in 4 (27%) of 15 infants with idiopathic SE. However, the significance of such figures is uncertain because most reports originate from specialized hospitals and referral centers. A lower proportion of severe cases would be expected in population studies.

The proportion of cases with neurologic or mental sequelae has been considerably less in later series (Shinnar et al., 1992; Maytal and Shinnar, 1990; Phillips and Shanahan, 1989; Dunn, 1988; Vigevano, 1986), and most residua now appear to be due to the underlying disorder. The incidence of hemiconvulsion–hemiplegia syndrome, which was once common, has decreased in industrialized countries (Arzimanoglou and Dravet, 2001; Roger et al., 1982).

Similarly, the risk of recurrent status following a first episode of status has decreased. According to Shinnar et al. (1992, 1997), new episodes occur mainly in symptomatic cases and in children with abnormal neurologic signs that predate the first status; these latter children account for 88% of the recurrences. Idiopathic or febrile SE in normal children is largely an isolated event. The recurrence risk for status in idiopathic cases was only 4% for initial idiopathic status and 3% for febrile status, but this rose to 11% for cases of acute symptomatic status and to 44% for remote symptomatic cases.

The improvement in prognosis of convulsive SE is at least partly related to more effective, faster treatment. Cases of severe sequelae of apparently idiopathic status continue to be observed in developing countries, and infants or children with prolonged seizures of whatever cause should receive immediate and appropriate therapy because status remains one of the most urgent emergencies in child neurology.

Several mechanisms may be operative in the genesis of sequelae, with the main issue being whether the convulsive activity itself, independent of the cause of the seizures, is able to produce brain damage. Strong arguments supporting the hypothesis that prolonged seizures, irrespective of their cause, are able to produce brain lesions exist both experimentally (Meldrum, 1978, 1983b; Ben-Ari et al., 1979; Blennow et al., 1978) and clinically (Sagar and Oxbury, 1987; Soffer et al., 1986). However, some authors have been unable to produce brain damage in experimental models (Brown and Babb, 1983), and cases of extremely prolonged SE without sequelae have been recorded in humans. Residual damage following febrile convulsions has been associated with long-lasting and lateralized seizures and with young age at onset (Aicardi and Chevrie, 1976), whereas short bilateral convulsions have not been followed by any neurologic or mental abnormalities. However, long-lasting unilateral febrile seizures in young infants may be the result of acquired acute encephalopathies and/or preexisting unrecognized brain damage (Nelson and Ellenberg, 1978; Chevrie and Aicardi, 1975).

Some of the brain damage incurred during status is at least partly caused by complications of the seizures (e.g., hypoxia or vascular collapse) (Glaser, 1983; Scheuer, 1992), and it is therefore preventable. Some of the lesions may be related to the epileptic discharge itself, regardless of the complicating factors (Aicardi and Chevrie, 1983). The significance of the neuropathologic lesions found in the brains of patients who have had SE remains controversial. Some authors (Roger et al., 1974; Radermecker et al., 1967) have noted that the lack of correlation among the duration, location, and intensity of seizures seen clinically with the extent of pathologic damage argues against the causal role of status. Some of the discrepancy may result from the different ages of the patients studied. Although Corsellis and Bruton (1983) were only able to find acute lesions attributable to status (other than causal ones) in 1 of 12 brains of adults who died following status, they could demonstrate acute damage in the brains of all 6 children younger than 3 years who died shortly after an episode of status.

OTHER TYPES OF GENERALIZED STATUS

Tonic Status Epilepticus

Tonic status is less common than tonic-clonic or clonic status. It occurs exclusively in children and adolescents with previous epilepsy, particularly in patients with Lennox-Gastaut syndrome (LGS) (Roger et al., 1974), most of whom have some degree of mental retardation. However, tonic status also may be observed in patients with epilepsy syndromes intermediate between a typical absence epilepsy and LGS. In some cases (Devinsky et al., 1991; Alvarez et al., 1981; Bittencourt and Richens, 1981), tonic status was precipitated by the intravenous injection of diazepam or clonazepam (Alvarez et al., 1981) for the treatment of absence status in children with LGS (Tassinari et al., 1972a). Oral clonazepam also can precipitate tonic status (Bourgeois and Wad, 1988).

Several episodes of tonic status commonly occur in the same patient. The duration of tonic status may be much longer than that of other convulsive types. In a series of 28 patients by Gastaut et al. (1967), the average duration of the episodes was 9 days. The serial tonic seizures are initially typical, although they tend to last longer (70 seconds) on average than do isolated tonic seizures (15 seconds). With the repetition of the attacks, they tend to become less conspicuous, with lessening of the tonic phenomena but aggravation of autonomic manifestation, especially bronchial secretion (Roger et al., 1974). After several hours, the attacks are often limited to slight eye deviation, with respiratory irregularities and marked tracheobronchial obstruction resulting from hypersecretion.

In some patients, the attacks may be attenuated from the start (Somerville and Bruni, 1983), or they may even be subclinical. In such cases, only polygraphic recordings can demonstrate the tachycardia, changes in respiratory rhythm, and occasional hypertonus of the trunk or neck muscles. In most patients, consciousness is moderately to severely impaired. The EEG demonstrates the successive tonic seizures. Interictal tracings may show diffuse slow waves or bursts of delta or theta activity (Lugaresi and Pazzaglia, 1975). Not uncommonly, tonic status is combined with absence status. In such cases, the fast activity characteristic of tonic attacks periodically interrupts the interictal spike-wave complexes (Fig. 16.1).

Tonic status is a serious condition; 4 of the original 28 patients collected by Roger et al. died (1974). Death now appears uncommon (Tassinari et al., 1983), but tonic status is often followed by a period of confusional state that may last several days. Neurologic sequelae have not been reported following tonic status.

Myoclonic Status Epilepticus

Myoclonic status, which is characterized by the incessant repetition of massive myoclonic jerks, is an uncommon condition (Gastaut, 1983; Roger et al., 1974). It may occur in patients with myoclonic epilepsy of adolescence or in children with a mixture of generalized tonic-clonic seizures and absences or massive myoclonias (Janz, 1991; Asconapé and Penry, 1984). In such cases, consciousness may be preserved despite continuous jerking for hours. The EEG in primary types of myoclonic status shows bursts of multiple spikes that are synchronous and symmetric over homologous regions of the scalp (Gastaut and Tassinari, 1975b; Gastaut et al., 1967). Myoclonic status also may be observed in patients with degenerative myoclonus epilepsy (see Chapter 7). In such cases, the myoclonus is often less regular, and it often alternates with brief atonic seizures, either generalized or limited to a single segment or group of muscles.

Episodes of prolonged erratic myoclonic jerking with some blurring of consciousness are often present in patients with Dravet syndrome (Dravet et al., 1992a; Dalla Bernardina et al., 1982), in those with "myoclonic astatic" epilepsy, and in some children with LGS (Beaumanoir and Dravet, 1992; Aicardi and Gomes, 1988). Such episodes may erroneously suggest the possibility of degenerative disease.

Acute hypoxic-ischemic encephalopathy, such as that occurring with cardiac arrest, is a common cause of myoclonic status in adults (Celesia et al., 1988), and it can occur in children. Shorvon (1994) preferred the term *myoclonic SE in patients with coma* for such cases, as they are associated with severe diffuse brain damage. Similar cases can result from metabolic insults, such as hypoglycemia; hepatic or renal failure; or intoxication with heavy metals. Physical trauma and inflammatory diseases are seldom a

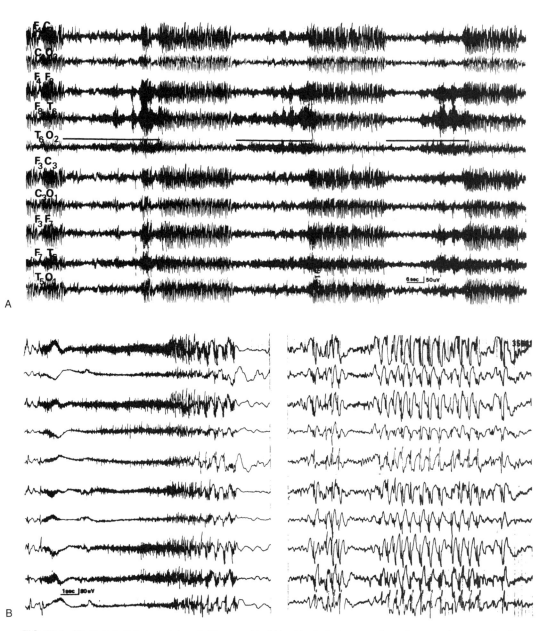

FIG. 16.1. Tonic and absence status. A 12-year-old girl had typical absences from 5 years of age and tonic axial seizures from 7.5 years of age. She had multiple episodes of absence status, some of which were interspersed with repeated tonic attacks. **Upper trace** (slow paper speed): brief tonic seizures (*underlined*) are separated by periods of high-voltage activity. **Lower trace** (normal paper speed): two samples of tracing obtained during the same recording session. **Left:** Detail of a tonic attack (clinically, tonic neck flexion, abduction of arms, and flexion of forearms with fists clenched). **Right:** High-voltage activity between tonic seizures consists of continuous slow spike-wave complexes (in the clinical observation, the child was confused and she did not respond appropriately even to simple commands). Electroencephalographic and clinical characteristics match with those of intermediate petit mal with some features of absence epilepsy and some of Lennox-Gastaut syndrome.

cause. Dialysis encephalopathy, which is observed in children undergoing extracorporeal depuration for renal failure, is typically marked by intense myoclonic activity (Foley et al., 1981).

Myoclonic status may also comprise one type of seizure activity that can be due to chemicals, such as massive doses of penicillin (Shorvon, 1994), and to intrathecally-introduced radiologic contrast agents (Aicardi and Chevrie, 1970). In the latter case, the prognosis is usually favorable.

A special form of myoclonic status has been reported in patients with fixed encephalopathy (Dalla Bernardina et al., 1992b, 2002). The myoclonic activity may be hardly detectable clinically in some cases, and a polygraphic recording may be required for demonstration. Angelman syndrome (Guerrini et al., 1996b) probably represents the most common cause. In such cases, EEG paroxysmal activity is asynchronous.

PARTIAL (OR FOCAL) CONVULSIVE STATUS EPILEPTICUS

Partial (or focal) convulsive SE applies only to those cases in which convulsive activity remains localized to a restricted segment of one side of the body, without generalization and diffusion to the whole of the affected side; a situation in which ipsilateral diffusion is seen corresponds to *unilateral status*. Admittedly, a complete separation between partial and unilateral status is arbitrary, but the clinical presentation of and consequences for strictly localized versus the more diffuse forms are quite different. These practical differences justify separating the two types. Partial somatomotor status may occur during an acute encephalopathic illness. In such cases, the seizures have a tendency to develop into secondarily generalized status (Roger et al., 1974). However, when partial motor status occurs in a chronic epileptic condition, the seizures tend to become more restricted in their extent. Even with narrowly localized seizures, autonomic disturbances and some impairment of consciousness may be present (Gastaut et al., 1967). When localized segmental myoclonus persists between partial somatomotor seizures, the resulting condition, which is known as Kojewnikow syndrome (see Chapter 10), may persist for months.

Partial convulsive status may also be symptomatic of a focal pathology; herpes encephalitis should be considered in all febrile cases. Several cases of SE of benign partial rolandic epilepsy have been reported (Colamaria et al., 1991; Boulloche et al., 1990; Roulet et al., 1989; Feldman, 1983a). These were marked by jerking of the corner of the mouth or cheek, salivation, swallowing difficulties, and absent speech, all of which are reminiscent of an anterior opercular syndrome (Roulet et al., 1989; Feldman, 1983a). The EEG in such cases shows intense paroxysmal activity that is augmented in sleep, during which continuous spike-waves can be noted (de Saint Martin et al., 1999, 2001) (see Chapter 10).

NONCONVULSIVE STATUS EPILEPTICUS

Nonconvulsive status almost always occurs in children with known epilepsy. It may be part of several epilepsy syndromes. Making a clear-cut differentiation between generalized and partial nonconvulsive SE on clinical or even electroclinical grounds is difficult and often arbitrary. The definition depends on the criteria that are applied (type of seizures and/or type of epilepsy and/or characteristics of EEG abnormalities and/or etiology).

Generalized Nonconvulsive Status Epilepticus

Generalized nonconvulsive SE is characterized clinically by variable degrees of clouding of mental processes, from simple slowing of ideation to complete unconsciousness, and electrically by bilateral discharges of spike-wave complexes (Jayakar and Seshia, 1991; Shorvon, 1987, 1994; Guberman et al., 1986; Gastaut, 1983; Porter and Penry, 1983; Roger et al., 1974).

Generalized nonconvulsive status has been variably termed *absence status* (Gastaut, 1983), *petit mal status* (Porter and Penry, 1983), *spike-wave stupor*, *epilepsia minoris continua*, or *epileptic twilight state* (Niedermeyer and Khalifeh, 1965). None of these terms is entirely satisfactory. *Absence status* may be inaccurate in cases in which only mild blunting of consciousness or slurred speech is present. *Petit mal status* implies a relationship with typical absence that does not exist in many cases, and terms like *minor epileptic status* or *twilight state* are nonspecific. Some authors distinguish between cases in which the loss of awareness is sufficiently abrupt and marked to resemble typical absences, even though they do admit that the degree of unawareness is rarely as profound as in brief typical absences, and those in which the disturbance of consciousness is less marked or in which is associated with other manifestations, such as myoclonic jerks or atonic attacks. These authors tend to relate typical absence status to the primary generalized epilepsies with typical absences and atypical absence status to LGS or secondary generalized epilepsies (Ohtahara et al., 1979). The clinical distinction between the two types, however, is often difficult, if not impossible, to make (Gastaut, 1983).

The situation is further compounded because, for some authors (Gastaut, 1983; Porter and Penry, 1983), the terms *absence* or *petit mal status* imply a clear change, both clinically and on EEG, at the time of the ictal event, whereas for others (Doose, 1983; Hess et al., 1971), they include less distinct states that are marked only by subtle behavioral alterations that may last for weeks or months without even necessarily being reversible.

Such differences in definition probably account for the various frequencies with which absence epilepsies or LGS are found in association with absence status. Roger et al. (1974) found that 69% of their patients had a history of typical absences, whereas Gastaut (1983) indicates that petit mal only exceptionally causes absence status. Similarly, Kruse (1968), Oller-Daurella (1973), and Doose (1983) state that LGS or "myoclonic astatic epilepsy" causes absence status much more commonly than does petit mal. LGS is commonly associated with *distinct* episodes of absence status, but the full range of transitions may be found between distinct episodes of absence status and prolonged bad periods during which paroxysmal EEG activity is continuous and mental efficiency is fluctuating, sometimes only during specific tasks (Erba and Cavazzuti, 1977).

Another nosologic issue is raised by the occurrence of episodes of status that are identical to those observed in primary or secondary generalized epilepsies in children with epilepsies of a clearly partial character, as the occurrence of partial seizures, fixed EEG foci, and localized lesions demonstrates. In such cases, the paroxysmal EEG activity during status is bilateral, although, at times, asymmetric, and deciding whether they should be classified as "partial" or "generalized nonconvulsive status" is difficult (see later discussion).

In 75% of cases, absence status occurs before the age of 20 years, and most take place during the first decade. Absence status is the first manifestation of epilepsy in only a small minority of patients (Porter and Penry, 1983). Even patients who have a history of typical absences rarely have pure absence epilepsy, and many develop tonic-clonic and/or myoclonic seizures (Porter and Penry, 1983; Roger et al., 1974; Andermann and Robb, 1972; Gastaut et al., 1967). Conversely, nonconvulsive status may follow generalized convulsions (Fagan and Lee, 1990).

The main clinical symptom of absence status is an impairment of consciousness that may vary from barely noticeable, which permits the automatic execution of the acts of everyday life (Matsuoka et al., 1986) or even the persistence of higher cognitive functions, which may only be slowed, to a severe impairment of consciousness, in which the patient is barely responsive. Complex automatisms may occur, and most epileptic fugues likely are manifestations of absence status (Roger et al., 1974). Motor manifestations occur in about half of the cases. These include bilateral or unilateral myoclonus and/or atonic phenomena that may be generalized, resulting in falls, head nods, sagging of the knees, or localized and clearly visible lapses of posture when the arms are extended. Rare cases may be marked predominantly by motor involvement, and these may present as ictal catatonia (Lim et al., 1986). The episodes of status are totally or partially amnesic.

The EEG shows continuous, bilaterally synchronous, symmetric epileptic activity of variable appearance. One type that features closely-spaced bursts of spike-wave complexes at 3 Hz resembling a succession of typical absences is unusual. In another type, brief bursts of 3-Hz spike-wave activity lasting less than 2 to 3 seconds occur in close succession. Less commonly, the continuous spike-wave activity occurs at a slower rhythm, and it is often irregular or arrhythmic. Another variant is slow high-amplitude background activity, usually over the frontal areas, with superimposed bursts of spike-wave complexes and occasional runs of fast (10-Hz) activity (Gastaut and Tassinari, 1975b; Roger et al., 1974; Gastaut and Broughton, 1972). Runs of fast spike-wave complexes at 4 to 6 Hz are occasionally seen (Porter and Penry, 1983). Absence status is not commonly associated with focal EEG or clinical manifestations (Janz, 1973).

The outcome of absence status is probably related more to the type and cause of the underlying epilepsy than to the duration of repetition of the episodes. Doose and Volzke (1979) argued that absence status is strongly correlated with the development of dementia in children with "myoclonic astatic epilepsy" (see Chapter 6), implying a causal relationship. Doose (1983) included hypsarrhythmia and the "bad periods" observed in LGS in their definition of absence status.

This is at odds with the experience of others (Beaumanoir and Dravet, 1992; Aicardi and Gomes, 1988), who have been unable to demonstrate a correlation between nonconvulsive status and mental outcome in children with LGS.

Whether continuous EEG discharges in deep structures without scalp concomitants may produce behavioral and/or cognitive alterations remains to be determined. Wieser (1983a, 1991) has recorded continuous paroxysms from the amygdala in four patients with severe psychiatric disturbances.

The diagnosis of generalized nonconvulsive status may be difficult. Intoxications should always be considered in cases of unexplained obtundation, and coma or confusion of metabolic origins is not rare in children. A rare, but difficult, problem is that of the cases of idiopathic stupor (Cirignotta et al., 1990; Tinuper et al., 1992), which may occur in a recurrent manner.

A new epileptic disorder associated with the *ring chromosome 20* has recently been described (Petit et al., 1999; Canevini et al., 1998; Inoue et al., 1997) as a recognizable entity; it consists of almost daily episodes of atypical absence status. The syndrome is characterized by mild to moderate mental deficiency, which manifests around the age of 6 years after initially normal development; a behavioral disorder; the lack of specific dysmorphic features; and epilepsy. The seizures usually begin in childhood, and they are reported as a fluctuating alteration of contact that lasts several minutes. These may be associated with automatic behavior, wandering, hallucinations, and an impression of fear. Short-lasting motor seizures and tonic-clonic seizures have also been reported. The ictal EEG recorded during nonconvulsive status shows high-amplitude, rhythmic slow activity, with superimposed spikes or spike-waves that predominate over the frontal regions.

Partial Nonconvulsive Status Epilepticus

Partial nonconvulsive SE is rarely reported in children, and it occurs in the course of temporal lobe or other lesional epilepsies. As Shorvon (1994) has stated, perhaps Hughlings Jackson was the first to report clearly a fugue state in temporal lobe epilepsy (Taylor, 1931), and the first case authenticated by EEG was reported by Gastaut et al. (1956). The incidence is poorly known, even in adults, but, according to Shorvon (1994), this form of status is more common in adults than other types of nonconvulsive status or even than tonic-clonic status. The terms *complex partial status* and *simple partial status*, which are regularly used in the literature, are theoretically differentiated by the presence or absence of alteration of consciousness. In fact, all intermediates from severe confusion to mild confusion to prolonged episodes of partial symptomatology (e.g., fear, blindness, and psychotic behavior) exist.

According to Gastaut and Tassinari (1975b), partial status with alteration of consciousness (termed *complex partial status* in the literature) can present in the following two forms: (a) frequently recurring partial seizures with alteration of consciousness and classic manifestations (see Chapter 10) but without full recovery of mental activity between individual seizures and (b) continuous long-lasting episodes of mental confusion and behavioral disturbances with or without automatisms. Engel et al. (1978) and Treiman and Delgado-Escueta (1983) have noted that many episodes of partial status with alteration of consciousness are characterized by cycling between the following two behavioral states: one of complete unresponsiveness, with staring, speech arrest, and stereotypic automatisms, and one of partial responsiveness, with complex, semipurposeful automatisms. From the EEG viewpoint, the two components of the cycles comprise, respectively, fast discharges over one or both temporal lobes and bilateral slow-wave activity this is often intermixed with low-voltage fast activity (Engel et al., 1978). However, the clinical and EEG picture is much more variable, and a number of patients display continuously abnormal behavior without cyclic variations. The EEG may exhibit almost any combination of more or less focal patterns, with shifting of paroxysmal activity from one side to the opposite at times (Ballenger et al., 1983; Maynard and Garrel, 1983; Treiman and Delgado-Escueta, 1983; McBride et al., 1981; McLachlan and Blume, 1980; Markand et al., 1978). The psychic manifestations of partial status with alteration of consciousness are almost indistinguishable from those of absence status, and the diagnosis rests largely on the ictal EEG recordings. However, typical absence status characteristically presents as a fluctuating confusional state with myoclonus, whereas confusion with psychotic states is suggestive of psychomotor status; confusion accompanied by euphoria and programming difficulties are seen mainly with frontal status.

Cases of partial seizures with bilateral spike-wave activity have been reported (Roger et al., 1974). However, bilateral paroxysmal activity can occur in children with partial epilepsies associated with focal brain lesions, especially frontal ones, and in cases of atypical benign partial epilepsy (see Chapter 10).

The authors have seen several children presenting with what appeared to be absence status with clouding of consciousness; innumerable atonic attacks; and, at times, erratic myoclonias. These episodes were associated with continuous or almost continuous bilateral paroxysmal EEG activity, and they lasted for several days (Fig. 16.2). The interictal EEG regularly showed a unilateral frontocentral focus of spikes and slow waves.

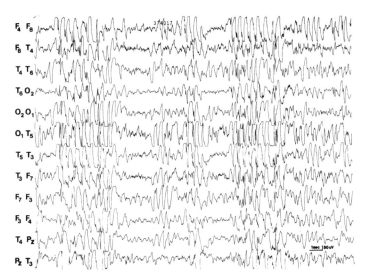

FIG. 16.2. Absence status. A 6-year-old boy had repeated episodes during which he would answer only in monosyllables and in which he appeared slightly confused. His head would nod repeatedly, at times for several hours. The electroencephalogram shows diffuse continuous, irregular, slow spike-wave complexes predominating over the right hemisphere. Brief intervals of more normal background tracing appear between high-amplitude paroxysmal bursts.

All children had hemiplegia or hemiparesis, and most had various degrees of mental retardation. All had localized congenital lesions on one side. Now, most such lesions are known to be primarily dysplastic (Guerrini et al., 1998f) (see Chapters 10 and 19).

The outcome of partial status with alteration of consciousness is imperfectly known because of the small number of reported cases, the underrecognition of episodes with spontaneous resolution, and incorrect diagnoses based on a misinterpretation of EEG abnormalities and definition problems (Kaplan, 2000). Profound memory deficit has been reported in adults (Collins et al., 1983; Engel et al., 1978). Transient neuroimaging abnormalities have been reported following partial status (Kramer et al., 1987b; Aicardi and Arzimanoglou, 1986; Sammaritano et al., 1985; Chevrie and Aicardi, 1972). They consist of localized areas of hypodensity with enhancement on computed tomographic scanning and increased T2-weighted signal on magnetic resonance imaging that is suggestive of focal edema. Such anomalies may persist for several days, and they should be distinguished from a causal lesion. Complex partial status has been observed as a complication of drug treatment, most notably cyclosporin A therapy (Appleton et al., 1989).

Depending on the location and propagation of the discharges, partial nonconvulsive status may also manifest as episodes of prolonged unmotivated fear, pro-

longed aphasia (Kanemoto and Janz, 1989; Kellerman, 1978; Roger et al., 1974), prolonged ictal blindness (SE amaurotics), or visual hallucinations. Prolonged ictal paralysis (somatoinhibitory status) is another form of nonconvulsive status that can be difficult to distinguish from Todd paresis (Tinuper et al., 1987). Nonconvulsive status may also take the form of a prolonged "aura" that is characterized by prolonged visceral or sensory symptoms (Manford and Shorvon, 1992). Among other lesional causes, the origin of such prolonged episodes may be a cortical dysplasia.

Borderlands of Status Epilepticus

Prominent psychic symptomatology with severe autistic or schizophrenic features and/or hallucinations have been observed in conscious adults and confirmed by concomitant scalp EEG or stereo-EEG recordings (Wieser, 1983a, 1991). This finding suggests the possibility that some of the psychoses observed in epileptic patients may actually represent nonconvulsive status (Wieser, 1991), even in the absence of scalp EEG paroxysms.

Prolonged postictal confusional states may follow discrete epileptic seizures (Biton et al., 1990; Fagan and Lee, 1990). Prolonged confusional states lasting 8 to 36 hours, often with psychotic features, may follow a tonic-clonic seizure or a cluster of attacks. The EEG is often grossly abnormal, so such cases can be regarded as episodes of status. Whether similar cases without paroxysmal EEG recordings are due to the same mechanism is unknown (Shorvon, 1994).

Mikati et al. (1985) reported children who presented with a picture of chronic encephalopathy with variable motor signs for months that was accompanied by marked regression of previously acquired skills and an occasional seizure. The condition was reversible. During the symptomatic period, more or less rhythmic diffuse slow waves were present in the EEG, and the neuroimaging showed no abnormalities. Whether such cases actually represent status is open to question. Similar or identical cases have been attributed to protracted encephalitis (Sebire et al., 1992).

The taxonomic situation of the "bad periods" observed in the course of LGS and some cases of myoclonic or polymorphic epilepsies is uncertain (see Chapters 4 and 5). The diagnosis of status in LGS is easy when a clear-cut and abrupt change occurs in the patient's behavior, but episodes lasting several days or weeks that start and end progressively and that include mildly decreased awareness may be difficult to interpret. Indeed, during such episodes, the EEG activity may not differ from that of "interictal" records (Beaumanoir et al., 1988).

Similarly, complete separation of nonconvulsive SE from "electrical SE" or "continuous spike-waves of slow sleep" and from epileptic aphasia (Landau-Kleffner syndrome) or even West syndrome raises insoluble taxonomic and nosographic problems (see Chapters 3 and 11).

Indeed, the continuous, intense EEG paroxysmal activity in such syndromes does not differ significantly from that observed in nonconvulsive status, and interpreting the behavioral and/or cognitive changes that accompany these syndromes as manifestations or consequences of "subclinical" nonconvulsive SE is tempting. The extreme of the spectrum may be represented by the cases of almost purely "electrical status" that cause only subtle psychic or sensory anomalies or that are completely devoid of symptoms (Shorvon, 1994).

DIAGNOSIS

Diagnosis of SE is not always easy. Although the diagnosis of *convulsive* status is unlikely to be missed, the duration of the seizures is often underestimated because the intensity of jerking tends to diminish with time so that localized twitching may become almost undetectable. The jerking may disappear altogether, even though paroxysmal EEG discharges still persist. Whether the treatment of purely electrical discharges should be pursued remains undetermined. Issues related to prolonged EEG discharges without

evident clinical symptoms in neonates are discussed in Chapter 12.

Pseudo-SE (Pakalnis et al., 1991; Shorvon, 1994) is extremely common in adults, and it is encountered in adolescents and older children (see Chapter 21). In most cases, the abnormal movements are of a thrashing or flailing character, but in a few patients, they may be more similar to true jerking. Features such as forced eye closure, its occurrence when the individual is observed, and a susceptibility to suggestion may be of considerable help. Vocalization is common, as are bizarre behavior and resistance to examination. If clinical doubt exists, an EEG can confirm the diagnosis by showing normal ictal tracings. Although the frequency of pseudo-SE is unknown, misdiagnosis is certainly common in routine hospital practice, leading to a vicious treatment cycle.

Nonconvulsive status is easily mistaken for drowsiness, inattention, or abnormal psychogenic behavior when the impairment of consciousness is mild. An occasional child may appear normal when he or she is first seen, but the parents notice a difference from the child's usual behavior. Abnormal movements, such as erratic jerking or head drops, are sometimes interpreted as tics, or they may be considered psychogenic. In fact, the converse error is possible, and pseudoabsences are not exceptional (North et al., 1990). In individual cases, minor status is either hardly identifiable, or may present in a very atypical way (e.g., with catatonia [Lim et al., 1986] or mutism [Fejerman and Di Blasi, 1987]).

Some abnormal movements of nonepileptic mechanism, such as prolonged jitteriness in infancy, may appear to mimic *partial motor status*. The authors have seen two infants with "recovery tremor" following the treatment of protein-calorie malnutrition who received a diagnosis of partial motor status because of the predominant localization of the tremor to one arm.

Prolonged occipital attacks with eye deviation, unconsciousness, and vomiting (Panayiotopoulos and Igoe, 1992) in partial epilepsies may mimic stroke or other severe insults of severe prognosis.

TREATMENT OF STATUS EPILEPTICUS

Convulsive Status Epilepticus

Convulsive status is a major emergency in the therapy of epilepsy because of its life-threatening character and the possibility of sequelae. Before considering therapy, the clinician must discard the possibility of psychogenic status, for which the intensive drug treatment applicable for true status is obviously not indicated and which would in fact be dangerous.

The main objectives of the treatment of convulsive status (Table 16.2) are threefold—(a) support of vital

TABLE 16.2. *Management of convulsive status epilepticus*

Stage	Procedure
Immediate management	1. Establish the diagnosis by clinical observation and start EEG as soon as possible, but do not delay treatment unless EEG verification of the diagnosis is necessary. Assessment and monitoring of vital functions. Secure airway. Establish i.v. catheter with normal saline[a]. Conduct blood sampling (glucose, electrolytes, urea, anticonvulsant levels). 2. Administer i.v. diazepam, 0.25–0.50 mg/kg, at no faster than 2 mg/min or i.v. lorazepam, 0.05–0.1 mg/kg (<2 mg/min). When an i.v. line is not available within the first 5–10 min, *do not delay treatment.* Use rectal administration of diazepam, (0.5–0.75 mg/kg), to a maximum of 20 mg. Rectal administration is very useful for home administration, particularly in children with frequent serial seizures.
Second stage or established status	*Steps 3 and 4 in all patients:* 3. Monitor vital functions and correction of disturbances. Secure airway (by tracheal intubation, if necessary). 4. Investigate the possible causes of status, especially any metabolic and infectious causes. Correct any metabolic derangement, particularly hypoglycemia (bolus injection of 30% glucose, 3–20 mL depending on age). 5. Administer 100 mg of pyridoxine i.v. (younger than 2 years). 6. Employ other treatments of cause if available (e.g., meningitis, encephalitis). *Steps 7 and 8, if seizures are not controlled within minutes of giving benzodiazepines:* 7. May repeat dose of diazepam but preferably pass on to step 8. 8. Administer i.v. fosphenytoin, 20 mg/kg phenytoin equivalent (fast push up to 150 mg phenytoin equivalents/min). If only phenytoin is available, give by slow i.v. push (<25–50 mg/min). If status persists, give phenobarbitone (loading dose, 20 mg/kg). In all cases monitor blood pressure and electrocardiogram. *Steps 9 to 11 for resistant status:* 9. Monitor EEG closely and ensure supervision by specialized medical and nursing personnel (in intensive care unit). 10. Consider available therapeutic agents, including paraldehyde (400 mg i.v., 200 mg/kg/h in 5% dextrose), sodium valproate (20 mg/kg as a bolus, followed by continuous infusion of 1 mg/kg/h), lidocaine (2 mg/kg i.v. as a bolus, followed by continuous i.v. infusion of 6 mg/kg/h), clonazepam as a bolus (0.25–0.50 mg repeated up to four times).
Third stage	11. When one or more of the above agents fail (step 10), the use of general anesthesia with i.v. barbiturates or halothane may be indicated. Neuromuscular blockade may be necessary for maintaining ventilation. EEG monitoring is imperative.

Abbreviations: EEG, electroencephalogram, i.v., intravenous.

The management procedures proposed in this table are not appropriate for absence status epilepticus, which may be exacerbated by phenytoin or even phenobarbital.

[a]Dextrose solutions may precipitate phenytoin. With fosphenytoin, either dextrose or saline is acceptable.

functions, (b) identification and treatment of causal or precipitating factors, and (c) termination of ictal activity.

A second point worth emphasizing is that status often has a prodromal stage, at least in those patients with previous epilepsy. Serial seizures or a sudden worsening in the habitual seizure pattern is a common warning. At this stage, the early use of diazepam, preferably intravenously, is often sufficient to prevent further seizures (Lombroso, 1989; Shorvon, 1994).

Once status is established, which generally occurs without warning in patients with an acute cause to their seizures, the patient should be hospitalized and closely monitored.

A high proportion of the complications of SE in humans result from such factors as systemic hypotension, lack of oxygen, and lactic acidosis (Scheuer, 1992; Brown and Hussain, 1991a; Kreisman et al., 1983). Devoting scrupulous attention to the acid-base balance and cardiorespiratory and pulmonary functioning is, therefore, mandatory (Treiman and Delgado-Escueta, 1980; Simon, 1985). While the child is being transported to the hospital, he or she should be placed in a lateral prone position to avoid aspiration and to facilitate a clear airway (Brown and Hussain, 1991b). A soft plastic oral airway should be taped in place. In the hospital, tracheal intubation is performed if the status is not rapidly controlled. Some authors advocate the routine administration of oxygen even before further clinical and laboratory investigations are performed. A secure venous line should be available for administration of fluids; for blood sampling for routine laboratory determinations, especially blood glucose, calcium, magnesium, and other electrolytes and for monitoring blood levels of AEDs. During status, hyperthermia occurs relatively frequently.

Saline, not glucose, should be given, because phenytoin may precipitate in a glucose solution. An intraarterial line should be avoided because the intraarterial injection of some antiepileptic agents, including the benzodiazepines, phenytoin, and chlormethiazole, may cause severe arterial spasm. A 50% glucose solution should be given if hypoglycemia is suspected, and intravenous pyridoxine (100 to 200 mg) should be administered systematically to infants younger than 24 months (Baxter, 2002; Mikati et al., 1991; Goutières and Aicardi, 1985; Bankier et al., 1983) at the onset of treatment and certainly before long-acting anticonvulsants are used (Goutières and Aicardi, 1985) to avoid missing the rare diagnosis of pyridoxine dependency. Emergency investigations include blood gas analyses, sugar and calcium levels, and blood levels of AEDs in all previously treated patients. Information from relatives concerning epilepsy history, drug regimen, and details on dose and last administration of ongoing antiepileptic treatment must eventually be obtained.

The identification of precipitating factors should be conducted at the same time as the treatment of status is initiated. The main precipitating factors in children include (a) acute CNS insult, especially meningoencephalitis; (b) metabolic disorders (most commonly those involving sodium, calcium, or glucose); (c) acute poisoning, whether accidental or therapeutic, with substances such as tricyclic antidepressant drugs (Messing et al., 1984), theophylline (Schwartz and Scott, 1974; Dunn, 1988), or piperazine; and (d) the withdrawal of chronic anticonvulsant drug therapy.

EEG monitoring is advised for patients who remain unconscious after the initial phase of treatment or who require prolonged therapy for refractory status. The suspected diagnosis of nonconvulsive status should be confirmed by EEG monitoring before the administration of other antiepileptic agents is pursued. EEG facilities and qualified personnel in emergency departments are required for optimal care. However, a lack of EEG facilities is no excuse for delaying treatment.

Symptomatic early therapy of SE includes mainly the benzodiazepines, especially diazepam, phenytoin or fosphenytoin, and phenobarbital. Other agents such as valproate, lidocaine, and anesthetic barbiturates are less commonly employed. Drug treatment in the prodromal (see earlier discussion) and early stages of status is relatively noncontroversial and highly effective. Recent retrospective studies have suggested that the prehospital treatment of status shortens the duration of the event and simplifies the subsequent management in the emergency department (Alldredge et al., 1995). The *recommended total dose* of the drug chosen must be administered at onset. In the later, more severe stages, the treatment becomes more difficult to apply, and it is less effective as time passes. Therefore, the most important part of the treatment is the most simple one, applied wherever the patient happens to be, rather than delaying therapy until late in the intensive care unit.

The drug used should be administered by a route enabling rapid and efficient absorption. This is best accomplished by intravenous administration. In the case of diazepam and perhaps of valproate, the rectal route may be used. The *intramuscular route is contraindicated*, except for midazolam, because the absorption is irregular and slow (Brown and Hussain, 1991b). This rule also applies to the intramuscular administration of fosphenytoin because therapeutic levels of both total and free phenytoin are not attained until as late as 30 minutes after injection (Uthman et al., 1996). An exception to the rule may be made only when an appropriate venous route is not possible.

Once the control of status is obtained, the decision for chronic treatment should be based on the general rules of epilepsy therapy (see Chapter 23 and 24). Even in cases of an initially refractory status, no proof exists indicating that the drug that controlled the status is necessarily the most appropriate for chronic treatment.

Benzodiazepines

Diazepam is the most often employed because it can easily be administered by either the venous or rectal routes (Tassinari et al, 1983; Fröscher, 1979; Dulac et al., 1978; Browne and Penry, 1973), it penetrates the brain almost immediately (Schmidt, 1985), and it is highly effective in terminating most types of status. Browne and Penry (1973) found that the long-lasting control of status was attained in 62% to 83% of patients and temporary control in an additional 13% to 27% (except myoclonic status). Less favorable results have been reported in status due to acute brain lesions. However, fat body tissues rapidly take up diazepam, which is highly lipid soluble, with a resulting decrease in the blood level of diazepam and the subsequent release of diazepam in the brain into the blood. In practice, this phenomenon is reflected both by the high incidence of recurrent seizures 15 to 30 minutes after administering diazepam (Fröscher, 1979) and by the occurrence of respiratory depression or even arrest that may occur after repeated doses when the release from fat tissue occurs. This occurs because diazepam and its metabolite, *N*-desmethyl diazepam, have relatively long half-lives (Woodbury et al., 1982).

At regular doses of diazepam, the toxicity is low (Strandjord, 1984), with the main danger being respiratory depression and, very seldom, cardiocirculatory depression. Respiratory arrest has rarely been seen in children and adolescents. The previous administration of barbiturates certainly increases the risk of respiratory depression, but, even in that circumstance, it remains small.

Diazepam is regarded by many authors (Strandjord, 1984; Fröscher, 1979; Duffy and Lombroso, 1978), including these writers, as the drug of first choice in the early treatment of SE. The possibility of administering the drug by the rectal route represents an important advantage for the initial treatment of status in small convulsing children. Diazepam may be given with caution to patients who have previously received a loading dose of a long-acting anticonvulsant drug (Aicardi, 1990b; Brown and Hussain, 1991b). Special caution should be exercised when phenobarbital is the loading drug. Diazepam is *not* indicated for patients with repeated seizures who have already received two or more injections of the drug or for those with brief seizures separated by relatively long intervals. It should not be given to patients in a postconvulsive coma (Brown and Hussain, 1991b).

Several authors (Treiman and Delgado-Escueta, 1980; Wilder, 1983) now consider diazepam not to be the first choice agent for the treatment of SE because of its short action and the rapid release of diazepam from the brain, especially when combined with the risk of respiratory arrest. Some authors, however, use diazepam if long-acting drugs fail to arrest status (Brown and Hussain, 1991b). Others have suggested the usage of diazepam in combination with phenytoin for all cases of status (Treiman and Delgado-Escueta, 1980). That technique takes advantage of the rapid penetration of diazepam into the brain, which prevents delay in treatment before therapeutic brain levels of phenytoin are achieved.

The usual dose of diazepam is 0.2 to 0.5 mg per kg in infants and children, and this is given as a single intravenous bolus. The dose may be repeated after 10 to 20 minutes. Injection of the smallest possible amount to control the seizures (0.2 to 0.5 mg every 2 to 5 minutes to a maximum of 5 mg in children younger than 5 years and 1 mg every 2 to 5 minutes to a maximum of 10 mg in older children) is satisfactory in many cases (Brown and Hussain, 1991b). Larger doses are usually tolerated without problems, but they should not be administered if no possibility of ventilatory support is available. Using the rectal route, doses of 0.5 to 1 mg per kg are effective (Knudsen, 1979; Dulac et al., 1978). With these doses, blood levels in excess of 0.3 to 2 μg per mL are obtained, but these decrease by 34% to 50% during the first 20 minutes after intravenous injection and by 62% to 72% during the first 2 hours after intravenous or rectal injection (Dulac et al., 1978). A continuous diazepam infusion of 0.1 mg per kg per hour for not more than a few hours has been used to maintain stable therapeutic levels (Treiman and Delgado-Escueta, 1980), but this generally is not now recommended.

If an intravenous infusion is administered, the solution should be freshly prepared, because diazepam is absorbed by polyvinyl chloride plastics. Furthermore, the infusion should be carefully mixed; 20 mg of diazepam should not be dissolved in less than 250 mL of solvent (4% dextrose, 0.18% sodium chloride) because of the danger of precipitation in higher concentrations (Shorvon, 1994).

Lorazepam has a longer duration of action than does diazepam (Shorvon, 1994). Human data indicate that the drug has a half-life of 13 to 15 hours and that it rapidly penetrates the CNS (Levy and Krall, 1984; Ameer and Greenblatt, 1981; Gluckman and Stein, 1978). Although reports had indicated that lorazepam may have less cardiorespiratory-depressant effects than diazepam, recent research has not confirmed this advantage. However, no secondary release occurs, and the drug does appear quite safe and effective (Giang and McBride, 1988; Deshmukh et al., 1986; Lacey et al., 1986; Leppik et al., 1983a), so it is recommended for early established status. The doses used in children have been on the order of 0.05 to 0.25 mg per kg (Lacey et al., 1986; Walker et al., 1979). Its efficacy is similar to that of diazepam.

Treiman et al. (1998) reported the results of a recent double-blind study in adults comparing four intravenous regimens for the treatment of either *overt generalized status,* which was defined as recurrent convulsions without complete recovery between seizures, or *subtle status,* which was defined as the stage of generalized convulsive status when the patient is in continuous coma but only subtle motor convulsions are seen. Patients were randomly assigned to receive intravenous treatment with lorazepam, phenobarbital, phenytoin, or diazepam followed by phenytoin. In the group of overt generalized status, lorazepam was successful in 65% of those who received it, phenobarbital in 58%, diazepam and phenytoin in 56%, and phenytoin in 44%. In the group of subtle status, no significant differences among the treatments were detected. In an intention-to-treat analysis, the differences among the treatment groups were not significant, among either the patients with overt SE or those with subtle SE.

Clonazepam appears to be roughly as efficient as diazepam (Tassinari et al., 1983; Congdon and Forsythe, 1980), but it has no major advantages. It may actually produce more bronchial and salivary secretion with their consequent risks. In an occasional patient, however, it may arrest status after diazepam has failed. The drug is best given by bolus injections of 0.5 mg over 30 seconds; these can be repeated if necessary. It should diluted with 1 mL of water immediately before injection.

Midazolam, a fast-acting benzodiazepine (Bell et al., 1991; Raines et al., 1990; Ghilain et al., 1988; Jawad et al., 1986), has the advantage of rapid absorption with intramuscular administration, and it is well suited for early phase or premonitory SE. At doses ranging from 0.15 to 0.3 mg per kg, midazolam has been shown to control convulsive seizure activity effectively (Bebin and Bleck, 1994). Recently, midazolam has been used for the treatment of refractory status (Parent and Lowenstein, 1994; Kumar and Bleck, 1992). The intramuscular administration of midazolam is as effective as that of intravenous diazepam in abolishing interictal spikes on EEG recordings (Leszczyszyn and Pellock, 2001). The drug is also used in children (Pellock, 1998), but the dosing of midazolam for status has not been established. An open-label, randomized, controlled study (Singhi et al., 2002) compared continuous midazolam with diazepam infusion for refractory convulsive SE in 40 children from 2 to 12 years of age. Refractory status was controlled in 18 (86%) and 17 (89%) patients in the midazolam and diazepam groups, respectively, and the median time to seizure control was similar (16 minutes). However, seizures recurred in more children in the midazolam group (57% versus 16% in the diazepam group; *p*<0.05).

Leszczyszyn and Pellock (2001) recommend a dose of 0.15 to 0.3 mg per kg. Thus, children younger than 6 months should receive an initial dose of 0.5 to 2 mg, and children 6 to 12 months of age, an initial intravenous dose of 1 to 4 mg. For children from 1 to 5 years of age, the initial dose ranges from 1.5 to 10 mg depending on the child's weight; it can be as high as 15 or 20 mg for older children.

For both diazepam and midazolam, the intranasal and buccal routes of administration have also been proposed (Fisgin et al., 2002; Wassner et al., 2001; Lahat et al., 2000).

Phenytoin and Fosphenytoin

Phenytoin alone (Albani, 1983; Wilder, 1983; Cranford et al., 1979) or in combination with diazepam (Treiman and Delgado-Escueta, 1980) is considered the drug of first choice in the treatment of status by several authorities. To control SE quickly and to prevent its recurrence, a high serum concentration is mandatory. This can be obtained only by giving a loading dose of the drug intravenously. Phenytoin is extremely effective for convulsive SE (Brown and Hussain, 1991b; Simon, 1985; Wilder, 1983), and it may be more effective than the benzodiazepines for patients with partial status (Tassinari et al., 1983), although this was not confirmed in a recent double-blind study (Treiman et al. 1998). Control can be achieved in 75% to 80% of patients with status with previous epilepsy but in lower percentages of those with symptomatic seizures (Leppik et al., 1983b). It can be used safely and efficaciously in infancy and childhood (Albani, 1983). One of its advantages is that it does not depress the level of alertness as much as the alternative drugs do, and it therefore permits a better evaluation of mental status. Combining phenytoin with the benzodiazepines is probably safer than phenobarbital if adjunctive therapy is required. The therapeutic range of phenytoin serum concentrations required for control of status is probably about 10 to 25 μg per mL (Brown and Hussain, 1991b; Turnbull et al., 1984). A loading dose of 10 to 20 mg per kg produce a therapeutic concentration for 6 to 24 hours in most patients. In children, blood level monitoring is necessary to determine the need for additional doses, as the metabolism of phenytoin may vary considerably in them, especially during the first few years of life (Aicardi, 1980c).

Intravenous phenytoin should be given at a maximum rate of 1 mg per kg per minute because of the risk of cardiorespiratory depression that is associated with faster administration (Albani, 1983). The drug should not be mixed with intravenous fluids because of the possibility of precipitation. The vein should be flushed with saline after the administration of phenytoin, as it is a highly basic substance. Penetration of phenytoin into the brain may take from a few minutes to as long as 20 to 60 minutes (Wilder, 1983; Wilder et al., 1977) to reach a peak level. In any case, the time necessary for infusion is such that peak blood and brain levels and maximum therapeutic effects cannot be obtained before 20 to 60 minutes (Treiman and Delgado-Escueta, 1980); therefore, the combination of phenytoin with diazepam is advantageous as the seizures may otherwise continue for a relatively long period before maximum brain uptake is achieved (Wilder, 1983; Wilder et al., 1977). Complications of phenytoin treatment include hypotension, cardiac arrhythmias, and respiratory arrest. Such complications are rare in children. No comparative data about the relative frequency of complications with diazepam and phenytoin are available at this time. The drug should not be used for patients with a known allergy to phenytoin.

In contrast to phenytoin, *fosphenytoin*, a phosphate ester prodrug of phenytoin, is freely soluble in aqueous solutions. The safety, tolerance, and pharmacokinetics of fosphenytoin following administration to patients with SE, patients with epilepsy, and neurosurgical patients have been studied (Browne et al., 1996; Uthman et al., 1996; Leppik et al., 1990). The conversion half-life is approximately 10 to 15 minutes, and the metabolism of the drug begins immediately upon introduction into the blood system. The prior administration of diazepam has no effect on the protein binding of fos-

phenytoin (Hussey et al., 1990). Doses of fosphenytoin are expressed as phenytoin equivalents, which correspond to the amounts of phenytoin released by the drug. Loading doses of fosphenytoin should be administered at 150 mg per minute when the rapid achievement of therapeutic levels of phenytoin is desired. When administered at 150 mg per minute, 1,200 mg of fosphenytoin (approximately 15 mg per kg) is bioequivalent, in terms of the rate and extent of systemic exposure to free phenytoin, to a 1,200 mg dose of phenytoin infused at the maximum recommended rate of 50 mg per minute. Thus, both drugs likely have a similar time to onset in controlling status. No clinically significant differences between the hypotensive or adverse cardiac effects of loading doses have been reported. In large clinical trials with *fosphenytoin*, the most common side effects have been related to the CNS; they include nystagmus, headache, ataxia, and somnolence. Infusion-site reactions (phlebitis and soft tissue damage) are less common with fosphenytoin (Lowenstein and Alldredge, 1998).

As part of larger studies concerning intravenous and intramuscular administration of fosphenytoin, a limited number of patients ranging from 5 to 18 years of age have been studied. In this group, no significant differences in efficacy, adverse effects, or pharmacokinetics have been demonstrated compared with adults of up to 40 years of age (Pellock, 1996). In young children, the initial intravenous administration of fosphenytoin should consist of 15 to 25 mg of phenytoin equivalents, with a rate of administration of up to 3 mg per kg per minutes. The mean dose for a child younger than 12 months is between 60 and 250 mg per kg of phenytoin equivalent; between 300 and 1,200 mg per kg of phenytoin equivalent should be administered to older children, based on the recommended dose of 20 mg per kg. Although the intramuscular administration should be avoided for the treatment of status, the ability to administer fosphenytoin by either route has important implications for facilitating administration in children in whom establishing intravenous access may be particularly difficult. Furthermore, the type of vessel needed for intravenous administration is significantly different (Pellock, 1996). Pharmacokinetic and safety studies are needed for neonates.

Phenobarbital

Phenobarbital is a powerful drug for the treatment of convulsive SE. However, in animals, maximum blood concentrations of phenobarbital do not occur until 20 minutes after intravenous administration

(Goldberg and McIntyre, 1983), and the penetration into the CNS may take 60 minutes or more. In human patients with SE, however, the distribution half-life of phenobarbital has been found to be less than 5 minutes, and patients treated in this study (Goldberg and McIntyre, 1983) stopped convulsing within a few minutes of administration, with peak serum concentrations of less than 15 µg per mL. This was speculatively attributed to the hypermetabolic activity in convulsing patients.

A major disadvantage of phenobarbital is the marked and prolonged sedative effects it produces. Respiratory depression and hypotension are also potential hazards, and tracheal intubation and artificial ventilation may be required when high doses of phenobarbital are used. The drug may be useful for patients with anoxic encephalopathy because phenobarbital reduces the metabolic rate of the brain. The recommended dose of phenobarbital has not been precisely determined. High loading doses are advised in neonates (see Chapter 12), whereas some authors have used much lower doses (3 to 5 mg per kg) in adults with SE (Goldberg and McIntyre, 1983). A second dose of equal magnitude may be given if the seizures persist 15 to 30 minutes after injection. Goldberg and McIntyre (1983) found that such doses, which usually produce serum levels of less than 15 mg/mL, were effective in controlling status. Larger doses of 10 to 20 mg per kg may be necessary (Crawford et al., 1988; Treiman and Delgado-Escueta, 1980). For refractory status, doses of 40 to 80 mg per kg can be used with respiratory support. Phenobarbital can be mixed with the usual intravenous solutions. The rate of administration should not exceed 60 mg per minute in adults. In the Veterans Affairs cooperative study, phenobarbital was found to be as efficacious in treating status as lorazepam and diazepam plus phenytoin, and it was a better first drug than phenytoin alone (Treiman et al., 1998).

Other Drugs

Other drugs are used mostly in cases of refractory SE (i.e., those statuses that cannot be controlled by adequate dosage of one or two of the three major drugs and/or by correction of precipitating factors).

Valproate or valproic acid can be administered by an oral (Barnes et al., 1976) or rectal (Vajda et al., 1978) route for the treatment of refractory convulsive status. Although some success has been achieved in a limited number of patients, valproate is, at best, an experimental agent for treatment of status. An intravenous preparation is now available. The dose suggested is 15 mg per kg, followed by 1 mg/kg per hour

(Giroud et al., 1993). Multicenter, controlled studies of intravenous valproate in SE are lacking, and further experience, probably with higher doses, is needed. In neonates, a metabolic screening may be necessary before administering sodium valproate for serial seizures or status.

Paraldehyde is sometimes used as a first drug, especially when no facilities for intravenous injection or resuscitation are available. Paraldehyde can probably control convulsive SE in a high proportion of both adult and pediatric patients. It may also control status when other agents fail, and it may be more effective for generalized than for partial SE. The intramuscular administration of paraldehyde can produce abscesses. The dose of paraldehyde for the treatment of SE is 0.1 to 0.15 mL per kg. The intravenous administration of paraldehyde may also be hazardous (Shorvon, 1994; Brown and Hussain, 1991b). Absorption by the oral route is slower than by the intramuscular route, and this route is best avoided in convulsing patients because of the risk of inhalation. The rectal route (paraldehyde diluted 2 to 1 in olive or cottonseed oil or in 200 mL of 0.9% sodium chloride) is often used because of the ease of administration (Lombroso, 1978). The risk of cardiorespiratory depression is small, but hypotension, pulmonary edema, and sterile abscesses may occur. Intravenous paraldehyde solution is no longer commercially available in the United States.

Chlormethiazole is still a popular mode of therapy in the United Kingdom, but it is not commonly used in other countries; its use is not licensed in the United States. It seems effective against convulsive status in children and adults (Shorvon, 1994; Browne, 1983a), even after the failure of other agents. The drug can cause respiratory and circulatory depression. Its action is rapid, and its clearance is initially fast because of redistribution into nonvascular compartments and accumulation, which makes prolonged infusion dangerous. After 24 to 48 hours, the half-life markedly increases; prolonged administration, therefore, carries the risk of sudden coma and cardiocirculatory collapse. Chlormethiazole is given as an intravenous infusion of 20 to 60 mg per minute, followed by a maintenance infusion of 4 to 8 mg per minute in a 0.8% solution. The rate of administration in children is 0.01 mL per kg per minute, increased every 2 to 4 hours until control is achieved or the child becomes drowsy. Prolonged use should be avoided.

Lidocaine seems effective against convulsive SE. However, the antiepileptic action of the drug is transient, lasting 20 to 30 minutes. Therefore, a continuous lidocaine infusion is usually necessary to avoid the recurrence of seizures. The initial dose is 1.5 to 2 mg per kg. If this dose is effective but a secondary recurrence of seizures occurs, a lidocaine infusion rate of 3 to 14 mg per kg per hour is recommended (Walker and Slovis, 1997; Radvanyi-Bouvet et al., 1990; Pascual et al., 1988; Browne, 1983a). The rate of infusion should be carefully controlled because high doses of lidocaine can precipitate convulsions.

Propofol is another short-acting intravenous anesthetic that can be administered by bolus or infusion (Brown and Levin, 1998; Stecker et al., 1998), but controlled studies for the use of the drug in children with status are not available. Propofol is extremely lipid soluble, and it is bound to plasma proteins at 97% to 98%. Its induction characteristics are similar to those of thiopentone, with a dose-related depression of consciousness and cardiovascular and respiratory function. In the patient who has not been previously medicated, the dose of propofol of 1 to 2 mg per kg is usually sufficient to induce anesthesia, and infusion rates of 6 to 12 mg per kg per hour are required to maintain anesthesia in surgery (Shorvon, 1994; Lowenstein and Alldredge, 1998). The drug is administered as a 1% solution in a 20-mL ampoule containing 10 mg per mL (i.e., 200 mg) as an emulsion. The regimen used in status consists of an initial bolus dose of 2 mg per kg that can be repeated if seizures continue, followed by an infusion of about 5 to 10 mg per kg per hour with the dose guided by the EEG. The infusion is typically maintained for 12 to 24 hours and is then withdrawn gradually. Intensive care unit facilities, assisted respiration, and EEG monitoring are required. Propofol has the advantage of a very rapid onset of action and recovery with only minor hemodynamic side effects. However, very little has been published on its use in status or on the effects of prolonged infusion in children. The drug commonly causes involuntary movements that should not be mistaken for convulsions. Seizures have been reported during the induction of anesthesia with propofol and with emergence from it (Mäkelä et al., 1993), but the importance of these proconvulsant effects in the management of SE is unknown (Lowenstein and Alldredge, 1998). A prolonged infusion in the large doses required in status results in marked lipemia, an accumulation of inactive glucuronide metabolites, and a metabolic acidosis, particularly in children, in whom doses as large as 9 to 15 mg per kg are usually required (Shorvon, 1994). Cases of severe metabolic acidosis and rhabdomyolysis have been recorded (Hanna and Ramundo, 1998; Parke et al., 1992).

In refractory status, after subanesthetic doses of other agents, *general anesthesia* is indicated as a last resort. It controls convulsive movements and reduces cerebral seizure activity and metabolic needs. This can be achieved with barbiturate or nonbarbiturate anesthetics. Inhalation anesthesia has a number of drawbacks, and it requires operative room environment (Opitz et al., 1983). *Halothane* depresses the cerebral metabolism, and it may increase intracranial pressure. *Isoflurane* has a consistent effect in suppressing EEG activity, a rapid action, and a short half-life, but its use has not been fully assessed.

Pentobarbital is used much more commonly (Van Ness, 1990; Osorio and Reed, 1989; Rashkin et al., 1987; Goitein et al., 1983). Intubation and artificial ventilation are necessary. Intravenous pentobarbital is first given as a bolus of 50 to 100 mg, with further doses of 25 to 30 mg every 2 to 3 minutes until the seizures are controlled or vital functions are impaired. The infusion should then be maintained at a rate sufficient to control seizure activity and to produce a burst-suppression pattern of EEG (Tasker et al., 1989). Accumulation with cardiovascular collapse is a risk of prolonged administration, and the doses and techniques of monitoring are essentially determined empirically.

Keeping certain general points in mind is essential. If status is caused by drug withdrawal, the immediate replacement of the missing drug is imperative, and this may be all that is required. Emergency treatment should be immediately followed by the initiation of an oral drug regimen by nasogastric tube to avoid the recrudescence of seizures upon the discontinuation of acute therapy. The administration of inadequate small doses initially, while intending to give the total recommended dose only if more seizures occur, is a mistake because this ignores the reality that controlling status at onset is easier. The intramuscular route should not be used except with midazolam. In exceptional cases, emergency resective surgery has been successfully used (Ma et al., 2001; Gorman et al., 1992).

Nonconvulsive Status Epilepticus

In *generalized nonconvulsive status*, the most effective agent is usually diazepam, which is administered intravenously at the same doses and with the same precautions as in convulsive status. Diazepam is effective in 80% to 100% of patients with nonconvulsive generalized status occurring in the setting of primary generalized epilepsy (Tassinari et al., 1983). The effect of diazepam may be transient, and several doses may be necessary at intervals of 15 to 30 minutes. An oral drug (ethosuximide or valproate) should be started while the diazepam is being administered if the status is the initial epileptic event. The effectiveness of diazepam for episodes of absence status that occur in the setting of secondary generalized epilepsies (LGS and atypical forms) is much more limited than for primary types. Tassinari et al. (1983) found that diazepam or other benzodiazepines terminated absence status in only 15% to 59% of secondary cases, compared with 90% to 100% of primary cases.

In a few patients, the benzodiazepines precipitate the transformation of absence status into tonic status, which may be more dangerous (Levy and Krall, 1984; Bittencourt and Richens, 1981). The use of benzodiazepines must be immediately abandoned if tonic manifestations occur or if an increase in fast, high-amplitude, 10-Hz paroxysmal activity is seen in the EEG. Phenytoin is not indicated in the treatment of absence status.

Some authors have advised the use of intravenous acetazolamide because it has few side effects and it can be effective (Brown and Hussain, 1991b). The dose of intravenous acetazolamide for absence status is 250 mg for children weighing less than 35 kg and 500 mg for those weighing more than 35 kg. Presumably, acetazolamide is effective only in the primary forms of absence status, for which diazepam is almost constantly efficacious.

The treatment of partial nonconvulsive SE does not differ fundamentally from that of convulsive status. Because the degree of emergency may be less, some authors prefer not to use intravenous benzodiazepines in such cases, and they begin treatment with intravenous phenytoin or phenobarbital (Browne and Penry, 1973). However, the benzodiazepines have given good results in 62% to 73% of cases of temporal lobe or psychomotor status (Tassinari et al., 1983; Browne and Penry, 1973).

Serial Seizures

Repetitive seizures do not meet all the criteria of SE. However, many cases of status are the end point of a series of epileptic events. No studies are available on when and how serial seizures should be treated. Many clinicians use intravenous diazepam, perhaps because of tradition rather than pharmacokinetics (Bleck, 1999). Some authors (Mitchell, 1996; Payne and Bleck, 1996) have suggested that lorazepam is a better choice because the anticonvulsant effect of a single dose of diazepam is quite brief (20 minutes), whereas that of lorazepam is much longer (approximately 4 hours), and because the risk of respiratory depression is potentially greater with diazepam. Midazolam may also be a drug of choice (Bleck, 1999).

In children known to have serial seizures that may lead to status or a generalized tonic-clonic seizure, parents should be give instruction in the use of rectal diazepam. In older children or adolescents, the authors often advise the occasional use of a single dose of oral clobazam (10 to 20 mg), which may eventually be repeated if serial seizures persist.

SUMMARY

SE is a condition characterized by the repetition of epileptic seizures at brief intervals without recovery of consciousness between the attacks or by prolongation of a seizure such that an enduring epileptic condition is produced. As many types of SE exist as there are types of epileptic seizures.

Convulsive tonic-clonic SE, whether generalized or unilateral, is the most common and most dangerous form. This type of status is caused by an acute or chronic encephalopathy in more than half the cases. Cryptogenic status is more common in infants and children than in adults. Approximately half of the cases of cryptogenic status are associated with fever, and they may represent prolonged febrile convulsions. Unilateral clonic SE is a common type in infancy and early childhood. It may not be associated with the presence of a focal lesion, and it may have the same causes as generalized status. Convulsive status may end in death, or it may leave severe mental and/or neurologic sequelae. Although most sequelae are due to the underlying disorder, the convulsive activity may contribute to or be responsible for some residua. Therefore, emergency treatment is imperative. The aims of treatment are (a) to maintain vital functions, (b) to diagnose and treat any precipitating condition, and (c) to terminate the convulsive activity as soon as possible. Intravenous diazepam alone often immediately arrests SE. The recurrence of the seizures is not uncommon, and this is best treated with loading doses of fosphenytoin, phenytoin, or phenobarbital. Lorazepam has a similar efficacy according to certain studies. The combination of diazepam or lorazepam and a loading dose of phenytoin or fosphenytoin is advocated by several authors as initial therapy of convulsive SE. Refractory cases may require the use of several drugs, with their attendant hazards of respiratory and circulatory depression, and these should be treated in an intensive care unit. In general, however, status should be treated promptly whenever it occurs, and it can probably be prevented in many patients by the prompt administration of diazepam. The rectal route is suitable for the early treatment of convulsive seizures that do not stop within a few minutes.

Convulsive tonic SE occurs mainly in patients with LGS. It may last several days, and it may be refractory to most drugs. Phenytoin may be the best drug for this condition.

Nonconvulsive SE includes generalized forms called *absence status* or *petit mal status*. These are characterized by variable degrees of clouding of consciousness that often is associated with more or less complex automatic or semipurposeful behaviors and by bilateral paroxysmal activity of the spike-wave type on the EEG. Absence status may be seen in epilepsies featuring typical absences, LGS, and various forms of myoclonic epilepsy. Clouding of consciousness can be so slight that prolonged episodes of status may be difficult to distinguish from the bad periods often observed during the course of such epileptic syndromes. Absence status does not produce death or neurologic sequelae. Its effect on intellectual function is controversial, although typical absence status is probably harmless in that regard. Treatment of absence status with the benzodiazepines is extremely effective for patients with primary generalized epilepsy. For patients with LGS, the benzodiazepines are much less efficacious, and they may induce tonic SE.

Partial nonconvulsive status is uncommon, and it can be difficult to distinguish from generalized nonconvulsive status without EEG studies. Transitional forms, with bilateral paroxysmal EEG activity diffusing from a localized area of brain damage, may be more common than the classic form in children. Treatment of partial nonconvulsive status is the same as that of convulsive SE.

17

Stimulus-Sensitive Epilepsies

Epileptic seizures are paroxysmal events, and many, if not most, are likely precipitated by known or unknown factors acting on a central nervous system (CNS) that is predisposed to the production of epileptic discharges by the presence of an organic lesion, a genetically determined neuronal hyperexcitability, or both. The known precipitating influences are quite varied. Aird (1988) indicated that 40 seizure-precipitating mechanisms are known, some 10 of which vary from hour to hour depending on habits and the daily activities of the patients. Tension states, alterations in the level of consciousness, sleep deprivation, disturbances of acid-base and water balances, drug withdrawal, proconvulsant drugs, and sensory stimuli all are important factors. Psychologic factors are probably common precipitants of certain types of seizures (Wolf and Inoue, 2002; Verduyn et al., 1988). Some may be specific, with a given psychologic situation regularly provoking seizures. More commonly, seizure-facilitating psychologic factors are nonspecific; these may include stress (Friis, 1990; Aird, 1988); excitation; or, conversely, inattentiveness and boredom (Papini et al., 1984). The regulation of such precipitating factors, both psychologic and otherwise, may play a significant role in the stabilization and improvement of epilepsy in selected patients. One estimation has indicated that such factors were of crucial importance in 17% of a group of refractory patients (Aird et al., 1984).

In some cases, specific stimuli regularly and reproducibly evoke seizures or facilitate their occurrence (Newmarck, 1983). These stimuli are of various natures, and some (e.g., hyperventilation) are routinely employed in the diagnosis of some forms of epilepsy (see Chapter 8). Seizures induced by specific sensory stimuli, which are often called *reflex epilepsy* (Zifkin et al., 1998), and, to a lesser extent, by specific psychic precipitants form a small but interesting set of seizure disorders. Such seizures may be broadly classified into two groups. The first group includes those patients in whom attacks are always or almost always evoked by a specific stimulus, such as flickering light, reading, and music. The second group consists of those who have spontaneous seizures in addition to

their stimulus-sensitive attacks. The second type is relatively common, and 5% to 6% of patients with epilepsy are estimated to have a seizure disorder that some specific sensory stimuli may exacerbate (Binnie and Jeavons, 1992). Such a distinction, however, is not absolute because the epilepsies of some patients may pass through successive stages during which seizures occur spontaneously or only after exposure to a specific stimulus. Stimulus-sensitive seizures are often clinically stereotyped, and they are associated with a consistent electroencephalographic (EEG) pattern that may be reproduced under laboratory conditions. However, the appearance of a well-defined EEG pattern with exposure to a given stimulus is not sufficient to characterize the associated seizures as "stimulus sensitive." Many patients, for example, exhibit a photoparoxysmal EEG response, although their actual seizures are not precipitated by light. This chapter considers only those cases in which specific stimuli are associated with clinical seizures, whether they are always precipitated by the specific stimulus or are associated with spontaneous seizures, not those in which stimuli evoke only an EEG response. Situation-related epilepsies, which are considered elsewhere in this book (see Chapter 15), differ from true stimulus-sensitive epilepsies by their mechanisms and mode of provocation because the seizures preferentially occur in specific circumstances.

Although some stimuli are closely associated with certain types of seizures (e.g., reading with jaw jerks or photic stimulation with generalized myoclonic jerks), no strong correlation between any one stimulus and a specific type of attack has been found, and the same stimulus may be effective in quite different clinical contexts. For example, photic stimulation can produce attacks in patients with structural brain lesions or metabolic disorders, as well as in those with idiopathic epilepsy.

In children and adolescents, visually evoked seizures are, by far, the predominant form of stimulus-sensitive epilepsy. Startle epilepsy is also relatively common; other stimuli only rarely provoke seizures.

PHOTOSENSITIVE EPILEPSIES AND OTHER EPILEPSIES RELATED TO THE VISUAL SYSTEM

Photosensitivity, also known as *visual sensitivity*, may be defined as an abnormal EEG or clinical response to flickering light (Kasteleijn-Nolst Trenité et al., 2001; Newmark and Penry, 1979). The purpose of this section is not a study of photosensitivity, which is essentially a laboratory finding established only by the use of an appropriate technique. Excellent reviews of this topic are available elsewhere, and they include discussions of the many necessary factors for light stimulation to be effective in the laboratory (Takahashi, 2002; Kasteleijn-Nolst Trenité et al., 2001; Guerrini et al., 1998d; Harding and Jeavons, 1994; Wilkins and Lindsay, 1985). The greatest clinical significance is attached to the *photoparoxysmal response*, also termed *photoconvulsive*. This is a paroxysmal; focal; or, most often, generalized discharge of spike-waves, polyspike-waves, or occasionally multiple spikes that is elicited by photic stimulation. Although the traditional belief was that epilepsy was more common if the *photoparoxysmal* response was continued for 100 ms or longer after the stimulus ends (Reilly and Peters, 1973), this has not been confirmed in more recent studies (Jayakar and Chiappa, 1990). The photoparoxysmal response should be separated from the *photomyoclonic response*, which is anteriorly located and is always associated with myoclonic jerks of the periocular muscles and muscles of the face that are time-locked to the flashes of intermittent photic stimulation (IPS) and are sometimes accompanied by vertical oscillations of the eyeballs (Kasteleijn-Nolst Trenité et al., 2001). The photomyoclonic response is blocked by eye opening, and it stops immediately after the stimulation is terminated. The frequency range of the flashes that is effective in triggering the photomyoclonic response is usually between 8 and 20 Hz. The photomyoclonic response is rarely seen in children. The current understanding indicates that it is an expression of cortical response within the spectrum of photic cortical reflex myoclonus (Artieda and Obeso, 1993).

Photosensitive epilepsies are characterized by the occurrence of *seizures* evoked by photic stimuli that occur under everyday environmental circumstances; these can be divided into two broad categories (Kasteleijn-Nolst Trenité et al., 2001; Harding and Jeavons, 1994; Wilkins and Lindsay, 1985; Newmark and Penry, 1979; Forster, 1977). The first category includes those patients who have seizures only in response to flickering lights that they encounter in a normal environment. The second includes those patients who have spontaneous seizures in addition to attacks evoked by flickering light. In both categories, self-induction of seizures may occur, but it is much more common in the first. Such patients belong to different categories.

Categories of Photosensitive Epilepsies

The first category includes *patients with a photoparoxysmal response in the EEG and no history of epileptic seizures*. A photoparoxysmal response has been estimated to occur in about 4% of normal children or adolescents (Eeg-Olofsson et al., 1971). In such individuals, the abnormal EEG response to photic stimulation is usually detected by chance during an EEG that is performed for reasons unrelated to epilepsy. The likelihood of these children for developing epilepsy is unknown, but it has been estimated as roughly 20% in young adults (Kasteleijn-Nolst Trenité et al., 2001). Higher rates are highly likely in children as the reaction to IPS may increase during adolescence, leading to clinical seizures (Kasteleijn-Nolst Trenité et al., 1994).

Patients with spontaneous seizures only, but a photoparoxysmal response in the EEG may belong to various epilepsy syndromes.

A photoparoxysmal EEG response can be observed in patients with various epilepsy syndromes that are characterized by spontaneous seizures (Table 17.1). In many such patients, no evidence indicates that, in addition to the spontaneous seizures, photic-induced attacks also occur.

Patients in whom an isolated visually induced seizure, with or without a photoparoxysmal response in the EEG, occurs are not uncommon, especially in young adolescents in whom a single seizure may occur in front of the television, while playing with video games, or in a dance club. Generalized tonic-clonic seizures or prolonged visual seizures that may or may not be followed by unresponsiveness and secondary generalization may occur (Hennessy and Binnie, 2000; Guerrini et al., 1994, 1997a). Although a visual trigger is highly probable when ictal visual symptoms are present, the absence of a photoparoxysmal response is not uncommon even in such circumstances (Ferrie et al., 1994).

Patients with only recurrent visually induced seizures, with or without a photoparoxysmal response in the EEG, often have generalized tonic-clonic seizures or myoclonic jerks (Fig. 17.1). Some may

TABLE 17.1. *Epileptic syndromen with visual sensitivity*

Generalized epilepsies
  IGE, in order of age:
    Benign myoclonic epilepsy of infancy (included late and reflex variants)
    Childhood absence epilepsy
    Juvenile absence epilepsy
    Juvenile myoclonic epilepsy
    GTCS on awakening
    IGE with practice-induced seizures, including primary reading epilepsy
    Visual sensitive IGE, including eyelid myoclonus with absences
  Cryptogenic generalized epilepsies: epilepsy with myoclonic astatic seizures
  Symptomatic generalized epilepsies
    Progressive myoclonus epilepsies
      Neuronal ceroidlipofuscinosis (late infantile, adult forms)
      Myoclonus epilepsy with ragged-red fibers
      Lafora disease
      Unverricht-Lundborg disease
    Gaucher (type III, neuronopathic form)
    Other forms
Focal epilepsies
  Idiopathic focal epilepsies
    Idiopathic photosensitive occipital lobe epilepsy
  Symptomatic and cryptogenic focal epilepsies
Undetermined epilepsies: severe myoclonic epilepsy of infancy (Dravet syndrome)
Situation-related and occasional seizures
  Strong provocative visual stimuli in patients with latent photosensitivity
  Alcohol withdrawal, drugs, vitamins, toxic drugs

Abbreviations: GTCS, generalized tonic-clonic seizures; IGE, idiopathic generalized epilepsy.

present with focal occipital seizures with prominent visual symptoms, with or without secondary generalization (Hennessy and Binnie, 2000; Guerrini et al., 1995). In some children, seizures are observed only during IPS in the EEG laboratory. Such seizures rarely are generalized tonic-clonic convulsions, partly because the IPS is stopped when a photoparoxysmal response lasts too long (Binnie and Jeavons, 1992). Jeavons and Harding (1975) reported children in whom absences were regularly induced by IPS. The absences were evoked by a narrow range of frequencies (usually less than 15 per second). The average age at onset in the affected patients, two-thirds of whom were girls, was 12 years, which considerably exceeds the average age of patients with usual absence seizures (see Chapter 8).

Patients with visually induced and spontaneous seizures, with or without a photoparoxysmal response in the EEG, may belong to different syndromes.

Pattern Sensitivity

Overview

The precipitation of seizures by visual patterns is commonly associated with photosensitivity. Viewing linear patterns evokes epileptiform discharges in 30% of photosensitive patients if the pattern is static and in 70% if the patterns oscillate in a direction orthogonal to the line orientation (Wilkins et al., 1979b). The presentation of patterns is seldom effective in individuals who do not demonstrate a photoparoxysmal EEG response to IPS (Binnie and Wilkins, 1997). Those patterns that have been reported to induce epileptic attacks generally are strongly contrasting and black and white (Stefansson et al., 1977), but the character of inducing patterns can be quite variable. The occurrence of paroxysmal EEG activity in pattern-sensitive patients depends on the spatial frequency, orientation, contrast, and size of the pattern (Wilkins et al., 1979b; Porciatti et al., 2000). Oscillating and phase reversal patterns are more epileptogenic than drifting or static patterns (Wilkins et al., 1979b; Binnie et al., 1985b). The physiologic abnormality underlying sensitivity to both IPS and pattern stimulation appears to be the inability of the visual cortex to process afferent inputs of high luminance contrast through the normal mechanisms of cortical gain control (Porciatti et al., 2000).

Striped tissues, escalator gratings, radiators, and rugs have been incriminated in precipitating attacks in these patients. The induced seizures are usually

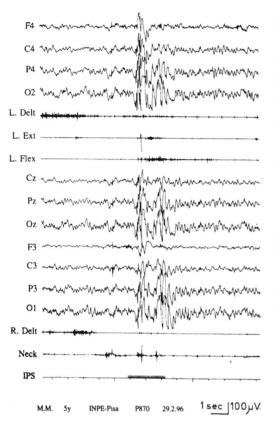

FIG. 17.1. Intermittent photic stimulation–induced generalized myoclonic jerks in a 5-year-old boy with myoclonic astatic epilepsy. A referential montage and a polygraphic recording are shown. Clinically, the child nods and briskly abducts his arms. The electroencephalogram shows a discharge of multiple spike-wave complexes that are generalized but that predominate posteriorly. Electromyographic myoclonic potentials are seen better on the wrist extensors and on the neck muscles.

tonic-clonic attacks, but absence seizures, myoclonic attacks, and partial seizures also occur (Dravet et al., 2002; Guerrini et al., 1995; Binnie and Jeavons, 1992; Newmark, 1983). Pattern-induced seizures are associated with sensitivity to flickering light in 70% to 100% of patients (Newmark and Penry, 1979; Stefansson et al., 1977). Adding a pattern to the lamps used for photostimulation may render them more effective in attack induction (Jeavons and Harding, 1975); however, only 2% of the patients of Jeavons and Harding (1975) had a history of pattern sensitivity, probably indicating that the effect of patterns may go unrecognized. Indeed, Binnie and Jeavons (1992) found that almost 20% of photosensitive patients re-

ported precipitation by visual patterns when they were carefully questioned.

In some families, pattern sensitivity seems to be genetically transmitted (Brinciotti et al., 1992). The phenomenon is most common in patients with otherwise normal neurologic status and in the context of idiopathic epilepsies, and it can induce generalized and focal seizures (Kasteleijn-Nolst Trenité et al., 2001; Binnie and Wilkins, 1997; Guerrini et al., 1995; Ricci and Vigevano, 1993). It is also common in children with Dravet syndrome (see Chapter 5).

Incidence and Triggering Factors

The prevalence of photosensitive epilepsy in the general population is unknown. In an EEG study of 223 normal school children from 12 to 16 years of age of which only the boys were chosen to avoid the possible influences of hormonal variations, 3 children (1.3%) showed a generalized photoparoxysmal response. None had a clear history of seizures. Jeavons and Harding (1975) found 181 patients with seizures that were induced only by flickering light, 151 in whom spontaneous seizures also existed, and 122 patients who had a photoparoxysmal response without light-induced seizures. Dreifuss and Seino (Dreifuss, 1985) found 16 patients with attacks induced by environmental flickering lights, 31 with seizures induced by IPS in the laboratory, and 158 with a photoconvulsive response but not light-induced seizures. However, the patients in these studies were selected for EEG examination on the basis of clinical findings as mentioned earlier, studies in an unselected pediatric population show a photoparoxysmal response in 4% of individuals (Eeg-Olofsson et al., 1971). Binnie and Jeavons (1992) mention that the incidence of photosensitive epilepsy is roughly 1 in 4,000. In Western countries, the most common precipitant is television (Kasteleijn-Nolst Trenité et al., 2002b; Jeavons and Harding, 1975), which was reported to cause seizures in 299 of 461 patients of Jeavons and Harding (1975). Other investigators have reported lower figures (Binnie and Jeavons, 1992; Mayr et al., 1987). Although these discrepancies may reflect different criteria (e.g., Jeavons and Harding [1975] included patients with single attacks and a photoconvulsive response) (Newmark, 1983), the role of television in inducing these attacks is related to both its diffusion and to the characteristic screen frequency (50-Hz main screen frequency in Europe; 60-Hz main screen frequency in the United States and in part of Japan) (Kasteleijn-Nolst Trenité et al.,

2001; Enoki et al., 1998; Harding and Jeavons, 1994). An outbreak of visually induced seizures was recently reported in Japan, where about 700 children and adolescents experienced photic-induced seizures while they were watching television broadcasting of a popular cartoon containing a scene with highly contrasting red-blue frames at 12 Hz (Harding, 1998; Takahashi and Tsukahara, 1998). Often children experience their first television-induced seizure while they are changing channels or are watching faulty channels, especially if they are close to the screen (Ricci et al., 1998). These children often use television for self-induction.

Computer screens may also cause photic-induced seizures. Their effectiveness as triggers is higher when they have a screen refresh rate of less than 70 Hz (Badinand-Hubert et al., 1998), especially when they are used for playing video games featuring highly contrasted, high-frequency stimuli (Kasteleijn-Nolst Trenité et al., 2002b; Ricci et al., 1998). Arcade video games have also been incriminated (Ferrie et al., 1994; Graf et al., 1994; Maeda et al., 1990). Some video games have been proven to be more provocative than standard television programs are (Kasteleijn-Nolst Trenité et al., 2002b). However, their efficacy in provoking seizures appears to be related to some specific features, including a bright background and flashing images. In addition, as has been observed with TV programs, playing the games on a 50-Hz television is significantly more provocative than is playing them on the 100-Hz television (Kasteleijn-Nolst Trenité et al., 2002b). Fatigue and stress have also been demonstrated to be cofactors in seizures precipitated during video game playing (Ferrie et al., 1994), but their role is difficult to demonstrate. Video game watching can also be provocative, although it is possibly less provocative than actually playing (Kasteleijn-Nolst Trenité et al., 2002b). Discotheque lighting and flickering sunlight are less common precipitants.

The peak age for photosensitivity occurs around puberty (Kasteleijn-Nolst Trenité et al., 2001). However, no general agreement exists on whether the photoparoxysmal response declines after that age. Harding et al. (1997) observed the persistence of photosensitivity with age, whereas Kasteleijn-Nolst Trenité et al. (1994) and Jeavons et al. (1986) observed a decrease after the age of 25 years. Patients with juvenile myoclonic epilepsy (JME) may represent a large subset that continues to be photosensitive (Kasteleijn-Nolst Trenité et al., 2001).

A strong genetic component underlies the photoparoxysmal response. Both dominant and multifactorial inheritance have been suggested by family studies (Doose et al., 1969; Davidson and Watson, 1956); however, a dominant mechanism with age-dependent, but not sex-dependent, penetrance seems most likely (Waltz and Stephani, 2000). A photoparoxysmal response is most likely in patients and relatives with spontaneous generalized epileptiform discharges, but this can also be seen in individuals with spontaneous focal seizures (Doose and Gerken, 1973). Patients with JME may present with a different type of photosensitivity trait that has a higher chance of photoparoxysmal response in relatives (Tsai et al., 1989).

Pure Photosensitive Epilepsies

Flickering light is the most common known trigger of epileptic seizures (Kasteleijn-Nolst Trenité et al., 2001; Zifkin et al., 1998; Newmark and Penry, 1979; Forster, 1977). Pure photosensitive epilepsy is found in 40% of photosensitive patients (Binnie and Jeavons, 1992), and this includes patients in whom seizures are provoked only by environmental flicker stimulation. Environmental stimuli include flickering sunlight, such as that occurring when one is traveling along an avenue of trees or past railings or riding in a car (not driving) along a tree-lined road, sunlight shining through the leaves of trees, the interruption of light by helicopter blades, the reflection of sunshine on snow or from ripples on water, cinema screens, and oscilloscopes. As was already mentioned, television is the predominant cause. Television-induced or video game–induced seizures do not seem to differ from the pure photosensitive seizures precipitated by other flickering lights. The age and gender of the patients are similar, as are the types of attacks and the EEG manifestations (Guerrini et al., 1998d; Jeavons and Harding, 1975). Precipitation of seizures by both television or video games and other flickering lights is common (Jeavons and Harding, 1975).

The most common type of seizure in pure photosensitive epilepsy is the generalized tonic-clonic attack. Myoclonic jerks, absences, and focal seizures are noticed in smaller groups of patients, with the proportions varying in the different studies (Kasteleijn-Nolst Trenité et al., 2001; Hennessy and Binnie, 2000; Guerrini et al., 1998d). Because these patients have normal neurologic and cognitive development and, according to classic studies, mostly generalized seizures (Harding and Jeavons, 1994), they have traditionally been classified as a special subgroup of idiopathic generalized epilepsy (Commission on Classification and Terminology of the International League Against Epilepsy, 1989). However, recent work has indicated that, in about 25% patients with clinical photosensitivity, the visually induced seizures are primarily focal (Kasteleijn-Nolst Trenité et al., 2002d; Hennessy and Binnie, 2000; Guerrini et al., 1995; Ricci and Vigevano, 1993; Tassinari et al., 1988). The clinical and EEG characteristics of these patients appear to be sufficiently homogeneous to suggest that a syndromic subgroup of *pure photosensitive idiopathic occipital lobe epilepsy*, typically with an onset in adolescence, exists (Engel, 2001; Guerrini et al., 1995).

The reflex seizures of this subgroup are characterized by a succession of visual symptoms, especially elementary visual hallucinations and blurring, followed by epigastric discomfort, vomiting, and ictal headache (Guerrini et al., 1995). The seizure duration is extremely variable, and secondary generalization can occur rapidly or after several minutes (Fig. 17.2). The underrecognition of such seizures may partly be due to the lack of attention given to early visual symptoms when rapid secondary generalization has obscured the initial manifestations (Hennessy and Binnie, 2000) and partly to a misdiagnosis of migraine when ictal activity does not spread above the sylvian fissure and no recognizable motor manifestations occur (Walker et al., 1995; Swanson and Vick, 1978). Some patients have developed this type of epilepsy after presenting with typical benign rolandic epilepsy at school age (Guerrini et al., 1997b). Focal seizures provoked by photic stimuli have also been reported in children with cerebral palsy, brain malformations, or ischemic occipital lesions, with or without spontaneous occipital seizures (Guerrini et al., 1994) (see later discussion).

The frequency of seizures in patients with pure photosensitive epilepsy is quite variable; it is closely related to the photosensitivity range and exposure to the trigger(s). Most patients have a narrow photosensitivity range, and, if they can manage to avoid environmental triggers, they experience infrequent seizures, which may even be single seizures. Drug treatment is not necessary in such patients. However, the few patients with a wide photosensitivity range are difficult to control, even with drug treatment, and they can become severely disabled by their frequent seizures and fear of encountering provocative stimuli in daily life (Guerrini et al., 1995).

In nearly all cases of pure photosensitive epilepsy, the EEG shows normal background activity and a photoparoxysmal response to IPS. Several types of photoparoxysmal responses have been described (Table 17.2). Bursts of generalized spike-wave complexes with a slow component at 3 to 3.5 Hz are the most usual response. Bursts of generalized polyspike-waves or polyspikes are also common (Newmark and Penry, 1979). These generalized discharges are often preceded by occipital spikes (Jeavons and Harding, 1975). In patients with visually induced focal seizures, the photoparoxysmal response is often, but not necessarily, confined to the posterior regions (Guerrini et al., 1995). Jeavons and Harding (1975) found "theta spike and wave" discharges in 7% of their patients, and irregular spike-wave discharges were also described. Some authors have included high-amplitude slow waves in the photoparoxysmal response, but these are rare and their significance is unknown. No type of photoparoxysmal response is specific for photic epilepsy. The resting EEG in pure photosensitive epilepsy is normal in approximately half of the patients. The remaining patients exhibit bursts of spike-wave activity that are generalized or are posteriorly located and that usually, although not necessarily, are related to the main type of photic-induced seizures. These bursts supervene on eye closure in approximately one-third of the patients (Guerrini et al., 1998d; Jeavons and Harding, 1975).

The age at onset of pure photosensitive epilepsy usually is between 8 and 19 years. Children younger than 5 and 6 years are rarely photosensitive (Kasteleijn-Nolst Trenité et al., 2002b). A significant female preponderance of about 1.5 to 1 has been noted in all of the reported series. A family history of pure photosensitive epilepsy or of a photoconvulsive response without seizures is common (Waltz and Stephani, 2000); identical twins are almost uniformly affected, and pedigrees with photosensitive epilepsy transmitted through three generations have been recorded (Newmark and Penry, 1979; Brinciotti et al., 1992). A dominant mode of genetic transmission has been suggested (Waltz and Stephani, 2000).

Visually Induced Seizures Associated with Spontaneous Seizures

Photosensitive epilepsy associated with spontaneous seizures is a common occurrence (Kasteleijn-Nolst Trenité et al., 2002a). According to Binnie and Jeavons (1992), 60% of patients with a photoparoxysmal EEG response experience spontaneous seizures; 33% have additional attacks precipitated by environmental visual stimulation; and 20% fail to report visually precipitated seizures.

The proportion of photosensitive subjects who do not suffer from epilepsy is unknown. Although a vast majority of patients who are found to be photosensitive on EEG examination have epilepsy, a high pro-

A

B

C

TABLE 17.2. *Classification of the EEG responses to intermittent photic stimulation*

EEG Response	Grade
Photic following	1
At flash rate	
At harmonics	
Orbitofrontal photomyoclonia	2
Posterior stimulus–dependent response	3
Posterior stimulus–independent responses	4
Limited to the stimulus train	
Self-sustaining	
Generalized photoparoxysmal response	5
Limited to the stimulus train	
Self-sustaining	
Activation of preexisting focus	6

Grade 3, 4, and 5 are generally described as photoparoxysmal responses.

The latter condition is, however, remarkable mainly for single posterior spikes evoked by each flash during slow (1 to 3 Hz) photic stimulation.

Except for these rare diseases, the presence of visually induced seizures with spontaneous seizures is associated with several common epilepsy syndromes (Table 17.1). Photosensitivity is especially common in adolescence (e.g., idiopathic generalized epilepsy of adolescence and JME) (see Chapter 6). Common features include age at onset, the presence of nocturnal seizures and attacks on awakening, a preponderance of female patients, small number of seizures in most patients, neurologic normality, and diffuse paroxysmal EEG abnormalities on a normal background tracing. A photoparoxysmal EEG response is common in idiopathic generalized epilepsy. Therefore, the question arises of whether visually induced epilepsy might represent the most photosensitive of the patients with idiopathic generalized epilepsy of adolescence.

portion of individuals in the general population with a photoparoxysmal response probably do not have epilepsy.

In patients with both photosensitivity and spontaneous seizures, the unprovoked seizures are mainly of the generalized tonic-clonic type, but myoclonic jerks like those observed in JME are more common than in pure photosensitive epilepsy. Of the patients in the series by Jeavons and Harding (1975), 55% had grand mal attacks, 15% had absences, and 8% had myoclonic seizures. Light-induced seizures may, on rare occasions, be seen in degenerative diseases, such as progressive myoclonic epilepsy in adolescents (Lafora body disease, type III Gaucher disease) (see Chapter 7) and neuronal ceroid lipofuscinosis in younger children (Harden and Pampiglione, 1982).

However, photosensitivity is not evenly distributed among the idiopathic generalized epilepsies. Wolf and Gooses (1986) identified photosensitivity in 31% of patients with JME, in 18% of those with childhood absences, in 13% of those with grand mal on awakening, and in only 7.5% of those with juvenile absence epilepsy. In addition, some genetically determined specificity seems to be present in photosensitive epilepsy. Light-induced epilepsy often has been observed in more than one family member (Waltz and Stephani, 2000; Brinciotti et al., 1992; Jeavons and Harding, 1975). Because, in contrast to the photoconvulsive response, seizures precipitated by light are uncommon, their presence in several members of these families or in identical twins suggests that this is a genetic trait.

FIG. 17.2. Intermittent photic stimulation (IPS)–induced occipital seizure in a 16-year-old boy. During IPS, seizure activity begins with an ictal discharge at the O2-Oz channel. Nineteen seconds after the beginning of IPS (*19'*), the patient claims to see "three rainbow-colored spots surrounded by a dark shadow" in the left visual field that then roll to the left. The seizure activity spreads progressively over the right occipito-posterior temporal area while transmitted waves are present contralaterally. From the second to the fifth minute after ictal electroencephalographic activity is recognized (2 to 5 minutes), the patient reports the spots have slowly faded while the shadow progressively covers the left visual field, producing left hemianopia. At the twelfth minute (*12'*), the seizure activity involves both occipitoposterior temporal areas, but it still predominates on the right; the patient reports complete blindness. At 15 minutes (*15'*), slow waves appear on the right, and the patient's eyes deviate tonically to the left. At 17 minutes (*17'*), the ictal discharge progressively slows to rhythmic spike and slow waves on the right, while it persists on the left. The patient's head deviates toward the left, but he is still completely responsive. At 18 minutes (*18'*), the patient's head returns to midline; he complains of a sudden headache and epigastric discomfort, and, at 20 minutes (*20'*), he retches. Ictal activity stops on the right hemisphere 18 minutes after seizure onset (*18'*), but it continues for a further 2 minutes on the left (*20'*). Continuous clinical testing revealed gradual postictal improvement of visual blurring. The patient recovered vision fully about 3 minutes after the end of the seizure, but he remained visually agnosic, only beginning to identify objects 6 minutes later.

The relationship of photosensitive epilepsy to absence epilepsy raises similar questions. Although absence epilepsy of adolescence (the nonpyknoleptic absences) is closely linked to JME and awakening grand mal, the incidence of photosensitivity is lower in this group, suggesting that additional genetic factors may be involved.

Doose (1979) found the inheritance of a photoconvulsive response to be independent of that of spikes and waves in the resting EEG recordings and during hyperventilation. The significance of such findings is obscured by the more or less restricted definitions that are accepted for photoconvulsive response and by the lack of distinction between patients with a photoparoxysmal response only and those who also have light-induced seizures in genetic studies.

Photosensitivity is common in Dravet syndrome (or severe myoclonic epilepsy), in which it was found in 71% of patients (Dravet et al., 1992a; Aicardi, 1991a). In this syndrome, a photoconvulsive response may appear during the first 2 years of life, even as early as 4 or 5 months of age. About 15% to 20% of children with benign myoclonic epilepsy or myoclonic astatic epilepsy present with IPS-induced myoclonic jerks. Photosensitivity is also common in the progressive encephalopathies with myoclonic epilepsy, such as Unverricht-Lundborg or Gaucher disease. Sensitivity to light is less common in the usual forms of symptomatic epilepsy than it is in idiopathic cases. However, even in patients with partial symptomatic epilepsies, it is not rare (Guerrini et al., 1998d; Binnie and Jeavons, 1992).

Eyelid Myoclonia With Absence and Self-Induced Photosensitive Epilepsies

Eyelid myoclonia with absence is regarded by some authors as a separate entity (Jeavons, 1982). The characteristic feature is that eye closure in the presence of light induces a clinical attack consisting of eyelid jerking with upward deviation of the eyes. The EEG shows spike-and-wave or polyspike-wave discharges on eye closure that are not present in the dark. Eyelid myoclonia, with or without absences, is also observed in the context of symptomatic epilepsies in children with mental retardation. The age at onset is earlier than that seen in the usual photic-induced epilepsies. Jeavons (1982) found a mean age at onset of 6 ± 2 years, which is well within the range of that of childhood typical absences.

Treatment with sodium valproate alone or in combination with ethosuximide is often effective, and it should be maintained for an indefinite duration as this epilepsy has a low tendency to remit spontaneously, although the course is imperfectly known.

Eyelid myoclonia with absence can probably be self-induced, although this is disputed (Duncan and Panayotopoulos, 1995a; Binnie et al., 1980). Differentiating spontaneous from self-induced eyelid myoclonia can be quite difficult.

Self-Induction of Photosensitive Epilepsy

Light-sensitive epilepsy is the most common type of self-induced epilepsy. Most patients stare at a source of bright light, most commonly the sun, and rapidly wave one hand with the fingers spread out in front of the eyes. In this manner, they are able to precipitate the seizures, primarily absences or myoclonic jerks. In some children, however, the hand waving is relatively slow and the fingers are not spread apart. Self-induction of seizures may be more common when the patients are emotionally stressed (Newmark and Penry, 1979). In some children, the intensity of the environmental light is influential, with the hand waving and seizures occurring much more commonly on bright sunny days (Green, 1966).

Most patients appear to be compulsively attracted to gaze at bright light sources, but most cannot explain this attraction. Only 13% admit to finding the sensation pleasurable (Tassinari et al., 1989a). Some authors have suggested that the movements of the hand may not be intentional but that, instead, they are a part of the ictal pattern (Ames and Saffer, 1983; Newmark and Penry, 1979). Ames and Saffer (1983), noting the slow rate of light interruption, the often unilateral stimulation, and the unusual associated eye and body positions, suggested that the hand movements were part of the seizure, rather than a triggering factor. However, Tassinari et al. (1989a, 1990) have convincingly shown that the intermittently interrupted light produced by the hand motion was the initiating event. These authors collected 170 cases of self-induced seizures, most of which occurred in children. About 30% of these patients were mentally retarded. Flickering light was the most effective trigger for the seizures, and the maneuvers used to produce flicker were waving a hand before the eyes, head shaking or nodding, and rhythmic blinking. The seizures that were induced were myoclonic in 58% of the patients. Impairment of consciousness was a feature in 92% of seizures, and it was the only manifestation of an attack in 32% of cases. Photic stimulation induced spike-wave bursts in three-fourths of the patients. Mental retardation was clear in 44% of patients.

Blinking at a source of light (Darby et al., 1980; Green, 1968) is another maneuver commonly used, and it may occasionally be combined with hand waving (Aicardi, 1994a). Blinking may also be part of the ictus, rather than an attempt to precipitate a fit (Ames and Saffer, 1983). In some patients, blinking may be associated with sudden movements of the neck that, at least in some cases, seem to precede the EEG discharge. In some children, myoclonic jerking of the eyelids is part of a complex, repetitive self-stimulation habit with deliberate fluttering of the eyes and hyperextension of the head in front of any bright light source, including IPS. In these circumstances, distinguishing between eyelid myoclonus and blinking for the purpose of self-inducing may be impossible.

Slow eye closure with extreme upward deviation of the eyes (Darby et al., 1980; Green, 1968; Tibbles and Prichard, 1965) is a common precipitating maneuver that is seen mainly in intelligent patients because it is much less conspicuous than hand waving and it is readily mistaken for a tic or for eyelid flutter accompanying an absence. When patients with photosensitivity are placed in a well-lit environment, 24% to 30% appear to engage in self-induction, particularly if they are stressed (Binnie and Jeavons, 1992; Darby et al., 1980). Diagnosing seizures that are self-induced by slow eye closure may be difficult. Combined video-EEG monitoring may be extremely useful because it can show that the eye movement precedes the discharge and that the oculographic artifact is larger and slower than normal eye closure. Often, a superimposed ocular tremor at about 6 Hz is present (Binnie and Jeavons, 1992). Other suggestive features include the rarity of eye closure in darkness, an increased frequency of the maneuver with stress, and a feeling of guilt when the behavior is discussed. Some patients report experiencing pleasurable sensations when they self-induce.

Some patients deliberately use the television set as a stimulator by blurring the image and making the hold unstable (Jeavons and Harding, 1975). Jeavons and Harding (1970) described 30 patients who appeared to be drawn toward the television screen until a seizure was provoked. A few appeared to enjoy the sequence and even admitted to switching on the television to obtain a seizure and/or a sensation. Most said they did not desire a seizure but that they were nevertheless attracted to the screen as soon as the set was turned on.

Features common to all patients with self-induced photosensitive seizures, except those mentioned in the paragraph immediately preceding, are a marked preponderance of girls, the rare occurrence of generalized tonic-clonic seizures, and the predominance of myoclonic and absence seizures (Newmark and Penry, 1979; Jeavons and Harding, 1975). Most patients have spontaneously occurring attacks in addition to self-induced fits, and mental retardation or psychiatric disturbances are common, especially among younger children. Self-induction has never been reported in patients with visually induced focal seizures.

Patients with self-provoked attacks are notoriously difficult to treat, and they are liable to be regarded as drug resistant, with consequent increases in the doses of drugs being administered. Proper identification is, therefore, important; if the medication is not successful in controlling the self-provoked seizures, it should be maintained at the lowest level appropriate for controlling other coexisting seizures.

Other Seizures Related to the Visual System but not to Flickering Lights

Eye Closure

The act of closing the eyes provokes seizure discharges in many patients, most of whom have spontaneous seizures (Terzano et al., 1983; Newmark and Penry, 1979). Rare patients have clinical seizures that are induced by eye closure. Newmark (1983) reviewed 14 reported cases, 11 of whom were below 15 years of age. Seven were mentally retarded, and 6 had spontaneous seizures. The induced attacks were absence seizures in 12 of the patients. A photoparoxysmal response was observed in only 6 of the 12 tested patients. In most cases, the seizures could be precipitated by eye closure, even in the dark, but passive closure was usually ineffective. Seizures that are induced by blinking in patients with no detectable photoparoxysmal response to IPS have also been reported by other authors (Kohno et al., 1987; Rafal et al., 1986).

Rare patients with prolonged periods of eye closure that, at times, can last a whole day have been recorded (Snead et al., 1983). During these periods, a certain degree of impairment of consciousness is present; the patients can respond when they are spoken to and can open their eyes in response to a strong command, but they immediately fall back to their previous state. When the eyes are closed, continuous paroxysmal activity is recorded, and the EEG returns to normal immediately upon opening of the eyes (Fig. 17.3).

Eye movements such as extreme lateral gaze (Schanzer et al., 1965) or convergence (Vignaendra

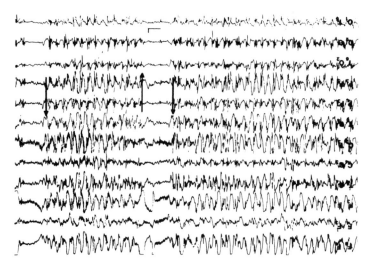

FIG. 17.3. Light-sensitive epilepsy, self-induced by keeping the eyes closed. Polyspike-wave complexes are present throughout the scalp when the eyes are closed (*downward arrow*), and they disappear on eye opening (*upward arrows*). The patient was able to induce episodes of status lasting hours by closing her eyes. However, the maneuver was only occasionally successful. Calibration: 1 second, 50 μV.

and Lim, 1978) may, in exceptional cases, induce seizures.

Differential Diagnosis of Visually Evoked Seizures

A common diagnostic problem is raised by seizures that appear while the child is watching television or playing video games. Not all seizures that occur in such circumstances are visually triggered, and some are not epileptic. A significant number of attacks, which may occur merely as a result of the long hours children spend watching television or playing video games, must be coincidental. Seizures also may be facilitated during television watching by drowsiness or sleep. Syncope can be induced as a result of the frightening character of certain images (Stephenson, 1978a). Self-induced seizures are often disregarded as tics or "bad habits," and they may go undiagnosed for years. In general, attacks of a relatively minor character, such as absences or brief myoclonic jerks, are underdiagnosed. On the other hand, recording a photoparoxysmal response with EEG is not sufficient evidence for photic-induced epilepsy or, indeed, for any epilepsy, even though it is necessary for making a diagnosis of photosensitive epilepsy. The clinician should remember that a photoparoxysmal response may not be present in a few of the patients who experience seizures in front of the television or while playing video games or who have

pattern-sensitive epilepsy. However, such patients usually have an abnormally enlarged visual-evoked potential on pattern stimulation (Guerrini et al., 1998d).

Those patients who present with prolonged visually-induced focal seizures characterized by a clustering of visual symptoms; headache; abdominal discomfort; and, sometimes, vomiting pose a particular problem. Such seizures are often misdiagnosed as migraine (Walker et al., 1995; Swanson and Vick, 1978), especially in patients with infrequently occurring attacks; in these individuals, recognizing the triggering role of television, computer screens, or bright lights can be difficult. Moreover, a slow spread of ictal activity, which is often seen in such patients, causes overt extraoccipital symptoms to appear when the patient is no longer facing the provoking stimulus (Guerrini et al., 1995). An important element in the differential diagnosis between elementary visual hallucinations of occipital seizures and those of migraine is that the seizures are predominantly characterized by circular or spherical multicolored patterns, as opposed to the predominantly black-and-white ictal patterns of migraine (Panayiotopoulos, 1994a). A few cases in which limbic seizures with abdominal discomfort and fear but no preceding visual symptoms were induced by photic stimuli have been recorded (Guerrini et al., 1998d; Isnard et al., 1998). In some children or adolescents in whom visually induced occipital seizures occur in the absence of an abnormal response to IPS, the clinical and EEG findings may be misleading, resulting in a misdiagnosis of the late onset variant of childhood epilepsy with occipital paroxysms (CEOP), in which, however, the reflex triggering of seizures does not occur.

Therapy of Visually Evoked Seizures

In a number of patients with pure photic-induced seizures, no drug treatment is necessary. This is especially applicable to television-induced and video game–induced epilepsy, in which the attacks are generally infrequent and preventive measures are relatively easy to take. Many patients are sensitive to the frequency of the mains supply (50 Hz in Europe, 60 Hz in North America), and they are thus affected by the flicker of the screen (Badinand-Hubert et al., 1998; Ricci et al., 1998). For such patients, this sensitivity appears to be reduced by the use of bright ambient lighting. Patients are recommended to remain a distance of 2.5 m from the screen *at all times* (Wilkins and Lindsay, 1985; Jeavons and Harding, 1975). A small table lamp should be placed on top of the television set, which should be in a well-lit room to reduce the contrast in illumination. A remote control should be used to adjust or switch channels, and, if the patient has to go near the set for some reason, he or she should cover one eye with the palm of his or her hand to prevent any light from entering the eye. Wilkins and Lindsay (1985) recommend, in addition, the use of polarizing glasses if seizures still occur when the child is watching a normally functioning television set from a conventional viewing distance. Some patients are sensitive to the linear pattern of the raster generating the television picture. This effect is present only when the patient is close enough to the screen for the raster pattern to be resolved (Binnie and Jeavons, 1992). This form of visual sensitivity is exacerbated by television viewing in a well-lit environment, so maintaining a distance to the screen of 2 m or more is the main preventive method. The use of optical filters has been suggested for the prevention of television-induced seizures (Takahashi et al., 2001).

Video games should be avoided by photosensitive children. However, playing video games on a 100-Hz television screen is much less provocative than is playing at 50 Hz (Kasteleijn-Nolst Trenité et al., 2002b). Other flickering lights may be more difficult to avoid. The flashing lights in discotheques may be dangerous even at relatively slow rates, although this remains controversial (Bergman et al., 1983; Jeavons

and Harding, 1975). The use of polarized glasses should be advised as they remove the reflected flicker produced by sunlight on water, snow, and wet surfaces.

In patients with spontaneous seizures in addition to those that are light-induced or in patients with marked light sensitivity, anticonvulsant therapy is necessary. The best results have been obtained with the use of sodium valproate (Jeavons and Harding, 1975). In one series in which this drug was used, photosensitivity was abolished in 54% of the cases and was markedly reduced in another 24% (Jeavons and Harding, 1970). The effect of treatment on long-term prognosis is uncertain (Jeavons et al., 1977). Valproate may abolish photosensitivity for up to several days despite waning blood levels (Rowan et al., 1979), and photosensitivity has developed in previously nonphotosensitive patients following valproate withdrawal (Ambrosetto and Tassinari, 1987). Ethosuximide and the benzodiazepines are also effective in some cases (Tassinari et al., 1990; Newmark and Penry, 1979). Photosensitivity may be abolished by the acute administration of several antiepileptic drugs, and the assessment of the effect of new antiepileptic therapies on the photoparoxysmal response following acute administration of a single dose has consequently been used as a test of their efficacy (Rimmer et al., 1987). A single dose of oral lamotrigine produces a clear narrowing in the photosensitivity range (Binnie et al., 1986). The acute administration of levetiracetam has an effect on both the photoparoxysmal EEG response and the photic-induced myoclonic jerks (Kasteleijn-Nolst Trenité et al., 1996).

Carbamazepine, phenytoin, and gabapentin are not effective for treating photosensitive patients (Hirsch et al., 2000).

A marked reduction in self-inducing behavior has been reported in photosensitive children following dopamine receptor agonist therapy (Kasteleijn-Nolst Trenité et al., 2002a; Clemens, 1988) and, paradoxically, with fenfluramine therapy (Boel and Casaer, 1996; Aicardi and Gastaut, 1986), which suggests that dopaminergic mechanisms are in some way involved in the self-provocation of seizures. Combination therapy with valproate and fenfluramine has been advocated in such cases (Boel and Casaer, 1996).

Conditioning therapies have received less extensive trials (Forster, 1977). After repetitive monocular stimulation, stimulation at out-of-range frequencies, or stimulation with a brightly lit background that does not produce a photoconvulsive response, the patient may be able to withstand stimuli that were previously epileptogenic. These results, however, are unclear, and the methods are very expensive and highly complex.

STARTLE EPILEPSY AND MOVEMENT-INDUCED SEIZURES

Startle-Induced Seizures

Startle-induced seizures are precipitated by sudden, unexpected stimuli, especially but not exclusively by sounds or proprioceptive stimuli that are capable of provoking a startle (Alajouanine and Gastaut, 1955). Startle epilepsy occurs only in patients with brain pathology. The abnormalities can be unilateral and can date back to the prenatal or perinatal period, or they can be more diffuse. They include porencephalic cysts, circumscribed atrophic lesions, rarely angiomas (Alajouanine and Gastaut, 1955), Sturge-Weber disease (Newmark, 1983), and focal cortical dysplasia (Manford et al., 1996b). Less commonly, diffuse or disseminated brain lesions have been reported, including perinatal asphyxia, encephalitis sequelae, methotrexate encephalopathy, Down syndrome, and other unclassified fixed encephalopathies (Aicardi, 1994a; Guerrini et al., 1990b, 1992b; Gimenez-Roldan and Martin, 1979).

The incidence of startle epilepsy is unknown, but the condition is rare. Undoubtedly, an element of surprise is usually at the origin of epileptic seizures (Forster, 1977; Chauvel et al., 1987). However, in many patients, both a startle reaction and a specific sensory stimulus seem to be necessary to induce an attack. Some patients may have startle seizures either only or predominantly with sounds while others respond only to proprioceptive or exteroceptive stimuli. Some patients are sensitive to many sudden stimuli, regardless of the specific nature of the stimulus. Most cases of startle epilepsy have their onset in infancy, childhood, or adolescence (Vignal et al., 1998; Forster, 1977; Alajouanine and Gastaut, 1955). Furthermore, most cases occur in children or adolescents with mild congenital hemiparesis that, in some, is associated with a slight intellectual deficit.

The seizures are usually frequent, and they are always precipitated by unexpected stimuli, such as a telephone ringing, a sudden noise, stumbling on a folded rug, or a tap on the shoulder. Even minor stimuli, such as a cough, a dropping teaspoon, or even somebody talking in a normal voice after a silence, may precipitate the attacks. The suddenness of the stimuli is essential, and expected stimuli, even those that are of high intensity, are ineffective. The seizures begin with a startle that is characterized clinically by a brief movement and flexion of the head, trunk, and limbs. This is followed by a tonic phase during which the limbs of the hemiparetic side stiffen, with flexion of the upper limb and extension or flexion of the lower limb. Oculocephalic adversion to the paretic side is observed. A fall may result, and a few clonic jerks are possible. Consciousness may be either spared or blurred during the seizure, which lasts only 10 to 20 seconds (Sàenz-Lope et al., 1984a; Alajouanine and Gastaut, 1955).

The EEG may show a sharp vertex artifact corresponding to the startle, followed by a flattening of background activity and the appearance of a rapid recruiting rhythm (Fig. 17.4). or, less often, a fast (10 to 15 Hz) recruiting rhythm. The latter rhythm, when present, is often followed by spike-wave discharges or polyspike-waves. Interictal records may be normal or display focal abnormalities.

Most patients also have spontaneous seizures that may precede or follow the induced attacks or alternate with them. The attacks are quite disturbing because of the falls and the resulting injuries. However, the overall prognosis is variable. The frequency of attacks tends to lessen with increasing age. The seizures may respond favorably to carbamazepine (Sàenz-Lope et al., 1984a) and, less commonly, clonazepam (Gimenez-Roldan and Martin, 1979). Most patients with focal lesions have average intelligence quotient (IQ) scores, permitting relatively satisfactory social integration if the seizures are controlled.

Bilateral startle-induced seizures are regarded as uncommon (Newmark, 1983). However, bilateral cases (Guerrini et al., 1990b; Sàenz-Lope et al., 1984a) were not uncommon in series including patients with diffuse encephalopathies (Guerrini et al., 1990b; Aguglia et al., 1984). In contrast with unilateral seizures, bilateral attacks occur in severely retarded patients, and the prognosis is poor. Often, such patients have Lennox-Gastaut syndrome (Guerrini et al., 1990b; Aguglia et al., 1984) and the attacks, which are often provoked by minor stimuli (Gimenez-Roldan and Martin, 1979), are the typical tonic seizures seen in the syndrome. These attacks are associated with similar seizures that occur spontaneously, as well as atypical absences and atonic seizures (Guerrini et al., 1990b, 1997c; Aguglia et al., 1984) (see Chapter 4). The interictal tracings often show a slow, disorganized background with bilateral frontal paroxysmal discharges and/or multifocal spike discharges. A tracing of slow spike-wave discharges that is similar to that observed in Lennox-Gastaut syndrome may be seen (Guerrini et al., 1990b; Sàenz-Lope et al., 1984a).

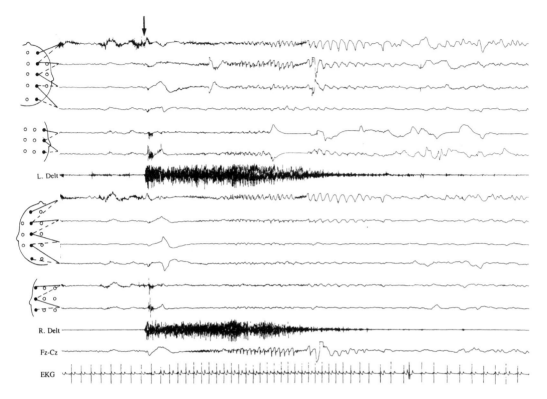

FIG. 17.4. A 20-year-old male patient with Down syndrome and startle epilepsy. A sudden, unexpected noise induces a tonic seizure lasting 15 seconds, accompanied by tachycardia; the patient who is sitting on the bed is projected violently backward. A sustained axial tonic contraction, which is visible on the deltoid muscles (*R* and *L Delt*), is accompanied on the electroencephalogram by a decremental event, followed by low-voltage fast activity with increasing amplitude and decreasing frequency that is well recognizable over the vertex and fronto-central electrodes and is more apparent on the right.

The mechanism of startle-induced seizures is disputed. External stimuli appear to trigger a normal or excessive startle reaction that, in turn, activates an epileptogenic area that may be located in or near the supplementary motor cortex via a volley of proprioceptive influxes (Chauvel et al., 1987; Lamarche and Chauvel, 1978). Interestingly, an increased startle reaction has been observed in patients with startle epilepsy that is independent of the startle-induced seizures (Sàenz-Lope et al., 1984a). Even though excessive startle reactions (so-called *syncinésie-sursaut*) (Alajouanine and Gastaut, 1955) may be associated with startle epilepsy, the condition can be easily separated from startle disease or hyperekplexia (Markand et al., 1984; Sàenz-Lope et al., 1984b; Andermann et al., 1980a), in which no evidence of a brain lesion is found (see Chapter 21). A history of rigidity in early infancy is common in hyperekplexia, and this should not be mistaken for a diplegic type of cerebral palsy.

Movement-Induced Seizures

Movement-induced seizures have some similarities with startle epilepsy because the attacks are usually induced by a rapid movement after a period of rest or by a sudden change in the pace of movement. Thus, the seizures occur when the patient has to rise from a sitting position or to do rapid movements on command (Lishman et al., 1962). The attacks can be prevented by slow preparation for the usually provoking movement. The movement itself, which sometimes is a specific movement, not the startle is the precipitating event, although differentiation from startle epilepsy is often difficult.

The attacks themselves differ from those of startle epilepsy. A bizarre feeling that is localized to the affected side or limb usually initiates them. They may be purely tonic, but, quite commonly, they include a writhing or athetotic component. Consciousness is preserved throughout the seizures. In rare patients, the seizures are induced by passive movements, percussion of deep tendon reflexes, or muscular tension, without a startle effect (Aicardi, 1994a; Aquino and Gabor, 1980; Oller-Daurella and Dini, 1970). According to Vignal et al. (1998), a combination of movement and sensory stimuli may be operating as a trigger in some patients. However, in a patient reported by Gabor (1974), the movement-induced seizures did not depend on peripheral sensory impulses. Volitional hyperextension of the neck and trunk was found to be a specific stimulus in an unusual case of gelastic seizures (Jacome et al., 1980). Generalization of movement-induced seizures is uncommon, but the cooccurrence of similar spontaneous seizures is common (Vignal et al., 1998).

The brain lesions in movement-induced seizures are localized in or near the rolandic cortex (Vignal et al., 1998; Falconer, 1963). The most commonly observed lesions include cortical dysplasia and tumors (Vignal et al., 1998).

True movement-induced seizures are rare (Vignal et al., 1998), and many reported cases might, in fact, have had kinesigenic paroxysmal dyskinesia (Lance, 1977), which generally is considered nonepileptic in nature (Guerrini et al., 2002b, 2002d; Fahn, 1994). Quite similar attacks have also been described in cases of hypoparathyroidism.

Ogunyemi et al. (1988) have indicated that exercise, rather than single movements, may be at the origin of seizures. However, patients with motor attacks that follow sustained motor activity likely have paroxysmal exercise-induced dyskinetic attacks (Bhatia et al., 1997), which may occur in isolation or in patients who also have true epileptic seizures (Guerrini et al., 2002b), including focal motor seizures (Guerrini, 2001; Guerrini et al., 1999b). In some patients with true movement-induced seizures, the repetition of a given movement, not the exercise, acts as a trigger (Vignal et al., 1998). Differentiating between true movement-induced seizures and exercise-induced dyskinesia in such patients may be even more difficult. Both types of attacks start with tonic posturing of the limbs involved in the triggering motor activity, and they may subsequently spread to contiguous segments without impairment of consciousness.

SEIZURES PROVOKED BY NONVISUAL SENSORY STIMULI

Somatosensory Stimuli

Somatosensory stimuli are rare precipitants of epileptic attacks. Stroking specific parts of the body induces clinical seizures or a characteristic paroxysmal activity in the EEG in a few patients (Vignal et al., 1998; Goldie and Green, 1959).

Myoclonic seizures precipitated by tapping the head, face, or, less often, other body parts occur in some patients, notably infants or young children (Ricci et al., 1995; Deonna and Despland, 1989; Revol et al., 1989; Callaghan et al., 1985). In well babies, these may be transient, disappearing without treatment. They present as myoclonic jerks of the limbs, especially of the upper limbs, and they are associated with bursts of irregular, fast (3 Hz or faster) spike-wave or polyspike-wave activity. They may represent a special form of "benign myoclonic epilepsy of infants" (Ricci et al., 1995; Dravet et al., 1992b); they are dealt with in more detail in Chapter 6.

Other sensory modalities are rarely effective (Tassinari et al., 1989a). A few cases have been described in which more than one sensory modality was effective (Daniele et al., 1987) or in which a combination of sensory stimulation and a specific related movement were necessary (Vignal et al., 1998; Aicardi, 1994a). Some children, especially those with brain damage, may discover a triggering sensorimotor sequence and may indulge in self-induction (Guerrini et al., 1992b). In severely affected patients, the self-inducing behavior may become compulsive. Different seizure types have been described, including epileptic spasms (Guerrini et al., 1992b).

Hot-water epilepsy may be related to sensory-precipitated seizures. Very few cases have been documented in the Western world, and these children have complex partial seizures that appear as soon as the body is immersed in hot water (Roos and Van Dijk, 1988; Shaw et al., 1988; Parsonage et al., 1976; Stensman and Ursing, 1971). In such patients, deciding whether the attacks are epileptic or syncopal in nature is difficult because the EEG accompanying them consists mainly of slow, more or less rhythmic, waves.

Mani et al. (1974) described a large number of Indian children and adolescents in whom generalized tonic-clonic seizures or complex partial seizures were precipitated when hot water was poured on their head. A large series that included several children was recently reported by Bebek et al. (2001), who emphasized the occurrence of complex partial seizures and simple partial seizures, both of which were induced while bathing and or could occur spontaneously; a pleasurable feeling that prompted self-induction; and a striking male preponderance. No ictal record was available, however, in this series. A few children with focal or diffuse cortical maldevelopment have been reported in whom immersion of specific body segments in hot water produced well-documented electroclinical focal seizures that originated from an area of cortical maldevelopment (Lee et al., 2000b; Bourgeois, 1999). Such cases might represent examples of sensory-induced focal seizures, and they may differ from the form of hot-water epilepsy described in India. The predisposition that children with Dravet syndrome have for presenting with seizures (usually clonic) when they are bathed in hot water is different from hot-water epilepsy; it is probably due to the same mechanisms that produce frequent, prolonged seizures during fever.

Auditory Stimuli

Auditory stimuli rarely precipitate seizures when they do not provoke a startle (Griffith and Karp, 1980). Intermittent sound stimulation may induce absence attacks in few patients (Gastaut and Pirovano, 1949). Music has precipitated complex partial seizures or secondarily generalized tonic-clonic seizures in several adult patients (Newmark, 1983; Newman and Saunders, 1980; Critchley, 1977). The mechanism of musicogenic epilepsy is unclear; several types of music may be responsible, and the musical stimulus may be related to other auditory stimuli, such as the sound of church bells (Poskanzer et al., 1962), or a specific human voice (Griffith and Karp, 1980). The role of emotions may be significant as well, and a prominent role for the right temporal lobe has been suggested (Genc et al., 2001). Musicogenic epilepsy induced by singing and reciting nursery rhymes has been reported in a child (Herskowitz et al., 1984).

SEIZURES INDUCED BY CERTAIN COMPLEX ACTIVITIES

Reading Epilepsy

Reading epilepsy has been reported mainly in adult patients; its onset occurs at a mean age of 17 to 18 years, and it is extremely rare before 12 years of age (Wolf and Inoue, 2002). In primary reading epilepsy, the attacks are precipitated only by prolonged reading, and no seizures are spontaneous (Wolf, 1992d; Merlis, 1974). The clinical presentation is so characteristic that this condition is considered an epileptic syndrome with a specific mode of provocation (Commission on Classification and Terminology of the International League Against Epilepsy, 1989). Reading aloud is more provocative than is silent reading, and understanding of the content is not essential (Wolf and Inoue, 2002).

Wolf (1992d) reviewed 111 published cases. The seizures begin with jerks involving the muscles in the somatic areas involved in the reading and talking, in-

cluding the jaw, lip, face, and throat. Such jerks may progress to a generalized tonic-clonic seizure if reading continues. A few patients may report visual symptoms as well. Temporoparietal involvement in the language-dominant hemisphere has been hypothesized on the basis of clinical (Wolf and Inoue, 2002) and ictal single photon emission tomography findings (Kücük et al., 1999). However, abnormal activity in the complex bilateral network subserving reading was suggested by Koepp et al. (1998), and a bilateral, although not generalized, onset has been more recently proposed (Wolf and Inoue, 2002). A family history of reading epilepsy is present in about 25% of patients with the disorder (Wolf and Inoue, 2002; Sàenz-Lope et al., 1985; Wilkins and Lindsay, 1985; Newmark, 1983). The male-to-female ratio is 1.8 to 1.

Secondary reading epilepsy (Sàenz-Lope et al., 1985; Newmark, 1983) includes those patients who have spontaneous seizures of various types in addition to those provoked by reading. Reading epilepsy certainly differs from the more common visually induced epilepsies. Only 20% of patients have a paroxysmal response to light (Newmark, 1983), and the interictal records are normal in most patients with primary reading epilepsy. The ictal recordings consist of bursts of theta or delta activity or brief discharges of bilateral or unilateral fast spike-wave complexes (Wolf and Inoue, 2002). Patients should be taught to stop reading to avoid major seizures when this becomes necessary. If the avoidance of the triggering situation is not possible, sodium valproate or clobazam treatment may be successful (Wolf and Inoue, 2002). Although complete remission of this disorder is very rare, a good prognosis seems relatively common (Radhakrishan et al., 1995).

Language-Induced Seizures

The term *language-induced seizures* is used to designate the rare disorder seen in patients whose seizures can be precipitated by reading, speaking, or writing. The disorder shares features with reading epilepsy, especially jaw myoclonus induced by reading (Cirignotta et al., 1986; Forster, 1977; Geshwind and Sherwin, 1967). In some patients, writing is an effective stimulus, and it may evoke absence attacks and/or myoclonic jerks, particularly in the hand that is writing. Language-induced seizures are variable in their provocation and expression, and they are less stereotypic than primary reading epilepsy (Terzano et al., 1983).

Thinking-Induced Seizures

Seizures induced by thinking is the name proposed by Wilkins et al. (1982) for seizures induced by elaborate mental activity of a complex nature, such as mathematical computation of certain types and manipulation of spatial information (e.g., playing chess), but not by retention of numerical information or short-term memory tasks. A such few cases have been reported (Senanayake, 1989; Anderson and Wallis, 1986; Cirignotta et al., 1980). The process of decision making rather than that of computation or the manipulation of abstract information may play a role in such cases (Crandall, 1982). The process of decision making, however, produces anxiety and stress, which may be an important but nonspecific trigger for the seizures (Newmark and Penry, 1979).

Eating Epilepsy

Eating epilepsy has been reviewed by Loiseau et al. (1986) and Fiol et al. (1986). The seizures do not appear to be secondary to motor masticatory movements, salivation, or sensory stimuli originating in the buccal cavity. The attacks are usually focal, and they may be caused by structural abnormalities such as tumors (Robertson and Fariello, 1979) or cortical dysplasia (Verdu and Ruiz-Falco, 1991). They may produce serious nutritional problems. Spontaneous attacks may coexist with induced ones. A familial case of eating epilepsy has been reported (Senanayake, 1990).

SUMMARY

Certain epileptic seizures are regularly precipitated by specific stimuli. Most of these stimuli are sensory in nature, but some are caused by complex activities involving several sensory systems or higher brain functions (e.g., reading epilepsy). Intermittent light is by far the most common sensory precipitant of seizures (photosensitive or visually sensitive epilepsy). IPS is also a potent precipitant of paroxysmal events in the EEG, which have been termed the photoparoxysmal response. This response is much more common than photic-induced attacks, and it may be observed both in epileptic patients without photic-induced seizures and in individuals without

epilepsy. The most common type of photosensitive epilepsy is represented by generalized tonic-clonic seizures that are precipitated by flickering light from either natural sources or, more commonly, artificial ones, mainly television screens. Photic-induced focal (occipital) seizures have been recently recognized as being much more common than was previously thought. They are probably underdiagnosed, and they may often be mistaken for migraine attacks. The seizures may always be precipitated by flickering light, or they may also occur spontaneously, especially in patients with generalized seizures. Visually sensitive epilepsy occurs mainly in preadolescents and adolescents. The generalized forms appear to be closely related to the primary generalized epilepsies that occur in the same age groups. Genetic factors are important in their etiology. Other forms of light-induced epilepsy may be observed in children, including absences occurring with eye closure (eyelid myoclonia with absence) and a variety of self-induced seizures in both mentally retarded and intellectually normal patients.

Startle provoked by auditory, tactile, proprioceptive, or other stimuli is the second most common cause of stimulus-sensitive seizures. In contrast with photosensitive epilepsy, which is observed mainly in patients without structural cerebral pathology, startle epilepsy occurs in patients with cerebral lesions, most of which originate in the prenatal or perinatal periods. Attacks precipitated by startle should be separated from movement-induced seizures, which are extremely rare; these are often confused with paroxysmal kinesigenic and exercise-induced dyskinesias.

Other less common precipitating factors include rare sensory stimuli and complex activities like eating, reading, computation, or decision making.

The physiopathology of stimulus-sensitive seizures, even of the best-defined and most common type (visually evoked seizures), is incompletely understood. A complex combination of factors is involved. Both the idiopathic and symptomatic forms of reflex epilepsies are characterized by the abnormal processing of afferent inputs to specific cortical areas or networks, leading to an exaggerated response.

18

Posttraumatic Seizures and Posttraumatic Epilepsy

Epilepsy develops in a small proportion of head-injured patients. Head trauma caused by street or traffic accidents is increasingly common in infancy, childhood, and adolescence, so posttraumatic epilepsy is an important condition in pediatrics. For many patients, posttraumatic epilepsy is the only serious sequel of their accident, but this supervenes only rarely, considering the high incidence of head injury.

The identification of those patients with head trauma who are at risk for epilepsy is desirable because then practical advice could be given to parents and patients regarding the lifestyle for the children at risk and, later, the choice of a profession and the problems of acquiring a driver's license. Reliable information is now available about epilepsy after civilian (nonmilitary) injury (Jennett and Teasdale, 1981; Jennett, 1973, 1974), but information about posttraumatic epilepsy in children is still limited (Weiner et al., 1991; Foulon and Noel, 1977; Kollevold, 1976; Jennett, 1973; Hendrick and Harris, 1968). The ability to predict better the occurrence of eventual epilepsy after head trauma also raises a question of the value of and indications for prophylactic treatment of children following head injuries.

The mechanisms underlying posttraumatic epileptogenesis remain unknown. Trauma that results from shearing of the axons could lead to the loss of inhibitory interneurons through anterograde transsynaptic degeneration (Saji and Reis, 1987). The release of aspartate or glutamate following trauma (Faden et al., 1989), the enhancement of reactive gliosis (Nieto-Sampedro, 1988), and the cellular responses to free radical oxidants that result from the release of hemoglobin or iron-containing heme into the brain all may contribute to epileptogenesis (Chandler, 2000).

From a clinical viewpoint, the occurrence of posttraumatic seizures is not a random event. Distinguishing seizures by when they occur relative to the trauma is customary; immediate seizures occur within 1 hour of the trauma (immediate or impact seizures), delayed early-onset seizures are defined as those occurring between 24 hours and 7 days after the trauma, and late-onset seizures supervene later, up to

months or years after the trauma. The significance of the timing of the seizures is not the same. Some ambiguity exists with respect to the terminology used in posttraumatic cases. For example, the earliest seizures often remain isolated, and, consequently, they should not be termed *epilepsy*, a term which is reserved for chronic recurrent seizures. The same applies to some of the early seizures; however, the term *early epilepsy* is often used for these. Likewise, many authors consider even a single seizure occurring in a patient with an antecedent of significant head injury late epilepsy (Annegers et al., 1980; Jennett, 1973). During the past few decades, several studies have emphasized the different significance of early posttraumatic seizures and late posttraumatic epilepsy (Jennett and Teasdale, 1981; Jennett, 1974), and this distinction is followed in this chapter.

INCIDENCE

The incidence of *early seizures* varies considerably with the type of injury sustained by the patient and among various series, probably as a result of the lack of agreement on terms, the composition of series, or other methodologic factors. The overall incidence following civilian head injury is between 2% and 2.5% in adults, which rises to 5% for hospitalized neurosurgical patients (Chandler, 2000). The figures are substantially higher in severely brain-injured patients (those with a Glasgow Coma Scale score of 8 or less), reaching 10% to 15% in adults (Temkin et al., 1990; Annegers et al., 1980) and 30% to 35% in children (Hahn et al., 1988). Annegers et al. (1980) found that this high risk was caused by an increased frequency of early epilepsy following severe head injury only. Other authors (Kollevold, 1976; Jennett, 1973; Hendrick and Harris, 1968) have reported that the higher incidence of early seizures in children was almost entirely the result of the greater propensity of young patients compared to adults to develop seizures after mild or trivial trauma. Thus, Kollevold (1976) indicated that frequency of early seizures in children and adults was, respectively, 4.2% and 0.9% following concussion, 5.4% and 5.8% following contusion, and 21% and 9.2% when an intracranial hematoma was present. The higher incidence of early posttraumatic seizures in children compared with adults can be accounted for by a much higher incidence of immediate (impact) seizures. The findings of Annegers et al. (1980) cast doubt on the reality of an increased frequency of seizures after mild head injury. Another confounding factor may be the high incidence of trivial trauma in childhood, so a coincidence between trauma and the onset of seizures cannot be excluded. Similar discrepancies have been found in various studies with respect to the influence of the type of head injury on the development of early epilepsy. Whereas Annegers et al. (1980) found an incidence of 31% for early seizures following severe trauma and of roughly 1% for mild and moderate trauma, Jennett (1973) did not notice a marked effect of the severity of the trauma on the frequency of early seizures as opposed to its effect on the incidence of late epilepsy. Referral patterns and methodologic differences probably account for such discrepancies.

The incidence of *late posttraumatic epilepsy* in children varies from 0.2% to 12%, which is slightly lower than the 1.3% to 15% commonly quoted for adults. The risk of late epilepsy also varies considerably with the severity of head trauma. It is greatly increased with hematoma requiring surgical evacuation, torn dura, and/or posttraumatic amnesia of 24 hours or more. The risk is 12% for severe trauma, 1.6% in moderate trauma, and only 0.6% in mild trauma (Annegers et al., 1980). The last figure is still significantly higher than the incidence of epilepsy in the general population.

Nonaccidental head injuries in infants raise specific problems. According to a recent study (Barlow et al., 2000), the incidence of seizures is much higher than that seen in accidental injuries. Of 44 children seen at one institution, 32 (73%) had early posttraumatic seizures. The average age was 5.9 months. The exact time of occurrence of seizures in such cases is difficult to ascertain, but the peak incidence was seen on the second day of hospitalization and all cases occurred before day 3. The incidence of late-onset epilepsy was also quite high, appearing in 22% of survivors. Six children died, and the outcome with regard to both survival and late epilepsy was strongly correlated with the severity of the injury. The incidence of early status epilepticus was also extremely high (13 patients), and 16 infants had intractable seizures.

EARLY ONSET SEIZURES

Features

Early onset seizures are those that occur during the first week following head trauma. They are mainly concentrated in the first 24 hours, during which period of time at least 50% of cases occur (Snoek et al., 1984; McQueen et al., 1983; Annegers et al., 1980; Hendrick and Harris, 1968). This is due mainly to the very high incidence of impact seizures (Chandler, 2000). As in adults, the incidence of posttraumatic seizures rises with the severity of the head injury. In children younger than 16 years, the proportion is even higher, with 80% of patients having fits within 24 hours of injury (Jennett, 1973). Approximately one-third of those patients with early posttraumatic epilepsy have seizures within 1 hour of the trauma. Most of the early seizures are focal, and, of these, 75% are partial motor attacks, even in children younger than 5 years. The remaining attacks are generalized (Caveness et al., 1979; Maijkowski, 1977; Jennett, 1974). Approximately one-third of patients have only one fit during the first week (Jennett, 1973). However, status epilepticus following head trauma is much more common in children than in adults. Status was observed in 29 (16%) of 177 children, compared with 22 (7.5%) of 288 adults in one series (Jennett, 1973), and the highest incidence (22.1%) was in those children younger than 5 years. Status may cause secondary brain damage resulting from hypoxia or ischemia, but it does not seem to be associated with an increased risk of late epilepsy beyond that associated with any type of early epilepsy (Grand, 1974; Jennett, 1973).

These early epileptic seizures should be distinguished from the paroxysmal manifestations that may occur in the hours following head trauma, including sudden blindness, aphasia, hemianopia, and disturbances of consciousness (Snoek et al., 1984; Oka et al., 1977). Convulsions may appear in children with such phenomena before recovery (Oka et al., 1977). Such accidents may be related to migraine or to the mechanism of the spreading depression of Leão (Oka et al., 1977).

Significance

The occurrence of early seizures should not mislead the clinician, resulting in a diagnosis of intracranial hematoma, nor should they be regarded as an indication for surgical intervention. Seizures are never the sole sign of a neurosurgical complication. However, seizures may confuse the clinical picture because they may be followed by focal signs and/or they may be associated with temporary alterations in consciousness. Early seizures *per se* do not indicate a need for chronic treatment. Anticonvulsant therapy for the first week or until the acute effects of head injury have abated is required.

However, an early seizure in an apparently mildly injured child identifies a group of patients whose injuries must be investigated further because a significant number are found to have more serious underlying brain injuries (Lee and Lui, 1992).

Most authors consider the major implication of early posttraumatic seizures to be the increased risk of late epilepsy (Weiss et al., 1983; Annegers et al., 1980; Caveness et al., 1979; Hendrick and Harris, 1968). The figures given vary greatly, ranging from 15% to 50% (Holmes, 1986; Caveness et al., 1979; Scherzer and Wessely, 1978; Maheshwari and Jeavons, 1975). However, Annegers et al. (1980) found no relationship between the occurrence of early seizures following severe or moderate injury and that of late epilepsy in children, as opposed to adults. On the contrary, Jennett (1975) found a fourfold increase in incidence of late epilepsy in patients with early seizures for children both older and younger than 5 years. In the same study (Holmes, 1986), focal seizures were associated with late epilepsy significantly less often (7.6% vs. 29%) than nonfocal seizures. However, early onset seizures may not be as strongly predictive of late-onset epilepsy in children as they are in adults.

LATE POSTTRAUMATIC EPILEPSY

All seizures that occur more than 1 week after head trauma are termed *late posttraumatic epilepsy*. The incidence of late-onset seizures is much lower than that of early seizures. The incidence is greatly increased with hematoma requiring surgical evacuation, torn dura, depressed fracture, and/or posttraumatic amnesia of 24 hours or more (Jennett, 1974). The overall incidence in children is slightly lower than that in adults (Jennett and Teasdale, 1981; Annegers et al., 1980); the incidence most commonly quoted for adults is roughly 5%. Lower figures have been reported by Annegers et al. (1980) and McQueen et al. (1983). The latter study, however, excluded those patients with early epilepsy, who, however, are at greatest risk of developing late seizures. According to Annegers et al. (1980), the risk of developing epilepsy within 5 years of a head injury varies greatly with the severity of trauma. The risk was 12% in the case of severe trauma, 1.6% in moderate trauma, and only 0.6% in mild trauma. The last

figure is not significantly higher than that for the incidence of epilepsy in the general population.

Features

Late epilepsy can develop at any time following trauma. However, the risk decreases with time, even though late or very late seizures (i.e., more than 5 or 10 years after injury) do occur. Up to 57% of epilepsies have their onset within 1 year of injury (Willmore, 1992). Caveness et al. (1979) reported that the onset of seizures occurred during the first months in 7% to 9% of cases, with the rate falling to 2% to 3% for the next 6 months and to 1% or less after that time period. In one series (Paillas and Bureau, 1982), the relative risk of developing late epilepsy compared with the general population was 13% for the first year, 4.4% for the next 4 years, and only 1.4% after 5 years. In children, the tendency of seizures to occur after free periods is longer than those in adults (Jennett, 1974). In one study (Paillas and Bureau, 1982), late epilepsy (i.e., after 5 years) was more common than early epilepsy (58% versus 14%). However, the number of children in this study was small (54 of 333 patients), and the occurrence of seizures may have been the reason for referral.

The seizures of late posttraumatic epilepsy are generalized, at least in appearance, more often than those of early epilepsy, and the frequency of generalized seizures varies from 60% (Jennett and Teasdale, 1981) to 80% (Paillas and Bureau, 1982) of cases. The incidence of focal features at the onset of generalized seizures is poorly known, but it is probably high. Caveness et al. (1979) found the ratio of focal to generalized seizures to be about 3 to 1; focal seizures tended to be more common than those that were generalized and to be associated with a higher frequency of seizures and a longer duration of the seizure period. Generalized seizures are more common with frontal lobe lesions (Paillas and Bureau, 1982). Complex partial seizures are observed in 20% to 75% of cases. In young children, a severe form of epilepsy that clinically is reminiscent of Lennox-Gastaut syndrome may occur following severe frontal head trauma (Niedermeyer et al., 1970). Status epilepticus may also be observed, especially with frontal lobe lesions (Janz, 1983).

The course of late epilepsy is unpredictable. Seizures remit spontaneously in approximately 50% of cases within 5 years (Paillas and Bureau, 1982). About 25% of patients with late-onset seizures have only one attack and 50% or more have fewer than four seizures (Temkin et al., 1995; Jennett, 1974). A total of 75% to 85% have their first seizure within 2 years of the head injury (Jennett, 1974). However, the relative benignity of posttraumatic epilepsy has been questioned. Jennett and Teasdale (1981) noted that 80% of their patients who were followed for 2 to 5 years after their first attack continued to have some fits and that one-third of them had frequent fits. An apparent remission was not uncommon during the first 2 years.

Predictors of Late Epilepsy

According to Jennett (1973), three factors dominate the prediction of late epilepsy. They include (a) the existence of early epilepsy, (b) the need to evacuate an intracranial hematoma within 2 weeks of injury, and (c) the presence of a depressed fracture. Patients with hematomas have a 35% risk of developing late epilepsy, and those with early epilepsy have a 19% to 25% risk. Patients with depressed fractures have varying risks depending on various combinations of the three factors. On the other hand, the risk of late epilepsy is extremely small in the absence of such factors (less than 2%), even in patients with a posttraumatic amnesia or coma lasting more than 24 hours. As was indicated, the precise figures vary with the type of referral. For example, the risk of epilepsy is extremely small in children with linear skull fractures, a common type of injury in that age-group.

The electroencephalogram (EEG) is only marginally useful for predicting the occurrence of late epilepsy (Courjon and Mauguière, 1982; Reisner et al., 1979; Scherzer and Wessely, 1978; Jennett, 1974). Tracings are often abnormal at the time of injury. Later, most recordings revert to normal, but this does not signify that late epilepsy will not occur. In a series of 453 patients who developed late epilepsy, Courjon and Mauguiere (1982) found that 40% had normal tracings during the period between the trauma and the first seizure. Conversely, localized abnormalities, including spikes or spike-wave complexes, do not necessarily indicate that posttraumatic epilepsy will occur. However, the persistence of focalized abnormalities usually is associated with late epilepsy, although localized paroxysmal anomalies can persist for 10 years or more without the patient ever developing seizures.

Computed tomographic or magnetic resonance imaging evidence of parenchymal damage or intracerebral hemorrhage is associated with a higher incidence of posttraumatic seizures (D'Alessandro et al., 1988; Hahn et al., 1988).

TREATMENT AND PHARMACOLOGIC PREVENTION OF POSTTRAUMATIC EPILEPSY

Aggressive treatment of early posttraumatic seizures is an essential part of the treatment of severe or moderate head injuries. Seizures in patients with head trauma are deleterious because they raise cerebral blood flow, favoring the development of brain edema; they increase metabolic demands; and they cause the release of excitotoxic neurotransmitters, thus increasing neuronal damage. In addition, movements resulting from seizures may cause further damage to patients with multiple injuries. For these reasons, antiepileptic agents must be given in the first week after head injury or until the acute effects have abated. Phenytoin (Temkin et al., 1990) and carbamazepine (Glötzner et al., 1983; McQueen et al., 1983) have been shown to be effective in the treatment of early seizures.

Anticonvulsant treatment of late seizures is probably indicated because three-fourths of patients who present with a first attack have more than one seizure.

Attempts at giving prophylactic therapy are based on the assumption that antiepileptic agents given early enough after trauma can prevent the development of an epileptic focus. This effect could take place through inhibiting the kindling phenomenon, although the existence of this phenomenon has not been demonstrated in the human brain. Servit and Musil (1981) reported 143 patients who received phenytoin for 3 to 5 years after head trauma. Only three developed seizures. In two, the attacks followed the discontinuation of treatment. On the other hand, 6 of 24 untreated patients exhibited seizures, 4 of them within 1 year of the trauma. This was an uncontrolled study, and the results could not be duplicated in several better controlled studies using several anticonvulsant agents, including sodium valproate (Janz, 1983; Penry et al., 1979; Rapport and Penry, 1972). A prospective, controlled study showed that carbamazepine has some effectiveness in the prevention of late epilepsy, although it does not affect the incidence of early seizures (Glötzner, 1981). However, the degree of protection that was afforded was modest, and more work is necessary before the prophylactic treatment of posttraumatic epilepsy can be advised. Temkin et al. (1990) showed that the use of phenytoin to suppress acute seizures in 404 adult patients treated prospectively following head injury was effective during the acute early period. On the other hand, no difference in the incidence of posttraumatic late epilepsy at 1 year after injury and in control groups was observed, and, by 2 years after the injury, seizures had occurred in 28% of treated patients as opposed to 21% of the controls. This occurred even though blood levels were maintained within the therapeutic range and were repeatedly controlled. This result has been since confirmed (Manaka, 1992). The actual practice of neurosurgeons is quite variable (Rapport and Penry, 1970). Even if an effective treatment were available, this would be indicated only in selected at-risk patients (Jennett and Teasdale, 1981), because the incidence of late epilepsy is quite low in most patients. The question about whether anticonvulsant drug prophylaxis is indicated in children who undergo neurosurgical operations is somewhat similar. In such situations, drug prophylaxis also appears to be possibly ineffective (Shaw and Foy, 1991).

SUMMARY

Posttraumatic epilepsy is an important condition in pediatrics because of the high incidence of head trauma in children.

Posttraumatic seizures are particularly common during the first week following trauma. Most of these early seizures are of the partial or focal type, and one-third of patients have only one attack. However, status epilepticus as a complication of head trauma is more common in children than in adults. Early posttraumatic epilepsy usually does not indicate the presence of a neurosurgical complication, but it is a predictor of late posttraumatic epilepsy, which is approximately four times more common in patients with early seizures than in those without.

Late posttraumatic epilepsy occurs in approximately 5% of patients. The maximum risk is concentrated within the first 2 years following trauma, but long seizure-free intervals may be more common in children than in adults. Complex partial seizures are especially common in late posttraumatic epilepsy, and the prognosis is probably more severe than was traditionally thought because four out of five patients still have seizures 2 years after their first attack.

The possibility of preventing late posttraumatic epilepsy by administering anticonvulsant agents prophylactically after head trauma has been a topic of much discussion. Recent work indicates that the effect, if any, of prophylactic therapy is marginal at best (Chandler, 2000).

Epilepsy as the Presenting Manifestation
of Structural Brain Lesions

Although epilepsy can be caused by a host of brain lesions of congenital or acquired origin, these causes are not reviewed in detail here; this chapter deals only with some of the organic causes of epilepsy that have been selected because of their diagnostic importance; their frequency; or the specific problems they pose regarding therapy, investigations to be performed, or genetic counseling. Selected causes include brain tumors, abnormalities of cortical development, tuberous sclerosis (TS), hippocampal sclerosis (HS), vascular malformations, Sturge-Weber syndrome, and cerebral palsy.

BRAIN TUMORS

Seizures can occur with both malignant and benign tumors, and they may be their first clinical manifestation. They may be caused by the effect of the tumor on the surrounding cortex; by associated lesions that may be contiguous to the tumor, such as cortical dysplasia (Prayson and Estes, 1995; Prayson et al., 1993), or by distant lesions involving especially the mesial temporal lobe. In the latter case (dual pathology), the respective roles of tumor and the other lesions remain a subject of dispute (Cendes et al., 1995). In rare cases, the tumor itself can be the origin of seizure discharges (Harvey et al., 1996; Munari et al., 1995).

Epileptic seizures in childhood are only seldom caused by brain tumors. In unselected series of children with epilepsy, only 0.2% to 0.3% had brain tumors (Livingston, 1972; Page et al., 1969), although a higher proportion of tumors has been found in some selected series, especially when epilepsies with partial seizures have been considered (Blume et al., 1982; Aicardi et al., 1970). Thus, Gilsanz et al. (1979) found three tumors among 169 children with apparently cryptogenic partial epilepsy (i.e., isolated seizure disorders without neurologic signs or concomitant disease). Aicardi et al. (1983) found three tumors among 274 children with apparently crypto-

genic partial epilepsy without neurologic signs or concomitant disease. Hauser et al. (1993) found an incidence of 1% in patients younger than 15 years, and Sander and Sillanpää (1998) found an incidence of 1% in those younger than 30 years. Only 2% of infants younger than 1 year with tumor present with a seizure. Seizures are uncommon in children with infratentorial tumors. On the other hand, epileptic seizures are the first manifestation of tumors of the cerebral hemispheres in one-fourth (Gilles et al., 1992) to half (Aicardi et al., 1970) of the cases in both children and adults.

Most tumors that give rise to seizures are benign; thus, an early diagnosis is important because many are amenable to surgical treatment. The problem is, therefore, selecting from the extremely large number of children with seizures those few whose attacks are likely to be caused by brain tumors, while minimizing the number of patients submitted to neuroimaging diagnostic procedures. Epilepsy also may be a consequence of the treatment (surgical or otherwise) of recognized brain tumors, but such epilepsies are not dealt with in this chapter.

Any type of tumor can give rise to seizures, but benign tumors are most often the cause of isolated epilepsy. Rapidly growing tumors usually present with focal deficits and/or intracranial hypertension. Low-grade gliomas, especially astrocytomas and oligodendrogliomas and mixed oligoastrocytomas, were mostly found in early studies (Aicardi et al., 1970). More recent studies have emphasized the role of neuronal glial tumors, especially *gangliogliomas and developmental neuroepithelial tumors* (DNTs), in the causation of chronic epilepsy; these may remain monosymptomatic in the form of recurrent partial seizures for many years. The frequency of the different types varies from center to center, and this may depend partly on the pathologic criteria used. At the Maudsley Hospital, London, Bruton (1988) found that, of 37 tumors from 249 temporal lobectomies, nine were gangliogliomas. Of 216 temporal lobectomies performed in Bonn, Germany, 75 contained tumors, of which 34 (45%) were gangliogliomas and 25 (33%) were astrocytomas (Wolf et al., 1993). The idea that, regardless of histologic diagnosis, indolent tumors associated with chronic epilepsy may constitute a distinct clinicopathologic group has been expressed (Fried et al., 1994). Likewise, Bartolomei et al. (1997) suggested that low-grade temporal and extratemporal tumors found in 45 patients shared many features with DNTs in terms of their clinical profile and course and that they may represent variants of DNTs (Pasquier et al., 2002). The latter are diagnosed especially in children and adolescents; they are often superficially located in the temporal lobe, and they tend to remain static over time. They often manifest as isolated partial seizures of early onset for quite long periods (Raymond et al., 1994b; Kirkpatrick et al., 1993; Daumas-Duport, 1988), although they may be associated with cognitive and behavioral deterioration in a few early cases (Neville et al., 1997). Their histologic appearance is heterogeneous, and their differential diagnosis may be difficult (Honavar et al., 1999). Gangliogliomas and gangliocytomas are closely related tumors that may occur even in neonates (Duchowny et al., 1989), and their total removal with subsequent seizure control is often feasible (Duchowny et al., 1996; Zeutner et al., 1994).

However, malignant tumors (high-grade astrocytomas) have been found in a few cases of long-standing epilepsy, which suggests that malignant changes may occur within benign tumors with time (Aicardi et al., 1970; Page et al., 1969).

Clinical and Electroencephalographic Features of Epilepsies Caused by Brain Tumors

The clinical and EEG features of the epilepsies that reveal tumors of the cerebral hemispheres in children are important to consider mainly in those patients in whom epilepsy is not immediately or very rapidly associated with other neurologic signs and symptoms or with signs of intracranial hypertension. In many patients with hemispheral tumors, epileptic seizures remain the sole clinical manifestation for a few months to many years (Spencer et al., 1984a). In one series (Aicardi et al., 1970), the mean interval between the first seizure and the diagnosis of a tumor was 5.6 years, and intervals as long as 20 years have been reported (Blume et al., 1982; Aicardi et al., 1970; Page et al., 1969; Lennox and Lennox, 1960). In the same series, 8% of patients were younger than 1 year and 19% younger than 2 years, and cases occurring in infancy or the neonatal period have been recorded (Duchowny et al., 1989; Rutledge et al., 1987). Most cases, however, occur in older children and adolescents (Kirkpatrick et al., 1993; Blume et al., 1982; Page et al., 1969). In mixed series of children and adults (Cascino, 1990; Boon et al., 1991), refractory epilepsy commonly is the sole manifestation of a tumor. Boon et al. (1991) found that 50 of 250 patients with intractable partial seizures had a detectable lesion on neuroimaging and that the lesion was neoplastic in 35 (70%). Most patients had an onset of seizures at adolescence (mean age of 13 years), and the mean duration of the epilepsy was 11 years. The lesions were located in the temporal lobe in 57% of patients. This series included four cases of hamartoma and three of ganglioglioma. Cascino (1990) and Cascino et al. (1993a) similarly reported that the seizures were refractory to drug treatment in 30 of their 45 patients. The widespread use of neuroimaging techniques has shortened the diagnostic delay considerably.

Partial seizures are more common than generalized seizures, but the latter are not uncommon. Several types of attacks are commonly associated, but generalized seizures can occur in isolation for months or years. Some seizures are described as "generalized" because of nonlocalizing symptoms, such as staring, eye blinking, generalized hypertonia, or hypotonia, are the expression of localized, often temporal discharges (Spencer et al., 1984a; Aicardi et al., 1970). Some types of seizures (e.g., complex partial seizures with olfactory hallucinations) are usually regarded as symptomatic of a tumor in a high proportion of cases (Penfield and Jasper, 1954), although this has been debated (Howe and Gibson, 1982). In the authors' experience, purely or predominantly sensory symptoms may often be associated with central tumors. In a series of 98 children with supratentorial astroglial tumors and seizures, partial seizures were part of the presentation in half of the cases, and they were the only complaint in 30% (Shady et al., 1994).

A tumor should be readily suspected when deterioration in personality or performance becomes evident or when progressive neurologic deficits or signs and symptoms of increased intracranial pressure appear. However, especially with developmental tumors, epilepsy often remains the only abnormality for long periods lasting up to several years (Duchowny et al., 1996; Raymond et al., 1994b). These tumors are often localized to the temporal lobe, especially its mesial aspect, but they may also arise from the frontal and other lobes. They are often resistant to drug therapy, and they are not associated with any neurologic sign or other symptoms.

Contrary to what is often stated, no pattern of seizure recurrence is indicative of a tumor, and patients with hemispheral tumors may have only occasional fits or seizures that respond favorably to drug therapy, at times for prolonged periods. Neurologic signs appear late, and the correct diagnosis should not await their appearance. Behavioral and/or intellectual deterioration, on the other hand, may be more precocious (Aicardi et al., 1970; Page et al., 1969). Blume et al. (1982) found that the likelihood of tumors was highest in patients with a normal intellect.

The electroencephalographic (EEG) abnormalities associated with brain tumors have been extensively reviewed (Daly and Markand, 1990; Hughes and Zak, 1987; Blume, 1982; Bancaud et al., 1973; Page et al., 1969). No EEG pattern is specific for tumors. Localized foci of polymorphic delta waves are the most suggestive, but these are often absent. Foci of sharp waves on a slow disorganized background are almost as common, and these are suggestive of an organic lesion. Focal spiking without significant changes in background tracing is not rare. The EEG anomalies associated with developmental tumors seem more diffuse than those associated with hippocampal atrophy (Hamer et al., 1999; Blume et al., 1982). Multifocal spiking may occur (Blume et al., 1982), and it seems relatively common in children. Bilateral synchronous discharges, either asymmetric or symmetric, have been reported in 10% to 25% of patients (Page et al., 1969; Madsen and Bray, 1966). A normal EEG is rare with tumors of the cerebral hemispheres (5% of patients), but it may be seen in 10% to 20% of patients with deep midline tumors or tumors of the parasagittal region (Hughes and Zak, 1987).

Several unusual epileptic presentations can occur in children with tumors. Infantile spasms are rarely caused by brain tumors (Kotagal et al., 1995a; Ruggieri et al., 1989), and this is also true for the Lennox-Gastaut syndrome (LGS) (Angelini et al., 1979). Two uncommon syndromes deserve special attention.

Diencephalic hamartomas may be responsible for a well-defined epileptic syndrome (Berkovic et al., 1988; Breningstall, 1985; Curatolo et al., 1984; Diebler and Ponsot, 1983; Matustik et al., 1981) that is characterized by gelastic (giggling) seizures with onset in the first 2 years of life. Such giggling attacks are usually frequently repeated. They are often associated with progressive mental retardation (Berkovic et al., 1988, 2003; Deonna and Ziegler, 2000), especially when the seizures evolve into secondary generalized attacks reminiscent of those in LGS (see Chapter 4).

Another rare syndrome of epilepsy arising from deep structures has recently been reported under the terms *cerebellar epilepsy* (Arzimanoglou, 1999; Harvey et al., 1996) or *subcortical epilepsy* (Arzimanoglou et al., 1999). It is due to a hamartomatous tumor located in the cerebellar peduncle and brainstem, and it is manifested by repeated brief attacks of hemifacial contracture from early life. Harvey et al. (1996) demonstrated that the attacks were associated with a typical epileptic discharge originating in the vicinity of or within the tumor. This lesion may be amenable to surgical therapy, which may control the seizures if the resection is complete (Harvey et al., 1996) (see Chapter 10).

Neuroimaging Findings in Brain Tumors

Modern neuroimaging has resulted in a considerable change in the circumstances of the diagnosis, although some tumors continue to be missed for substantial periods. This occurs especially when only a computed tomographic (CT) scan is performed, particularly when the tumors involve the temporal lobe because of the common presence of bone artifacts in that area. Missing a tumor also can result from a failure to use contrast enhancement, which should be used routinely in this clinical context, or from the use of less than optimal machines. In the series of Spencer et al. (1984a), the initial CT scan was not diagnostic in 5 of 20 patients. Two of the CT scans were misinterpreted, but three were normal, even in retrospect, demonstrating that repeat examination may be necessary in some cases.

Magnetic resonance imaging (MRI) is clearly preferable to CT (Commission on Neuroimaging of the International League Against Epilepsy, 1997), and MRI should be the first imaging investigation performed for epilepsy. A CT scan may be used in special indications, especially for the demonstration of calcifications, which are better visualized with CT than with MRI.

Neither CT nor MRI are indicated in children with only generalized epilepsy of the idiopathic type because the yield of imaging in such patients is extremely low (Harwood-Nash, 1983; Varma et al., 1983). These include the primary generalized epilepsies of adolescence, various types of myoclonic epilepsy of late childhood, and typical absence epilepsy. Imaging is also unnecessary in typical cases of partial benign epilepsy with rolandic focus. If the physician does not feel secure enough about his or her ability to diagnose benign partial epilepsy or one of the other syndromes for which neuroradiologic examination is not indicated, imaging should be conducted. On the other hand, the clinician need not wait before obtaining an imaging study as long as he or she is not dealing with a child who has an occasional seizure because tumors can be detected even at a very early stage. Certainly, neuroimaging has made the diagnosis of brain tumors easier at an earlier stage.

MRI has considerably improved the diagnosis of small tumors. The possibility of using different planes of imaging has considerable value for the detection of small lesions such as those in the hippocampus. Several sequences should be used, including fluid-attenuated inversion recovery (FLAIR) images, thin cuts, three-dimensional acquisition, reformatting in different planes, and gadolinium enhancement. In most cases, this should distinguish tumors from dysplastic and inflammatory lesions. However, distinguishing peritumoral edema from the tumor itself may remain difficult, thus making the delimitation of the lesion difficult. Repeating the examination after a few months can be necessary when doubt about the nature and a possible change in volume of the lesion exist.

Astrocytomas usually present as areas of increased signal, often with cystic formation (Fig. 19.1). Oligodendrogliomas involve the white matter, with possible infiltration of the neighboring cortex. Gangliogliomas may not show well on T1-weighted sequences, but they do appear as an area of increased signal that usually involves both the gray and the white matter (Duchowny et al., 1996; Sutton et al., 1983).

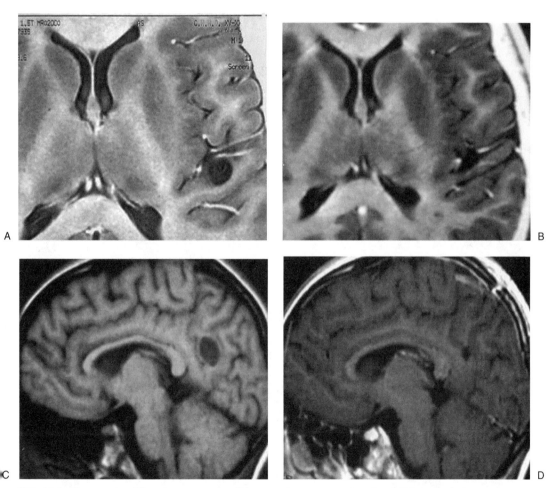

FIG. 19.1. Preoperative **(A)** and postoperative **(B)** magnetic resonance imaging (MRI) scan of a 7-year-old boy who presented with partial motor seizures related to the presence of an astrocytoma. He has been seizure free since surgery. Preoperative **(C)** and postoperative **(D)** MRI scans of an astrocytoma responsible for gyratory seizures in a 12-year-old girl. (Courtesy of Pr. Sainte-Rose, Hospital Necker, Paris, France.)

Dysembryoplastic neuroepithelial tumors are well demarcated, often multilocular, lesions that may be cystic and/or calcified (Figs. 19.2 and 19.3). They mostly involve the cortex, although they may be associated with edema of the white matter or they may impinge on it. They may be found in any lobe, but they most often involve the mesial or external aspects of the temporal lobe. They may enhance with gadolinium, and, occasionally, they may be visible after only contrast enhancement (Raymond et al., 1994b; Pasquier et al., 2002). When they are located near the inner table of the skull, they usually expand the overlying calvarium.

Finally, attention should be paid to the detection of other lesions, the so-called *dual pathology* (Cendes et al., 1995; Raymond et al., 1994a; Levesque et al.,

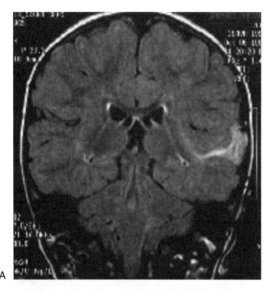

A

FIG. 19.2. A, B: Histologically confirmed dysembryoplastic neuroepithelial tumor (DNET) (magnetic resonance imaging and positron emission tomography), localized over the left posterior temporal gyrus, in a 2.5-year-old boy who presented with an episode of status followed by aphasia. No seizures were observed during the following 12 months. However, aphasia persisted despite intensive speech therapy. A left temporal spike-wave focus was present in all of the interictal electroencephalograms. Furthermore, long-duration recordings evidenced sequences of attenuation of the focus that were followed by rhythmic theta activity of low amplitude and flattening without any accompanying clinical signs. Two months later, clinical seizures were observed again. He was operated on at the age of 4 years (partial gyrectomy with complete excision of the DNET), and he has been seizure free for the last 18 months. His language acquisition has rapidly progressed back to normal.

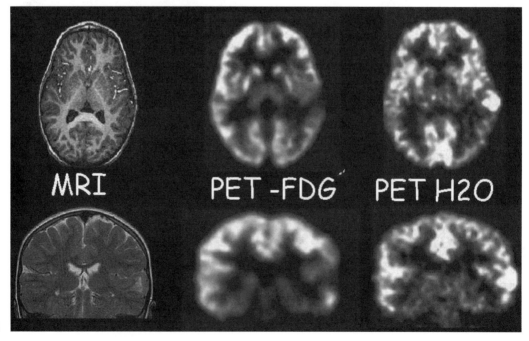

B

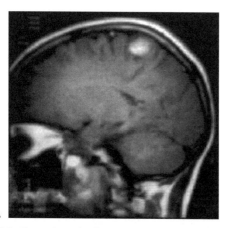 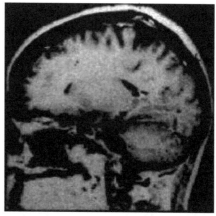

A   B

FIG. 19.3. Dysembryoplastic neuroepithelial tumor in a 9-year-old girl who presented with episodes of twitching and contraction of the right calf. The episodes could be associated with hypoesthesia of the leg, difficulty controlling movement, or even postictal paresis. A neurologic examination showed no abnormalities. After surgery **(right)**, she remained seizure free. (Courtesy of Dr. Philippe Kahane, Grenoble University Hospital, France.)

1991). The second lesion is usually HS, but other abnormalities are possible. Cendes et al. (1995) found hippocampal atrophy in 23 (14%) of 167 patients (both adults and children) with partial seizures that was mostly temporal. The frequency of dual pathology in this series was 2% in tumors, as opposed to 9% in vascular malformations and 25% in neuronal migration defects. Although the precise significance of dual pathology is still unclear, it should be detected and its role discussed when a surgical operation is being contemplated.

The common practice of imaging has uncovered some new diagnostic problems, especially those raised by the discovery of localized, more or less rounded areas of signal change, which may or may not represent indolent gliomas. When doubt persists, repeated imaging or biopsy of the lesion may be indicated. A signal change on MRI may be due to changes in blood–brain barrier permeability following seizures (Yaffe et al., 1995), and the investigations should resolve whether this is due to brain edema, hence emphasizing the need for follow-up examinations in cases of doubt.

Treatment

The treatment of epilepsy caused by brain tumors consists primarily of treating the tumor when it is clearly an aggressive, growing lesion. When the epilepsy is isolated, the treatment of seizures begins with antiepileptic agents, followed by treatment of the underlying tumor, usually by surgical resection. In most cases of indolent tumors, especially in dysembryoplastic neuroepithelial tumors and similarly behaving tumors, no other treatment is indicated because these are benign lesions that seldom, if ever, raise oncologic problems. However, not all tumors, including indolent ones, are always resectable; in such cases, partial resection may be successful. Monitoring of the lesion by follow-up MRI is probably acceptable when the prospect of resection is poor (Duchowny et al., 1998).

Excellent results have been reported after complete resection of the lesion, especially small indolent tumors, without specific attempts at the removal of the epileptogenic area (Boon et al., 1991; Cascino, 1990; Hirsch et al., 1989; Drake et al., 1987). In a large series of children with small glial tumors, Hirsch et al. (1989) reported control of epilepsy in 86% of their patients. The results were particularly satisfactory for those patients with the more benign pathologies in temporal, rather than extratemporal, epilepsy (Cascino et al., 1993a). In a series of 49 patients with alien tissue lesions, Bruton (1988) observed complete relief in 4 of 5 patients with a ganglioglioma and in 10 of 11 of those with mixed glial lesions, some of which would probably now be considered dysembryoplastic neuroepithelial tumors. Similar results were reported by Kirkpatrick et al. (1993).

Whether lesionectomy alone represents the optimal therapy remains a topic of debate. The relationship between a tumor and the origin of epileptic seizures is complex (Bancaud et al., 1973). Epileptic activity may not arise within the tumor itself, which is electrically silent when depth electrodes are inserted into it; rather, it may originate in the modified surrounding neural tissue (Engel, 1982a; Talairach and Bancaud, 1974; Falconer and Cavanagh, 1959). The question arises, therefore, of the removal of both the tumor tissue and the epileptogenic area that have been previously located by neurophysiologic studies (Cascino, 1990; Taft and Cohen, 1971). Some investigators think complete tumor resection, including additional resection of the epileptogenic area as determined by electrophysiologic investigation, electrocorticography (EcoG), or depth electrodes, is more effective. Cascino et al. (1992c) treated 23 patients by computer-assisted lesionectomy; 17 of them (74%) had a greater than 90% reduction in seizures, and 13 (56%) had an Engel grade 1 outcome. Boon et al. (1991) studied 50 patients (38 with tumors) who had a lesionectomy only; 83% were seizure free, and 11% had a greater than 90% reduction of seizures. Berger et al. (1991) used EcoG to achieve complete resection of the epileptogenic area in 45 adult patients with glial tumors; 41 (91%) became seizure free. Jooma et al. (1995) treated adults with lesionectomy, with only 3 patients becoming seizure free, whereas, of the 14 who had lesionectomy plus resection of the epileptogenic area as defined by corticography, 13 became seizure free. Montes et al. (1995) used lesionectomy alone in 18 children, 16 of whom (89%) were rendered seizure free. Although the current data are difficult to interpret because of methodologic problems, the resection of the epileptogenic area appears logical, especially because certain tumors (dysembryoplastic ones) are often associated with areas of dysplasia that may well be epileptogenic (Raymond et al., 1994b; Prayson et al., 1993).

Overall, the best outcome for seizure relief is when the tumor can be excised completely. The prognosis can probably be improved if the epileptogenic cortex defined by electrophysiologic studies is removed with the tumor. However, even partial resection may, in some cases, give good seizure control.

ABNORMALITIES OF CORTICAL DEVELOPMENT

Abnormal cortical development is increasingly recognized as a cause of both epilepsy and developmental disabilities (Vigevano et al., 2003). Histologically proven developmental brain abnormalities are observed in up to 25% of children with intractable seizures (Kuzniecky and Powers, 1993). Most such abnormalities may now be detected with MRI. However, some cortical malformations, or cortical dysplasias, remain undetectable even with the best imaging techniques. Although such information can detect

even very slight structural alterations, it does not always provide a precise indication of the pathologic nature of the lesion. The use of generic terms, such as *dysplasias* (Robain, 1996) or *malformations* of cortical development (Barkovich et al., 2001) or of the cerebral cortex, appears more appropriate whenever the exact nature of the developmental lesion is unclear on MRI and pathologic studies are unavailable. More specific terms may be used with highly characteristic MRI patterns (Barkovich, 1996).

Abnormalities of the cerebral cortex may be diffuse, or they may involve discrete cortical areas. The development of the cerebral cortex involves three distinct, but overlapping, processes, including neuronal and later glial proliferation, neuronal migration, and cortical organization. Cortical malformations can originate from abnormalities of any or all of these processes. Often, classifying cortical dysplasias according to their supposed mechanism is difficult because some dysplasias (e.g., polymicrogyria) may represent distinct histologic types of abnormalities and because different pathologic processes can coexist in the same macroscopic lesion (e.g., heterotopia and polymicrogyria). In fact, defects in one mechanism (e.g., differentiation) can cause secondary disturbances because the abnormal cells do not migrate or differentiate normally.

Certain malformations are genetically determined (Guerrini and Carrozzo, 2001a), and, for others, a genetic origin has been hypothesized. Some may be linked to prenatal insults (Sarnat, 1992; Friede, 1989). In most cases, however, the cause remains unknown. Some malformations are more epileptogenic than others. In specific forms, the epileptogenesis appears to originate from the intrinsic properties of the dysplastic tissue (Guerrini et al., 1999a; Mattia et al., 1995). The following sections review the most common disorders of cortical development and the characteristics of the associated epilepsy and EEG patterns.

Anomalies Related to Abnormal Proliferation and Differentiation of Neurons and Glia

Hemimegalencephaly

In hemimegalencephaly (HME), one cerebral hemisphere is enlarged and structurally abnormal, with a thick cortex, wide convolutions, and reduced sulci. The abnormality is strictly unilateral (Robain and Gelot, 1996). Laminar organization is absent in the cortex, and the demarcation between gray and white matter is poor. Giant neurons (up to 80 µ in diameter) are found throughout the cortex and the underlying white matter. In about 50% of patients, large bizarre cells, which are also termed *balloon cells*, are also observed (Robain and Gelot, 1996). HME is probably a heterogeneous condition.

HME may be associated with many disorders (see Table 1.3) (Guerrini et al., 1999a), but it can also occur in isolation. The clinical spectrum of HME includes cases with severe epileptic encephalopathy beginning in the neonatal period (Robain et al., 1988) and a few patients who may have a normal cognitive level (Guerrini et al., 1996a; Fusco et al., 1992), with or without epilepsy. The typical presentation is with hemiparesis, hemianopia, mental retardation, and early onset seizures. The most severely affected children have almost continuous seizures beginning in the neonatal period (Fig. 19.4), accompanied or followed by infantile spasms and a burst-suppression

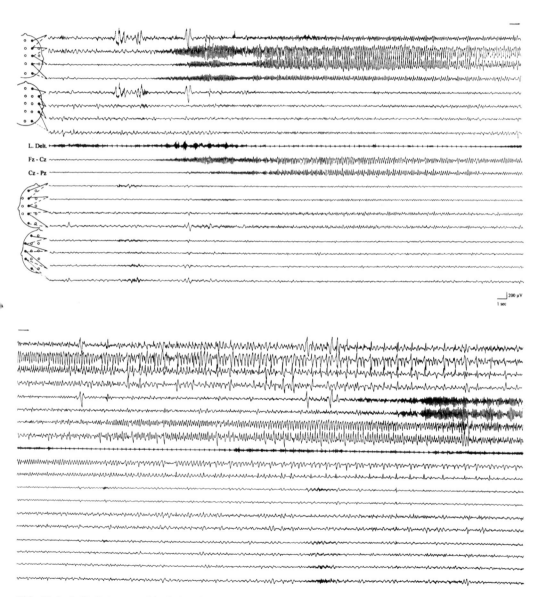

FIG. 19.4. A, B: Seizure activity in hemimegalencephaly. Three-month-old boy (corresponds to Fig. 19.7H) with electrical status epilepticus. Continuous subclinical seizure activity with multiple sites of origin within the malformed hemisphere.

pattern on the sleep EEG (Vigevano et al., 1996; Paladin et al., 1989). A high mortality rate, often due to status epilepticus, is present in the first months or years of life (Robain et al., 1988; Tijam et al., 1978). The survivors have severe cognitive and motor impairment (Trounce et al., 1991). Early hemispherectomy (Di Rocco, 1996) or hemispherotomy (Villemure and Mascott, 1995) might prevent life-threatening seizures or the deleterious interference on the healthy hemisphere (Vigevano et al., 1989a; King et al., 1985). A higher degree of recovery of neuropsychologic function is achieved in patients who are operated on at a young age.

Focal Cortical Dysplasia

Histologic abnormalities reminiscent of those encountered in HME may be restricted to one cerebral lobe, or they may involve a segment measuring only a few centimeters (Taylor et al., 1971). These discrete cortical malformations were initially described by Taylor et al. (1971) in surgically resected tissue from an epilepsy surgery series. The abnormal area is not usually sharply delineated from the adjacent tissue (Robain, 1996; Taylor et al., 1971). The term *focal cortical dysplasia* has been used to refer to a wide range of alterations of the cortical mantle. A recent neuropathologic review of a large epilepsy surgery series (Tassi et al., 2002) proposed separating focal cortical dysplasia into the following subtypes: (a) architectural dysplasia, which is characterized by abnormal cortical lamination and ectopic neurones in white matter; (b) cytoarchitectural dysplasia characterized by giant neurofilament-enriched giant neurones in addition to altered cortical lamination; and (c) Taylor-type cortical dysplasia with giant dysmorphic neurones and balloon cells associated with cortical laminar disruption. Such abnormalities probably originate at different times in embryogenesis (Barkovich et al., 2001). In the series by Tassi et al. (2002), patients with architectural dysplasia had a lower seizure frequency than did those with cytoarchitectural and Taylor-type dysplasia.

Focal cortical dysplasia may occur in any part of the cortex (Guerrini, 1997; Guerrini et al., 1992c; Kuzniecky et al., 1992a; Palmini et al., 1991c). The lesions may be quite extensive (see Figs. 3.3 and Fig. 10.3), rendering complete removal impossible in many patients (Olivier et al., 1996; Palmini et al., 1991b). MRI may be unrevealing in up to 34% of patients (Tassi et al., 2002; Desbiens et al., 1993). Distinctive signal alterations on T2-weighted (Fig. 19.5) or FLAIR images are present in most patients with

Taylor-type dysplasia, and they are often associated with focal areas of cortical thickening, simplified gyration, blurring of the gray-white limit, or rectilinear boundaries between gray and white matter (Tassi et al., 2002; Kuzniecky, 1996; Bergin et al., 1995). Focal hypoplasia with MRI abnormalities is often found in architectural dysplasia (Tassi et al., 2002). Discrete areas of dysplasia may be associated with widespread minor structural changes of undetermined significance in an undetermined proportion of cases (Sisodiya et al., 1995). Progress in MRI techniques may allow the recognition of subtle areas of dysplasia that are often missed by more conventional studies (Bastos et al., 1999; Sisodiya et al., 1999). Dysplasias involving the mesial temporal lobe are usually accompanied by abnormal development of the hippocampal formation, which sometimes occurs as an isolated anomaly (Baulac et al., 1998).

Neuropathologic and electrophysiologic studies of dysplastic tissue have shown that some dysplasias are intrinsically epileptogenic with continuous or prolonged spike discharges on corticography or depth recordings (Mattia et al., 1995; Palmini et al., 1995). Such discharges might be due to abnormalities of circuitry; these have been demonstrated in some cases (Spreafico et al., 1998; Ferrer et al., 1992).

The *clinical presentation* in focal cortical dysplasia is typically that of intractable focal epilepsy developing at a variable age but generally before the end of adolescence, although neonatal onset has been reported (Guerrini et al., 1996c; Palmini et al., 1991c). Infantile spasms are common (Dulac et al., 1996; Chugani et al., 1990), but no other age-related epilepsy syndromes are usually observed. Partial status epilepticus has been frequently reported (Palmini et al. 1995; Desbiens et al., 1993; Guerrini et al., 1992c), and, when the location is in the precentral gyrus, the case is often complicated by epilepsia partialis continua (Aicardi, 1994b; Kuzniecky and Powers, 1993; Ferrer et al., 1992; Kuzniecky et al., 1988). Unless the dysplastic area is large, these patients do not suffer from severe neurologic deficits.

The interictal EEG shows focal, often rhythmic epileptiform discharges in about half the patients (Gambardella et al., 1996). These EEG abnormalities (Fig. 19.6) are highly suspicious, they are located over the epileptogenic area, and they are related to the continuous epileptiform discharges recorded with EcoG (Palmini et al., 1995). Most patients with EcoG ictal discharges who have complete removal of the discharging tissue become seizure free or they have a more than 90% reduction in major seizures. None of

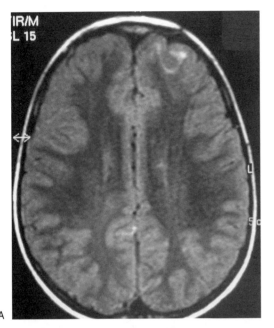

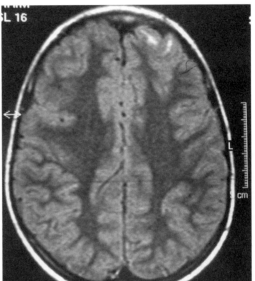

A   B

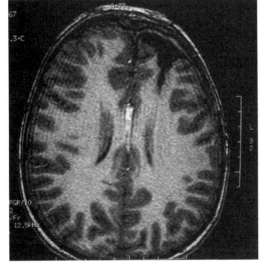

C

FIG. 19.5. Taylor-type dysplasia (T2) (preoperative and postoperative). Right frontal Taylor-type dysplastic lesion (A, B) in a boy who presented at the age of 3 years with a low number (not more than 10) of episodes characterized by the arrest of ongoing activity and some automatisms. When he was on vigabatrin, he remained seizure free for more than 24 months, and the drug was discontinued. He remained without treatment for 16 months, at which time his epilepsy relapsed. The seizures occurred very frequently. During this same period, he underwent severe behavioral deterioration and regression of school performance. Electroencephalograms (EEGs) showed the previously present right frontal focus, but diffusion of the EEG abnormalities was also present. The previously used and new antiepileptic drugs did not allow control of seizures. After the behavioral deterioration was taken into account, he was operated on 6 months after the relapse (C). He has been seizure free since that time, and he has no behavioral problems.

the patients with persistence of discharging tissue had a favorable outcome (Palmini et al., 1995).

The different histologic subtypes of focal cortical dysplasia may carry different chances of seizure freedom after surgery. According to Tassi et al (2002), who used depth electrodes in most cases, patients with Taylor-type dysplasia had the best outcome, with 75% becoming seizure free (Engel class Ia), compared with 50% of those with cytoarchitectural dysplasia and 43% of those with architectural dysplasia.

The area of resection is perhaps better defined in patients with Taylor-type dysplasia, possibly due to the distinctive interictal epileptiform discharges (Palmini et al., 1995), which can be captured by depth electrodes (Munari et al., 1996).

However, the clinical and electrophysiologic features reported in focal cortical dysplasia and HME are biased because they originate from epilepsy surgery centers at which the most severe cases are seen. In the authors' experience, some patients with

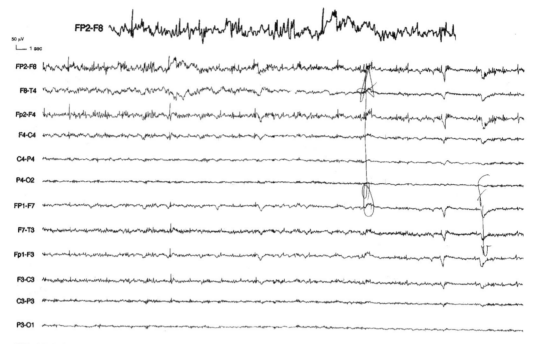

FIG. 19.6. Interictal electroencephalographic abnormalities (Fp2-F8) related to the presence of a right frontal cortical dysplasia. (Courtesy of Dr. Pierre Thomas, Nice University Hospital, France.)

well-controlled seizures show focal dysplastic lesions on MRI that are identical to those present in patients with histologically proven focal dysplasia.

Schizencephaly

Schizencephaly (cleft brain) consists of a full-thickness unilateral or bilateral cleft of the cerebral hemispheres with communication between the ventricle and the pericerebral subarachnoid spaces. The cortex surrounding the cleft is comprised of *polymicrogyria*, which also covers the lips of the fissure and extends along the walls of the cleft all the way to the ventricular surface (Ferrer, 1984) and which is probably responsible for the epilepsy. The walls of the clefts may be widely separated (open-lip schizencephaly) (Fig. 19.7A) or closely apposed (closed-lip schizencephaly) (Fig. 19.7B). The clefts may be located in any region of the hemispheres, but, by far, they are most commonly located in the perisylvian

FIG. 19.7. A: Unilateral open-lip schizencephaly. T1-weighted axial magnetic resonance imaging (MRI) scan shows that a large cleft in the left hemisphere spans from the subarachnoid space to the lateral ventricle. Cortical thickening with abnormal folding is present in the contralateral hemisphere. **B:** Unilateral closed-lip schizencephaly shown on a T1-weighted coronal MRI scan. A thin cleft in the left hemisphere spans from the subarachnoid space to the lateral ventricle. **C:** T1-weighted axial section scan shows the bilateral periventricular nodular heterotopia caused by an *FLN1* gene mutation (7627del8). Nodules of gray matter presenting the same signal as the normal cortex line the lateral ventricles. The young woman is from a family with multiple affected women with focal epilepsy and a borderline cognitive level. **D:** LIS1 lissencephaly (deletion). T2-weighted axial section showing a simplified gyral pattern and a thick cortex that, especially in the posterior brain, is completely smooth. Four-year-old boy with epileptic spasms. **E:** XLIS lissencephaly. FSPGR axial MRI scan shows a simplified gyral pattern with a severely thickened cortex with a prominent frontal involvement in a two-year-old boy with a missense mutation of the *DCX* gene. **F:** Tuberous sclerosis in a 22-year-old female patient with symptomatic generalized epilepsy and mental retardation. PD-weighted axial MRI scan shows that multiple cortical lesions representing cortical tubers are clearly visible in both frontal lobes and in the left parietal lobe.

(continued on page 296)

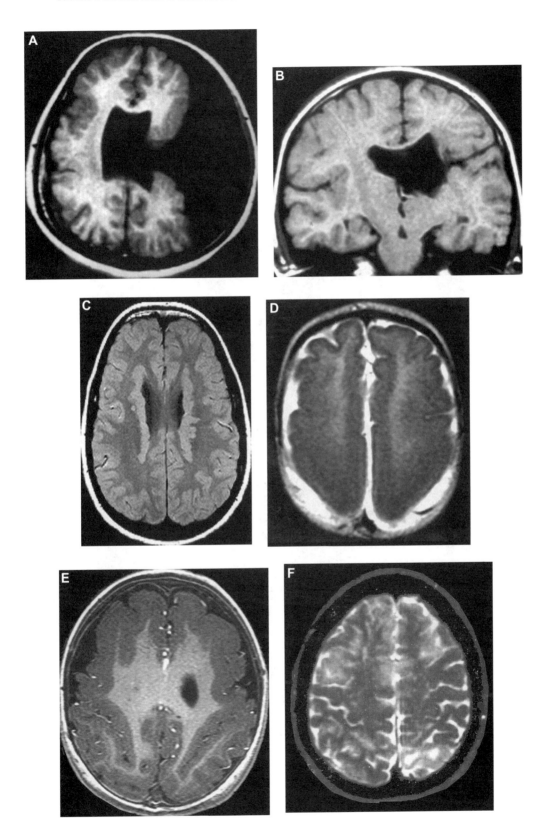

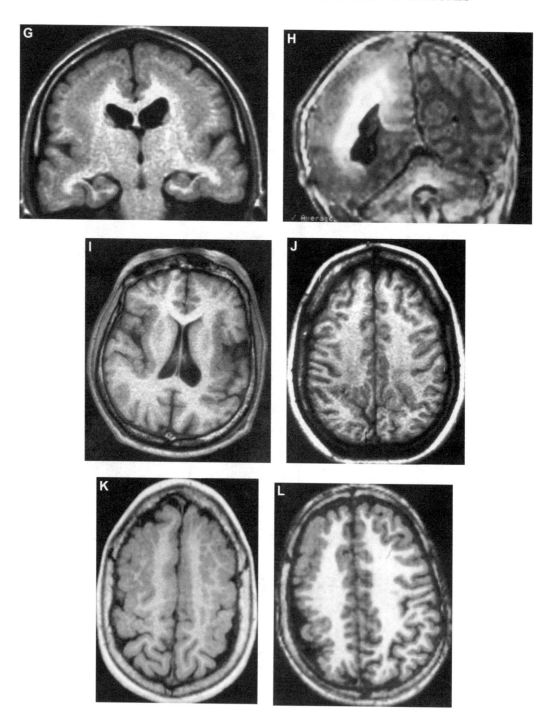

area (Barkovich and Kjos, 1992). The bilateral clefts are usually symmetric in location but not necessarily in size. Unilateral clefts are sometimes associated with a localized cortical abnormality in the contralateral hemisphere. Septooptic dysplasia (agenesis of the septum pellucidum and optic nerve hypoplasia) is observed in some patients (Barkovich and Norman, 1988). No agreement exists on whether schizencephaly should be classified as an abnormality of neuron proliferation (Barkovich et al., 2001), and establishment of the time of origin of the developmental abnormality during embryonic development is extremely difficult.

Although schizencephaly is sporadic in most cases, familial occurrence (Hosley et al., 1992) and a specific genetic origin are possible in some cases. Several sporadic patients and two siblings of both sexes who harbored a germline mutation in the homeobox gene *EMX2* have been described (Granata et al., 1997; Brunelli et al., 1996). However, at present, the role of the *EMX2* gene in causing schizencephaly is still unclear, as is the possible pattern of inheritance and the practical usefulness that mutation detection in an individual with schizencephaly would have in terms of genetic counseling.

Clinical findings include partial seizures that are present in most patients (81% of patients in one large review) (Granata et al., 1996) that usually begin before 3 years of age; these are more frequent in bilateral than unilateral cases. Bilateral cases are also associated with severe neurologic abnormalities, whereas unilateral cases are associated with hemiplegia or they may occur in otherwise normal individuals (Barkovich and Kjos, 1992). Surgical treatment

for medically resistant seizures is difficult, although some patients may experience worthwhile seizure reduction (Leblanc et al., 1996). In patients with bilateral lesions, resective surgery is not indicated.

Anomalies Caused by Abnormal Neuronal Migration

This category of malformations is represented by isolated neuronal cells or their agglomerates (heterotopia) in an abnormal site because of failure to reach their final destination during neuronal migration.

Nodular Heterotopia

Bilateral periventricular nodular heterotopia (BPNH) consists of confluent and symmetric subependymal nodules of gray matter located along the superolateral walls of the lateral ventricles that extend from the frontal horns to the trigones, particularly along the ventricular body (Fig. 19.7C). The malformation is mainly seen in females, often showing a familial distribution that is consistent with X-linked dominant transmission (Dobyns et al., 1996; Dubeau et al., 1995; Huttenlocher et al., 1994). Mutations of the filamin-1 gene (*FLN1*) (Moro et al., 2002; Sheen et al., 2001; Fox et al., 1998) have been observed in almost all X-linked pedigrees, and they are often associated with epilepsy in females with normal or borderline intelligence quotients and with prenatal or early postnatal lethality in males (Moro et al., 2002; Dobyns et al., 1996). Very few male patients with BPNH and epilepsy caused by mild *FLN1* mutations have been recorded (Sheen et al., 2001).

FIG. 19.7. *(Continued.)* **G:** Subcortical band heterotopia. T1-weighted coronal slice MRI scan showing a thick diffuse band of heterotopic cortex with a simplified gyral pattern. Twenty-year-old woman with drug-resistant focal epilepsy and the *DCX* gene mutation (N200K). **H:** Hemimegalencephaly in a 3-month-old boy with intractable seizures (same patient as in Fig. 19.4). MRI, SE, coronal section. The right hemisphere is enlarged, with a thickened cortex and smooth surface. No digitations occur between the gray and white matter. High-signal intensity is seen in the white matter throughout the right hemisphere. **I:** Bilateral perisylvian polymicrogyria. The T1-weighted axial section shows open sylvian fissures overlaid by an irregular and thick cortex in a 16-year-old male patient with faciopharyngoglossomasticatory diplegia, mild mental retardation, and Lennox-Gastaut syndrome. **J:** Bilateral parasagittal parietooccipital polymicrogyria. T1-weighted MRI scan showing irregular thickening and infolding of the cortex at the mesial parietooccipital junction in a 15-year-old girl with complex partial seizures. **K:** Bilateral frontal polymicrogyria in a 10-year-old boy with spastic quadriparesis, moderate mental retardation, and focal epilepsy. T1-weighted MRI axial section demonstrates the polymicrogyric cortex with irregular bumpy aspect involving all of the gyral pattern anterior to the precentral gyri. His seizures have been in remission for some years. **L:** Unilateral polymicrogyria shown on T1-weighted MRI axial section. The right hemisphere is smaller than the left, and the subarachnoid space overlying the right hemisphere is enlarged. The cortex on the right is irregular, with areas of thickening, in this 8-year-old boy with left hemiparesis, moderate mental retardation, atypical absences, and partial motor seizures in the context of epilepsy with continuous spike-wave activity during sleep.

However, most patients of both sexes having BPNH are sporadic, without *FLN1* mutations. The genetic recurrence risk for women with X-linked BPNH is 50% for daughters; it is unknown but is presumably much lower for severely affected sons (Moro et al., 2002), with an increased rate of miscarriages.

Several other syndromes featuring BPNH, mental retardation, and often epilepsy have been described in boys, but these always occur sporadically (Guerrini and Dobyns, 1998; Dobyns et al., 1997). In some such syndromes, the malformation may result from small chromosomal rearrangements involving the *FLN1* gene (Fink et al., 1997), but other genes causing BPNH probably exist (Guerrini and Carrozzo, 2001a).

The *clinical phenotype* ranges from asymptomatic individuals to patients with seizures and a normal cognitive level or mild to severe delay (Guerrini and Carrozzo, 2001b). The EEG may be normal, or it can show interictal discharges that are often located over the temporal regions (Dubeau et al., 1995). Depth electrode studies have demonstrated that the seizure activity may originate within the heterotopic cortex (Munari et al., 1996). Dubeau et al. (1995) studied 33 patients with *periventricular* and *subcortical nodular heterotopia*, 29 (88%) of whom had presented with seizures, mainly partial attacks with temporoparietooccipital auras. The seizures began between the age of 2 months and 33 years, and they were intractable in 27 patients (82%). BPNH was observed in nine patients. Dubeau et al. (1995) and Li et al. (1997) showed that temporal lobectomy, which did not include the area of heterotopia in seven, did not result in any significant improvement despite EEG findings in the temporal area.

Lissencephaly (Classic Lissencephaly or Type I Lissencephaly) and Subcortical Band Heterotopia

Lissencephaly and subcortical band heterotopia (SBH) constitute the *agyria-pachygyria-band spectrum* (Barkovich et al., 2001; Aicardi, 1991d). Both malformations can be caused by mutations of the *LIS1* gene (LIS1 lissencephaly) and the *DCX* gene (XLIS lissencephaly) (Des Portes et al., 1998; Gleeson et al., 1998; Sossey-Alaoui et al., 1998). *Lissencephaly* (smooth brain) is characterized by absent (agyria) or decreased (pachygyria) surface convolutions, producing a smooth cerebral surface (Fig. 19.7D and 19.7E) (Friede, 1989). *SBH* comprises the mild end of the agyria-pachygyria-band spectrum (Fig. 19.7G and 19.7H) (Barkovich et al., 1994). In this malformation, the cerebral convolutions appear to be either normal or mildly broad, but, just beneath the cortical ribbon, a thin band of white matter separates the cortex from the bands of gray matter.

In *lissencephaly*, the cerebral cortex is abnormally thick, usually measuring 10 to 15 mm and consisting of four layers. Additional abnormalities include hypoplasia of the corticospinal tracts, heterotopia of the inferior olives, and mild dysplasia of the cerebellar cortex. Transitional forms may include frontal pachygyria, which merges with posterior SBH in some patients, and partial frontal or posterior bands (Barkovich et al., 2001). The prevalence of lissencephaly was found to be 11.7 per one million births (1 in 85,470) (De Rijk-van Andel et al., 1991).

In *SBH*, which is also called *double cortex syndrome*, a band of gray matter of variable thickness is separated from the cortex by a rim of white matter. The cortex may be normal or pachygyric. The band is sometimes continuous and uniform, or it may be prominent in or confined to the anterior or posterior part of the brain. SBH is much more common in females.

Genetic Data

Most cases of lissencephaly occur without any associated malformations outside the brain (isolated lissencephaly sequence [ILS]), and some belong to more complex malformation syndromes. The best known is *Miller-Dieker syndrome* (MDS), which also features facial abnormalities (Dobyns et al., 1991); it is caused by large deletions of the *LIS1* gene, which maps to chromosome 17p13.3, and its contiguous genes (Chong et al., 1997). About 80% of the cases of ILS are caused by mutations of the *LIS1* and *DCX* genes (Fogli et al., 1999; Gleeson et al., 1998; Dobyns et al., 1993). LIS1 lissencephaly occurs in both sexes, and its occurrence is sporadic. XLIS lissencephaly occurs only in boys, and it may be inherited from females with SBH who carry *DCX* gene mutations. Children with *DCX* mutations have anteriorly predominant lissencephaly, whereas children with *LIS1* mutations and MDS have posteriorly predominant lissencephaly (Dobyns et al., 1999b). When MDS is suspected or the lissencephaly is more severe posteriorly (Fig. 19.7D), a standard chromosome analysis and on fluorescent *in situ* hybridization (FISH) assay on 17p13.3 are indicated. A chromosome analysis shows visible deletions or other rearrangements in about two-thirds of children with MDS (Dobyns et al., 1991), whereas the chromosomes are usually normal in ILS. FISH studies show submicroscopic deletions in more than 90% of children with MDS and in about 40% of those with ILS (Pilz et al., 1998). If a deletion is not found, *LIS1* gene sequencing should be performed. In boys in whom the MRI shows more severe lissencephaly in the frontal lobes (Fig. 19.7E), sequencing of the *DCX* gene is indicated (Guerrini and Carrozzo, 2001b). Recent work has suggested that mild forms of pachygyria and epilepsy in which the patients have normal MRI scans may result from mild mutations of the *LIS1* and *DCX* genes (Guerrini et al., 2003c; Leventer et al., 2001).

X-linked lissencephaly in hemizygous males and SBH in heterozygous females in the same family (Pinard et al., 1994) constitute a distinct genetic entity that is linked to mutation of the *DCX* gene (Matsumoto et al., 2001). However, sporadic SBH may be genetically heterogeneous because only about 60% of patients carry *DCX* mutations (Gleeson et al., 2000a). Maternal germline or mosaic *DCX* mutations may occur in about 10% of cases of either SBH or X-linked lissencephaly (Gleeson et al., 2000b). SBH in the rare affected boys has been associated with missense mutations of *DCX* or *LIS1* (Guerrini et al., 2003c; Pilz et al., 1998).

DCX gene sequencing is indicated in both female and male patients with SBH whenever genetic counseling is advisable (Guerrini and Carrozzo, 2001b). The recurrence risk for carrier females is high; 50% of their sons will have lissencephaly, and 50% of their daughters will have SBH. Brain MRI is less reliable than mutation analysis for determining the carrier status (Guerrini and Carrozzo, 2001b).

Clinical Features

All patients with *lissencephaly* have early developmental delay and eventual profound or severe mental retardation. Rare patients with pachygyria may have moderate mental retardation. Other neurologic manifestations include early diffuse hypotonia and later spastic quadriplegia. The lifespan is less than 10 years in most patients. Seizures occur in more than 90% of patients, with onset before 6 months of age in about 75%. About 80% of children have infantile spasms in the first year of life. Later, most children have various seizure types, including focal motor and generalized tonic seizures, atypical absences, and atonic seizures (Guerrini et al., 1996c; Gastaut et al., 1987; Dulac et al., 1983c). The characteristic EEG changes include diffuse fast rhythms (Hakamada et al., 1979) and high-amplitude rhythmic activity, which has a high diagnostic specificity but low sensitivity (less than 50%) (Quirk et al., 1993).

Mental retardation and epilepsy are also present in patients with *SBH*. Children with gyral abnormalities may have more severe ventricular enlargement, thicker heterotopic bands, and a significantly earlier seizure onset (Barkovich et al., 1994). About 90% of reported patients with SBH have epilepsy, and about 50% of them have a form of generalized epilepsy, often with characteristics of LGS (Barkovich et al., 1994; Ricci et al., 1992; Palmini et al., 1991a; Livingston and Aicardi, 1990). Intractable seizures were seen in 65% of patients.

Epilepsy in SBH may be due to local epileptogenesis. Using depth electrodes, Morrell et al. (1992) demonstrated that epileptiform activity may originate directly from the heterotopic neurons, independently of the activity of the overlying cortex.

Aicardi Syndrome

Aicardi syndrome (Aicardi et al., 1965, 1969b) is a complex malformation that includes the following: (a) a thin unlayered cortex, (b) diffuse unlayered polymicrogyria with fused molecular layers, and (c) nodular heterotopias in the periventricular region and the centrum semiovale (Billette de Villemeur et al., 1992; Ferrer et al., 1986), in addition to agenesis of the corpus callosum. The syndrome is exclusively observed in females, with the exception of two males with two X chromosomes that have been reported (Aicardi, 1996); it, therefore, is thought to be due to an X-linked gene that is lethal in the hemizygous male. It occurs sporadically, although one case of two sisters that have been affected has been published (Molina et al., 1989).

The clinical and neuroimaging features include severe mental retardation, infantile spasms, chorioretinal lacunae, agenesis of the corpus callosum, and a high rate of early death (Menezes et al., 1994). Additional malformations include choroid plexus cysts; ependymal cysts, especially around the third ventricle; colobomata; and *vertebral and costal abnormalities*.

Spasms were the only seizure type in 88 (47%) of 184 reported patients. In 35% of patients, the spasms were associated with partial seizures (Cahan and Engel, 1986). Hypsarrhythmia is observed in roughly 18% of patients (Aicardi, 1996). The interictal EEG abnormalities are typically asymmetric and asynchronous ("split-brain EEG"), with or without suppression bursts during wakefulness and sleep. The seizure and EEG patterns change little, if at all, over time, and the seizures are almost always resistant.

Anomalies Related to Abnormal Cortical Organization

Disorders of abnormal cortical organization, mainly faulty layering, result from the disruption of the late stages of cortical formation, but they may also be partly caused by the abnormal late migration of cells and/or premigration abnormalities of the precursor cells, preventing the proper establishment of normal cortical architecture. They include several types.

One type is the cortical dysplasia with abnormal cortical lamination, without neuronal atypies and balloon cells (Tassi et al., 2002). Another major form, which is observed in children with epilepsy and developmental disabilities, is *polymicrogyria* (Guerrini, 1999). A milder form, the significance of which is less clear, has been termed *microdysgenesis* (Meencke, 1985).

Polymicrogyria

Polymicrogyria designates the appearance of an excessive number of small and prominent convolutions separated by shallow and enlarged sulci that give the cortical surface a lumpy aspect (Friede, 1989). On direct brain inspection and MRI, recognizing polymicrogyria or distinguishing it from pachygyria is often impossible because the microconvolutions are packed and their molecular layers fused (Guerrini et al., 1992c). However, polymicrogyria often alters the gyral pattern (Barkovich, 1996; Raybaud et al., 1996).

Two types of polymicrogyria are recognized. In *unlayered polymicrogyria*, only one wavy band of neurons that does not follow the profile of the convolutions and has no laminar organization is present (Ferrer and Catala, 1991). Unlayered polymicrogyria may be focal (Becker et al., 1989; Galaburda et al., 1985), multilobar, or diffuse (Billette de Villemeur et al., 1992). It is probably a migration disorder (thirteenth to eighteenth week of gestation), and it may be genetically determined (Billette de Villemeur et al., 1992).

In *four-layered polymicrogyria*, two neuronal layers occur under the molecular layer and are separated by an intermediate layer with many fibers and few cells (Harding, 1997). Four-layered polymicrogyria is often focal. This type of polymicrogyria has been suggested to be the possible result of a perfusion failure limited to one or more arterial vascular beds, occurring between the twentieth and the twenty-fourth week of gestation (Friede, 1989). However, unlayered and four-layered polymicrogyria may also coexist in

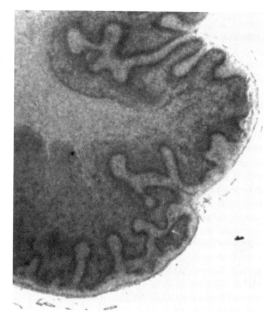

FIG. 19.8. Magnification of a cortical specimen showing many small microgyri with fused surfaces. Microscopic examination shows the four-layered polymicrogyria (thinner cortex) merging with unlayered polymicrogyria (thicker cortex).

the same brain (Fig. 19.8), indicating that they may comprise a single spectrum (Harding, 1997).

The *clinical manifestations* associated with polymicrogyria vary in relation to the extent of the cortical abnormality, ranging from severe encephalopathies with spastic quadriparesis, profound mental retardation, and intractable epilepsy to normal individuals with selective impairment of higher order neurologic functions (Cohen et al., 1989b; Galaburda et al., 1985).

Various polymicrogyria syndromes have been identified using MRI (Barkovich et al., 1999; Guerrini, 1999). They are covered in the following sections.

Bilateral Perisylvian Polymicrogyria

Bilateral perisylvian polymicrogyria bilaterally involves the gray matter that borders the lateral fissure, which, in typical cases, is almost vertical and in continuity with the central or postcentral sulcus (Fig. 19.7I). The cortical abnormality is usually symmetric (Fig. 19.9), but its extent is variable (Kuzniecky et al., 1993a; Guerrini et al., 1992b). Polymicrogyria may

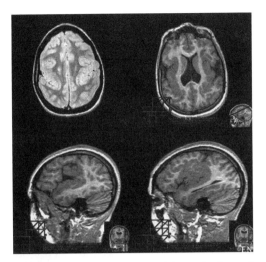

FIG. 19.9. Typical bilateral perisylvian polymicrogyria in a 12-year-old girl with disturbances in facial and buccal motility, very mild mental retardation, and rare clonic jerks of the arms.

be four layered (Kuzniecky et al., 1993a) or unlayered (Becker et al., 1989).

Familial cases have been reported, with possible autosomal recessive (Andermann and Andermann, 1996), X-linked dominant (Borgatti et al. 1999) and X-linked recessive (Yoshimura et al., 1998) inheritance, indicating genetic heterogeneity (Guerreiro et al., 2000). A locus for X-linked bilateral perisylvian polymicrogyria maps to Xq28 (Villard et al., 2002). Recent reports of an association with chromosome 22q11.2 deletions in some patients with extensive perisylvian polymicrogyria (Bingham et al, 1998) makes FISH analysis for 22q11.2 an essential investigation in patients with such malformation (Guerrini and Carrozzo, 2001b).

Bilateral perisylvian polymicrogyria has also been reported following complicated pregnancies (e.g, in children born from monochorionic, diamniotic twin pregnancies that were complicated by twin-to-twin transfusion syndrome with the death of one of the twins between the tenth and eighteenth week of gestation) (Van Bogaert et al., 1996). In such cases, the malformation could result from ischemic injury secondary to the hemodynamic changes induced by death of the co-twin. Parabiotic twin syndrome has also been associated with focal polymicrogyria involving the parietooccipital cortex (Larroche et al., 1994; Sugama and Kusano, 1994).

The clinical features are often distinctive (Kuzniecky et al., 1993a; Guerrini et al., 1992b), with faciopharyngoglossomasticatory diplegia and language impairment ranging from mild dysarthria to complete absence of speech. Almost all patients have mental retardation, and most have epilepsy. Seizures, often atypical absences, tonic or atonic drop attacks, and tonic-clonic seizures, present as an LGS in many cases. Some patients (26%) have partial seizures that predominantly involve the perioral or facial muscles. The clinical spectrum of bilateral perisylvian polymicrogyria is broad, including infantile spasms; resistant partial seizures; and variable degrees of encephalopathy, sometimes with very early onset.

Bilateral Parasagittal Parietooccipital Polymicrogyria

This malformation (Fig. 19.7J) has been reported in unrelated patients with partial epilepsy (Guerrini et al., 1998c).

Bilateral Perisylvian and Parietooccipital Polymicrogyria

In some cases, perisylvian polymicrogyria extends posteriorly, with the sylvian fissure being prolonged across the entire hemispheric convexity up to the mesial surface of the hemispheric convexity. Most patients have severe epilepsies (Pupillo et al., 1996) with characteristics similar to those of the bilateral perisylvian syndrome, or they may have partial epilepsies with seizure onset in the occipital or parietal lobes.

Bilateral Frontal Polymicrogyria

Bilateral frontal polymicrogyria, a recently described type (Guerrini et al., 2000a) (Fig. 19.7K), has been observed in children with developmental delay or mild spastic quadriparesis and epilepsy. Most of the reported cases have been sporadic, but occurrence in the offspring of consanguineous parents and in siblings suggests autosomal recessive inheritance. A locus for this malformation has been mapped to chromosome 16q12.2-21 (Piao et al., 2002). Epilepsy, which is seen in most patients, consists mainly of partial seizures and atypical absences.

Unilateral (Hemispheral) Polymicrogyria

Large areas of the polymicrogyric cortex involving a whole hemisphere or a major proportion of one hemisphere, usually in the perisylvian region, are often associated with hypoplasia of the affected hemisphere (Fig. 19.7L). This abnormality may be associated with a suggestive clinical syndrome (Guerrini et al., 1996d). In a series of 20 patients, 75% had seizures and mild to moderate hemiparesis, and 70% had mild to moderate mental retardation. In patients with interictal EEG abnormalities and seizures involving the motor cortex, hemiparesis has been observed to worsen with worsening of the interictal epileptiform abnormalities or seizures (Guerrini et al., 1996c).

The age at seizure onset and epilepsy severity are quite variable (Guerrini et al., 1996d). The most common seizure types are partial motor seizures (73%), atypical absences (47%), generalized tonic-clonic seizures (27%), and complex partial seizures (20%). In some cases, *electrical status epilepticus* of slow sleep (ESES) or epilepsy with continuous spike-waves of slow sleep (CSWS) develops (Caraballo et al., 1999; Guerrini et al., 1996a, 1998f; Pascual-Castroviejo, 1992).

The association between the abnormality and clinical syndrome has subsequently been confirmed by others (Caraballo et al., 1999) (see Fig. 11.1). The condition is usually detected between ages 2 and 10 years, and it may last for months to years. The epilepsy outcome in patients with polymicrogyria does not differ from that seen in patients with other etiologies or cryptogenic ESES–CSWS (i.e., the seizures and EEG abnormalities disappear, but cognitive and behavioral disturbances often endure).

Microdysgenesis

Microdysgenesis consists of variable anomalies, including increased cellular density in the molecular layer, heterotopic neurons in the subcortical white matter, and failure of normal lamination (Hardiman et al., 1988; Meencke, 1985). It may exist in isolation, or it may be associated with macroscopical dysplasias in adjacent or distant cortical areas. Similar anomalies may be found also in the brains of neurologically normal individuals, so their significance remains in dispute (Lyon and Gastaut, 1985). Meencke (1989) found microdysgenesis in 223 (38%) of 591 brains of epileptic persons, as opposed to only 442 (6%) of 7,374 control brains; furthermore, the changes were severe in 12% of the epileptic brains, as opposed to 2% of control brains. This suggests a relationship with clinical epilepsy, but more information is needed on this issue.

Dual Pathology

A special problem is raised by the so-called *dual pathology* that occurs in patients in whom an area of cortical dysplasia is associated with unilateral or bilateral hippocampal volume loss, as assessed by MRI volumetric studies (Ho et al., 1998; Raymond et al., 1994a). Although the onset of epilepsy in childhood is quite common, a history of childhood febrile convulsions seems much less common than that observed in individuals with isolated hippocampal volume loss (Raymond et al., 1994a). The possible coexistence of cortical dysplasia with hippocampal structural abnormalities implies that careful imaging of additional potentially epileptogenic abnormalities is essential when patients with either hippocampal volume loss or cortical dysplasia who are candidates for epilepsy surgery are evaluated.

Surgical Management of Cortical Dysplasias

The surgical management of cortical dysplasis depends on the extension of lesions. Many children who are considered for surgical treatment of focal epilepsy have a lobar or multilobar area of abnormal cortical development. The pathologic substrate is usually of the type underlying focal cortical dysplasia and HME (Mischel, 1995; Taylor et al., 1971). Children with polymicrogyria may also be suitable surgical candidates if their lesions are unilateral and if no evidence of diffuse epileptogenesis or of a self-limiting, age-related epilepsy syndrome is suggested by clinical or EEG evidence (Guerrini et al., 1999a). Bilateral or diffuse dysplasias that generate atonic-tonic seizures may be amenable to callosotomy (Kuzniecky et al., 1994b; Guerrini et al., 1992a). Surgical resection for the limited areas of cortical dysplasia only uncommonly leads to complete seizure control, probably because of the extent of the lesions or their multiplicity. According to Palmini et al. (1995), the only significant factor for the prediction of the outcome is the extent of the resection. In this study, 78% of their patients who underwent resection of more than 50% of the lesion had a good outcome, although only 1 became seizure free.

However, better results have been published more recently (Tassi et al., 2002). Positron emission tomography (PET) and single photon emission CT (SPECT) may help define the extent of the dysplastic epileptogenic cortex (Juhász et al., 2001a; Chugani et al., 1990). Although colocalization of the structural abnormality and epileptogenic activity may considerably help in planning the area of the resection, the relationships among the macroscopic abnormality, microscopic changes, and the area of seizure origin may be highly complicated (Li et al., 1997), and depth electrode studies may be preferred in some patients (Tassi et al., 2002; Chassoux et al., 2000; Munari et al, 1996).

TUBEROUS SCLEROSIS

TS or TS complex (TSC) is a multisystemic disorder involving primarily the central nervous system, the skin, and the kidney (Gomez, 1988). The condition bears a close relationship to cortical dysplasias, from which the individual lesions may be impossible to differentiate. A prevalence of 1 in 10,000 to 1 in 30,000 has been reported. The classic clinical triad of mental retardation, epilepsy, and "adenoma sebaceum" (facial angiofibromas) is present in only one-third of the cases.

The characteristic brain lesions are *cortical tubers* (Fig. 19.7F), subependymal nodules, and giant cell tumors. Cortical tubers are the lesions directly related to epileptogenesis.

The pathologic changes observed in cortical tubers are remarkably similar to those seen in focal Taylor-type cortical dysplasia (Robain, 1996; Taylor et al., 1971), which is, however, not associated with any of the other features of TS and which has no known familial distribution. Some investigators had described dysplasia as the "formes frustes" of TS (Palmini et al., 1991b; Andermann et al., 1987). In actuality, such anomalies should be considered distinct from this disease.

TSC is transmitted as an autosomal dominant trait with variable expression. Its recurrence in the offspring of nonaffected parents has rarely been reported, and it is thought to be related to low expressivity or gonadal mosaicism. Between 50% and 75% of all cases result from new mutations.

Two genes, *TSC1* and *TSC2*, have been identified. The TSC1 gene (Van Slegtenhorst et al., 1997) mapping to 9q34 encodes a protein named *hamartin*. The gene mapping to chromosome 16p13.3, *TSC2*, (European Chromosome 16 Tuberous Sclerosis Consortium, 1993) encodes a protein named *tuberin*. TSC genes are thought to act as tumor suppressors (Carbonara et al., 1994).

No obvious phenotypic differences have been found in the families linked to the *TSC1* or the *TSC2* gene mutations, although patients with TSC1 mutations have been suggested to have less severe epilepsy and cognitive impairment (Dabora et al., 2001).

In infants and children, the seizures are the most common presenting symptom of TSC. They usually begin in the first 2 years of life, with 63% beginning before 1 year of age (Gomez, 1988) and 70% before 2 years (Abo et al., 1983). Infantile spasms are the most common seizure type in the first year of life, and these are sometimes preceded by partial seizures (Dulac et al., 1984; Chevrie and Aicardi, 1977). They differ clinically and electroencephalographically from classic infantile spasms with typical hypsarrhythmia (Curatolo, 1996; Dulac et al., 1984).

Other types of epilepsy, especially focal seizures, may occur in infants and young children. Roger et al. (1984) found 63 of 126 children (50%) with West syndrome and 63 (50%) with other types, mainly partial epilepsies or LGS. Of the latter 63 patients, 42 had their first seizure before 2 years of age (22 [28%] partial epilepsies, 22 [28%] other types), and a poor outcome was strongly related to this early onset, especially when these patients presented with infantile spasms. In the group of partial epilepsies, the initial seizures were mainly simple partial motor and unilateral seizures, often associated with generalized seizures (tonic or atonic). The course of epilepsy was severe in about one-third of patients.

Waking EEGs show multifocal or focal spike discharges and irregular focal slow activity. (Curatolo, 1996; Dulac et al., 1984). The abnormalities increase during sleep. Atypical hypsarrhythmia that is often asymmetric is present in one-third of patients. Video-EEG monitoring and analysis of the EEG patterns in patients presenting with partial motor seizures and infantile spasms may suggest a focal origin of the latter (Curatolo, 1996; Dulac et al., 1984). Later in life, the EEG abnormalities are similar to what is observed in LGS. Diffuse spike-wave discharges are common in partial epilepsies in childhood TS, and they are related to secondary bilateral synchrony.

MRI studies may show some correlation between the number and the location of the tubers and epilepsy. Curatolo and Cusmai (1988) thought that the largest tuber corresponds to the main EEG focus, both in patients with partial epilepsy and in those with infantile spasms.

Mental retardation is common in TS; it is seen much more often in patients who have had seizures, especially those children with early onset epilepsy (Gomez, 1988; Roger et al., 1984). In addition to mental subnormality, autistic features or other deviant behavior, such as hyperkinesia or aggressiveness, are common in patients with TS and a history of infantile spasms (Jambaqué et al., 1991; Hunt and Dennis, 1987).

The *diagnosis* of TS should always be suspected in children with epilepsy, especially with the presence of infantile spasms or a history of familial seizures or other neurologic or mental disorders. A careful examination of the skin for the cutaneous stigmata of the condition is mandatory.

MRI demonstrates the tubers much better than CT, and it usually indicates the presence of several lesions that are not detectable by CT scanning (Curatolo, 1996; Gomez, 1988).

The *pharmacologic management* of epilepsy in TS is usually difficult, and drug resistance is common (Erba and Duchowny, 1990). Several investigators (Mackay et al., 2002) have reported excellent results; they advise the use of vigabatrin for the treatment of infantile spasms due to TS (see Chapter 3). Surgical resection of a tuber can be successful if a single epileptogenic focus can be identified (Sivelle et al., 1995; Bebin et al., 1993). Anterior callosotomy can markedly reduce the drop attacks (Garcia-Flores, 1987).

HIPPOCAMPAL SCLEROSIS

Definitions

The terms *HS*, *Ammon horn sclerosis*, and *mesial temporal sclerosis* (MTS) are used almost interchangeably. However, structural changes patterns differ subtly among these entities. The term *MTS* comprises structural abnormalities in the hippocampus, amygdala, and entorhinal cortex, whereas the term *HS* designates gliosis and neuronal loss that particularly affects the CA1 and CA4, or Sommer sectors; the dentate gyrus; and the subiculum. The term *Ammon horn sclerosis* designates abnormalities restricted to the areas CA1 and CA4. Amygdalar sclerosis may also be part of the process of MTS (Hudson et al., 1993), but this is always accompanied by HS (Cendes et al., 1993c). However, the term *HS* is widely used, and it is often applied to patients whose abnormalities are not limited to the hippocampus. In this section, *HS* is used with this meaning. *Dual pathology* is defined as the presence of a hippocampal structural abnormality, usually HS, plus an extrahippocampal, usually developmental, lesion in the same patient (Levesque et al., 1991).

HS is unilateral in about 80% of patients (Jackson et al., 1993a; Kuzniecky et al., 1992a; Berkovic et al., 1991a; Margerison and Corsellis, 1966). Concomitant atrophy of the homolateral temporal neocortex is common (Kuzniecky and Jackson, 1995b).

HS or atrophy is the most extensively studied abnormality related to temporal lobe epilepsy at all ages. HS used to be considered uncommon in chil-

dren with focal seizures. However, MRI studies of children with "temporal lobe epilepsy" have demonstrated HS in 21% of those younger than 15 years with new-onset epilepsy (Harvey et al., 1996) and in 57% of those from 2 to 17 years of age with refractory seizures (Harvey et al., 1995; Grattan-Smith et al., 1993). Moreover, neuropathologic studies of resected temporal lobes in pediatric epilepsy surgery series found HS in 60% of patients (Davidson and Falloner, 1975). In a few infants, HS can be detected by MRI within the first months (DeLong and Heinz, 1997) or first 2 years of life (Harvey et al., 1995; Nohria et al., 1994).

Clinical Features

Mohamed et al. (2001) comprehensively described a series of 34 children and adolescents in whom HS had been diagnosed with MRI and confirmed pathologically after temporal lobe resection. The age at seizure onset ranged from 4 months to 14 years (mean of 3.8 years). The *seizure symptomatology* included an epigastric aura in most, followed by decreased responsiveness and awareness and oral or gestural automatisms. The initial symptoms, which were reported in a minority, included gustatory, affective psychic, somatosensory, and "indescribable" sensations. The automatisms were usually subtle and moderate in children, and they were more prominent in adolescents. In this series, a dual pathology was observed in 11 (79%) of 14 patients for whom adequate surgical specimens were available. On the whole, the clinical EEG imaging findings and the postsurgical seizure outcome were considered similar to those reported in adults, with 78% of children being seizure free and 12% having rare seizures.

The severity of the hippocampal atrophy, as determined by MRI volumetric analysis, is significantly related to proportionally low values in the Wechsler logical memory percent retention score in adults (Lencz et al., 1992; Sass et al., 1990) and the same is probably true in the pediatric age. Right-sided HS has been associated with a reduced potential for learning spatial material, even in the absence of severe epilepsy, in a group of children with HS and a history of prolonged febrile seizures (Brizzolara et al., 2001). Vargha-Khadem et al. (1992b) reported a child with seizure onset at the age of 4 years who had subsequent severe declarative memory impairment. The MRI demonstrated bilateral mesial temporal lobe sclerosis and hippocampal atrophy. Beardsworth and Zaidel (1994) have assessed memory for faces preoperatively and postoperatively in children and adolescents with right and left temporal lobe epilepsy, most of whom had HS; they found that right-sided lateralization was accompanied by a significantly impaired delayed memory for faces both preoperatively and postoperatively.

DeLong and Heinz (1997) have suggested that early onset bilateral HS following convulsive status is causally linked with infantile autism.

Neuropathology

Pathologic studies (Cascino, 1990; Margerison and Corsellis, 1966) have shown that the most common lesional pattern is that of Ammon horn sclerosis, including primary nerve cell loss in the CA1 and CA4 sections of the hippocampus and less severe damage in the CA3 and CA2 regions. Less common patterns include widespread cell loss in the hippocampus (total Ammon horn sclerosis) and cell loss limited to the end folium (end-folium sclerosis). The severity of cell loss may vary, but it usually is more than 50% in association with gliosis (Sagar and Oxbury, 1987; Babb et al., 1984). Additional characteristic features associated with HS include the sprouting of mossy fibers in the fascia dentata and the selective loss of somatostatin-containing and neuropeptide Y–containing neurons (De Lanerolle et al., 1992; Sutula, 1990). The synaptic changes that result from neuronal cell loss, sprouting, and the establishment of an altered circuitry may result in hypersynchronization and hyperexcitability.

Pathophysiology

Arguments supporting a causative role for HS in mesial temporal lobe epilepsy have been presented in numerous papers (Sagar and Oxbury, 1987; Falconer, 1976; Ounsted et al., 1966; Falconer et al., 1964). However, HS may also be a secondary phenomenon, as shown by its presence in temporal lobe specimens that also demonstrate extensive congenital abnormalities such as cortical dysplasias or tumors (Shields et al., 1992a; Levesque et al., 1991) and by its occurrence in patients with a primary epileptogenic area outside the temporal lobe (Cook et al., 1992).

The evidence that repeated, prolonged, generalized, or unilateral seizures can produce HS, with or without other atrophic lesions, in additional areas of the temporal lobe or in other lobes is discussed in Chapter 14.

Although most of the epilepsies with seizures of mesial temporal origin are not preceded by febrile seizures (Nelson and Ellenberg, 1978, 1983), retrospective studies and rare prospective observations have demonstrated that the sequence of prolonged febrile seizure followed by temporal lobe epilepsy does exist, no matter what its mechanism and frequency (Scott et al., 2002; Van Landingham et al., 1998; DeLong and Heinz, 1997; Abou-Khalil et al., 1993; Cendes et al., 1993a; Kuks et al., 1993).

Likely, only injury occurring within a crucial developmental window is able to cause a reorganization of the internal hippocampal circuits with the consequent disruption of the balance between inhibitory and excitatory mechanisms (Sutula et al., 1989). Many authors have indicated that noxious events, such as prolonged febrile seizures, between the ages of 3 months and 5 years are particularly harmful (Wieser et al., 2000; Corsellis and Bruton, 1983; Ounsted et al., 1966). Additional remote neurologic insults in early childhood, including trauma or meningoencephalitis, represent risk factors for developing MTS (Trenerry et al., 1993). Scott et al. (2002) analyzed T1-weighted and T2-weighted structural imaging and T2-weighted relaxometry, volumetric measurements, and proton magnetic resonance spectroscopy in 16 children with HS, half of whom had a history of prolonged (more than 30 minutes) febrile convulsions. In the whole group, sclerosis of the horn of Ammon had been confirmed histologically after temporal lobe resection. Those children with a history of prolonged febrile convulsions had significantly smaller hippocampi and a higher T2-weighted relaxation time ipsilateral to the side of seizure onset. Ipsilateral-to-contralateral ratios for these parameters were also significantly more asymmetric in this group. These findings suggest that more severe hippocampal damage and a more unilateral disorder occur in children with a history of prolonged febrile convulsions (Scott et al., 2002). Reports that patients with such a history have a better outcome after temporal lobectomy are in accord with this observation (Abou-Khalil et al., 1993).

Genetic factors probably play a secondary role in the etiology of HS. Studies on identical twins have shown nonconcordance (Jackson et al., 1998). However, an increased frequency of febrile seizures is seen in relatives of individuals with HS (Abou-Khalil et al., 1993), and studies on familial temporal lobe epilepsy suggest that familial HS may be underreported (Cendes et al., 1998). Genetically determined, sporadic (Baulac et al., 1998) or familial (Fernandez et al., 1998), subtle malformations of mesial temporal lobe structures have been reported on MRI studies. Such subtle malformations would predispose the individual to HS and/or temporal lobe epilepsy, often, but not necessarily, through febrile seizures. Such subtle abnormalities include small hippocampus with blurred internal pattern, incomplete folding with abnormal medial location, globular shape, and verticalization of the hippocampus and heterotopia.

A unifying view on the pathogenesis of HS suggests that a brain insult, such as prolonged febrile seizures or another injury, would produce damage to the hippocampus only in the presence of preexisting factors that make such a structure vulnerable. Such factors are represented by developmental lesions (Fernandez et al., 1998) or a specific genetic predisposition (Kanemoto et al., 2000). Certainly, additional unidentified factors must be involved.

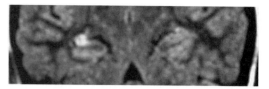

FIG. 19.10. Hippocampal sclerosis in a 10-year-old girl with a history of one episode of febrile status epilepticus. The age at onset of the partial seizures was 6 years. The magnetic resonance imaging scan (coronal section, T1, 0.5T) shows hippocampal atrophy on the right. Memory testing showed specific visuospatial memory impairment.

Neuroimaging

MRI is far superior to CT for the detection of HS (Jackson et al., 1993a, 1993b). The best morphologic evaluation of the hippocampal region is obtained by using cuts in two orthogonal planes along the long axis of the body of the hippocampus and at a right angle to this (Jackson et al., 1993a), thus avoiding oblique images of the hippocampus, which can be difficult to interpret because of partial-volume effects. The MRI features include a T1-weighted signal decrease, a T2-weighted or FLAIR signal increase (Fig. 19.10), hippocampal atrophy (Fig. 19.11), and the disruption of the internal morphologic structure of the hippocampus with failure to differentiate white matter from cortical structures. At least one of these abnormal features was present in 93% of cases in one series (Jackson et al., 1990), even though all four features were found in only 39%.

Using thin slices, hippocampal volume assessment can detect up to 90% of cases of HS (Jack et al., 1989, 1990), compared with about 80% by visual assessment (Kuzniecky and Jackson, 1995b). Hippocampal

volume loss correlates with the side of seizure onset and with HS, as resected tissue specimens have demonstrated (Cendes et al., 1993a, 1993b; Jack et al., 1992). MRI-based hippocampal volume measurements are the most reliable noninvasive investigation for determining the site of the lesion, thus suggesting that of seizure onset (Spencer et al., 1993). Normally, both hippocampi are of equal volume; any asymmetry of more than a few percent is abnormal (Jack et al., 1992). However, volumetric assessment also has limitations because it relies on a subjective definition of the hippocampal boundaries and on side-to-side comparison, which may fail to detect bilateral changes (Kuzniecky and Jackson, 1995b). In addition, hippocampal volumes as determined by preoperative MRI may be normal in a small subgroup of patients with an abnormal signal in one hippocampus and pathologically proven HS (Jackson et al., 1994).

Quantitative MRI may be used to detect hippocampal gliosis (Scott et al., 2002; Jackson et al., 1994). Quantitative MRI measurements of the T2 relaxation time may permit the recognition of unilateral or bilateral involvement in patients with apparently normal

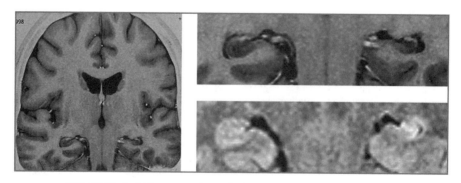

FIG. 19.11. Left hippocampal atrophy in a child with temporal epilepsy.

MRI scans obtained by classic techniques (Jackson et al., 1994). The atrophic-gliotic changes may be limited to one part of the hippocampal formation (Bertram et al., 1990) or to patchy areas, or they may extend to other parts of the temporal cortex, often predominating in the anterior segment of the first temporal gyrus (Mathieson, 1975; Cavanagh and Meyer, 1956), but they may involve other temporal gyri and even structures outside the temporal lobe (insula; frontobasal and opercular cortex, a lesion termed *pararhinal sclerosis*).

OTHER SELECTED LESIONS

Epilepsy and Vascular Malformations

Arteriovenous Malformations

Epilepsy is present in 8% (Hladky et al., 1994) to 20% (Humphreys et al., 1996; Aicardi et al., 1990) of patients with arteriovenous malformations (AVMs). Epileptic seizures may also occur at the time of rupture and bleeding and after surgery. The seizures are mainly partial ones.

The diagnosis of AVMs can almost always be made by CT scan, and angiography is probably not necessary for diagnosis when enhanced CT scan results are normal. Small, partially thrombosed AVMs can mimic small brain tumors (Aicardi et al., 1990; Kelly et al., 1978). An MRI is more specific than a CT scan (Gomori et al., 1986; Lemme-Phlagos et al., 1986). However, according to some studies, cryptic lesions may be missed in as many as 25% of patients, (Ormson et al., 1986).

Cavernous Angiomas

Cavernous angiomas or cavernomas are a more common cause of isolated seizures than are AVMs. They represent 10% to 20% of cerebrovascular malformations, and they cause seizures or, less commonly, focal neurologic signs or stroke. Although the lesions are usually hemispheral, cavernomas may occur in the brainstem, spinal cord, skin, and retina. Multiple cavernomas may be present (Fig. 19.12).

Epilepsy is usually the sole manifestation of cavernomas for very long periods, and it may appear at any age from infancy to adulthood. About 65% to 79% of patients with cavernomas present with seizures (Moran et al., 1999; Kattapong et al., 1995). However, cavernomas are a rare cause of newly diagnosed epilepsy in children. In a community-based study, only one case in 488 unselected patients was detected

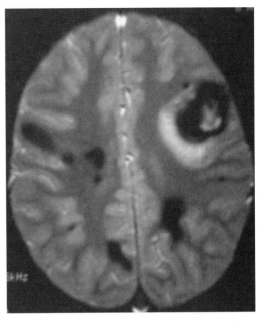

FIG. 19.12. Multiple cavernomatosis in a 7-year-old boy who has presented with purely aphasic seizures since the age of 6 years. The left frontoparietal cavernoma is the bigger one.

with CT or MRI scan (Berg et al., 2000). The seizures are focal in type, and they are often difficult to control.

The diagnosis may be difficult. Calcifications of the angioma are seen on CT scans in about half of patients. CT scan may also show changes in density ranging from edematous to hematoma like. The MRI features of cavernous malformations are distinctive (Zimmerman et al., 1991; Farmer et al., 1988), consisting of a central focus of mixed signal intensity surrounded by a rim of low signal due to the paramagnetic effect of hemosiderin, which becomes more evident on T2-weighted images. Angiography is usually normal. The appearance of new cavernomas has been seen in a few patients (Labauge et al., 2001; Kattapong et al., 1995).

Cavernous angiomas are often a familial autosomal dominant condition (Aicardi, 1992a; Rigamonti et al., 1988; Dobyns et al., 1987). A locus for familial cavernous angiomatosis was initially mapped to chromosome 7q (*CCM1* locus) (Marchuk et al., 1995), where the *Kritl* gene was subsequently shown to harbor mutations both in familial cases (Laberge-le Couteulx et al., 1999; Davenport et al., 2001) and in some sporadic patients (Lucas et al., 2001). Two additional loci (*CCM2* and *CCM3*) have been identified in other families (Craig et al., 1998). In affected families, seizures occur in 69% of patients and in 64% of symptomatic first-degree relatives (Rigamonti et al., 1988).

Treatment Issues

Surgical treatment of refractory epilepsy caused by vascular malformations is indicated when the size and location of the lesion do not represent an unreasonable risk. The results of surgery for vascular abnormalities are variable. Some investigators have reported very high success rates (Murphy, 1985), whereas, in some series, the results on epilepsy were disappointing. Thus, Cascino et al. (1993a) found that only 5 of 11 patients with vascular malformations became seizure free, compared with 9 of 11 tumor cases. In the authors' experience (Aicardi, 1992a; Aicardi et al., 1990), resective surgery for small cavernomas has given excellent results, but the treatment of AVMs is much less satisfactory.

A review of the literature suggests that about 85% of patients in whom cavernomas are resected are rendered seizure free, regardless of the site of the lesion (Moran et al., 1999). Patients with a shorter duration of epilepsy have a higher chance of becoming seizure free. Oxbury and Polkey (2000) reported that 7 of 16 patients treated by lesionectomy or temporal lobectomy and followed for a mean of 3.2 years were rendered seizure free. Gamma-knife surgery for the treatment of cavernomas located in highly functional areas has given interesting results (Régis et al., 2000a). A total of 26 (53%) of 49 patients with a follow-up of more than 1 year were seizure free, and a significant decrease in the number of seizures was achieved in 10 other patients (20%). The complications were minor. The lesions, however, can be multiple, and more may perhaps develop after operation for a first lesion.

Sturge-Weber Syndrome

Sturge-Weber syndrome is a nonfamilial phakomatosis with a potentially progressive course. The syndrome consists of a venous angioma of the leptomeninges in all patients that is accompanied by nevus flammeus of the skin supplied by the trigeminal nerve (port-wine stain) in 90% of the cases and, less often, by choroidal angioma and glaucoma. The facial and leptomeningeal angioma are usually ipsilateral, but both can be bilateral (Gilly et al., 1977; Bolthauser et al., 1976). Angiomatosis more frequently occurs in the occipital region, but it can be localized anywhere and it can involve an entire hemisphere.

Epilepsy is the most common and the earliest manifestation. Roughly 70% of patients with epilepsy have their first seizure within the first year of life, and, in about 20%, the onset of seizures is between the ages of 1 and 3 years (Erba and Cavazzuti, 1990; Rochkind et al., 1990; Dulac and Roger, 1980; Gilly et al., 1977). However, the age at seizure onset may vary from birth to 23 years of age (Sujansky and Conradi, 1995). The early seizures are triggered by fever in about one-third of patients (Revol et al., 1984), and they are often long lasting, usually consisting of unilateral status epilepticus. Bilateral involvement is correlated with an earlier seizure onset and a worse developmental prognosis. Large series of Sturge-Weber syndrome with epilepsy (Arzimanoglou and Aicardi, 1992; Erba and Cavazzuti, 1990; Ogunmekan et al., 1989; Hoffman et al., 1979) have shown that most seizures were simple partial or complex partial in type, with frequent secondary generalization. Unilateral convulsive status was observed in 11 of the 23 patients of Arzimanoglou and Aicardi (1992), and it was followed by permanent hemiplegia in 6 patients.

The diagnosis of the condition is generally obvious in a patient presenting with epileptic seizures. In some cases, however, the pial angiomatosis is present without a facial angioma, and, in other patients, the pial angioma may be bilateral, while the facial nevus is unilateral (Aicardi, 1992a; Gomez and Bebin, 1987). Epilepsy in Sturge-Weber syndrome is strongly associated with the occurrence of the neurologic features of the syndrome (Hoffman et al., 1979).

Hemiplegias of Sturge-Weber syndrome often appear after an episode of serial seizures or unilateral status epilepticus that generally occurs during the first year of life (Arzimanoglou and Aicardi, 1992). They are, therefore, acquired hemiplegias that closely resemble those observed in the hemiconvulsion–hemiplegia–epilepsy (HHE) syndrome (see Chapter 10). The cortex underlying the angioma appears to be made more susceptible to the anoxia produced by seizure activity because of the abnormal circulation in the angioma, which is probably related to the abnormal development of the venous system and the absence of the superficial cortical veins (Aylett et al., 1999; Terdjman et al., 1991). Some authors have also reported temporary hemiplegia that is not preceded by epileptic seizures (Arzimanoglou et al., 2000; Dulac and Roger, 1980; Gilly et al., 1977). A temporary circulatory deficit or subclinical ictal activity can be responsible for these transitory phenomena, which often present with headache, vomiting, and other features reminiscent of migraine.

The presence of epilepsy makes the prognosis worse. Gomez and Bebin (1987) showed that mental retardation was absent in all 25 patients without seizures, compared with only 21 of 76 patients with epilepsy. However, even seizures of early onset are not necessarily a predictor of intractable epilepsy. The epilepsy was benign in about one-fourth of the patients in one study (Erba and Cavazzuti, 1990), and it could be controlled with antiepileptic drugs in 40% to 50% of patients in others (Sujansky and Conradi, 1995; Arzimanoglou and Aicardi, 1992). Deterioration after bouts of status epilepticus and neurologic deterioration with progressive parenchymal atrophy can occur even if the epilepsy is not severe (Arzimanoglou and Aicardi, 1992). Thus, surgery seems required in up to 40% of the affected children in some series (Arzimanoglou and Aicardi, 1992; Erba and Cavazzuti, 1990).

The *interictal EEG* in Sturge-Weber syndrome shows focal or unilateral depression of the background activity over the area of the leptomeningeal angiomatosis (Sassover et al., 1994; Gilly et al., 1977; Breuner and Sharbrough, 1976). Polymorphic delta slowing is the next most common EEG abnormality, and, when it is unilateral, it correctly lateralizes the angiomatosis (Arzimanoglou et al., 2000; Arzimanoglou and Aicardi, 1992). Focal epileptiform abnormalities are uncommon in infants, even in those with frequently occurring seizures (Sassover et al., 1994). Bilateral epileptiform abnormalities occur early in cases with bilateral lesions, but these usually do not appear until after 3 years of age in cases with unilateral lesions (Chevrie et al., 1988; Revol et al., 1984; Rosen et al., 1984). Bilateral paroxysmal activity may be associated with the occurrence of apparently generalized seizures, including occasional infantile spasms (Chevrie et al., 1988; Fukuyama and Tsuchiya, 1979). Such cases may respond well to resective surgery despite the presence of bilateral EEG abnormalities (Chevrie et al., 1988; Rosen et al., 1984).

Determining whether the pial angioma is strictly unilateral and what its extent is in order to plan the necessary resection precisely is crucial. An enhanced CT scan does not outline the superficial angiomatosis, but it does demonstrate cortical enhancement due to postepileptic increases in the blood–brain barrier permeability. SPECT or PET scan has been used to demonstrate a significant reduction in blood flow and glucose metabolism in the resting state (Chiron et al., 1989; Chugani et al., 1989).

Gadolinium-enhanced MRI demonstrates the angioma (Fig. 19.13), but it should be performed distant (no less than 3 weeks) from an episode of status to avoid images due to the intracortical leakage following blood–brain barrier alterations, which do not correlate well with the extent of the angioma (Terdjman et al., 1991; Elster and Chen, 1990; Sperner et al., 1990). Both short echo and long repetition time and/or echo-time studies should be conducted. In addition, gradient-echo sequences are helpful for demonstrating the presence of microcalcifications (Kuzniecky and Jackson, 1995b).

Rapid and vigorous treatment of incipient episodes of status epilepticus with antiepileptic drugs is essential to prevent postconvulsive damage. *Resective surgery* (hemispherectomy, lobectomy, or circumscribed cortical resection) gives satisfactory results in selected cases (Arzimanoglou, 1997; Aicardi, 1992a; Arzimanoglou and Aicardi, 1992; Erba and Cavazzuti, 1990; Ito et al., 1990; Rosen et al., 1984; Hoffman, et al., 1979). Lesionectomy is indicated for lesions limited to one lobe or less (Arzimanoglou et al., 2000). Hemispherectomy can be performed in cases with more extensive lesions and in children with preexisting hemiplegia. In a recent study of 20 patients treated with different approaches, including callosotomy in 1, hemispherectomy in 5, and cortical resection in 14, 13 became seizure free; almost all benefited from the surgery despite the variability in age at seizure onset and the type of operation (Arzimanoglou et al., 2000). In the patients treated with le-

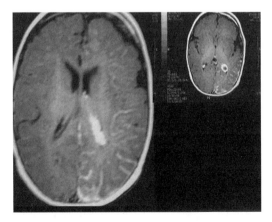

FIG. 19.13. Gadolinium-enhanced magnetic resonance imaging scan in a boy with Sturge-Weber syndrome. The pial angioma stands out clearly after injection. Note the signs of frontal atrophy and enlargement and the angiomatous appearance of the left choroid plexus.

sionectomy, visually guided complete resection of the pial angioma and underlying cortex appeared sufficient, and no better results were obtained with intraoperative corticography. In the same series, complete seizure control was achieved in all five patients with hemiparesis treated with hemispherectomy. Surgically treated patients have significantly better seizure control. The earlier the surgery is with respect to seizure onset, the lower is the chance of increased neurologic deterioration (Arzimanoglou et al., 2000; Hoffman, 1997; Ogunmekan et al., 1989). Hemispherectomized patients did not differ statistically with regard to motor function from conservatively treated children, and they had a much higher incidence of normal or borderline intelligence (Rochkind et al., 1990).

Epilepsy and Cerebral Palsy

Cerebral palsy (CP) is the most common neurologic disorder associated with epilepsy. The frequency of epilepsy in CP varies from between 15% and 60% of patients (Stephenson, 1998; Hadjipanayis et al., 1997; Aksu, 1990) but differs with the type. In the series of Hadjipanayis et al. (1997), it was present in 50% of children with quadriplegia, 47% of those with hemiplegia, but only 27% of those with spastic diplegia. The frequency of epilepsy is highest (80%) in children with acquired postconvulsive hemiplegia (Aicardi et al., 1969a). Only about 25% of patients with dyskinetic CP have seizures; these are more common in the dystonic types than they are in the athetoid or dyskinetic forms, in which 32% and 11%, respectively, of patients have seizures (Kyllerman, 1981). The incidence of epilepsy in preterm infants with diplegia was as low as 11% in one series (Amess et al., 1998), probably as a result of the predominance of deep white matter lesions in such cases.

All types of seizures may occur with CP. Partial motor attacks are most common in children with hemiplegia (73%), whereas generalized seizures predominate in dystonic or quadriplegic cerebral palsy, in which they represent 75% of seizure types. Infantile spasms are observed in more than 15% of patients (Hadjipanayis et al., 1997). Startle epilepsy is mainly observed in children with congenital hemiparesis (Chauvel et al., 1992b).

The onset of epilepsy in patients with CP is usually early. In one series, 50% of patients had an onset before 2 years of age, although the onset was usually later in those patients with hemiplegia (3 to 5 years of age).

The course of epilepsy in these patients tends to be severe. Delgado et al. (1996) found that only 69 (13%) of 531 patients with both CP and epilepsy achieved a remission lasting 2 years or more. In other series, a higher remission rate of 30% to 40% has been observed, but this sometimes has been reached only after many years. However, relatively benign epilepsies can be seen in children with CP, especially those with hemiparesis (Goutières et al., 1972).

Epilepsy associated with CP considerably aggravates the total disability of these patients because of the inconvenience of the seizures and the increased social rejection, so its effect is multiplicative rather than simply additive. Moreover, epilepsy is an index of the severity of the condition, and associated disabilities and mental retardation are much more common in patients with both CP and epilepsy than in those without seizures. Both neurologic difficulties and mental retardation tend to be more severe when seizures are also present. In patients with hemiplegic CP, the presence of epilepsy is clearly associated with more severe, increasing cognitive difficulties. Vargha-Khadem et al. (1992a) showed that such patients function at lower levels in both intelligence and memory than do children with the same form of CP without seizures. The decrease in achievement seems to be directly correlated with the occurrence of epilepsy rather than with the extent of brain damage because, as a group, the patients with small lesions and epilepsy do less well than those with larger lesions without epilepsy. Uvebrandt (1988) found epilepsy to be five times more common in hemiplegic patients with mental retardation than in those with normal intellect, and Goutières et al. (1972) reported that 71% of their hemiplegic children with epilepsy were mentally retarded, compared with 29% of those without epilepsy.

Epilepsy associated with CP is not always refractory to drug treatment. However, severe cases are common, and they may require surgical treatment.

Epilepsy and Mitochondrial Disorders

Epilepsy is an important symptom of mitochondrial disorders. It may be an early manifestation of the disorders and, sometimes, their most apparent clinical feature. In a series of 31 patients with recurrent and apparently unprovoked seizures associated with primary mitochondrial diseases (Canafoglia et al., 2001), seizures were the first symptom in 53%. However, generalized myoclonic seizures were present in only five patients with the clinical features of the syndrome of myoclonic encephalopathy with ragged-red fibers (MERRF) due to an A8344 C to G mitochondrial DNA point mutation or in "overlap" syndromes of MERRF and mitochondrial myopathy, encephalopathy, lactic acidosis, and strokelike episodes (MELAS) syndrome (Aicardi, 1992a). In such cases, the myoclonus is often photosensitive. In one case (Garcia Silva et al., 1987), the myoclonus was mainly sensitive to eye closure before it became movement induced, as is often present in MERRF. Photoparoxysmal EEG responses have been observed in these disorders and in occasional patients with Leigh syndrome (Canafoglia et al., 2001).

The most common type of seizures is partial motor (71% of patients in the series by Canafoglia et al. [2001]), in association with focal or multifocal EEG paroxysms. An atypical phenotype was seen in 70% of patients with epilepsy, and their mitochondrial diseases were difficult to classify. In MELAS, epilepsia partialis continua is relatively common (Montagna et al., 1988; Chevrie et al., 1987), but the clinical presentation of epilepsy in mitochondrial disorders may be quite variable (Tulinius and Hagne, 1991).

In a large family with maternally inherited mitochondrial disease, myoclonus, partial seizures, and generalized tonic-clonic seizures were observed in different members. The age at onset was infancy for three patients and adulthood in the remainder (Torbergsen, 1991). Infantile onset of progressive myoclonic epilepsy due to a mitochondrial defect has been reported (Harbord et al., 1991). At least some of the cases of Alpers disease, particularly those associated with liver disease (Harding, 1990), are likely due to mitochondrial defects (Bicknese et al., 1992). In such cases, multifocal myoclonus may occur over long periods lasting several days, and continuous partial epilepsy is common in the late stages of the illness.

The diagnosis of a mitochondrial disorder should always be considered in unexplained cases of myoclonic epilepsy, epilepsia partialis continua, and partial seizures.

SUMMARY

Brain tumors are an uncommon cause of chronic epilepsy in children. Nevertheless, hemispheric tumors are often manifested by epileptic seizures that may remain the sole symptom for prolonged periods, and epilepsies caused by tumors manifest mostly with isolated focal seizures. Generalized seizures and bilateral synchronous EEG abnormalities are present in a proportion of patients with a tumor, and no single clinical or EEG feature permits the complete exclusion of a brain tumor as a cause of epilepsy in a particular patient. Tumors causing epilepsy are mostly benign developmental tumors, especially gangliogliomas and DNTs, whose surgical resection often gives excellent results.

Cortical dysplasias are a common cause of epilepsy that is often refractory. Their diagnosis has now been made much easier by MRI, which also shortens the time to diagnosis. Diffuse abnormalities of cortical development are usually the cause of severe epilepsy, mental retardation, and intractability. However, some abnormalities, such as bilateral periventricular heterotopias, may be asymptomatic, or they may be associated with a relatively mild phenotype. Focal cortical developmental anomalies are revealed by epilepsy, whether or not they are associated with cognitive problems. Interestingly, they may also be a common cause of infantile spasms. Surgical resection, when this is feasible, can control the seizures, but the results are still less favorable than those in small tumors but the patients do tend to improve. The diagnosis of a cortical development disorder and of the type causing it is essential because an increasing number of genetically transmitted forms is known.

Tuberous sclerosis, although it is a distinct condition, is closely related to cortical dysplasias. Epilepsy in TS is usually difficult to control, especially in the early onset cases, and only a few cases are amenable to surgical therapy.

Sturge-Weber syndrome is a cause of severe seizures, often in the form of status epilepticus occurring in the first year of life. Complete and early surgical resection of the pial angioma often results in the patient becoming seizure free. Vascular malformations are not a common cause of epilepsy. Cavernomas, the most common type, are often familial. Surgical treatment is possible in some cases.

Cerebral palsy is often associated with various types of seizures. Epilepsy in many cases complicates the treatment and aggravates the handicap of the affected children.

20

Genetics

The prominent role of genetic factors in the causation of epilepsy has been suspected for centuries based on the observations of familial aggregation but, in spite of extensive research, its definition has been elusive. A complete review of the genetic contribution to epilepsy is not possible because epilepsy is a heterogeneous condition in which many causative factors may intervene. The basic mechanisms of the epilepsies involve many of the neural processes that have been recognized in the normal brain, making the number of genes that could be involved in epileptogenesis quite high (Anderson et al., 2002). Although the study of rare epilepsy syndromes with single gene inheritance has recently permitted the discovery of several genes involved in epileptogenesis, most common genetic epilepsies do not follow familial patterns of aggregation consistent with simple inheritance.

The genetically determined epilepsies may be divided into the following two major subgroups: those that originate directly from the functional consequences of a defective gene product on neuronal excitability and those secondary to structural brain abnormalities. Many of the genetically determined epilepsies belonging to the latter category are actually associated diseases, some of which have specific inheritance mechanisms. These associated conditions may have mendelian inheritance, or they may be a derivative of chromosomal abnormality syndromes. The main mendelian disorders associated with epilepsy (Table 20.1) have already been covered in other chapters of this book (see Chapter 19); these are only mentioned briefly here.

In many circumstances, the distinction between idiopathic and symptomatic genetic epilepsies may be artificial. For example, genetic factors that are prominent in the etiology of the idiopathic epilepsies also reportedly influence the likelihood of developing posttraumatic epilepsy (Jennett, 1975). Some gene mutations may only decrease the seizure threshold, therefore increasing the individual's susceptibility to environmental factors (Ottman, 1997). Ion channel mutations are another example. Although they are thought to affect neuronal excitability only, they can cause severe epileptic encephalopathies, such as occurs in Dravet syndrome, in which the mental retardation could suggest a symptomatic origin.

GENERAL CONSIDERATIONS

Clinical and electroencephalographic (EEG) studies in families have provided interesting evidence about the importance of the interaction between specific genetic factors and environmental determinants consistent with a polygenic inheritance model.

Studies on twins have demonstrated much higher concordance rates in monozygotic than in dizygotic pairs (Ottman, 1997). Even considering that most such studies have been performed without particular attention to the specific epilepsy type or syndrome, these rates overwhelmingly favored the presence of a shared genetic susceptibility in identical twins when idiopathic ("intact") cases were considered (70% versus 6% of dizygotic twins) (Lennox, 1960).

First-degree relatives of individuals with epilepsy have an increased genetic susceptibility to show epileptiform EEG abnormalities and seizures (Andermann, 1982). For example, up to 50% of the siblings and offspring of patients with what has been termed *benign rolandic epilepsy* also have rolandic spikes; however, only 12% develop epilepsy (Bray and Wiser, 1965a, 1965b). The relatives of children with absence epilepsy (Metrakos and Metrakos, 1966) have also been reported to have a high incidence of generalized paroxysmal EEG abnormalities. Such an observation indicates that, in at least a minority of patients, non-specific factors act by transforming the individual's genetic predisposition into overt seizures. Annegers et al. (1982b) estimated that the standardized morbidity ratios for unprovoked seizures in the relatives of individuals with idiopathic childhood-onset epilepsy were 2.5 in siblings and 6.7 in offspring. More distant relatives did not have an increased risk of unprovoked seizures. A later study of the same patient population found that morbidity ratios for the offspring were 3.4 (Ottman, 1997). A study of siblings and children of individuals with symptomatic focal epilepsy came to complementary conclusions, as EEG abnormalities were present in 20%, seizures in 7%, and epilepsy in 4% (Andermann and Straszak, 1982). Therefore, the

TABLE 20.1. *Main mendelian disorders and chromosomal abnormalities associated with epilepsy*

Disorder	Gene	Chromosomal Mapping and/or Chromosome(s) Involved	Epilepsy (%)
Lafora disease	EPM2A	6q23.25	100
Unverricht-Lundborg disease	EPM1	21q22.3	100
Ceroid lipofuscinosis (recessive)	CLN1, CLN2, CLN3, CLN	1p32, 11p15.5, 513q21.1-32, 16p12.1	100
Galactosialidosis	GLB2	20q13.1	100
Gangliosidosis GM1 type 1	GLB1	3p21.33	100
Type III Gaucher disease	GBA	1q21	100
Aicardi	—	Xp22	100
Miller-Dieker/ILS	LIS1	17p13.3	100
XLAG and XL infantile spasms	ARX	X	100
Wolf-Hirschhorn syndrome (4p-)	—	4p-	100
Ring chromosome 20	—	20 ring	100
Ring chromosome 14	—	14 ring	100
Angelman syndrome	UBE3A	15q11–q13	90–100
Inv Dup (15) syndrome	—	15q tetrasomy	90–100
SBH/XL lissencephaly	DCX	Xq22.3	90–100
Periventricular nodular heterotopia	FLN1	Xq28	80–100
Tuberous sclerosis	TSC1/TSC2	9q24/16p13.3	60–100
Rett syndrome	MECP2	Xq28	70
Familial cavernous angiomas	unknown	7q	70
Alpha-thalassemia mental retardation	XH2	Xq13.3	45
Fragile X	FMR1	Xq27.3	28–45
Trisomy 21 (Down syndrome)	—	21	12–40

Abbreviations: ILS, isolated lissencephaly sequence; SBH, subcortical band heterotopia; XL, X linked; XLAG, X-linked lissencephaly with ambiguous genitalia.

inheritance of nonspecific predisposing factors may act by increasing the chances that acquired epileptogenic factors will cause seizures or epilepsy even in the relatives of patients with acquired lesions, though this occurs to a much lesser degree than that observed in the relatives of patients with idiopathic epilepsy.

The relatives of patients with early onset epilepsy have a higher risk of developing seizures than do the relatives of those with later onset epilepsy (Anderson et al., 1991), which is in keeping with the high frequency of epilepsies of genetic origin in young children. The possible presence of a gradient of risk in first-degree relatives was suggested by Lennox (1947), with the highest risk being present in the relatives of probands with an onset before 4 years of age. Other factors that enhance the risk of epilepsy in offspring include a mother who is affected, which confers a higher risk than an affected father (9% versus 3%), and an age at onset of epilepsy in the affected parent of younger than 20 years (Ottman, 1997).

Hauser et al. (1986) observed that the risk for epilepsy in relatives of probands with febrile convulsions is increased to an extent similar to that in the relatives of probands with epilepsy. A history of both febrile convulsions and epilepsy in the proband implies an even greater risk for relatives, suggesting a higher genetic load that favors the cooccurrence of both manifestations. However, potentially epileptogenic environmental and behavioral factors may be equally shared within the same family, making many studies of familial aggregation of limited use in estimating the specific role of genetic factors (Ottman, 1997).

IDIOPATHIC GENERALIZED EPILEPSIES WITH COMPLEX INHERITANCE

A multifactorial inheritance seems to be operative in most of the common forms of epilepsy. This type of genetic influence can act in conjunction with environmental factors in determination of the phenotype. Studies in which the specific epilepsy syndromes in probands and relatives have been taken into account have provided a more precise estimate of the magnitude of the genetic influences. A high incidence of epilepsy was observed in the siblings of probands with myoclonic astatic epilepsy (MAE) (13% to 20%), childhood absence epilepsy (CAE) (5% to 10%), and juvenile myoclonic epilepsy (JME) (5% to 7%) (Beck-Mannaggetta et al., 1989). The risk for offspring of individuals who had CAE, JME, and grand mal on awakening was estimated to be at about 7%. The offspring of individuals with a history of absence epilepsy were also found to carry a higher risk than the offspring of parents with other types, not only for absence seizures but also for other seizure types in the study of Ottman et al. (1989).

The relatives of probands with specific idiopathic syndromes have a tendency to develop the same type of epilepsy (Beck-Mannaggetta and Janz, 1991), although not necessarily the same syndrome. In the Italian League Against Epilepsy concordance study (Italian League Against Epilepsy Genetic Collaborative Group, 1993), which was conducted on 72 families of probands with idiopathic generalized epilepsy in which more than three individuals were affected, multiple types of idiopathic generalized epilepsy were observed in 75% of the families. However, the concordance for the epilepsy syndrome in the identical twin pair study of Berkovic et al. (1998) was 94%.

A major difficulty that arises in the study of the genetic basis of the epilepsies derives from the poor correspondence between genotype and phenotype. Studies on monogenic epilepsies have discovered that *reduced penetrance* is common with epilepsy genes, thus implying that mutation carriers may be unaffected (Ottman, 1997). Reduced penetrance is even more difficult to demonstrate in polygenic epilepsies. *Locus* (or genic) *heterogeneity* (i.e., the possibility that mutations at different loci may underlie the same syndrome) implies that different families with the same syndrome may harbor mutations of different genes. For example, the generalized epilepsy with febrile seizures plus (GEFS+) spectrum of phenotypes has been linked to mutations of the *SCN1A*, *SCN1B*, and *GABR1A* genes in different families

(Meisler et al., 2001). *Allelic heterogeneity* is observed when different alleles at the same locus cause different syndromes, so families or individuals with different syndromes have different mutations of the same gene. For example, many children with Dravet syndrome with mutations of the *SCN1A* gene have truncating mutations (Nabbout et al., 2003; Claes et al., 2001), whereas missense mutations of the same gene have been detected in individuals with milder phenotypes within the GEFS+ spectrum.

EPILEPSIES WITH SINGLE GENE INHERITANCE

Over the last several years, the recognition of families in which epilepsy phenotypes, which are comparable to those observed in the common idiopathic epilepsies but which are segregated in a mendelian fashion, has led to genetic linkage studies and the identification of a number of loci (Table 20.2). Causative genes, mostly those for the ion channels, have been identified for a number of these conditions (Meisler et al., 2001; Lerche et al., 2001) (Table 20.3). Although single gene epilepsies account for only about 1% of the epilepsy population (Ottman, 1997), they have been instrumental to understanding the molecular genetic mechanisms of epileptogenesis that may also be operative in the more common idiopathic epilepsies with complex inheritance. Some nonprogressive syndromes of epilepsy associated with other paroxysmal neurologic disorders, such as myoclonus and dystonia (Guerrini et al., 1999b, 2001b; Szepetowski et al., 1997), suggest that the

TABLE 20.2. *Genetic epilepsy syndromes with simple inheritance (gene unknown)*

Mode of Transmission	Linkage
Autosomal dominant	
Adolescent-onset idiopathic generalized epilepsy	8p12, 18q12, 5p
Autosomal dominant cortical myoclonus and epilepsy	2p11.1-q12.2
Autosomal dominant nocturnal frontal lobe epilepsy	15q24
Autosomal dominant rolandic epilepsy with speech dyspraxia	—
Benign familial infantile convulsions	19q, 16p, 2q24
Benign rolandic epilepsy	15q24
Childhood absence epilepsy	8q24
Familial mesial temporal lobe epilepsy	—
Familial adult myoclonic epilepsy	8q23.3-24.1
Familial partial epilepsy with variable foci	22q11-q12
Febrile seizures	8q13, 19p, 5q14-15
Idiopathic generalized epilepsy	3q26, 14q23, 2q36, 16p12-p11
Infantile convulsions and paroxysmal coreoathetosis	16p12-11.2
Juvenile myoclonic epilepsy	6p21, 5q14
Partial epilepsy with pericentral spikes	4p15
Autosomal recessive	
Familial idiopathic myoclonic epilepsy	16p13
Rolandic epilepsy–exercise-induced dystonia–writer's cramp	16p12-11.2

TABLE 20.3. *Known idiopathic epilepsy genes in 2003*

Gene	Function	Locus	Inheritance/ MIM	Type of Mutations	Epilepsy Syndrome	Seizure Types
GABRA1 GABA$_A$ α_1-receptor subunit	Partial inhibition of GABA-activated currents	5q34	AD/606904	Missense	AD JME	TCS, myoclonic, absence
GABRG2 GABA$_A$ receptor γ subunit	Rapid Inhibition of GABAergic neurons	5q31	AD/604233	Missense, truncation	FS, CAE, GEFS+	Febrile, absence, TCS, myoclonic, clonic, partial
SCN2A Sodium channel α_2 subunit	Fast sodium influx initiation and propagation of action potential	2q24	AD/604233	Missense	GEFS+ BFNIC	Febrile, afebrile generalized tonic and TCS
SCN1A Sodium channel α_1 subunit	Somatodendritic sodium influx	2q24	AD/604233	Missense	GEFS+ SMEI	Febrile, absence, myoclonic, TCS, partial
SCN1B Sodium channel β_1 subunit	Coadjuvate and modulate a subunit	19q13	AD/604233	Missense	GEFS+	Febrile, absence, tonic-clonic, myoclonic
KCNQ2 Potassium channel	M current interacts with *KCNQ3*	20q13	AD/602235	Missense	BFNC	Neonatal convulsions
KCNQ3 Potassium channel	M current interacts with *KCNQ2*	8q24	AD/121201	Missense	BFNC	Neonatal convulsions
CHRNA4 Acetylcholine receptor α_4 subunit	Presynaptic; nicotinic current modulation; interacts with β_2 subunit	20q13	AD/600513	Missense	ADNFLE	Sleep related focal seizures
CHRNB2 Acetylcholine receptor β_2 subunit	Presynaptic; nicotinic current modulation; interacts with α_2 subunit	1p21	AD/605375	Missense	ADNFLE	Sleep related focal seizures
LGI1 Leucine-rich, glioma activated	Disregulates homeostasis, interactions between neurons and glia?	10q24	AD/600512	Missense	ADPEAF	Partial seizures with auditory or visual hallucinations
CLCN2 Voltage-gated chloride channel	Neuronal chloride efflux	3q26	AD	Stop codon, splicing, missense	IGEs	TCS, myoclonic, absence

Abbreviations: AD, autosomal dominant; ADNFLE, autosomal dominant nocturnal frontal lobe epilepsy; ADPEAF, autosomal dominant partial epilepsy with auditory features; BFNC, benign familial neonatal convulsions; BFNIC, benign familial neonatal-infantile convulsion; GEFS+, generalised epilepsy with febrile seizures plus; MAE, myoclonic astatic epilepsy; SMEI, severe myoclonic epilepsy of infancy; TCS, tonic-clonic seizures; XL, X linked. Modified from Guerrini et al., 2003b.

same genetic mechanisms of channel dysfunction known to be operative in the single gene epilepsies may be part of the cause in these cases as well.

Generalized Epilepsy with Febrile Seizures Plus and Mutations of the Voltage-Gated Sodium Channel Subunit Genes

The collection of large dominant pedigrees with about 60% penetrance that feature heterogeneous epilepsy phenotypes, including febrile seizures (FSs) that often persist beyond the age of 6 years (FS+), generalized tonic-clonic (GTC) seizures, absence, and myoclonic seizures, led to the concept of GEFS+ (Wallace et al., 1998; Scheffer and Berkovic, 1997). These types of seizures may occur in isolation, most often in FS+ individuals who have no other seizure types, or they may be combined in variable phenotypes that are often mild but that, in very rare cases (Berkovic and Scheffer, 2001), may also include intractable syndromes, such as MAE and severe myoclonic epilepsy (Dravet syndrome).

A locus for the GEFS+ spectrum has been mapped to chromosome 19q13 (Wallace et al., 1998) to which the voltage-gated sodium channel β_1 subunit gene (*SCN1B*) had been assigned. A missense mutation of this gene (C121W) has been found in two unrelated families (Wallace et al., 1998, 2002). *In vitro* functional studies (voltage-clamp recording on *Xenopus laevis* oocytes) showed changes consistent with the loss of function. In particular, the mutant protein failed to accelerate the recovery of the associated α subunit from inactivation (Wallace et al., 1998). Co-expression of mutant and wild type β subunits with the α subunits caused an intermediate inactivation rate (Moran and Conti 2001), which arose from the competitive binding of the inactive mutant subunit with the α subunit, accounting for dominant inheritance. In heterozygotes, the association of inactive β subunits with α subunits generates a persistent sodium current, rendering the neurons hyperexcitable and making them apt to initiate firing with small depolarizations (Meisler et al., 2001).

Two GEFS+ families with linkage to chromosome 2q24-33 were found to harbor missense mutations of the sodium channel α subunit gene *SCN1A* (Escayg et al., 2000). Both mutations affected highly conserved residues coding for the putative voltage sensor of the transmembrane region of the channel. Functional studies have shown that these mutations have different functional consequences. One (R1648H) accelerated the recovery from inactivation, with consequent neuronal hyperexcitability. The other (T875M) in-

creased the slow inactivation mode, with consequent reduction of the whole channel protein accessible for opening (Escayg et al., 2000).

The most common mutations found in GEFS+ families are estimated to be those involving *SCN1A*, which accounted for 5.6% of the cases in a large series (Escayg et al., 2000).

An R187W mutation of the *SCN2A* gene has been reported in a single family (Sugawara et al., 2001).

The γ-aminobutyric acid A (GABA$_A$) receptor γ_2 subunit gene has also been shown to be involved in the pathogenesis of GEFS+ (Baulac et al., 2001; Wallace et al., 2001a), confirming the locus heterogeneity for this spectrum of epilepsy phenotypes.

Dravet Syndrome (Severe Myoclonic Epilepsy of Infancy) and Mutations of the Voltage-Gated Sodium Channel Subunit Genes

In severe myoclonic epilepsy of infancy (SMEI) (Dravet et al., 1992a), the relatives of the affected individuals have an elevated incidence of epilepsy (Benlounis et al., 2001; Singh et al., 2001), although a clear familial distribution for the syndrome is rare. The association of seizures with febrile episodes suggested that it may be analogous to GEFS+ and prompted mutation screening for *SCN1A* in a small series of affected children (Claes et al., 2001). All were shown to carry *de novo* frameshift or nonsense mutations leading to null alleles with complete loss of function. In two subsequent studies, Ohmori et al. (2002) detected mutations of the *SCN1A* gene in 24 of 29 patients with SMEI and Sugawara et al. (2002) in 10 of 14; these included deletion, insertion, missense, and nonsense mutations. These were *de novo* mutations because none of the parents were carriers. In a large series including approximately 100 patients, mutations of the *SCN1A* gene were observed in one-third of the children and, surprisingly, in a few unaffected or mildly affected parents as well (Nabbout et al., 2003). The variable frequency of mutations in various series and the high frequency of epilepsies of various types that is found in the families of these patients are as yet unexplained (Fujiwara et al., 2003) The genotype–phenotype correlation in this syndrome is probably much more complex than has been previously thought, and mutations in additional genes or strong environmental factors may be needed for the phenotype to manifest. SMEI has also been observed in association with an inherited *GABRG2* mutation within a GEFS+ pedigree (Harkin et al., 2002).

Missense mutations in three sodium channel genes (*SCN1A*, *SCN1B* and *SCN2A*) most often cause the same spectrum of usually mild epilepsy phenotypes, while loss-of-function mutations of one of these genes (*SCN1A*) usually causes a more severe phenotype. However, the phenotypes associated with missense mutations of these genes may sometimes be severe, including some cases with Dravet syndrome or a picture reminiscent of MAE. Genetic heterogeneity may result from either variable expression of some genes or allelic heterogeneity (Meisler et al., 2001).

Febrile Seizures and Idiopathic Generalized Epilepsy with Variable Phenotypes Associated with Mutations of the Ligand-Gated γ-Aminobutyric Acid-A Receptor Subunit Genes

The GABA$_A$ receptor is a ligand-gated Cl$^-$ channel that functions as a pentameric assembly of homologous subunits α, β, χ, δ, and π that mediate fast synaptic inhibition in the brain. Several subtypes of each subunit exist. The main GABA$_A$ receptor isoform in the brain consists of α$_1$, β$_2$, and γ$_2$ subunits. Mutations causing reduced activity are expected to cause neuronal hyperexcitability, and they may lead to seizure activity.

Mutations of the gene encoding the γ$_2$ subunit (*GABRG2*) have been observed in a few pedigrees (Kananura et al., 2002; Baulac et al., 2001; Wallace et al., 2001a) with a GEFS+ phenotype, including one in which some individuals had absence epilepsy.

Recently, a mutation in the α$_1$ subunit of the GABA$_A$ receptor gene was described in a large family with dominant JME (Cossette et al., 2002). JME represents up to 25% of all idiopathic generalized epilepsies (Genton et al., 1994), and it has a common familial distribution. However, with the exception of this family, this syndrome has proven difficult to assign to consistent loci because of its uncertain inheritance pattern(s) (Greenberg et al., 2000).

Benign Familial Neonatal Convulsions and Potassium Channels

Benign familial neonatal convulsions (BFNCs) (see Chapter 12) represent one of the first disorders for which candidate regions were identified by linkage analysis. Although two loci had been mapped to chromosomes 8q24 and 20q13.3 (Lewis et al., 1993; Leppert et al., 1989), several years elapsed before the causative genes were identified as the voltage-gated potassium channel genes *KCNQ3* (Charlier et al., 1998) and *KCNQ2* (Biervert et al., 1998; Singh et al., 1998). *KCNQ2* and *KCNQ3* are widely represented in the brain, and they have similar expression patterns (Biervert et al., 1998). They belong to a subfamily of proteins, all of which are characterized by six transmembrane regions, a pore domain, and a long C-terminus.

KCNQ2 and *KCNQ3* interact to generate slowly activated potassium conductance that contributes to subthreshold neuronal excitability and responsiveness to synaptic inputs (Meisler et al., 2001). In particular, their activity may reduce the number of action potentials by countering the inward flow of ions that is triggered by neuronal signals (Steinlein, 2001). Functional studies of the heterozygous expression of the truncated and wild type KCNQ2 and KCNQ3 proteins in the *Xenopus* oocytes has shown a reduction of currents, resulting in neuronal hyperexcitability (Steinlein, 2001). Coexpression of *KCNQ2* and *KCNQ3* produces currents that are more than tenfold larger than those seen in homomeric channels alone, which implies the formation of KCNQ2/KCNQ3 heteromers (McNamara, 1999). Since a single copy of the mutant gene is sufficient to produce BFNCs, the implication is that a 25% loss of the heteromeric KCNQ2/KCNQ3 channel function is sufficient to determine critical neuronal hyperexcitability (Schroeder et al., 1998).

Why BFNCs are restricted to the first weeks or months of life remains difficult to understand. One possibility is that the immature newborn brain is more vulnerable to mild changes in neuronal excitability. Alternatively, mutated KCNQ2/KCNQ3 channels may be replaced with other potassium channel subunits that are upregulated after the first months of life (Steinlein, 2001).

Nocturnal Frontal Lobe Epilepsy and the Nicotinic Receptors

Autosomal dominant nocturnal frontal lobe epilepsy (ADNFLE) (see Chapter 10) is characterized by brief seizures during sleep. A genetic etiology can be established in only a small minority of patients with nocturnal frontal lobe epilepsy.

The condition is autosomal dominant with incomplete penetrance that may be due to an unrecognized mild form in obligate carriers. Multiple loci have been associated with the presence ADNFLE in large pedigrees. The first locus was assigned to chromosome 20q13.2 (ADNFL1) in a large Australian family (Phillips et al., 1995), a second locus (ADNFL2) was localized to chromosome 15q24 (Phillips et al., 1998), and, more recently, a third locus (ADNFL3) was mapped to chromosome 1p21 in a 23-member three-generation family (Gambardella et al., 2000).

The genetic causes of ADNFLE are, thus far, homogeneous, as the two genes responsible for ADNFL1 and

ADNFL3 that have been identified belong to the neuronal nicotinic acetylcholine receptor (nAChR) family. Different mutations of the α_4 subunit (*CHRNA4*) have been found in several ADNFL1 pedigrees (Hirose et al., 1999; Steinlein et al., 1995a, 1997). ADNFL3 is caused by mutations of the β_2 isoform of the nAChRs (Phillips et al., 2001; De Fusco et al., 2000). The gene associated with ADNFL2 has not been identified thus far.

The observation of the increased sensitivity to carbamazepine of the mutant *CHRNA4* receptor compared with wild type receptors (Picard et al., 1999) is supported by clinical evidence demonstrating that patients with ADNFLE often show a good response to this drug. Most of the patients with nocturnal frontal lobe epilepsy represent sporadic cases, and why *de novo* mutations, which might account for at least some of the sporadic cases, are rare remains to be established (Phillips et al., 2000). Most families with nocturnal frontal lobe epilepsy do not show mutations of the candidate genes (Picard et al., 2000).

Absence Epilepsy Associated with Mutations of Calcium Channel Genes

The calcium channel α_{1A} and β_4 genes were considered potential candidates for human absence epilepsy following observations of mutant mouse models with absence epilepsy (Meisler et al., 2001). Scattered reports have pointed out a possible role for calcium channel mutations in human epilepsy, although these do occur in association with other disorders and in small pedigrees. An α_{1A} mutation was described in a patient with seizures, mental retardation, and episodic ataxia (Jouvenceau et al., 2001). Nonsense mutations of the calcium channel β_4 subunit gene *CACNB4* were detected in a woman with JME and in a family with generalized epilepsy and episodic ataxia. In spite of these reports, the role and functional mechanisms of calcium channel gene mutations in human epilepsy must still be fully determined.

Autosomal Dominant Partial Epilepsy with Auditory Features and Leucine-Rich Glioma-Inactivated 1 Gene Mutations

This form of monogenic focal epilepsy, which is characterized by seizures with sensory symptoms, has been linked to chromosome 10 (Ottman et al., 1995). Its typical manifestations include ictal auditory hallucinations, such as ringing or humming. In addition, other individuals may have visual hallucinations or other sensory (olfactory, vertiginous) symptoms (Winawer et al., 2000). Recently, the responsible

gene, the leucine-rich glioma-inactivated 1 gene (*LGI1-epitempin*), was identified (Kalachikov et al., 2002; Morante-Redolat et al., 2002). Silencing of both of the alleles of the *LGI1* gene, which is expressed ubiquitously in neuronal tissue, is common in several high-grade gliomas (Chernova et al., 1998). The functional inactivation of one allele product (i.e., haploinsufficiency) leads to partial epilepsy with auditory features.

Thus far, *LGI1* is the only epilepsy gene for an idiopathic form of epilepsy that does not belong to a family of voltage-gated or ligand-gated ion channels. The LGI1 protein harbors a repeat of 44 amino acid residues termed the epilepsy-associated repeat (EAR) domain that is common to another protein MASS1, which is mutated in one murine model of audiogenic epilepsy (Scheel et al., 2002).

X-Linked Infantile Spasms and Aristaless-Related Homeobox Gene Mutations

The syndrome of X-linked infantile spasms is characterized by the onset of spasms in boys between the ages of 2 to 6 months, and it is usually accompanied by hypsarrhythmic EEG and developmental arrest (Stromme et al., 1999). It has been identified only in families with more than one affected boy, so its real frequency is not yet known. It may partially account for the predominance of males in infantile spasms.

The initial mapping pointed to the Xp11.4-Xpter region, where mutations of the Aristaless-related homeobox gene (*ARX*) were subsequently found (Stromme et al., 2002). The mutations have included a recurrent expansion of polyalanine tracts and a truncation. The polyalanine expansions of ARX have also been found in unrelated X-linked neurologic disorders, including syndromic and nonspecific mental retardation and epilepsy and a form of dystonia. This phenotypic variability is difficult to explain. A severe loss of function of *ARX* has been associated with X-linked lissencephaly and ambiguous genitalia, a brain malformation syndrome that is also associated with infantile spasms (Kitamura et al., 2002). The knockout mouse model shows aberrant tangential migration and differentiation of GABAergic interneurons.

GENETICALLY DETERMINED SYMPTOMATIC EPILEPSIES AND CHROMOSOMAL ABNORMALITY SYNDROMES

About 237 single trait disorders and numerous chromosomal abnormalities have been associated with epilepsy (Online Mendelian Inheritance in Man, 2002). In only a few, is the association consistent and highly characteristic. In most cases, the epilepsy appears in a variable percentage of patients, suggesting that seizure susceptibility may be multifactorial or that it is not merely linked to the genetically determined structural or biochemical abnormalities. Because brain dysfunction in these disorders is almost always extensive and neuropathologic changes are complex, understanding which of these changes are more directly responsible for epileptogenesis is difficult. Table 20.1 shows a list of the main genetic disorders that are of special importance because of their high frequency or universal association with epilepsy. The progressive myoclonic epilepsies, developmental abnormalities of the cerebral cortex, tuberous sclerosis, and neurofibromatosis are covered elsewhere in this book (see Chapters 7 and 19). Other disorders such as Rett syndrome (Aicardi, 1998a) and the alpha-thalassemia mental retardation syndrome (Guerrini et al., 2000c), are not dealt with in detail because, in spite of their frequent association with epilepsy, they do not seem to feature specific electro-clinical features isolating them from the symptomatic epilepsies. In this section, only the chromosomal abnormality syndromes that are consistently associated with epilepsy are considered.

Virtually all of the known chromosomal abnormalities lead to anatomofunctional impairment of the central nervous system, and most are accompanied by mental retardation. However, although the risk of epilepsy is greater in patients with chromosomal disorders than it is in the general population (Holmes, 1987a), such genetic disorders do not represent a common cause of epilepsy *per se* (Jennings and Bird, 1981). The techniques of high-resolution chromosome banding, fluorescent in situ hybridization (FISH), and molecular genetics will certainly increase the number of cases that will be associated with small chromosomal rearrangements.

Chromosomal abnormality syndromes are not necessarily complicated by epilepsy. However, these syndromes do have a high probability of causing intractable seizures, leading to further severe disability in children who are already impaired. In a proportion of the cases, they show characteristic features that may lead to suspicion of a specific effect at certain loci (Singh et al., 2002).

Most chromosomal abnormality syndromes are duplication syndromes (duplication of a segment of chromosome), deletion syndromes (absence of a segment), and breakpoint disruption syndromes (only one or a few genes are disrupted) (Singh et al., 2002).

Trisomy 21 (Down Syndrome)

Down syndrome (DS) has an approximate incidence of 1 in 650 births (Smith and Berg, 1976). In 95% of patients, the cause is a nondisjunction of chromosome 21 during meiosis, while, in about 4%, an unbalanced translocation occurs. Approximately 1% of patients are mosaics, and these show a less severe phenotype. The region, which, if it is "triplicated," results in the typical phenotype, maps to 21q22.3 (Delabar et al., 1993). The risk of bearing a child with DS increases with increasing maternal age and very young maternal age (Jones, 1988).

Some neuropathologic features, such as the number of small granule cells (mainly GABAergic interneurons) and the tendency to develop the neuropathologic changes typical of Alzheimer disease in all individuals 35 years or older, probably are significant (Friede, 1989).

The incidence of epilepsy in children with DS has been estimated as 1.4% (Tatsuno et al., 1984). However, the overall prevalence of epilepsy increases with age, reaching 12% in patients older than 35 years (Veall, 1974). A biphasic distribution was observed by Pueschel et al. (1991), with 40% of patients having seizures since their first year of life and 40% experiencing their first seizure during their third decade. This trend may be related to early medical complications, such as hypoxic-ischemic encephalopathy and congenital heart disease (Stafstrom et al., 1991), and to the development of the neuropathologic changes typical of Alzheimer disease (Friede, 1989). In a large retrospective study (Stafstrom et al., 1991), 62% of patients with DS experiencing seizures had a specific etiology that, in most instances, was related to common medical complications, such as hypoxic-ischemic perinatal suffering, hypoxia from congenital heart disease, or infection. In that study, febrile seizures had a low frequency (0.9%) in comparison to that seen in the general population, as other investigators (Guerrini et al., 1993a, 1997d) have also noted. When only cases without known causes were considered, 2.5% of patients presented with seizures. GTC seizures predominated in the group with known etiology, as well as in that with unknown etiology. Myoclonic seizures and infantile spasms with hypsarrhythmia were also common, with the latter predominating in the idiopathic group. Partial seizures usually occurred in those patients with an identifiable etiology. The prognosis for recurrent seizures varied with the etiology. Those patients whose seizures were related to cardiovascular disease were usually well controlled with anticonvulsants. Neonates with hypoxic-ischemic injury had poor outcomes. Patients with idiopathic seizures generally had good outcomes. The authors concluded that children with DS have an increased susceptibility to seizures early in life and that superimposed systemic illness increased that risk.

In a review of studies in which population estimates were available, spasms occurred in 0.6% to 13% of children with DS, representing 4.5% to 47% of all seizures (Stafstrom and Konkol, 1994). Infantile spasms probably represent the most common seizure type in DS, and these appear without any evidence of additional brain damage in most children. The prognosis is usually good with regard to seizure control. Remission has been obtained using conventional antiepileptic drugs (AEDs), adrenocorticotropic hormone (ACTH), or steroids without relapse of seizures (Guerrini et al., 1997d) or with the later onset of age-related generalized seizure disorders that are amenable to pharmacologic control (Silva et al., 1996). Conversely, the spasms proved resistant in most of the patients who suffered hypoxic insults, subsequently progressing to other forms of intractable epilepsy (Stafstrom and Konkol, 1994; Guerrini et al., 1993a) (see Chapter 3).

The occurrence of reflex seizures in the context of startle epilepsy seems particularly common (Pueschel and Louis, 1993; Guerrini et al., 1990a; Sàenz-Lope et al., 1984; Gimenez-Roldan and Martin, 1980). The age at seizure onset is variable, and, usually, no evidence of etiologic factors other than DS is present. Most of the patients that have been described present with "pure" forms of reflex epilepsies, and almost all seizures are precipitated by acoustic or tactile stimuli. However, the epileptic syndrome varies in type and severity, with a predominance of Lennox-Gastaut syndrome (LGS)-type patterns.

LGS has been well documented in DS, but it does not appear common. Its *de novo* appearance at a mean age of 10 years without being preceded by other forms of epilepsy is quite characteristic (Guerrini et al., 1993a). In rare instances, LGS follows infantile spasms.

Angelman Syndrome

Angelman syndrome (AS) has a prevalence of about 1 in 12,000 to 1 in 20,000 in the general population (Steffenburg et al., 1996), accounting for up to 6% of all cases with severe mental retardation and epilepsy (Kyllerman, 1995). The main clinical features of AS may not be apparent early in life. All patients have developmental delay that becomes apparent by 6 to 12 months of age; microcephaly; severely impaired expressive language; ataxic gait; tremulousness of limbs;

and a typical behavioral profile, including a happy demeanor, hypermotoric behavior, and short attention span. About 90% have epilepsy (Viani et al., 1995; Zori et al., 1992; Angelman, 1965).

A deletion involving the maternally inherited chromosome 15q11-q13, which encompasses a cluster of GABA receptor subunit genes, is seen in 70% of patients; chromosome 15 paternal uniparental disomy (UPD) is seen in 5%; a mutation in the imprinting centre, a transcriptional regulatory element, occurs in 5%; intragenic mutations of the *UBE3A* gene are found in 10%. A few patients have no detectable genetic abnormality. The few cases of familial recurrence of AS show either imprinting center or *UBE3A* mutations (Guerrini et al., 2003).

Neuroimaging does not reveal conspicuous central nervous system anomalies, and only scant neuropathologic data are available. Small temporal and frontal lobes with disorganized and irregular gyri, irregular distribution of the neurons in layer 3, and minor heterotopia in both the cerebrum and the cerebellum have been observed in two patients (Kyriakides et al., 1992; Jay et al., 1991).

Viani et al. (1995) reviewed 155 cases in the literature; of these, 130 (84%) had experienced seizures. The first seizures occur between the ages of 3 months and 20 years (Guerrini et al., 1996b; Viani et al., 1995; Sugimoto et al., 1994; Matsumoto et al., 1992; Zori et al., 1992). The first seizures are often precipitated by fever (Sugimoto et al., 1994; Matsumoto et al., 1992). Cases of infantile spasms are very rare. Complex partial seizures with eye deviation and vomiting, possibly indicating an occipital lobe origin, have been estimated to occur frequently (Viani et al., 1995). Atypical absences, myoclonic seizures, GTC, and unilateral seizures are among the main ictal patterns (Guerrini, et al., 1996b; Viani et al., 1995; Sugimoto et al., 1994; Matsumoto et al., 1992). More than half the patients suffer from episodes of decreased alertness and hypotonia that can last days or weeks; these have been described as nonconvulsive status epilepticus (Sugimoto et al., 1994; Matsumoto et al., 1992). Often, concomitant mild jerking, which may or may not be rhythmic, is present (Dalla Bernardina et al., 1992d; Guerrini et al., 1996b), which is typical of myoclonic status. The polygraphic recordings reveal diffuse, slow irregular spike-wave complexes at about 2 Hz, that, in some patients, are accompanied by myoclonic potentials time-locked to the EEG spikes. This clinical and EEG pattern has also been termed myoclonic status in nonprogressive encephalopathies (Dalla Bernardina et al., 1992b). In other patients, the myoclonus may remain erratic, having no apparent relationship to EEG discharges. The myoclonic jerks typically cease during sleep (Guerrini et al., 1996b; Viani et al., 1995). Myoclonic status is rare after the age of 6 years. In addition to myoclonic seizures or status, patients with AS exhibit quasicontinuous, multifocal rhythmic cortical myoclonus at about 11 Hz that mainly involves the hands and face, producing a mild jerking or twitching that is easily mistaken for tremor (Guerrini et al., 1996b).

Individuals with chromosome 15q11-q13 deletions have a more severe clinical picture, and they are more prone to the development of severe epilepsy. Uniparental disomy is probably associated with a milder phenotype (Minassian et al., 1998a).

Although the seizures generally are difficult to treat in infancy and early childhood, they are usually less severe in later childhood (Zori et al., 1992), although complete seizure remission is rare (Laan et al., 1997). The exact percentage of patients who continue to suffer seizures as adults is unknown.

Episodes of myoclonic status or of nonconvulsive status can usually be stopped by the intravenous injection of benzodiazepines (Guerrini et al., 1996b; Viani et al., 1995), although they frequently relapse (Matsumoto et al., 1992). Chronic treatment with benzodiazepines is fairly effective for controlling myoclonus. Particularly effective is the combination of clobazam and valproic acid (VPA) for the long-term treatment of epilepsy (Viani et al., 1995; Guerrini et al., 1996b). VPA and ethosuximide (ESM) used together are also effective in patients presenting with recurrent myoclonic status (Dalla Bernardina et al., 1992b). Myoclonus and absence seizures may worsen with treatment with carbamazepine or vigabatrin (Kuenzle et al., 1998; Viani et al., 1995). In those patients in whom cortical myoclonus is particularly disabling, it may be treated with generous doses of piracetam with good results (Guerrini et al., 1996a).

About 80% of cases of AS are identified through the methylation test, which allows the detection of the deletion, UPD, and IC mutations. Mutation analysis of the *UBE3A* gene should be performed when the methylation test result is negative.

Syndrome of Inverted Duplication of Pericentromeric Chromosome 15

The inverted duplication of pericentromeric chromosome 15 (inv-dup 15) is the most common of the so-called ESACs (extra structurally abnormal chromosomes) syndromes, accounting for about 50% of supernumerary marker chromosomes (Hook and Cross, 1987). The origin of the duplicated chromosome 15 is

maternal in all cases (Robinson et al., 1993). The severity of the clinical picture varies according to the presence of a 15p or 15q tetrasomy (Torrisi et al., 2001). Patients with large inv-dup(15) extending to q15, which contains the Prader-Willi and/or AS region, usually have severe epilepsy, mental retardation, autistic-like behavior, and minor dysmorphic features (Borgatti et al., 2001; Takeda et al., 2000; Cabrera et al., 1998; Battaglia et al., 1997). A clinical presentation as infantile spasms in children with minor dysmorphic features has been reported in some patients, whereas LGS with an extremely poor outcome has been observed by several authors (Torrisi et al., 2001; Takeda et al., 2000; Cabrera et al., 1998; Battaglia et al., 1997). Focal epilepsy has also been reported (Borgatti et al., 2001).

Milder presentations with mild mental retardation, generalized epilepsy with an onset in adolescence of absence seizures, and an interictal pattern of generalized spike-wave discharges have been reported even in patients with large duplications (Chifari et al., 2002). Various genetic mechanisms beyond the size of chromosomal duplication have been hypothesized to explain the clinical heterogeneity, including a dosage effect of genes located within the duplication (Chifari et al., 2002; Torrisi et al., 2001). Because a mild epilepsy phenotype is possible, the need to rule out inv-dup(15) as a possible, though rare, cause of "cryptogenic" or seemingly idiopathic generalized epilepsy has been suggested (Chifari et al., 2002). The derivation of a marker chromosome is easily determined by FISH analysis.

Fragile X Syndrome

Both sexes may be affected, but the phenotype is notably more severe in males. One in 1,000 females are estimated to be carriers (Blomquist et al., 1983). The chromosome analysis shows a "fragile" site at Xq27.3 when cells are grown in a folic-deprived medium. The condition results from a dynamic mutation in heritable unstable DNA (Richards and Sutherland, 1992), due to variation in the copy number of a trinucleotide repeat p(CGG)n within the *FMR1* gene. This fragile site is termed FRAXA. Transmission through families is consistent with an X-linked, semidominant condition.

The prevalence of epileptic seizures is thought to be about 25% in affected individuals (Wisniewski et al., 1991). According to Wisniewski et al. (1991), the seizures usually appear before the age of 15 years, and they tend to disappear during the second decade of life. The epilepsy is usually not severe. In most patients, the seizures are fairly rare, or they are controlled with simple drug regimens (Guerrini et al., 1992a, 1993a; Musumeci et al., 1991; Wisniewski et al., 1991). Severe childhood epilepsy syndromes are extremely rare.

The most frequently mentioned seizure types are GTC (Finelli et al., 1985). In one series, most patients experienced their first seizure between ages 2 and 12 years (Guerrini et al., 1993a). The main seizure types were GTC, complex partial, or focal motor seizures. The background EEG activity is slow (Musumeci et al., 1991; Wisniewski et al., 1991). An EEG pattern of midtemporal spikes that is possibly age related and is similar to the waveform of benign rolandic epilepsy has been described in affected males, with or without seizures (Musumeci et al., 1991). This EEG pattern has been confirmed in various series, although only in a minority of patients (Guerrini et al., 1993a; Wisniewski et al., 1991). The variety in seizure types in the fragile X syndrome may reflect the extreme clinical polymorphism resulting from the variability of amplification of the trinucleotide repeat among patients (Fu et al., 1991).

Most fragile X males show their fragile site in 5% to 50% of their lymphocytes. Normal transmitting males usually do not express the fragile site. Similarly, while fragile X females with mental impairment do express their fragile site, female carriers do not express the fragile site. Normal chromosomes contain 6 to 52 copies of the p(CGG)n repeat in the *FMR1* gene, whereas males with more than 200 copies are affected (full mutation). Normal transmitting males have 50 to 200 copies (premutation). Females bearing the premutation are normal, and they do not express the fragile site. These premutations tend to expand when they are transmitted to offspring through female carriers. The premutation and the full mutation can be detected by Southern blot analysis. A few patients with fragile X harboring deletions in *FMR1* have also been described (Quan et al., 1995).

Partial Monosomy 4p (4p− or Wolf-Hirschhorn Syndrome)

About 85% of 4p− cases are sporadic events, and the remaining 15% result from translocations (Stengel-Rutkowski et al., 1984). The deletion of band 4p16 appears to be necessary for the full expression of the phenotype. The main clinical features include low birth weight, severe mental retardation, congenital heart defects, microcephaly, hypertelorism, downward slanting of the eyes, epicanthus, preauricular dimples, a carplike mouth, cleft lip and/or palate, a weak cry, and a midline scalp defect. In at least one-third of patients, death occurs during the first year of life be-

cause of the severe systemic malformations, cardiac failure, or pulmonary infection. Main structural brain abnormalities include micrencephaly, an abnormal gyral pattern, gray matter heterotopia, and dysplasia of the nuclear structures (Gottfried et al., 1981).

Between 70% and 100% of patients with 4p− syndrome have epilepsy (Battaglia et al., 1999; Guerrini et al., 1997d). Seizure onset usually occurs within the first year of life, between 6 and 12 months of age in most patients. Partial motor or unilateral seizures or status, myoclonic status, and GTC seizures are the most commonly reported types of attacks (Battaglia et al., 1999; Sgrò et al., 1995). A characteristic electroclinical pattern is observed in most patients who, after the onset of focal motor or GTC seizures in the first year of life, develop frequent episodes of atypical absences that are triggered by eye closure and are accompanied by mild myoclonus (Sgrò et al., 1995). These episodes are accompanied by generalized atypical slow spike-wave complexes, although the interictal EEG shows multifocal or diffuse discharges predominating over the centroparietal and occipital regions. Although little information about treatment is available, in the authors' experience, the seizures observed in 4p− syndrome can be effectively controlled by VPA, either alone or in combination with ESM. Carbamazepine administration, on the other hand, may cause worsening of seizures. In spite of the early severity of the epilepsy, its long-term outcome seems good; in the series of Battaglia et al. (1999), seizures were reported to disappear with age.

Molecular studies have assigned the critical region to be within 4p16.3 (Anvret et al., 1991). Genes encoding for a cluster of $GABA_A$ subunit receptors are located on chromosome 4p13-4q11, and the α_2 and β_1 genes are included in the critical region. A reduction of the gene product could, therefore, contribute to the high epileptogenicity of this syndrome, similar to the observations in patients with AS who carry a chromosome 15q11-q13 deletion.

Standard chromosome analysis detects deletions involving the 4p16.3 band, the haploinsufficiency of which has been reported in all individuals with the syndrome. However, FISH studies may be necessary to detect submicroscopic deletions or cryptic translocations (Battaglia et al., 1999).

Ring Chromosome 20

Ring chromosome 20 (r20) is a rare chromosomal disorder that has been increasingly recognized because of its strong association with epilepsy, which occurs in all cases with specific characteristics. In most cases, the locus of fusion between the deleted short and long arm of the ring chromosome is p13q13 or p13q13.3 or p13q13.33 (Singh et al., 2002). Although some patients may have microcephaly, mild to moderate mental retardation, and behavioral abnormalities (Porfirio et al., 1987), the lack of specific phenotypic features in most individuals makes diagnosing the disorder difficult.

Several reports have emphasized the peculiarities of epilepsy in patients with r20. Seizure onset occurs between infancy and age 14 years (Singh et al., 2002). The typical presentation is with repetitive episodes of a confusional state that last from several minutes to 30 minutes, which have also been described as *complex partial status* or *nonconvulsive status*, during which patients appear confused and unresponsive to a variable degree. Motionlessness, staring, complex automatisms, or wandering has been described (Singh et al., 2002; Inoue et al., 1997). Perioral jerking and eyelid myoclonus appear during such episodes in some patients (Petit et al., 1999; Inoue et al., 1997). The attacks are almost always drug resistant, and they often occur daily (Singh et al., 2002; Lancman et al., 1993). Hyperventilation, specific mental activities, or adverse psychologic situations play a triggering role in some children (Roubertie et al., 2000). The description of more than 30 cases of r20 associated with epilepsy has progressively clarified the uniqueness of the electroclinical presentation of the syndrome (Singh et al., 2002). However, such prolonged seizures still have a high risk of being misinterpreted as behavioral nonepileptic manifestations if video-EEG diagnostic support is not available, especially in small children (Inoue et al., 1997). Partial motor seizures, complex partial seizures, and GTC seizures have also been reported.

The interictal EEG has been described as normal in some patients, but it often shows interictal spikes over the frontotemporal regions. Ictal EEG during nonconvulsive status shows long bursts or trains of rhythmic theta waves and high-amplitude, 2-Hz to 3-Hz, rhythmic notched slow waves with frontal predominance (Petit et al., 1999; Canevini et al., 1998; Inoue et al., 1997). Typical spike-wave discharges are rarely seen. Frontal lobe ictal onset was recorded in one patient with subdural electrodes during typical confusional episodes (Inoue et al., 1997). The prominent role of subcortical structures in the genesis of the typical ictal pattern has been hypothesized on the basis of ictal single photon emission computed tomography studies (Biraben et al., 2001a). The electroclinical picture of r20 is highly characteristic, and every child presenting with similar clinical and EEG features should have a karyotype study conducted.

The loss of telomeric material on both arms of chromosome 20 can usually be identified by molecular cytogenetic techniques (Brandt et al., 1993). The chromosomal abnormality can occur in a mosaic fashion. Most cases are sporadic, but a few familial cases have been reported (Canevini et al., 1998). Although the severity of mental impairment seems to correlate with the percentage of mosaicism, that of the epilepsy does not (Inoue et al., 1997). In the presence of clinical and EEG manifestations that are highly characteristic of r20, some have suggested that at least 100 mitoses should be examined because the percentage of lymphocytes carrying the chromosomal abnormality may be low (Roubertie et al., 2000).

Ring Chromosome 14

Ring chromosome 14 (r14) is a rare chromosomal abnormality that has consistently been associated with seizures. Reviews of reported cases have suggested that early onset epilepsy that is often intractable is a constant feature of the syndrome but that it does not have typical clinical or EEG features (Singh et al., 2002). GTC seizures, myoclonic seizures, and complex partial seizures have been reported in these patients (Lippe and Sparkes, 1981; Schmidt et al., 1981).

The general clinical features include moderate to severe mental retardation, microcephaly, and facial dysmorphism, with a narrow, elongated face and retrognathia (Rethore et al., 1984). Ocular abnormalities, including cataracts and retinal pigmentation, have been observed in about 50% of patients (Zelante et al., 1991). Most patients show a mosaic chromosomal abnormality. Familial occurrence is possible (Matalon et al., 1990). No indication exists regarding the brain histopathology that underlies such a severe neurologic presentation, and neuroimaging seems to be of little help (Ono et al., 1999).

Klinefelter syndrome (XXY Syndrome)

The prevalence of seizures in Klinefelter syndrome (KS) ranges from 2% to 10% in major series (Guerrini et al., 1997d). In four patients with KS with seizures reported by Elia et al. (1995), the early onset of febrile seizures or other variable seizure types has been observed, consistently with presentations of low severity. Some patients with generalized epilepsy with absence or GTC seizures, as well as 3-Hz spike-wave EEG pattern, have been reported (Genton et al., 1992; Bolthauser et al., 1978). However, most patients have partial epilepsy that usually responds to AEDs (Guerrini et al., 1997d).

Trisomy 12p

Trisomy of the short arm of chromosome 12 can be caused either by a malsegregation of a balanced parental chromosomal rearrangement or by *de novo* occurrence (Allen et al., 1996).

Trisomy 12p is characterized clinically by severe mental retardation, early hypotonia, turricephaly, flat occiput, short neck, round facies with prominent cheeks, prominent forehead, hypertelorism, epicanthal folds, and other dysmorphic facial features. In addition, lateralized microgyria, internal hydrocephalus, cortical dysplasia, and ectopic glial tissue in the leptomeninges were reported by Nielsen et al. (1977).

Most seizure patterns reported are generalized convulsive, whether febrile or not, or myoclonic. Particularly striking was the finding of generalized 3-Hz spike-wave discharges in four patients, three of whom had childhood-onset myoclonic absences or myoclonic seizures that appeared well controlled by AEDs (Elia et al., 1995; Guerrini et al., 1990a).

SUMMARY

Considerable evidence indicates that genetic factors can strongly influence epileptogenesis. Because "epilepsy" is not truly a disease but rather a symptom of multiple heterogeneous diseases, various categories are also expected from a genetic viewpoint. Separating epilepsies caused by brain abnormalities or damage (symptomatic epilepsies) from idiopathic epilepsy not associated with an obvious brain lesion is usual.

The symptomatic epilepsies, in turn, may be due to both acquired factors and congenital conditions or to either alone; these congenital conditions may be genetically determined or they may result from prenatal insults. Acquired factors are often prominent, but this does not exclude a genetic influence. When they are due primarily to genetic factors, the symptomatic epilepsies may not only be the expression of mendelian disorders that are associated with epilepsy, but they may also feature other neurologic abnormalities or, more often, they may have a multifactorial inheritance in which both genetic and environmental influences are operative. Only some such disorders are consistently associated with epilepsy and show characteristic electroclinical features.

Epilepsies that are isolated or that clearly are the prominent feature can also be due to acquired factors, which are often difficult to determine, or they can be predominantly the result of genetic factors. The genetic influences on epilepsy are best, but not exclusively, observed in the idiopathic epilepsies in which specific genetic factors have, however, not been identified in the large majority of patients. The relationship of the phenotype with the genotype is not straightforward. Both locus (genic) heterogeneity (i.e., several genes producing the same clinical picture) and allelic heterogeneity (i.e., several mutations at the same locus with different clinical syndromes) are common. In addition, modifying genes and other complex mechanisms may further compound the issue. Genetic heterogeneity and gene–environment interactions appear to operate in many circumstances, making research of the specific epilepsy genes a difficult task.

The recent identification of mutations of specific genes in families with different mendelian epilepsy syndromes (monogenic epilepsies) is of great theoretical interest, but these represent only a very small proportion of the epilepsies and they are not of great practical help for the determination of the prognosis or for genetic counseling, except in rare families. On the other hand, the monogenic epilepsies have shed light on some aspects that may explain how genes may influence epileptogenesis and that may, in the future, be applicable to the study of the multifactorially inherited epilepsies, which form the bulk of cases. They have also increased the awareness of the extent of genetic and phenotypic heterogeneity.

Chromosomal abnormality syndromes are an important cause of epilepsies that virtually always occur in association with other neurologic and/or mental anomalies. Only some such syndromes are consistently associated with epilepsy, and, in some of them, epilepsy may be the presenting symptom. Careful chromosomal studies should be performed systematically when "cryptogenic" epilepsies are being investigated.

Despite these recent progresses in the genetics of epilepsy, the determination of the prognosis and especially of the need for genetic counseling, is still essentially based on the collection of statistical data from clinical studies. The results are clearly quite imprecise, especially because most studies have not considered the clinical heterogeneity of the epilepsies. Only recently have attempts been made to determine the outcome and genetic risks according to epilepsy syndromes, which should increase the predictive power. However, a number of uncontrolled factors, such as the variable expression in families, the possible genetic heterogeneity, and the variations in severity, render prediction hazardous.

Clearly, only the delineation of epileptic *entities* rather than *syndromes* with progress in the understanding of the mechanisms of multifactorial inheritance will permit a better approach to the problems raised by the epilepsies.

Diagnosis and Differential Diagnosis

POSITIVE DIAGNOSIS

History Taking

"Careful and detailed history taking remains the cornerstone of accurate diagnosis" (O'Donohoe, 1985). History taking should be performed in a methodical and comprehensive manner, but flexibility in practical modalities is an absolute requirement when the clinician is dealing with children. The questions asked should be adapted to each individual, and the doctor should take advantage of the opportunities that arise in conversation rather than following a preestablished order. All relevant points should be covered by the end of the session.

In children, the history is usually obtained from the parents, but data from patients, even when they are young, may be useful because subjective feelings during seizures may be of great importance. Data from other witnesses has to be integrated as well; professional witnesses, such as doctors and nurses, are sometimes less valuable than lay persons because of their preconceived ideas about what a seizure should be like. The history taking may require more than one session because new memories and questions may arise after the first questioning. Care should be taken not to accept previous accounts, even those from professionals, without a critical examination of them, and the clinician must attempt to verify and critically consider all witness accounts (Stephenson, 1990).

Now, a home videotape of the episodes may be available, and such a resource is invaluable. The parents should be encouraged to attempt to obtain one; however, many important points cannot be decided on this basis alone because of the inherent problems with home videotaping, including angles and obstructing persons, and because consciousness cannot be assessed. Careful history taking, therefore, remains essential. As Jeavons (1983b) noted, "the diagnosis is as good as the history."

The questioning should seek a history of both the complaint (seizures) and the person. The circumstances surrounding the occurrence of the attacks and the possible precipitating factors are of great importance. Seizures regularly precipitated by stimuli such as pain and emotion strongly suggest nonepileptic

phenomena. A full description of the seizures, including aura, reconstitution of the whole ictal sequence, and postictal phenomena, is essential. The physician must adapt his or her language to the cultural level of the parents, and he or she should also ask the parents to act out or mimic the attacks (sometimes, he or she can help them by demonstrating the types of movements for which he or she is searching), which may be of considerable benefit.

The manner of asking questions is essential. The questions should be precise without leading the parents, and providing the parents with multiple terms from which they can select those that seem applicable to the description of their child's seizures can often be useful. Beginning with descriptions of the last attack and the worst attack is often important (Aicardi and Taylor, 1998).

Questions regarding the person with seizures should include his or her developmental history, a detailed drug history, a determination of the impact of seizures on the life of the child and the family, and their level of understanding of the disease.

Neurologic and General Examination

Overview

A *complete neurologic and general examination* is mandatory. It should especially involve the skin, on which stigmata such as achromic spots, hemangiomas, or other abnormalities may be essential diagnostic clues; the eyes; and anthropometric data, particularly head circumference. Neurologic signs, principally those of cerebral palsy, are important for the diagnosis and prognosis. A rapid assessment of the patient's competence both cognitively and socially is also essential.

Electroencephalography

Electroencephalographic (EEG) data are important for confirming the epileptic nature of seizures and, if possible, for making a precise diagnosis of epilepsy syndrome. Some patterns, such as the foci of delta waves suggestive of a structural lesion or the bilateral spike-waves suggestive of idiopathic origin, may help in the search for a cause. However, one must remember that epilepsy is a clinical disorder, so its diagnosis does not depend primarily on EEG findings, no matter how important they may be.

In most cases, simple, "standard" EEG recordings are sufficient. The current techniques of digital recording allow reformatting, as well as having other practical advantages. In children, all tracings should include sleep, even though, in most cases, the recording of sleep onset and the first phases of sleep may be sufficient. Other routine facilitating maneuvers include intermittent photic stimulation (IPS) (Kasteleijn-Nolst Trenité et al., 1987, 1999; Harding and Jeavons, 1994; Wilkins and Lindsay, 1985) and hyperventilation (Blume, 1982). Sleep and the use of routine stimulants increase the positivity rate of routine EEG from 60% to roughly 90% (Mizrahi, 1984; Gastaut and Broughton, 1972).

Both hyperventilation and photic stimulation are effective mostly in generalized epilepsies and in approximately one-third of focal epilepsies. However, hyperventilation should be avoided in patients with sickle cell disease, moyamoya disease, and strokes because of the increased risk of aggravating brain hypoxia (Lin et al., 2000; Allen et al., 1976). More sophisticated techniques, such as polygraphy with simultaneous recording of the electromyography, an electrocardiogram (ECG), a respirogram, and an electrooculogram, can provide valuable data in selected patients, especially for precisely classifying seizures or for their differential diagnosis.

Additional nonconventional electrodes (nasoethmoidal, pharyngeal, and sphenoidal) are widely used in some centers for the presurgical investigation of patients with complex partial seizures (Oxbury et al., 2000; Lüders et al., 1989b; Wieser and Elger, 1987), but they are used less often in children (Alvarez et al., 1983). Closely spaced additional electrodes may also be useful for better localizing and defining the electrical field of transients (Blume, 1982).

The correct recognition of epileptiform transients is a crucial prerequisite for an EEG-established diagnosis. A number of EEG graphical elements may resemble these more or less closely. Epileptiform transients include the so-called psychomotor variant pattern, six-per-second spike-waves and 14-6 positive spikes, wicket spikes, and small sharp waves (Blume, 1982). Hypnagogic bursts (Alvarez et al., 1983) are probably the most commonly misdiagnosed EEG pattern in children younger than 5 years, in whom they are often interpreted as bursts of spike-waves.

In about 10% of patients with epilepsy, EEG with routine stimulations and short sleep recording is negative. The sensitivity can be increased by long-duration (24 to 48 hours) recording (particularly overnight or nap records) and sleep deprivation (Dalla Bernardina et al., 1985b; Degen and Degen, 1984).

Long-duration records can be obtained at home with the use of EEG cassettes (Ebersole, 1998; Crandall et al., 1983; Ebersole and Leroy, 1983) or telemetry, or they may be conducted in the laboratory. Invasive EEG techniques are not considered in this text. Video-EEG recording has become an essential tool because it allows the clinician to review clinical phenomena that are often difficult to analyze because of their brevity, as well as to correlate them with the simultaneous EEG study. This method is routinely used in presurgical evaluation. However, no interaction with unattended patients is possible, and, even if the EEG correlates permit the clinician to assign significance to relatively trivial events, the limitations mentioned for videotapes apply to video-EEG as well.

The specificity of interictal EEG is relatively low, especially when stimulations are used. IPS gives a positive result in the form of photoparoxysmal reaction in 5% to 8% of children (Eeg-Olofsson et al., 1971), and sleep may also decrease the specificity and induce graphical elements that can simulate epileptic paroxysms in the absence of epilepsy, making the interpretation of sleep figures and their differentiation from true paroxysms more difficult.

Various types of EEG epileptiform paroxysms can be observed in the interictal EEGs of 5% to 8% of nonepileptic children when an adequate sleep record is obtained. These paroxysmal abnormalities can include generalized spike-wave discharges (9% in the series by Eeg-Olofsson et al. [1971]) and focal spikes or sharp waves that closely resemble those in children with rolandic epilepsy. Cavazzuti et al. (1980) found such spikes in 2.4% of school children from 6 to 14 years of age in Modena, Italy. Eeg-Olofsson et al. (1971) found spike foci in 1.9% of a sample of well children in Stockholm, Sweden. At follow-up, only a small proportion of those children in whom the EEG paroxysms were discovered but who had no clinical history of seizures later developed epilepsy (Cavazzuti et al., 1980). Such abnormalities may be a marker of a genetic susceptibility to seizures. Thus, "characteristic" EEG paroxysms are several times more common than *all forms* of epilepsy. The coincidence of finding such common EEG abnormalities with equally common clinical paroxysmal events, such as syncope, breath-holding spells (BHSs), or migraine, is, on a purely statistical basis, not unexpected. This precludes making a diagnosis of epilepsy based solely on the EEG in the absence of convincing clinical manifestations (see "Differential Diagnosis"). Conversely, a normal interictal EEG does not exclude the diagnosis of epilepsy, when the clinical history is convincing.

The ictal EEG is obviously much more specific. It is pathognomonic when it is associated with the clinical phenomena. In a few cases, however, paroxysmal discharges closely resembling those of seizures may be recorded (e.g., patients who have experienced severe head trauma) (Courjon and Mauguière, 1982). Less rarely, the ictal discharges may be atypical, thus making them difficult to interpret. This may be the case for ictal flattening or for low-amplitude rapid rhythms, which may easily escape recognition.

Finally, genuine epileptic seizures can occur without EEG paroxysms being detectable on the scalp records. This may occur, for example, in cases of frontal epilepsy (Picard et al., 2000; Oldani et al., 1998; Scheffer et al., 1995a) or in other focal seizures originating in parts of the brain that are remote from the electrodes or that are deeply located (Blume, 1982). Therefore, even a negative ictal EEG does not absolutely rule out epilepsy, although it should certainly lead to the consideration of other possibilities.

The occurrence of *abnormal EEG discharges* in the absence of simultaneous clinical seizures raises a delicate issue. Some of these discharges have been associated with detectable disturbances of cognition or behavior or both (Massa et al., 2001; Binnie, 1990; Kasteleijn-Nolst Trenité et al., 1988, 1990; Binnie et al., 1981, 1987). Precise neuropsychologic testing has demonstrated disruptions of attention, especially with discharges of generalized spike-waves, and memory or of other cognitive functions with focal spikes that are closely correlated with the EEG paroxysms. Such phenomena, which are termed *transient cognitive impairments*, could be regarded as minimal electroclinical seizures. However, the practical significance of this phenomenon must still be fully assessed, although, in some cases, it has been demonstrated to interfere with the patient's activities (Aarts et al., 1984).

A similar problem can be raised by the association of intense and continuous (or almost continuous) paroxysmal EEG activity with lasting cognitive or behavioral dysfunction or deterioration even in the absence of seizures. Some investigators have proposed that this type of deterioration may be regarded as a form of prolonged "seizure" or status and that it may be the direct consequence of the epileptic disturbance that is expressed by the EEG abnormalities (Deonna, 1996). Examples include continuous spike-waves of

slow sleep (or electrical status epilepticus of slow sleep) and Landau-Kleffner syndrome (Beaumanoir, 1992). Hypsarrhythmia and intense spike-wave activity in Lennox-Gastaut syndrome have been similarly interpreted by many investigators (see Chapter 3).

A close relationship between cognitive disturbances and EEG discharges is suggested by the coinciding times of occurrence of both phenomena, the possible parallels between the intensity of EEG and clinical anomalies, and the observation that the clinical anomalies do not seem to disappear as long as the EEG paroxysms have not cleared (Aicardi, 1999a; Engel and Pedley, 1998; Deonna, 1996; Morrell et al., 1995). Deonna (1996) suggested using the term *cognitive epilepsy* to describe such occurrences. The significance of these is of practical importance because efforts at controlling the EEG activity might also check the neuropsychologic disturbances, even though this has not been demonstrated. This dilemma is further discussed in Chapters 3, 4, and 11.

Other Laboratory Tests

Other laboratory tests play only a minor role in the diagnosis of seizures and epilepsy. Prolactin is released following generalized (Fisher et al., 1991) and some focal (Bilo et al., 1988; Molaie et al., 1988; Sperling et al., 1986b) seizures, but this does not occur with pseudoseizures. Thus, determining the level of serum prolactin within an hour of a seizure can help establish its true nature. However, hypoxic attacks can also result in prolactin release, so the practical value of the test is limited. An increase in creatine kinase levels is seen after generalized seizures only, and it is related to muscle activity.

DIFFERENTIAL DIAGNOSIS

Definition of Epilepsy and Diagnosis Issues

This section is concerned with differentiating epileptic seizures and epilepsy from other nonepileptic, paroxysmal clinical events. Epilepsy is characterized by the repetition of unprovoked seizures, so, even though the diagnosis of an epileptic seizure does not establish that of epilepsy, it is crucially important. A diagnosis of epilepsy requires that the repeated seizures are unprovoked (Engel and Pedley, 2001). A commonly used definition of *repetition* is the occurrence of two or more events that are not part of the same episode. This epidemiologic definition is of relatively little help in clinical practice. The notion of chronicity that is associated with epilepsy implies a "sufficient" duration, which clearly is arbitrary. Conversely, some single clinical episodes occurring in association with characteristic EEG patterns (e.g., in rolandic epilepsy) may well be considered to fulfill, for all practical purposes, the major criteria for epilepsy if not for treatment.

The requirement of unprovoked seizures also is in need of more precision. Some triggers, such as photic stimulation, and a vast number of precipitating factors, such as reading or cognitive or language activities, are conventionally included in the group of the so-called *reflex epilepsies*, whereas others, such as fever, are not, even though they demonstrate the individual's special sensitivity to seizures.

The differential diagnosis of epilepsy is of utmost importance because of its personal and social consequences for the affected individual, so it must be made only on solid evidence. The differential diagnosis of individual epilepsy syndromes is briefly considered in the preceding chapters. The present discussion is limited to considerations relevant to the diagnosis of epilepsy in general.

Epilepsy is, unfortunately, grossly overdiagnosed. Jeavons (1983b) found that 20% to 25% of patients referred to his epilepsy clinic did not have epileptic seizures. Likewise, Metrick et al. (1991) reported that 10% to 20% of children who had been referred with a diagnosis of refractory epilepsy actually had nonepileptic attacks. Because an incorrect label of epilepsy can have profound and regrettable consequences on a child's schooling, social life, and employment, such misdiagnoses must be avoided.

Jeavons (1983b) listed the most common misdiagnoses in 200 patients. Syncopes accounted for 44% of errors, psychiatric disturbances for 20%, BHSs for 11%, migraine and night terrors for 6% each, and miscellaneous conditions for 11%. The main reasons for misdiagnosis were an inadequate history, the presence of a family history of epilepsy or a history of febrile seizures, an "abnormal EEG," and misinterpretation of clonic movements or incontinence as being inherently epileptic. Jeavons (1983b) also stressed the obvious but often overlooked fact that nonepileptic seizures may occur in epileptic patients who are being treated and, therefore, that any seizure in a "known epileptic" should not necessarily be interpreted as a recurrence. In a series composed entirely of children, Robinson (1984) found that the diagnosis of epilepsy was doubtful in 94 of 201 patients referred to his outpatient clinic with a possible diagnosis of epilepsy, and 75 children were proved to have some other kind of episodic attack. The most com-

mon nonepileptic paroxysmal disorders in his series were BHSs, fainting, migraine, and dizziness or vertigo. Metrick et al. (1991) found that the most common cause of a misdiagnosis of epilepsy in children was an unusual reaction to stimuli that included an arrest of ongoing activity, stereotypic behavior, and/or abnormal movements. The main types of nonepileptic attacks are considered in "Main Differential Diagnoses" below (Pranzatelli and Pedley, 1991; Stephenson, 1990; Aicardi, 1988c).

Underdiagnosis of epilepsy is much less common. However, the wrong diagnosis of nonepileptic seizures can be made in those patients who have atypical manifestations that are wrongly thought to be of psychogenic origin, who exhibit some abnormal paroxysmal movements, or who, as in cases of familial frontal epilepsy, present with nocturnal seizures that, not infrequently, are interpreted to be parasomnias (Oldani et al., 1998). In a few cases, the possible diagnosis of epilepsy may not be considered in patients presenting with mainly cognitive or behavioral symptoms; however, a sleep EEG may reveal intense paroxysmal activity. Some of these have rare, subtle seizures, and others may not have any seizures at all. The term *cognitive epilepsy* has been proposed for such cases (Deonna, 1996), emphasizing the notion that cognitive and/or behavioral manifestations can be regarded to be the direct consequence of the epileptic activity and that they represent an equivalent to seizures. Even though some uncertainty still exists about the exact significance of such cases because both EEG changes and clinical manifestations may also be regarded as being due to the same basic dysfunction that is as yet undetermined (Holmes et al., 1981), the recognition of these EEG abnormalities is of definite diagnostic and possibly therapeutic value.

Some abnormal paroxysmal motor events may not be recognized as epileptic because of their unusual characteristics. This may be true for some patients with seizures in the supplementary motor area (Kaplan, 1975), in whom these may be regarded as psychogenic pseudoseizures (Kawazawa et al., 1985), and for some with nocturnal familial frontal epilepsy, which is often misdiagnosed as parasomnias or behavior disorders (Oldani et al., 1996, 1998).

Main Differential Diagnoses

Anoxic Seizures

Although the use of the term *anoxic seizures* is not correct because some degree of oxygenation does persist, it is commonly used and thus is employed here. Anoxic seizures comprise a heterogeneous group of paroxysmal events that include a loss or attenuation of consciousness and variable other sensorimotor phenomena. Cortical anoxia that is sufficient to provoke syncope may occur under a number of the following circumstances: bradycardia with a heart rate of less than 40 beats per minute or tachycardia with more than 150 beats per minute, asystole of more than 4 seconds, systolic pressure of less than 50 mm Hg, or a jugular venous O_2 concentration of less than 20 mm Hg. Obstructive apnea may occasionally be seen in children with a palatal malformation (Fig. 21.1).

Severe decorticate rigidity, when it ensues, is caused by the loss of corticoreticular inhibition of certain brainstem structures involved in the control of muscle tone (Gastaut, 1974). On the EEG, increasing degrees of cortical anoxia produce slowing of the frequency of the dominant cortical rhythms. If the decorticate state is reached (convulsive syncope), complete electrical silence with an isoelectric recording occurs. Convulsive syncope seems to be more common than generally assumed; it has been observed in 42% of prospectively studied blood donors who fainted (Lin et al., 1982) and in an even higher proportion of young adults who fainted as a result of the Valsalva maneuver (Schmidt and Lampert, 1990). With the resumption of sufficient blood flow, the slow waves reappear; they may be synchronous with a few jerks of the limbs (Gastaut, 1974; Lombroso and Lerman, 1967) (Fig. 21.2). Normal rhythms return rapidly, and very little postictal abnormality is observed.

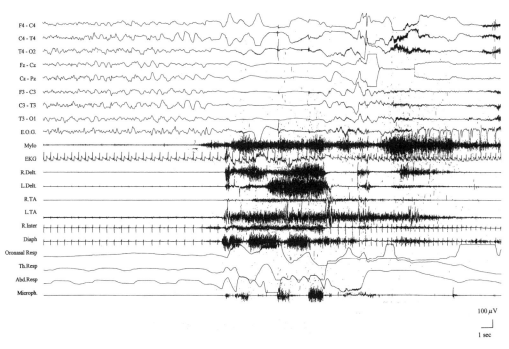

FIG. 21.1. An 8-year-old boy with pachygyria and repeated short convulsive episodes upon falling asleep that were mistakenly interpreted as serial tonic seizures. Video-electroencephalographic (EEG) and polygraphic recording and measure of O_2 and CO_2 saturation showed the following sequence. Mechanic obstruction of the soft palate causes an obstructive apnea (oronasal respiratory activity is not visible, but thoracic and abdominal respiratory acts are visible), with severe oxygen desaturation, progressive slowing of background EEG activity, and complete flattening lasting about 12 seconds that is accompanied by a tonic contraction (convulsive syncope). Some violent respiratory acts interrupt the apnea and ensure recovery of oxygen saturation with cessation of tonic muscular activity while the EEG shows slow-wave activity, followed by the recovery of background EEG rhythms. Treatment with a positive airway pressure device was accompanied by the disappearance of such episodes.

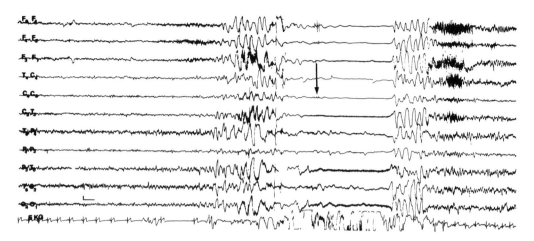

FIG. 21.2. Convulsive syncopal attack. Marked slowing of electrocardiogram, probably followed by cardiac arrest (*artifacts*), is accompanied first by slowing of electroencephalographic (EEG) background rhythm, then by a burst of high-voltage slow waves, and eventually by flattening of the EEG. The resumption of cardiac beats is accompanied by a second burst of slow waves, followed by the progressive return of a normal EEG. Extensor rigidity and opisthotonus appeared at the end of the first burst of slow wave (*arrow*). Calibration: 1 second, 50 µV.

Reflex Anoxic Seizures and Breath-Holding Spells

Reflex anoxic seizures (RASs) and BHSs are probably pathophysiologically distinct phenomena. RASs are usually the result of a temporary asystole that is of reflex origin, and BHSs feature cyanosis and grunting that suggest the presence of expiratory apnea with intrapulmonary blood shunting and a mismatch of ventilation and perfusion (Stephenson, 1990; Southall et al., 1985). The clinical differences between them can, however, be minimal if they even exist. RASs and BHSs may often coexist in the same child, with differing mechanisms for different episodes; there is no absolute proof that they differ essentially (Stephenson, 2001).

The overall frequency of RASs and BHSs, which occur in about 4% of children, is high. Lombroso and Lerman (1967) found that 19% of cases were of the pallid type, probably due to the reflex anoxic mechanism, and 76% were cyanotic, which is suggestive of BHSs. The onset mostly occurs in infants and toddlers between 6 and 18 months of age, but a very early onset in the first days of life can be seen.

Reflex Anoxic Seizures. Classic RASs are typically precipitated by pain, often due to a bump on the head. The toddler may begin to cry, but the crying is rapidly interrupted by a loss of consciousness and tone, resulting in a fall that may be slow and progressive or abrupt. When the asystole lasts more than a few sec-

onds, hypertonia of the trunk and limbs sets in and opisthotonus, a rare manifestation of epileptic seizures, is common. A few jerks and eye deviation, either upward or downward, are common (Engel and Pedley, 1998; Lempert et al., 1994; Lin et al., 1982). The child is pale, and, occasionally, the parent may note the absence of pulse. After a variable period (usually 30 to 60 seconds), the child returns to consciousness, and the hypertonia resolves. In some cases, a genuine, usually clonic, epileptic seizure immediately follows the tonic episode (Stephenson, 2001; Battaglia et al., 1989; Aicardi et al., 1988). Such seizures, which have been termed *anoxic epileptic seizures,* may be of long duration, and cases of resulting status epilepticus have been recorded (Emery, 1990; Stephenson, 1990). Conversely, a true epileptic seizure may result in severe hypoxia as a consequence of the interference of the discharge with the respiratory control mechanisms; this is the so-called *epileptic anoxic seizure* (Stephenson, 1983). However, this rarely causes a misdiagnosis of epilepsy.

Atypical features such as lateral body incurvation and postictal confusion are common. In older children, auras, which usually consist of an unpleasant feeling of discomfort but which may occasionally be quite complex, including hallucinations and automatisms that are sometimes elaborate, may complicate the diagnostic problem (Stephenson, 2001).

The consistent presence of a precipitating factor is a major characteristic, but this may be difficult to elicit; it often escapes detection with perfunctory questioning. Older children and adolescents tend to be reluctant to tell "strange stories," thus adding to the difficulties. Contrary to the common belief, RASs can occur not only when an individual is standing or sitting but also when one is lying down, so the individual's position does not rule out the diagnosis.

Recording of an event may be of help in some cases; events can be precipitated by compression of the eyeballs, but eyeball pressure is not advised routinely. Provoking a cardiac arrest of more than 2 seconds (positive oculocardiac reflex) is suggestive but not diagnostic of RASs, and the maneuver is justified only in rare, difficult cases.

The natural precipitating factors are extremely varied. Pain and emotional triggers are most common in infants and toddlers. The occurrence of reflex anoxic attacks may be facilitated by fever (Stephenson, 1976; Gastaut, 1974; Gastaut and Gastaut, 1958). Stephenson (1976) found that 142 (23%) of 630 children with a history of "febrile convulsions" had a markedly positive response to eyeball pressure, especially those with a history of tonic rather than clonic attacks. He suggested that, in these children, the febrile seizures might have had an anoxic rather than an epileptic mechanism. In older children, the precipitating factors can include emotions, the sight of blood, standing in a confined atmosphere, venipuncture, and injections.

Specific factors may be responsible in some cases; these can include hot baths (Patel et al., 1994) (see Chapter 17), combing one's hair (Stephenson, 1990; Igarashi et al., 1988), or stretching (Pelekanos et al., 1990). These can also precipitate cardioinhibitory syncopes in adults, and the mechanisms of both are similar or identical (Stephenson, 1990).

In the most severe cases, prolonged ambulatory cardiac monitoring can be useful in showing the actual frequency and duration of the events. In rare cases, cardiac pacing has been used (Stephenson, 1990). Except in very rare cases in which an associated underlying condition was present, no deaths are known to have been caused by RAS; in most patients, no treatment besides reassurance is necessary.

Breath-holding spells. BHSs are closely related to RASs. Distinguishing them from RASs is often difficult, although their clinical presentation may differ. In BHSs, the child cries vigorously for a prolonged manner period of time and then blocks expiration, with resulting cyanosis, limpness, and loss of consciousness. ECG recording shows bradycardia replacing the initial tachycardia, with slowing and sometimes flattening on the EEG.

Gastaut and Broughton (1972) distinguished *sobbing spasms* from the usual cyanotic breath-holding. In such cases, the infant sobs for a prolonged period of time until he or she is out of breath, without apnea. Cerebral hypoxia results from poor gas exchange. Although the sequence of events in breath-holding attacks is unmistakable, a surprising number of diagnostic errors are seen, especially with the convulsive type. Errors are also seen when the initial phase of crying or sobbing is lacking and the apnea intervenes early or even after a single gasp.

Both BHS and RAS seems to have a definite familial tendency (Lugaresi et al., 1973).

Unusual types of reflex anoxic seizures. Paroxysmal events resulting from a mechanism similar to that of RASs may occur with special precipitating factors or in patients with an underlying basal disorder.

Syncopes induced by a Valsalva maneuver sometimes occur as a result of tricks that are occasionally still practiced by schoolboys (the "fainting lark" trick). Gastaut et al. (1987c) drew attention to a peculiar type of self-induced seizure that they observed in 10 mentally retarded children. The attacks were stereotyped, starting with apnea and overinflation of thorax, followed by loss of consciousness with pallor and, at times, a fall. The same phenomenon may be observed in intellectually normal children with relatively mild behavioral disturbances (Fig. 21.3).

The authors have observed two girls of normal or borderline intelligence who induced several dozen attacks daily that mimicked atypical absences. The attacks could produce a fall. In one of the patients, some of the induced syncopes were followed by a typical (epileptic) absence that was apparently triggered by anoxia (Aicardi et al., 1988). The mechanism seemed to be a Valsalva maneuver producing brain anoxia (Schmidt and Lampert, 1990). Tassinari et al. (1976) described "absences" with or without falls in two patients in whom the apnea seemed to result from hyperventilation, and a similar mechanism may occur in many patients with marked and prolonged hyperventilation (Mangin et al., 1982), particularly in girls with Rett syndrome (Hagberg et al., 1983), in whom the syncopes induced by hyperventilation may mimic epileptic seizures (Arzimanoglou et al., 1995). Distinguishing such phenomena from absences or complex partial seizures may be difficult, and polygraphic recording may be required.

In the severe form of hyperekplexia (or excessive startle disease), this uncommon condition can give rise to typical RASs that are precipitated by sudden stimuli and that may even result in sudden death. The

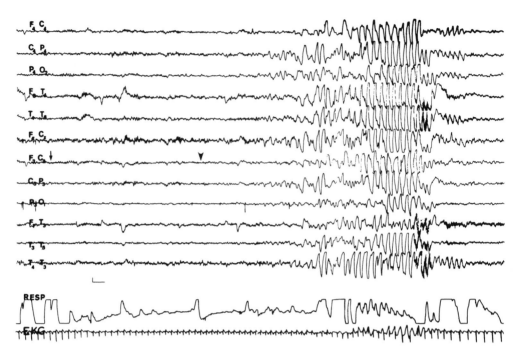

FIG. 21.3. Self-induced syncope in a 9-year-old girl. From 6 years of age, this girl had multiple daily episodes of "absence" during which she would stare, turn pale or slightly cyanotic, and appear unresponsive. In some attacks, muscle tone was lost, with a resulting fall to the ground. All of the attacks were preceded by inflation of the thorax. The attacks occurred almost exclusively when she was inactive or bored. Anticonvulsant therapy was ineffective. When she was given fenfluramine, her self-induced attacks disappeared. The attack started with apnea (*RESP*) with thoracic inflation (*arrow*); 18 seconds later, a burst of high-voltage slow waves appeared while the child became pale and unresponsive (*arrowhead*). After a few seconds, normal respiration was resumed and consciousness returned. Changes in the appearance of the electrocardiogram probably correspond to the modification in the electrical axis of the heart, and they are regularly present in such cases (Aicardi et al., 1988). Calibration: 1 second, 50 μV.

attacks can be terminated by the forced flexion of the head and trunk, which can be lifesaving (Vigevano et al., 1989b). The disorder occurs in two forms. In addition to the excessive startle, the major form features marked hypertonia from birth, which disappears during sleep, and violent, repetitive jerks of the limbs on falling asleep (Andermann et al., 1980a) that may manifest on resolution of hypertonia after the first year of life. Touching the child's nose often precipitates an apneic attack. The disorder is dominantly inherited in most cases, although recessive transmission and sporadic cases have been recorded (Aicardi, 1998d; Andermann et al., 1988). A mutation in the α_1 subunit of the glycine receptor appears to be responsible for the disease (Ryan et al., 1992). Cases of secondary hyperekplexia may be more common than the primary type. The same excessive startle response is present, but neurologic signs, especially those in the form of major spasticity, are present.

Quite similar episodes have been described in the rare syndrome of *familial rectal pain* (Engel and Pedley, 1998; Elmslie et al., 1996; Schubert and Cracco, 1992). Syncopal episodes have also been described in some patients with alternating hemiplegia; these may occur in association with paralytic attacks or in isolation (Aicardi, 2001), and they may be quite extensive.

Cardiogenic Syncopes

Syncopes of cardiac origin are much more rare than RASs in childhood. They may be caused by structural heart defects, particularly aortic stenosis, but they are mainly due to rhythm disturbances resulting from surgical interference with the intrinsic heart conduction system or to genetic conditions, especially sick sinus syndrome and prolonged QT syndrome (Zareba et al., 1998).

The cardiogenic syncopes include the Romano-Ward syndrome, which is dominantly inherited (Gospe and Choy, 1989; Horn et al. 1986a), and the Jervell-Lange-Nielsen syndrome, a recessively inherited condition which features an associated sensorineural deafness (Jervell and Lange-Nielsen, 1957). In all such cases, the syncopes are usually of the convulsive type, and, in the essentials, they are similar to Adams-Stokes attacks.

The QT syndromes, which can be due to several types of ionic channel dysfunction, are relatively common. The syncopal episodes can closely mimic epileptic seizures, and this misdiagnosis is not uncommon (Gordon, 1999; Pacia et al., 1994). Nonetheless, diagnosing the prolonged QT syndromes correctly is important because sudden death can occur and the placement of a pacemaker can be lifesaving. The clinician should therefore have a high index of suspicion, especially when the syncopes occur during sleep or they are precipitated by sudden emotion, effort, or noise and when the individual has a history of chest pain or a family history of sudden death. However, in most cases, the events have no special precipitants, so systematic simultaneous recording of the ECG and the EEG and the *measurement* of the corrected QT (QTc) interval are highly recommended. Prolonged recording of the ECG and exercise testing may be indicated in selected cases, especially when a history of familial syncopes or sudden death is present (Aicardi, 1998d, Nousiainen et al., 1989). However, occasional cases of cardiac syncope with normal QTc have been recorded (Brucker et al., 1984).

Other events of cardiac origin, such as episodes of hyperpnea in cyanotic heart diseases, rarely mimic epilepsy, although they may end in loss of consciousness.

"Near-Miss" Sudden Death and Apparent Life-Threatening Events in Infants

Young infants, particularly those younger than 6 months, are often referred with a diagnosis of epilepsy for dramatic episodes of change in color, respiratory rate disturbances, or bradycardia. Some of these may be accompanied by dystonic posturing and opisthotonus, and they are often preceded by restlessness and an apprehensive look. Some may be due to episodes of gastroesophageal reflux (Pranzatelli and Pedley, 1991; Spitzer et al., 1984), which can be diagnosed by pH measurements and/or manometry and radiology.

Others may be episodes of "near-miss" sudden infant death, particularly those that occur during sleep.

Some of these episodes can produce such a severe degree of hypoxia that brain damage results; these can manifest with epileptic attacks or status epilepticus (Constantinou et al., 1989; Aubourg et al., 1985) immediately following the hypoxic events, so a misdiagnosis of epilepsy can result. Conversely, severe epileptic seizures can result in a state suggestive of sudden infant death when the seizure is not recognized. Suffocation is probably a major mechanism for sudden infant death. It may also be a part of Munchausen syndrome by proxy, in which the infant is being pressed against the perpetrator, usually the mother (Stephenson, 1990). A careful study of the circumstances and history can suggest the diagnosis, which is often quite difficult to prove. The authors have found that such rather ill-defined episodes of severe malaise are a common reason for referral to a specialized epilepsy unit in infants younger than 6 months.

Paroxysmal Attacks Caused by Toxic Agents

The possibility of acute toxicity, especially that related to drugs, should always be considered in children, especially toddlers. This is an important diagnostic problem because the emergency treatment of toxic absorption differs from that of seizures, yet some toxic agents can generate epileptic seizures (e.g., tricyclic antidepressants) or acute dystonic episodes that are often misinterpreted as seizures, making differentiation more difficult. The drugs most commonly responsible for dystonic episodes are psychotropic agents, such as phenothiazines or butyrophenones (Pranzatelli, 1996), and metoclopramide (Casteels-van Daele, 1981), but other agents are continuously being added to the list. More often, however, coma is the major or sole clinical manifestation. In all such cases, meticulous history taking should attempt to establish the possibility of toxicity, but this may be extremely difficult.

Endogenous toxicity resulting from metabolic disturbances, especially hypoglycemia and hypocalcemia, must always be considered. Glycemia, calcemia, and plasma electrolytes should be systematically determined. Hypocalcemia in young children is manifested by real seizures more often than by classic tetany (Aicardi, 1998d).

Pseudoepileptic Seizures and Other Psychiatric Manifestations

In the experience of Jeavons (1983b), acute psychiatric manifestations represented the second most common cause of an incorrect diagnosis of epilepsy. In most cases, the resemblance to epileptic seizures is only superficial, and episodes such as attacks of anxiety, acute phobic episodes, fugues, and feelings of derealization, do not usually pose major diagnostic problems. However, panic attacks are sometimes mistaken for epilepsy (Genton et al., 1995b), and hallucinations due to schizophrenia or schizophrenia-like states due to substance abuse may be difficult to separate from some types of nonconvulsive status epilepticus. Munchausen syndrome by proxy may be a cause of "psychogenic" seizures, which may pose great diagnostic difficulties. The mother may invent a sophisticated history of seizures (Meadow, 1984, 1991), sometimes even teaching the child that he or she has epilepsy and encouraging him or her to invent episodes as well (Croft and Jervis, 1989).

Attacks of rage may occur in adolescents and older children; these may be associated with postictal sleep and some apparent obscuration of consciousness. However, the aggressiveness is clearly directed and provoked, even though by slight motives, which differs from what occurs in patients with complex partial seizures fighting against restraint.

Pseudoepileptic seizures, also called *pseudoseizures*, *nonepileptic seizures*, *hysterical seizures*, or *psychogenic seizures*, have been the subject of much recent interest (Lesser, 1985; Lesser et al., 1983; Gulick et al., 1982; Riley and Roy, 1982; Dreifuss et al., 1981; Holmes et al., 1980). They are more common in young adults than in children, but, not infrequently, they are observed in adolescents and even in children as young as 4 to 6 years (Holmes et al., 1980; Finlayson and Lucas, 1979). They are often associated with true epileptic attacks in the same patient (Metrick et al., 1991). However, 6 of the 17 patients of Holmes et al. (1980) had only pseudoepileptic attacks, and others have reported a similar experience (Goitein et al., 1983; Lesser et al., 1983). Pseudoepileptic seizures in patients who have had previous epileptic fits mimic real fits more closely than those occurring in patients without preceding epileptic experiences. Pseudoepileptic seizures can mimic generalized tonic-clonic or tonic seizures.

They can occur in children with impaired neurodevelopment (Neill, 1990), but they are more common in normally developing children. They can be observed following head injury (Westbrock et al., 1998), and they have even been observed after successful epilepsy surgery (Parra et al., 1998). This has also been seen in two of the authors' patients; in adults, they can occur immediately after a true epileptic attack (Devinsky, 1998).

Pseudoepileptic seizures can mimic generalized tonic-clonic or tonic seizures. More rarely, the motor manifestations remain unilateral or partial. Commonly, the seizures express themselves by coordinated activity reminiscent of that seen in complex partial seizures. In a few cases, pseudoepileptic attacks manifest only with unresponsiveness, often in association with the loss of postural tone (Gulick et al., 1982). In one series of 21 children (Wyllie et al., 1991), 10 had episodes of unresponsiveness, generalized limb jerking, and thrashing movements, and 6 had episodes of staring and unresponsiveness. Most children were responsive immediately after the paroxysm.

Pseudoseizures masquerading as absences have also been observed in 18 children with hyperventilation syndrome (North et al., 1990). Responsiveness may actually be altered during hyperventilation and may be accompanied by the appearance of rhythmic slow waves at 3 Hz. However, the spikes are not associated with the lack of responsiveness (Epstein et al., 1994).

In most cases, pseudoseizures are relatively easy to recognize. They differ from true epileptic fits in several ways. The episodes are usually preceded by dizziness, funny feelings, unilateral or bilateral numbness, and similar sensations. The ictal movements are not true clonias but rather a spectrum of movements ranging from quivering to uncontrolled flailing of the extremities. In most cases, the movements are coordinated in nature, and they are bilaterally symmetric. The onset is not as sudden as that seen in epileptic attacks, and the motor activity often gradually builds up to a paroxysm. The diagnosis may, however, be difficult when the parents panic during the attacks, subsequently preventing them from being able to give a precise description of the events.

Pseudoseizures with semipurposeful movements may simulate complex partial seizures. However, the activity also has a progressive onset, and it is often theatrical or violent, with loud screaming or shouting that is different from the vocalization that can accompany complex partial seizures of temporal lobe origin; similar vocalization may, however, occur with frontal lobe seizures. Generally pseudoseizures are not as stereotyped as true epileptic attacks (Meierkord et al., 1991; Lesser, 1985; Dreifuss et al., 1981). However, the notion that most repetitive stereotyped behaviors are organic attacks may be faulty because, in a few patients, pseudoseizures may have stereotypic patterns (Cohen and Suter, 1982; Gulick et al., 1982).

A postictal state is uncommon in pseudoseizures. Most patients become immediately responsive at the end of their fits, and, even during the attacks, most patients avoid painful stimuli and resist trials at opening their lids (Lesser, 1985). Urination is uncommon but it may occur, and the same applies to tongue biting or self-injury. Pseudoepileptic seizures never occur during sleep, and they occur only infrequently when the patient is alone. They are often provoked by observation and especially by suggestion, which is best accomplished with EEG recording (Wilkus et al., 1984; Cohen and Suter, 1982).

A special problem is posed by the occurrence of *pseudostatus epilepticus* or repetitive pseudoseizures (Shorvon, 1994; Schmidt and Lampert, 1990; Levitan and Bruni, 1986). This syndrome is not rare in adults. It may actually be more common than true status. Episodes of pseudostatus may also be observed in children, and 64% of the patients of Metrick et al. (1991) had a history of "status." Such patients have 10 to 20 attacks that resemble tonic-clonic seizures within a 24-hour period; these attacks are usually separated by intervals of full alertness, which distinguishes them from true status. However, such intervals are often masked by the administration of massive amounts of sedative drugs; some patients are referred to intensive care units, and they may even be intubated and artificially ventilated. Video-EEG monitoring is particularly helpful in such patients because the absence of epileptic discharges under such circumstances rules out status epilepticus.

Females are predominately found in most series of pseudoseizures (Lesser, 1985). The psychiatric background of patients with pseudoepileptic seizures is variable. A hysteric personality is found in only some cases and malingering is uncommon, so the use of the term *hysteric attack* should be avoided. The vast majority of patients with pseudoseizures are receiving drug therapy, and pseudoseizures should always be considered in cases of "intractable epilepsy" (Aicardi, 1988a). Once the diagnosis has been established, the previous drug treatment should be rapidly discontinued. In the series of Metrick et al. (1991), the antiepileptic drugs were withdrawn in eight patients, and the dose was reduced in another nine. The outcome was also favorable in the patients of Wyllie et al. (1991), in which 14 of the 18 followed for more than 18 months were doing well. Some form of psychiatric treatment seems beneficial (Lesser, 1996; Holmes et al., 1980), at least in the short term. When both pseudoseizures and epileptic attacks coexist, establishing the diagnosis usually results in a considerable decrease in the frequency of attacks.

The 43 patients studied by Lancman et al. (1994) had an average age of 12.4 years at onset and of 15 years when the condition was diagnosed. Twenty-one

of them (49%) received antiepileptic agents. The average duration of the attacks was 5.6 minutes, and only a minority had only staring seizures.

The diagnosis may be particularly difficult because, in some patients with true epileptic seizures, especially those affecting the supplementary motor area, the clinical manifestations may be so bizarre that they wrongly suggest the possibility of pseudoseizures (Stores et al., 1991; Fusco et al., 1990; Kanner et al., 1990).

In all cases of psychogenic seizures, the ictal EEG does not show paroxysmal discharges, but the interictal record may be paroxysmal in epileptic patients who also have pseudoseizures. Conversely, in some frontal seizures, the ictal EEG may remain normal. Recording of an ictal discharge during a clinical event is diagnostic of a true seizure. Prolonged cassette or video-EEG recording can be particularly useful.

The induction of seizures by suggestion (Devinsky, 1998; Lancman et al., 1994) may be helpful, but this must be performed after fully explaining the procedure to both the patient and the family.

Hyperventilation Syndrome

Hyperventilation syndrome is fairly common, particularly in adolescent girls. Hyperpnea is defined as an increase in the rate and depth of respiratory movements, whereas hyperventilation implies that the ventilatory effort is greater than the metabolic needs. In many subjects, hyperventilation is not a continuously symptomatic state; rather, it is characterized by recurrent symptoms with or without provocative stresses. Patients with the full hyperventilation syndrome breathe with rapid, shallow, irregular breaths, whereas those who complain primarily of their inability to obtain satisfyingly deep breaths hyperventilate with deep sighing respirations (Brodtkorb et al., 1984; Magarian, 1982). Although common presenting complaints in hyperventilators include mainly dyspnea, chest pain, and lightheadedness, syncope and pseudoabsence spells are not uncommon (Magarian and Olney, 1984). These should not be mistaken for epileptic seizures, especially since the rhythmic, high-amplitude slow waves at 3 Hz may resemble spike-wave discharges (Epstein et al., 1994).

The diagnosis depends on a high index of suspicion and on the presence of the typical symptoms, which often include myalgias, thoracic pain, and dyspnea. The diagnosis may be difficult when hyperventilation is responsible for unilateral sensory and, rarely, motor symptoms (Blau et al., 1983). Rebreathing in a plastic or paper bag permits control of the symptoms of impending attacks to be achieved quickly, and this has both diagnostic and therapeutic value. Hyperventilation in children and adolescents, however, should alert the physician to the presence of family discord and significant psychologic disturbances (Joorabchi, 1977). Reassurance therapy alone is often ineffective, and many patients go on to hyperventilate and to show chronic anxiety as adults (Herman et al., 1981).

Paroxysmal Movement Disorders, Paroxysmal Vertigo, and Torticollis

Benign Paroxysmal Vertigo and Paroxysmal Torticollis

Benign paroxysmal vertigo (Basser, 1964) occurs in children from 1 to 5 years of age who have no neurodevelopmental impairment. The episodes occur without warning, and they usually last 1 minute or less. The onset is sudden; the child may cry out, cling to nearby persons or objects, and turn pale. A fall often results, but no loss of consciousness or amnesia occurs. The child may talk about a sensation of rotation, and unsteadiness is commonly observed. Nystagmus is sometimes described by witnesses. The attacks are usually infrequent (one to five per year), but, in a few cases, they may occur repeatedly. They tend to disappear by 5 to 7 years of age, and they leave no sequelae.

Paroxysmal torticollis (Deonna and Martin, 1981) is probably related to paroxysmal vertigo, and both almost certainly reflect vestibular dysfunction. It is less likely to be misdiagnosed as epilepsy because of its long duration with preserved consciousness (Fernandez-Alvarez and Aicardi, 2001). The episodes may last hours or days, and they are usually associated with vomiting, instability, and a tendency to veer to one side and sometimes with truncal incurvation and unilateral stiffness. Other forms of vertigo are uncommon in children, and epileptic vertigo is clearly an exceptional occurrence.

Paroxysmal Movement Disorders and Episodic Ataxias

These include multiple conditions that may be related to epilepsy on the one hand and to disorders of movement on the other. The mechanisms are probably multiple, but, in some cases, the conditions are probably due to the dysfunction of ionic channels ("channelopathies") (Griggs and Nutt, 1995).

The *episodic ataxias* are easy to differentiate from epileptic seizures, especially episodic ataxia type 2 (Baloh et al., 1997), a calcium channel disease in which the attacks are often prolonged and in which nystagmus and cerebellar signs are often present. The disease often responds to acetazolamide, which interrupts or prevents the attacks. Episodic ataxia type 1, which is caused by a gene that maps to chromosome 12p13, is a potassium channel disease. Clinically, it is characterized by brief attacks lasting seconds to minutes and by the interictal persistence of continuous myokymia (Brunt and van Werden, 1990). It may also respond to acetazolamide.

The *paroxysmal dyskinesias* are much more difficult to distinguish from some forms of epilepsy. They are characterized by the sudden occurrence of transient attacks of extrapyramidal movements that may be dystonic or choreoathetotic and that usually are localized to one side of the body. In most patients, the attacks are precipitated by sudden movement (kinesigenic dyskinesias). The patient's consciousness is preserved, but the bizarre, often writhing, and sometimes ballic movements superficially suggest the diagnosis of epilepsy, a diagnosis that, in the authors' experience, is often made. The attacks are usually brief. In many cases, they occur without precipitants. The ictal EEG, when it is recorded, is normal. The attacks are usually frequent, up to 100 per day, but their frequency commonly decreases with age. The disorder usually responds favorably to antiepileptic drugs, such as carbamazepine or phenytoin. Most cases are familial, with a dominant inheritance and reduced penetrance. A locus has been mapped to the pericentromeric region of chromosome 16. A second locus (EKD2) that maps to 16q13-q22 has been recently found, indicating genetic heterogeneity (Valente et al., 2000).

The less common paroxysmal dyskinesias include the paroxysmal choreoathetosis of Mount and Reback (Fernandez-Alvarez and Aicardi, 2001; Bressman et al., 1988), which has been linked to chromosome 2q31-36. In this condition, the attacks, which are not precipitated by movement, are usually of long duration. In an intermediate type, the attacks are triggered by prolonged exercise (Lance, 1977). The relationship between the paroxysmal dyskinesias and epilepsy is complex, as the occurrence of both epileptic seizures and dyskinesia in some patients shows. These include cases of infantile convulsions that, years later, are followed by paroxysmal dyskinesia (Szepetowski et al., 1997); individuals with rolandic epilepsy associated with writer's cramp and episodic dyskinesia (Guerrini et al., 1999b), both of which are linked to the centromeric region of chromosome 16; and those with episodic ataxia type 1 linked to a potassium channel gene on chromosome 12q13 who also have generalized epilepsy (Eunson et al., 2000). This association suggests strongly a role for channel dysfunction in at least some types of epilepsy (see Chapter 13). Likewise, some cases of paroxysmal dyskinesia have been associated with ictal paroxysmal discharges that have been recorded intracranially over the supplementary motor area (Lombroso, 2000), again suggesting a close relationship between these phenomena.

A similar association may be seen in *alternating hemiplegia of children* (Aicardi, 2001), in which the epileptic seizures can be associated with the characteristic paralytic and dystonic episodes and with variable autonomic manifestations in approximately half the cases. Because the initial episodes are often dystonic and one sided and they are followed by a hemiplegia lasting hours to days, the diagnosis of partial epilepsy with Todd palsy is usually made. However, antiepileptic agents are generally ineffective, although flunarizine decreases the frequency and severity of attacks in 50% of children.

Other Movement Disorders That May Pose a Diagnostic Problem

Myoclonus, which is often a manifestation of epilepsy (see Chapter 6), can also be nonepileptic (Guerrini, 2002d). *Infantile sleep myoclonus* occurs in otherwise normal infants in the first weeks or months of life (Di Capua et al., 1993; Resnick et al., 1986). The jerks involve mainly the limbs, often occurring in clusters that may last several minutes; they occur repeatedly over periods of up to several hours, to the point that the condition can be misdiagnosed as status epilepticus. The jerks immediately disappear when the infant is awakened (Alfonso et al., 1995), and they never affect the face and only rarely the trunk. They disappear spontaneously at no later than 6 months of age.

Benign infantile myoclonus occurs in some normally developing infants at around 3 to 8 months of age. The attacks may mimic infantile spasms, and they often occur in clusters; however, no developmental arrest occurs, and the EEG remains normal (Pachatz et al., 1999; Dravet et al., 1986). Individual jerks look more closely like shudders, and they are often precipitated by emotional stimuli (Pachatz et al., 2002). Shuddering attacks consisting of mild stiffening of the upper limbs with very fine, low-amplitude, rapid (8 to 10 Hz) oscillatory movements with preservation of full consciousness have also been reported as a distinct phenomenon (Holmes and Russman, 1986). These have been said to herald the later development of essential tremor (Vanasse et al., 1976), although this seems to be quite unusual.

Except for complex tics such as those observed in Tourette syndrome, *tics* seldom raise a diagnostic issue (Fernandez-Alvarez and Aicardi, 2001). The term *myoclonic tics*, which is sometimes used, describes the few cases that may resemble myoclonus. The sudden head movements seen in children with congenital ocular motor apraxia (Harris et al., 1996; Zee et al., 1977) have been sometimes mistaken for myoclonic jerks (Altrocchi and Menkes, 1960).

Ritualistic movements, stereotypies, and head banging rarely pose a problem, although, in rare cases, stereotypies have been shown to be regularly associated with paroxysmal EEG abnormalities (Deonna et al., 2001). Infantile masturbation is common in the first few years, especially in girls, some of whom are referred with a suspected diagnosis of complex partial seizures (O'Donohoe, 1985; Livingston, 1972). The child is commonly found with thighs tightly adducted or crossed and is lying down or rocking herself backward and forward while perspiring with a staring glare. Such minor episodes are harmless, and they spontaneously disappear. No treatment, except reassurance to the parents, is needed.

Episodes of Altered Responsiveness

Daydreaming is a common source of erroneous diagnoses of absence epilepsy. However, episodes of daydreaming clearly differ from absences by the lack of sudden onset and termination and by the persistence of responsiveness to stimuli of sufficient intensity.

Paroxysmal disturbances of consciousness may be the predominant or even the only manifestation of epilepsy. These may occur as brief episodes or a prolonged state, as in some types of nonconvulsive status epilepticus (see Chapter 16). However, isolated disturbances of awareness or responsiveness are caused much more often by the ingestion of toxics or drugs or by intermittent metabolic disorders.

Migraine and Periodic Syndrome

Like epilepsy, complicated migraine is characterized by paroxysmal symptoms of central nervous dysfunction, such as paresthesias, scotomata, mental dulling, and pareses, in addition to headache, nausea, and vomiting. Such symptoms may pose a difficult diagnostic problem between migraine and epilepsy, and the relationship of the two conditions has been discussed extensively (Andermann and Lugaresi,

1985). Although migraine and epilepsy are basically different disorders, some syndromes (e.g., occipital epilepsy with continuous spike-wave [Panayiotopoulos, 1994a; Gastaut, 1992; Newton and Aicardi, 1983; Camfield et al., 1978]) share characteristics of both diseases. In most cases, however, the diagnosis is relatively easy to establish with careful questioning of the patient. In rare patients, headache may be the most prominent manifestation of the epilepsy (Bladin, 1987; Laplante et al., 1983; Young and Blume, 1983; Swaiman and Franck, 1978).

The most common error in making the diagnosis is to attribute wrongly the initial phenomena of migrainous attacks, such as phosphenes, hemianopia or amaurosis, micropsia, tinnitus or vertigo, and localized or bilateral paresthesias, to epilepsy. Such phenomena are usually, but not always, followed by headache and vomiting. If no headache occurs, the phenomena are easily interpreted as epileptic. The initial phenomena in migraine, however, are recognizably different from those that are observed in partial epileptic seizures. Paresthesias, for example, spread much more slowly in migraine than they do in epilepsy, and they tend to have a cheirooral distribution. A careful description of the visual phenomena is of great diagnostic value. In migraine, the visual phenomena are not colored, and they tend to present as broken lines (fortification spectra) or undulating patterns, whereas, in occipital epilepsy, they are often brightly colored, presenting in the form of circles or balls (Panayiotopoulos, 1994a).

Complex distortions of perception, such as "micropsia," an impression of changes in the size or shape of the body or of part of it or of surroundings that are abnormally close or distant, constitute the "Alice in Wonderland" syndrome (Golden, 1979). This may be confused with the hallucinations or illusions observed in complex partial seizures, but it much more commonly is a feature of migraine. The persistence of a normal consciousness throughout the attacks, the throbbing nature of the headache, and the long duration of the cephalagia are important features favoring migraine. However, in some migrainous attacks, especially in basilar artery migraine, a brief loss of consciousness may be observed (Pranzatelli and Pedley, 1991; Golden, 1979; Lapkin and Golden, 1978). More prolonged confusional episodes and transient amnesia that fulfill the criteria for transient global amnesia (Haas and Ross, 1986) may also occur; together, these may be misinterpreted as nonconvulsive status epilepticus (Gascon and Barlow, 1970). The association of migrainous symptoms and true epileptic manifestations is observed in a few patients,

either in different attacks or as parts of the same seizure (Fig. 21.4). Epileptic phenomena can include clonic jerks, head and eye deviation, or complex partial seizures following a migrainous "aura," especially a visual one.

EEG abnormalities, mainly slow waves, are common during or immediately after a migrainous attack (Barlow, 1984; Slatter, 1968). Paroxysmal interictal abnormalities are rare. Spike foci may be the result of ischemia and even infarction of the brain following the repeated episodes of vasoconstriction that are associated with the attacks of migraine. This occurrence, however, is extremely rare, and it is unlikely to account for the high proportion of abnormal interictal EEG records found in migrainous patients (Kinast et al., 1982; Westmoreland, 1979; Lapkin et al., 1977; Hockaday and Whitty, 1969). Most of these abnormalities are, however, nonspecific, so the relationship between epilepsy and migraine remains controversial. The incidence of epilepsy in migrainous persons is higher than would be expected by chance, and the incidence of migraine in patients with epilepsy slightly exceeds that seen in controls.

Attacks of hemiplegic migraine should be differentiated from postictal paralysis and the rare inhibitory seizures (Hanson and Chodos, 1978). Its relationship with alternating hemiplegia of children remains an item of debate (Andermann et al., 1995).

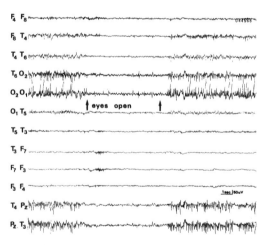

FIG. 21.4. Electroencephalogram of a 15-year-old boy with both migrainous and epileptic attacks. This patient had five partial clonic seizures between the ages of 4 and 10 years. Since the age of 7 years, he has also had attacks of classic migraine with visual auras. The arrest of continuous spike activity by eye opening was repeatedly demonstrated between 6 and 15 years of age.

The *periodic syndrome,* which may be closely related to migraine, includes the syndrome of episodic recurrent abdominal pain and the syndrome of cyclical vomiting. Both are common in children, but, in an overwhelming majority of patients, neither are related to epilepsy. In fact, they should raise the suspicion of metabolic disorders, such as intermittent hyperammonemia, or of a gastrointestinal abnormality more than that of a neurologic problem.

Abdominal epilepsy is rare. It is a nonconvulsive disorder occurring principally in children (O'Donohoe, 1985). The pain of abdominal epilepsy is of brief duration (a few minutes), and it is often accompanied by borborygmi, vomiting, pallor or redness of the face, and profuse perspiration. The pain is periumbilical in location, it is usually colicky in nature, and it is severe. In most cases, it is accompanied by other features suggestive of epilepsy, especially altered consciousness and brief, simple automatisms. The EEG abnormalities associated with abdominal seizures include bilateral spike-wave, polyspike-wave, low-voltage fast patterns, and 10-Hz fast rhythms (Feldman, 1983a; Gastaut and Tassinari, 1975a; Papatheopailou et al., 1972). In cases in which the abdominal pain is isolated, the demonstration of one of these typical epileptic patterns coinciding with the time of the clinical attacks is necessary to establish the diagnosis of abdominal epilepsy (Feldman, 1983a). The mere presence of interictal spiking is not enough to make a def-

inite diagnosis. The presence of the so-called 14-6 positive spikes is a normal phenomenon in many young patients that has no diagnostic value (Eeg-Olofsson et al., 1971; Lombroso et al., 1966).

Cyclic vomiting, when it is not accompanied by other more typical epileptic symptoms, is probably never of epileptic nature. A relationship with migraine is more common, with cyclic vomiting being regularly followed by typical migrainous attacks (Feldman, 1983a).

Paroxysmal Disturbances Occurring During Sleep

The most common pediatric disorders of sleep are the non–rapid eye movement (REM) parasomnias (Guilleminault and Brooks, 2001; Guilleminault et al., 1988; Guilleminault and Lugaresi, 1983). These events occur during slow sleep at the time of arousal from stage 3 and/or 4 sleep, and they are thought to arise when the arousal is incomplete. Some can raise delicate diagnostic problems, and they are not uncommonly misdiagnosed as epileptic events.

Night terrors (pavor nocturnus) are the most common condition in this group that may raise diagnostic issues with epilepsy (Fig. 21.5). Night terrors usually occur between the ages of 18 months and 5 years (Dravet, 1992b; Dimario and Emery, 1987; Tassinari, 1976). They supervene most commonly in the first few hours of sleep. The child starts screaming and

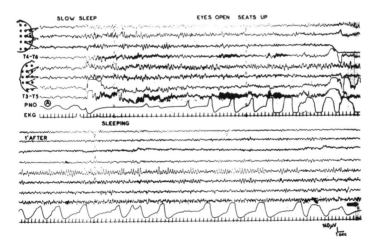

FIG. 21.5. Epileptic seizure mimicking an episode of night terror in a 6-year-old boy who also had similar episodes of fear when he was awake. More prolonged seizures were associated with masticatory or swallowing motions, but the brief attacks consisted exclusively of an expression of intense fear as the child suddenly awoke and sat up on his couch. Differentiation from an episode of night terror was easy because of the history of diurnal seizures and the occurrence of more prolonged and more characteristic episodes. In most cases, the reverse situation prevails (i.e., common night terrors are misdiagnosed as epileptic seizures).

then generally sits up and looks terrified. Although the child seems awake, he or she does not recognize the parents and continues to cry in spite of their attempts to comfort. The episode lasts only a few minutes, and the child goes back to sleep with no memory of the event. Night terrors often occur every night for periods of time and then disappear without apparent reason. Polygraphic recordings (Gastaut and Broughton, 1972) have shown that the episodes of night terror occur during intense arousal from deep slow-wave sleep and that they are not accompanied by any EEG paroxysms. They may persist to the age of 8 years in half of the affected children and to adolescence in one-third (Dimario and Emery, 1987).

Nightmares in children may produce a quite similar picture, with the main difference being that they take place during REM sleep. Both nightmares and night terrors are often erroneously diagnosed as epileptic events (Fischler, 1962). Partial seizures do often occur in sleep, but they are associated with stereotypic behavior, such as alimentary automatisms (e.g., smacking or swallowing) and they are generally less spectacular in their initial manifestations (Fig. 21.5). Night terrors are a benign condition that is self-limited and that does not necessitate drug treatment, only firm reassurance that the child will outgrow the condition (O'Donohoe, 1985; Guilleminault and Lugaresi, 1983).

Somnambulism (sleepwalking) occurs in about 15% of children from 5 to 12 years of age. It is marked by an incomplete arousal that permits some semipurposeful activity without clear consciousness or memory of the event. The patient rises from the bed as if he or she is awake and can walk or climb stairs, but he or she appears more or less confused; in most cases, the person does not answer questions or answers them rather distantly. The episodes are usually brief, lasting a few minutes, and the activity in which the child engages is of a simple type, such as going to the bathroom.

Night terrors, nightmares, and sleepwalking are disorders of arousal. EEG recordings in all of the cases that have been studied (Pranzatelli and Pedley, 1991; Gastaut and Broughton, 1972) show that the episodes mostly occur during the deep stages of slow sleep. They are associated with an incomplete awakening that is often accompanied by intense autonomic and muscular activation. Sleepwalking and night terrors occur together in more than half the cases, and they share the same genetic predisposition (Dimario and Emery, 1987).

Violent manifestations may occur in older children and adolescents in REM sleep motor disorder and in the so-called nocturnal paroxysmal dystonia (Lu-

garesi and Cirignotta, 1981). The latter may occur as either brief or prolonged attacks that may last several minutes, and they consist of dystonic, often writhing, and violent movements. Considerable evidence indicating that nocturnal paroxysmal dystonia is actually a manifestation of frontal lobe epilepsy has now accumulated (Tinuper et al., 1990). Frontal lobe seizures occur electively during sleep, and they often feature violent movements, such as pedaling, flinging arms, and sometimes shouting. They are of short duration, and they do not include a postictal phase that is manifest clinically. The syndrome of familial nocturnal frontal lobe epilepsy (Picard et al., 2000; Oldani et al., 1998; Scheffer et al., 1995a) is particularly interesting in this regard because the clinical manifestations may easily be interpreted as parasomnias and because several relatives for whom a diagnosis of "sleep disorder" may have already been made may be affected. Even EEG recording of the seizures may not solve the problem because the interictal and even the ictal EEG can be normal or nonspecific.

Other paroxysmal phenomena occurring during sleep may occasionally suggest the possibility of epilepsy. These include hypnagogic hallucinations, which are brief episodes of auditory, visual, or proprioceptive hallucinations or distortions of perception that occur in transition between wakefulness and sleep, and some abnormal movements, especially sleep myoclonus (see Chapter 6). Rhythmic movement of the head (*jactatio capitis nocturna*) or the body, especially rocking, is common in normal children. Such phenomena seldom raise diagnostic difficulties, however.

Narcolepsy is uncommon in prepubertal children (Guilleminault and Pelayo, 1998), but it may occur as early as 2 years of age. The characteristic episodes of sudden sleep and the associated daytime sleepiness do not suggest epilepsy, but the cataplectic attacks may well be misinterpreted. They consist of sudden falls that are often precipitated by pleasant emotions. These may be complete or "partial," featuring knee buckling or head and shoulder dropping, thus mimicking astatic seizures. However, consciousness is fully preserved, and sleepiness is usually present, although the cataplexy may remain isolated for some time at the onset (Guilleminault and Pelayo, 1998). In some patients, the episodes of amnesic automatism may simulate complex partial seizures (Schenk and Mahowald, 1992; Aldrich, 1990). The diagnosis can be confirmed by polysomnography results. The multiple sleep latency test (MSLT) demonstrates the occurrence of sleep-onset REM sleep episodes and a short sleep latency (Guilleminault and Pelayo, 1998). Almost all patients (respectively, 46 and 45 of 46 children in the series by Guilleminault and Pelayo [1998]) express the human leukocyte antigen class II antigens DQw6 and DRw11. Preliminary evidence suggests that the cerebrospinal fluid level of hypocretin-1 may be abnormally low in some narcoleptic patients (Nishino et al., 2000).

Apneic episodes may, in some cases, result in loss of consciousness that can be difficult to interpret. In one personal case, a diagnosis of epilepsy was made on the basis of such syncopal episodes in an infant with congenital alveolar ventilation syndrome (Guilleminault et al., 1982), in which the central ventilatory drive is depressed during slow sleep. Apneas also result in nocturnal insomnia that, in turn, may be responsible for episodes of daytime "microsleep."

SUMMARY

A host of paroxysmal conditions can simulate epileptic seizures in children. Indeed, the overdiagnosis of epilepsy is all too common in spite of the disastrous effect of the wrongly attributed label of epilepsy on children's lives. Probably 20% to 30% of patients sent to specialized epilepsy clinics with a diagnosis of possible epilepsy are found to suffer from other, mostly benign conditions. The most common of these include syncopes, faints, and breath-holding attacks. Sleep disorders, which are also of a benign nature, are another common cause of error. The incorrect interpretation of the EEG or its interpretation without considering the clinical history represents another source of erroneous diagnoses of epilepsy. Less commonly, the reverse error—the exclusion of the diagnosis of epilepsy on the basis of a normal EEG—is made.

Most diagnostic errors can be avoided by careful history taking, which remains the major step in diagnosis. Physicians must recognize that many nonepileptic conditions are associated with loss of consciousness or with other paroxysmal symptoms. Nonepileptic paroxysmal events can be properly diagnosed by clinical means in a vast majority of the cases. The clinician should remember that enuresis, the occurrence of a few clonic jerks, or tongue biting is not pathognomonic for epileptic seizures. Similarly, a preceding diagnosis of seizure disorder, febrile or nonfebrile, is not sufficient evidence for attributing paroxysmal events of a dubious nature to epilepsy.

The EEG may be of great help in difficult cases or for a more precise classification of seizures, but one cannot emphasize too strongly that, in no case, should a diagnosis of epilepsy rest only on EEG grounds. Especially in children, paroxysmal EEG abnormalities (e.g., rolandic spikes or a paroxysmal reaction to IPS) are often unassociated with any clinical abnormality. In such cases, antiepileptic treatment should not be given, a rule that also applies to patients who have paroxysmal EEG abnormalities and nonepileptic disturbances, such as behavior or learning disorders.

In general, in doubtful situations, deferring the diagnosis of epilepsy until the evidence is sufficiently clear is preferable. In severe cases, the diagnosis does not remain in doubt for any length of time. On the other hand, when the diagnosis of epilepsy seems dubious, usually starting treatment on an emergency basis is not necessary.

In some forms of epilepsy, particularly those cases in which brief atypical seizures or unusual manifestations (e.g., petit mal status) are the sole paroxysmal phenomena, the diagnosis of an epileptic condition may be missed for long periods. The clinician must keep in mind the possibility of epilepsy for patients with odd or unusual behavior, especially when it is episodic, and he or she should apply appropriate techniques, such as cassette recording or telemetry. In such cases, EEG evidence is of considerable diagnostic help.

22

General Aspects of Prognosis

The prognosis for children with epileptic seizures depends largely on the type of epilepsy syndrome responsible for the attacks. Throughout this book, the concept that different epilepsy syndromes have different outcomes has been emphasized, so a global study of prognosis for childhood epilepsies mainly reflects the distribution of the various epilepsy syndromes in the studied samples. However, an overview of the prognostic aspects of the epilepsies of children in general may be of interest for several reasons. First, not all of the epilepsies can be separated into definite syndromes, so a significant proportion of cases remain unclassified. In such cases, some general method for assessing prognosis is required. Second, global studies of prognosis provide at least some idea of the magnitude of the problems raised by the convulsive disorders of children and of the needs of the community with regard to these individuals. Finally, studies of the global prognosis of childhood epilepsy have shown that certain factors (e.g., frequency of seizures, presence or absence of neurologic or mental deficits, type of seizure, and duration of seizures) have a strong correlation with the outcome of epilepsy. Such factors have a predictive value, not only for unclassified cases of epilepsy but also for some cases belonging to well-defined syndromes. The ready applicability of the factors of prognosis justifies their study.

For many years, the prognosis of epilepsy was considered poor. Rodin (1989) characterized epilepsy as a chronic condition with an average rate of long-term control of 32% in children and 28% in adults. This gloomy outlook was probably due to the patients who were studied, as they were from institutions rather than the general population, as well as to multiple other biases (Sander and Sillanpää, 1998). Indeed, the discrepancy between the lifetime prevalence rate for epilepsy of 2% to 5% in most epidemiologic surveys (Hauser et al., 1993) and the concomitant prevalence rate for active epilepsy of about 0.5% implies that most patients have a favorable outcome.

As Robinson (1984) pointed out, use of evidence from the literature is particularly difficult in studies of prognosis. The differences among studies are often large, and they reflect the manner in which selection biases influence the patient population of particular series and the different proportion of various syndromes in different series. In addition, few studies are concerned specifically with childhood epilepsy, and several series have included mixed populations of adults and children, so some caution must be exercised in applying the results to children. Furthermore, the diagnosis of epilepsy can be difficult, and the inclusion of nonpileptic seizures and a lack of recognition of "minor" attacks are both common. Both can influence the results, as can different rates of reporting by patients or families (Sander et al., 1998). Several investigators have emphasized the importance of the temporal aspects of seizure disorders on relapse and remission rates (Annegers et al., 1986; Elwes et al., 1984, 1985; Elwes and Reynolds, 1981). Patients with long-standing epilepsy are likely to continue to have seizures, whereas "fresh" patients with only two or few seizures have seizures that are much more likely to remit. The results, therefore, vary with the proportion of this type of patient. Moreover, chronic cases are referred more often to specialized units, whereas "fresh" cases are often treated locally. As a result, series from specialized centers give a more pessimistic view of the prognosis.

Another reason for the differences in the results is the variable interval separating the first seizure from entry into the studies. When this interval is prolonged, a proportion of the original patients may have experienced another seizure, and these individuals are therefore not suitable for inclusion. This leads to the underestimation of the true recurrence rate of a first seizure. In one adult series (Hirsch et al., 1991a), the rate was 15% for patients who entered the study within 8 weeks of their first seizure, compared with 50% in those who registered within 4 weeks.

PROGNOSIS FOR SEIZURE RECURRENCE AND REMISSION

The prognosis of seizures is of primary importance because the occurrence of attacks influences all aspects of the individual's quality of life. The problem presents differently in patients who have experienced a first epileptic seizure and those with established recurrent epilepsy. These two situations are considered successively.

Recurrence Rate after a First Seizure

The evidence in this regard is conflicting, with an estimated recurrence risk that varies from 27% to 81% (Hopkins et al., 1988) (see Chapter 15).

In series including adults or children, the rate is generally lower in series from the general population than it is in hospital-based series (Hopkins et al., 1988). The issue is complex because time factors (i.e., how early after the event the patient is seen), the circumstances of occurrence (i.e., how certain is the absence of precipitating factors), antecedents (personal and familial), and the type of seizure and syndrome are involved. This section considers only those cases in which the first seizure is of the generalized or localized motor type, is unprovoked, and does not take place at the time of an acute disorder.

Recent studies focusing exclusively on children have shown that the risks vary with the type of seizure and the presence or absence of neurologic and electroencephalographic (EEG) abnormalities (Berg and Shinnar, 1991; Shinnar et al., 1990; Boulloche et al., 1989; Arts et al., 1988; Camfield et al., 1985b; Hirtz et al., 1984). Recurrence was seen in 87 (52%) of 168 children after an average of 32 months in one series (Camfield et al., 1985b). In this series, the risk was highest for patients with sylvian (rolandic) seizures (70% when the EEG was normal and 97% when it was abnormal); next highest for patients with other types of partial seizures, whether simple or complex (50% to 83% depending on type, EEG, and results of neurologic examination); and lowest for patients with generalized tonic-clonic seizures (30% when no EEG or neurologic anomalies were found and 63% when both neurologic and EEG abnormalities were present). Roughly similar figures have been found in other studies (Berg and Shinnar, 1991; Shinnar et al., 1990; Boulloche et al., 1989; Arts et al., 1988), but lower figures (e.g., 16% at 1 year and 27% at 3 years [Annegers et al., 1979a]) and higher figures (e.g., 67% and 78% at 1 and 3 years, respectively [Hart et al., 1990]) have been recorded in mixed adult and children series. Recent work has shown that EEG results can reliably identify children with very high (those with paroxysmal abnormalities) or very low recurrence rates (those with normal EEG) (Hirtz et al., 2000; Shinnar et al., 1994).

Discrepancies among the figures that are given likely result from sampling and methodologic differences; some patients with an isolated seizure may never be seen in a specialized center or even by a doctor (Costeff and Avni, 1982), which may result in an apparent increase in recurrence rate. On the other hand, some series may include children with nonepileptic seizures, thus lowering the recurrence rates because these are not likely to be followed by continuing epilepsy.

Notwithstanding such methodologic difficulties, a sizable proportion of children with a first seizure (approximately 40% to 60%) do not experience a recurrence over the duration of follow-up. Moreover, the occurrence of a second episode, even though this arbitrarily defines epilepsy, does not signify that the child will develop a chronic incapacitating disorder.

The relatively high incidence of isolated epileptic seizures in adolescents, especially those of a partial motor or complex type, is discussed in Chapter 15. When a single seizure or a cluster of seizures occurs in an adolescent, the overall prognosis is favorable, with a likelihood for remaining seizure free of 67% after 5 years and 76% after 10 years. With simple partial seizures and a normal EEG, 100% of patients remain seizure free after 3 years. The figure is slightly lower (89%) for patients with complex partial seizures and a normal EEG (King et al., 1999; Loiseau and Orgogozo, 1978).

Approximately 20% of children with rolandic seizures have only one attack, as retrospective studies have shown (Ambrosetto et al., 1987; Beaussart and Faou, 1978; Loiseau and Beaussart, 1973; Beaussart, 1972).

The aforementioned figures have an obvious impact on the decision to treat. The decision should be discussed with the patients and parents because no firm evidence-based decision is possible when the clinician is facing the individual patient. Certainly, abstaining from therapy is reasonable when the risk of recurrence is low.

Outcome for Seizures in Patients with Confirmed Epilepsy

For the purpose of epidemiologic study, *epilepsy* is defined as the occurrence of at least two spontaneous (unprovoked) seizures that do not supervene in the same episode and that are not related to fever or an acute disorder. This definition is purely operational. However, patients who experience two seizures may have a higher risk of recurrence than do those with a first seizure, but they do not necessarily develop chronic epilepsy. Of those patients who experienced a second seizure, 79% went on to have at least a third seizure, even though they usually received antiepileptic agents (Camfield and Camfield, 2000). In a cohort of adults, Hauser and Hersdoffer (1990) and Hauser et al. (1990) noted that the recurrence rate after a second seizure was 65%, and 63% of those with a third seizure also experienced a fourth. In fact, including patients who had already experienced a second seizure in their study of the recurrence risk in patients who had experienced a first seizure resulted in only a minor increase in relapse rate (Hauser et al., 1990).

Remission Rate

Most studies of seizure outcome deal with treated epilepsy, even though the highly variable modalities of therapy and patient compliance are almost universally unreported. Figures for the recurrence rate in newly diagnosed epilepsy vary between 35% and 57% in the literature (Hart et al., 1990; Sander and Shorvon, 1987; Annegers et al., 1979).

In series of childhood epilepsy, more than half the patients were seizure free after a 10-year or longer follow-up. Actual figures at that point range between 51% (Sillanpää, 2000) and 82% (Oka et al., 1989). In a long (12 years), prospective, follow-up study of 119 children, Brorson and Wranne (1987) found an overall terminal remission rate of 64%. The 3-year terminal remission rate was 89% if the child's neurologic status was normal but 49% if the patient had "mental retardation" and/or abnormal neurology. In a study including both children and adults (Annegers et al., 1979), the remission rates were 42%, 61%, and 70% after follow-ups of 1 year, 10 years, and 15 years, respectively. In several long-term, prospective studies, Sillanpää (1990, 2000) and Sillanpää et al. (1998a) found 5-year terminal remission rates of 48% at 10 years, 56% at 20 years, 60% at 30 years, and 70% at 40 years. Interestingly, these studies included a sample of children with epilepsy that was typical of the child population in a well-defined, representative catchment area of Finland. About half the patients who were in remission were not on medication. The remission rate depended on the etiology of the seizures, with the 5-year terminal remission rates for idiopathic, cryptogenic, and remote symptomatic seizures being 95%, 68%, and 45%, respectively (Sillanpää, 2000). Another recent prospective study (Cockerell et al., 1997) found a 3-year terminal remission rate of 66% and a 5-year rate of 46% in children younger than 16 years after a 9-year follow-up. However, other studies have found a less favorable outcome. Ellenberg et al. (1984) found that 344 (67%) of their 513 children with epilepsy, excluding those with febrile convulsions and seizures associated with acute systemic disorders, still had seizures at the age of 7 years. Methodologic differences, especially in the criteria of inclusion and duration of follow-up, are probably important (Beghi and Tognoni, 1988; Goodridge and Shorvon, 1983a).

Excluding children with obvious associated brain damage, the overall prognosis for the seizures in those with "ordinary" uncomplicated epilepsy (Camfield and Camfield, 2000) is good in 70% to 80% of cases (Sillanpää et al., 1998a; Sander, 1993). Even lesional epilepsies can remit. Huttenlocher and Hapke (1990) followed 155 children, 145 of whom were not operated on, with refractory epilepsy that was not due to a progressive central nervous system disorder or tuberous sclerosis; 61% had mild to moderate retardation, and 39% were of borderline intelligence. Good seizure control in these children increased by roughly 4% yearly starting about 4 years after onset of epilepsy, and only one-fourth of those followed for 18 years or more continued to have more than one seizure per year. Even 1.5% of the children with mental retardation achieved control during each year of follow-up, but 70% still had seizures after 18 years. Similar results have been reported by Goulden et al. (1991). However, achieving control of such severe epilepsies by drug treatment takes often inordinately long periods of time, so surgery should be considered early when the seizures continue despite therapy.

Factors associated with structural brain pathology and the propensity toward intense seizures, such as age at onset and frequency of seizures, indicate a higher likelihood of persistence (Table 22.1). A symptomatic cause of epilepsy is especially ominous. Conversely, a rapid response to therapy is an important predictor of lasting remission with an odds ratio for remission of 2.22 to 1. Indeed, in a prospective, multifactorial study of 792 adults and children with seizures, McDonald et al. (2000) found that the single most important prognostic factor for remission was the number of seizures in the initial period of the disease. However, the number and the resistance of seizures might be related to the etiology. Complex partial seizures or atonic attacks herald a difficult epilepsy with odd ratios of remission of 0.26 to 1 and 0.28 to 1, respectively (Sillanpää, 2000).

The significance of the EEG as a predictor of outcome has been variably interpreted (Shinnar et al., 1994; Theodore et al., 1984b; Todt, 1984; Emerson et al., 1981; Rowan et al., 1980), which is hardly surprising because the tracings are not obtained under standard conditions and they represent only brief samples of the total EEG activity. The likelihood of obtaining patterns of prognostic value, if any are pre-

TABLE 22.1. *Probability of recurrences of seizures with the presence or absence of certain factors*

Factor	Low Probability	High Probability
Abnormalities on neurologic examination[a]	Absent	Present
Intellectual function[b]	Normal	Disturbed
Demonstrable brain lesion[b]	Absent	Present
Number of seizures	One	Multiple
Age at onset[a]	≥3–4 yr	<3 yr
Duration of uncontrolled seizures[b]	Brief	Long
Response to therapy[b]	Rapid	Slow/absent
Frequency of seizures[c]	Low	High
Tonic and/or atonic[a] seizures, episodes of status, complex partial seizures[c]	Absent	Present
Electroencephalogram[a]	Normal or normalized rapidly with treatment	Persistently abnormal
Treatment	Regularly taken	Irregular

[a]Significant factor.
[b]Major factor.
[c]Significance uncertain.

sent, varies with the number of recordings and the recording conditions. A normal EEG is a favorable omen (Shinnar et al., 1994). Sleep tracings and special recording techniques, such as long-duration tracings in a laboratory, or free conditions, especially when they are coupled with video recording, improve the value of EEG. However, no absolute relationship between the EEG and the recurrence of seizures exists.

An early age at onset has been associated with a poor outcome in most studies (Sillanpää, 2000; Todt, 1984; O'Leary et al., 1981) but not in that of Ellenberg and Nelson (1978), whose study was limited to children younger than 7 years. Epilepsies with onset in infancy and early childhood often have a severe course. Overall, a combination of favorable factors, especially the absence of brain damage, normal intelligence and neurologic examinations, and a rapid response to therapy, predicts an absence of seizures in the long term with a probability of 90% to 95% (Sillanpää, 2000).

The *remission rate in untreated patients* does not differ substantially from that of drug-treated newly diagnosed patients (Sillanpää, 2000; Annegers et al., 1979), varying between 16% and 43%. The remission rate in both treated and untreated patients increases with time. Patients who are left untreated because of the unavailability of drugs in some developing countries achieve a remission rate of about 50% (Shorvon and Farmer, 1988). One randomized trial showed no improvement in long-term outcome with treatment after first seizure as opposed to after later generalized

tonic-clonic seizures (Musico et al., 1997). However, rapid control of seizures can be obtained in 70% to 80% of previously untreated children (Sillanpää, 2000), indicating that drug treatment is significant. No compelling evidence indicates that early treatment is of value in the prevention of chronic epilepsy or later intractability (Sillanpää, 2000).

Relapse Rate on Withdrawal of Drug Treatment

Most epilepsies remit with antiepileptic drug (AED) treatment. Because of the possible inconvenience of prolonged therapy, the withdrawal of drugs is often considered when a substantial remission has been obtained. The required time of remission depends on the epilepsy syndrome; however, this is not universally agreed upon (Arts et al., 1988). Relapses can occur in 11% to 41% of patients (Berg and Shinnar, 1994). In a mixed, controlled study of 1,013 patients in remission, the risk for relapse for those without treatment was 41% within 2 years, compared with 22% for those randomized to continuing treatment (MRC Antiepileptic Drug Withdrawal Group, 1991). The risk is greatest in the 1 to 2 years after discontinuation.

The risk for relapses is higher in patients with a structural brain lesion, abnormal neurologic signs, learning difficulties, a long history of seizures before remission, the occurrence of more than one seizure type, and some epilepsy syndromes. The relapse rate tends to be lower in children than in adults (Sander, 1993). Most relapses usually are controlled by the resumption of the previous treatment. An abnormal EEG is a predictor of relapses, with the relative risk being 1.45 (range of 1.18 to 1.99) (Shinnar et al., 1994).

PROGNOSIS FOR INTELLIGENCE AND SOCIAL ADJUSTMENT

Intelligence

The intellectual abilities of children with epilepsy depend essentially on the cause of the disorder. Children with idiopathic epilepsy usually have normal or even superior intelligence, except in some rare types. However, subtle cognitive and language dysfunctions can be detected in some idiopathic syndromes, such as epilepsy with rolandic spikes (Massa et al., 2001; Deonna et al., 2000a; Staden et al., 1998; Weglage et al., 1997). These may partly be related to the occurrence of transient cognitive impairment (TCI) (Kasteleijn-Nolst Trenité et al., 1988; Binnie et al., 1987) occurring at the time of EEG discharges or to an undetermined maturation defect of the brain (Doose and Baier, 1989). On the contrary, those with brain lesions do significantly worse, although this does vary to some degree. In Finland, 23% to 41% of children with epilepsy had an intelligence quotient (IQ) less than 70 (Sillanpää, 1990, 2000). Special education, whether in institutions or in the community, was required for 30%. However, the need for institutionalization was seldom, if ever, due to the epilepsy; it was due instead to the associated retardation and neurologic disability. Clearly, the cause of epilepsy is the major factor, but the epilepsy itself is important because it multiplies the effect of the existing disabilities rather than simply adding to them.

Learning difficulties of variable severity are present in 5% to 50% of children with seizures. Complex partial seizures seem particularly noxious in this regard (Schoenfeld et al., 1999). Schoenfeld et al. (1999) found that children with complex partial seizures, no comorbid conditions, and a normal magnetic resonance imaging (MRI) scan were inferior to the controls in all seven cognitive domains studied, indicating the presence of a relatively diffuse cognitive deficit. An early age at onset was significantly associated with cognitive difficulties, whereas the frequency of seizures was a predictor of behavioral problems.

Cognitive and behavioral problems are relatively stable in most children with epilepsy. In his classic study, Rodin (1968) found a low intelligence in children with brain lesions, whereas, in "pure" epilepsy,

the IQ was within normal limits, although the curve of IQ was shifted to the left. In the whole group, a mild, irregular downward trend was present, and significant loss was seen in only some cases. Sillanpää (2000) found some deterioration in 60% of his patients, and Bourgeois et al. (1983b) identified decreases in IQ in 11% of their children.

When deterioration is present, it is usually mild to moderate. It is probably related not only to multiple factors, including biological ones among which repeated head trauma resulting from seizures may play a role, but also and perhaps predominantly to sociocultural and psychologic difficulties, low expectations and low self-esteem, and the side effects of drug treatment. The cumulative damage from seizures remains a disputed issue. Experimental research has demonstrated the possibility of neuronal loss, dendritic changes, modifications in the number and regulation of receptors and neurotransmitters, and changes in connectivity, but whether these occur in humans, particularly in children (Holmes, 1991a; Moshé, 1993), except in the case of prolonged seizures, is as yet not fully documented. In general, short seizures do not appear to have a major effect on gross development, and only children with catastrophic seizures are severely retarded (Camfield and Camfield, 2000).

Austin et al. (1999) compared the academic achievements of 98 children with nonlesional epilepsy and 96 with chronic asthma over 4 years, assessing them in the following five areas: composite, reading, mathematics, language, and vocabulary. The children with epilepsy did worse in all five achievement areas. Those with inactive or low-severity epilepsy had mean scores within the range of the national United Kingdom scores, whereas those with severe epilepsy were behind. The performance scores were unchanged over the 4-year study period. Though these results are encouraging overall, they clearly point to the problems associated with severe seizure disorders.

A much more severe and rarer type of cognitive and/or behavioral deterioration occurs in certain specific groups of syndromes, particularly in infants and young children. Examples include the West and Lennox-Gastaut syndromes; severe myoclonic epilepsy of infants; and syndromes with continuous EEG paroxysmal activity, such as electrical status epilepticus of slow sleep and Landau-Kleffner syndrome. Remarkably, in these syndromes, deterioration can occur even in the absence of clinical seizures or in the face of only mild seizure activity. Although the causes and mechanisms of this *epileptic deterio-*

ration are not known, the paroxysmal activity seen in the EEG almost certainly plays an important role. This is shown by the temporal coincidence between the paroxysmal EEG and deterioration, as the latter never disappears as long as the EEG remains grossly abnormal. This is further supported by the similar localization of the maximum EEG abnormalities and the neuropsychologic deficits (e.g., aphasia and temporal paroxysms in Landau-Kleffner syndrome, autism and executive function deficits with frontally predominant spike-waves [Tassinari et al., 1971]) and by the (sometimes) concomitant fluctuations in the severity of both the clinical and EEG disturbances (Billard et al., 1990). Some hypothetical mechanisms for this deterioration are considered elsewhere in this book (see Chapter 11). Although the evidence indicting paroxysmal activity is incomplete and the possibility exists that other mechanisms (e.g., vascular factors [Cross et al., 1997]) may also be responsible, its probable role justifies determined attempts to control not only the seizures but also the paroxysmal activity, the most striking manifestation of which is found on the EEG.

To a certain extent, the long-lasting clinical manifestations of epileptic deterioration can be regarded as an extension of the short-lasting cognitive dysfunctions that occur concomitantly with the brief epileptic discharges known as TCIs (Kasteleijn-Nolst Trenité et al., 1988; Binnie et al., 1987).

When the paroxysmal activity is continuous or quite prolonged, the cognitive and behavioral deterioration may represent a form of "subclinical" nonconvulsive status epilepticus. Deonna (1996) has labeled such situations *cognitive epilepsy*, a term that implies a direct relationship between the EEG and clinical manifestations. The same relationship is implied by the term *epileptic encephalopathy* (Engel, 2001). However, the persistence of the deterioration beyond the period during which the paroxysmal EEG activity persists seems to indicate that such activity can produce lasting changes in brain function, probably through the changes in brain circuitry that are possible in the young, developing, plastic brain. Whether such an effect can be prevented by current therapies is a fascinating dilemma. Although the efficacy of prevention has not been proven, the attempts at prevention by vigorous treatment are probably justified (see Chapters 3, 4, 5, and 6).

AEDs may play a role in cognitive and behavioral problems of children with epilepsy (Bourgeois, 1998; Calandre et al., 1990; Trimble, 1990a; Aldenkamp et al., 1987; Thompson et al., 1987; Hirtz and Nelson, 1985). Some investigators have thought that the in-

fluence of anticonvulsant drugs has been underestimated (Thompson and Trimble, 1982).

The evaluation of the possible deleterious effects of drugs is particularly important because these can be avoided by careful use. Reports in the literature have suggested that persons with epilepsy may display various cognitive impairments, including impoverished memory, reduced attentional capacity (Stores, 1971, 1978, 1981), and mental slowness (Corbett, 1991; Trimble and Corbett, 1980). The exact role played by drugs in such deficits has been variously assessed because of methodologic problems (Hirtz and Nelson, 1985). Studies in volunteers (Trimble, 1990a; Trimble and Cull, 1988) have shown that "AEDs did have a measurable, generally detrimental, effect on test performance, although differences between the drugs were apparent." Phenytoin and, to a lesser extent, the benzodiazepines and valproate do affect results on some tests of memory, mental processing, and speed; in these, the effects achieve significance only when the demands of the tasks are increased. Carbamazepine affected only motor, but not mental, speed.

Studies in institutionalized epileptic patients have shown that mental functioning generally is improved by a reduction in the number of drugs used even when blood levels are not in the toxic range for any of the individual medications; however, high doses and high serum levels do produce more impairment than lower ones (Thompson and Trimble, 1982). Significant decreases in IQ have been observed in patients receiving anticonvulsant drugs (McLachlan, 1987; Zaret and Cohen, 1986; Thompson and Trimble, 1983). The greatest decreases in IQ were observed in patients with the highest blood levels of AEDs, especially when phenytoin was used. On average, carbamazepine again had fewer adverse effects on mental processing and memory than did phenytoin or valproate (Bourgeois et al., 1983b, 1998; Lesser et al., 1986; Ambrosetto et al., 1985). Phenobarbital and primidone may also have detrimental effects on cognitive function in addition to their influence on behavior, although remarkably few studies on these drugs are available (Thompson and Trimble, 1983; Viani et al., 1977; Reynolds, 1975). The long-term effects of the newer AEDs have yet to be fully determined (see Chapter 24); lamotrigine seems to be the drug with the fewest cognitive and behavioral side effects.

These results are, however, not easy to interpret. The decrease in IQ may not result from treatment but may simply be associated with mental deterioration, especially in more severe cases in which the patients require higher drug dosages. However, the combination of data on the acute effects of the drug in volunteers and those on the decreases in IQ with long-term treatment in institutionalized epileptics gives weight to a direct role of anticonvulsants, especially phenytoin. On the other hand, alternative explanations cannot be discarded. Corbett (1991) reported preliminary data of marked decreases in IQ (up to 30 points or more) in institutionalized children, most of whom were not on phenytoin or other "depressive" drugs.

At this stage, the effects of most drugs may have been overemphasized (Aldenkamp et al., 1987), and antiepileptic agents likely are not a major factor in the mental deterioration of children with epilepsy. The possible effect of phenobarbital on intelligence (Farwell et al., 1990) has not been confirmed. Nonetheless, some agents may have a major effect on cognitive functions in individual patients. Moreover, some drugs can have a relatively specific effect on the thought process. For example, topiramate may produce language and thought disturbances in some children (Reife, 1996; Reife et al., 1995).

Social Adjustment

Social adjustment depends not only on the cognitive level but also on specific learning difficulties and psychiatric factors. The lifetime prevalence of psychotic disorders varies from 3% to 5% (Jalava and Sillanpää, 1998; Okuma and Kumashiro, 1981). Camfield et al. (1993) found behavioral disturbances that were sufficiently pronounced to require mental health consultation in 22% of normally intelligent patients with childhood-onset epilepsy. Jalava and Sillanpää (1998) found that 39 (41%) of 94 patients followed for 35 years had psychiatric disorders of any type, versus 12 (12%) of 99 matched general population controls. Three percent of these patients had a psychotic disease, and none was observed in the controls. The odds ratio for all psychiatric disorders in people with epilepsy versus controls was 4.0 (confidence interval [CI] of 1.6 to 10).

Education

Young adults with childhood-onset epilepsy living in the community fail to go beyond the primary educational level more often than do controls (20% versus 2%). Only 33% to 49% of children with uncomplicated epilepsy attain an upper secondary education level, with or without a university degree, compared with 68% to 77% of matched controls (Aldenkamp et al., 1990; Aldenkamp, 1983). Even those patients with childhood-onset idiopathic epilepsy that is in remission and who are taking no medication achieved only a primary education more often than the controls (56% versus 23%). Thus, the impact of even benign epilepsy on the quality of life of children is quite substantial, and sociopsychologic factors are important in this field.

Additional specific difficulties are also a factor. Aldenkamp et al. (1990) encountered different types of problems in children with epilepsy. Mental slowness was sometimes marked, and memory and attention deficits also played a role. These deficits were most prominent in children taking polytherapy.

The predictors of academic failure include the age of the child at onset of epilepsy, lifetime seizure frequency, and multiple seizure types (Seidenberg et al., 1986).

Employment

In the long follow-up study of Sillanpää (1990), more than 50% of adults with childhood-onset epilepsy were able to work, and 60% were actually employed—30% were white-collar employees, 34% were manual workers, and 36% were unemployed. These figures reflect the societal attitudes toward epilepsy and the limited vocational education training that 74% of patients versus 95% of matched controls had obtained. Of these patients, 42% thought they had been stigmatized because of their epilepsy and that they had been denied opportunities.

The risk of unemployment is increased in those with an organic etiology, associated difficulties, or both. Psychoneurotic behavior and poor results of short-term treatment are strong predictors of employment difficulties. Accidents and sickness absences are not more common among people with epilepsy than among their fellow employees (Scampler and Hopkins, 1980). The prognosis for social adjustment was good in 62% of the Japanese children participating in the multicenter study (Okuma and Kumashiro, 1981), and, in an additional 9%, the social adjustment was almost normal.

Clearly, behavioral difficulties can be more important than seizures for the overall social outcome. However, the trend is for children with fits that are difficult to control to accumulate multiple handicaps.

In one very long-term study (Sillanpää, 2000), 60% of adults with childhood-onset epilepsy were well adjusted and were completely independent in the activities of daily living, while 15% required only little assistance. Of the remainder, 21% percent were dependent on continual assistance and support by other persons. Only 4% to 15% of those with uncomplicated epilepsy report that their condition influences their way of life (Jalava and Sillanpää, 1997; Jalava et al., 1997).

Of patients with childhood-onset epilepsy, 35% were not married or cohabiting versus 10% of controls. However, the figures for those with idiopathic epilepsy that was in remission and who were off medication was lower at 30% (Sillanpää, 2000). The fertility rate was significantly lower in those with epilepsy than in the controls. The self-estimation of the quality of life was generally good in the whole group, but it was poor in patients with persistent seizures and in those on polypharmacy (Baker et al., 1997; Hanai, 1992).

MORTALITY IN EPILEPSY

Patients with epilepsy suffer an excess mortality at all ages (Tomson and Forsgren, 2003; Hauser et al., 1980; Zielinski, 1975). In a series devoted exclusively to childhood epilepsy, mortality during the first 10 years after onset was 5.7%, and another 2.9% of the patients died between 11 and 12 years after onset (Kurokawa et al., 1982).

More recent studies have confirmed these data (Breningstall, 2001). Trevathan et al. (1997) reported that 4% of their epileptic population died before 11 years of age. An Australian study found a mortality rate of 3 per 1,000 individuals, compared with 0.23 per 1,000 in control children (Harvey et al., 1993c).

Mortality is much higher in those epilepsies with an onset before the age of 1 year, in symptomatic epilepsy, and in infantile spasms than it was in epilepsies with grand mal seizures. Excess mortality is also present in population-based studies. In a review of the literature, Harvey et al. (1993c) found the mean estimate of death in epileptic children younger than 15 years was approximately 5 per 1,000 children. Children with secondary epilepsy accounted for 94% of all deaths (Harvey et al., 1993c). The standardized mortality ratio was 2.5 in a British study involving both children and adults (Cockerell et al., 1994, 1997). Higher mortality ratios were found for the younger patients in the Rochester group study (Annegers and Coan, 1999; O'Donoghue and Sander, 1997) and in a Finnish study (Sillanpää, 2000), in which the ratio was 6.23 per 1,000 person-years with a large excess in patients with symptomatic epilepsies. By and large, the overall mortality among patients of all ages is two to three times that of the general population (O'Donoghue and Sander, 1997). Although the causes of death are quite variable, sudden unexpected death, accidents, and suicide deserve special consideration.

Sudden Unexpected Death in Epilepsy

The excessive frequency of sudden unexpected death in epilepsy (SUDEP) was initially suggested by autopsy studies of causes of death among patients with epilepsy, especially those in young subjects. In one study (Shorvon, 1997), SUDEP accounted for 63% of the deaths in epileptics.

The criteria for a diagnosis of SUDEP are a nontraumatic, unwitnessed death occurring in a patient with epilepsy who had previously been relatively healthy and in whom no cause of death is found even after a thorough postmortem examination (Annegers and Coan, 1999; Leestma, 1990; Leestma et al., 1984). Many SUDEPs are probably seizure related (i.e., they occur during or shortly after a seizure when no evidence of status epilepticus is found and no other explanation for death exists). This is supported by the finding in a case–control study that the risk of SUDEP in adolescents and adults was 10 times higher in patients with frequent (more than 50 per year) seizures (Nilsson et al., 1997) and that it was greater in those with frequent changes of drugs and doses and in those with early onset epilepsies. The occurrence of sudden death only in patients with seizure recurrence, whereas it did not occur in those patients who became seizure free after successful surgery, may further suggest this (Sperling et al., 1999).

SUDEP accounts for 7.5% to 17% of the excess mortality ratio in patients with epilepsy (Lathers and Schraeder, 1990). It occurs more often in patients with severe epilepsy and generalized seizures. In children, SUDEP was responsible for 10% of deaths among those between 2 and 20 years of age in one study (Keeting and Knowles, 1989) and for 12% of deaths in young children in another study (Harvey et al., 1993c). The incidence might be greatest in children and adolescents, although this has been disputed (Nashef et al., 1995a, 1995c). Sudden death in epilepsy may be due to several mechanisms, including suffocation, pulmonary edema, and cardiac arrhythmias probably related to brainstem involvement in the discharge, but no single mechanism has been proved (Breningstall, 2001).

Role of Accidents in Mortality

Overall, the rate of accidents among persons with epilepsy does not differ significantly from that in the rest of the population (Hauser et al., 1980), but relatively few reliable data are available (Tomson and Forsgren, 2003). In adults and probably in children, a small group of accident-prone people accounts for most of the accidents among persons with epilepsy (Sonnen, 1991). In general, the fear of accidents is likely excessive given the current data. However, Wirrell et al. (1996) reported that the rate of serious injury as a direct result of a seizure was 15% in a cohort of 59 children with absence epilepsy followed to at least 18 years of age. These authors felt the risk was minimal with most other types of seizure. Hauser et al. (1980) attributed 12 of 185 deaths to accident in a prospective cohort study, whereas only 4.9 were statistically expected. Krohn (1963) found that 12 (11%) of 107 deaths in people with epilepsy were due to seizure-related accidents.

Head traumas are more common in some children with atonic or tonic seizures, in whom this may represent a major problem. Skull and face protection is essential in such cases. However, very serious injuries are uncommon. Of the 12,626 seizures associated with falls that were recorded in a center for children and adolescents, 766 resulted in significant head injuries, with 422 requiring simple dressing and 341 requiring sutures. One skull fracture and two intracranial hemorrhages were observed (Russel-Jones and Shorvon, 1989).

The incidence of drowning is roughly four times greater in children with epilepsy than in the general population. Most frequently, the drowning occurs at home, as occurred in 11 of the 14 deaths studied by Krohn (1963). The relative risk of drowning for children with epilepsy from 5 to 19 years of age, compared with that of the general population, was considerably increased, reaching 1,309.9 (CI of 157.1 to 10,819.1) for bathtub drowning and 54.1 (CI of 27.1 to 107.8) for swimming pools. The risk was not increased in children younger than 5 years, probably due to the careful supervision of small children.

Burns occurring during or immediately after a seizure are a significant hazard. In one study (Spitz, 1992), 25 (12%) of 244 patients with epilepsy suffered such an accident. The most severe burns occurred during showering.

INDIVIDUAL FACTORS RELATED TO PROGNOSIS

Most cases of childhood epilepsies run a favorable course. A recent collaborative study in children, adolescents, and adults, 68% of whom were younger than 19 years and 11% than 4 years, found the cumulative probability of a 1-year remission of 62% at 1 year after the initiation of treatment, 81% at 2 years, 92% at 3 years, and 98% at 5 years. The probabilities of a 2-year and a 3-year remission at 5 years were 92% and

78%, respectively (Cockerell et al., 1997). Despite these optimistic figures, severe cases do occur, so methods of improving prognostic abilities clearly are of interest.

The prediction of the outcome of epilepsy in a specific individual can be improved by two methods, the results of which are largely complementary. Because different epilepsy syndromes have widely diverse outcomes (Jallon, 2003), making a syndromic diagnosis is clearly desirable. In some cases, such a diagnosis permits an accurate prognosis (e.g., benign rolandic epilepsy), as the previous chapters have described. In a sizable proportion of cases, however, making a diagnosis of a syndrome leaves a significant degree of uncertainty regarding the outlook. This is the case for many of those with myoclonic or grand mal epilepsy, and a complementary approach that can help reduce the spectrum of possibilities is of obvious importance.

The probability of a favorable outcome is increased significantly when all or some of the following factors are present:

1. Absence of abnormalities at neurologic examination;
2. Normal intellectual function;
3. Absence of a demonstrable brain lesion;
4. Occurrence of only one type of seizure;
5. Relatively brief duration of uncontrolled seizures and a good response to antiepileptic treatment;
6. Late onset of seizures (i.e., after 3 or 4 years of age);
7. Low frequency of seizures;
8. Absence of certain types of attacks, especially tonic and/or atonic seizures, and of *episodes* of status epilepticus; possibly the absence of complex partial seizures as well;
9. Normality of the EEG at the start of treatment or the disappearance of EEG abnormalities with therapy;
10. Rapid response to therapy
11. Regular compliance with antiepileptic treatment.

Conversely, the absence of these factors is associated with a lower probability of remission, and some specific factors, such as tonic seizures or spasms, can be a cause for concern, even though they do not always herald a poor outcome.

The significance of the EEG as a predictor of outcome has been variably interpreted (Shinnar et al., 1994; Gross-Tsur and Shinnar, 1993; Theodore et al., 1984b; Todt, 1984; Rowan et al., 1980), which is hardly surprising given the variations in timing and duration of recordings. The persistence of paroxysmal discharges is worrying, whereas a normal sleep EEG is favorable.

Combining the favorable factors listed earlier may permit a more accurate prediction of the outcome. Sillanpää (2000) has shown that the combination of one type of seizure only, a good response to treatment, a normal development, and no occurrence of status epilepticus predicts, in the long term, an absence of seizures with a probability of 90% or 95%.

Interestingly, the same factors that predict seizure control are also associated with a favorable outlook for educational and social adjustment. Thus, the degree of predictability of a number of cases of childhood epilepsy is relatively high, and a definite syndrome diagnosis is not always necessary. Separating relatively favorable cases from severe ones in whom a combination of impairments and consequent disabilities can be very disabling is generally possible. The former group, which comprises some 70% to 80% of cases of uncomplicated epilepsy in the community, represents a majority. The remaining 20% to 30% have problems with control, associated disabilities, or both. A whole spectrum of outcomes between two extremes can be obtained.

Relatively Benign Epilepsies

Another way to approach the prognosis of epilepsy of childhood is to attempt to delineate those recognizable epilepsy syndromes that run a consistently predictable course so that recognition of a particular syndrome enables the clinician to provide a firm, specific prognosis. That approach has recently received great attention, especially for predicting a benign outcome. "Benign" epilepsy syndromes have thus been defined, the best recognized of which are idiopathic partial epilepsy of childhood with rolandic (or centrotemporal) spikes or rolandic epilepsy (see Chapter 10).

The term *benign* implies an invariably favorable outcome, even in the absence of treatment, with ultimate and definitive remission before adulthood and the absence of severe or exceedingly disturbing seizures and of the associated serious intellectual or behavioral disturbances. It also implies that early recognition is possible with reasonable certainty. Rolandic epilepsy fulfills these conditions satisfactorily, even though rare exceptions and minor neurodevelopmental abnormalities are sometimes present.

Other "benign" epilepsy syndromes have been proposed. They include benign occipital epilepsy (Panayiotopoulos and Igoe, 1992; Panayiotopoulos, 1989b), benign affective epilepsy (Dalla Bernardina et al., 1992a), benign frontal epilepsy, and benign my-

oclonic epilepsy of infants (Dravet et al., 1992b). The actual benignity and, indeed, the delineation of some of these syndromes are still uncertain, and the possibility of early diagnosis has not been firmly established. In some, behavioral disturbances or learning difficulties can occur (Weglage et al., 1997). Thus, among the 26 patients with "benign affective epilepsy" who were initially reported by Dalla Bernardina (1992a), 5 continued to have seizures during adolescence or early adulthood, and one of these was found to harbor a brain tumor.

Indeed, many of the "benign" syndromes have been isolated in retrospective studies because of their favorable outcome without comparing these cases with the original population from which they had been drawn. The delineation of benign epilepsy syndromes should make them clearly recognizable at onset or shortly thereafter; furthermore, their benignity should be verified in prospective, long-term studies. In addition, their diagnosis should permit a significant improvement in predictive accuracy, compared with a classic study of the factors linked to the prognosis. Such criteria are seldom fulfilled, and, in many cases, a factorial approach is as precise as, and is easier to apply than, the syndromic one.

Severe Epilepsies

Severe epilepsies form the other end of the spectrum. As has been indicated, these often combine the characteristics of being difficult to control with additional deficits, and they are commonly associated with structural brain abnormalities. Such cases account for 20% to 40% of all epilepsies, and a significant fraction of these are resistant to AED therapy.

Intractable Epilepsies

Intractable epilepsies have been the subject of many studies, especially with the development of epilepsy surgery (Aicardi, 1988a; Schmidt, 1986a; Juul-Jensen, 1963). However, no single clear-cut definition of intractability has been formulated. Whereas Juul-Jensen (1963) broadly defined intractable epilepsy as an epilepsy that did not respond to "relevant" therapy, other investigators have tried to define the limits of intractability precisely using practical terms (Gilman et al., 1994; Schmidt, 1986a). Schmidt (1982, 1986a) has proposed that medical intractability is a graded, rather than an "all or none," phenomenon with cases ranging from mildly to highly resistant to therapy.

Indeed, intractability is not a purely biological phenomenon. The decision on whether an epilepsy should be considered intractable must take into account the desires of the patient and family, the lifestyle of the patient, the patient's views about the risks and side effects of treatment, and the limitations of treatment. The endpoint of therapy must be clearly defined, and the possible means for attaining this endpoint, whether medical or surgical, as well as the balance of risks, must be explained thoroughly to the patient and/or family.

Because of these uncertainties, estimating the frequency of intractable epilepsy is not possible, although this problem is obviously crucial. An early prediction of intractability is obviously of clinical importance, but, given the above variables, it may be difficult. Recently, Berg et al. (2001) tried to identify children likely to develop intractable seizures prospectively; 60 of their 613 patients met the criteria for intractable epilepsy during follow-up. After adjustment for the epilepsy syndrome, the initial seizure frequency, focal EEG slowing, and a history of acute symptomatic or neonatal status epilepticus were significantly associated with an increased risk of intractability. Only 2.7% of children with idiopathic epilepsy became intractable. Half the children with intractable epilepsy had nonidiopathic localization-related epilepsy syndromes.

Before accepting the diagnosis of intractability, the physician should exclude causes of *apparent* intractability (Table 22.2), which results from the misdiagnoses of nonepileptic seizures, the type of seizures, or the epilepsy syndrome (e.g., confusion between absences and complex partial seizures) or from a failure to detect an underlying cause, such as a tumor or progressive brain disease. Errors leading to incorrect therapy should also be considered (see Chapter 24).

The problems of *surgically* intractable epilepsies are considered in Chapter 25. Once more, this is a graded phenomenon because cases can be unfit for resective surgery but may possibly be amenable to palliative operations.

SUMMARY

The prognosis for children with epilepsy depends largely on the type of epilepsy syndrome in the particular patient. However, certain general predictors of prognosis exist. These predictors are usually valid for the long-term recurrence of seizures and for the mental and neurologic prognosis.

TABLE 22.2. *Causes of apparent intractability in childhood epilepsy*

Cause	Examples
Erroneous diagnosis of epilepsy	Pseudoseizures and peudostatus epilepticus
	Syncopes of cardiac or other origin
	Other nonepileptic attacks, e.g., paroxysmal dystonia and other movement disorders, migraine, and paroxysmal sleep disturbances
Erroneous diagnosis of type of epilepsy	Absence seizures mistaken for complex partial seizures and vice versa with resultant inefficacy of drugs
Failure to detect underlying central nervous system disease	Brain tumors
	Progressive degenerative disease
	Metabolic disease
Failure to detect precipitating factor	Sleep deprivation
	Use of certain drugs, alcohol
	Light stimulation (e.g., videogames)
	Erratic lifestyle
Errors in management	Noncompliance
	Use of inappropriate drug, such as drugs with potential aggravating effect (e.g., carbamazepine or vigabatrin in primary generalized seizures)
	Use of inappropriate dosage
	Usually too low (some patients may need *supratherapeutic* blood levels)
	Occasionally too high (e.g., phenytoin or clonazepam precipitating seizures)
	Inappropriate timing of doses
	Inappropriate drug associations (because of pharmacokinetic or pharmacodynamic interactions)
	Failure to use all available major drugs

The factors associated with a favorable outlook include an absence of neurologic and mental abnormalities; a limited number of seizures, especially those of grand mal type; the presence of a single type of seizure; and rapid control of seizures. They also include the absence of certain types of seizure, particularly of tonic and atonic attacks. A relatively late age at onset (after the age of 2 or 3 years) is also favorable, and a family history of epilepsy generally is unimportant. When all of these favorable factors are present, a complete remission of seizures may be expected in most patients. The risk of recurrences after the discontinuation of treatment depends on the same factors as the remission of seizures. Conversely, factors associated with a poor prognosis include an organic cause of the seizures; the presence of mental and/or neurologic abnormalities; and the existence of several types of seizure, including frequent grand mal attacks and/or tonic and atonic seizures.

The most useful investigation for establishment of prognosis is the EEG, which is of value for determining the risk of recurrence and for refining the precise diagnosis, especially with regard to syndromes. Imaging studies may also be helpful, but this is probably true only in selected cases.

Apparently intractable epilepsies can result from errors of diagnosis or management. True intractability is primarily associated with specific syndromes of generalized epilepsy or with partial epilepsies of lesional origin. A regular reassessment of children with apparently intractable seizures is essential because the cause may not be immediately detectable.

Certain epilepsy syndromes have an extremely high incidence of remission that approaches 100%; these are known as *benign epilepsies*. However, the concept of benign epilepsy must not be applied too broadly if it is to retain its value in clinical neurology. At this moment, only benign epilepsy with centrotemporal foci fully qualifies for inclusion in this group.

The possible adverse effects of drugs on mental functioning that have been described in institutionalized patients are probably less likely to occur with present-day drugs. Careful monitoring and the parsimonious use of drugs that may depress the patient's mental functioning are nonetheless advised.

23

General Principles of Management

The management of epilepsy can be conceived only as a global therapeutic strategy applied to individual patients. The management of the epilepsies of childhood has a wider scope than the sole prevention of both seizures and the other consequences of paroxysmal neurophysiologic dysfunction. The epilepsies are socially handicapping disorders, and even a single seizure occurring in certain circumstances may have disastrous effects. The impact of epilepsy on every aspect of both the child's and the family's life is considerable (Carpay et al., 1996, 1997; Hoare and Russel, 1995; Collings, 1990; Levin et al., 1988). Recurrent seizures severely disrupt the personal and social life of the patients, and uncontrolled epilepsy may definitively compromise both the physical safety and the overall quality of life of the affected children or adolescents. The risks of physical injury are real. Death, especially sudden death, has a higher incidence in the epileptic population than it does in the general population (Sperling et al., 1999; Nashef et al., 1995a, 1995b) (see Chapter 22).

The unpredictable character of the seizures represents a considerable burden in everyday life, and this applies even to those patients whose seizures are well controlled by drug therapy. Recent studies (Birbeck et al., 2002) have provided clear-cut evidence supporting the assertion that health-related quality-of-life improvement was consistently evident only among those patients achieving seizure freedom. The long-term outcome must also be considered, and appropriate advice on what the indications for treatment are must be sought (Sillanpää, 2000).

In addition to the obvious problems posed by overt seizures, *apparent subclinical epileptic activity* may, in some patients, profoundly disturb their mental functioning. This is seen in children with prolonged episodes of nonconvulsive status epilepticus. In addition, such an effect may possibly occur in those with major paroxysmal electroencephalographic (EEG) abnormalities that are unassociated with clinical seizures or that are accompanied only by infrequent and apparently minor attacks, such as those observed in the syndrome of continuous spike-wave paroxysms of slow sleep (Chapter 11); Landau-Kleffner syndrome; and the so-called atypical cases of rolandic

epilepsy, despite the usually benign course of this syndrome (De Saint Martin et al., 2001; Massa et al., 2001).

Subclinical epileptic activity may have undesirable effects, at least in some patients. Several reports have indicated that isolated paroxysms or brief EEG bursts could interfere with ongoing cognitive processes (Aldenkamp et al., 1992; Kasteleijn-Nolst Trenité et al., 1988, 1990; Siebeling et al., 1988; Aarts et al., 1984). Such *transient cognitive impairments* may be global, especially with bilateral spike-wave discharges, which mostly affect the level of awareness, or more specialized for left or right hemisphere functions, as occurs in focal discharges (Kasteleijn-Nolst Trenité et al., 1988, 1990; Stores, 1971, 1980).

In addition, under certain circumstances, recurrent brief seizures may produce brain damage, and repeated stimulation by the frequent seizures and/or EEG discharges might, in itself, be conducive to an epileptic state. This is in concordance with the view that seizures are a self-perpetuating phenomenon (Shorvon, 1984). Such an effect could result from kindling (Goddard et al., 1969), but, more probably, it is due to different, as yet undefined mechanisms (Lado et al., 2002; Nehlig et al., 1999).

Therefore, *all reasonable efforts* should be made to prevent seizures and the other effects of epileptic activity. Treatment is clearly indicated in children with clinical seizures if the likelihood of recurrences is high (see Chapters 15 and 22). The indications for antiepileptic treatment for children with subclinical epileptic activity are more difficult to define. "Treatment of the EEG" is, in principle, not desirable in asymptomatic patients. Nonetheless, when cognitive difficulties or deterioration appear in a child with paroxysmal EEG discharges, treatment may be considered, even in the absence of classic seizures. At this time, however, no dogmatic statement can be made regarding this (Arzimanoglou, 2002b; Guerrini et al., 2002a). Children who are not initially treated for asymptomatic EEG discharges should receive regular neuropsychologic evaluation so that a slowly progressive decline of intellectual performances can be detected. In some cases, the interference of infraclinical discharges with mental functioning has been clearly demonstrated to represent a major problem, and, after therapy was instituted, all difficulties were corrected. A librarian who was a patient of Aarts et al. (1984) had subclinical discharges that appeared only when he was concentrating on his work. When these were controlled, he was able to resume work efficiently. In patients with language disturbances (the Landau-Kleffner syndrome), these do not usually disappear as long as the ongoing EEG paroxysms remain uncontrolled, and controlling the continuous paroxysmal activity during sleep may result in an improvement in language function (Deuel and Lenn, 1997).

However, the control of seizures and especially of EEG paroxysmal activity should not be obtained by compromising the intellectual and physical capabilities of the patients. All antiepileptic drugs (AEDs) can have unfavorable effects on behavior and/or the learning processes (Aldenkamp, 2001; Trimble, 1990a; Aldenkamp et al., 1987, 1990), and heavy treatment may result in a severe deficit of attention and cognitive skills (Meador, 2001). The treatment *must*, therefore, remain compatible with a normal family and social life.

For many children, the sociopsychologic factors far outweigh the mere problem of seizure prevention. Epilepsy goes far beyond simply having fits, a concept that the clinician should keep in mind when he or she is planning comprehensive care for the individual patient. The aim of treatment is an improvement in the patient's global quality of life. Control of seizures may be useless or it may even have a negative effect because epilepsy is a chronic illness that comes to dominate the life of patients and to constitute, in some cases, their pivotal interest and justification (Taylor, 1993; Trostle et al., 1989; Viberg et al., 1987; Betts, 1983).

TREATMENT OPTIONS

AEDs are the most commonly used therapy for epilepsy. All AEDs have some potential side effects, so the indications for their use should be carefully weighed as one of the main objectives is controlling seizures without producing drug-related undesirable effects. In the last decade, about 10 new AEDs have become available. However, the overall efficacy of both the old and the new drugs is moderate at best. In a recent study (Kwan and Brodie, 2000), only 331 individuals (63%) in a cohort of 525 patients were seizure free. The situation for infants and children is even more serious as a number of epilepsy syndromes remain difficult to treat. Adrenocorticotropic hor-

mone and steroids can be used as antiepileptic agents for special indications, and they may be more effective than the usual AEDs (Deonna, 1991; Lerman et al., 1991; Marescaux et al., 1990). When the newer drugs are compared with conventional AEDS, the newer drugs are certainly tolerated better, but their potential side effects are not negligible (Marson et al., 1996).

Recent evidence suggests that various epilepsy syndromes respond differently to AEDs (Arzimanoglou, 2002b). Therefore, a more precise diagnosis and a better understanding of the mechanisms of action of AEDs enable physicians to use AEDs more specifically and more effectively (Aicardi and Arzimanoglou, 1996). The patient's characteristics, including age at onset, seizure frequency, EEG data, and the findings of imaging studies, provide diagnostic pointers that permit the physician to reach a diagnosis of the *syndrome* and to choose the most appropriate AED for the individual patient. However, the specificity of AEDs is relatively limited, and, often, pharmacotherapy is begun with an agent with a broad spectrum of activity that is appropriate for the primary seizure type. Indeed, several antiepileptic agents have a similar or identical effectiveness for one particular form of epilepsy. Therefore, the eventual side effects and the difficulties in the practical handling of the drug play an essential role in the choice of a therapeutic agent. Cost must also be a consideration (Guerrini et al., 2001; Arzimanoglou et al., 1998)

The drug-induced exacerbation of seizures is a clinical problem that is often unrecognized or overlooked. Although further studies evaluating the prevalence of this phenomenon and investigating its mechanisms are required, a review of existing data (Guerrini et al., 1998c; Perucca et al., 1998) implicated the following two separate processes: (a) a nonspecific manifestation of drug intoxication due to excessive doses or polypharmacy or (b) a specific adverse action of a drug on specific seizure types or in certain epilepsy syndromes.

Carbamazepine has been reported to precipitate or to exacerbate a variety of seizures (myoclonic or absence), particularly in patients with idiopathic generalized epilepsies. In focal epilepsies, on the other hand, a recent report (Corda et al., 2001) suggests that aggravation by the drug is uncommon. Phenytoin and vigabatrin also have been implicated in the worsening of generalized seizures, whereas gabapentin has been associated with precipitating myoclonic jerks. Benzodiazepines have been reported to precipitate tonic seizures, especially in patients with Lennox-Gastaut syndrome (LGS) (see Chapter 24).

For some children, choosing not to treat the seizures may be appropriate. This *no-treatment option* may apply to provoked seizures, to those occurring in the context of an intercurrent disease, to almost all simple febrile seizures, to cases of rolandic epilepsy in whom seizures are rare, and to adolescents with isolated seizures (Camfield and Camfield, 2000; Wyllie, 1994).

Nondrug or nonconventional therapies include dietetic treatment, especially the ketogenic diet (Freeman et al., 1998; Prasad et al., 1996), and the use of immunoglobulins (Echenne et al., 1991; Illum et al., 1990; Arizumi et al., 1987).

Emphasis should be placed on the avoidance of stimuli that are capable of inducing seizures. According to Aird (1988), no fewer than 40 different stimuli can precipitate seizures, but the proportion of seizures that are induced by stimuli is poorly known (see Chapter 17). A range of figures from 5% to more than 50% has been given (Fenwick, 1992). These apply mainly to adults, and they include those seizures provoked by tense or stressful situations. In children, the roles of boredom and inattention as precipitants are well known (Olsson, 1990; Aird, 1988). Therefore, prohibiting many activities may indeed be counterproductive, and these children should be encouraged to lead an active life. According to Dahl et al. (1985, 1988), some children (12 of 18 of their patients) could identify situations in which the risk for seizure occurrence was low, and such knowledge should be used advantageously when it is available. These authors also found that some children were capable of identifying the onset of paroxysmal activity and of preventing the development of a seizure by countermaneuvers; Pritchard et al. (1985) found the same in 7 of 71 adults with complex partial seizures. Various forms of therapy, including self-control, relaxation, desensitization, or psychotherapy, have been used in an attempt to decrease seizure frequency (Fenwick, 1992).

In the past decade, considerable work has been dedicated to *epilepsy surgery* in young patients (Lüders and Comair, 2001; Bureau et al., 1998; Tuxhorn et al., 1997a), and epilepsy surgery programs have been launched in most major pediatric centers (Lüders and Comair, 2001; Engel, 1993; Duchowny et al., 1993). New concepts and techniques have led to the earlier and more frequent use of surgical therapy for children with partial epilepsy. Procrastination in the hope that new AEDs or new combinations of drugs will become efficacious is not justified for some forms of epilepsy (Duchowny, 1999), which can often be recognized from onset or after a relatively short course (Aicardi,

1997). Surgery for epilepsy is now a realistic therapeutic option. A recent study (Salanova et al., 2002) evaluating the surgical outcome, complications, and late mortality in a group of 215 adolescent and adult patients with temporal lobe epilepsy showed that 89% became seizure free or they had seizures only rarely. No mortality due to surgery was observed. Late mortality did occur in patients with persistent seizures (standardized mortality ratio [SMR] of 7.4), but the mortality for those who became seizure free was much lower (SMR, 1.7) and was similar to that of the general population. The presurgical evaluation must be started early, and it should be conducted at an experienced epilepsy center. Palliative surgery (e.g., commissurotomy and subpial transections) may be useful when resective surgery is not possible (see Chapter 25). In patients in whom surgery is not an option and major AEDs have failed, vagus nerve stimulation could be offered as a possibility (see Chapter 24). Newer techniques (e.g., gamma-knife surgery, deep brain stimulation) are under investigation (Régis et al., 2000a; Velasco et al., 1995).

ASSESSMENT AND GENERAL PATIENT MANAGEMENT

Management is concerned not only with the rational aspects of the disease but also has to take into account the misunderstandings, erroneous opinions, and prejudice that are deeply rooted even in modern societies (Eadie and Bladin, 2001). The parents of children with epilepsy and the affected children must understand the nature of the unpredictable attacks, and they should know the best manner of handling them. They should be fully informed in terms they can understand of the nature of the disorder, its general mechanisms, and its possible causes. The misperceptions that epilepsy is a psychiatric disease and that it is one form of mental illness should be firmly dispelled. The rarity of a brain tumor as the origin of seizures should be emphasized, and the parents should be brought to understand that epileptic seizures are just a symptom of many brain dysfunctions, some of which are quite benign and often transient. Whenever direct explanations to the child are possible, these should also be given to him or her directly.

A full explanation of the aims and shortcomings of therapy, information on the possibility and the significance of the side effects of the treatment, and an indication of the probable duration of therapy and the problems that may be encountered upon discontinuation are imperative. The parents and/or patients should be encouraged to keep a detailed calendar of seizures, drug modifications, and eventual adverse events, particularly during periods of major changes in treatment. The interruption of a prescribed drug because the parents think that a single course of treatment was all the child needed is a common phenomenon that often results from a lack of information. The parents must be informed that efficacy of a given drug can be determined only after a relatively long period of seizure control and that breakthrough seizures do not necessarily indicate the drug's lack of efficacy. As is true with all chronic disorders, much depends on the establishment of a good relationship between the patient and the physician. Doctors should not lose sight of the fact that they are only advisors and that the parents and patients actually implement treatment.

Patient and Parent Education

Providing education and support for parents is essential; in addition, they should be given counseling and help with educational and school problems and the management of behavioral difficulties. Although the need for information for the parents and patients seems obvious, it is not always fulfilled. In one study (Mittan et al., 1982), 53% of patients considered epilepsy their primary personal problem, 55% thought seizures could cause brain damage, and 66% believed that putting something in their mouth was necessary to prevent "tongue swallowing." One-third of these adult patients felt that sports, strenuous physical activity, dancing, loud music, or movies could be dangerous for them. Such misconceptions may be as responsible for the social stigma as the low level of education (Rodin, 1989) and employment (Sillanpää, 1990), and they may be to blame for the restricted lifestyle of many adult epileptic persons (Nakken, 1999; Steinhoff et al., 1996; Sonnen, 1991). Specialized nurses and other paramedical personnel who specialize in epilepsy management can be of great help to parents and children. They shoud be in an integral presence in all specialized epilepsy centers.

A precise diagnosis of the seizure type(s) and especially of the epilepsy syndromes is often difficult at the onset of the disorder because it mainly depends on description, which may not be possible before some time has elapsed. Parents and other family members must be educated about the importance of the eventual lateralizing signs, the duration of the seizure and its differentiation from the postictal state, and the detection of precipitating factors. All of the necessary information cannot usually be communicated in a single session, and repetition and reinforcement are usually required. When the parents' descriptions are not clear enough or when the clinician is looking for precise symptoms (e.g., ictal aphasia, hemideficit, and automatisms), the parents should be strongly encouraged to make homemade videos.

Risks in Daily Life

Providing counseling about the *risks faced by children with epilepsy* is an integral and essential part of the general management of children with epilepsy, but this is not always easy because relatively little factual information is available in this respect. In general, the available studies in adults (Sonnen, 1980) indicate that accidents, whether in traffic or at work, are rarer in persons with epilepsy than they are in the general population (Nelen et al., 1988), perhaps because the affected persons tend to limit their activities. Those that do occur are, however, concentrated in a small group of patients in which they tend to be rather common (Sonnen, 1991).

In children, dangerous types of epilepsy are uncommon; those that are dangerous include LGS and syndromes with myatonic seizures. Only in such severe cases are special precautions required at home; these include barriers at staircases, flat or round hooks or door handles, shields for sources of heat, soft carpets, and radiator covers. The bathroom doors should not have a lock because more persons with epilepsy drown while bathing than in a swimming pool (Sonnen, 1980, 1991), and the showers should be equipped with thermostatically controlled faucets that prevent hot-water burns. The patients and families must be informed of the possibility that patients with epilepsy will have accidents and instructed in what adequate measures should be applied. However, the tendency toward exaggerated protectionism must be avoided because the ensuing social isolation will have considerable consequences on the child's social integration.

Participation in most sports, including contact sports and skiing, does not appear inordinately dangerous in most patients. Swimming can be practiced with one-to-one supervision in swimming pools or in shallow seaside. Lake or river swimming is discouraged because supervision is difficult (Arzimanoglou, 2002a). Car driving is usually not a consideration in patients younger than 16 years. Cycling, particularly the use of motorbikes, may pose a difficult safety problem because, although it is undoubtedly dangerous, prohibiting this is hard, especially in the countryside where not using bikes may relegate the individual to confinement at home.

In general, a lifestyle that is as normal as possible is of utmost importance for children and adolescents with epilepsy, and a reasonable increase of risks should be accepted. The doctor should discuss this in detail with each patient and family on an individual basis so that an acceptable balance between risks and excessive prohibitions can be achieved.

Assessment of Possibilities and Schooling Issues

A full assessment of the actual potentials of children with epilepsy is essential in order to define their strong points and weaknesses and to adjust counseling and therapy accordingly. This is even more crucial because epilepsy is often only one part of a more complex disability. Although most children with epilepsy are not mentally retarded and they have no major behavioral problems, 20% to 30% of them do have some degree of mental retardation, usually as a result of the cerebral lesion that is also responsible for their seizures. Cerebral palsy frequently accompanies seizures, and it often is associated with cognitive problems as well (see Chapter 19). An association between epilepsy and psychiatric disease also exists (De Toffol, 2001; Stagno, 2001; Trimble, 1991). Psychiatric difficulties, which may affect the whole family (Hoare, 1984a, 1984b), have multiple causes. Some are secondary to environmental or personal problems that are related to the epilepsy (Hoare, 1984b), and others result at least partly from the epileptic activity itself or the cause of the epilepsy.

Epilepsy occurs in 30% to 40% of autistic patients before 30 years of age (Gillberg, 1998). Slightly less than half of these experience various epilepsy types, including infantile spasms, with onset in early childhood. Such cases raise difficult therapeutic issues because the effects of the various deficits generally are multiplicative rather than additive.

In some cases, *subtle neuropsychologic disturbances* may be suspected. Whether these should be searched for systematically is uncertain. However, a neuropsychologic evaluation is indicated for cases in whom regression, stagnation, or unexplained school failure are seen. This applies in cases of benign epilepsies as well.

Approximately 10% of children with epilepsy *acquire mental retardation* (Lesser et al., 1986; Bourgeois et al., 1983b) after the onset of seizures. *Deterioration* in children with epileptic disorders can be due to several causes. Drug toxicity, school absences, low expectations (Long and Moore, 1979), and other sociopsychologic factors undoubtedly play a role. The deleterious effects of status epilepticus are well recognized (Aicardi and Chevrie, 1970, 1983). The effects, if any, of brief seizures remain a matter of conjecture,

but they may not be negligible (Lesser et al., 1986). Finally, deterioration in a small proportion of patients, mainly those who are young, is associated with continuous or long-lasting periods of marked EEG paroxysmal abnormalities, even in the absence of clinical seizures; this deterioration may be directly related to that activity. Psychiatric disease is common in such cases. Although the causes of the deterioration and the possible role of continuous subclinical activity are poorly understood, this type of situation, which is associated with several epilepsy syndromes (e.g., LGS, West syndrome, electrical status epilepticus of slow sleep, Landau-Kleffner syndrome, and the so-called epileptic encephalopathies), requires specific therapeutic measures (see Chapters 3, 4, and 11).

The possible effects of seizures and epilepsy on schooling must be explained to the parents and school personnel. No simple answers may be available for these complex problems, particularly when the epilepsy is not related to an underlying neurologic disorder. Parents may have a tendency to attribute all of the difficulties that the child encounters to the antiepileptic medication. This can be a cause, but all other possibilities must be considered. It is rarely possible to pinpoint the cause of behavioral problems without having a global view of the child's situation. The treating physician should elicit information from the parents, the school, and other involved parties and consider with the parents what can be done to break the cycle of deterioration—perhaps a change in drugs or dosage, perhaps moving to a different school, or perhaps by just counseling the parents (Green, 1985). This is one of the most difficult areas for the parents, and, even when the mental retardation is obvious, they need time to accept it.

Normal school attendance should be the rule for children and adolescents with a normal mental level. A study in the United Kingdom, however, found that only 43 (67%) of 64 children with epilepsy attended ordinary school at the age of 11 years and only 37 (58%) at the age of 15 years (Verity and Ross, 1985). Moreover, children with epilepsy who attend ordinary schools often have school-related problems. Holdsworth and Whitmore (1974) found that about 43 (50%) of 85 children with epilepsy were considered to function at a below-average level by their teachers and that about 13 (15%) had fallen seriously behind. The fear of seizures and a lack of information about what to do in emergencies are often at the origin of the systematic exclusion from school. Providing information to teachers must become one of the primary tasks of family associations.

Learning difficulties are more prevalent in children with epilepsy than they are in the general population

(Ayala et al., 2001; Sillanpää, 1973, 2000; Aldenkamp et al., 1990), and early recognition and implementing appropriate steps for their treatment are important, an approach that does not differ from that in nonepileptic children. In selected cases, long-term EEG monitoring in conjunction with neuropsychologic assessment may be indicated. This may indicate that subclinical discharges affect the child's performance, raising the issue of prophylactic drug therapy (Binnie et al., 1990; Kasteleijn-Nolst Trenité et al., 1988, 1990; Siebeling et al., 1988; Aarts et al., 1984).

Underachievement in school is quite common in epileptic patients (Seidenberg et al., 1986; Pazzaglia and Pazzaglia, 1976). In children with uncomplicated epilepsy, a final upper secondary education level, with or without a university degree, was achieved as adults by 33% to 49%, compared with 68% to 77% of matched controls (Jalava et al., 1997). In addition to psychosocial factors, a left-sided focus (Kasteleijn-Nolst Trenité et al., 1990; Stores, 1980) and memory impairment may contribute to educational difficulties. Finally, the prospects for the employment of patients with uncontrolled epilepsy remain rather gloomy (Sillanpää, 2000). Only a small proportion of them receive a university education (Sillanpää, 1990; Fraser and Clemmons, 1989), and as many as 30% to 50% are unemployed. These poor results testify not only to the reality that epilepsy is indeed a real source of learning difficulties when it is severe but also to the unfairness of society toward persons with epilepsy. Little doubt exists that a significant part of their problems is due to prejudice, ignorance, and neglect.

BASIC GUIDELINES FOR CHRONIC TREATMENT

The natural history of untreated epilepsy is not well understood. The only factual basis for prescribing AEDs is the possibility of reducing the risks attendant to seizures because, in most cases, treatment clearly has no preventive effects on the long-term occurrence of seizures (see Chapter 21). However, the possibility that treatment may help prevent the deterioration associated with prolonged severe epileptic activity, even in the absence of seizures, may be an additional, if as yet unproven, justification for treatment (Aicardi, 1999a).

The institution of chronic treatment must respect at least the following four basic principles, and it should not be guided by the irrational fear that the clinician may have of seizures.

First, chronic treatment should be started only when the physician is satisfied that the patient's attacks are truly epileptic seizures. Prescribing an AED as a clinical test for confirming a diagnosis of epilepsy is a medical error. As Chapter 21 indicates, the overdiagnosis of epilepsy is not rare, and, when an erroneous diagnosis is made, it often has disastrous consequences, including the "justification" of prolonged drug treatment and exposing the child to the sociopsychologic consequences of such a diagnosis. Such errors should be avoided by carefully assessing those patients who are being considered for treatment with clinical and ancillary examinations.

In general, an EEG is indicated for all suspect cases, except febrile seizures. The diagnostic EEGs should not be performed as part of an emergency examination. Available clinical data on the paroxysmal phenomena justifying the performance of the EEG should be transmitted to the neurophysiology department. Sleep recordings are easily obtained in children, and they are essential for making a diagnosis. At least one sleep EEG should be systematically requested for almost all newly diagnosed childhood epilepsies. In order to obtain 20 to 30 minutes of sleep recording, the parents must be advised on how to prepare their child, especially when the patient is older than 6 to 7 years. Sleep EEGs should not be considered as one of the ancillary investigations but rather as an essential tool for the diagnosis and treatment of epilepsy. Therefore, every effort should be made to work together to obtain an informative EEG, including a sleep recording. Nevertheless, the physician must keep in mind (a) that a significant proportion of patients with epilepsy can have a normal EEG recording, even when hyperpnea, photic stimulation, sleep recording, and sleep deprivation are used (Degen and Degen, 1984), and (b) that, conversely, an abnormal or even a paroxysmal EEG is not sufficient to reach a diagnosis of epilepsy, let alone to indicate the need of chronic therapy. The conjunction of clinical phenomena compatible with the diagnosis is an absolute requirement. The diagnostic yield of the interictal EEG can be augmented by the performance of multiple EEG recordings or by increasing the duration of the EEG.

The *second principle* is that chronic treatment should not be started without ensuring that the seizures are not caused by a progressive, sometimes treatable condition. Failure to recognize such a disease not only leads to persistent seizures in many cases but also results in a missed opportunity for catching severe brain disorders in their early stages, of which seizures can be the initial warnings. In addition to conducting a complete history and physical examination, laboratory examinations and imaging are indicated in many cases. In the physical examination, special attention should be devoted to the skin in a search for signs of possible neurocutaneous disorders; to the eyes in a search for signs of intracranial hypertension or disturbances of eye movements; and to routine, but often neglected, measures such as measuring blood pressure.

The authors' practice is to require neuroimaging examinations for patients with epilepsy that is not a classic primary generalized epilepsy, whether absence epilepsy, juvenile myoclonic epilepsy, or isolated awakening grand mal (see Chapters 6, 8, and 9); a typical case of rolandic epilepsy (see Chapter 10); or a case of epilepsy due to old, previously known lesions (e.g., cerebral palsy) in which no new sign is present. Asking for brain imaging of patients who have had a first seizure is not unreasonable when the seizure is focal and is unexplained, even though such persons cannot be diagnosed as having epilepsy and, in general, they should not receive treatment. After a seizure, however, imaging can only be considered an emergency investigation in exceptional cases. In fact, only when accompanying symptoms, such as signs of intracranial hypertension, the rapid installation of a hemideficit, fever, and a confusional state, are present is emergency investigation justified as a diagnostic tool for a treatable disorder. All other lesions related to a partial seizure are detected much better by a good magnetic resonance imaging (MRI) examination performed at a distance from the event.

Several published studies (Anslow, 1991; Aicardi et al., 1983a) have shown that the "yield" of a computed tomographic (CT) scan for epilepsy is relatively high, but only a small proportion of the abnormalities detected are essential for defining a treatment strategy (Riela and Penry, 1990; Aicardi et al., 1983a; Yang et al., 1979; Gastaut and Gastaut, 1976), with most lesions that are seen being of an atrophic character (Anslow, 1991). CT scanning is better than MRI for demonstrating calcified tissue, which is of interest in conditions such as tuberous sclerosis. However, CT is much less sensitive than MRI, and it has little value as a first-line imaging modality for intractable epilepsy (Anslow and Oxbury, 2000). For situations in which access to MRI is limited because of its cost or other reasons, a CT scan provides sufficient information for general therapeutic care; the indications for MRI are limited to intractable partial epilepsies with a normal CT scan or to presurgical cases. After a seizure, CT scanning can be helpful in the few cases in which emergency imaging is indicated.

An MRI allows a precise study of brain morphology (Kuzniecky and Jackson, 1995b) because it per-

mits use of several planes of cut and provides a more precise separation and definition of white and gray matter, as well as information about the structure of the tissues; gliosis and dysplasias do not produce the same signals as the normal components of the brain. The superiority of MRI for the diagnosis of atrophy; gliosis, especially that of the hippocampus (Jackson et al., 1993b; Cascino et al., 1992a, 1992b; Jack et al., 1992); migration disorders; and other brain malformations is overwhelming (Briellmann et al., 2003; Cascino and Jack, 1996; Cook and Stevens, 1995; Sisodiya et al., 1995; Berkovic et al., 1991a; Palmini et al., 1991d; Kuzniecky et al., 1987, 1988). In industrialized countries, MRI has progressively replaced the CT scan in the routine examination for partial nonidiopathic or generalized symptomatic epilepsies. However, a normal routine MRI often cannot eliminate the possibility of the presence of a small focal lesion or dysplasia. Undoubtedly, the results are more useful when the investigation is being performed to support or falsify a previously formulated diagnostic hypothesis. The clinical semiology must be taken into account, particularly when the clinician is looking for small lesions (e.g., a small hypothalamic hamartoma is strongly suspected with gelastic seizures, or a vigorous search for a minute dysplastic lesion should be prompted by recurrent intractable focal seizures).

Aside from imaging and EEG, few laboratory examinations are useful in the initial assessment of a child with epilepsy. Biochemical examinations are indicated only when a metabolic disease is suspected. Indeed, isolated epilepsy is only rarely the presenting manifestation of a metabolic disease, even though rare conditions such as Lafora disease or Unverricht-Lundborg disease may have a close resemblance to generalized epilepsy at their initial stage.

The *third principle* is that the goal of treatment should be the prevention of further epileptic seizures; it is therefore indicated only when the recurrence risk is of a "sufficient" magnitude. The risk has the following two elements: the likelihood of seizure recurrence and the risk that recurrent seizures have for the patient. The latter risk must be assessed individually for each affected patient, whereas the former can be, to some extent, evaluated statistically.

As Chapter 22 indicates, variation is seen between series of adults and children in the risk of recurrent attacks after a first unprovoked seizure. Most surveys give figures of about 40% to 60%. Such figures suggest that patients may not need to be treated after a single unprovoked seizure but that they probably should be treated after the second attack because the risk increases after the second event. This does not, however, apply to those seizures that are virtually always recurrent, such as atonic or absence seizures, or to epilepsy syndromes such as juvenile myoclonic epilepsy. However, some evidence indicates that whether an epilepsy may become an active, ongoing problem may be determined early in the history of the disorder (Berg et al., 1996, 2003; Jallou, 2003; Ko and Holmes, 1999; Cockerell et al., 1997; Shorvon, 1984; Reynolds et al., 1983). If this can be determined, early treatment (i.e., from the first seizure) may conceivably improve the long-term prognosis. Indeed, a delay in commencing treatment in adults has been correlated with a reduced chance of the successful withdrawal of therapy, even after 5 years, in one study, and the chance of controlling epilepsy appears to be significantly less in those patients whose seizures are not controlled within 2 years of onset. Similarly, Rodin (1968) found that the shorter the duration of epilepsy is before treatment is begun, the better the chance is of obtaining a long-term remission. However, none of the available studies provides definite proof because the aforementioned findings can be explained by the observation that patients with the most severe epilepsies tend to have more fits in the early stages of their disorder, as well as a smaller likelihood of achieving complete remission. However, the view that late treatment may be an important factor in the emergence of intractable epilepsy is plausible. Therefore, one may argue that treatment after the first seizure may be justified, at least in selected patients, although no evidence indicates that the prevention of a second seizure decreases the risk of occurrence of later chronic epilepsy. In actuality, the decision of whether to treat depends more on the desires of the patient and family and on the resulting risks in the lifestyle of the individual patient. In children regarded as having refractory partial symptomatic or cryptogenic epilepsy, the possibilities for a definite surgical solution must be evaluated early in the course of the disease (see Chapter 25).

The *fourth principle* is that, whenever possible, a diagnosis of a specific syndrome should be made. Identifying a specific syndrome can provide essential clues regarding the choice of drug in some cases (Arzimanoglou, 2002b), the duration or modalities of treatment, and the necessary investigations. Thus, a diagnosis of juvenile myoclonic epilepsy is a strong indication for valproate as the first-choice agent. The diagnosis of rolandic epilepsy is a virtually absolute guarantee that a relatively short period of treatment with a low dosage of a single drug will suffice and that no investigation except an EEG is required. The correct diagnosis of epilepsy syndromes also offers considerable help with the decisions to start antiepileptic therapy after a first seizure or to discontinue treatment after a period of remission. However, a syndromic diagnosis is often not possible at onset, even in cases with recurrent seizures. In such cases, a large spectrum AED (e.g., lamotrigine or valproate) can be prescribed initially, but investigations for a precise diagnosis must still be pursued.

SUMMARY

Although most epilepsies of childhood require drug treatment, some benign forms may not mandate chronic therapy, and infrequent seizures require other types of therapy. Treatment should be started soon whenever delay might harm the child. However, the treatment of epilepsy is rarely an emergency, and taking the time to confirm the diagnosis and to reflect on it is probably wiser, because an incorrect decision to treat has serious implications. Whatever treatment is chosen, the careful assessment of patients is mandatory. This should include the consideration not only of the seizures and the underlying brain disorder, if present, but also of the various aspects of the impact of epilepsy on the patient's cognitive functions and behavior, as well as of the overall effect of the disease on the functioning of the child and the family in the social and school environment.

The specificity of the available AEDs is relatively limited. However, growing evidence indicates that the effects of certain drugs on childhood epilepsies are partly linked to the specific type of epilepsy or epilepsy syndrome. Most, but not all, types of epilepsy can be classified into categories that are conceptually meaningful. Likewise, it is logical to set treatment targets and to estimate the risks according to the main syndromic groups. The treatment should then be adjusted to each patient's clinical characteristics. Specific contraindications, including the aggravation of some seizure types by an inappropriate drug choice or a paradoxical reaction, should be considered.

One major emphasis in the management of epilepsy is on disseminating information to the patients and family. This information should be complete, it should be adapted to their level of understanding, and, although it should be given in a positive manner, it should be objective. The patients and/or family must understand that the "absolutely safe and certain to be efficacious" drug does not exist. The goal of treatment is to achieve the best possible balance between effectiveness and unpleasant side effects. The understanding and cooperation of patients and families is clearly decisive for the success of therapy, and, for this, a good relationship between the physician and the patient is required.

The goal of therapy should certainly be to control the seizures. In some cases, the suppression of paroxysmal EEG activity may be a target, although the limits of this type of therapy are imprecise. Because having epilepsy entails more than just having seizures, every effort should be made to help the patients have lives that are as normal as possible and to support their integration as full members of the community.

24

Medical Treatment

The propensity of individuals with epilepsy to have seizures varies considerably from patient to patient and in the same patient at different times. In most patients, the increased susceptibility can be mitigated or suppressed by antiepileptic agents when used in adequate doses. Since 1990, new drugs have become available that have broadened the clinician's ability to choose the most appropriate drug for each patient. Despite this, recent studies in adolescents and adults have shown that roughly 60% of patients are controlled on monotherapy with the first or second choice antiepileptic drug (AED), whereas the remainder are refractory to one or several combinations. However, most of the new agents are better tolerated than the older compounds. Certain patients with epilepsy have benefited from the introduction of new AEDs. The best choice for each patient results from a combination of the available clinical data on the individual and an understanding of the pharmacologic characteristics, indications, and potential adverse effects of each AED.

DRUG TREATMENT

Overview

Drug treatment is the major form of therapy for a vast majority of children with seizure disorder. Like any other therapy for epilepsy, drug treatment should follow the general principles of management outlined in Chapter 23. This chapter is concerned with a survey of the AEDs, their metabolism and action in the body, and their indications and mode of practical use.

Most of today's knowledge about the efficacy and mode of action of AEDs has been obtained in animals. A host of potential anticonvulsant agents has been developed and tested in animal models of experimental seizures, and a number have been found effective in the treatment of human epilepsy. Only a few, however, have withstood extensive clinical trials and the test of time sufficiently well to become part of the therapeutic armamentarium against the epilepsies. During the last decade, many randomized, controlled studies have been performed, primarily in adults but sometimes in children as well. Regularly

updated, excellent books dedicated to AEDs testify to the explosion of knowledge in this field (Levy et al., 2002; Wyllie, 2001).

Clinical experience has shown that AEDs can control a high proportion of cases of human epilepsy. Moreover, it has demonstrated that certain types of human epileptic seizures respond better to some drugs than to others, even though the correlations between the seizure type and a potentially effective drug are far from perfect (Eadie and Tyrer, 1989). Various epilepsy syndromes also respond differently to AEDs (Arzimanoglou, 2002b). Despite the lack of specificity of existing AEDs, clinical practice has shown that a precise diagnosis, when combined with a better understanding of the mechanisms of action of AEDs, permits their more specific and more effective use. Patient characteristics, including age at onset, seizure frequency, electroencephalographic (EEG) data, and the findings of imaging studies, provide diagnostic clues that enable the physician to reach a syndrome diagnosis and to choose the most appropriate AED for each patient.

The *mode of action* of AEDs is beyond the scope of this book, so only a few basic notions are offered (Rogawski, 2002; Sills and Brodie, 2001). Epileptogenesis does not originate in a single neuron but rather in neuronal pools that have an inherited or an acquired tendency to produce high-frequency bursts of spike discharges (Najm et al., 2001; Prince and Connors, 1986). These bursts are then transmitted along axons, and, when a sufficient volume of neural tissue has been activated, a clinical seizure results. Therefore, clinical seizures may be prevented either by lowering the excitability of the pacemaker neuronal pools or by preventing the spread of epileptogenic spike bursts from the pools. Either mechanism may be at work, depending on the drug used, but the prevention of the burst propagation is more significant for most of the conventional anticonvulsants (Fromm, 1985). This applies especially to primidone (PRM), phenytoin (PHT), carbamazepine (CBZ), and diazepam (Levy et al., 2002; Eadie and Tyrer, 1989), whereas some drugs, especially the barbiturates, act mainly by raising the seizure threshold. These presumably act on "epileptic" neurons within the focus.

Anticonvulsant drugs usually bind to specific receptors in the brain. *Receptors* are tissue molecules with which drugs form various types of physicochemical bonds through which they exert their therapeutic action. In general, the magnitude of drug effect is related to the number of receptor sites occupied by drug molecules (Goldstein et al., 1975). The mode of action of an individual drug apparently is closely related to its site of binding (Levy et al., 2002; Eadie and Tyrer, 1989). PHT, CBZ, and lamotrigine (LTG), for example, act selectively on sodium channels (Kuo, 1998), thus preventing repetitive firing of neuronal action potentials, consequently inhibiting the spread of epileptic activity. Other drugs appear to act primarily on synaptic transmission. This action may be presynaptic (e.g., by increasing concentration of γ-aminobutyric acid [GABA] as a result of a decreased catabolism of this compound, as is the case with γ-vinyl-GABA, or by decreasing reuptake within the synaptic cleft), synaptic, or postsynaptic (e.g., binding to specific receptors, thus modifying their excitability). The latter mechanism may involve GABAergic synapses by increasing their activity as a major inhibitory cortical system or excitatory synapses by decreasing the activity of glutamatergic excitatory transmission. Ultimately, all AEDs appear to act on ion channels, although in some cases, the effect is mediated indirectly (Rogawski, 2002).

Within the limits of current knowledge about the mechanisms of action, most AEDs can be categorized by their mechanisms into several broad categories. Those that act mainly as *voltage-dependent sodium channel blockers* include PHT, CBZ, oxcarbazepine (OXC), and LTG. Agents like vigabatrin (VGB) and tiagabine potentiate GABAergic inhibition by enhancing the synaptic availability of GABA. Barbiturates, such as phenobarbital (PB), augment the function of GABA$_A$ receptors, and they have additional effects on the calcium and other ion channels. Benzodiazepines, although they enhance only a subset of GABA$_A$ receptors, are broad-spectrum agents. Ethosuximide seems to act by affecting T-type calcium channels. Valproate, gabapentin (GPT), felbamate (FBM), topiramate (TPM), zonisamide, and levetiracetam (LEV) appear to have novel mechanisms (or, perhaps, a combination of mechanisms) of action; these may possibly affect the calcium channels and glutamate receptors, as well as conventional targets, including sodium channels and GABA receptor systems (Rogawski, 2002). Extensive discussions of the mechanisms of action of drugs are available (Bialer et al., 2002; Levy et al., 2002; Eadie and Tyrer, 1989; Meldrum, 1983a).

Basic Notions on the Pharmacokinetics of Antiepileptic Drugs

Treatment with anticonvulsant agents has long been empirically guided. Recently, the development of clinical pharmacokinetics has enabled the accurate study of the metabolism of drugs through the development of techniques for measuring minute amounts in body fluids. As a result, a large body of new knowledge has been gained about the metabolism of AEDs, their effects relative to the doses given, and the interactions between anticonvulsants and other pharmaceuticals administered to the same patient (Meldrum, 1983a; Morselli, 1977).

A number of new concepts have stemmed from pharmacokinetic knowledge, such as the value of monotherapy versus polypharmacy and, in particular, the concept of effective or optimal blood levels of anticonvulsants (Kutt, 1985; Richens, 1982).

The concept of *optimal blood levels* has often been misinterpreted, to the point that many physicians believe that blood levels outside the therapeutic range are without value and that all prescriptions of an AED should aim for blood levels within that range. The falsity of this interpretation has been amply documented (Levy et al., 2002; Perucca, 2000; Mattson et al., 1992; Brodie, 1990; Eadie and Tyrer, 1989; Holmes, 1987; Vajda and Aicardi, 1983). The concept of a therapeutic range is statistical, applying only to populations rather than to individual patients. In some patients, the upper or lower limits of individual therapeutic range may lie outside the accepted values, and no effort should be made to achieve therapeutic values in patients who are clinically controlled, even though they are outside the "therapeutic" or optimal range, if they have no clinical evidence of toxicity (Brodie, 1990; Vajda and Aicardi, 1983). Blood levels are only one link in the chain of pharmacokinetic processes that occur between ingestion of a drug and that drug then reaching its site of action where it exerts its pharmacodynamic effects. The important factor is, therefore, its concentration at the receptor sites in the central nervous system (CNS).

The concept of an optimal range of a drug applies only if the drug is not irreversibly bound to its receptor and/or if it has active metabolites (Chadwick, 1988; Vajda and Aicardi, 1983). Thus, measuring the blood levels of VGB is pointless because this drug is irreversibly bound to GABA transaminase. Likewise, the determination of the blood levels of CBZ or the benzodiazepines is open to criticism because these agents do have active metabolites that may become highly significant clinically when interference from other pharmaceuticals increases the levels of metabolites (Agbato et al., 1986).

The value of blood-level estimations is that, for most AEDs, the blood levels are well correlated with the brain levels (Vajda and Aicardi, 1983; Sherwin et al., 1973), and the relationship between blood and brain levels is much closer than that between the dosage that was ingested and the blood levels. Blood levels are, therefore, related to therapeutic action. However, exceptions do exist (Kutt, 1985). In addition, the correlation between blood and brain levels has been verified only on a relatively rough level (e.g., in the white or gray matter), and little research has been conducted on local variations, especially in and around epileptic foci or epileptogenic lesions (Monaco et al., 1985; Baron et al., 1983; Munari et al., 1982a).

Blood levels of AEDs are the result of a series of processes (Fig. 24.1). Most anticonvulsants are administered orally and are absorbed rapidly and usually fairly completely (Table 24.1). Once the drugs are absorbed, they enter the circulation. In the blood, they are variably bound to proteins. The level of protein-bound drugs is in constant equilibrium with that of the free drugs. Only the free fraction can diffuse across the blood–brain barrier to reach the receptor sites. The free fraction of a drug can be altered by various factors (Bourgeois, 2001). The first is the displacement of the drug from its binding sites by another drug or other chemicals, such as bilirubin (Morselli, 1977) or free fatty acids. Other factors include pregnancy or age (e.g., infancy or elderly patients). The distribution of drugs varies (Table 24.1),

with the apparent volume of distribution depending particularly on the lipid solubility of particular agents. Some AEDs, such as the benzodiazepines, have volumes of distribution that are greater than the total body water, thus indicating binding to tissue constituents, active transport into cells, or accumulation in storage areas. Others have volumes of distribution equal to or approaching that of total body water, while valproic acid (VPA) has a volume of distribution close to that of the extracellular water.

Anticonvulsants leave the blood by the following two mechanisms: (a) biotransformation to inactive or, less commonly, active metabolites and (b) excretion through the kidney, intestine, sweat, or tears. "Biotransformation" is an enzymatic process resulting mainly from hepatic microsomal activity. This, in turn, depends on the genetic makeup and gender of the patient, on the one hand, and on a number of extraneous factors such as diet and interaction with other drugs that induce the synthesis of microsomal drug-metabolizing enzymes, on the other. Interference also may result from inhibition of the metabolism of one drug by another through various mechanisms (Kutt, 1985; Perucca and Richens, 1980). The excretion of drug also can be altered by such factors as urinary pH level, urine flow, or the glomerular filtration rate.

The apparent *plasma half-life of a drug* is defined as the time it takes for the plasma level to decline to 50% of its previous value. The decline usually occurs exponentially. The average plasma half-lives of the main anticonvulsant drugs are indicated in Table 24.1. Considerable variations exist, and these values are

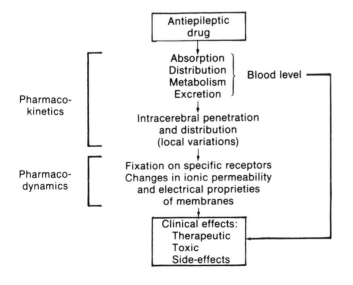

FIG. 24.1. Schematic representation of the successive steps from ingestion of an antiepileptic drug to its clinical effects. The steps from absorption through brain entry and distribution represent the pharmacokinetics of a drug; the later steps with the resulting changes in membrane properties and excitability represent the pharmacodynamic phase of drug action. Note that some of the unwanted effects of antiepileptic drugs may be a direct result of the drug present in blood (e.g., liver toxicity, skin rashes, or interference with other drugs), whereas the therapeutic effects require the presence of the drug at its site of action in the brain.

TABLE 24.1. *Main pharmacokinetic data on anticonvulsant drugs*

Drug	Oral Availability[a]	T_{max} (h)[a,b]	Protein Binding (%)[a]	Plasma Half-Time (h)	Apparent VD (L/kg)	Optimal Range[c]	
						µg/mL	µmol/L
Carbamazepine	75–85	2–24	70–80	$35.6 \pm 15.3^{c,d}$	1.20 ± 0.45	4–12	17–51
Clobazam	87	1.3–1.7	82–90	16–48.6	194 (Ch)	NA	NA
Clonazepam	95	2–3 (Ch)	86	28 ± 4.6 (Ch)	2.1 ± 0.6 (Ch)	NA	NA
Diazepam	75	1–2	95	10–20	2.6 ± 0.5 (Ch)	NA	NA
Ethosuximide	100	1–4	0	30	0.7	40–100	300–750
Felbamate	NA	NA	22–25	16–22	0.756	NA	NA
Gabapentin	35–57	2–3	0	5–7	50–58	NA	NA
Lamotrigine	70	2–4	55	$19–30^f$	0.9–1.5	NA	NA
Levetiracetam	>95	1.3	0	5–7 (Ch)	0.5–0.7	NA	NA
Oxcarbazepine	89	1.3 ± 0.2	60	3.1 ± 1.5	11.5	NA	20–200
Phenobarbital	80	2–10	50	37–73	0.9	10–30	45–130
Phenytoin	80–95	4–12	90	20	0.65	10–20	40–80
Primidone	90	0.5–4	10	5–10	0.6–1	5–12	23–55
Sodium valproate	100	$1–3^e$	90	7–15	0.2	50–100	345–690
Tiagabine	>90	0.5–2	>95	4.5–8.1	NA	NA	NA
Topiramate	81–95	1–3	9–17	21	40–60	NA	NA
Vigabatrin	60–80	1–4	0	0.6–10	5–7	NA	NA
Zonisamide	NA	2.4–5.8	40–60	50–88	1.8	NA	NA

Abbreviations: Ch, children; NA, not applicable in clinical practice, T_{max}, time of maximal concentration; VD, volume of distribution.
[a] Data derived mainly from adult studies.
[b] Time to maximum blood level following a single dose.
[c] Indicative value only (see text).
[d] Higher figure values for single dose.
[e] Enteric-coated preparations have an average T_{max} of 6–8 hr.
[f] Considerably prolonged when combined with valproate. Decreased when combined with inducers.

only a general indication. Moreover, the half-life can be influenced by a number of factors affecting excretion and/or biotransformation. For example, the half-life of many drugs tends to decrease, often considerably, as a result of the microsomal enzymatic induction that is provoked by the administration of the drug itself (autoinduction) or by that of another drug (Perucca and Levy, 2002; Bourgeois, 1988, 1992; Eadie and Tyrer, 1989; Bourgeois and Wad, 1988).

The time course of drug concentrations in different fluids or tissues can be fitted to mathematical models that are used for interpreting the plasma concentration pattern obtained in a given patient. Many pharmacokinetic processes, especially excretion and biotransformation of a drug, are said to be first order. In that situation, the elimination process varies directly with the plasma concentration of the drug, and a linear relationship between the dosage and serum levels is observed. When the elimination is independent of the concentration or dose that is administered, the process is said to be "zero order." Many drugs convert from first-order to

zero-order kinetics when their concentration becomes sufficiently high to saturate their enzyme or transport mechanism. That change is clinically significant when PHT is being used because the saturation point is within the average therapeutic concentration range. When saturation is attained, minimal incremental increases in dose produce considerable increases in plasma levels, with attendant toxicity.

As has already been indicated, *variability is the rule rather than the exception for most pharmacokinetic processes.* Part of this variability is intrinsically determined. For example, the following two populations exist with regard to the speed of hydroxylation of PHT: slow and fast hydroxylators (Eadie and Tyrer, 1989; Richens, 1982). A considerable part of the variation results from extraneous processes, among which interactions, especially drug interactions, are important (Kutt, 1984). Interactions can take place at any step from absorption to interaction with specific receptors. Among antimicrobial agents, chloramphenicol may cause the accumulation of PHT and PB, and isoniazid may cause PHT, CBZ, and PRM to accrue. Erythromycin may cause the buildup of CBZ. Among antiulcer agents, antacids may reduce PHT concentration, whereas cimetidine may cause the accumulation of PHT, CBZ, and diazepam. Salicylates displace strongly bound drugs such as PHT, diazepam, or VPA from the binding sites in plasma proteins, which may lead to some decline of the total plasma level and a corresponding increase in the unbound drug percentage. However, only a few of these interactions are clinically significant, necessitating the adjustment of drug dosages. In children, one important example is the toxicity produced by the coadministration of CBZ and some antibiotics, especially triacetyloleandomycin (Mesdjian et al., 1980) and erythromycin (Goulden et al., 1986), which considerably increase the levels of CBZ.

The timing of ingestion of valproate relative to meals, as well as the composition of the meals, markedly influences the absorption of that drug (Loiseau et al., 1982; Lévy et al., 1981) and the time at which peak and trough plasma levels are achieved. The galenic form of drugs can also significantly influence their bioavailability and rate of absorption (Issakainen and Bourgeois, 1987; Wyllie et al., 1987b; Hodge et al., 1986), and poor preservation of drugs may also be responsible for variations. Thus, storing PHT and CBZ in a hot and humid place can reduce their bioavailability by up to 50% (Cloyd, 1991). Extremely rare cases of malabsorption of AEDs have been recorded (Gilman et al., 1988). These may be important, especially with short half-life drugs, for determining the optimal time for sampling blood for a plasma level determination. Following a gastrostomy, one of the authors' patients who was on slow-release sodium valproate experienced a relapse of seizures. The competition of drugs for protein-binding sites may produce significant interaction when both of the agents that are used are strongly protein bound. Valproate can displace PHT from its albumin sites, with resultant increases in free fraction. At that point, the determination of the PHT blood levels, in which both free and protein-bound fractions are measured, does not give a true picture of the pharmacokinetic situation because the active (free) fraction is abnormally high relative to the total level. Toxicity may result if the PHT dose is increased without taking that phenomenon into account (Richens, 1982; Perucca and Richens, 1980). At a second stage, the increases in the free fraction augment the clearance of PHT, thus reestablishing the original equilibrium, often with a lower total level of the pharmaceutical in the blood (Perucca and Richens, 1980).

The determination of blood levels of free drugs rather than the total blood level (free plus protein-bound fractions) may obviate some of these difficulties (Herngren et al., 1991; Gianelli et al., 1988; Agbato et al., 1986; Lévy and Schmidt, 1985). However, the technique for such a determination is more complicated (Pacifici and Viani, 1992), so a measurement of the free levels of AEDs has not supplanted total level determination, except in special circumstances such as pregnancy, hypoalbuminemia, and hepatic or renal failure (Lévy and Schmidt, 1985). An indirect approach to the determination of free drug level is by using biological fluids other than blood for determination. Tears and, in particular, saliva levels have been studied and are used in several places (Drobitch and Svensson, 1992; Knott, 1983; Kristensen et al., 1983). Although these are relatively protein-free fluids, their concentration of AEDs may vary with the secretion rate and other factors, and sampling may be more difficult (Bäckman et al., 1987).

The induction of microsomal drug-metabolizing enzymes can result in drug interference. The clinical significance of this type of interference is usually limited (Perucca and Levy, 2002; Patsalos and Lascelles, 1982; Perucca and Richens, 1980). However, CBZ may reduce the blood levels of PHT and vice versa, partly through that type of interaction (Bourgeois, 1988; Browne et al., 1988b), and many interactions of at least some clinical significance are known (Pippenger, 1987; Pisani et al., 1987; Patsalos and Lascelles, 1982). The failure of oral contraceptives has been attributed to anticonvulsants in some patients. Probably, the most predictable interaction necessitating dosage adjustment is the accumulation of PB that is caused by valproate (Kutt, 1984). The most significant interactions result from the inhibition of the metabolism of one drug by another. This occurs with the coadministration of PB and valproate, in which valproate produces an average increase of 30% in the blood levels of PB (Scheyer, 2002). PRM concentrations, as well as the derived PB concentrations, increase when valproate is added. However, large variations ranging from 0% to more than 100% can be observed in individual patients.

Valproate blocks the glucuronidation of LTG and results in the increased concentration of LTG, so the dose used should be cut to about half when such a combination is prescribed. On the other hand, the metabolism of LTG, like that of many other drugs, is accelerated with combined use with other inducing anticonvulsants, so the dose may need to be increased when these are used together.

Pharmacokinetic interactions can be evaluated rather easily by measuring changes in blood concentrations. However, measuring the so-called *pharmacodynamic interactions*, which manifest by a change in the pharmacologic response in the absence of changes in blood levels, objectively has proven much more difficult (Perucca and Levy, 2002). Pharmacodynamic interactions may be expressed negatively (additive neurotoxicity), usually leading to the appearance of CNS side effects in patients on polytherapy, even when the doses and blood levels of individual AEDs are in the low range (Besag et al., 1998). The combination of drugs on an empirical basis also produces some favorable interactions, providing a superior therapeutic index. Clinical evidence is convincing for the combination of valproate with ethosuximide for the control of refractory absence seizures (Rowan et al., 1983) and for valproate with LTG in patients with generalized epilepsies (Arzimanoglou et al., 2001; Brodie and Yuen, 1997; Panayiotopoulos et al., 1993) or partial seizures (Pisani et al., 1999). Potential advantages have been reported for other combinations, but the evidence is mostly anecdotal and interindividual variation can be considerable (Perucca and Levy, 2002).

In children, an additional and major source of variability is the *age of the patient*. Age influences all aspects of drug metabolism (Dodson, 1983, 1987b; Morselli et al., 1983). The absorption of AEDs, except CBZ, is usually faster in infants and young children than in adults (Dodson, 1987a). The half-lives of most anticonvulsants are quite prolonged in newborn babies during the first 1 to 3 weeks of life, and they shorten dramatically thereafter over the first 2 or 3 months of life. High metabolic levels are maintained during the first years of life. At 10 to 15 years, a marked metabolic slowing to adult values often occurs (Dodson, 1987b). This slowing may be progressive, or, on some occasions, it may be quite sudden (Morselli, 1977). The evolution of drug metabolism explains why intoxication is common in neonates receiving repeated doses of anticonvulsants over the first days of life, whereas, a few days or weeks later, maintaining adequate therapeutic levels may be difficult or even impossible (Arzimanoglou and Aicardi, 2001). This also accounts for the higher doses per unit of weight or surface area that are required in children compared with adults. Finally, the slowing of metabolism at the time of adolescence may account for the relative frequency of overdosage at that period of life despite the increase in body weight.

Other sources of variability in the doses required and the blood levels necessary to control the seizures

depend on the *individual variations* in the severity of epilepsy, pharmacologic tolerance, and other unknown causes.

Significant changes can occur also with stress (e.g., trauma or surgery), which can increase the metabolism of drugs, such as valproate or CBZ, consequently diminishing their blood level; however, the effectiveness is not necessarily diminished when CBZ is used because the increased level of the epoxide is also active and potentially toxic (Cloyd, 1991). Febrile illnesses can also alter PHT clearance (Leppik et al., 1986).

Reciprocally antiepileptic agents, many of which are strong microsomal inducers, can alter the metabolism and efficacy of simultaneously used drugs (Perucca and Levy, 2002). For example, one important interference is seen in patients who receive corticosteroids to avoid rejection of a transplant, in whom the acceleration of the catabolism of steroids may lead to acute rejection (Pentella et al., 1982). In such cases, the use of noninducing drugs, such as valproate, LTG, GPT, or the benzodiazepines, is advised. The same type of problem may present with the combined use of warfarin and some anticonvulsant drugs, including CBZ, PB, and PHT, which induce warfarin (Levy et al., 2002). The interference of anticonvulsants with the metabolism of vitamin D has resulted in decreases in calcium fixation, thereby repeatedly causing the occurrence of osteomalacia or rickets (Chung and Ahn, 1994; Offerman et al., 1979). This does, however, not appear to be of major clinical importance in ambulatory children for whom no increase in vitamin D administration is recommended (Ala-Houala et al., 1986). In institutionalized patients, the routine administration of vitamin D supplementation may be indicated.

The considerable magnitude of individual variations from all sources is one of the reasons that rigid schemes or protocols cannot be established for the treatment of the epilepsies of childhood.

PB, PHT, and CBZ are potent inducers of drug metabolism, and their administration is usually associated with decreases in levels of CBZ (heteroinduction and autoinduction), cyclosporine, oral contraceptives, and corticosteroids. OXC, TPM, and FBM have a narrower spectrum of enzyme-inducing activity, but they have also been found to reduce the blood levels of steroid and oral contraceptives (Perucca and Levy, 2002).

GENERAL GUIDELINES FOR DRUG TREATMENT

As has been explained, the control of seizures by drugs depends on the use of those drugs that are appropriate for the patient's seizure types, on the prescription of doses that are sufficient to maintain effective levels of drugs at their site of action in the brain, and on their actual ingestion and retention by the patient. Whenever possible, the initial drug choice must be based on a specific syndromic diagnosis (Aicardi and Arzimanoglou, 1996). During the last decade, considerable knowledge has accumulated regarding the special efficacy of certain drugs in specific syndromes or epilepsies in which the underlying mechanisms are assumed to be similar (Arzimanoglou, 2002b). The treatment is always long lasting, ranging from a minimum duration of 1 or 2 years to lifelong.

All antiepileptic agents produce *side effects* that may seriously hamper the patient's activities. These side effects range from acute intoxication with disturbances of consciousness (Meador, 1994, 2001; Martin et al., 1999; Weaver et al., 1988; Zaret and Cohen, 1986; Larrieu et al., 1985) or, exceptionally, death (Leestma et al., 1997; Murphy et al., 1987; Stone and Lange, 1986) to subtle chronic toxicity with protean manifestations (Gerber et al., 2000; Weig and Pollack, 1993; Appleton et al., 1990; McLachlan, 1987; Pellock, 1987; Kaplan et al., 1982; Dravet et al., 1980; Joyce and Gunderson, 1978; McLeod et al., 1978) or to apparently minor but sometimes psychologically and socially disabling effects such as acne, excessive weight gain (De Toledo et al., 1997; Dinesen et al., 1984; Egger and Brett, 1981), or weight loss (Potter et al., 1997). Allergic or idiosyncratic reactions are also common, and these may rarely be responsible for fatalities (Fernandez-Calvo et al., 2000; Schlienger et al., 1998; Kaufman et al., 1997; Brown, 1988; Gilhus and Matte, 1986).

The cognitive effects of anticonvulsants (Aldenkamp, 2001; Meador, 1994, 2001; Aldenkamp et al., 1993) are particularly worrying, and no drug appears to be completely exempt from unfavorable cognitive or behavioral effects, even though these may be more marked with some agents (e.g., PB) than with others (e.g., sodium valproate, CBZ, or GPT). The relative effects of the newer AEDs have yet to be fully determined. No cognitive effects were found with LTG in one study (Smith et al., 1993), and several studies using quality-of-life measures reported a beneficial effect of LTG on patient perception of psychologic well-being (Brodie et al., 1995; Smith et al., 1993). In 25 healthy adults participating in a double-blind randomized crossover design study, LTG produced significantly fewer cognitive and behavioral effects than did CBZ (Meador et al., 2001). Psychomotor slowing, language problems, and difficulty

with memory are reported with TPM (Martin et al., 1999). The word-finding difficulty seen in both children and adults is unique to TPM (Meador et al., 2001).

Finally, the *possibility of teratogenicity* when treatment is prolonged to the reproductive age must be taken into account when long-term treatment is being prescribed to female adolescents (Morrell, 2002; Tettenborn et al., 2002; Kaneko et al., 1988; Janz et al., 1982). The older AEDs (benzodiazepines, PHT, PB, CBZ, and valproate) are associated with a risk of major fetal malformations, including cleft lip and palate and cardiac defects. The incidence of these major malformations in infants born to mothers taking AEDs is 4% to 6%, compared with 2% to 4% for the general population. Neural tube defects occur in 1% to 2% of infants exposed to valproate and in 0.5% to 1% of those exposed to CBZ (Omtzigt et al., 1992; Rosa, 1991). All authors have agreed and recent studies have confirmed (Holmes et al., 2001) that the risks of malformations are highest in those fetuses exposed to multiple AEDs and in those exposed to higher doses. Little information regarding effects of newer AEDS on the developing human fetus is yet available. For some, substantial data are accumulating (Tennis and Eldridge, 2002), but more than 2,000 prospective pregnancies are needed to detect a drug effect that occurs in 4% to 8% of exposed fetuses (Morrell, 2002). The teratogenic potential of AEDs will be better defined when global prospective registries are developed to record pregnancy outcomes after AED exposure (Beghi et al., 2001).

Clinicians following adolescent girls for their epilepsy must be aware that the malformations associated with AEDs are all generated in the first trimester of pregnancy and that neural tube defects are formed by day 28 after conception. Pre-conception counseling is thus essential. Modifications of the ongoing treatment should take place before conception to allow optimal therapy with the lowest possible dose, preferably of monotherapy. The type(s) of seizures must be taken into account. For example, if generalized tonic-clonic seizures in a patient with juvenile myoclonic epilepsy are well controlled with an average dose of LTG but some myoclonic jerks persist, not adding any other medication, at least until the end of the first trimester, might be preferable.

In some cases, AEDs may produce a *paradoxical increase in seizure frequency* (Guerrini et al., 1998c, 2002c; Perruca et al., 1998). CBZ is contraindicated in patients with absence epilepsy and juvenile myoclonic epilepsy (Sozuer et al., 1996; Callaghan and Noetzel, 1992; Shorvon et al., 1978), but, in some cases, its use might be necessary for the control of tonic-clonic seizures resistant to other available drugs. It should also be used with caution in patients with a mixed seizure disorder, particularly in those with a combination of atonic, tonic-clonic, myoclonic, and atypical absence seizures and generalized bilateral EEG discharges (Perucca et al., 1998). VGB or GPT may be responsible for an increase in the frequency of typical absences and/or myoclonias. An aggravating effect has been reported when LTG is administered in young children with Dravet syndrome (Guerrini et al., 1998e). The aggravation of absence or myoclonic seizures with the use of PHT has also been reported, but the overall number of cases is lower than that recorded with CBZ.

In view of the problems associated with the chronic treatment with AEDs (American Academy of Pediatrics Committee on Drugs, 1995; Aldenkamp et al., 1993; Schmidt, 1989; Herranz et al., 1988; Oxley et al., 1983), much depends on the intelligent cooperation of the patient and his or her family and on their understanding of the problems posed by the disorder. Therefore, the nature of the problem should be explained in simple terms, and the necessity for prolonged supervision should be made clear. Treatment is a reasonable compromise between benefits and toxicity (i.e., between control of seizures and side effects), and that essential aspect should be understood by families.

It is important to warn parents at the outset of initiating anticonvulsant medication that modifying the dosage to find the best dose for the individual child is often necessary and that trying a different or additional medication if the first drug fails to control seizures is also not uncommon. This may help parents to accept later changes with less anxiety and fewer doubts about the competence of their physician than if they are not warned from the beginning.

Especially during the period of initiation and equilibration of drug therapy, an accurate record of the frequency of the patient's seizures and response to drugs is essential. The establishment of calendars or graphs should be strongly encouraged because memory is a highly selective process and is subject to many faults. Parents commonly state that the occurrence of seizures in their children is related to certain cyclic or psychic events, although written records often clearly indicate that no real relationship exists. When information is lacking, the patient and his or her family must be taught how to identify and describe the important signs and symptoms. Home videotapes of the paroxysmal events are increasingly becoming available, and these are often of great as-

sistance. Parents should be encouraged to record their children's attacks.

The *combination of two or more AEDs* for the treatment of epilepsy was common until the early 1980s to the point that many of the available AED preparations contained fixed-ration combinations of two agents, usually PB and PHT. Based on data from a controlled study assessing the value of CBZ and PHT monotherapy, Shorvon et al. (1978) were the first to challenge this practice. During the last 20 years, the use of a *single drug* (monotherapy) has been preferred to polypharmacy (Perucca and Levy, 2002; Heller et al., 1989; McGowan et al., 1983; Reynolds et al., 1981; Reynolds and Shorvon, 1981), and, certainly, in the overwhelming majority of patients, no valid reason exists for *starting* treatment with two or more drugs. Several studies have shown that 70% to 90% of newly diagnosed common forms of epilepsy can be controlled with a single agent (Da Silva et al., 1989; Heller et al., 1989; Forsythe and Sills, 1984; Reynolds and Shorvon, 1981; Strandjord and Johannessen, 1980), and recent active-control monotherapy trials of the new AEDs have confirmed the existing data. The use of a single agent is generally associated with fewer and easier to recognize side effects than polypharmacy, and the opportunity for drug interactions is lower. Additionally, with the use of two or more drugs, the blood levels of one or all of the agents are commonly inadequate; the adjustment of the blood level of one drug to the so-called *optimal range* in such cases often results in control (Reynolds and Shorvon, 1981; Viani et al., 1977).

Conversely, a *reduction from polypharmacy to monotherapy* is often possible without the exacerbation of seizure frequency or a loss of control (Holmes, 2002; Albright and Bruni, 1985; Shorvon and Reynolds, 1980). Children with mental impairment are particularly at risk of overtreatment, and institutionalized patients are frequently left on a sedative barbiturate or a benzodiazepine in addition to their AED regimen, even though the seizures persist. Recent studies have shown that, despite the significant number of side effects associated with PB, the drug continues to be widely used, in both institutions and outpatient settings (Rochat et al., 2001). Pellock and Hunt (1996) attempted to discontinue or to reduce the use of AEDs in 244 institutionalized patients. The percentage of patients receiving monotherapy increased from 37% to 58% with no observed loss of seizure control. Converting a patient to monotherapy from polytherapy is more difficult than maintaining the patient on monotherapy. The reduction of drugs is time consuming and it must be directed by skillful child neurologists, but the quality of life and alertness of these patients certainly benefit from the adjustment.

Drug combinations should be used only after correct dosages of single drugs have been used long enough to make an adequate assessment. The duration of such periods depends on the pharmacokinetics of the drug used and on other poorly understood factors. Thus, the full effect of certain drugs may be obtained only after 2 or 3 months of administration (Vajda and Aicardi, 1983), whereas with others, such as VGB, the effect, if any, is rapidly obtained (Herranz et al., 1991). In the case of failure of a first drug, substitution with another drug is preferable to adding another drug. However, the temporary association of a second drug to a first agent that has been unsuccessful may be preferable to simple crossover because this avoids some of the withdrawal problems. When control is obtained after the addition of a second drug, withdrawal of the first agent may be attempted to verify that the second drug rather than a combination of both was actually the effective agent.

No consensus exists on the number of monotherapy trials that should be attempted before combination therapy is introduced. The authors believe that at least two appropriate AEDs at the maximally tolerated dose must be tried. Evidence from open clinical trials in adolescents and adults (Kwan and Brodie, 2000, 2001) has shown that the full control of seizures is only rarely obtained from a third drug when the first two have failed. This probably applies to children as well. However, the occurrence of two types of seizures in the same patient that require different therapy (Perucca and Levy, 2002; Aird et al., 1984) (e.g., Lennox-Gastaut syndrome or Dravet syndrome) sometimes justifies the early introduction of combination therapy. Even in such cases, however, the use of some modern drugs with a large spectrum of action (e.g., valproate, LTG, TPM, LEV) may obviate the need for polytherapy (Arzimanoglou, 2002b).

The *progressivity of changes in dosage* in the initiation or withdrawal of any drug is essential. The first drug or successive drugs should be introduced at low dosages. The dose should be increased gradually until control is obtained or the limit of tolerance is reached.

Many physicians systematically adjust the dose until it is within the so-called *optimal range* of blood levels. However, keeping the dose as low as possible is preferable, as long as clinical control is gained, even if the blood levels remain "subtherapeutic." The latter method is difficult to apply to patients with infrequent seizures because ensuring that control has been obtained is difficult. *However, physicians must be aware that, even when a drug is used within the so-called therapeutic range, the control of seizures is the sole criterion of efficacy.* Because of the possible effects of AEDs on intelligence and development (Meador, 2001; Thompson, 1991; Thompson et al., 1981, 1987; Thompson and Trimble, 1981, 1982, 1983), the use of small doses may be especially important.

Most *recurrences* occur within 3 months of the first seizure; patients who have had no fit during that period can probably be maintained on a low dose, regardless of the blood levels. However, the dilemma should be understood by the parents, and their agreement should be obtained. The dose is, of course, increased if further fits supervene.

When the first drug that is tried has failed, the plasma level may have to be verified before switching to another drug. Side effects may develop even at relatively low levels at the beginning of treatment. Tolerance may develop later, so abandoning an effective drug because of transient difficulties should be avoided. The *lack of efficacy of a drug* should be clearly established before it is abandoned. However, if no side effects develop in the absence of control, the recommendation is to increase blood levels above the so-called *therapeutic range*, provided this is done with caution and proper surveillance. The fear of chronic toxicity tends to limit this practice. Reports suggesting that high levels of certain AEDs might be associated with significant decreases in intelligence quotients (IQs) in the chronic treatment of epilepsy (Thompson et al., 1987; Zaret and Cohen, 1986) are worrisome in this regard, although the results are not unanimous (Dodrill and Wilensky, 1992). The impact of CBZ and valproate monotherapy on cognitive function was minimal, compared with the pretreatment baseline performance (Prevey et al., 1996). Effects on cognition are a matter of concern with the use of PB and especially PHT because of their chronic toxicity and their possible adverse effects on brain development and intellectual performance (Trimble, 1990a). In the authors' opinion, increasing the doses of AEDs to the highest possible level is perhaps safer with the newer antiepileptic agents, such as LTG or GPT. Comparable studies in adults support this position (Meador, 2001; Meador et al., 1999; Brodie et al., 1995). Drowsiness may be observed with high doses of GPT (Leach et al., 1997), and hyperactivity has also been reported in children (Lee et al., 1996). More experience is needed before firm conclusions are formulated.

Ineffective drugs should be withdrawn progressively, except in the case of dangerous reactions. This gradual tapering should be combined with the progressive introduction of a second drug or should follow the introduction of the second drug, whether or not control has been achieved (Aird et al., 1984). The authors' practice is to discontinue the ineffective drug over 1 to 3 months. Thus, for a brief duration, the two drugs are given simultaneously.

CHOICE OF ANTIEPILEPTIC DRUGS

The *choice of drug* depends first on the type(s) of seizure the patient is experiencing (Arzimanoglou, 2002b; Guerrini et al., 2002a). However, the specificity of any given drug for a particular type of seizure is not very great (Aicardi and Arzimanoglou, 1996; Verity et al., 1995; Chadwick, 1987; Chadwick and Turnbull, 1985; Mattson et al., 1985), and only rough directions can be given. Randomized, controlled trials comparing two or more AEDs used as first choice monotherapy either are lacking, or they cover only very short periods of treatment, thus rendering any definite conclusion rather arbitrary.

The lack of direct comparative evidence has led to a number of metaanalysis studies (Marson et al. 2000, 2001, 2002; Tudur et al., 2001, 2002; Taylor et al., 2001). In most of these studies, no significant differences were found in seizure outcome. However, the specific effects of each drug on certain syndromes, particularly those expressing with several types of seizures, and especially on individual patients cannot be ascertained by these studies. During the last decade, clinical practice has shown that, in given situations, there are stronger indications for some drugs than for others (see earlier discussion).

In difficult cases, several drugs must be used in succession on the basis of the data provided in Table 24.2 and then modified by a process of trial and error, as the clinical results in individual patients dictate. The efficacy on the EEG does not need to parallel the clinical efficacy strictly, and subclinical epilepsy that is associated with intense paroxysmal EEG activity tends to be resistant to most conventional antiepileptic agents.

The effectiveness of AEDs against the main types of seizures or syndromes is indicated in Tables 24.2 and 24.3. In general, from the standpoint of effectiveness, AEDs can be divided into the following three broad categories:

(a) those active only against generalized nonconvulsive seizures (absences) and certain myoclonic seizures, a category that includes ethosuximide and its related compounds and the diones;

(b) those active against a wide range of seizure types, whether generalized or partial, a group including the benzodiazepines, sodium valproate, LTG, TPM, and probably LEV; and

(c) those that are mainly active against partial seizures, including GPT, VGB, tiagabine, PB, PHT and its related compounds, PRM, CBZ, and pheneturide.

This classification is somewhat simplified, and variations among the individual drugs do exist within the three groups.

Phenobarbital and Phenytoin

Phenobarbital (PB) and phenytoin (PHT) belong to the first generation of AEDs. PB is an effective anticonvulsant against tonic-clonic and focal seizures. The drug is ineffective against absence or atonic seizures or infantile spasms, or it may even worsen them. Behavioral disturbances are commonly observed in children. Cognitive function disturbances, with memory problems or compromised school performance, have been regularly reported. Whenever possible, the use of PB in children should be avoided. The drug is still used in neonates (see Chapter 12). This choice is not based on its proven superiority. It is founded on many years of familiarity with the drug by pediatricians and is related to the lack of controlled studies and injectable formulations of newer AEDs. PHT remains a drug of choice for the treatment of partial and generalized tonic-clonic seizures. Acute toxic effects (e.g., ataxia, nystagmus, incoordination) are dose related and relatively frequent. Chronic adverse effects, such as gingival hyperplasia, hirsutism, and coarsening of the facies, should be kept in mind when prescribing the drug as a chronic treatment, particularly in children. Neuropathy and cerebellar degeneration may occur with long-term use. In neonates, adequate blood levels may be difficult to obtain. For a complete review of indications and adverse effects, see Levy et al. (2002:489–540 [for PB], 551–610 [for PHT]).

Carbamazepine

CBZ, along with VPA, belongs to the second generation of AEDs, which are considered to have less neurotoxicity than the older drugs, such as PHT, PB, and PRM. CBZ, which has been available since the early 1960s, is prescribed as a first-line drug for children with partial seizures. It is effective as single-drug treatment and in combination therapy. The titration rate should always be slow, and even moderate dosages may be sufficient. Common adverse events include ataxia, diplopia, and rash (Pellock, 1987). Its efficacy in other types of seizures is controversial. An increase in generalized tonic-clonic seizures and absences and the precipitation of atonic and myoclonic seizures in children with symptomatic or cryptogenic generalized epilepsies have been reported. For a complete review of indications and adverse effects, see Levy et al. (2002:262–272, 285–297).

Sodium Valproate

Sodium valproate (or VPA) is an established anticonvulsant that has withstood the test of time. It is a large-spectrum AED, whose use is indicated for the treatment of all types of seizures, and it has an extremely low potential for seizure exacerbation. It is the drug of first choice for myoclonic seizures and absences, and its use is almost systematic in combination therapies for the treatment of severe epilepsy syndromes, such as Lennox-Gastaut syndrome or Dravet syndrome. Weight gain and tremor are rather common side effects.

VPA is contraindicated in patients with hepatic disease, significant hepatic dysfunction, or mitochondrial disorders. Routine monitoring of liver enzymes during VPA therapy is a common practice, and, often, some elevation of the transaminases is seen. This finding is of no value for predicting hepatic failure, and the diagnosis of hepatotoxicity depends mostly on the early recognition of the clinical features, including nausea, vomiting, anorexia, and lethargy. The highest risk of fatal hepatotoxicity is found in infants younger than 3 years (Bryant and Dreifuss, 1996), which suggests that VPA therapy should be avoided in this age-group if this is at all possible. Potentially fatal acute hemorrhagic pancreatitis has been reported, and this possibility should be investigated in cases manifesting with abdominal pain, nausea, vomiting, or anorexia. Comedication with TPM has been reported to be a risk for VPA-induced hyperammonemic encephalopathy (Hamer et al., 2000). However, severe adverse effects are rare.

The titration should be slow (10 to 15 mg per kg per day at weekly intervals up to a dose of 30 to 50 mg/kg per day) and twice daily administration is recommended. In the authors' experience, this is possible for most cases, even with the use of the oral syrup or immediate-release formulations. Measurement of the VPA blood levels can be valuable in selected cases, but the results must be interpreted cautiously. No good correlation has been demonstrated between VPA levels and clinical efficacy at a given time, and the VPA levels fluctuate considerably during a 24-hour period because of its short half-life. For a complete review of the indications and adverse effects, see Levy et al. (2002:808–817, 837–851).

Lamotrigine

LTG, a broad-spectrum AED, is chemically unlike other current anticonvulsants. It acts partly by blocking voltage-dependent and use-dependent sodium channels, thus stabilizing the neuronal membrane. It inhibits the excessive release of excitatory amino acids (e.g., glutamate), although other actions have been proposed (Leach et al., 2002; Messenheimer et al., 2000).

LTG has been proven effective as both add-on therapy and monotherapy (Sander et al., 1990a, 1990b). Thirteen studies have demonstrated its efficacy in 1,096 children with a variety of seizure types. Efficacy and safety have been reported in children and adolescents with partial-onset seizures (Schlumberger et al., 1994), a finding that was confirmed by a placebo-controlled, parallel group trial (Duchowny et al., 1999). Statistically, more of the LTG-treated patients had a reduction in the frequency of all types of major seizures, drop attacks, and tonic-clonic seizures in a double-blind study of adjunctive LTG treatment in children and adolescents with Lennox-Gastaut syndrome (Motte et al., 1997). Open studies have confirmed the efficacy of LTG or the LTG–valproate combination in this syndrome (Arzimanoglou et al., 2001; Pisani et al., 1999). The authors now tend to use this combination as early as possible in the treatment of children with an onset reminiscent of Lennox-Gastaut syndrome or in epilepsies characterized by myoclonic astatic seizures. A paradoxical aggravating effect has been reported (Guerrini et al., 1998e) in young children with Dravet syndrome.

VPA strongly interferes with the metabolism of LTG, producing a marked elevation of its blood levels, so the dose should be reduced (roughly halved) when the drug is combined with valproate. LTG monotherapy at a median dose of 5 mg per kg per day fully controlled typical absence seizures in 30 (71%) of the 42 children who completed the dose escalation in a double-blind, placebo-controlled study (Franck et al., 1999). In cases of intractable absence epilepsy, moderate dosages of a VPA–LTG combination should usually be tried.

The principal, usually mild to moderate adverse effects associated with LTG in the various studies included dizziness and diplopia, which were seen more frequently in the presence of CBZ; tremor, which occurred more frequently in the presence of VPA;

TABLE 24.2. *Indications, suggested dose, side effects, and toxicity of antiepileptic drugs*

Drug	Indication	Usual Dose (Oral)	Number of Daily Doses	Side Effects	Serious Toxicity
Acetazolamide	Absences; partial and tonic-clonic	10 mg/kg/d <1–12 mo, 20–30 mg/kg/d >1 yr	2	Drowsiness; headache; acidosis; polyuria	Renal calculi
Carbamazepine	Partial and tonic-clonic seizures[a]	10–20 mg/kg/d	2–3[b]	Ataxia, diplopia, rashes	Aplastic anemia (rare)
Clobazam	Adjunctive therapy for partial and generalized seizures; NCSE; LKS[f]	10–20 mg/d	1–3	Sedation; may worsen tonic status	—
Clonazepam	Status epilepticus; all forms	0.1–0.2 mg/kg/d	2–3	Fatigue, drowsiness, hypotonia, behavior disturbances, salivary and bronchial hypersecretion	Respiratory depression (only i.v. route)
Diazepam	All forms, mainly acute treatment of status	0.25–1.5 mg/kg/d, 0.01–0.25 mg/kg i.v., 0.25–0.5 mg/kg (rectal)		Hypotonia, drowsiness	Respiratory depression (only i.v. route)
Ethosuximide	Absences, myoclonic seizures, NCSE	20–30 mg/kg/d	1–2	Gastric discomfort, hiccups, rash, blurred vision, headache	Aplastic anemia (rare)
Felbamate	Partial, tonic-clonic, atonic, myoclonic seizures, and atypical absences	15–45 mg/kg/d	2	Somnolence, anorexia, gastric discomfort, nervousness	Aplastic anemia (300 per million adult patients treated); hepatotoxicity (164/million)
Gabapentin	Partial seizures[a]	30–60 mg/kg/d	2–3[b]	Somnolence, dizziness, weight gain	Almost never
Lamotrigine	Partial and all types of generalized seizures[c]	5–15 mg/kg/d[d], 1–5 mg/kg/d[e]	2	Dizziness; diplopia; ataxia; somnolence; rash	Stevens-Johnson syndrome; Lyell syndrome
Levetiracetam	Partial seizures; tonic-clonic seizures; probably large spectrum	20–40 mg/kg/d	2	Somnolence; asthenia; psychotic events (rare)	Of recent use not allowing full knowledge
Nitrazepam	Infantile spasms; syndromes with multiple types of seizures; myoclonic epilepsies	0.25–1 mg/kg/d	2	Hypotonia, drowsiness, hypersalivation	
Oxcarbazepine	Partial and tonic-clonic seizures[a]	20–40 mg/kg/d	2	Somnolence; headache; ataxia; hyponatremia; rash	
Phenobarbital	Partial and tonic-clonic seizures[a]	3–5 mg/kg/d <5 yr; 2–3 mg/kg/d >5 yr	2 or 1 at bedtime	Behavior disturbances, drowsiness, rash; may affect cognitive function; systemic toxicity	Hypersensitivity reactions (rare)

Drug	Indication	Dosage		Adverse effects
Phenytoin	Partial and tonic-clonic seizures[a]	8–10 mg/kg/d <3 yr; 4–7 mg/kg/d >3 yr	2	Ataxia, diplopia, nystagmus, acne, gum hypertrophy, hirsutism; cognitive and sedative effects; peripheral neuropathy	Megaloblastic anemia, lymphoma, encephalopathy, choreoathetosis
Primidone	Partial and tonic-clonic seizures[a]	10–20 mg/kg/d	2–3[b]	Behavior distubances, drowsiness, rash; may affect cognitive function	Anemia (rare)
Sodium valproate	All types of seizures	15–40 mg/kg/d	2–3[b]	Nausea and epigastric pain, tremor, alopecia, weight gain, hyperammonemia	Encephalopathy, hepatitis and pancreatitis (rare)
Sulthiame	Partial seizures	5–15 mg/kg/d	2	Ataxia, paresthesia	—
Tiagabine	Partial seizures[a]	0.5–2 mg/kg/d	2	Dizziness, abdominal pain, nervousness; difficulty with concentration	NCSE
Topiramate	All types of seizures	3–9 mg/kg/d, slow titration	2	Weight loss, renal calculi, paresthesias; cognitive dysfunction (mental-slowing and word-finding difficulty)	
Vigabatrin	Infantile spasms; partial seizures	20–80 mg/kg/d; Spasms: 100–150 mg/kg/d	2	Excitation; drowsiness; weight gain	Psychosis (rare); visual field defects (40%; not always clinically detectable)
Zonisamide	Partial and tonic-clonic seizures; atypical absences	4–8 mg/kg/d	2	Somnolence; dizziness; ataxia; abdominal discomfort; psychomotor slowing; oligohidrosis; weight loss	Psychiatric disorders

Abbreviations: LKS, Landau-Kleffner syndrome; NA, not applicable; NCSE, nonconvulsive status.

[a]May have a paradoxical effect in idiopathic generalized epilepsies.
[b]In clinical practice, administering twice is possible. See text.
[c]May not be efficacious or aggravate myoclonic seizures in some juvenile myoclonic epilepsy patients.
[d]Child on enzyme inducers.
[e]Child on valproate. Slow titration.
[f]The authors often use clobazam during transitory aggravation of a severe epilepsy or as intermittent treatment in generalized idiopathic epilepsies (juvenile myoclonic epilepsy) as well as to stop serial seizures.

TABLE 24.3. *Main drugs for various types of epilepsy*

Type of Epilepsy	Drugs
Idiopathic generalized epilepsies with tonic-clonic seizures	*Valproate,* lamotrigine, topiramate, primidone, phenobarbital
Generalized epilepsies with myoclonic seizures	*Valproate,* ethosuximide, benzodiazepines, topiramate, lamotrigine[a]
Generalized epilepsies with typical absences	*Valproate,* ethosuximide, lamotrigine, benzodiazepines
Epilepsies with secondarily generalized tonic-clonic seizures	All drugs except ethosuximide
Secondary generalized epilepsies with tonic-atonic seizures and/or atypical absences	*Valproate, lamotrigine,* topiramate, benzodiazepines, carbamazepine, phenytoin, vigabatrin, ACTH and/or corticosteroids, felbamate[a]
West syndrome	*Vigabatrin,* ACTH and/or corticosteroids, nitrazepam, valproate
Idiopathic partial epilepsies	*Valproate,* gabapentin, carbamazepine
Symptomatic partial epilepsies	*Carbamazepine, Valproate,* gabapentine, lamotrigine, topiramate, levetiracetam, vigabatrin[a], primidone, phenobarbital
Continuous spike-waves of slow sleep (electrical status epilepticus of slow sleep and Landau-Kleffner)	*Clobazam,* ethosuximide, sulthiame, ACTH and/or corticosteroids
Dravet syndrome	*Valproate,* clobazam, stiripentol, topiramate

Note: The drugs usually considered as first choice are in italic type. Order of preference is only approximate and depends on various factors (see appropriate chapters).
Abbreviation: ACTH, adrenocorticotropic hormone.
[a]See comments in Table 24.2.

ataxia; and nausea. Skin rashes occurred in approximately 5% of patients treated with the drug, but their incidence can be minimized by starting with a low dose that is slowly escalated over several weeks (Messenheimer, 1998; Dooley et al., 1996). The rashes usually are mild, although, in a small number of patients, they may be life threatening as they may occur in the form of Stevens-Johnson and Lyell syndrome. For a complete review of the indications and adverse effects of LTG, see Levy et al. (2002: 388–402, 408–416).

Gabapentin

GPT, a chemical derivative of GABA, was thought to mimic the actions of GABA at inhibitory synaptic receptors in the brain. Subsequent studies have, however, shown that GPT is inactive at $GABA_A$ and $GABA_B$ receptors, although it does increase the synthesis and nonvesicular release of GABA, and that it probably possesses multiple mechanisms of action (Sills and Brodie, 2001). The drug is approved for adjunctive or monotherapy treatment of partial seizures.

Two pediatric studies have been reported. The first, a 12-week multicenter, double-blind study, evaluated the efficacy and tolerability of add-on GPT in pa-

tients from 3 to 12 years of age with refractory partial seizures (Appleton et al., 1999a), and the second evaluated the drug over a 6-month period in 237 children (Appleton et al., 2001). All of the children received GPT at doses of 24 to 70 mg per kg per day. For all partial seizures, the median percentage change in seizure frequency was −34%, and the overall responder rate was 34%. A more recent study (Ouellet et al., 2001) reported on the pharmacokinetics of GPT in infants and children and concluded that, on a weight basis, 33% larger doses are required in children younger than 5 years to achieve the same exposure as in older children.

GPT may increase typical and atypical absences or myoclonias. Serious adverse events are extremely rare. In children, especially in those with chronic epilepsy and static encephalopathy, behavioral changes characterized by the acute onset of aggression, hyperactivity, and impulsive behavior have been reported. Weight gain is not rare. The safety and tolerability profile of the drug, along with the absence of pharmacokinetic interactions, are strong advantages that favor its use for the treatment of newly diagnosed partial epilepsies, as well as in usually benign idiopathic partial epilepsies (Bourgeois et al., 1998).

Topiramate

TPM has multiple pharmacologic effects. The drug modulates the voltage-dependent sodium ion channels, potentiates GABA-mediated inhibitory neurotransmission, blocks the excitatory neurotransmission mediated by non–*N*-methyl-D-aspartate receptors, modulates voltage-gated calcium ion channels, and inhibits brain carbonic anhydrase (White, 2002). Coadministration with the enzyme-inducing AEDs, such as PHT or CBZ, can be expected to result in a twofold to threefold increase in TPM clearance, and these interactions can be clinically significant. Furthermore, oral contraceptive effectiveness may be compromised in the presence of TPM.

Several controlled studies have provided evidence for efficacy of TPM in partial epilepsies, both in adults and in children (Elterman et al., 1999). In long-term, open-label extension studies, the mean TPM dose in children was 9 mg per kg per day. In the authors' experience, doses greater than 5 mg per kg per day are only rarely tolerated. The drug has also been evaluated for the control of primary generalized tonic-clonic seizures and as an adjunctive treatment for patients with Lennox-Gastaut syndrome (Sachdeo et al., 1999). Of 82 patients who experienced drop attacks and who received TPM for 6 months or more, 55% had a reduction of more than 50% in the drop attacks. A reduction of 75% was experienced by 35%, and 15% became free of drop attacks for at least 6 months. The clinical efficacy and the broad spectrum of TPM have been shown in a number of open studies and case reports. Ongoing monotherapy studies in children have provided similar results.

Thus far, the most important adverse effect of TPM is cognitive dysfunction, which is evidenced by mental slowing and word-finding difficulty and which can be quite significant. Other side effects include weight loss, which may be substantial, and paresthesias.

Based on clinical experience, the recommendation is that TPM should be started at a low dose and titrated slowly to clinical response. For a review of indications and adverse effects of TPM, see Levy et al. (2002:740–752, 760–764).

Oxcarbazepine

OXC is essentially a prodrug. The percentage of patients achieving complete seizure control with OXC is comparable to that of patients taking CBZ; OXC may, however, be associated with fewer adverse effects. The drug may reduce LTG concentrations while increasing those of PHT. OXC induces oral contraceptives. The drug shows comparable efficacy to PHT and VPA as well as to CBZ as monotherapy for partial-onset seizures. Hyponatremia that rarely is clinically relevant is observed in more than 25% of children treated with OXC (Holtmann et al., 2002).

OXC is indicated for the control of partial seizures. A total of 267 children with partial epilepsy from 3 to 17 years of age were enrolled in an add-on, randomized, placebo-controlled study (Glauser et al., 2000b); 41% of the patients treated with OXC (30 to 46 mg per kg per day orally) experienced a more than 50% reduction from baseline in partial seizure frequency over 28 days, compared with a reduction of only 22% in children treated with placebo ($p=0.0005$).

The common adverse effects in previously untreated patients include somnolence, headache, dizziness, nausea, apathy, and rash. For a review of indications and adverse effects of OXC, see Levy et al. (2002:470–475, 479–486).

Levetiracetam

LEV is the *S*-enantiomer of the ethyl analog of piracetam. Its mechanism of action has not yet been characterized. The efficacy of LEV as adjunctive therapy for localization-related epilepsies has been established by three multicenter studies, and monotherapy studies are ongoing. Anecdotal data suggest that the drug has a broad spectrum of action (Brodie and French, 2003), including efficacy against myoclonic seizures, photosensitivity, and generalized tonic-clonic seizures (Kasteleijn-Nolst Trenité and Hirsch, 2003; Genton and Gelisse, 2000). An open-label study with adjunctive LEV (20 to 40 mg per kg per day) for the treatment of partial seizures in 24 children was conducted; in 52%, the seizure frequency decreased by more than 50%, and 2 patients remained seizure free during the entire evaluation period (Glauser et al., 2002). In the authors' limited experience, the results in children with refractory partial epilepsy confirm the results of studies in adults. The drug is well tolerated, but somnolence is a relatively common side effect. Rare cases presenting with psychotic events are on record (Youroukos et al., 2003). For a review of indications and adverse effects of LEV, see Levy et al. (2002:432–441, 442–447).

Vigabatrin

VGB (γ-vinyl-GABA) is an irreversible inhibitor of the enzyme GABA transaminase, which catalyzes the catabolism of the inhibitory neurotransmitter GABA. VGB therefore considerably increases the levels of GABA in the brain and cerebrospinal fluid (Richens,

1991). The drug is extremely active in the treatment of partial epilepsies in adults (Sivenius et al., 1991b; Cocito et al., 1989; Tartara et al., 1989; Browne et al., 1987) and in children (Lortie et al., 1997; Nabbout et al., 1997; Uldall et al., 1991; Livingston et al., 1989; Luna et al., 1989a), but it may also be effective as therapy for other types, including infantile spasms (Elterman et al., 2001; Appleton et al., 1999b; Aicardi et al., 1996; Chiron et al., 1990) (see Chapter 3). It may be particularly effective against symptomatic spasms, especially those that are caused by tuberous sclerosis (Chiron et al., 1990, 1991a, 1997; Vigevano and Cilio, 1997). For the treatment of infantile spasms, the most effective dosage has been found to be 100 to 150 mg per kg per day. For partial seizures, 2 to 3 g per day is considered the effective dosage in adults, and it ranges from 45 to 150 mg per kg in children. The titration of VGB is relatively easy, and it must be discontinued slowly to avoid rebound seizures (Arzimanoglou, 1994).

The drug does not cause enzyme induction, and it does not interact significantly with most drugs. Sedation, fatigue, and weight gain are the most commonly reported side effects. Psychosis and depression have been noted in some studies, and hyperactivity has been reported in children (Sander et al., 1991b). The first reports suggesting irreversible impairment of visual fields in patients on chronic VGB therapy appeared only 16 years from onset of use (Mackenzie and Klistorner, 1998). Several retrospective studies, including studies of patients who received VGB monotherapy, have confirmed these data (Kalviainen et al., 1999). The overall prevalence of the visual impairment is approximately 20% to 40%, and it is twice as high in men as it is in women. The prevalence of symptomatic cases, however, is much lower, possibly in the vicinity of 1% (Wild et al., 1999). Visual field constriction has also been reported in children (Vanhatalo et al., 1999, 2002; Gross-Tsur et al., 2000). Visual field perimetry tests cannot be performed in young children, and alternative techniques using visual evoked potentials are being developed (Harding et al., 2002). Although several questions remain, the available evidence suggests that visual field loss is less likely to occur after the first 4 years of continuous treatment (Wild et al., 1999).

The authors still consider VGB a first-line drug for infantile spasms because if a response to the drug occurs, it is usually observed within 1 to 2 weeks. Once the infantile spasms are under control, the VGB treatment period may then be reduced to a few months, which considerably reduces the risk of developing a visual field defect. In partial epilepsies that are in-

tractable to other AEDs, the use of VGB still has a place. However, the need for a regular ophthalmologic examination and the availability of a considerable number of new AEDs have limited its use to the most refractory cases. For a complete review of the indications for its use and the adverse effects, see Levy et al. (2002:855–863).

Felbamate

FBM is a drug of interest, particularly because it may be effective in patients with secondary generalized epilepsies. Its efficacy for both partial and generalized epilepsies has been established in adjunctive and monotherapy studies, and its initial clinical toxicity profile suggested an acceptable risk. However, the subsequent identification of life-threatening aplastic anemia and hepatotoxicity has limited its use to severe drug-resistant epilepsies.

Recently published updates (Pellock, 1999; Pellock and Brodie, 1997) have reported that 34 patients have contracted FBM-associated aplastic anemia, with 13 known fatalities. The overall FBM-associated aplastic anemia risk is estimated as being between 27 and 209 per million versus 2 to 2.5 per million in the general population. Prior AED hypersensitivity, cytopenia, and immune disease significantly increase the risk. FBM-associated aplastic anemia has not been reported in children younger than 13 years. Hepatic failure is much less common, occurring with an overall risk that is similar to that associated with valproate, but children younger than 5 years have been affected. Human leukocyte antigen studies and the recent identification of the reactive metabolite atropaldehyde suggest that high-risk patients could be identified. The efficacy profile of FBM should encourage further investigations to allow improved use.

Other Agents

Other new agents of potential value that are as yet incompletely tested or are not commercially available include zonisamide, stiripentol (Chiron et al., 2000), and a number of compounds in various stages of development (Bialer et al., 2002; Levy et al., 2002; Wyllie, 2001).

Clobazam is often effective in difficult cases (Sheth et al., 1995; Heller et al., 1988; Koepden et al., 1987; Schmidt et al., 1986b). However, the development of tolerance is a major problem with the benzodiazepines, and the loss of initial effectiveness is often observed within a few weeks or months. This phenomenon is related to the downregulation of benzodiazepine receptors in the brain (Specht et al., 1989; Kammerman,

1985). The same phenomenon may also account for the problems associated with the withdrawal of benzodiazepine therapy, especially with the common occurrence of withdrawal seizures (Hauser et al., 1989; Specht et al., 1989; Schmidt, 1985), so the use of benzodiazepines as a chronic treatment for epilepsy should always proceed with caution. The authors often use clobazam to cover periods of increased seizure susceptibility (e.g., titration of a new AED and occasionally after a short night's sleep).

In addition to the main drugs discussed here, minor drugs can occasionally be useful for individual cases (Battaglia et al., 1991; Oles et al., 1989; Binnie et al., 1985a; Gibberd et al., 1982; Berchou et al., 1981; Wilensky et al., 1981). Favorable results are sometimes obtained with second-line agents (Dasheiff et al., 1986), such as *chlorazepate* (Fuji et al., 1987; Naidu et al., 1986), *methsuximide* (Tennison et al., 1991), *sulthiame* (Rating, 2000; Rating et al., 2000; Green et al., 1974), *phenacemide* (Coker, 1986), and even *bromides* (Ernst et al., 1988). In refractory cases, all of the available agents should be tried (Aicardi, 1988a). They have been considered with the discussion of the treatment of the particular types of epilepsy, so they are not discussed in this chapter.

SELECTION OF THE FIRST DRUG

The *selection of the first drug* depends as much on the likely side effects and the greater or lesser difficulties in handling the drug as it does on efficacy. Any choice is necessarily arbitrary because neither the efficacy nor the side effects of any drug are entirely predictable (Mikati and Browne, 1988). Extensive reviews of the side effects of AEDs are available (Levy et al., 2002; Wyllie, 2001; Eadie and Tyrer, 1989). Many authors tend to avoid the use of PB in children because of its undesirable behavioral effects. PHT does not provoke similar behavioral disturbances, but its use is difficult because of its unpredictable pharmacokinetics, which makes relatively frequent blood-level determinations mandatory. In addition, PHT has a long list of undesirable side effects, many of which may have an insidious onset over many years. It also may be responsible for lowering IQs under certain conditions (Trimble, 1990a). The use of PRM represents a form of polytherapy because it is metabolized into two compounds, PB and phenylethylmalonamide.

With many drugs, repeated blood counts and hepatic tests are advised, although their value as predictors of serious side effects has never been established (Pellock and Wilmore, 1991; Evans et al., 1989; Cam-

field et al., 1986). Such tests may do more to protect the physician in the medicolegal arena than to safeguard the patient from toxicity. Indeed, leukopenia or elevation of transaminases rarely, if ever, heralds the occurrence of pancytopenia or liver failure, which can supervene abruptly even a few days after normal test results have been obtained. On the other hand, such abnormalities often lead to the discontinuation of effective therapy with disastrous results for the control of seizures.

Within each broad category of agents, an order of preference can be established that varies with the country, depending on the drugs available, health authority regulations, economic factors, and medical habits. Patients with the same epilepsy syndromes may well receive different drugs because of their country of residence or the preferences of their doctors. Table 24.3 indicates commonly accepted drugs for various forms of epilepsy.

Determining whether some drugs are more specifically indicated in specific epilepsy syndromes would be helpful. During the last 5 years, some data for the comparison of different drugs in different syndromes have become available (Arzimanoglou, 2002b). Most of the literature on this subject, however, deals with comparisons between drugs in extremely broad types of epilepsy (e.g., generalized tonic-clonic seizures or "partial" seizures), rather than in more specific syndromes. Considerably more work is necessary before definitive statements can be made in this regard.

CHOICE OF THE SECOND DRUG

The choice of a second drug is governed by the same general rules as those for the selection of a first agent. All physicians experienced in the care of epileptic patients have their own preferred sequence of drugs, depending not only on the type of epileptic seizure or syndrome but also on their personal habits and preferences. Alternative drugs are best used as single agents; after a crossover period, the modalities and duration of these depend on the case in question. Alternative single-drug therapy may lead to control of refractory epilepsies in 15% to 20% of patients (Kwan and Brodie, 2001; Schmidt and Richter, 1986).

The *addition of a second drug* (on rare occasions, of more than one drug) is justified when single drugs have failed or when seizures recur after the discontinuation of a drug that was found ineffective when used alone and control had been achieved when the patient received the ineffective drug in combination with a second drug. When patients are receiving two or more drugs, a determination of blood levels may be advisable because of possible drug interactions. It is often assumed that, when low blood levels of one drug or both drugs are found, dosages should be modified accordingly or that the agent with a low concentration can be withdrawn (Shorvon and Reynolds, 1980). Although that is often the case, many exceptions are known, and the discontinuation of one of a combination of drugs because of low blood levels may result in the resumption of seizures (Richens, 1982).

Theoretically, it is preferable to use combinations of drugs with different mechanisms of action (Brodie and Mumford, 1999). An agent that acts primarily on membrane conductance, such as CBZ, should therefore be combined with one that has a predominantly synaptic mechanism of action, such as sodium valproate. Alternatively, agents that act on different synapses (e.g., VGB on GABAergic synapses) can logically be associated. However, the current knowledge of the mechanisms of action of the various drugs, most of which have more than one primary action, is still too incomplete to allow the rational application of such an approach (Perucca, 1996).

The *choice of an association depends* mostly on clinical assessment of how drug combinations behave with regard to both their efficacy and their unwanted side effects (Bourgeois, 1988; Bourgeois and Wad, 1988). From both points of view, drug associations can have an additive effect or a supraadditive effect, or no change from the effects of each individual drug may be seen. Desirable associations are those in which the increase in the therapeutic effects is greater than that of the unwanted effects, regardless of whether this results from true synergism or from an additive therapeutic effect without augmentation of side effects.

In general, care should be taken to avoid certain combinations, particularly the association of drugs that have similar side effects that may be additive when used together. For example, PB and clonazepam may produce marked sedation. Similarly, combining PB with drugs such as PRM that are metabolized in large part to PB is unwise.

Combinations of three or more drugs are only rarely indicated, and their efficacy remains to be demonstrated (Reynolds and Shorvon, 1981). If they are used at all, the multiple associations should be carefully monitored both clinically and with the determination of blood levels. Studies have shown that, in such cases, excessively high levels of one drug, usually PB, and subtherapeutic levels of the others are commonly found (Morselli et al., 1980).

ADMINISTRATION OF ANTIEPILEPTIC DRUGS

The modalities of administration of the AEDs depend largely on their pharmacokinetic properties. The frequency of drug administration is partly dependent on the drug half-life. For anticonvulsants with long half-lives, such as PB, one dose per day is usually sufficient (Strandjord and Gilhus, 1984; Davies et al., 1981; Walson et al., 1980), except in young infants with a very fast metabolism. PHT may be given once a day for adults, but it should probably be used as two daily doses for children. Ethosuximide also may be given as a single daily dose, but its gastric side effects make dividing the daily dose into two halves desirable.

CBZ, after an initial period of relatively slow elimination, has a short half-life, so its levels fluctuate rather widely over 24 hours (Rey et al., 1979; Porter, 1987). In addition, the side effects may be clinically detectable at the time of highest blood levels (Riva et al., 1984). In such cases, administration in three or even four divided doses could be advisable. Repeated administration is, however, highly inconvenient from both the practical and psychologic points of view, and this may well be unreliable because the child may dispense with the midday dose to avoid taking drugs in public. With virtually all drugs, including CBZ, this can usually be avoided, and the results of twice-a-day administration of that drug seem satisfactory.

With VPA, the situation is probably more complex. In most children, the half-life of the drug is indeed brief, which seems to imply a need repeated administration because of the rapid and marked fluctuations of blood levels (Loiseau et al., 1982), which are only partly avoided by the use of enteric-coated tablets. Some reports have, however, suggested that the anticonvulsant effect is maintained even at low blood levels (Rowan et al., 1979, 1981), and the use of a single daily dose has been advocated by some (Covanis and Jeavons, 1980; Stefan et al., 1984). The development of slow-release preparations of CBZ and sodium valproate has simplified this issue. Most of the newer drugs can be administered twice a day.

For all drugs, even when slow-release preparations are available, the authors prefer a twice-a-day administration because this also helps to avoid low concentrations of the ongoing treatment in instances in which the patients forget to take the medication.

Another consequence of the different pharmacokinetics of anticonvulsants is that the time required for the drug to become stabilized at those blood levels that are usually effective varies considerably. In principle, the achievement of stable blood levels requires approximately four times the plasma half-life of each agent (Richens, 1982). This duration may be even longer when the doses are gradually increased over several weeks, as frequently occurs when the patient's tolerance is being evaluated (Aird et al., 1984). This is one reason why a delay of at least 3 or 4 weeks should occur before an anticonvulsant with a long half-life is replaced with another agent.

Even excluding the treatment of status epilepticus, the administration of drugs by routes that allow rapid absorption may be helpful. Kriel et al. (1991) reported that the home use of rectal diazepam is useful in the treatment of breakthrough serial and prolonged seizures in children on maintenance AEDs. Its use has been associated with significant decreases in the use of emergency hospital services (Carlson et al., 1988). The authors also advise the occasional use of clobazam for patients presenting with serial seizures.

MONITORING OF ANTIEPILEPTIC TREATMENT

In the case of well-controlled epilepsy, regular *clinical supervision* is the only essential measure. Asking the patient specifically about side effects may be necessary because some patients do not mention temporary diplopia or vertigo, which they have come to consider a normal phenomenon. The search for side effects is especially difficult in infants or mentally retarded children (Eadie and Tyrer, 1989; Aicardi, 1980c) because marked mental and physical slowing may be erroneously attributed to seizures rather than to therapy. Moreover, the adverse effects of anticonvulsants may be particularly likely to occur in patients with a damaged brain. In school-aged children, a normal performance should be expected when the child's intellectual level is normal. Slowing of or decreases in school performance should always raise the possibility of a maladjustment to therapy and should prompt the monitoring of blood levels.

The *determination of blood levels of anticonvulsant drugs* has been an important step in the progress of antiepileptic therapy. A number of methods are now available (Jøhannessen and Tomson, 2000), and measurement of AED levels has been extended to other biological fluids, such as tears or saliva (Knott, 1983; Paxton et al., 1983; Monaco et al., 1981; Rylance and Moreland, 1981). Methods for the determination of the concentration of free drugs (non–protein bound) in plasma have been developed (Monaco et al., 1984; Paxton et al., 1983; Vajda and Aicardi, 1983), but these have not yet become standard prac-

tice. The determination of free drug concentrations may be useful in special circumstances, particularly with liver or renal disease. Measurements of anticonvulsants in saliva or tears, which have the advantage of avoiding needle sampling, may have limitations because of pH differences (Eadie and Tyrer, 1989), and they have not replaced whole blood levels in clinical practice.

Whatever methods are used, the particular laboratory processing the tests must have a quality-control scheme in place because studies have shown the unreliability of a number of determinations (Griffiths et al., 1980; Pippenger et al., 1978). The limitations of blood levels have been discussed earlier in this chapter. The clinician should keep in mind that some severe epilepsies require "supraoptimal" doses, whereas benign syndromes may be controlled at levels well below those that are recommended (Schmidt et al., 1986a; Turnbull et al., 1983, 1984).

Because the long-term side effects and toxicity of AEDs in developing children are largely unknown and since subtle effects may occur even at drug levels within the optimal range, using the lowest possible dose of anticonvulsant drug that prevents seizures, regardless of the plasma levels, is strongly recommended. Therefore, the number of therapeutic levels is as great as the number of patients (Lesser et al., 1984), which seriously limits the value and indications for blood-level measurements of anticonvulsant drugs (Meijer, 1991).

In one prospective study, 79 adult patients with idiopathic generalized tonic-clonic seizures receiving PB or PHT who were found to have "subtherapeutic" levels of these drugs were randomly allotted to the following two groups: one in which an attempt was made to push the level to the "therapeutic" zone and one in which no effort was made to adjust blood levels. No differences were seen with respect to the frequency of seizures, but more side effects were observed in the first group (Woo et al., 1988).

The main indications for obtaining blood levels include the following:

1. Persistence of seizures despite a correctly prescribed therapy;
2. Presence or suspicion of toxic effects;
3. Occurrence of "breakthrough" seizures in previously well-controlled patients;
4. Use of several drugs, whether anticonvulsants or others, that are likely to interfere with one another;
5. Use of drugs with a relatively low therapeutic ratio (i.e., when therapeutic doses are close to toxic

doses) or of drugs with which saturation kinetics can occur, especially PHT;

6. When the age of the patient or the presence of mental and/or physical handicap is such that the usual clinical manifestations of toxicity are difficult or impossible to elicit;
7. In patients of young age, especially during the first days or weeks of life, because large swings in blood levels and resulting inefficacy or toxicity are common, particularly with certain drugs;
8. Before changing to another agent when the prescribed drug is ineffective.

The *time of sampling* is important when drugs with a short half-life are being used. With such drugs, the interpretation of the results is possible only if the time of absorption and the time of sampling are known. Even so, the results are not necessarily comparable from one determination to the next because of day-to-day fluctuations in metabolism. Comparisons may be particularly difficult when enteric-coated preparations are used, because large variations occur in release (Loiseau et al., 1982). In general, when toxicity is suspected, sampling at the time of the likely maximal blood level is best. Conversely, if a low blood level is suspected because of ineffective treatment, sampling at the time of the likely trough level is recommended. With drugs that have a short half-life, the use of blood-level determinations to check the patient's compliance is subject to limitation. The use and absorption of the drug within the 24 hours before appointment can result in reasonably high blood levels, whereas this problem does not arise with anticonvulsants of long half-life because their level gradually builds over several days. The occurrence of breakthrough seizures demands a thorough investigation and determination of plasma levels. The diagnosis of the seizure type should be reconfirmed because misdiagnosis (e.g., of syncope for grand mal seizures or of complex partial seizures for absences) not uncommonly leads to the use of inappropriate drugs and resultant treatment failure. A search for possible provoking factors, such as stress, lack of sleep, or an underlying brain disorder, is in order if no other cause is found.

The use of EEG for monitoring of antiepileptic treatment has not been systematically studied. Information on particular epilepsy syndromes has been given in their corresponding chapters. In general, the EEG has only a secondary role in the regulation of drug treatment, because the objective is not to clear the EEG of paroxysmal activity but rather to free the patient from seizures. In many epilepsy syndromes, a marked dissociation between EEG and clinical abnor-malities can be observed. Attempts at suppressing all paroxysmal EEG activity should be discouraged because they often lead to useless overdosage.

DISCONTINUATION OF DRUG TREATMENT

In 30% to 75% of children with epilepsy, the complete control of seizures is obtained with drug treatment, and the question of how long treatment should be maintained arises. The factors associated with a favorable or unfavorable outcome in such cases are discussed in Chapter 22. Matricardi et al. (1989) followed 425 children who had been seizure free for 2 years for an average of 8 years. Of these, 375 (88%) remained seizure free. Relapses occurred in 21% of the mentally retarded children but in only 11% of those who were mentally normal. They supervened within 3 years of the discontinuation of therapy in 98% of patients, and 88% of the children who relapsed were seizure free at cutoff. An organic cause, the need for more than one AED, and an abnormal EEG were associated with multiple relapses. Over the past 25 years, prospective and retrospective studies involving more than 6,000 children and adolescents have addressed the issue of remission and relapse rates after the withdrawal of AEDs. An exhaustive bibliography and a discussion of existing data can be found in a recent review by Shinnar and Gross-Tsur (2001).

In general, the same factors that are associated with the likelihood of obtaining a remission are also associated with a high probability of maintaining the seizure-free state after the discontinuation of therapy. No agreement exists, however, concerning the time at which the discontinuation of treatment can be considered, the precise method for the cessation of treatment, or the selection of candidates for the discontinuation of therapy (Pedley, 1988; Gordon, 1982).

In the authors' experience, patients with epilepsy syndromes of proven or probable lesional origin and those that are known to be refractory to treatment, such as Lennox-Gastaut syndrome or severe myoclonic epilepsy, should be treated for very long periods (more than 5 years) after the last seizure. In such cases, late relapses are not uncommon. In epilepsy syndromes of lesser severity, mainly those that do not result from structural brain damage, the interruption of treatment can be considered earlier. A seizure-free period of 4 years is often advised (Holowach-Thurston et al., 1982; Rodin, 1968). Most authors think that shorter seizure-free periods—in the vicinity of 2 years (Shinnar et al., 1985; Janz and Sommer-Burkhardt, 1976)—could be sufficient in a significant proportion of patients (Arts et al., 1988;

Callaghan et al., 1988; Bouma et al, 1987; Robinson, 1984; Emerson et al., 1981).

In actuality, the timing of discontinuation of treatment should probably vary with the individual epilepsy syndromes, as well as with other factors. In typical absence epilepsy of childhood, for example, a seizure-free period of 18 months or 2 years is probably sufficient, especially if the EEG has reverted to normal. In the case of benign epilepsy with centrotemporal focus, the timing of the discontinuation of treatment should probably vary with both the duration of the seizure-free period *and* the age of the patient. In such cases, treatment can be more easily stopped in a child between the ages of 9 and 10 years than in a child from 5 to 6 years of age because spontaneous remission often occurs about the end of the first decade. In most cases, however, a short treatment period of about 18 months will suffice. On the contrary, in adolescents with juvenile myoclonic epilepsy and/or awakening generalized tonic-clonic seizures, a prolonged period of effective treatment is mandatory. Such primary generalized epilepsies are easily controlled by therapy, but they commonly relapse after periods of 10 years or more (Gastaut et al., 1973b; Roger and Tassinari, 1973). Similarly, epilepsies of early onset probably deserve protracted periods of treatment because of their usual severity (Aicardi, 1980c).

When a discontinuation of therapy is contemplated, an EEG recording should be obtained. Most authors have reported that the risk of a relapse is greater for those patients with paroxysmal EEGs than for those with normal tracings, although agreement on this point is not complete (Berg et al., 1994; Shinnar et al., 1985; Todt, 1984; Emerson et al., 1981; Annegers et al., 1979a). Some authors have, however, reported prolonged remissions in patients with marked EEG abnormalities (Oller-Daurella and Marquez, 1972), and some authors tend to treat as long as the EEG remains paroxysmal. Others continue treatment for another year and then discontinue the drugs no matter what is seen on the EEG recordings. In most epilepsy syndromes, a normal EEG is not, in the authors' view, a prerequisite for discontinuation of treatment. This is especially applicable to benign rolandic epilepsy in which the EEG may normalize, on an average, 2 years after the last seizure. No evidence indicates that puberty has any significance in the decision to stop treatment.

The abrupt discontinuation of an AED may result in status epilepticus (Chadwick, 1985; Aminoff and Simon, 1980; Janz, 1969), so this is contraindicated. Almost all authors agree that the withdrawal of anticonvulsants should be gradual based on clinical experience, and they indicate that relapses are common even after slow discontinuation. Withdrawal over a period of 6 months to 1 year is often advised (Juul-Jensen, 1964, 1968). Nonetheless, Holowach-Thurston et al. (1982) has withdrawn treatment over a 3-month to 9-month period and Emerson et al. (1981) over a 3-month period without apparent adverse effects. On the other hand, Groh (1975) and Todt (1984) have found that the discontinuation of treatment over periods of less than 6 months is associated with an increased rate of relapse. The authors' practice is to advise slow discontinuation over 3 to 12 months. The withdrawal of drugs such as PB and the benzodiazepines requires special caution because the occurrence of withdrawal seizures seems particularly common with these agents.

The occurrence of one or, less often, two seizures after the withdrawal of therapy raises a difficult problem. Many epileptologists accept that such seizures may be *withdrawal seizures* rather than relapses and that they therefore may not be an indication for the resumption of treatment (Spencer et al., 1981). While some patients do remain seizure free in the absence of therapy after such "withdrawal seizures," the incidence of this is not known, and the very notion of withdrawal attack is purely empirical. On the other hand, the psychologic effect of a seizure occurring with the discontinuation of treatment is quite severe. The authors' practice is to warn the patient and his or her parents of the possibility of such an incident; to tell them that the seizure might well remain isolated; and to advise them not to resume therapy if an attack occurs; this approach gives them the choice to act otherwise if they are too afraid of a second seizure. Others resume the original treatment for a period of 6 months. Fits that occur more than 2 to 3 months after withdrawal should be regarded as relapses. The resumption of treatment for a long period is then generally indicated.

In all cases, the decision must be made in close collaboration with the patient and his or her family. The discontinuation of a chronic therapy is an emergency in only exceptionally rare cases, and the most suitable period for discontinuation must be chosen, taking into account the patient's age, lifestyle, employment, or education status. The patient must be ready to accept the risks of such a trial. The authors believe that, whenever possible, a withdrawal trial should be conducted while the patient is still young and is living in a protected environment. Adolescents with well-controlled epilepsies are regularly tempted to discontinue treatment. To avoid abrupt experimental withdrawal, the risks must be explained. General guidelines for progressive discontinuation must be discussed.

INTRACTABLE EPILEPSY

The term *intractable epilepsy* is poorly defined. Some authors apply the term to cases that continue to be active despite "relevant" therapy, but what constitutes "relevant therapy" varies considerably in terms of both the agents used and the duration of trials. Schmidt (1986a) proposes that intractability is a graded, rather than an all-or-none, phenomenon. Many clinicians would consider that epilepsies that are not controlled with any first-line AED or with combinations of two major agents could be termed *intractable*. In addition, apparent intractability may result from many causes. As O'Donohoe (1985) noted, epilepsy proves to be intractable in a number of patients for reasons that have little to do with actual failure of the medication.

Epilepsy may be intractable because a serious associated brain disease is present (Semah et al., 1996). Brain tumors are one possible cause, but any structural lesion of the brain in an epileptogenic (low-threshold) area is likely to lead to difficulties with seizure control. Intractability is also the norm in partial epilepsies related to focal cortical dysplasias or hippocampal sclerosis. Seizure-free intervals may be observed, but relapses are usual. Such patients are early candidates for surgical treatment. The disposal of a considerable number of AEDs is not a valid reason for considering intractable epilepsies to be only those that have remained resistant to all existing AEDs. Diffuse lesional brain disease, often occurring in association with motor and mental handicap, is a common cause of refractory epilepsy in children. Finally, many progressive degenerative disorders of the brain may present with intractable epilepsy, and seizures will seriously compound the increasing problems of such patients.

Another cause of intractable epilepsy is improper treatment that may result from the physician prescribing the wrong drug or the right drug in incorrect amounts. Improper treatment often results from the attitude of the patient and family when, for example, they arbitrarily modify the prescribed treatment or they move from doctor to doctor without accepting the need for the long process of initiation and careful adjustment of therapy. This attitude may result from a lack of explanation on the part of the doctor, thus emphasizing the necessity of obtaining the understanding and confidence of the family from the start. Adolescents pose a special problem as they may reject any form of drug treatment or in whom a disorganized way of life may lead to poor seizure control. The importance of regular medication cannot be overemphasized, and the frequency of poor compliance has been repeatedly demonstrated. Irregular or improper therapy is all the more regrettable because the epilepsy may not always be intractable from the start but it may become so because of the lack of control over long periods (Elwes et al., 1985). Careful and rigorous treatment is, therefore, an absolute necessity (Rodin et al., 1982).

Medically intractable epilepsy can be amenable to effective surgical treatment (see Chapter 25), especially in patients with partial epilepsies. The most severe cases may be both medically and surgically intractable. Even in difficult cases in which the seizures cannot be totally controlled, diminishing their number, severity, or consequences may be possible, which again indicates the relative or at least graded significance of the term *intractability*.

Intractable epilepsy in childhood is often observed with certain epilepsy syndromes, especially Lennox-Gastaut syndrome. With Dravet syndrome, Lennox-Gastaut syndrome might account for 70% of the intractable epilepsies of childhood. The difficulty of controlling the fits in such cases has already been emphasized, as has the danger of overtreating these patients. Overtreatment with PHT (Troupin and Ojemann, 1975), CBZ (Snead and Hosey, 1985; Johnsen et al., 1984; Shields and Saslow, 1983), and clonazepam (Alvarez et al., 1981) may increase the frequency of seizures or induce particular types of attacks, especially tonic or myoclonic seizures. For such cases, referral to specialized units, which have technical capacities and considerably more manpower, is certainly justified. Several reports have shown that intensive monitoring (Thirumalai et al., 2001; Porter, 1983b; Theodore et al., 1983c; Sutula et al., 1981; Penry and Porter, 1977) improves the outlook for some patients. Another large group of intractable epilepsy consists of the severe partial epilepsies of childhood. These differ from the partial epilepsies in adults as they more often are due to extensive and early acquired lesions and because they are usually associated with cognitive and/or behavioral difficulties that can be progressive.

Both the intractable secondary generalized epilepsies and the severe partial ones are sometimes referred to as the "catastrophic epilepsies" of childhood. These represent a major therapeutic challenge in childhood epilepsy.

OTHER AGENTS USED IN TREATMENT OF SOME FORMS OF EPILEPSY

Adrenocorticotropic Hormone and Corticosteroids

Adrenocorticotropic hormone (ACTH) and corticosteroids are commonly used in the treatment of some forms of epilepsy (Snead and Martien, 2001), especially West syndrome (see Chapter 3) and Lennox-Gastaut syndrome (see Chapter 4). Some investigators have also found them useful in the management of other types of severe epilepsy (Snead et al., 1983). The results are difficult to evaluate because of the heterogeneity in the reported series, the methods of assessment, and the case selection. Indeed, the whole problem of the effect of ACTH on seizure susceptibility in the developing brain has not been completely solved (Baram, 1993, 2001; Holmes and Weber, 1986), but the empirical use of hormonal therapy is helpful in selected cases of severe epilepsy (De Vivo, 1983).

Hormonal therapy has particularly been recommended for the therapy of epilepsies associated with intense paroxysmal EEG activity, such as that observed in the Landau-Kleffner syndrome or in electrical status epilepticus of slow sleep. These syndromes tend to be refractory to conventional AEDs, and they may better respond to ACTH or steroids (Deonna, 1991; Lerman et al., 1991; Marescaux et al., 1990). However, no controlled, prospective study has been conducted, and the variable natural history of these syndromes, as well as the realization that any apparent effect of treatment may appear only after several months, makes totally excluding coincidence difficult. Although clinical experience justifies the use of ACTH or corticosteroids, further study of the dose and duration of therapy is needed.

As they do in the treatment of West syndrome, the techniques of treatment vary in such cases. Both ACTH (natural or synthetic) and corticosteroids are used, although the latter are generally preferable for long-term treatment. Doses of 1.5 to 3 mg per kg per day of prednisolone or "equivalent" doses of other steroids are commonly used. Such treatment requires close medical supervision.

Immunoglobulins

Immunoglobulins have been introduced in the therapeutic armamentarium against the epilepsies because of the possible relationship of some epileptic syndromes with immunologic phenomenon (see Chapters 3 and 4). The indications have included West syndrome, Lennox-Gastaut syndrome, and severe epilepsies not belonging to these syndromes (Etzioni et al., 1991; Rapin et al., 1988; Arizumi et al., 1987). The efficacy of immunoglobulins remains to be demonstrated, as only anecdotal reports are available. Although intravenous immunoglobulins may represent a valuable resource for some drug-refractory epilepsies and their effectiveness has important

pathogenetic implications, controlled studies with the systematic monitoring of immunologic markers are needed to define more precisely the indications for use and to optimize the administration protocols (Villani and Avanzini, 2002).

NONDRUG TREATMENTS

Ketogenic Diet

The *ketogenic diet* has long been advocated for the treatment of refractory seizures (Livingston, 1972). More recently, several practical methods for achieving a ketogenic diet have become available, including the use of medium-chain triglycerides in particular. Reviews and comparisons of the ketogenic diets are available (Nordli and De Vivo, 2001; Prasad et al., 1996; Woody et al., 1988a; Sills et al., 1986; Gordon, 1977; Huttenlocher, 1976). Only one prospective study of 150 children between the ages of 1 to 16 years is available; these children presented with more than two seizures per week despite adequate therapy with at least two anticonvulsant medications. They were treated with the ketogenic diet and were followed for a minimum of 1 year (Freeman et al., 1998). The children (mean age of 5.3 years) averaged 410 seizures per month before the diet despite an exposure to a mean of 6.2 AEDs. Three months after the initiation of the diet, 83% of those who had started remained on the diet, and 34% had a more than 90% decrease in seizures. At 6 months, 71% still remained on the diet, and 32% had a more than 90% decrease in seizures. At 1 year, 55% remained on the diet, with 27% having a more than 90% decrease in seizure frequency. Most of those who discontinued the diet did so because it was either not effective enough or it was too restrictive, while 7% stopped because of intercurrent illness.

The mechanisms of action of the diet are not known, but the role played by a high concentration of ketone bodies in the blood has been demonstrated (Huttenlocher, 1976). Several problems are associated with the use of ketogenic diets, including diarrhea, vitamin deficiency, and difficulties in making the diet acceptable. The degree of success achieved by various researchers is variable. The regimen has been effective in a significant proportion of children with myoclonic or atonic seizures and in some cases of the Lennox-Gastaut syndrome (Schwartz et al., 1983b), although other authors believe that its use is no longer justified in view of the available drug therapy. However, drug-resistant cases deserve a full trial of the diet, especially cases of myoclonic epilepsy. Epilepsy syndromes for which treatment with the ketogenic diet can be considered include early infantile epileptic encephalopathy, Lennox-Gastaut syndrome, intractable myoclonic-astatic epilepsy, and other forms of refractory generalized cryptogenic or symptomatic epilepsies. The diet has also been used for the treatment of severe partial epilepsies.

The ketogenic diet is generally safe but not risk free. It may have devastating effects, particularly during its initiation, in children with inborn errors of metabolism (Nordli and De Vivo, 2001) (i.e., in those children who may present with forms of epilepsy considered amenable to such a treatment). No comparative study of the ketogenic diet has been published, and little information about its possible long-term adverse effects is available. The diet seems to be primarily used for relatively short periods (6 months to 1 year), but further information is needed. However, the ketogenic diet has been maintained for periods of several years, especially in patients with neuroglycopenia (De Vivo et al., 1991), without major problems in growth or biological equilibrium.

Behavioral Methods of Seizure Control

Behavioral methods of seizure control have been reviewed in detail (Ramaratnam et al., 2001; Fenwick, 1994). Psychologic methods for treatment of epilepsy include reward management, self-control, psychophysiologic treatment, relaxation therapy, cognitive behavior therapy, EEG biofeedback, and educational interventions. Psychotherapy of various types has given only minimal results, but it may improve behavior globally.

As Chapter 23 discussed, a complete treatment of epilepsy involves not only medication but also educating patients about their brain and its functioning. Psychologic support to the patients and their family is often neglected because of a dearth of resources and specialized personnel. However, controlled studies assessing whether the treatment of epilepsy with psychologic methods is effective in reducing seizure frequency are not available. A recent review of the existing data clearly concluded that, in view of the methodologic deficiencies and limited number of patients studied, no reliable evidence supporting the use of these treatments is available and further trials are needed (Ramaratnam et al., 2001). The importance of avoiding or regulating seizure-inducing factors can-

not be overstressed, and systematic inquiry into that aspect of the problem should be conducted.

SUMMARY

The potential for drug therapy of the epilepsies has increased significantly during the past decade. New agents have became available, and a considerable amount of factual data has emerged from well-designed controlled studies that included patients with relatively well-defined types of seizures or epilepsy. The mode of action of antiepileptic agents has been largely clarified. Most act by blocking the transmission of repetitive firing along axons, but some are active at the synaptic level by increasing inhibitory transmission or hindering excitatory transmission. A number of broad-spectrum AEDs are now available.

All AEDs have side effects, and their use should, therefore, be limited to the smallest amount of as few drugs as possible. A better knowledge of the pharmacokinetics of drugs has permitted their more rational use, and the monitoring of blood levels of AEDs has become routine practice. Though blood-level measurements are useful in certain circumstances, they are not a substitute for clinical judgment; and the aim of treatment is to render the patient seizure free with minimal side effects, not to achieve a predetermined "therapeutic" blood-level value.

AEDs may have some specificity for action against certain forms of epilepsy or epilepsy syndromes; thus, the selection of the correct agent is important. Whenever possible, the use of one drug is preferable to polypharmacy, which is more difficult to monitor and is effective only in a relatively small proportion of cases and which also has more side effects.

Treatment with AEDs should not usually be started at the first seizure, and it should be maintained for variable durations depending on the epilepsy syndrome. In specific cases, conventional AEDs are not effective. Some of these cases may respond to unconventional agents, such as corticosteroids and/or ACTH, or to nondrug therapies, such as the ketogenic diet. The efficacy of other agents, such as immune globulins, has not been demonstrated. Surgery has become a more accessible solution for a growing number of patients, and, in cases of partial epilepsy, it should be considered an early option.

In the last decade, considerable work has been dedicated to epilepsy surgery in young patients. At least in specialized centers, *epilepsy surgery in children is no longer considered a treatment of last resort* when all else has failed. Although an overwhelming majority of children are still treated with drugs, many with satisfactory results, and a few more can benefit from various nondrug therapies (see previous chapters), surgery is being increasingly used for patients resistant to medical treatment. Its indications, techniques, and results have received considerable attention (Lüders and Comair, 2001; Bureau et al., 1998; Tuxhorn et al., 1997a; Engel, 1993).

Surgical treatment is still used for only a relatively small proportion of children with difficult-to-control seizures. The usual delay from the onset of seizure intractability to surgery is still in the range of 12 to 15 years at most centers (Wyllie and Bingaman, 2001). The lack of a sufficient number of specialized epilepsy centers has also resulted in unacceptable delays. This may prove harmful, particularly for children who could benefit from the early elimination of or significant reduction in their seizures, which would result in better social integration. Physicians must be aware of the new concepts and techniques that allow the earlier safe use of surgical therapy for children with epilepsy.

The spectrum of surgical possibilities for early onset epilepsy has rapidly widened to include not only the focal epilepsies but also more diffuse types or specific etiologies. New categories of patients who might benefit from surgical methods have been identified (Duchowny, 1999; Engel and Shewmon, 1992). The small number of persons with epilepsy currently undergoing surgical treatment could increase considerably, even though a significant proportion (12% to 25%) present with types of secondary generalized epilepsy that may not be as easily amenable to surgical treatment. Approximately 5,000 new surgical candidates are seen in the United States each year. Although most of these are adults, the recent trend toward earlier intervention will undoubtedly increase the number of children and adolescents considered for surgery.

Only the general aspects of surgical treatment are discussed here. The details of presurgical evaluation, operative techniques, and results are available in a host of specialized books and articles (Lüders and Comair, 2001; Wyllie, 2001; Engel et al., 1997; Engel, 1993; Lüders, 1992; Spencer and Spencer, 1991; Wieser and Elger, 1987). The rapidly growing volume of articles and books (Oxbury et al., 2000; Bureau et al., 1998; Wyllie, 2000; Duchowny, 1999; Tuxhorn et al., 1997a; Duchowny et al., 1992) dealing with epilepsy surgery in children testifies to the increasing interest in early intervention (Moshé and Shinnar, 1993).

The *aims of surgical treatment* are no different from those of any other form of therapy. The ultimate goal is improving the quality of life (QoL) for patients. Control of seizures is the major factor in the QoL (Vickrey et al., 1995), and surgery appears to be a most effective method for achieving complete control. Even when full control has not been achieved, surgery can still greatly improve QoL by significantly reducing the frequency of seizures or limiting the clinical manifestations and practical consequences of uncontrolled attacks (e.g., by suppressing dangerous falls or preventing the generalization of partial seizures). Surgical therapy may also reduce the excessive side effects of drugs, especially those on cognitive or behavioral development. Surgery likely also prevents the aggravation of epilepsy through secondary epileptogenesis or the extension of epileptogenic areas as a consequence of an initially focal paroxysmal activity (Morrell, 1989; Morrell et al., 1989) and thus lessens the noxious effects of epileptic activity, whether clinical or subclinical (Spencer, 1988), although this has not been proven.

IDENTIFICATION OF POTENTIAL SURGICAL CANDIDATES

The first concern is determining whether the seizures are medically intractable (see Chapter 22). This may not be easy because *intractability* may be difficult to define (Shields, 1997). A full review of the drug history is, therefore, the initial step. This should determine whether the drugs that are most likely to be useful for a particular form of epilepsy have been tested. However, testing *all possible drugs* is not advisable, because this process would be excessively long when surgery is a reasonable possibility. Furthermore, increasing evidence indicates that drug therapy is likely to fail to achieve control of the attacks when two of the major drugs have not obtained satisfactory results (Kwan and Brodie, 2000).

The *duration* of medical trials is a critical point. Although no patient should be operated on without a full, initial attempt at controlling seizures with drugs, the consequences of years of disabling seizures and high doses of antiepileptic medication during a period of neurologic and psychosocial development must be weighed against the risks of surgery. Many investigators now think that intractable epilepsy can be recognized early (Berg et al., 2003; Jallon, 2003; Shinnar and Pellock, 2002; Shinnar et al., 2000); they have indicated that making a decision on surgical therapy should not exceed a duration of 1 or 2 years (Mohamed et al., 2001; Engel and Shewmon, 1992; Kotagal and Lüders, 1992).

The timing of surgery partly depends on the probable effectiveness of the operation available for each particular patient. When a highly efficacious operation is available for the epilepsy of a particular patient, the duration of the medical therapy should be shortened; for instance, in the case of mesial temporal epilepsy without complicating factors, which is controlled by drugs only infrequently, surgery is highly effective. In such cases, surgery without long delays may be preferable to medical therapy, after a short trial has failed to achieve full control of seizures (Engel and Shewmon, 1992). The presence of cognitive and/or behavioral deterioration in association with intense epileptic electroencephalographic (EEG) activity, even in the absence of seizures, is now regarded by many investigators as an indication for early surgery with the hope of preventing further cognitive loss (Arzimanoglou, 2002b; Aicardi, 1997, 1999a; Roulet-Perez et al., 1998; Neville et al., 1997; Shewmon et al., 1997; Deonna, 1996).

Epileptic seizures must be disabling before surgical treatment can be considered. However, what constitutes a disabling seizure disorder is not clearly defined, as this is largely dependent on individual factors, such as lifestyle, psychosocial environment, and personal expectations. Again with the improving risk–benefit ratios of surgery, the growing tendency is to offer surgery for refractory seizures that are less obviously disabling.

CONTRAINDICATIONS TO SURGICAL TREATMENT

Some forms of epilepsy such as the primary generalized epilepsies and the idiopathic focal epilepsies of childhood are absolute contraindications to surgical treatment. As indicated later in this chapter, epilepsies

caused by diffuse brain damage are a contraindication to resective surgery, but they may be amenable to palliative surgery in selected patients. Surgery is also contraindicated when the epilepsy is due to an underlying progressive brain disease unless the disease is itself amenable to surgical therapy (e.g., brain tumors).

A severely dysfunctional family or a failure of parents and patients to understand the goals and limitations of surgery is also a contraindication to surgery. Surgery is also contraindicated if it cannot be integrated into a program of rehabilitation.

Another contraindication is the unavailability of a specialized center. Epilepsy surgery mandates a multidisciplinary approach that requires special skills (e.g., neurologists, neuropsychologists, neuroradiologists, neurosurgeons, and nuclear medicine specialists) and sophisticated instruments and materials that cannot be improvised. The indications for surgery depend on a sophisticated *global evaluation* that can delineate the epileptogenic zone or lesion and can propose a resection that includes the epileptogenic cortex while avoiding unacceptable cognitive or neurologic sequelae. For most cases, the experience of the neurosurgeon in epilepsy surgery might be of considerable importance. In addition, epilepsy centers should offer postoperative rehabilitation programs.

Mental retardation of a severe degree is *not an absolute contraindication* to surgical treatment if a realistic hope exists that the operation may give sufficient improvement such that the care of the epileptic person is transformed and/or his or her QoL and that of the persons in charge are improved satisfactorily. However, the person and the family must fully understand the limitations of this type of indication in which the objectives are narrowly limited.

Moderate mental retardation is not a contraindication because the occurrence of seizures in a retarded child may considerably increase his or her practical problems and may make the overall management much more difficult (Herman and Austin, 1993; Taylor, 1993). Even if partial control of the seizures is attainable, it may transform desperate situations.

A psychiatric disorder is usually a contraindication to surgery, but it is not a common problem in young children. In adolescent patients, permanent psychosis should discourage the use of surgical treatment, but repeated postictal psychosis is not a contraindication (Taylor, 1993).

TYPES OF AVAILABLE SURGICAL TREATMENT

Several operations are available for the treatment of epilepsy (Table 25.1). The following two major

TABLE 25.1. *Available operations for surgical treatment of patients with epilepsy*

Resective surgery	Palliative surgery
Simple removal of lesion ("lesionectomy")	Anterior callosotomy (50%–75%)
Limited cortical resections	Complete callosotomy
Amygdalohippocampectomy[a]	Commissurotomy (including callosotomy
Lobectomy (mainly temporal) (may be standard or tailored)	plus anterior and/or hippocampal
Multilobar resections	commissure)
Hemispherectomy (conventional, modified, hemidecortication)	Amygdalohippocampectomy[a]
	Multiple subpial transections

[a]May be either resective or palliative (see text).

categories of surgical therapy are used: (a) *resective surgery*, in which the object is to remove the cortical neuronal pool that is responsible for generation of the seizures, thereby obtaining full seizure control, and (b) *palliative or functional surgery*, which does not aim at complete seizure control. The latter leaves the epileptogenic area(s) in place but aims to interrupt or limit the propagation of the seizure discharges, thus limiting their clinical manifestations and consequences.

Resective surgery can range from small cortical resections to hemispherectomy. The latter operation has been modified to avoid leaving a large intracranial cavity, which is thought to have been associated with the development of late complications. These consisted mainly of hemosiderosis and hydrocephalus as a result of repeated bleeding in the operative cavity (Rasmussen, 1973). Currently, various methods of functional hemispherectomy (Villemure et al., 1993; Rasmussen and Villemure, 1989) or hemispherotomy (Villemure and Mascott, 1995; Delalande et al., 1992), in which disconnection is more prominent than excision, are preferred.

Palliative surgery (Polkey, 2003) is mostly represented by *callosotomy*, whether of the anterior half or two-thirds of this structure or complete (Blume, 1997; Gilliam and Wyllie, 1997). Complete callosotomy generally is performed after an anterior callosotomy fails to control seizures rather than as a first-choice procedure (Spencer, 1988; Spencer et al., 1987a). *Subpial transection* is another palliative operation (Andrews et al., 1989; Morrell et al., 1989), consisting of multiple subpial cortical incisions that attempt to interrupt the horizontal fibers through which the epileptic discharge is thought to propagate without severing the vertical effector connections, thus avoiding a loss of function of the area where the transection is performed (Morrell et al., 1995, 1997). This technique allows operation on the "eloquent" cortex (e.g., in language or primary motor areas).

Other palliative techniques include *vagus nerve stimulation*, which requires placement of a stimulator under the skin. In this technique, an electrode is wrapped around the left vagus nerve, so that adjustable pulsed stimuli can be applied (Crumrine, 2000; Ben-Menachem et al., 1999; Schachter and Saper, 1998). The technique is now often used in the treatment of resistant epilepsy that is not otherwise amenable to surgical therapy. Most of the studies that have been published concern adult patients with refractory epilepsy. In children, the results are encouraging with reduced seizure frequency, particularly in the epileptic encephalopathies (Polkey, 2003; Wheless and Maggio, 2002; Majoie et al., 2001; Parker et al., 2001). In addition to requiring an operation and the possible complications that may result from the presence of foreign material, the method is unfortunately costly. Which seizure types or epilepsy syndromes will benefit most from vagus nerve stimulation remains to be defined.

The role of *gamma-knife radiosurgery* in the treatment of cortical–subcortical cavernous angiomas and hypothalamic hamartomas is undergoing evaluation (Régis, 2001; Régis et al., 2000a, 2000b). Another technique that is still experimental is deep brain stimulation (Benabid et al., 2002; Chabardes et al., 2002; Fisher et al., 1997), the results of which are still too recent to draw conclusions. An extensive review of the palliative techniques, their indications, and results has recently been published (Polkey, 2003).

Some overlap exists between resective and palliative surgery. For example, *amygdalohippocampectomy* (Wieser and Yasargil, 1987; Yasargil et al., 1985) is most commonly used as a type of resective surgery for the treatment of mesial temporal epilepsy, but it may also be employed as palliative therapy for relieving seizures produced by inoperable brain tumors in posterior parts of the temporal lobe through removal of the mesial structures that amplify and stabilize epileptic discharges of neocortical or extratemporal origin (Wieser, 1988). The two categories are, therefore, not mutually exclusive. Subpial transection, for example, can be combined with lobectomy or limited cortical resections (Morrell et al., 1989; Polkey, 1989).

Although anterior temporal lobectomy is still the most commonly performed operation (Mohamed et al., 2001; Kotagal and Lüders, 1994; Duchowny et al., 1992; Mizrahi et al., 1990; Engel, 1987), other procedures, such as extratemporal cortical resections (Shewmon et al., 1990; Duchowny et al., 1989), multilobar resections (Shewmon et al., 1990, 1997; Wyllie, 1996; Lüders et al., 1993b), hemispherectomy, and callosotomy are increasingly being performed. This is due to the realization that seizures in children frequently have an extratemporal origin and to the growing awareness of the widely disseminated damage present in many such cases.

It has long been known (Rasmussen 1975a, 1975b) that the *best results of resective surgery* are in patients in whom a definite lesion is present in the resected brain tissue, not only in tumors but also in atrophic or dysplastic lesions, in which complete control of seizures may be achieved in more than 80% of patients (Munari et al., 2000). The simple removal of an epileptogenic lesion without attempts to define and remove the epileptogenic area (lesionectomy) has been shown to produce control of seizures in a significant proportion of the patients (Munari et al., 2000; Bourgeois et al., 1999b; Cascino et al., 1993; Boon et al., 1991; Hirsch et al., 1989). However, it appears that, in certain cases, the delineation and removal of the epileptogenic area associated with the lesion improves the outcome of lesionectomy (Jooma et al., 1995; Montes et al., 1995; Berger et al., 1993; Cascino et al., 1992b). The current experience confirms that the complete resection of the *epileptogenic area* is the major condition for a satisfactory surgical result, emphasizing the importance of the presurgical evaluation of the exact location and extent of the epileptogenic zone (Munari et al., 2000, 1985; Cascino et al., 1996; Garcia et al., 1994; Engel, 1993).

REQUIREMENTS FOR RESECTIVE SURGERY

The requirements for resective surgery vary with the type of resection considered. Basic requirements for all cases are (a) that the epileptogenic area be localized to the territory whose removal is contemplated, (b) that no other *independent* epileptogenic area exists in those areas that are not included in the planned resection, and (c) that any possible deficit resulting from resection be *acceptable*.

What constitutes an acceptable deficit is difficult to define, and this varies considerably with the patients and the circumstances. The difficulty of satisfying these requirements varies with the type of resection. The basic principle is that the different modalities of the investigation (neurologic and neuropsychologic examination; imaging; scalp video-EEG; and, when necessary, other electrophysiologic techniques) should give convergent data that point to a single localization of the epileptogenic zone (Munari et al., 1999a; Engel and Shewmon, 1992; Shewmon et al., 1990; Fish et al., 1989).

The extent of the *epileptogenic zone* may vary greatly. It seldom is narrowly localized; in most cases, it is best conceptualized as a network of abnormally behaving neurons that are distributed within a relatively large brain volume. Indeed, the definition of the epileptogenic zone is difficult. The best definition would be the smallest volume of brain whose resection causes the disappearance of seizures, but such a definition can be satisfied only after, rather than before, surgery. The epileptogenic zone differs from the *ictal onset zone*, which is the area of the cortex where seizures are initiated, as this may not be sufficient for sustaining seizure activity. It also differs from the *symptom-producing zone* and the *zone of functional alteration*. The former usually exceeds the limits of the epileptogenic zone because the seizure propagates to remote areas. The latter, which is defined as the area of cortex that presents evidence (e.g., by EEG, positron emission tomography [PET], or single photon emission computed tomography [SPECT]) of dysfunction, usually does not fully coincide with the epileptogenic area. The same applies to the *irritative zone* (i.e., the area over which paroxysmal activity is recorded) and to the *lesional zone*, which is anatomically defined (Lüders and Comair, 2001; Duchowny et al., 1997; Talairach et al., 1974; Bancaud et al., 1973). In practice, any lesional and ictal onset zone should always be removed, but the delimitation of what constitutes the epileptogenic area remains an unsolved problem.

Large multilobar resections (Shields et al., 1992a) and especially hemispherectomy (Tuite et al., 2000; Vigevano and Di Rocco, 1990; Lindsay et al., 1987) tend to make the precise definition of the epileptogenic area less important, although large lesions may raise problems. The main issues in such cases are to make sure that the abnormal area is entirely confined within a single hemisphere and that the postoperative deficit will not be more disabling than the preoperative dysfunction or that, at the very least, it will not create any new *severe* disability.

The problems posed by limited resections are much more difficult, and all possible sources of information may be required in difficult cases.

PRESURGICAL EVALUATION OF CHILDREN

The presurgical evaluation has the same bases in children as it does in adults; most methods are applicable, although the mapping of the epileptogenic area with depth or surface electrodes under general anesthesia is considered more difficult by most clinicians. The detailed consideration of the existing methods is beyond the scope of this book, and the reader is referred to the extensive literature available (Kahane et al., 1998, 2002; Lüders and Comair, 2001; Wyllie, 2000; Minotti et al., 1998; Duchowny et al., 1997; Engel, 1993; Chauvel et al., 1992a; Lüders, 1991; Wieser and Elger, 1987). Some general guidelines are, however, given here.

The presurgical assessment of a patient is a stepwise process. (Table 25.2). Congruence among the results of the clinical history and the definition of seizure pattern, the neuropsychologic evaluation and neuroradiology, scalp EEG (interictal and ictal), and, in selected cases, other supporting tests (e.g., ictal or interictal SPECT and PET) is sought. All of the available data must be reviewed and analyzed by an experienced multidisciplinary group.

The importance of the EEG has repeatedly been emphasized (Quesney, 1992; Bancaud et al., 1965, 1973), especially that of the ictal EEG (Lüders et al., 1989a; Duchowny, 1988). Thus, long-lasting EEG recordings by telemetry or cassette recording are of considerable help as they multiply the probability of obtaining seizures. *Combined video-EEG recording* is an integral and essential part of the arsenal of a presurgical unit (Foley et al., 1995, 2000; Mizrahi, 1999; Raymond et al., 1999; Engel, 1993; Duchowny, 1988; Duchowny et al., 1988). However, this does not obviate the need for direct clinical interaction (e.g., questioning and testing) between the patient and the physician during the seizure; this is necessary to determine the presence of ictal aphasia, hemianopia, and tonic posturing and the level of awareness, amnesic retention, and internal consciousness (Wieser and Kausel, 1987; Bancaud et al., 1973). Spontaneous seizures are of particular interest because induced seizures or seizures precipitated by the withdrawal of drugs may differ from habitual attacks (Marks et al., 1991; Marciani et al., 1985). Although the ictal EEG recording is a major element in the presurgical investigation, some investigators have questioned its necessity in selected cases (Cendes et al., 2000, 2002; Kahane et al., 2002). The use of additional or special electrodes is variably appreciated, but sphenoidal electrodes may be helpful.

Neuropsychologic assessment is used both to determine the general level of functioning of surgical candidates and to evaluate the localization of cerebral dysfunction separately (Oxbury, 2000; Jones-Gotman, 1991; Rausch, 1987). These tests should include several measures of memory, divided according to whether they tap largely into verbal or nonverbal skills. Deficits on tests of verbal learning and memory support dominant lobe dysfunction. Deficits in nonverbal learning and memory indicate the involvement of the nondominant hemisphere (Thompson, 1991; Rausch, 1987). Language skills and memory abilities are also assessed. Their results may indicate the presence of an extratemporal disturbance. Successive hemianesthesia of the two cerebral hemispheres, which is elicited by the injection of a barbiturate into the internal carotid artery, is performed as part of a presurgical investigation (*Wada test*) for determining language and memory dominance (Jones-Gotman et al., 1997; Kotagal, 1997; Silfvenius et al., 1997; Dodrill et al., 1993). This is difficult to perform in children of any age, and it is impossible to interpret in children younger than 8 years. A standardized approach for children is not established, and the test is indicated only in rare selected cases. In cooperative children, the use of functional magnetic resonance imaging (fMRI) is now possible; this helps to determine the location of language areas with increasing

---

TABLE 25.2. *Presurgical investigations for resective surgery*

To Be Performed in All Cases	To Be Performed in Selected Cases
Detailed history taking	Functional imaging (SPECT, PET, fMRI)
Definition of clinical seizure pattern	Intracranial EEG recordings (acute/chronic)
Video EEG (ictal and interictal)	Wada test (intracarotid amytal) (see text)
Neuropsychologic assessment	
High resolution morphologic imaging (MRI)	

Abbreviations: EEG, electroencephalogram; MRI, magnetic resonance imaging; fMRI, functional MRI; PET, positron emission tomography; SPECT, single photon emission computed tomography.

precision by demonstrating the increase in local blood flow in the language areas (Gaillard, 2001). fMRI may be particularly valuable in lesional cases, in which these areas may have been relocated because of the presence of damage or abnormal tissue.

Structural neuroimaging is now the most important investigation in the presurgical evaluation of children. The computed tomographic (CT) *scan* generally has been superseded by MRI, the major imaging procedure for cases of epilepsy (see Chapter 19). Using appropriate techniques (Briellmann et al., 2003; Kuzniecky and Jackson, 1995; Jackson et al., 1993a), MRI demonstrates better than any other method the presence of abnormalities of the temporal lobe, especially mesial temporal sclerosis or the loss of gray-white matter demarcation of the temporal pole (Ryvlin et al., 2002), as well as abnormalities of cortical development. However, some of the developmental abnormalities are rather subtle and difficult to visualize. A clinical hypothesis based on seizure semiology and EEG data helps provide orientation for the investigation. A routine MRI may not be sufficient, and a high-quality investigation, including thin slices, fluid-attenuated inversion recovery imaging (FLAIR), and three-dimensional volume acquisitions, is strongly recommended.

Whether hippocampal sclerosis may be secondary to the involvement of the mesial temporal structures in discharges originating in other lobes remains an open question (Fish et al., 1991). It is well known, however, that discharges of frontal or occipital origin propagate easily to the temporal limbic formations, but the evidence showing that they may generate anatomic lesions is far from complete. Indirect arguments can be drawn from the relatively common association of hippocampal and neocortical lesions, realizing a dual pathology (Levesque et al., 1991).

Although results vary among centers, with some frequently finding hippocampal sclerosis (Wieser, 1987) and others considering it an uncommon lesion (Spencer et al., 2001; Duchowny et al., 1993; Harvey et al., 1993b), there is general agreement that extrahippocampal lesions and extratemporal abnormalities are more common in children than in adults, constituting the most common lesion in this age-group (Wyllie et al., 1998; Arruda et al., 1996; Shields et al., 1993). MRI is the best tool for the detection of extrahippocampal lesions, whether temporal or extratemporal (Cascino et al., 1993; Cook et al., 1992). However, not all of these lesions are detectable, even by the best MRI techniques. Dysplasias, the most common lesions, may not show on MRI scans in a variable proportion of patients (Palmini et al., 1991d)

(see Chapter 19), particularly those dysplasias located in the frontal lobe.

Currently, high-quality MRI is capable of demonstrating brain lesions in a majority of candidates for epilepsy surgery, and operation should be considered reluctantly in situations in which the MRI scan is completely normal when an adequate machine and technique are used. Very often, MRI is a definitive examination, at least for deciding the side and general area of operation. The continuous development of new and better MRI techniques will likely lead to the vast majority of, if not all, epileptogenic lesions eventually becoming detectable, thus allowing more precise and effective surgery to be performed.

The place of *functional imaging* in presurgical assessment has not yet been completely defined. Both PET and SPECT are performed to identify or to confirm the ictal focus in presurgical evaluations and to identify eloquent cortical regions to be spared during surgery (Gaillard, 2001; Nobre and Rao, 2000). PET carries the additional potential for quantitatively studying the neurochemical alterations during epilepsy.

Positron emission tomography scanning most often uses 18-fluorodeoxyglucose (FDG) or flumazenil to determine the presence and location of areas of hypermetabolism or hypometabolism (Chugani et al., 1997). A good correspondence among areas of interictal hypometabolism, brain damage, and zones of abnormal EEG activity has been demonstrated, and PET undoubtedly has a place in the assessment of selected cases (Ryvlin et al., 1998). Some investigators (Muzik et al., 2000; Arnold et al., 1997; Chiron et al., 1993; Chugani et al., 1990, 1992) have used the technique extensively in the presurgical study of severe childhood epilepsies of the infantile spasms type (see Chapter 3), and they have claimed that PET can demonstrate localized abnormal areas that are not detectable by MRI and whose removal may lead to control of seizures. However, FDG PET provides less reliable localization and a lower yield in patients with extratemporal epilepsy. The drawbacks of PET include its cost; the use of radioactive material with the attendant ethical problems in childhood; and the time required for data acquisition, which makes it mainly a method of interictal study. It is currently used less often than SPECT. Furthermore, the results in children must be interpreted with caution, because abnormal glucose use may be less common and less profound in children with new-onset partial seizures than it is in adults with chronic partial epilepsy (Gaillard et al., 2002; Snead et al., 1996).

Single photon emission computed tomography uses a less expensive material, but it has a lower level of resolution and does not allow quantification. It assesses local cerebral blood flow, which is usually decreased interictally in the area of epileptogenic brain damage and is increased in the same area at the time of a seizure (Kaminska et al., 2003; Harvey et al., 1993a, 2002; Chiron et al., 2001; Cross et al., 1995; Harvey and Berkovic, 1994). Interictal scanning shows a hypometabolic area in approximately 60% of patients with focal epilepsy with a satisfactory level of congruence with other methods. Ictal studies using technetium-99m (^{99m}Tc) hexamethylpropyleneamine oxime or, more recently, the ^{99m}Tc ethyl cysteinate dimer, which is more stable and which can, therefore, be kept in solution, allow rapid injection at the onset of a seizure. These radioactive tracers are immediately taken up by lipid membranes, thus allowing the actual scanning to be performed within a few hours after injection. Ictal SPECT, particularly ictal-interictal substraction SPECT images coregistered to MRI, is a helpful technique (Chiron et al., 2001) despite the logistic issues raised by the necessity of injecting the tracer within 40 seconds of the onset of a seizure, making concomitant recording of the EEG mandatory. It remains a particularly useful presurgical investigation in children with partial epilepsy, especially those in whom hippocampal sclerosis, cortical dysplasia, or inflammatory disease is the underlying pathology. Recent studies have suggested that regional cerebral blood flow studies add little information in the investigation of children with seizures secondary to benign tumors or cerebral infarcts or in whom hemispherectomy is the option (Hartley et al., 2002).

Regional cerebral blood flow investigations demonstrate a sequence of a focal increase in blood flow in the epileptogenic area with secondary hypoperfusion in the same territory (Rowe et al., 1991; Stefan et al., 1990a). In adult patients with temporal lobe epilepsy, the immediate postictal period is characterized by focal hypometabolism with the persistence of high flow in the anteromesial aspect of the temporal lobe. With correct technical conditions, this method seems highly reliable, especially for temporal lobe seizures, but the timing of the injection is critical because secondary increases in blood flow may occur at a distance from the primary focus, especially in frontal lobe seizures (Stefan et al., 1990a).

The development of new MRI techniques (*magnetic resonance spectroscopy* [MRS] and *diffusion-weighted imaging*) and their applications in patients with epilepsy should allow an improved understanding of the pathophysiologic mechanisms involved in epilepsy. Use of the noninvasive proton MRS in conjunction with the existing diagnostic techniques ap-

pears to be potentially useful for localizing epileptic foci in children suffering from either temporal or extratemporal seizures, despite the age-dependent variation in MRS-detectable metabolites (Thian, 1997). *Functional magnetic resonance imaging* has been primarily used to identify the motor and sensory cortices, as well as the areas involved in language and memory functions, that should be spared during epilepsy surgery. Although evaluation of ictal activity with fMRI is not likely to be feasible because of head movements, this technique may be able to localize the source and spread of ongoing abnormal neural activity that appears on the EEG as interictal spikes (Nobre and Rao, 2000). Certain methods make EEG measurement during MRI safe, and ultrafast fMRI permits monitoring of the EEG between image acquisitions (Ives et al., 1993).

Intracranial EEG recording remains the gold standard for the localization and definition of the extent of the epileptogenic zone (Jayakar and Duchowny, 1997; Bancaud and Talairach, 1975; Bancaud et al., 1965). The removal of this zone is mandatory if seizure control is to be obtained (Paolicchi et al., 2000; Duchowny et al., 1998). Because of its complexity, the possibility of complications and the difficulties or even impossibility to perform this in young and retarded children, it cannot be considered a routine technique. Indeed, when all other investigations are concordant, at least in some localizations (e.g., the temporal lobe), it can be dispensed with in many cases, especially in children with mesial temporal lobe epilepsy in whom both EEG data and typical MRI characteristics are present (Cendes et al., 2000; Cascino et al., 1996). On the other hand, acute or chronic invasive (intracranial) recording is clearly necessary in discordant cases and in all those in which ambiguity persists regarding the localization and extension of the area to be removed. The frequency of use depends partly on the type of patients in each center. Semiinvasive methods, especially foramen ovale electrodes (Wieser and Morris, 1997; Wieser and Siegel, 1991), are used in special, less common situations to provide relatively limited information.

Considerable disagreement still exists over the best methods of intracranial recordings. *Depth electrodes* that are stereotactically implanted are the most appropriate for seizures of deep origin (e.g., amygdala and hippocampus) (Lüders and Comair, 2001; Wyllie, 2001; Bureau et al., 1998; Engel, et al., 1997; Spencer et al., 1997; Bancaud et al., 1973). They explore only a small cerebral volume, so the activation of one electrode may only mean that a discharge that may come from a distant area has reached it. Therefore, an hypothesis regarding the location and propagation of the discharge must be established beforehand so that the number of electrodes can remain limited. *Grids or strips* can cover a wide area, but they cannot be used to explore such regions as the mesial temporal lobe. Adequate exposure through a craniotomy is required and the operative procedure is rather complex. Subdural hemorrhage or infection may theoretically occur.

The *method to be used thus depends on the preoperative hypothesis* regarding the likely origin and propagation of the seizures in a particular patient; no "ready-made" techniques can be satisfactory. In general, with any type of invasive EEG recording, the relationship among paroxysmal discharges, the lesion, and the epileptogenic area is not a simple one (Engel et al., 1990; Bancaud and Talairach, 1975), and the evidence from intracranial recordings must be compatible with that of other sources (Munari et al., 2000), the most important of which are the clinical features of the habitual seizures and the results of imaging studies.

Two important points must be emphasized. First, the *various presurgical evaluation techniques are highly interdependent*. For example, the number of seizures that need to be recorded can be much lower when several localizing methods give similar unequivocal results. Second, *any discordance in the results of the various methods considerably decreases the chances of a good outcome*. In one study (Fish et al., 1989), even one discordant datum was associated with a favorable result in only 3 (16%) of 19 cases, compared with 53 (54%) of 99 concordant cases.

The requirements for hemispherectomy or large multilobar resections include the evaluation of the probable deficit resulting from such resections, especially on the global development of children to be operated on (Freeman et al., 1997; Vargha-Khadem and Mishkin, 1997).

No adverse effects on the development of language have been noted when hemispherectomy is performed for the treatment of prenatal or perinatal lesions or even for postnatally acquired lesions when the operation is performed before the age of 5 years, no matter the side on which the operation is performed (Vargha-Khadem et al., 1991). The control of seizures may actually improve the mental outlook, as epilepsy has been shown to be strongly associated with low intellectual performance in patients with congenital hemiplegia (Vargha-Khadem et al., 1992a).

REQUIREMENTS FOR PALLIATIVE SURGERY

The requirements for palliative surgery are less stringent than those for resections, but a dearth of information still exists regarding the long-term consequences of callosotomy, which is the most commonly performed palliative operation. Although, in most patients, the disconnection syndrome that is produced has relatively few practical consequences (Lassonde et al., 1991), the long-term subtle effects on address, hand coordination, and cognitive functions are not known. Therefore, the indications for callosotomy should be conservative. Immediate complications may occur (Polkey, 2000, 2003; Arzimanoglou et al., 1994; Blume, 1997), and mutism, which is virtually always transient, is common and sometimes frightening (Spencer, 1988).

Discrepant opinions exist regarding which patients are most likely to respond to callosotomy. Whereas most investigators agree that drop attacks, whether tonic or atonic, are the best indication (Polkey, 2003; Arzimanoglou et al., 1994; Nordgren et al., 1991; Oguni et al., 1991b; Spencer et al., 1985; Gates et al., 1984), some authors think that cases in which evidence indicates an anterior unilateral origin of the seizures especially benefit from the procedure (Spencer, 1988), although this is not a universal experience (Pinard, 1991). Some investigators have suggested that evidence of mixed laterality for handedness and language may be associated with a greater risk of bimanual incoordination after the operation (Gilliam and Wyllie, 1997).

OUTCOME OF SURGERY

The outcome of surgery depends primarily on the selection of surgical candidates and the type of outcome measurement used. Overall figures obtained from different centers operating on different types of patients are meaningless and difficult to compare (Munari et al., 1999a). The best results are obtained in patients with temporal lobe epilepsy with fully congruent data and a small resectable lesion. Excellent results can be obtained following excisional surgery in well-selected infants and young children with intractable seizures (Bittar et al., 2002; Duchowny et al., 1998; Mukahira et al., 1998). In a series of 75 patients younger than 12 years who underwent excisional surgery, the complete resection of the lesion and the electrographically abnormal region was the main determinant of outcome after focal resections (Paolicchi et al., 2000). Similar results following simple complete lesionectomy have been reported by Bourgeois et al. (1999b).

The Cleveland Clinic Group (Wyllie et al., 1998) studied seizure outcome in 136 pediatric patients with a mean postoperative follow-up of 3.6 years (range of 1 to 7.5 years), in which 62 children were compared with 74 adolescents. Extratemporal or multilobar resections and hemispherectomies had a similar frequency among children and adolescents, but these procedures strongly predominated in infancy (90% of patients were from 0 to 2 years of age). The remaining patients had temporal resection. Cortical dysplasia and low-grade tumor were the most common causes, and hippocampal sclerosis was rare. Overall, a seizure-free outcome was achieved for 69% of adolescents, 68% of children, and 60% of the infant subgroup. Seizure-free outcome was more common after temporal resection (56 [78%] of 72) than after extratemporal or multilobar resection (26 [54%] of 48; 41 of 48 with a focal lesion on MRI), and among patients with tumor (36 [82%] of 44) versus cortical dysplasia (16 [52%] of 31). The frequency of seizure-free outcome after epilepsy surgery was similar for infants, children, and adolescents, and it was comparable with the results from adult series.

Between 70% and 85% of patients with intractable partial epilepsy may remain controlled after surgery (Salanova et al., 2002; Bizzi et al., 1997; Elwes et al., 1991; Hirsch et al., 1991a, 1991b; Duchowny, 1989; So et al., 1989b; King et al., 1986; Talairach and Szikla, 1980; Engel et al., 1975). Patients with large lesions, which can rarely be totally removed, have a less favorable outcome, with a less than 50% success rate (Palmini et al., 1991b). However, a significant reduction in the frequency of seizures is often obtained, which may considerably improve the patient's quality of life.

Particularly in children with *focal cortical dysplasias*, for which the chances for medical control of their seizures are known to be low (Lortie et al., 2002) and which have an impact on cognitive functioning (Klein et al., 2000), recent studies have suggested a better outcome following early surgery (Kral et al., 2003; Kloss et al., 2002). Complete resection of the dysplastic lesion is significantly correlated with favorable seizure outcome (Kloss et al., 2002; Kameyama et al., 2001; Chassoux et al., 2000). Tassi et al. (2002) recently reported a series of 52 patients operated on for drug-resistant partial epilepsy related to architectural dysplasia (31 patients), cytoarchitectural dysplasia (6 patients), or Taylor-type cortical dysplasia (15 patients). Patients with Taylor-type dysplasia had the best outcome, with 75% remaining seizure free (Engel class Ia) after at least 1 year of follow-up, compared with 50% of cytoarchitectural dysplasia and 43% of architectural dysplasia patients who were seizure free.

The surgical treatment of *temporal lobe epilepsy* in childhood is very gratifying (see previous discus-

sion). Children with purely mesial temporal lesions and hippocampal sclerosis can undergo surgery after noninvasive monitoring (Spencer et al., 2001; Tuxhorn et al., 1997a), and the results that are obtained are similar to those reported in adults (Cendes et al., 2002; Arruda et al., 1996; Garcia et al., 1994). The Cleveland group (Mohamed et al., 2001) studied 34 children and adolescents who had anteromesial temporal resection. Overall, 78% of patients remained free of seizures at their latest available follow-up (mean of 2.6 years), and another 13% had only rare seizures. On histopathology, an unexpectedly high frequency of dual pathology with mild to moderate cortical dysplasia and hippocampal sclerosis was seen in 79% of children and adolescents. A high incidence of dual pathology in children with temporal lobe epilepsy has also been reported by other authors (Bocti et al., 2003). Dysembryoplastic neuroepithelial tumors are a common associated finding (Hennessy et al., 2001). Only preliminary data are available concerning the cognitive outcomes of temporal lobectomy in children and adolescents (Gleissner et al., 2002; Westerveld et al., 2000).

Poorer results are found in patients with frontal epilepsy, poorly congruent preoperative data, and no definite pathology, for whom success rates of 10% or less are likely. In general, *frontal lobe resections* are associated with, at most, 50% good outcomes (Chodkiewicz et al., 1988; Wyllie et al., 1987a), and the absence of a definite lesion has a highly unfavorable significance (Chauvel et al., 1992a; Fish et al., 1989; Talairach and Bancaud, 1974; Talairach et al., 1974). In children with frontal resectable neoplastic lesions, the outcome is excellent and is comparable to that of temporal lobe epilepsy surgery (Kral et al., 2001).

A globally better outcome is also observed in some children with intractable epilepsy caused by *multiple* or *diffuse* lesions, such as tubers (Karenfort et al., 2002) or leptomeningeal angiomatosis (Arzimanoglou et al., 2000; Arzimanoglou, 1997).

Hemispherectomy controls the seizures in more than 80% of patients (Tinuper et al., 1988; Lindsay et al., 1987; Verity et al., 1982). Any previous hemiplegia may be increased, but proximal movements of the limb and ambulation usually remain possible. Devlin et al. (2003) reported on the clinical course and outcome of 33 children who underwent hemispherectomy between 1991 and 1997. The median age at surgery was 4.25 years. The underlying pathology was developmental in 16, including 10 with hemimegalencephaly; acquired in 11 (mostly infarcts or trauma), and progressive in 6 children (4 with Rasmussen encephalitis, 2 with Sturge-Weber syndrome). At follow-up, 52% were seizure free, 9% experienced rare seizures, and 30% showed a more than 75% reduction in seizures. Seizure freedom was highest in those with acquired pathology (82%), followed by those with progressive pathology (50%) and those with developmental pathology (31%). The global outcome was worthwhile in all groups. Hemiplegia remained unchanged following surgery in 22 of 33 children, it was improved in 5, and it was worse in 6. No significant cognitive deterioration or loss of language occurred, and four children showed significant cognitive improvement. Behavioral improvement was reported in 92% of those who had behavior problems preoperatively. In a personal series of patients with Sturge-Weber syndrome submitted to hemispherectomy, 100% remained seizure free (Arzimanoglou et al., 2000).

In a recent study (Park et al., 2002), the frequency and prognostic features of *acute postoperative seizures* within the first postoperative week were determined in 148 patients (mean age at surgery was 13 years; range of 5 months to 18 years). Acute postoperative seizures were experienced by 25% of the patients in this cohort. Statistically significant ($p < 0.05$) risk factors for acute postoperative seizures included the following: the presence of other types of seizures, extratemporal surgery, postoperative fever, non–temporal lobe epilepsy, and postoperative interictal epileptiform activity. At the last follow-up, those patients who did not experience acute postoperative seizures had a significantly greater chance of being seizure free (80% versus 51%; $p < 0.001$).

The outcome of *nonresective surgery* should be assessed differently. For callosotomy, which is the most commonly performed operation of this type, no control of seizures can be expected (Blume et al., 1993). In some cases, partial seizures may be worsened by callosotomy (Spencer et al., 1984b). The frequency with which callosotomy prevents dangerous drop attacks by transforming them into partial seizures or gentle slow falls remains uncertain because of the heterogeneity of most series. Pinard (1991) found a significant decrease in seizure frequency following anterior callosotomy in one-third of 26 children with severe epilepsy. A two-stage complete callosotomy was associated with a decrease in the number and severity of seizures in five additional patients who had not benefited from anterior callosotomy. Oguni et al. (1991b) also found the operation helpful for children with Lennox-Gastaut syndrome and other forms of secondary generalized epilepsy in a large but mixed series of patients of different ages and with different forms of epilepsy, and the authors' results were similar (Arzimanoglou et al., 1994).

The available results from different studies suggest that children should be considered for surgical evaluation *at whatever age* they manifest with severe, intractable, disabling epilepsy. Epilepsy surgery in children has now become a realistic therapeutic option. It is not to be considered as a treatment of last resort when all else has failed.

SUMMARY

Surgery is an effective therapy for some forms of medically intractable epilepsy, but it is not applicable to all resistant cases and strict conditions must be fulfilled for its application. These include the reasonable certainty that medical treatment will remain unsuccessful; a sufficient likelihood that the epilepsy is severe enough to disrupt the patient's existence; the patient's informed agreement and understanding; and the availability of adequate technologic and human means, including facilities for a multidisciplinary approach and postoperative rehabilitation.

The most usual and effective type of surgery is the resection of epileptogenic brain tissue (epileptogenic area), which requires that a single lesion is present, that it is located to a cortical area that can be removed without producing unacceptable functional deficits, and that it is precisely localized by various techniques. Resective surgery can also be applied, with some reservations, to extensive lesions that necessitate multilobar resection or hemispherectomy, provided the balance of expected deficits and the advantages drawn from seizure control clearly favors of the latter. Palliative operations, mainly callosotomy, may help some patients with particularly disruptive seizure types, even though only the disappearance of the most unacceptable seizures is expected, not seizure control. Encouraging results have also been reported using vagus nerve stimulation.

The preoperative evaluation of candidates for surgery is the essential step. In recent years, neuroimaging has contributed considerably to the better selection of patients. The demonstration of a single clearly characterized and localized lesion is apparently a predictor of good surgical outcome. Functional imaging techniques are becoming increasingly important for the localization and delimitation of the zones to be resected.

The essential principle remains that information obtained by several methods should be concordant if favorable results are to be expected. Any incongruency is associated with a marked decrease in the quality of outcome.

References

Aarts JP, Binnie CD, Smit AM, et al. 1984. Selective cognitive impairment during focal and generalized epileptiform EEG activity. *Brain* 107:293–308.

Aarts WF, Visser LH, Loonen MC, et al. 1988. Follow-up of 146 children with epilepsy after withdrawal of antiepileptic therapy. *Epilepsia* 29:244–250.

Abe T, Kobayashi M, Araki K, et al. 2000. Infantile convulsions with mild gastroenteritis. *Brain Dev* 22:301–306.

Abo K, Morikawa T, Fujiwara T, et al. 1983. Tuberous sclerosis and epilepsy. In: *Advances in epileptology*, XIVth Epilepsy International Symposium. New York: Raven Press, 105–111.

Abou-Khalil BW, Siegel GJ, Sackellares JC, et al. 1987. Positron emission tomography studies of cerebral glucose metabolism in chronic partial epilepsy. *Ann Neurol* 22:480–486.

Abou-Khalil B, Andermann E, Andermann F, et al. 1993. Temporal lobe epilepsy after prolonged febrile convulsions: excellent outcome after surgical treatment. *Epilepsia* 34:878–883.

Abram HS, Turk WR. 1997. Lennox-Gastaut syndrome. In: *Management of epilepsy in children: the need for consensus*. Consensus in Child Neurology. Hamilton, Ontario: Decker Periodicals, 10–15.

Acharya N, Wyllie E, Lüders HO, et al. 1997. Seizure symptomatology in infants with localization-related epilepsy. *Neurology* 48:189–196.

Acharya JN, Wyllie E, Lüders HO. 2000. Hypomotor seizures. In: Lüders HO, Noachtar S, eds. *Epileptic seizures*. Philadelphia: Churchill Livingstone, 484–488.

Adams CB. 1983. Hemispherectomy—a modification. *J Neurol Neurosurg Psychiatry* 46:617–619.

Adams RD, Brunwald E. 1980. Faintness, syncope and episodic weakness. In: Isselbacher KJ, ed. *Harrison's principles of internal medicine*, 9th ed. New York: McGraw-Hill.

Adams DJ, Lüders H. 1981. Hyperventilation and 6-hour EEG recording in evaluation of absence seizures. *Neurology* 31:1175–1177.

Adams C, Hwang PA, Gilday DL, et al. 1992. Comparison of SPECT, EEG, CT, MRI and pathology in partial epilepsy. *Pediatr Neurol* 8:97–103.

Addy DP. 1986. Nosology of febrile convulsions. *Arch Dis Child* 61:318–320.

Adler J, Erba G, Winston KR, et al. 1991. Results of surgery for extratemporal partial epilepsy that began in childhood. *Arch Neurol* 48:133–140.

Afifi A, Corbett JJ, Thompson HS, et al. 1990. Seizure-induced miosis and ptosis: association with temporal lobe magnetic resonance imaging abnormalities. *J Child Neurol* 5:142–146.

Agathonikou A, Panayiotopoulos CP, Giannakodimos S, Koutroumanidis M. 1998. Typical absence status in adults: diagnostic and syndromic considerations. *Epilepsia* 39:1265–1276.

Agbato OA, Elyas AA, Patsalos PN, et al. 1986. Total and free serum concentrations of carbamazepine and carabamazepine-10,11-epoxide in children with epilepsy. *Arch Neurol* 43:1111–1116.

Aguglia U, Tinuper P, Gastaut H. 1984a. Startle-induced epileptic seizures. *Epilepsia* 25:712–720.

Aguglia U, Tinuper P, Farnarier G, et al. 1984b. Etat d'absence à prédominance EEG unilatérale: à propos d'une observation privilégiée. *Rev Electroencephalogr Neurophysiol Clin* 14:241–246.

Aicardi J. 1973. The problem of the Lennox syndrome. *Dev Med Child Neurol* 15:77–81.

Aicardi J. 1976. Les convulsions unilatérales de l'enfant. *Concours Médical* 98:921–928.

Aicardi J. 1979. Benign epilepsy of childhood with rolandic spikes. *Brain Dev* 1:71–73.

Aicardi J. 1980a. Course and prognosis of certain childhood epilepsies with predominantly myoclonic seizures. In: Wada JA, Penry JK, eds. *Advances in epileptology*, Xth Epilepsy International Symposium. New York: Raven Press, 159–163.

Aicardi J. 1980b. Myoclonic epilepsies. *Research and Clinical Forums* 2:47–55.

Aicardi J. 1980c. Seizures and epilepsy in children under two years of age. In: Tyrer JH, ed. *The treatment of epilepsy*. Lancaster, England: MTP Press, 203–250.

Aicardi J. 1982a. Childhood epilepsies with brief myoclonic, atonic or tonic seizures. In: Laidlaw J, Richens A, eds. *A textbook of epilepsy*. Edinburgh: Churchill Livingstone, 88–96.

Aicardi J. 1982b. Les myoclonies dans les maladies dégénératives du système nerveux central chez l'enfant. *Rev Electroencephalogr Neurophysiol Clin* 12:15–20.

Aicardi J. 1983a. Complex partial seizures in childhood. In: Parsonage M, Grant RHE, Craig AG, et al., eds. *Advances in epileptology*, XIVth Epilepsy International Symposium. New York: Raven Press, 237–242.

Aicardi J. 1983b. The benign epilepsies of childhood. In: Rose CF, ed. *Research progress in epilepsy*. London: Pitman, 231–239.

Aicardi J. 1985a. Epileptic syndromes in childhood. Overview and classification. In: Ross E, Reynolds E, eds. *Paediatric perspectives on epilepsy*. Chichester: John Wiley, 65–71.

Aicardi J. 1985b. The medical management of neonatal and infantile seizures and of febrile seizures. In: Porter R, Morselli PL, eds. *The epilepsies*. London: Butterworth-Heinemann, 206–226.

Aicardi J. 1986a. *Epilepsy in children*. New York: Raven Press.

Aicardi J. 1986b. Myoclonic epilepsies of infancy and childhood. In: Fahn S, Marsden CD, Van Woert MH, eds. *Myoclonus*. Advances in neurology, Vol. 43. New York: Raven Press, 11–31.

Aicardi J. 1986c. Treatment of infantile spasms. In: Schmidt D, Morselli PL, eds. *Intractable epilepsy: experimental and clinical aspects*. New York: Raven Press, 147–156.

Aicardi J. 1988a. Clinical approach to the management of intractable epilepsy. *Dev Med Child Neurol* 30:429–440.

Aicardi J. 1988b. Epileptic syndromes in childhood. *Epilepsia* 29:S1–S5.

Aicardi J. 1989. Current management of infantile spasms. *International Pediatrics* 4:188–192.

Aicardi J. 1990a. Epilepsy in brain-injured children. *Dev Med Child Neurol* 32:191–202.

Aicardi J. 1990b. Neonatal myoclonic encephalopathy and early infantile epileptic encephalopathy. In: Wasterlain CG, Vert P, eds. *Neonatal seizures* New York: Raven Press, 41–49.

Aicardi J. 1991a. Myoclonic epilepsies in childhood. *International Pediatrics* 6:195–200.

Aicardi J. 1991b. Neonatal seizures. In: Dam M, Gram L, eds. *Comprehensive epileptology*. New York, Raven Press.

Aicardi J. 1991c. Secondary bilateral synchrony in patients with partial epileptogenic lesions. In: Ohtahara W, Roger J, eds. *New trends in pediatric neurology*. Okayama: Okayama University Medical School, 37–46.

Aicardi J. 1991d. The agyria-pachygyria complex: a spectrum of cortical malformations. *Brain Dev* 13:1–8.

Aicardi J. 1992a. *Diseases of the nervous system in childhood*. London: MacKeith Press.

Aicardi J. 1992b. Early myoclonic encephalopathy (neonatal myoclonic encephalopathy). In: Roger J, Bureau M, Dravet C, et al., eds. *Epileptic syndromes in infancy, childhood and adolescence*, 2nd ed. London: John Libbey, 13–23.

Aicardi J. 1992c. Epilepsy and inborn errors of metabolism. In: Roger J, Bureau M, Dravet C, et al., eds. *Epileptic syndromes in infancy, childhood and adolescence*, 2nd ed. London: John Libbey, 97–102.

Aicardi J. 1994a. *Epilepsy in children*, 2nd ed. New York: Raven Press.

Aicardi J. 1994b. The place of neuronal migration abnormalities in child neurology. *Can J Neurol Sci* 21: 185–193.

Aicardi J. 1995. Typical absences in the first two years of life. In: Duncan J, Panayiotopoulos C, eds. *Typical absences and related epileptic syndromes*. London: Churchill Communication Europe, 284–288.

Aicardi J. 1996. Aicardi syndrome. In: Guerrini R, Andermann F, Canapicchi R, et al., eds. *Dysplasias of cerebral cortex and epilepsy*. Philadelphia: Lippincott-Raven, 211–216.

Aicardi J. 1997. Paediatric epilepsy surgery: how the view has changed. In: Tuxhorn I, Holthausen H, Boenigk H, eds. *Paediatric epilepsy syndromes and their surgical treatment*. London: John Libbey, 3–7.

Aicardi J. 1998a. *Diseases of the nervous system in children*, 2nd ed. Cambridge: Cambridge University Press.

Aicardi J. 1998b. Epilepsy and other seizure disorders. In: *Diseases of the nervous system in childhood*, 2nd ed. London: MacKeith Press, 575–637.

Aicardi J. 1998c. Paroxysmal disorders other than epilepsy. In: *Diseases of the nervous system in childhood*. London: MacKeith Press, 638–663.

Aicardi J. 1999a. Epilepsy: the hidden part of the iceberg. *Eur J Paediatr Neurol* 3:197–200.

Aicardi J. 1999b. Pyridoxine-responsive epilepsy. In: Kotagal P, Lüders H, eds. *The epilepsies*. New York: Academic Press, 443–448.

Aicardi J. 2000. Atypical semiology of rolandic epilepsy in some related syndromes. *Epileptic Disord* 2:S55–S59

Aicardi J. 2001. Alternating hemiplegia in children. In: Guerrini R, Aicardi J, Andermann F, Hallett M, eds. *Epilepsy and movement disorders*. Cambridge: Cambridge University Press, 379–392.

Aicardi J. 2001a. Dreamy state: a case report from the selected writings of John Hughlings Jackson. *Brain* 1874. *Epileptic Disord* 3:51–54.

Aicardi J, Arzimanoglou A. 1986. Images tomodensitométriques d'allure tumorale observées lors de certaines épilepsies de l'enfant. *Journées Parisiennes de Pédiatrie*. Paris: Flammarion, 133–138.

Aicardi J, Arzimanoglou A. 1996. Treatment of childhood epilepsy syndromes. In: Shorvon SD, Dreifuss FE, Fish D, Thomas D, eds. *The treatment of epilepsy*. London: Blackwell Science, 199–214.

Aicardi J, Baraton J. 1971. A pneumoencephalographic demonstration of brain atrophy following status epilepticus. *Dev Med Child Neurol* 13:660–667.

Aicardi J, Chevrie JJ. 1970. Convulsive status epilepticus in infants and children: a study of 239 cases. *Epilepsia* 11:187–197.

Aicardi J, Chevrie JJ. 1971. Myoclonic epilepsies of childhood. *Neuropédiatrie* 3:177–190.

Aicardi J, Chevrie JJ. 1976. Febrile convulsions: neurological sequelae and mental retardation. In: Brazier MA, Coceani F, eds. *Brain dysfunction in infantile febrile convulsions*. New York: Raven Press, 247–257.

Aicardi J, Chevrie JJ. 1978. Les spasmes infantiles. *Arch Fr Pediatr* 35:1015–1023.

Aicardi J, Chevrie JJ. 1982a. Atypical benign epilepsy of childhood. *Dev Med Child Neurol* 24:281–292.

Aicardi J, Chevrie JJ. 1982b. Epilepsy in infants. Clinical and prognostic aspects. In: Wise G, Blaw ME, Procopis PG, eds. *Topics in child neurology*, vol. II. New York: Spectrum, 73–83.

Aicardi J, Chevrie JJ. 1983. Consequences of status epilepticus in infants and children. In: Delgado-Escueta AV, Wasterlain CG, Treiman DM, Porter RJ, eds. *Status epilepticus: mechanisms of brain damage and treatment*. Advances in neurology, Vol. 34. New York: Raven Press, 115–125.

Aicardi J, Chevrie JJ. 1986. *Treatment of Lennox-Gastaut syndrome*. In: Schmidt D, Morselli P, eds. *Intractable epilepsy*. New York: Raven Press.

Aicardi J, Chevrie JJ. 1993. The Aicardi syndrome. In: Lassonde M, ed. *Callosal agenesis: the natural split-brain*. New York: Plenum.

Aicardi J, Gastaut H. 1985. Treatment of self-induced photosensitive epilepsy with fenfluramine. *N Engl J Med* 313:1419.

Aicardi J, Gomes AL. 1988. The Lennox-Gastaut syndrome: clinical and electroencephalographic features. In: Niedermeyer E, Degen D, eds. *The Lennox-Gastaut syndrome*. New York: Alan R. Liss, 25–46.

Aicardi J, Gomes AL. 1989. The myoclonic epilepsies of childhood. *Cleve Clin J Med* 59:S34–S39.

Aicardi J, Gomes AL. 1992. Clinical and EEG symptomatology of the "genuine" Lennox-Gastaut syndrome and its differentiation from other forms of epilepsy in early childhood. In: Degen R, ed. *The benign localized and generalized epilepsies of early childhood*. Amsterdam: Elsevier, 185–193.

Aicardi J, Goutières F. 1973. Les thromboses veineuses intracrâniennes: complications des déshydratations aiguës du nourrisson. *Arch Fr Pediatr* 30:809–830.

Aicardi J, Goutières F. 1978. Encéphalopathie myoclonique néonatale. *Rev Electroencephalogr Neurophysiol Clin* 8:99–101.

Aicardi J, Newton R. 1987. Partial epilepsy of childhood with occipital spike-wave complexes: the range of clinical manifestations. In: Andermann F, Lugaresi E, eds. *Migraine and epilepsy*. London: Butterworth-Heinemann, 111–124.

Aicardi J, Ohtahara S. 2002. Severe neonatal epilepsies with suppression-burst pattern. In: Roger J, Bureau M, Dravet CH, et al., eds. *Epileptic syndromes in infancy, childhood and adolescence.* London: John Libbey Ltd., 33–44.

Aicardi J, Taylor DC. 1998. History and physical examination. In: Engel J, Pendley TA, eds. *Epilepsy: a comprehensive textbook.* Philadelphia: Lippincott-Raven, 805–810.

Aicardi J, Lefebvre J, Lerique-Koechlin A. 1965. A new syndrome: spasms in flexion, callosal agenesis, ocular abnormalities. *Electroencephalogr Clin Neurophysiol* 19: 609–610.

Aicardi J, Weinman S, Chevrie JJ, et al. 1967. Les spasmes en flexion du nourrisson. Etude de l'excrétion urinaire des 17-hydroxy-cortico-stéroides et do taux de sécrétion du cortisol an cours de leur traitement par l'ACTH. *Arch Fr Pediatr* 24:521–530.

Aicardi J, Amsli J, Chevrie JJ. 1969a. Acute hemiplegia in infancy and childhood. *Dev Med Child Neurol* 11: 162–173.

Aicardi J, Chevrie JJ, Rousselie F. 1969b. Le syndrome agénésie calleuse, spasmes en flexion, lacunes chorioré-tiniennes. *Arch Fr Pediatr* 26:1103–1120.

Aicardi J, Praud E, Bancaud J, et al. 1970. Epilepsies cliniquement primitives et tumeurs cérébrales chez l'enfant. *Arch Fr Pediatr* 27:1041–1055.

Aicardi J, Goutières F, Challamel JM, et al. 1972. Hémiplégies cérébrales infantiles. Séméiologie, étiologie et pronostic. *Rev Electroencephalogr Neurophysiol Clin* 2:95–100.

Aicardi J, Goutières, F, Arsenio-Nunes ML, et al. 1977. Acute measles encephalitis in children with immunosuppression. *Pediatrics* 59:232–239.

Aicardi J, Plouin P, Goutières F. 1978. Les céroïdelipofuschinoses. *Rev Electroencephalogr Neurophysiol Clin* 8:149–160.

Aicardi J, Murnaghan K, Gandon Y, et al. 1983. Efficacité de la tomodensitométrie dans les épilepsies de l'enfant: problèmes posés par son utilisation. *J Neuroradiol* 10: 127–129.

Aicardi J, Gastaut H, Mises J. 1988. Syncopal attacks compulsively self-induced by Valsalva's maneuver, associated with typical absence seizures. *Arch Neurol* 45: 923–925.

Aicardi J, Revol M, Boon M, et al. 1990. Malformations vasculaires intracrâniennes et épilepsie. *Pédiatrie* 45: S217–S221.

Aicardi J, Mumford JP, Dumas C, Wood S. 1996. Vigabatrin as initial therapy for infantile spasms: a European retrospective survey. Sabril IS Investigator and Peer Review Groups. *Epilepsia* 37:638–642.

Aird RB. 1988. The importance of seizure-inducing factors in youth. *Brain Dev* 10:73–76.

Aird RB, Masland RL, Woodbury DM. 1984. *The epilepsies—a critical review.* New York: Raven Press.

Aird RB, Masland RL, Woodbury DM. 1989. Hypothesis: the classification of epileptic seizures according to systems of the CNS. *Epilepsy Res* 3:77–81.

Ajmone-Marsan C, Abraham K. 1960. A seizure atlas. *Electroencephalogr Clin Neurophysiol* 15:1–215.

Ajmone-Marsan C, Goldhammer L. 1973. Clinical ictal patterns and electrographic data in cases of partial seizures of frontal-central-parietal origin. In: Brazier MA, ed. *Epilepsy: its phenomena in man.* New York: Academic Press, 236–260.

Ajmone-Marsan C, Ralston BL. 1957. *The epileptic seizure: its functional morphology and diagnostic significance.* Springfield, IL: Charles C Thomas Publisher.

Aksu F. 1990. Nature and prognosis of seizures in patients with cerebral palsy. *Dev Med Child Neurol* 32:661–668.

Al Eissa YA. 1995. Febrile seizures: rate and risk factors of recurrence. *J Child Neurol* 10:315–319.

Al Shawan SA, Singh B, Riela AR, et al. 1996. Hemisomatic spasms in children. *Neurology* 44:1322–1333.

Ala-Houala M, Korpela R, Koivikko M, et al. 1986. Long-term anticonvulsant therapy and vitamin D metabolism in ambulatory pubertal children. *Neuropediatrics* 17: 212–216.

Alajouanine A, Gastaut H. 1955. La syncinésie-sursaut et l'épilepsie-sursaut à déclenchement sensoriel ou sensitif inopiné. *Rev Neurol (Paris)* 93:29–41.

Albala BJ, Moshé SL, Okada R. 1984. Kainic acid-induced seizure: a developmental study. *Dev Brain Res* 3: 139–148.

Albani M. 1983. Phenytoin in infancy and childhood. In: Delgado-Escueta AV, Wasterlain CG, Treiman DM, Porter RJ, eds. *Status epilepticus: mechanisms of brain damage and treatment.* Advances in neurology, Vol. 34. New York: Raven Press, 457–464.

Albright P, Bruni J. 1985. Reduction of polypharmacy in epileptic patients. *Arch Neurol* 42:797–799.

Aldenkamp AP. 1983. Epilepsy and learning behaviour. *Adv Epileptol* 14:221–229.

Aldenkamp AP. 2001. Effects of antiepileptic drugs on cognition. *Epilepsia* 42:46–49.

Aldenkamp AP, Alpherts WC, Moerland MC, et al. 1987. Controlled release carbamazepine: cognitive side-effects in patients with epilepsy. *Epilepsia* 28:507–514.

Aldenkamp AP, Alpherts WC, Dekker MJ, et al. 1990. Neuropsychological aspects of learning disabilities in epilepsy. *Epilepsia* 31:S30–S34.

Aldenkamp AP, Gutter T, Beun AM. 1992. The effect of seizure activity and paroxysmal electroencephalographic discharges on cognition. *Acta Neurol Scand* 86: 111–121.

Aldenkamp AP, Alpherts WC, Blennow G, et al. 1993. Withdrawal of antiepileptic medication in children—effects on cognitive function: the Multicenter Holmfrid Study. *Neurology* 43:41–50.

Aldrich MS. 1990. Narcolepsy. *N Engl J Med* 323:389–394.

Alemayehu S, Bergey GK, Barry E, et al. 1995. Panic attacks as ictal manifestations of parietal lobe seizures. *Epilepsia* 36:824–830.

Alfonso I, Papazian O, Aicardi J, et al. 1995. A simple maneuver to provoke benign neonatal sleep myoclonus. *Pediatrics* 96:1161–1163.

Alfonso I, Alvarez LA, Gilman J, et al. 2000. Intravenous valproate dosing in neonates. *J Child Neurol* 15: 827–829.

Alfonso I, Papazian O, Litt R, et al. 2001. Single photon emission computed tomographic evaluation of brainstem release phenomenon and seizures in neonates. *J Child Neurol* 15:56–58.

Aliberti V, Grünewald RA, Panayiotopoulos CP, Chroni E. 1994. Focal electroencephalographic abnormalities in juvenile myoclonic epilepsy. *Epilepsia* 35: 297–301.

Alldredge BK, Wall DB, Ferriero DM. 1995. Effect of prehospital treatment on the outcome of status epilepticus in children. *Pediatr Neurol* 12:213–216.

Allen JP, Imbus CE, Powars DR, et al. 1976. Neurologic impairment induced by hyperventilation in children with sickle cell anemia. *Pediatrics* 58:124–126

Allen JW, Oxley J, Robertson MM, et al. 1983. Clobazam adjunctive treatment in refractory epilepsy. *BMJ* 286: 1246–1247.

Allen TL, Brothman AR, Carey JC, et al. 1996. Cytogenetic and molecular analysis in trisomy 12p. *Am J Med Genet* 63:250–256.

Altrocchi RH, Menkes JA. 1960. Congenital ocular motor apraxia. *Brain* 83:579–588.

Alvarez N, Hartford E, Douet C. 1981. Epileptic seizures induced by clonazepam. *Clin Electroencephalogr* 12: 57–65.

Alvarez N, Lombroso CT, Medina C, et al. 1983. Paroxysmal spike and wave activity in drowsiness in young children: its relationship to febrile convulsions. *Electroencephalogr Clin Neurophysiol* 56:406–413.

Alvarez LA, Shinnar S, Moshé SL. 1987. Infantile spasms due to unilateral cerebral infarcts. *Pediatrics* 79: 1024–1026.

Ambrosetto G. 1992. Unilateral opercular macrogyria and benign childhood epilepsy with centrotemporal (rolandic) spikes: report of a case. *Epilepsia* 33: 499–503.

Ambrosetto G, Gobbi G. 1975. Benign epilepsy of childhood with rolandic spikes, or a lesion? EEG during a seizure. *Epilepsia* 16:793–796.

Ambrosetto G, Tassinari CA. 1987. Photosensitivity related to valproate withdrawal. *J Neurol Neurosurg Psychiatry* 50:1709–1710.

Ambrosetto G, Tassinari CA. 1990. Antiepileptic drug treatment of benign childhood epilepsy with rolandic spikes: is it necessary? *Epilepsia* 31:802–805.

Ambrosetto P, Ambrosetto G, Michelucci R, Bacci A. 1983. Sturge-Weber syndrome without port-wine facial nevus: report of two cases studied by CT. *Childs Brain* 10: 387–392.

Ambrosetto G, Tinuper P, Baruzzi A. 1985. Relapse of benign partial epilepsy of children in adulthood: report of a case. *J Neurol Neurosurg Psychiatry* 48:90.

Ambrosetto G, Giovanardi Rossi P, Tassinari CA. 1987. Predictive factors of seizure frequency and duration of antiepileptic treatment in rolandic epilepsy: a retrospective study. *Brain Dev* 9:300–304.

Ameer B, Greenblatt DJ. 1981. Lorazepam: a review of its clinical pharmacological properties and therapeutic uses. *Drugs* 21:161–200.

American Academy of Pediatrics Committee on Drugs. 1995. Behavioral and cognitive effects of anticonvulsant therapy. *Pediatrics* 96:538–540.

Ames FR, Saffer D. 1983. The sunflower syndrome: a new look at "self-induced" epilepsy. *J Neurol Sci* 59:1–11.

Amess PN, Baudin J, Townsend J, et al. 1998. Epilepsy in very preterm infants: neonatal cranial ultrasound reveals a high-risk subcategory. *Dev Med Child Neurol* 40:724–730.

Aminoff MJ, Simon RP. 1980. Status epilepticus: causes, clinical features and consequences in 98 patients. *Am J Med* 69:657–666.

Aminoff MJ, Simon RP, Wiedemann E. 1984. The hormonal response to generalized tonic-clonic seizures. *Brain* 107:569–578.

Amir N, Saalev RS, Steinberg A. 1986. Sleep patterns in the Lennox-Gastaut syndrome. *Neurology* 36:1224–1226.

Anand BK, Dua S. 1956. Circulatory and respiratory changes induced by electrical stimulation of limbic system (visceral brain). *J Neurophysiol* 19:393–400.

Andermann F. 1967. Absence attacks and diffuse neuronal disease. *Neurology* 17:205–212.

Andermann E. 1982. Multifactorial inheritance of generalized and focal epilepsy. In: Anderson VE, Hauser WA, Penry JK, et al., eds. *Genetic basis of the epilepsies.* New York: Raven Press, 355–374.

Andermann F. 1991. *Chronic encephalitis and epilepsy: Rasmussen's syndrome.* London: Butterworth-Heinemann, 295.

Andermann F, Andermann E. 1988. Startle disorders of man: hyperekplexia, jumping and startle epilepsy. *Brain Dev* 10:213–222.

Andermann E, Andermann F. 1996. Genetic aspects of neuronal migration disorders. In: Guerrini R, Andermann R, Canapicchi R, et al., eds. *Dysplasias of cerebral cortex and epilepsy.* Philadelphia: Lippincott-Raven, 11–15.

Andermann F, Berkovic SF. 2001. Idiopathic generalized epilepsy with generalized and other seizures in adolescence. *Epilepsia* 42:317–320.

Andermann F, Lugaresi E, eds. 1985. *Migraine and epilepsy.* London: Butterworth-Heinemann.

Andermann F, Oguni H. 1990. Do epileptic foci in children migrate? *Electroencephalogr Clin Neurophysiol* 76:96–99.

Andermann F, Robb JP. 1972. Absence status: a reappraisal following review of 38 patients. *Epilepsia* 13:177–187.

Andermann E, Straszak M. 1982. Family studies of epileptiform EEG abnormalities and photosensitivity in focal epilepsy. In: Akimoto H, Kazamatsuri H, eds. *Advances in epileptology,* XIIIth Epilepsy International Symposium. New York: Raven Press, 105–112.

Andermann F, Keene DL, Andermann E, et al. 1980a. Startle disease or hyperexplexia: further delineation of the syndrome. *Brain* 103:985–997.

Andermann F, Mathieson G, Wilkinson RD, et al. 1980b. Amygdaloid melanosis: a form of neurocutaneous melanosis associated with partial complex seizures. In: Canger R, Angeleri F, Penry JK, eds. *Advances in epileptology,* XIth Epilepsy International Symposium. New York: Raven Press, 115–122.

Andermann F, Olivier A, Melanson D, et al. 1987. Epilepsy due to focal cortical dysplasia with macrogyria and the forme fruste of tuberous sclerosis: a study of 15 patients. In: Wolf P, Dam M, Janz D, Dreifuss FE. *Advances in epileptology,* XVIth Epilepsy International Symposium. New York: Raven Press, 35–38.

Andermann F, Rasmussen TB, Villemure JG. 1992. Hemispherectomy: results for control of seizures in patients with hemiparesis. In: Lüders HO, ed. *Epilepsy surgery.* New York: Raven Press, 625–632.

Andermann F, Aicardi J, Vigevano F, eds. 1995. *Alternating hemiplegia of childhood.* New York: Raven Press.

Anderson VE, Hauser WA. 1990. Genetics. In: Dam M, Gram L, eds. *Comprehensive epileptology.* New York: Raven Press, 57–76.

Anderson NE, Wallis WE. 1986. Activation of epileptiform activity by mental arithmetic. *Arch Neurol* 43:624–626.

Anderson VE, Wilcox KJ, Hauser WA, et al. 1988. A test of autosomal dominant inheritance in febrile convulsions. *Epilepsia* 29:705–706.

Anderson VE, Hauser WA, Olafsson E, et al. 1990. Genetic aspects of the epilepsies. In: Sillanpää M, Dam M, Johanessen SI, et al., eds. *Epilepsy from infants to young adults*. Pietersfield, United Kingdom: Wrightson Biomedical Publishing Ltd.

Anderson VE, Rich SS, Hauser WA, et al. 1991. Family studies of epilepsy. In: Anderson VE, Hauser WA, Leppik IE, et al., eds. *Genetic strategies in epilepsy research*. New York: Elsevier; 89–103.

Anderson E, Berkovic S, Dulac O, et al. 2002. ILAE Genetics Commission Conference Report: molecular analysis of complex genetic epilepsies. *Epilepsia* 43:1262–1267.

André M, Boutray MJ, Dubruc O. 1986. Clonazepam pharmacokinetics and therapeutic efficacy in neonatal seizures. *Eur J Clin Pharmacol* 305:585–589.

André M, Matisse N, Vert P, et al. 1988. Neonatal seizures—recent aspects. *Neuropediatrics* 19:201–207.

Andrew RD. 1991. Seizure and acute osmotic change: clinical and neurophysiological aspects. *J Neurol Sci* 101:7–18.

Andrewes DG, Tomlinson L, Elwes RD, Reynolds EH. 1984. The influence of carbamazepine and phenytoin on memory and other aspects of cognitive function in new referrals with epilepsy. *Acta Neurol Scand Suppl* 69: 23–30.

Andrewes DG, Bullen JG, Tomlinson L, et al. 1986. A comparative study of the cognitive effects of phenytoin and carbamazepine in new referrals with epilepsy. *Epilepsia* 27:128–134.

Andrews R, Morrell F, Whisler WN. 1989. Subpial cortical transection in Landau-Kleffner syndrome [Abstract]. *Ann Neurol* 26:469a.

Andrews PI, Dichter MA, Berkovic SF, et al. 1996. Plasmapheresis in Rasmussen's encephalitis. *Neurology* 46: 242–246.

Angelini L, Broggi G, Riva D, et al. 1979. A case of Lennox-Gastaut syndrome successfully treated by removal of a parietotemporal astrocytoma. *Epilepsia* 20:665–669.

Angelman H. 1965. "Puppet" children: a report on three cases. *Dev Med Child Neurol* 7:681–683.

Annegers JF, Coan SP. 1999. SUDEP: overview of definitions and review of incidence data. *Seizure* 8:347–352.

Annegers JF, Hauser WA, Elveback LR, et al. 1976. Seizure disorders in offsprings of parents with a history of seizures. *Epilepsia* 17:1–9.

Annegers JF, Hauser WA, Elveback LR. 1979a. Remission of seizures and relapses in patients with epilepsy. *Epilepsia* 20:729–737.

Annegers JF, Hauser WA, Elveback LR, Kurland LT. 1979b. The risk of epilepsy following febrile convulsions. *Neurology* 29:297–303.

Annegers JF, Grabow JD, Groover RV, et al. 1980. Seizures after head trauma: a population study. *Neurology* 30: 683–689.

Annegers JF, Hauser WA, Anderson VE. 1982a. Risk of seizures among relatives of patients with epilepsy: families in a defined population. In: Anderson VE, Hauser WA, Sing C, Porter R, eds. *The genetic basis of the epilepsies*. New York: Raven Press, 151–159.

Annegers JF, Hauser WA, Anderson VE, et al. 1982b. The risks of seizure disorders among relatives of patients with childhood onset epilepsy. *Neurology* 32:174–179.

Annegers JF, Shirts SB, Hauser WA, et al. 1986. Risk of recurrence after an initial unprovoked seizure. *Epilepsia* 27:43–50.

Annegers JF, Hauser WA, Shirts SB, et al. 1987. Factors prognostic of unprovoked seizures after febrile convulsions. *N Engl J Med* 316:493–498.

Annegers JF, Hauser WA, Beghi E, et al. 1988. The risk of unprovoked seizures after encephalitis and meningitis. *Neurology* 38:1407–1410.

Annegers JF, Blakley SA, Hauser WA, et al. 1990. Recurrence of febrile convulsions in a population-based cohort. *Epilepsy Res* 5:209–216.

Ansink BJ, Sarphatie H, van Dongen HR. 1989. The Landau-Kleffner syndrome—case report and theoretical considerations. *Neuropediatrics* 20:170–172.

Anslow P. 1991. CT scanning in temporal lobe epilepsy. In: Dam M, Gram L, eds. *Comprehensive epileptology*. New York: Raven Press, 351–358.

Anslow P, Oxbury J. 2000. Diagnostic neuroradiology. In: Oxbury J, Polkey CH, Duchowny M, eds. *Intractable focal epilepsy*. Philadelphia: WB Saunders, 297–309.

Antony JH, Hawke SH. 1983. Phenobarbital compared with carbamazepine in prevention of recurrent febrile convulsions. *Am J Dis Child* 137:892–895.

Antunes NL. 2001. The spectrum of neurologic disease in children with systemic cancer. *Pediatr Neurol* 25: 227–235.

Anvret M, Nordenskjold M, Stolpe L, et al. 1991. Molecular analysis of 4p deletion associated with the Wolf-Hirschhorn syndrome moving the "critical segment" towards the telomere. *Hum Genet* 86:481–483.

Anziska B, Cracco RQ. 1977. Changes in frequency and amplitude in electrographic seizure discharges. *Clin Electroencephalogr* 8:206–210.

Apley J. 1975. *The child with abdominal pain*. London: Blackwell.

Appleton RE. 1995a. Vigabatrin in the management of generalized seizures in children. *Seizure* 4:45–48.

Appleton RE. 1995b. Eyelid myoclonia with absences. In: Duncan JS, Panayiotopoulos CP, eds. *Typical absences and related syndromes*. London: Churchill Communication Europe, 213–220.

Appleton RE, Farrell K, Teal P. 1989. Complex partial status epilepticus associated with cyclosporin A therapy. *J Neurol Neurosurg Psychiatry* 52:1068–1071.

Appleton RE, Farrell K, Applegarth DA, et al. 1990. The high incidence of valproate hepatotoxicity in infants may relate to familial metabolic defects. *Can J Neurol Sci* 17:145–148.

Appleton RE, Panayiotopoulos CP, Acomb A, et al. 1993. Eyelid myoclonia with typical absences: an epilepsy syndrome. *J Neurol Neurosurg Psychiatry* 56:1312–1316.

Appleton R, Fichtner K, LaMoreaux L, et al. 1999a. Gabapentin as add-on therapy in children with refractory partial seizures: a 12-week, multicentre, double-blind, placebo-controlled study. Gabapentin Paediatric Study Group. *Epilepsia* 40:1147–1154.

Appleton RE, Peters AC, Mumford JP, et al. 1999b. Randomised, placebo-controlled study of vigabatrin as first-line treatment of infantile spasms. *Epilepsia* 40: 1627–1633

Appleton R, Fichtner K, LaMoreaux L, et al. 2001. Gabapentin as add-on therapy in children with refractory partial seizures: a 24-week, multicentre, open-label study. *Dev Med Child Neurol* 43:269–273.

Aquino A, Gabor AJ. 1980. Movement-induced seizures in nonketotic hyperglycemia. *Neurology* 30:600–604.

Arizumi M, Baba K, Hibio S, et al. 1987. Immunoglobulin therapy in the West syndrome. *Brain Dev* 9:422–425.

Arnold S, Schlaug G, Holthausen H, et al. 1997. FDG-PET in childhood temporal lobe epilepsy of different artiologies. In: Tuxhorn I, Holthausen H, Boenigk H, eds. *Paediatric epilepsy syndromes and their surgical treatment.* London: John Libbey, 274–281.

Arroyo S, Lesser RP, Awad IA, et al. 1993. Subdural and epidural grids and strips. In: Engel J, ed. *Surgical treatment of the epilepsies*, 2nd ed. New York: Raven Press, 377–386.

Arruda F, Cendes F, Andermann F, et al. 1996. Mesial atrophy and outcome after amygdalo-hippocampectomy temporal removal. *Ann Neurol* 40:446–450.

Arseni C, Botez MI, Maretsis M. 1966. Paroxysmal disorders of the body image. *Psychiatr Neurol Basel* 151: 1–14.

Artieda J, Obeso JA. 1993. The pathophysiology and pharmacology of photic cortical reflex myoclonus. *Ann Neurol* 34:175–184.

Arts WF, Visser LH, Loonen MC, et al. 1988. Follow-up of 146 children with epilepsy after withdrawal of antiepileptic therapy. *Epilepsia* 29:244–250.

Arts WE, Halley DJ, Lindhout D. 1991. Benign familial neonatal convulsions. *Clin Neurol Neurosurg* 93: 352–355.

Arzimanoglou A. 1994. Vigabatrin and complex partial status. *Seizure* 3:79–80.

Arzimanoglou A. 1996. Hemifacial spasm or subcortical (infratentorial) epilepsy: a case report of a child with Goldenhar's syndrome and a pontomedullary junction lesion. In: Arzimanoglou A, Goutières F, eds. *Trends in child neurology: a festschrift for Jean Aicardi.* Paris: John Libbey Eurotext, 43–51.

Arzimanoglou A. 1997. The surgical treatment of Sturge-Weber syndrome with respect to its clinical spectrum. In: Tuxhorn I, Holthausen H, Boenigk H, eds. *Paediatric epilepsy syndromes and their surgical treatment.* London: John Libbey, 353–363.

Arzimanoglou A. 2001a. Epilepsies avec des myoclonies chez l'enfant et l'adolescent: démarche diagnostique. *Epilepsies* 13:137–146.

Arzimanoglou A. 2001b. Sports and epilepsies. *Epileptic Disord* 4:S163–S167.

Arzimanoglou A. 2002. Treatment options in paediatric epilepsy syndromes. *Epileptic Disord* 4:217–225.

Arzimanoglou A. 2003. Prognosis of Lennox-Gastaut syndrome. In: Jallon P, ed. *Prognosis of epilepsies.* Paris: John Libbey Eurotext, 277–288.

Arzimanoglou A, Aicardi J. 1992. The epilepsy of Sturge-Weber syndrome: clinical features and treatment in 23 patients. *Acta Neurol Scand Suppl* 140:18–22.

Arzimanoglou A, Aicardi J. 2001. Seizure disorders of the neonate and infant. In: Levene MI, Chervenak FA, Whittle M, eds. *Fetal and neonatal neurology and neurosurgery.* London: Churchill Livingstone, 647–656.

Arzimanoglou A, Dravet CH. 2001. Hemiconvulsion-hemiplegia-epilepsy syndrome. Available at: http://www. medlink.com/. Accessed October, 2003.

Arzimanoglou A, Gérardin V, Maszkowski J, Bidaut LM. 1993. Lamotrigine in patients with childhood onset intractable epilepsy [Abstract]. *Epilepsia* 34:113.

Arzimanoglou A, Sainte-Rose C, Goutières F, Aicardi J. 1994. Corpus callosotomy for seizures in children [Abstract]. *Epilepsia* 35:122.

Arzimanoglou A, Bourgeois M, Goutières F, Aicardi J. 1995. Epilepsy in Rett syndrome [Abstract]. *Epilepsia* 36:S238.

Arzimanoglou A, Prudent M, Salefranque F. 1996. Epilepsie myoclono-astatique et épilepsie myoclonique bénigne du nourrisson dans une même famille: quelques réflexions sur la classification des épilepsies. *Epilepsies* 8:307–315.

Arzimanoglou A, Thomas P, Durisotti C, et al. 1998. Tentative d'évaluation des coûts médico-sociaux des epilepsies. In: Bureau M, Kahane P, Munari C, eds. *Epilepsies partielles graves pharmacorésistantes de l'enfant: stratégies diagnostiques et traitements chirurgicaux.* Paris: John Libbey Eurotext, 87–97.

Arzimanoglou A, Salefranque F, Goutières F, et al. 1999. Hemifacial spasm or subcortical epilepsy? *Epileptic Dis* 1:121–125.

Arzimanoglou AA, Andermann F, Aicardi J, et al. 2000. Sturge-Weber syndrome: indications and results of surgery in 20 patients. *Neurology* 55:1472–1479.

Arzimanoglou A, Kulak I, Bidaut-Mazel C, et al. 2001. Optimal use of lamotrigine in clinical practice: results of an open multicenter trial in refractory epilepsy. *Rev Neurol* 157:525–536.

Arzimanoglou A, Sachs PH, El Maleh M, et al. 2002. Monosomy 1p36 microdeletion syndrome associated with epilepsy and polymicrogyria [Abstract]. *Epilepsia* 43:S167.

Asano Y, Yoshikawa T, Kajita Y, et al. 1992. Fatal encephalitis/encephalopathy in primary human herpes virus-6 infection. *Arch Dis Child* 67:1484–1485.

Asano Y, Yoshikawa T, Suga S, et al. 1994. Clinical features of infants with primary human herpesvirus 6 infection (exanthum subitum, roseola infantum). *Pediatrics* 93:104–108.

Asano E, Chugani DC, Muzik O, et al. 2000. Multimodality imaging for improved detection of epileptogenic foci in tuberous sclerosis complex. *Neurology* 54:1976–1984.

Asano E, Chugani DC, Juhász C, et al. 2001. Surgical treatment of West syndrome. *Brain Dev* 23:668–676.

Asanuma H, Wakai S, Tanaka T, et al. 1995. Brain tumors associated with infantile spasms. *Pediatr Neurol* 12: 361–364.

Asarnow RF, Lo Presti C, Guthrie D, et al. 1997. Developmental outcomes in children receiving resection surgery for medically intractable infantile spasms. *Dev Med Child Neurol* 39:430–440.

Asconapé J, Penry JK. 1984. Some clinical and EEG aspects of benign juvenile myoclonic epilepsy. *Epilepsia* 25:108–114.

Asher DM, Gajdusek DC. 1991. Virologic studies in chronic encephalitis. In: Andermann F, ed. *Chronic encephalitis and epilepsy: Rasmussen's syndrome.* Boston: Butterworth-Heinemann, 147–158.

Askenasi A, Snead OC III. 1991. Infantile spasms secondary to a brain tumor. *J Child Neurol* 6:180–182.

Aso K, Watanabe K, Negoro T, et al. 1987. Visual seizures in children. *Epilepsy Res* 1:246–253.

Atkins MR, Terrell W, Hulette CM. 1995. Rasmussen's syndrome: a study of potential viral etiology. *Clin Neuropathol* 14:7–12.

Aubourg P, Dulac O, Plouin P, et al. 1985. Infantile status epilepticus as a complication of 'near miss' sudden infant death. *Dev Med Child Neurol* 27:40–48.

Austin JK, Huberty TJ, Huster GA, Dunn DW. 1999. Does academic achievement in children with epilepsy change over time? *Dev Med Child Neurol* 41:473–479.

Autret E, Billard C, Bertrand P, et al. 1990. Double-blind randomized trial of diazepam versus placebo for prevention of recurrence of febrile seizures. *J Pediatr* 117: 490–494.

Avanzini G, Beaumanoir A, Mira L, eds. 2001. *Limbic seizures in children*. London: John Libbey.

Avoli M, Gloor P. 1994. Physiopathogenesis of feline generalized epilepsy: the role of thalamocortical mechanisms. In: Malafosse A, Genton P, Hirsch E, et al., eds. *Idiopathic generalized epilepsies*. London: John Libbey, 111–121.

Avrahami E, Weiss-Peretz J, Cohn DF. 1987. Focal epileptic activity following intravenous contrast material injection in patients with metastatic brain disease. *J Neurol Neurosurg Psychiatry* 50:221–223.

Awad IA, Rosenfeld J, Ahl J, et al. 1991. Intractable epilepsy and structural lesions of the brain: mapping, resection strategies and outcome. *Epilepsia* 32:179–186.

Ayala GF, Elia M, Cornaggia CM, et al., eds. 2001. Epilepsy and learning disabilities: Proceedings of the Workshop on Epilepsy and Learning Disabilities. *Epilepsia* 42(Suppl. 1):1–61.

Aykut-Bingol C, Bronen RA, Kim JH, et al. 1998 Surgical outcome in occipital lobe epilepsy: implications for pathophysiology. *Ann Neurol* 44:60–69.

Aylett S, Neville BG, Cross JH, et al. 1999. Sturge-Weber syndrome: cerebral haemodynamics during seizure activity. *Dev Med Child Neurol* 41:480–485.

Babb TL, Halgren E, Wilson C, et al. 1981. Neuronal firing patterns during the spread of an occipital lobe seizure to the temporal lobes in man. *Electroencephalogr Clin Neurophysiol* 51:104–107.

Babb TL, Brown WJ, Pretorius J, et al. 1984. Temporal lobe volumetric cell densities in temporal lobe epilepsy. *Epilepsia* 25:729–740.

Bachman DS. 1982. Use of valproic acid in treatment of infantile spasms. *Arch Neurol* 39:49–52.

Bachman DS. 1983. Late-onset pyridoxine-dependency convulsions. *Ann Neurol* 14:692–693.

Bachman DS, Hodges FJ III, Freeman JM. 1976. Computerized axial tomography in chronic seizure disorders of childhood. *Pediatrics* 58:828–832.

Bäckman E, Dahlström G, Eeg-Olofsson O, Bertler A. 1987. The 24 hour variations of salivary carbamazepine and carbamazepine 10,11-epoxide concentrations in children with epilepsy. *Pediatr Neurol* 3:327–330.

Backstrom T. 1976. Epileptic seizures in women related to plasma estrogen and progesterone during the menstrual cycle: a clinical study. *Acta Neurol Scand* 54:321–347.

Bacon C, Scott D, Jones P. 1979. Heatstroke in well-wrapped infants. *Lancet* 1:422–425.

Bacon CJ, Hierons AM, Mucklow J, et al. 1981a. Placebo-controlled study of phenobarbitone and phenytoin in the prophylaxis of febrile convulsions. *Lancet* 2:600–603.

Bacon CJ, Cranage JD, Hierons AM, et al. 1981b. Behavioural effects of phenobarbitone and phenytoin in small children. *Arch Dis Child* 56:836–840.

Badinand-Hubert N, Bureau M, Hirsch E, et al. 1998. Epilepsies and video games: results of a multicentric study. *Electroencephalogr Clin Neurophysiol* 107: 422–427.

Baker G, Jacoby A, Buck D, et al. 1997. Quality of life of people with epilepsy: a European study. *Epilepsia* 38: 353–362.

Baldy-Moulinier M. 1986. Inter-relationships between sleep and epilepsy. In: Pedley JA, Meldrum BS, eds. *Recent advances in epilepsy*, Vol. 3. Edinburgh: Churchill Livingstone, 37–55.

Baldy-Moulinier M, Touchon J, Billiard M, et al. 1988. Nocturnal sleep study in the Lennox-Gastaut syndrome. In: Niedermeyer E, Degen R, eds. *The Lennox-Gastaut syndrome*. New York: Alan R. Liss, 243–260.

Bale JF, Fountain T, Shaddy R. 1984. Phenylpropanolamine-associated CNS complications in children and adolescents. *Am J Dis Child* 133:683–685.

Ballenger CE III, King DW, Gallagher BB. 1983. Partial complex status epilepticus. *Neurology* 33:1545–1552.

Baloh RW, Yue Q, Furman JM, et al. 1997. Familial episodic ataxia: clinical heterogeneity in four families linked to chromosome 19q. *Ann Neurol* 41:8–16.

Bamberger E, Matthes A. 1959. *Anfälle im Kindesalter*. Basel: Karger.

Bancaud J. 1969. Les crises épileptiques d'origine occipitale (étude stéréo électroencéphalographique). *Rev Otoneuroophthalmol* 41:299–311.

Bancaud J. 1985. Kojewnikow's syndrome (epilepsia partialis continua) in child. In: Roger J, Dravet C, Bureau M, et al., eds. *Epileptic syndromes*. London: John Libbey, 286–298.

Bancaud J. 1987. Clinical symptomatology of epileptic seizures of temporal origin. *Rev Neurol (Paris)* 143: 392–400.

Bancaud J, Talairach J. 1975. Macro-stereo-electro-encephalography in epilepsy. In: *Handbook of EEG and clinical neurophysiology*, Vol. 10B. Amsterdam: Elsevier, 3–10.

Bancaud J, Talairach J. 1992. Semiology of frontal lobe epilepsy seizures in man. In: Chauvel P, Delgado-Escueta AV, Halgren E, et al., eds. *Frontal lobe seizures and epilepsies*. New York: Raven Press, 3–58.

Bancaud J, Bonis A, Morel P, et al. 1961. Epilepsie occipitale à expression "rhinencéphalique" prévalente (corrélations électrocliniques à la lumière des investigations fonctionnelles stéréotaxiques). *Rev Neurol* 105:219–220.

Bancaud J, Talairach J, Bonis A, et al. 1965. *La stéréoélectroencéphalographie dans l'epilepsie*. Paris: Masson.

Bancaud J, Bonis A, Talairach J, et al. 1970. Syndrome de Kojewnikow et accès somato-moteurs (étude clinique, EEG, EMG et SEEG). *Encéphale* 59:392–438.

Bancaud J, Talairach J, Geier S, et al. 1973. *EEG et SEEG dans les tumeurs cérébrales et l'epilepsie*. Paris: Edifor.

Bancaud J, Talairach J, Morel P, et al. 1974. "Generalized" epileptic seizures elicited by electrical stimulation of the frontal lobe in man. *Electroencephalogr Clin Neurophysiol* 37:275–282.

Bancaud J, Talairach J, Geier S, et al. 1976. Manifestations comportementales induites par la simulation électrique du gyrus cingulaire antérieur chez l'homme. *Rev Neurol (Paris)* 132:705–724.

Bancaud J, Bonis A, Trottier S, et al. 1982. L'épilepsie partielle continue: syndrome et maladie. *Rev Neurol (Paris)* 138:803–814.

Bancaud J, Brunet-Bourgin F, Chauvel P, et al. 1994. Anatomical origin of *déjà vu* and vivid "memories" in human temporal lobe epilepsy. *Brain* 117:71–90.

Bankier A, Turner M, Hopkins IJ. 1983. Pyridoxine dependent seizures—a wider clinical spectrum. *Arch Dis Child* 58:415–418.

Baram TZ. 1993. Pathophysiology of massive infantile spasms: perspective on the putative role of the brain adrenal axis. *Ann Neurol* 33:231–236.

Baram TZ. 2001. What are the reasons for the strikingly different approaches to the use of ACTH in infants with West syndrome? *Brain Dev* 23:647–648.

Baram TZ, Mitchell WG, Tournay A, et al. 1996. High-dose corticotropin (ACTH) versus prednisone for infantile spasms: a prospective, randomized, blinded study. *Pediatrics* 97:375–379.

Bare MA, Burnstine TH, Fisher RS, et al. 1994. EEG changes during simple partial seizures. *Epilepsia* 35: 715–720.

Barkovich AJ. 1995. *Pediatric neuroimaging*. 2nd ed. New York: Raven Press.

Barkovich AJ. 1996. Magnetic resonance imaging of lissencephaly, polymicrogyria, schizencephaly, hemimegalencephaly, and band heterotopia. In: Guerrini R, Andermann F, Canapicchi R, et al., eds. *Dysplasias of cerebral cortex and epilepsy*. Philadelphia: Lippincott-Raven, 115–119.

Barkovich AJ. 2002. Magnetic resonance imaging: role in the understanding of cerebral malformations. *Brain Dev* 241:2–12.

Barkovich AJ, Chuang SH. 1990. Unilateral megalencephaly: correlation of MR imaging and pathological characteristics. *Am J Neuroradiol* 11:523–531.

Barkovich AJ, Kjos BO. 1992. Nonlissencephalic cortical dysplasias: correlation of imaging findings with clinical deficits. *Am J Neuroradiol* 13:95–103.

Barkovich AJ, Norman D. 1988. MR imaging of schizencephaly. *AJR Am J Roentgenol* 150:1391–1396.

Barkovich AJ, Chuang SH, Norman D. 1988. MR of neuronal migration anomalies. *Am J Radiol* 150:179–187.

Barkovich AJ, Jackson DE, Boyer RS. 1989. Band heterotopias: a newly recognized neuronal migration anomaly. *Radiology* 171:455–458.

Barkovich AJ, Koch TK, Carrol CL. 1991. The spectrum of lissencephaly: report of ten patients analyzed by magnetic resonance imaging. *Ann Neurol* 30:139–146.

Barkovich AJ, Guerrini R, Battaglia G, et al. 1994. Band heterotopia: correlation of outcome with magnetic resonance imaging parameters. *Ann Neurol* 36:609–617.

Barkovich AJ, Rowley HA, Andermann F. 1996. MR in partial epilepsy: value of high-resolution volumetric techniques. *Am J Neuroradiol* 11:44–48.

Barkovich AJ, Hevner R, Guerrini R. 1999. Syndromes of bilateral symmetrical polymicrogyria. *AJNR Am J Neuroradiol* 20:1814–1821

Barkovich AJ, Kuzniecky RI, Jackson GD, et al. 2001. Classification system for malformations of cortical development: update 2001. *Neurology* 57:2168–2178.

Barlow CF. 1984. *Headaches and migraine in childhood*. Clinics in Developmental Medicine, No. 91. London: Spastics International Medical Publications.

Barlow KM, Spowart JJ, Minns RA. 2000. Early posttraumatic seizures in non-accidental head injury: relation to outcome. *Dev Med Child Neurol* 42:591–594.

Barnes SE, Bland D, Cole AP, et al. 1976. The use of sodium valproate in a case of status epilepticus. *Dev Med Child Neurol* 18:236–238.

Barnes D, McDonald WI, Landon DN, et al. 1988. The characterizations of experimental gliosis by quantitative nuclear magnetic resonance imaging. *Brain* 111:83–94.

Barnhart TD, Newsom JW, Crawley JW, et al. 1969. Long-term prognosis of petit mal epilepsy. *Electroencephalogr Clin Neurophysiol* 27:549–550.

Baron JC, Roeda D, Munari C, et al. 1983. Brain regional pharmacokinetics of ^{11}C labeled diphenylhydantoin: positron emission tomography in humans. *Neurology* 33:580–585.

Barone SR, Kaplan MH, Krilov LR. 1995. Human herpes virus-6 infection in children with first febrile seizures. *J Pediatr* 127:95–97.

Barry E, Sussman NM, Bosley TM, et al. 1985. Ictal blindness and status epilepticus amauroticus. *Epilepsia* 26: 577–584.

Barth PG. 1987. Disorders of neuronal migration. *Can J Neurol Sci* 14:1–16.

Bartolomei JC, Christopher S, Vives K, et al. 1997. Low grade gliomas of chronic epilepsy: a distinct clinical and pathological entity. *J Neurooncology* 34:79–84.

Barton NW, Brady RO, Dambrosia JM, et al. 1991. Replacement therapy for inherited enzyme deficiency—macrophage-targeted glucocerebrosidase for Gaucher's disease. *N Engl J Med* 324:1464–1470.

Baruzzi A, Procaccianti G, Tinuper P, Lugaresi E. 1988. Antiepileptic drug withdrawal in childhood epilepsies: preliminary results of a prospective study. In: Faienza C, Prati GL, eds. *Diagnostic and therapeutic problems in pediatric epileptology*. Amsterdam: Elsevier, 117–123.

Basser LS. 1964. Benign paroxysmal vertigo. *Brain* 87: 141–152.

Bastos AC, Comeau RM, Andermann F, et al. 1999. Diagnosis of subtle focal dysplastic lesions: curvilinear reformatting from three-dimensional magnetic resonance imaging. *Ann Neurol* 46:88–94.

Bate L, Gardiner M. 1999. Genetics of inherited epilepsies. *Epileptic Disord* 1:7–20.

Bate L, Williamson M, Gardiner M. 2000. The major susceptibility locus for juvenile myoclonic epilepsy on chromosome 15q. In: Schmitz B, Sander T, eds. *Juvenile myoclonic epilepsy: the Janz syndrome*. Petersfield: Wrightson Biomedical Publishing, 181–195.

Battaglia A, Guerrini R, Gastaut H. 1989. Epileptic seizures induced by syncopal attacks. *J Epilepsy* 2:137–145.

Battaglia A, Ferrari AR, Guerrini R. 1991. Double-blind placebo-controlled trial of flunarizine as add-on therapy in refractory childhood epilepsy. *Brain Dev* 13:217–222.

Battaglia A, Gurrieri F, Bertini E, et al. 1997. The inv dup(15) syndrome: a clinically recognizable syndrome with altered behaviour, mental retardation, and epilepsy. *Neurology* 48:1081–1086.

Battaglia A, Carey JC, Cederholm P, et al. 1999. Natural history of Wolf-Hirschhorn syndrome: experience with 15 cases. *Pediatrics* 103:830–836.

Bauer G, Benke T, Bohr K. 1988. The Lennox-Gastaut syndrome in adulthood. In: Niedermeyer E, Degen R, eds. *The Lennox-Gastaut syndrome*. New York: Alan R. Liss, 317–328.

Bauer J, Schuler P, Feistel H, et al. 1991. Blindness as an ictal phenomenon: investigations with EEG and SPECT in two patients suffering from epilepsy. *J Neurol* 238:44–46.

Baulac M, De Grissac N, Hasboun D, et al. 1998. Hippocampal developmental changes in patients with partial epilepsy: magnetic resonance imaging and clinical aspects. *Ann Neurol* 44:223–233

Baulac S, Gourfinkel-An I, Picard F, et al. 1999. A second locus for familial generalized epilepsy with febrile seizures plus maps to chromosome 2q21-q33. *Am J Hum Genet* 65:1078–1085.

Baulac S, Huberfeld G, Gourfinkel-An I. 2001. First genetic evidence of GABA_A receptor dysfunction in epilepsy: a mutation in the γ2-subunit gene. *Nat Genet* 28:46–48.

Baumgartner C, Doppelbauer A, Lischka A, et al. 1995. Benign focal epilepsy of childhood—a combined neuroelectric and neuromagnetic study. In: Baumgartner C, Deecke L, Stroink G, et al., eds. *Fundamental research and clinic applications*. Amsterdam: Elsevier, 39–42.

Baumgartner C, Flint R, Tuxhorn I, et al. 1996. Supplementary motor area seizures: propagation pathways as studied with invasive recordings. *Neurology* 46:508–514.

Baykan-Kurt B, Gokyigit A, Parman Y, et al. 1999. Eye closure related spike and wave discharges: clinical and syndromic associations. *Clin Electroencephalogr* 30:106–110.

Baxter P. 1999. Epidemiology of pyridoxine dependent and pyridoxine responsive seizures in the UK. *Arch Dis Child* 81:431–433.

Baxter P. 2002. Pyridoxine dependent and pyridoxine responsive seizures. In: Baxter P, ed. *Vitamin responsive conditions in paediatric neurology*. London: MacKeith Press, 109–165.

Baxter P, Aicardi J. 1999. Neonatal seizures after pyridoxine use. *Lancet* 354:2002–2003.

Baxter PS, Gardner-Medwin D, Barwick DD, et al. 1995. Vigabatrin monotherapy in resistant neonatal seizures. *Seizure* 4:57–59.

Baxter P, Griffiths P, Kelly T, et al. 1996. Pyridoxine-dependent seizures: demographic, clinical, MRI and psychometric features, and effect of dose on intelligence quotient. *Dev Med Child Neurol* 38:998–1006.

Beardsley RS, Freeman JM, Appel FA. 1983. Anticonvulsant serum levels are useful only if the physician appropriately uses them: an assessment of the impact of providing serum level data to physicians. *Epilepsia* 24:330–335.

Beardsworth ED, Adams CB. 1988. Modified hemispherectomy for epilepsy: early results in 10 cases. *Br J Neurosurg* 2:73–84.

Beardsworth ED, Zaidel DW. 1994. Memory for faces in epileptic children before and after brain surgery. *J Clin Exp Neuropsychol* 16:589–596.

Bernasconi A, Andermann F, Andermann E. 2002. Hyperreflexia: genetics and culture bound stimulus-induced disorders. In: Guerrini R, Aicardi J, Andermann F, et al., eds. *Epilepsy and movement disorders*. Cambridge: Cambridge University Press, 151–164.

Beaumanoir A. 1981. Les limites nosologiques du syndrome de Lennox-Gastaut. *Rev Electroencephalogr Neurophysiol Clin* 11:468–473.

Beaumanoir A. 1983. Infantile epilepsy with occipital focus and good prognosis. *Eur Neurol* 22:43–52.

Beaumanoir A. 1985. The Lennox-Gastaut syndrome. In: Roger J, Bureau M, Dravet C, et al., eds. *Epileptic syndromes in infancy, childhood, and adolescence*. London: John Libbey, 89–99.

Beaumanoir A. 1992. The Landau-Kleffner syndrome. In: Roger J, Bureau M, Dravet C, et al., eds. *Epileptic syndromes in infancy, childhood and adolescence*. London: John Libbey, 231–243.

Beaumanoir A. 1995. Continuous spike and waves during sleep, electrical status epilepticus during slow sleep, acquired epileptic aphasia and related conditions. In: Beaumanoir A, Bureau M, Deonna T, et al., eds. *Con-

tinuous spike and waves during slow sleep*. London: John Libbey, 217–223.

Beaumanoir A, Dravet C. 1992. The Lennox-Gastaut syndrome. In: Roger J, Bureau M, Dravet C, et al., eds. *Epileptic syndromes in infancy, childhood and adolescence*. London: John Libbey, 115–132.

Beaumanoir A, Nahory A. 1983. Les épilepsies bénignes partielles: 11 cas d'épilepsie partielle frontale à évolution favorable. *Rev Electroencephalogr Neurophysiol Clin* 13:207–211.

Beaumanoir A, Ballis T, Varfis G, et al. 1974. Benign epilepsy of childhood with rolandic spikes. *Epilepsia* 15:301–315.

Beaumanoir A, Foletti G, Magistris M, et al. 1988. Status epilepticus in the Lennox-Gastaut syndrome. In: Niedermeyer E, Degen R, eds. *The Lennox-Gastaut syndrome*. New York: Alan R. Liss, 283–299.

Beaumanoir A, Bureau M, Deonna T, et al., eds. 1995. *Continuous spikes and waves during slow sleep*. London: John Libbey.

Beaussart M. 1972. Benign epilepsy of children with rolandic (centro-temporal) paroxysmal foci: a clinical entity. Study of 221 cases. *Epilepsia* 13:795–811.

Beaussart M. 1981. Crises épileptiques après guérison d'une EPR (épilepsie à paroxysmes rolandiques). *Rev Electroencephalogr Neurophysiol Clin* 11:489–492.

Beaussart M, Faou R. 1978. Evolution of epilepsy with rolandic paroxysmal foci: a study of 324 cases. *Epilepsia* 19:337–342.

Bebek N, Gurses C, Gokyigit A, et al. 2001. Hot water epilepsy: clinical and electrophysiologic findings based on 21 cases. *Epilepsia* 42:1180–1184.

Bebin EM. 1998. Additional modalities for treating acute seizures in children: overview. *J Child Neurol* 13: S23–S26.

Bebin EM, Bleck TP. 1994. New anticonvulsant drugs. Focus on flunarizine, fosphenytoin, midazolam, and stiripentol. *Drugs* 48:153–171.

Bebin EM, Kelly PJ, Gomez M. 1993. Surgical treatment in cerebral tuberous sclerosis. *Epilepsia* 34:651–657.

Becker PS, Pixon AM, Troncoso JC. 1989. Bilateral opercular polymicrogyria. *Ann Neurol* 25:90–92.

Beck-Mannagetta G, Janz D. 1991. Syndrome-related genetics in generalized epilepsy. In: Anderson VE, Hauser WA, Leppik IE, et al., eds. *Genetic strategies in epilepsy research*. New York: Elsevier, 105–111.

Beck-Mannagetta G, Janz D, Hoffmeister U, et al. 1989. Morbidity risk for seizures and epilepsy in offspring of patients with epilepsy. In: Beck-Mannagetta G, Anderson VE, Doose H, Janz D, eds. *Genetics of the epilepsies*. Berlin: Springer-Verlag, 119–126.

Bednarek N, Motte J, Soufflet C, et al. 1998. Evidence of late-onset infantile spasms. *Epilepsia* 39:55–60.

Beghi E, Tognoni G. 1988. Prognosis of epilepsy in newly referred patients: a multicenter prospective study. Collaborative Group for the Study of Epilepsy. *Epilepsia* 29:236–243.

Beghi E, Annegers JF; Collaborative Group for the Pregnancy Registries in Epilepsy. 2001. Pregnancy registries in epilepsy. *Epilepsia* 42:1422–1425.

Bejsovec M, Kulenda Z, Ponca E. 1967. Familial intrauterine convulsions in pyridoxine dependency. *Arch Dis Child* 42:201–207.

Bell DM, Richards G, Dhillon S, et al. 1991. A comparative pharmacokinetic study of intravenous and intramuscular midazolam in patients with epilepsy. *Epilepsy Res* 10:183–190.

Bellman MH. 1983. Infantile spasms. In: Pedley TA, Meldrum BS, eds. *Recent advances in epilepsy*, Vol. 1. Edinburgh: Churchill Livingstone, 113–138.

Bellman MH, Ross EM, Miller DL. 1983. Infantile spasms and pertussis immunisation. *Lancet* 1:1031–1034.

Benabid AL, Minotti L, Koudsie A, et al. 2002. Antiepileptic effect of high-frequency stimulation of the subthalamic nucleus (corpus luysi) in a case of medically intractable epilepsy caused by focal dysplasia: a 30-month follow-up: technical case report. *Neurosurgery* 50:1385–1391.

Ben-Ari Y, Tremblay E, Ottersen OD, et al. 1979. Evidence suggesting secondary epileptogenic lesions after kainic acid: pre-treatment with diazepam reduces distance but not local brain damage. *Brain Res* 165:362–365.

Ben-Ari Y, Tremblay E, Riche D, et al. 1981. Electrographic, clinical and pathological alterations following systemic administration of kainic acid, bicuculline or pentetrazol: metabolic mapping using the deoxyglucose method with special reference to the pathology of epilepsy. *Neuroscience* 6:1361–1391.

Ben-Ari Y, Cherubini E, Krnjevic K. 1988. Changes in voltage dependence of NMDA currents during development. *Neurosci Lett* 94:88–92.

Benlounis A, Nabbout R, Feingold J, et al. 2001. Genetic predisposition to severe myoclonic epilepsy in infancy *Epilepsia* 42:204–209.

Ben-Menachem E, Hellstrom K, Waldton C, et al. 1999. Evaluation of refractory epilepsy treated with vagus nerve stimulation for up to 5 years. *Neurology* 52:1265–1267.

Bennett HS, Selman JE, Rapin I, et al. 1982. Nonconvulsive epileptiform activity appearing as ataxia. *Am J Dis Child* 136:30–32.

Berchou RC, Rodin E, Russell ME. 1981. Clorazepate therapy for refractory seizures. *Neurology* 31:1383–1385.

Berg AT, Shinnar S. 1991. The risk of seizure recurrence following a first unprovoked seizure: a quantitative review. *Neurology* 41:965–972.

Berg AT, Shinnar S. 1994. Relapse following discontinuation of antiepileptic drug: a meta-analysis. *Neurology* 44:601–608.

Berg AT, Shinnar S. 1996. Unprovoked seizures in children with febrile seizures: short-term outcome. *Neurology* 47:562–568.

Berg AT, Shinnar S. 1997. Do seizures beget seizures? An assessment of the clinical evidence in humans. *J Clin Neurophysiol* 14:102–110.

Berg AT, Shinnar S, Hauser WA, et al. 1990. Predictors of recurrent febrile seizures: a motor-analytic review. *J Pediatr* 116:329–337.

Berg AT, Shinnar S, Hauser WA, et al. 1992. A prospective study of recurrent febrile seizures. *N Engl J Med* 327:1122–1127.

Berg AT, Shinnar S, Shapiro ED, et al. 1995. Risk factors for a first febrile seizure: a matched case-control study. *Epilepsia* 36:334–341.

Berg AT, Levy SR, Novotny EJ, et al. 1996. Predictors of intractable epilepsy in childhood: a case-control study. *Epilepsia* 37:24–30.

Berg AT, Testa FM, Levy SR, et al. 2000. Neuroimaging in children with newly diagnosed epilepsy: a community-based study. *Pediatrics* 106:527–532.

Berg AT, Shinnar S, Levy SR, et al. 2001. Early development of intractable epilepsy in children. *Neurology* 56:1445–1452.

Berg AT, Langfitt J, Shinnar S, et al. 2003. How long does it take for partial epilepsy to become intractable? *Neurology* 60:186–190.

Bergamasco B, Benna P, Ferrero P, et al. 1984. Neonatal hypoxia and epileptic risk: a clinical perspective study. *Epilepsia* 25:131–136.

Berger MS, Ghatan S, Geier JR, et al. 1991. Seizure outcome in children with hemispheric tumors and associated intractable epilepsy: the role of tumor removal combined with seizure foci resection. *Pediatr Neurosurg* 17:185–191.

Berger MS, Ghatan S, Haglund MM, et al. 1993. Low-grade gliomas associated with intractable epilepsy: seizure outcome utilizing electrocorticography during tumor resection. *J Neurosurg* 79:62–69.

Berger A, Diener W, Schaestele M, et al. 1997. Complex partial seizures in early infancy with benign outcome [Abstract]. *Epilepsia* 38:48.

Bergin PS, Fish DR, Shorvon SD, et al. 1995. Magnetic resonance imaging in partial epilepsy: additional abnormalities shown with the fluid attenuated inversion recovery (FLAIR) pulse sequence. *J Neurol Neurosurg Psychiatry* 58:439–443.

Bergman I, Painter MS, Crumrine PK. 1982. Neonatal seizures. *Semin Perinatol* 6:54–67.

Bergman I, Painter MJ, Hirsch RP, et al. 1983. Outcome of neonates with convulsions treated in an intensive care unit. *Ann Neurol* 14:642–647.

Berkovic SF, Andermann F. 1986. The progressive myoclonus epilepsies. In: Pedley TA, Meldrum BS, eds. *Recent advances in epilepsy*, Vol. 3. Edinburgh: Churchill Livingstone, 157–187.

Berkovic SF, Scheffer IE. 1997. Epilepsies with simple gene inheritance. *Brain Dev* 19:13–18.

Berkovic SF, Scheffer IE. 2001.Genetics of the epilepsies. *Epilepsia* 42(Suppl. 5):16–23.

Berkovic SF, Andermann F, Carpenter S, et al. 1986. Progressive myoclonus epilepsies: specific causes and diagnosis. *N Engl J Med* 315:296–305.

Berkovic SF, Andermann F, Andermann E, et al. 1987. Concept of absence epilepsies: discrete syndromes or biological continuum. *Neurology* 37:993–1000.

Berkovic SF, Andermann F, Melanson D, et al. 1988. Hypothalamic hamartomas and ictal laughter: evolution of a characteristic epileptic syndrome and diagnostic value of magnetic resonance imaging. *Ann Neurol* 23:429–439.

Berkovic SF, Howell RA, Hopper JL, et al. 1990. A twin study of epilepsies. *Epilepsia* 31:813.

Berkovic SF, Andermann F, Olivier A, et al. 1991a. Hippocampal sclerosis in temporal lobe epilepsy demonstrated by magnetic resonance imaging. *Ann Neurol* 29:175–182.

Berkovic SF, Howell RA, Hopper JL, et al. 1991b. Generalized epilepsies: genetics as revealed by twins [Abstract]. *Neurology* 41:127.

Berkovic SF, Newton MR, Chiron C, et al. 1992. Single photon emission tomography. In: Engel J, ed. *Surgical treatment of the epilepsies*, 2nd ed. New York: Raven Press.

Berkovic SF, Cochins J, Andermann E, et al. 1993. Progressive myoclonus epilepsies: clinical and genetics aspects. *Epilepsia* 34:S19–S30.

Berkovic SF, Howell A, Hay DA, et al. 1994a. Epilepsies in twins. In: Wolf P, ed. *Epileptic seizures and syndromes*. London: John Libbey, 157–164.

Berkovic SF, Howell A, Hopper JL. 1994b. Familial temporal lobe epilepsy: a new syndrome with adolescent/adult onset and a benign course. In: Wolf P, ed. *Epileptic seizures and syndromes*. London: John Libbey, 257–260.

Berkovic SF, McIntosh A, Howell RA, et al. 1996. Familial temporal lobe epilepsy: a common disorder identified in twins. *Ann Neurol* 40:227–235.

Berkovic SF, Howell RA, Hay DA, et al. 1998. Epilepsies in twins: genetics of the major epilepsy syndromes. *Ann Neurol* 43:435–445.

Berkovic SF, Arzimanoglou A, Kuzniecky R, et al. 2003. Hypothalamic hamartoma and seizures: a treatable epileptic encephalopathy. *Epilepsia* 44:969–973.

Berney TP, Osselton JW, Kolvin I, et al. 1981. Effect of discotheque environment on epileptic children. *BMJ* 282: 180–183.

Bertram EH, Lothman EW, Lenn NJ. 1990. The hippocampus in experimental chronic epilepsy: a morphometric analysis. *Ann Neurol* 27:43–48.

Besag FM, Berry DJ, Pool F, et al. 1998. Carbamazepine toxicity with lamotrigine: pharmacokinetic or pharmacodynamic interaction? *Epilepsia* 39:183–187.

Bethune P, Gordon K, Dooley J, et al. 1993. Which child will have a febrile seizure? *Am J Dis Child* 147:35–39.

Betts TA. 1983. The psychological management of epilepsy. In: Rose CF, ed. *Research progress in epilepsy*. London: Pitman, 315–325.

Beun AM, Beintema DJ, Binnie CD, et al. 1984. Epileptic nystagmus. *Epilepsia* 25:609–614.

Bhatia KP, Soland VL, Bhatt MH, et al. 1997. Paroxysmal exercise-induced dystonia: eight new sporadic cases and a review of the literature. *Mov Disord* 12:1007–1012.

Biagioni E, Bartalena L, Boldrini A, et al. 2000. Electroencephalography in infants with periventricular leukomalacia: prognostic features at preterm and term age. *J Child Neurol* 15:1–6.

Bialer M, Johannessen SI, Kupferberg HJ, et al. 2002. Progress report on new antiepileptic drugs: a summary of the Sixth Eilat Conference. *Epilepsy Res* 51:31–71.

Bianchi A, Italian League Against Epilepsy Collaborative Group. 1995. Study of concordance of symptoms in families with absence epilepsies. In: Duncan JS, Panayiotopoulos CP, eds. *Typical absences and related syndromes*. London: Churchill Communication Europe, 328–337.

Bianchine JW. 1970. The nevus sebaceus of Jadassohn. *Am J Dis Child* 120:223–228.

Bicknese AR, May W, Hickey WF, et al. 1992. Early childhood hepatocerebral degeneration misdiagnosed as valproate hepatotoxicity. *Ann Neurol* 32:767–775.

Bien CG, Widman G, Urbach H, et al. 2002. The natural history of Rasmussen encephalitis. *Brain* 125:1751–1759.

Biervert C, Schroeder BC, Kubish C, et al. 1998. A potassium channel mutation in neonatal human epilepsy. *Science* 279:403–406.

Bignami A, Zeppella M, Benedetti P. 1964. Infantile spasms with hypsarrhythmia: a pathological study. *Helv Paediatr Acta* 19:326–332.

Bignami A, Maccagnani F, Zappella M, et al. 1966. Familial infantile spasms associated with leukodystrophy. *J Neurol Neurosurg Psychiatry* 29:129–134.

Bilgic B, Baykan B, Gürses C, et al. 2001. Perioral myoclonia with absence seizures: a rare epileptic syndrome. *Epileptic Disord* 3:23–27.

Billard C, Autret A, Laffont F, et al. 1981. Aphasie acquise de l'enfant avec épilepsie: à propos de 4 observations avec état de mal infraclinique du sommeil. *Rev Electroencephalogr Neurophysiol Clin* 11:457–467.

Billard C, Dulac O, Diebler C. 1982. Ramollissement cérébral ischémique du nouveauné. *Arch Fr Pediatr* 390:677–683.

Billard C, Santini JJ, Tassy J, et al. 1984. Les crises épileptiques accidentelles de l'enfant. *Arch Fr Pediatr* 41: 629–632.

Billard C, Autret A, Lucas B, et al. 1990. Are frequent spikewaves during non-REM sleep in relation with an acquired neuropsychological deficit in epileptic children? *Neurophysiol Clin* 20:439–453.

Billette de Villemeur T, Chiron C, Robain O. 1992. Unlayered polymicrogyria and agenesis of the corpus callosum: a relevant association? *Acta Neuropathol* 83: 265–270.

Bilo L, Meo R, Striano S. 1988. Serum prolactin evaluation after "minor" generalized seizures by EEG. *J Neurol Neurosurg Psychiatry* 51:308–309.

Bingham PM, Lynch D, McDonald-McGinn D, et al. 1998. Polymicrogyria in chromosome 22 deletion syndrome. *Neurology* 51:1500–1502.

Binnie CD. 1991. Long-term monitoring. In: Dam H, Gram L, eds. *Comprehensive epileptology*. New York: Raven Press, 339–349.

Binnie CD, Jeavons PM. 1992. Photosensitive epilepsies. In: Roger J, Bureau M, Dravet C, et al., eds. *Epileptic syndromes of infancy, childhood and adolescence*, 2nd ed. London: John Libbey, 299–305.

Binnie CD, Wilkins AJ. 1997. Visually induced seizures not caused by flicker (intermittent light stimulation). *Adv Neurol* 75:123–138.

Binnie CD, Darby CE, De Korte RA, et al. 1980. Self-induction of epileptic seizures by eye closure: incidence and recognition. *J Neurol Neurosurg Psychiatry* 43: 386–389.

Binnie CD, Rowan AJ, Overweg J, et al. 1981. Telemetric EEG and video monitoring in epilepsy. *Neurology* 31: 298–303.

Binnie CD, de Beukelaar F, Meijer JW, et al. 1985a. Open dose-ranging trial of flunarizine as add-on therapy in epilepsy. *Epilepsia* 26:424–428.

Binnie CD, Findlay J, Wilkins AJ. 1985b. Mechanisms of epileptogenesis in photosensitive epilepsy implied by the effects of moving patterns. *Electroencephalogr Clin Neurophysiol* 61:1–6.

Binnie CD, van Emde Boas W, Kasteleijn-Nolste Trenité DG, et al. 1986. Acute effects of lamotrigine (BW430C) in persons with epilepsy. *Epilepsia* 27:248–254.

Binnie CD, Kasteleijn-Nolst Trenité DG, Smit AM, et al. 1987. Interactions of epileptiform EEG discharges and cognition. *Epilepsy Res* 1:239–245.

Binnie CD, Channon S, Marston D. 1990. Learning disabilities in epilepsy: neurophysiological aspects. *Epilepsia* 31:S2–S8.

Biraben A, Chauvel P. 1997. Falls in epileptic seizures with partial onset. In: Beaumanoir A, Andermann F, Avanzini G, et al., eds. *Falls in epileptic and non-epileptic seizures during childhood*. London: John Libbey, 125–135.

Biraben A, Allain H, Scarabin JM, et al. 2000. Exacerbation

of juvenile myoclonic epilepsy with lamotrigine. *Neurology* 55:1758.

Biraben A, Odent S, Lucas J, et al. 2001a. Chromosome 20 en anneau et épilepsie: diversité des crises étudiées en vidéo-EEG. Un mécanisme sous-cortical d'épileptogénèse est-il au premier plan? *Epilepsies* 13:9–15.

Biraben A, Taussig D, Thomas P, et al. 2001b. Fear as the main feature of epileptic seizures. *J Neurol Neurosurg Psychiatry* 70:186–191.

Birbeck GL, Hays RD, Cui X, et al. 2002. Seizure reduction and quality of life improvements in people with epilepsy. *Epilepsia* 43:535–538.

Bird TD. 1987. Genetic considerations in childhood epilepsy. *Epilepsia* 28:S71–S81.

Bishop DV. 1985. Age of onset and outcome in 'acquired aphasia with convulsive disorder' (Landau-Kleffner syndrome). *Dev Med Child Neurol* 27:705–712.

Biton V, Gates JR, dePadua Sussman L. 1990. Prolonged postictal encephalopathy. *Neurology* 40:963–966.

Bittar RG, Rosenfeld JV, Klug GL, et al. 2002. Resective surgery in infants and young children with intractable epilepsy. *J Clin Neurosci* 2:142–146.

Bittencourt PR, Richens A. 1981. Anticonvulsant-induced status epilepticus in Lennox-Gastaut syndrome. *Epilepsia* 22:129–134.

Bizzi JW, Bruce DA, North R, et al. 1997. Surgical treatment of focal epilepsy in children: results in 37 patients. *Pediatr Neurosurg* 26:83–92.

Bjerre I, Corelius E. 1968. Benign familiar neonatal convulsions. *Acta Paediatr Scand* 57:557–561.

Bladin PF. 1987. The association of benign rolandic epilepsy with migraine. In: Andermann F, Lugaresi E, eds. *Migraine and epilepsy*. Boston: Butterworth-Heinemann, 145–152.

Blau JN, Wiles CH, Solomon FS. 1983. Unilateral somatic symptoms due to hyperventilation. *BMJ* 286:1108.

Bleasel AF, Lüders HO. 2000. Tonic seizures. In: Lüders HO, Noachtar S, eds. *Epileptic seizures: pathophysiology and clinical semiology*. Philadelphia: Churchill Livingstone, 389–411.

Bleasel A, Morris H 3rd. 1996. Supplementary sensorimotor area epilepsy in adults. In: Lüders H, ed. *Supplementary sensorimotor area*. Advances in neurology, Vol. 70. Philadelphia: Lippincott-Raven, 271–284.

Bleasel A, So N, Van Ness P, et al. 1993. The clinical syndrome of seizures arising from supplementary motor area [Abstract]. *Epilepsia* 34(Suppl. 6):54.

Bleasel A, Kotagal P, Kankirawatana P, Rybicki L. 1997. Lateralizing value and semiology of ictal limb posturing and version in temporal lobe and extratemporal epilepsy. *Epilepsia* 38:168–174.

Bleck TP. 1999. Management approaches to prolonged seizures and status epilepticus. *Epilepsia* 40:S59–S63.

Blennow G, Starck L. 1986. High-dose B₆ treatment in infantile spasms. *Neuropediatrics* 17:7–10.

Blennow G, Brierley JB, Meldrum BS, Siesjo BK. 1978. Epileptic brain damage: the role of systemic factors that modify cerebral energy metabolism. *Brain* 101:687–700.

Blennow G, Heijbel J, Sandstedt P, Tonnby B. 1990. Discontinuation of antiepileptic drugs in children who have outgrown epilepsy: effects on cognitive function. *Epilepsia* 31:S50–S53.

Blom S, Heijbel J. 1975. Benign epilepsy of children with centro-temporal foci: discharge rate during sleep. *Epilepsia* 16:133–140.

Blom S, Heijbel J. 1982. Benign epilepsy of children with centrotemporal EEG foci: a follow-up study in adulthood of patients initially treated as children. *Epilepsia* 23:629–632.

Blom S, Heijbel J. 1989. Benign epilepsy of childhood with centrotemporal spikes. In: Beck-Mannagetta G, Anderson VE, Doose H, et al. *Genetics of the epilepsies*. Berlin: Springer-Verlag, 67–72.

Blom S, Heybel J, Bergfors PG. 1972. Benign epilepsy of children with centro-temporal EEG foci: prevalence and follow-up study of 40 patients. *Epilepsia* 13:609–619.

Blom S, Heybel J, Bergfors PG. 1978. Incidence of epilepsy in children: a follow-up study three years after the first seizure. *Epilepsia* 19:343–350.

Blomquist HK, Gustavson KH, Holmgren G, et al. 1983. Fragile X syndrome in mildly retarded children in a northern Swedish country. *Clin Genet* 24:393–398.

Blume WT. 1978. Clinical and electroencephalographic correlates of the multiple independent spike foci pattern in children. *Ann Neurol* 4:541–547.

Blume WT. 1982. *Atlas of pediatric electroencephalography*. New York: Raven Press.

Blume WT. 1988. The EEG features of the Lennox-Gastaut syndrome. In: Niedermeyer E, Degen R, eds. *The Lennox-Gastaut syndrome*. New York: Alan R. Liss, 159–176.

Blume WT. 1989. Clinical profile of partial seizures beginning at less than four years of age. *Epilepsia* 30:813–819.

Blume WT. 1991. Occipital lobe epilepsies. In: Lüders H, ed. *Epilepsy surgery*. New York: Raven Press, 167–171.

Blume WT. 1992. Uncontrolled epilepsy in children. *Epilepsy Res Suppl* 5:19–24.

Blume WT. 1997. Corpus callosotomy: a critical review. In: Tuxhorn I, Holthausen H, Boenigk H, eds. *Paediatric epilepsy syndromes and their surgical treatment*. London: John Libbey, 815– 829

Blume WT, Dreyfus-Brisac C. 1982. Positive rolandic sharp waves in neonatal EEG: types and significance. *Electroencephalogr Clin Neurophysiol* 53:277–282.

Blume WT, Pillay N. 1985. Electrographic and clinical correlates of secondary bilateral synchrony. *Epilepsia* 26:636–641.

Blume WT, Young GB. 1987. Ictal pain: unilateral, cephalic, and abdominal. In: Andermann F, Lugaresi E, eds. *Migraine and epilepsy*. Boston: Butterworth—Heineman, 235–248.

Blume WT, Whiting SE, Girvin JP. 1991. Epilepsy surgery in the posterior cortex. *Ann Neurol* 29:638–645.

Blume WT, David RB, Gomez MR. 1973. Generalized sharp and slow wave complexes—associated clinical features and long-term follow-up. *Brain* 96:289–306.

Blume WT, Girvin JP, Kaufmann JC. 1982. Childhood brain tumors presenting as chronic uncontrolled seizure disorder. *Ann Neurol* 12:538–541.

Blume WT, Yong GB, Lemieux JF. 1984. EEG morphology of partial epileptic seizures. *Electroencephalogr Clin Neurophysiol* 57:295–302.

Blume WT, Aicardi J, Dreifuss FE. 1993. Syndromes not amenable to resective surgery. In: Engel J, ed. *Surgical treatment of the epilepsies*, 2nd ed. New York: Raven Press, 103–118.

Bobele GB, Bodensteiner JB. 1990. Infantile spasms. *Neurol Clin* 8:633–645.

Bocti C, Robitaille Y, Diadori P, et al. 2003. The pathological basis of temporal lobe epilepsy in childhood. *Neurology* 60:191–195.

Bodensteiner JB, Brownsworth RD, Knadik JR, et al. 1988. Interobserver variability in the ILAE classification of seizures in childhood. *Epilepsia* 29:123–128.

Boel M, Casaer P. 1989. Continuous spikes and waves during slow sleep: a 30 months follow-up study of neuropsychological recovery and EEG findings. *Neuropediatrics* 20:176–180.

Boel M, Casaer P. 1996. Add-on therapy of fenfluramine in intractable self-induced epilepsy. *Neuropediatrics* 27: 171–173.

Bolthauser E, Wilson J, Hoare RD. 1976. Sturge-Weber syndrome with bilateral intracranial calcification. *J Neurol Neurosurg Psychiatry* 39:429–435.

Bolthauser E, Meyer M, Deonna T. 1978. Klinefelter's syndrome and neurological disease. *J Neurol* 219:253–259.

Bonanni P, Parmeggiani L, Guerrini R. 2002. Different neurophysiologic patterns of myoclonus characterize Lennox-Gastaut syndrome and myoclonic astatic epilepsy. *Epilepsia* 43:609–615.

Boneschi FM, Barker-Cummings C, Lee JH, et al. 2002. Four new families with autosomal dominant partial epilepsy with auditory features: clinical description and linkage to chromosome 10q24. *Epilepsia* 43:60–67.

Boniver C, Dravet C, Bureau M, Roger J. 1987. Idiopathic Lennox-Gastaut syndrome. In: Wolf P, Dam M, Janz D, Dreifuss FE, eds. *Advances in epileptology*, XVIth Epilepsy International Symposium. New York: Raven Press, 195–200.

Boon PA, Williamson PD, Fried I, et al. 1991. Intracranial, intraaxial, space-occupying lesions in patients with intractable partial seizures: an anatomoclinical, neuropsychological, and surgical correlation. *Epilepsia* 32: 467–476.

Boone KB, Miller BL, Rosenberg L, et al. 1988. Neuropsychological and behavioral abnormalities in an adolescent with frontal lobe seizures. *Neurology* 38:583–586.

Borgatti R, Triulzi F, Zucca C, et al. 1999. Bilateral perisylvian polymicrogyria in three generations. *Neurology* 52:1910–1913.

Borgatti R, Piccinelli P, Passoni D, et al. 2001. Relationship between clinical and genetic features in 'inverted duplicated chromosome 15' patients. *Pediatr Neurol* 24:111–116.

Bossi L, Munari C, Stoffels C, et al. 1984. Somatomotor manifestations in temporal lobe seizures. *Epilepsia* 25:70–76.

Boulloche J, Leloup P, Mallet E, et al. 1989. Risk of recurrence after a single unprovoked generalized tonic-clonic seizure. *Dev Med Child Neurol* 31:620–632.

Boulloche J, Husson A, Le Luyer B, Le Roux P. 1990. Dysphagie, troubles du langage et pointes-ondes centrotemporales. *Arch Fr Pediatr* 47:115–117.

Bouma P, Peters AC, Arts RJ, et al. 1987. Discontinuation of antiepileptic therapy: a prospective study in children. *J Neurol Neurosurg Psychiatry* 50:1579–1583.

Bouma PA, Bovenkerk AC, Westendorp RG, et al. 1997. The course of partial epilepsy of childhood with centrotemporal spikes: a meta-analysis. *Neurology* 48:430–437.

Bour F, Chiron C, Dulac O, et al. 1986. Caractères électrocliniques des crises dans le syndrome d'Aicardi. *Rev Electroencephalogr Neurophysiol Clin* 16:341–353.

Bourgeois BF. 1986. Antiepileptic drug combinations and experimental background: the case of phenobarbital and phenytoin. *Naunym Schmiedebergs Arch Pharmacol* 333:406–411.

Bourgeois BF. 1988. Problems of combination drug therapy in children. *Epilepsia* 29:S20–S24.

Bourgeois BF. 1992. Childhood epilepsy: pharmacological considerations. *Acta Neurol Scand Suppl* 140:23–27.

Bourgeois BF. 1998. Antiepileptic drugs, learning and behavior in childhood epilepsy. *Epilepsia* 39:913–921.

Bourgeois BF. 1999. A retarded boy with seizures precipitated by stepping into the bath water. *Semin Pediatr Neurol* 6:151–157.

Bourgeois B. 2001. Pharmacokinetics and pharmacodynamics of antiepileptic drugs. In: Wyllie E, ed. *The treatment of epilepsy*, 3rd ed. Philadelphia: Lippincott Williams & Wilkins, 729–739.

Bourgeois BF, Wad N. 1988. Combined administration of carbamazepine and phenobarbital: effect on anticonvulsant activity and neurotoxicity. *Epilepsia* 29:482–487.

Bourgeois BF, Dodson WE, Ferrendelli JA. 1983a. Primidone, phenobarbital and PEMA. I: Seizure protection, neurotoxicity and therapeutic index of individual compounds in mice. II: Seizure protection, neurotoxicity and therapeutic index of various combinations in mice. *Neurology* 33:283–290, 291–295.

Bourgeois BF, Prensky AL, Palkes HS, et al. 1983b. Intelligence in epilepsy: a prospective study in children. *Ann Neurol* 14:438–444.

Bourgeois BF, Beaumanoir A, Blajev B. 1987. Monotherapy with valproate in primary generalized epilepsies. *Epilepsia* 28:S8–S11.

Bourgeois BF, Aicardi J, Goutières F. 1993. Alternating hemiplegia in infants. *J Pediatr* 122:673–679.

Bourgeois B, Brown L, Pellock J, et al. 1998. Gabapentin (Neurontin) monotherapy in children with benign childhood epilepsy with centrotemporal spikes (BECTS): a 36-week, double-blind, placebo-controlled study. *Epilepsia* 39:163.

Bourgeois M, Sainte-Rose C, Cinalli G, et al. 1999a. Epilepsy in childhood shunted hydrocephalus. *J Neurosurg* 90:274–281.

Bourgeois M, Sainte-Rose C, Lellouch-Tubiana A, et al. 1999b. Surgery of epilepsy associated with focal lesions in childhood. *J Neurosurg* 90:833–842.

Bout F, Plouin P, Jalin C, et al. 1983. Les états de mal unilatéraux au cours de la période néonatale. *Rev Electroencephalogr Neurophysiol Clin* 13:162–167.

Bower BD. 1980. Epilepsy in childhood and adolescence. In: Tyrer JH, ed. *The treatment of epilepsy*. Lancaster, United Kingdom: MTP Press, 251–273.

Boyd SG, Harden A, Egger J, et al. 1986. Progressive neuronal degeneration of childhood with liver disease ("Alpers' disease"): characteristic neurophysiological features. *Neuropediatrics* 17:75–80.

Braathen G, Theorell K, Persson A, et al. 1988. Valproate in the treatment of absence epilepsy in children: a study of dose-response relationships. *Epilepsia* 29:548–552.

Braham J, Hertzeanu H, Yahini JH. 1981. Reflex cardiac arrest presenting as epilepsy. *Ann Neurol* 10:277–278.

Branch CE, Dyken PR. 1979. Choroid plexus papilloma and infantile spasms. *Ann Neurol* 5:302–304.

Brandt NJ, Rasmussen K, Brandt S, et al. 1974. D-glyceric acidemia with hyperglycinemia: a new inborn error of metabolism. *BMJ* 4:334–336.

Brandt CA, Kierkegaard O, Hindkjaer J, et al. 1993. Ring chromosome 20 with loss of telomeric sequences detected by multicolour PRINS. *Clin Genet* 44:26–31.

Bray P, Wiser WC. 1964. Evidence for a genetic etiology of

temporal central abnormalities in focal epilepsy. *N Engl J Med* 271:926–933.

Bray PF, Wiser WC. 1965a. Hereditary characteristics of familial temporal-central focal epilepsy. *Pediatrics* 36:207–211.

Bray PF, Wiser WC. 1965b. The relation of focal to diffuse epileptiform EEG discharges in genetic epilepsy. *Arch Neurol* 13:233–237.

Breningstall GN. 1985. Gelastic seizures, precocious puberty, and hypothalamic hamartoma. *Neurology* 35:1180–1183.

Breningstall GN. 2001. Mortality in pediatric epilepsy. *Pediatr Neurol* 25:9–16.

Brenner RP, Atkinson R. 1982. Generalized paroxysmal fast activity: electroencephalographic and clinical features. *Ann Neurol* 11:386–390.

Bressman SB, Fahn S, Burke RE. 1988. Paroxysmal nonkinesigenic dystonia. *Adv Neurol* 50:403–413.

Brett EM. 1966. Minor epileptic status. *J Neurol Sci* 3:52–75.

Brett EM. 1988. The Lennox-Gastaut syndrome: therapeutic aspects. In: Niedermeyer E, Degen R, eds. *The Lennox-Gastaut syndrome.* New York: Alan R. Liss, 317–339.

Breuner RP, Sharbrough FW. 1976. Electroencephalographic evaluation in Sturge-Weber syndrome. *Neurology* 26:629–632.

Bridgers SL, Ebersole JS, Ment LR, et al. 1986. Cassette electroencephalography in the evaluation of neonatal seizures. *Arch Neurol* 43:49–51.

Bridgers SL, Wade PB, Ebersole JS. 1989. Estimating the importance of epileptiform abnormalities discovered on cassette electroencephalographic monitoring. *Arch Neurol* 46:1077–1079.

Briellmann RS, Pell GS, Wellard RM, et al. 2003. MR imaging of epilepsy: state of the art at 1.5 T and potential of 3 T. *Epileptic Disord* 5:3–20.

Brinciotti M, Trasatti G, Peliccia A, et al. 1992. Pattern-sensitive epilepsy: genetic aspects in two families. *Epilepsia* 33:88–92.

Brizzolara D, Brovedani P, Casalini C, et al. 2001. Neuropsychological outcome following prolonged febrile seizures associated with hippocampal sclerosis and temporal lobe epilepsy in children. In: Jambaqué I, Lassonde M, Dulac O, eds. *Neuropsychology of childhood epilepsy.* New York: Kluwer Academic/Plenum Publishers, 121–130.

Brna PM, Gordon KE, Dooley JM, et al. 2001. The epidemiology of infantile spasms. *Can J Neurol Sci* 28:309–312.

Brockhaus A, Elger CE. 1995. Complex partial seizures of temporal lobe origin in children of different age groups. *Epilepsia* 36:1173–1181.

Brod SA, Ment L, Ehrenkranz RA, et al. 1988. Predictors of success for drug discontinuation following neonatal seizures. *Pediatr Neurol* 4:13–17.

Brodie MJ. 1990. Established anticonvulsants and treatment of refractory epilepsy. *Lancet* 336:350–354.

Brodie MJ. 1992. Lamotrigine. *Lancet* 339:1397–1400.

Brodie MJ, French JA. 2003. Role of levetiracetam in the treatment of epilepsy. *Epileptic Disord* 5:S65–S72.

Brodie MJ, Mumford JP. 1999. Double-blind substitution of vigabatrin and valproate in carbamazepine-resistant partial epilepsy. 012 Study Group. *Epilepsy Res* 34:199–205.

Brodie MJ, Yuen AW. 1997. Lamotrigine substitution study: evidence for synergism with sodium valproate? 105 Study Group. *Epilepsy Res* 26:423–432.

Brodie MJ, Richens A, Yuen AW. 1995. Double-blind comparison of lamotrigine and carbamazepine in newly diagnosed epilepsy. *Lancet* 345:476–479.

Brodtkorb E, Sulg I, Gimse R. 1984. The hyperventilation syndrome. *Acta Neurol Scand* 69(Suppl. 98):395–397.

Broglin D, Delgado-Escueta AV, Walsh GO, et al. 1992. Clinical approach to the patient with seizures and epilepsies of frontal origin. In: Chauvel P, Delgado-Escueta AV, Halgren E, et al., eds. *Frontal lobe seizures and epilepsies.* New York: Raven Press, 59–88.

Bromfield EB, Dambrosia J, Devinsky O, et al. 1989. Phenytoin withdrawal and seizure frequency. *Neurology* 39:905–909.

Brorson LO, Wranne L. 1987. Long-term prognosis in childhood epilepsy: survival and seizure prognosis. *Epilepsia* 28:324–330.

Broughton R, Nelson R, Gloor P, et al. 1973. Petit mal epilepsy evolving to subacute sclerosing panencephalitis. In: Lugaresi E, Pazzaglia P, Tassinari CA, eds. *Evolution and prognosis of epilepsies.* Bologna: Aulo Gaggi, 63–72.

Brown JK. 1973. Convulsions in the newborn period. *Dev Med Child Neurol* 15:823–846.

Brown JK. 1988. Valproate toxicity. *Dev Med Child Neurol* 30:121–125.

Brown WJ, Babb TL. 1983. Effects of repeated seizures on hippocampal neurons in the cat. In: Delgado-Escueta AV, Wasterlain CG, Treiman DM, Porter RJ, eds. *Status epilepticus: mechanisms of brain damage and treatment.* Advances in neurology, Vol. 34. New York: Raven Press, 161–168.

Brown A, Horton J. 1967. Status epilepticus treated by intravenous infusions of thiopentone sodium. *BMJ* 1:27–28.

Brown JK, Hussain IH. 1991a. Status epilepticus. I: Pathogenesis. *Dev Med Child Neurol* 33:3–17.

Brown JK, Hussain IH. 1991b. Status epilepticus. II: Treatment. *Dev Med Child Neurol* 33:97–109.

Brown LA, Levin GM. 1998. Role of propofol in refractory status epilepticus. *Ann Pharmacother* 32:1053–1059.

Brown JK, Minns RA. 1980. Epilepsy in neonates. In: Tyrer JH, ed. *The treatment of epilepsy.* Lancaster, United Kingdom: MTP Press, 161–202.

Brown JK, Cockburn F, Forfar JO. 1972. Clinical and chemical correlates in convulsions of the newborn. *Lancet* 1:135–139.

Brown P, Steiger MJ, Thompson PD, et al. 1993. Effectiveness of piracetam in cortical myoclonus. *Mov Disord* 8:63–68.

Browne TR. 1983a. Paraldehyde, chlormethiazole, and lidocaine for treatment of status epilepticus. *Adv Neurol* 34:509–517.

Browne TR. 1983b. Tonic-clonic (grand mal) seizures. In: Browne TR, Feldman RG, eds. *Epilepsy: diagnosis and management.* Boston: Little, Brown and Company, 51–59.

Browne TR, Mirsky AF. 1983. Absence (petit mal) seizures. In: Browne TR, Feldman RG, eds. *Epilepsy: diagnosis and management.* Boston: Little, Brown and Company, 61–74.

Browne TR, Penry JK. 1973. Benzodiazepines in the treatment of epilepsy. *Epilepsia* 14:277–310.

Browne TR, Penry JK, Porter RJ, et al. 1974. Responsiveness before, during and after spike wave paroxysms. *Neurology* 24:659–665.

Browne TR, Dreifuss FE, Penry JK, et al. 1983a. Clinical and EEG estimates of absence seizure frequency. *Arch Neurol* 40:469–472.

Browne TR, Feldman RG, Buchanan RA, et al. 1983b. Methsuximide for complex partial seizures: efficacy, toxicity, clinical pharmacology, and drug interactions. *Neurology* 33:414–418.

Browne TR, Mattson RH, Penry JK, et al. 1987. Vigabatrin for refractory complex partial seizures: multicenter single-blind study with long-term follow-up. *Neurology* 37:184–189.

Browne TR, Szabo MT, Evans JE, et al. 1988a. Phenobarbital does not alter phenytoin steady-state serum concentration or pharmacokinetics. *Neurology* 38:639–642.

Browne TR, Szabo MT, Evans JE, et al. 1988b. Carbamazepine increases phenytoin serum concentration and reduces phenytoin clearance. *Neurology* 38:1146–1150.

Browne TR, Mattson RH, Penry JK, et al. 1991. Multicenter long-term safety and efficacy study of vigabatrin for refractory complex partial seizures: an update. *Neurology* 41:363–364.

Browne TR, Kugler AR, Eldon MA. 1996. Pharmacology and pharmacokinetics of fosphenytoin. *Neurology* 46: S3–S7.

Brucker JT, Garson A, Gillette PC. 1984. A family history of seizures associated with sudden cardiac death. *Am J Dis Child* 138:866–868.

Brunelli S, Faiella A, Capra V, et al. 1996. Germline mutations in the homebox gene EMX2 in patients with severe schizencephaly. *Nat Genet* 12:94–96.

Brunon AM, Mauguière F, Courjon J. 1978. Evolution à long terme des épilepsies survenant avant l'âge de deux ans. *Bolletino Lega Italiana contre l'Epilepsia* 22/23: 165–172.

Brunt ER, van Werden TN. 1990. Familial paroxysmal kinesigenic ataxia and continuous myokymia. *Brain* 113:1361–1382.

Bruton CJ. 1988. *The neuropathology of temporal lobe epilepsy.* Maudsley Monograph No. 31. Oxford: Oxford University Press.

Bryant AE 3rd, Dreifuss FE. 1996. Valproic acid hepatic fatalities. III: U.S. experience since 1986. *Neurology* 46: 465–469.

Buchanan N. 1996. The use of lamotrigine in juvenile myoclonic epilepsy. *Seizure* 5:149–151.

Buehler BA, Delimont D, Van Waes M, et al. 1990. Prenatal prediction of the risk of the fetal hydantoin syndrome. *N Engl J Med* 322:1567–1572.

Bureau M. 1995a. Continuous spikes and waves during slow sleep (ESES): definition of the syndrome. In: Beaumanoir A, Bureau M, Deonna T, et al., eds. *Continuous spikes and waves during slow sleep: electrical status epilepticus during slow sleep.* London: John Libbey, 17–26.

Bureau M. 1995b. Outstanding cases of ESES and LKS: analysis of the data sheets provided by the participants. In: Beaumanoir A, Bureau M, Deonna T, et al., eds. *Continuous spikes and waves during slow sleep: electrical status epilepticus during slow sleep.* London: John Libbey, 213–216.

Bureau M, Kahane P, Munari C, eds. 1998. *Epilepsies partielles graves pharmaco-résistantes de l'enfant: stratégies diagnostiques et traitements chirurgicaux.* Paris: John Libbey Eurotext.

Bureau M, Cokar O, Maton B, et al. 2002. Sleep-related, low-voltage rolandic and vertex spikes: an EEG marker of benignity in infancy-onset focal epilepsy. *Epileptic Disord* 4:15–22.

Bureau M, Tassinari CA. 2002. The syndrome of myoclonic absences. In: Roger J, Bureau M, Dravet C, et al., eds. *Epileptic syndromes in infancy, childhood, and adolescence,* 3rd ed. London, Paris: John Libbey Ltd., 305–312.

Burke CJ, Tannenberg AE. 1995. Prenatal brain damage and placental infarction—an autopsy study. *Dev Med Child Neurol* 37:555–562.

Burke JR, Winfield MS, Lewis KE, et al. 1994. The Haw Rives syndrome: dentatorubropallidoluysian atrophy (DRPLA) in an African American family. *Nat Genet* 7: 289–296.

Burnstine TH, Vining EP, Uematsu S, Lesser RP. 1991. Multifocal independent epileptiform discharges in children: ictal correlates and surgical therapy. *Neurology* 41:1223–1228.

Bye AM, Foo S. 1994. Complex partial seizures in young children. *Epilepsia* 35:482–488.

Bye AM, Cunningham CA, Chee KY, Flanagan D. 1997. Outcome of neonates with electroencephalographically identified seizures, or at risk of seizures. *Pediatr Neurol* 16:225–231.

Cabrera JC, Marti M, Toledo L, et al. 1998. West's syndrome associated with inversion duplication of chromosome 15. *Rev Neurol (Spain)* 26:77–79.

Caffi J. 1973. Zur Frage klinischer Anfallformen bei psychomotorisher Epilepsie. *Schweiz Med Wochenschr* 103:469–475.

Cahan LD, Engel J Jr. 1986. Surgery for epilepsy: a review. *Acta Neurol Scand* 73:551–560.

Calandre EP, Dominguez-Granados R, Gomez-Rubio M, et al. 1990. Cognitive effects of long-term treatment with phenobarbital and valproic acid in school children. *Eur Neurol* 81:504–506.

Calderon-Gonzalez R, Hopkins I, McLean WT Jr. 1966. Tap seizures: a form of sensory precipitation epilepsy. *JAMA* 198:521–523.

Callaghan DJ, Noetzel MJ. 1992. Prolonged absence status epilepticus associated with carbamazepine therapy, increased intracranial pressure and transient MRI abnormalities. *Neurology* 42:2198–2201.

Callaghan N, O'Hare J, O'Driscoll D, et al. 1982. Comparative study of ethosuximide and sodium valproate in the treatment of typical absence seizures (petit mal). *Dev Med Child Neurol* 24:830–836.

Callaghan N, Kenny RA, O'Neill B, et al. 1985. A prospective study between carbamazepine, phenytoin and sodium valproate as monotherapy in previously untreated and recently diagnosed patients with epilepsy. *J Neurol Neurosurg Psychiatry* 48:639–644.

Callaghan N, Garrett A, Goggin T. 1988. Withdrawal of anticonvulsant drugs in patients free of seizures for two years—a prospective study. *N Engl J Med* 318:942–946.

Camfield CS, Camfield PR. 1981. Behavioral and cognitive effects of phenobarbital in toddlers. In: Nelson KB, Ellenberg JH, eds. *Febrile seizures.* New York: Raven Press, 203–210.

Camfield PR, Camfield CS. 1987. Neonatal seizures: a commentary on selected aspects. *J Child Neurol* 2:244–251.

Camfield PR, Camfield CS. 2000. Treatment of children with "ordinary" epilepsy. *Epileptic Disorder* 2:45–51.

Camfield PR, Dooley JM. 1987. Multiple brief nontemporal

focal seizures in well children: a benign epilepsy syndrome with apparent cure in some by very short course of anticonvulsants [Abstract]. *Ann Neurol* 22:414A.

Camfield PR, Metrakos K, Andermann F. 1978. Basilar migraine, seizures, and severe epileptiform EEG abnormalities. *Neurology* 28:584–588.

Camfield PR, Camfield CS, Shapiro SH, Cummings C. 1980. The first febrile seizure—antipyretic instruction plus either phenobarbital or placebo to prevent recurrence. *J Pediatr* 97:16–21.

Camfield PR, Gates R, Ronen G, et al. 1984. Comparison of cognitive ability, personality profile, and school success in epileptic children with pure right versus left temporal lobe EEG foci. *Ann Neurol* 15:122–126.

Camfield PR, Camfield CS, Dooley JM, et al. 1985a. Epilepsy after a first unprovoked seizure in childhood. *Neurology* 35:1657–1660.

Camfield PR, Camfield CS, Smith ED, et al. 1985b. Newly treated childhood epilepsy: a prospective study of recurrences and side-effects. *Neurology* 35:722–725.

Camfield PR, Camfield CS, Smith ED, et al. 1986. Asymptomatic children with epilepsy: little benefit from screening for anticonvulsant induced liver, blood or renal damage. *Neurology* 36:838–841.

Camfield CS, Camfield PR, Smith E, et al. 1989a. Home use of rectal diazepam to prevent status epilepticus in children with convulsive disorders. *J Child Neurol* 4:125–126.

Camfield P, Camfield C, Dooley MB, et al. 1989b. A randomized study of carbamazepine versus no medication after a first unprovoked seizure in childhood. *Neurology* 39:851–852.

Camfield PR, Dooley J, Gordon K, et al. 1991. Benign familial neonatal convulsions are epileptic. *J Child Neurol* 6:340–342.

Camfield C, Camfield P, Smith B, et al. 1993. Biologic factors as predictors of social outcome of epilepsy in intellectually normal children: a population-based study. *J Pediatr* 122:869–873.

Canafoglia L, Franceschetti S, Antozzi C, et al. 2001. Epileptic phenotypes associated with mitochondrial disorders. *Neurology* 56:1340–1346.

Canevini M, Mai R, Di Marco C, et al. 1992. Juvenile myoclonic epilepsy of Janz: clinical observations in 60 patients. *Seizure* 1:290–298.

Canevini MP, Sgro V, Zuffardi O, et al. 1998. Chromosome 20 ring: a chromosomal disorder associated with a particular electroclinical pattern. *Epilepsia* 39:942–951.

Cao A, Cianchetti C, Signorini E, et al. 1977. Agenesis of the corpus callosum, infantile spasms, spastic quadriplegia, microcephaly and severe mental retardation in three siblings. *Clin Genet* 12:290–296.

Caplan C, Guthrie D, Mundy P, et al. 1992. Non-verbal communication skills of surgically treated children with infantile spasms. *Dev Med Child Neurol* 34:499–506.

Caplan R, Guthrie D, Korno S, et al. 1999. Infantile spasms: the development of nonverbal communication after epilepsy surgery. *Dev Neurosci* 21:165–173.

Capovilla G, Beccaria F. 2000. Benign partial epilepsy in infancy and early childhood with vertex spikes and waves during sleep: a new epileptic form. *Brain Dev* 22:93–98.

Capovilla G, Giordano L, Tiberti S, et al. 1998. Benign partial epilepsy in infancy with complex partial seizures (Watanabe's syndrome): 12 non-Japanese new cases. *Brain Dev* 20:105–111.

Capovilla G, Gambardella A, Romeo A, et al. 2001a. Benign partial epilepsies of adolescence: a report of 37 new cases. *Epilepsia* 42:1549–1552.

Capovilla G, Rubboli G, Beccaria F, et al. 2001b. A clinical spectrum of the myoclonic manifestations associated with typical absences in childhood absence epilepsy. A video-polygraphic study. *Epileptic Disord* 3:57–62.

Caraballo R, Fontana E, Michelizza B, et al. 1989. Carbamazepina, 'assenze atipiche', 'crisi atoniche' e stato di PO continua del sonno (POCS). *Bolletino Lega Italiana contre l'Epilepsia* 66/67:379–381.

Caraballo R, Cersósimo R, Galicchio S, Fejerman N. 1997. Epilepsies during the first year of life. *Rev Neurol* 25 (Spanish):1521–1524.

Caraballo R, Cerosimo R, Fejerman A. 1999. A particular type of epilepsy in children with congenital hemiparesis associated with unilateral polymicrogyria. *Epilepsia* 40:865–871.

Carbonara C, Longa L, Grosso E, et al. 1994. 9q34 loss of heterozygosity in a tuberous sclerosis astrocytoma suggests a growth suppressor-like activity also for the TSC1 gene. *Hum Mol Genet* 3:1829–1832.

Carlson AM, Cloyd JC, Kriel RL, et al. 1988. An evaluation of rectally administered diazepam at home: use and cost-benefit analysis [Abstract]. *Ann Neurol* 24: 320A.

Carpay HA, Arts WF, Vermeulen J, et al. 1996. Parent-completed scales for measuring seizure severity and severity of side effects of antiepileptic drugs in childhood epilepsy: development and psychometric analysis. *Epilepsy Res* 24:173–181.

Carpay HA, Vermeulen J, Stroink H, et al. 1997. Disability due to restrictions in childhood epilepsy. *Dev Med Child Neurol* 39:521–526.

Carrazana EJ, Lombroso CT, Mikati M, et al. 1993. Facilitation of infantile spasms by partial seizures. *Epilepsia* 34:97–109.

Carter S. 1964. Diagnosis and treatment: management of the child who has had one convulsion. *Pediatrics* 33: 431–434.

Cascino GD. 1990. Epilepsy and brain tumors: implications for treatment. *Epilepsia* 31:S37–S44.

Cascino GD, Jack CR Jr, eds. 1996. *Neuroimaging in epilepsy: principles and practice.* Boston: Butterworth-Heinemann.

Cascino GD, Jack CR, Parisi JE, et al. 1991. Magnetic resonance imaging-based volume studies in temporal lobe epilepsy: pathological correlations. *Ann Neurol* 30: 31–36.

Cascino GD, Jack CR, Hirschorn KA, Sharbrough FW. 1992a. Identification of the epileptic focus: magnetic resonance imaging. *Epilepsy Res Suppl* 5:95–100.

Cascino GD, Jack CR Jr, Parisi JE, et al. 1992b. MRI in the presurgical evaluation of patients with frontal lobe epilepsy and children with temporal lobe epilepsy: pathologic correlation and prognostic importance. *Epilepsy Res* 11:51–59.

Cascino GD, Kelly PJ, Sharbrough FW, et al. 1992c. Long-term follow-up of stereotactic lesionectomy in partial epilepsy: predictive factors and electroencephalographic results. *Epilepsia* 33:639–644.

Cascino GD, Boon P, Fish DR. 1993a. Surgically remediable lesional syndromes. In: Engel J, ed. *Surgical treatment of the epilepsies*, 2nd ed. New York: Raven Press, 77–86.

Cascino GD, Hulihan JF, Sharbrough FW, et al. 1993b. Parietal lobe lesional epilepsy: electroclinical correlation and operative outcome. *Epilepsia* 34:522–530.

Cascino GD, Treverry MR, So EL, et al. 1996. Routine EEG and temporal lobe epilepsy—relation to long term EEG monitoring, quantitative MRI, and operative outcome. *Epilepsia* 37:651–656.

Cassidy S, Gainey A, Holmes G, et al. 1983. Infantile spasms in Down syndrome: an unappreciated association [Abstract]. *Am J Hum Genet* 35:82A.

Casteels-van Daele M. 1981. Metoclopramide poisoning in children. *Arch Dis Child* 56:405–406.

Cavanagh JB. 1958. On certain small tumors encountered in the temporal lobe. *Brain* 81:389–405.

Cavanagh JB, Meyer A. 1956. Aetiological aspects of Ammon's horn sclerosis associated with temporal lobe epilepsy. *BMJ* 2:1403–1407.

Cavanagh NP, Bicknell J, Howard F. 1974. Cystinuria with mental retardation and paroxysmal dyskinesia in 2 brothers. *Arch Dis Child* 49:662–664.

Cavazzuti GB. 1973. Infantile spasms with hypsarrhythmia. In: Lugaresi E, Pazzaglia P, Tassinari CA, eds. *Evolution and prognosis of epilepsies*. Bologna: Aulo Gaggi, 109–113.

Cavazzuti GB. 1975. Prevention of febrile convulsions with dipropylacetate (Depakine). *Epilepsia* 16:647–648.

Cavazzuti GB. 1980. Epidemiology of different types of epilepsy in school age children of Modena (Italy). *Epilepsia* 21:57–63.

Cavazzuti GB, Cappella L, Nalin A. 1980. Longitudinal study of epileptiform EEG patterns in normal children. *Epilepsia* 21:43–55.

Cavazzuti GB, Ferrari P, Laba M. 1984. Follow-up study of 482 cases with convulsive disorders in the first year of life. *Dev Med Child Neurol* 26:425–437.

Cavazzuti GB, Ferrari P, Galli V, et al. 1989. Epilepsy with typical absence seizures with onset during the first year of life. *Epilepsia* 30:802–806.

Caveness WF, Meirowski AM, Rish BL, et al. 1979. The nature of post-traumatic epilepsy. *J Neurosurg* 50:545–553.

Celesia GG, Grigg MM, Ross E. 1988. Generalized status myoclonus in acute anoxic and tonic-metabolic encephalopathies. *Arch Neurol* 45:781–784.

Cendes F, Andermann F, Dubeau F, et al. 1993a. Early childhood prolonged febrile convulsions, atrophy and sclerosis of mesial structures, and temporal lobe epilepsy: an MRI volumetric study. *Neurology* 43:1083–1087.

Cendes F, Andermann F, Gloor P, et al. 1993b. Atrophy of mesial structures in patients with temporal lobe epilepsy: cause or consequence of repeated seizures? *Ann Neurol* 34:795–801.

Cendes F, Andermann F, Gloor P, et al. 1993c. MRI volumetric measurement of amygdala and hippocampus in temporal lobe epilepsy. *Neurology* 43:719–725.

Cendes F, Cook MJ, Watson C, et al. 1995. Frequency and characteristics of dual pathology in patients with lesional epilepsy. *Neurology* 45:2058–2064.

Cendes F, Lopes-Cendes I, Andermann E, et al. 1998. Familial temporal lobe epilepsy: a clinically heterogeneous syndrome. *Neurology* 50:554–557.

Cendes F, Li LM, Watson C, et al. 2000. Ictal recording mandatory in temporal lobe epilepsy? Not when the interictal electroencephalogram and hippocampal atrophy coincide. *Arch Neurol* 57:497–500.

Cendes F, Kahane P, Brodie M, Andermann F. 2002. The mesio-temporal lobe epilepsy syndrome. In: Roger J, Bureau M, Dravet C, et al., eds. *Epileptic syndromes in infancy, childhood and adolescence*, 3rd ed. London: John Libbey, 513–530.

Cerullo A, Marini C, Carcangiu R, et al. 1999. Clinical and video-polygraphic features of epileptic spasms in adults with cortical migration disorder. *Epileptic Disord* 1:27–33.

Chabardes S, Kahane P, Minotti L, et al. 2002. Deep brain stimulation in epilepsy with particular reference to the subthalamic nucleus. *Epileptic Disord* 4:83–93.

Chadwick D. 1985. The discontinuation of antiepileptic therapy. In: Pedley TA, Meldrum BS, eds. *Recent advances in epileptology*. Edinburgh: Churchill Livingstone, 111–124.

Chadwick DW. 1987. Valproate monotherapy in the management of generalized and partial seizures. *Epilepsia* 28:S12–S17.

Chadwick DW. 1988. Overuse of monitoring of blood concentrations of antiepileptic drugs. *BMJ* 294:723–724.

Chadwick D. 1991. Epilepsy after first seizures: risks and implications. *J Neurol Neurosurg Psychiatry* 54:385–387.

Chadwick D. 1992. Gabapentin. In: Pedley TA, Meldrum BS, eds. *Recent advances in epileptology*. Edinburgh: Churchill Livingstone, 211–221.

Chadwick DW, Turnbull DM. 1985. The comparative efficacy of anticonvulsant drugs for partial and tonic-clonic seizures. *J Neurol Neurosurg Psychiatry* 48:1073–1077.

Chadwick D, Reynolds EH, Marsden CD. 1976. Anticonvulsant-induced dyskinesias: a comparison with dyskinesias induced by neuroleptics. *J Neurol Neurosurg Psychiatry* 39:1210–1218.

Chadwick D, Shaw MD, Foy P, et al. 1984. Serum anticonvulsant concentrations and the risk of drug-induced skin eruptions. *J Neurol Neurosurg Psychiatry* 47:642–644.

Chamberlain MC. 1996. Nitrazepam for refractory infantile spasms and the Lennox-Gastaut syndrome. *J Child Neurol* 11:31–34.

Chan S, Chin SS, Nordli DR, et al. 1998. Prospective magnetic resonance imaging identification of focal cortical dysplasia, including the non-balloon cell subtype. *Ann Neurol* 44:749–757.

Chandler C. 2000. Posttraumatic seizures and posttraumatic epilepsy. In: Oxbury J, Polkey C, Duchowny M, eds. *Intractable focal epilepsy*. London: WB Saunders, 185–193.

Chandy MJ, Rajshekhar V, Ghosh S, et al. 1991. Single small enhancing lesions in Indian patients with epilepsy: clinical, radiological and pathological considerations. *J Neurol Neurosurg Psychiatry* 54:702–705.

Chang YC, Guo NW, Huang CC, et al. 2001. Neurocognitive attention and behavior outcome of school-age children with a history of febrile convulsions: a population study. *Epilepsia* 41:412–420.

Chaplin ER, Goldstein GW, Norman D. 1979. Neonatal seizures, intracerebral hematoma and subarachnoid hemorrhage in full-term infants. *Pediatrics* 63:812–815.

Charlier C, Singh NA, Ryan SG, et al. 1998. A pore mutation in a novel KQT-like potassium channel gene in an idiopathic epilepsy family. *Nat Genet* 18:53–55.

Charlton MH. 1975. Infantile spasms. In: Charlton MH, ed. *Myoclonic seizures*. Amsterdam: Excerpta Medica.

Chassoux F, Devaux B, Landre E, et al. 2000. Stereoelectroencephalography in focal cortical dysplasias: a 3D approach to delineating the dysplastic cortex. *Brain* 123:1733–1751.

Chauvel P, Louvel J, Lamarche M. 1978. Transcortical reflexes and focal motor epilepsy. *Electroencephalogr Clin Neurophysiol* 45:309–318.

Chauvel P, Vignal JP, Liégeois-Chauvel C, et al. 1987. Startle epilepsy with infantile brain damage: the clinical and neurophysiological rationale for surgical therapy. In: Wieser HG, Eiger CE, eds. *Presurgical evaluation of epileptics.* Berlin: Springer-Verlag, 306–307.

Chauvel P, Dravet C, Dileo M, et al. 1991. The HHE syndrome. In: Lüders H, ed. *Epilepsy surgery.* New York: Raven Press, 183–196.

Chauvel P, Delgado-Escueta AV, Halgren E, et al. 1992a. *Frontal lobe seizures and epilepsies.* New York: Raven Press.

Chauvel P, Trottier S, Vignal JP, et al. 1992b. Somatomotor seizures of frontal lobe origin. In: Chauvel P, Delgado-Escueta AV, Halgren E, et al., eds. *Frontal lobe seizures and epilepsy.* New York: Raven Press, 185–232.

Chauvel P, Kliemann F, Vignal JP, et al. 1995. The clinical signs and symptoms of frontal lobe seizures: phenomenology and classification. In: Jasper HH, Riggio S, Goldman-Rakic PS, eds. *Epilepsy and the functional anatomy of the frontal lobe.* Advances in neurology, Vol. 66. New York: Raven Press, 116–126.

Chayasirisobhon S, Rodin EA. 1981. Atonic-akinetic seizures [Abstract]. *Electroencephalogr Clin Neurophysiol* 50:225.

Chee MW. 2000. Versive seizures. In: Lüders HO, Noachtar S, eds. *Epileptic seizures: pathophysiology and clinical semiology.* Philadelphia: Churchill Livingstone, 433–438.

Chen LS, Wang N, Lin ML. 2002. Seizure outcome in intractable partial epilepsy of children. *Pediatr Neurol* 26: 282–287.

Chernova OB, Somerville RP, Cowell JK. 1998. A novel gene, LGI1, from 10q24 is rearranged and downregulated in malignant brain tumors. *Oncogene* 17:2873–2881.

Cherubini E, Galarsa JL, Ben-Ari Y. 1991. GABA: an excitatory transmitter in early postnatal life. *Trends Neurosci* 14:515–519.

Chevrie JJ, Aicardi J. 1967. Facteurs étiologiques des spasmes en flexion du nourrisson. Etude de 81 cas. *Arch Fr Pediatr* 24:511–520.

Chevrie JJ, Aicardi J. 1971. Le pronostic psychique des spasmes infanties traités par l'ACTH ou les corticoïdes. Analyse statistique de 78 cas suivis plus d'un an. *J Neurol Sci* 12:351–357.

Chevrie JJ, Aicardi J. 1972. Childhood epileptic encephalopathy with slow spike-wave. A statistical study of 80 cases. *Epilepsia* 13:259–271.

Chevrie JJ, Aicardi J. 1975. Duration and lateralization of febrile convulsions. Etiological factors. *Epilepsia* 16: 781–789.

Chevrie JJ, Aicardi J. 1977. Convulsive disorders in the first year of life: etiologic factors. *Epilepsia* 18:489–498.

Chevrie JJ, Aicardi J. 1978. Convulsive disorders in the first year of life: neurologic and mental outcome and mortality. *Epilepsia* 19:67–74.

Chevrie JJ, Aicardi J. 1979. Convulsive disorders in the first year of life: persistence of epileptic seizures. *Epilepsia* 20:643–649.

Chevrie JJ, Aicardi J. 1986. The Aicardi syndrome. In: Pedley TA, Meldrum BS, eds. *Recent advances in epilepsy,* Vol. 3. Edinburgh: Churchill Livingstone, 189–210.

Chevrie JJ, Aicardi J, Goutières F. 1987. Epilepsy in childhood mitochondrial myopathy. In: Wolf P, Dam M, Janz D, et al., eds. *Advances in epileptology,* The XVIth Epilepsy International Symposium. New York: Raven Press, 181–184.

Chevrie JJ, Specola N, Aicardi J. 1988. Secondary bilateral synchrony in unilateral pial angiomatosis: successful surgical treatment. *J Neurol Neurosurg Psychiatry* 51: 663–670.

Chevrie-Muller C, Chevrie JJ, Le Normand MT, et al. 1991. A peculiar case of acquired aphasia with epilepsy in childhood. *J Neurolinguistics* 6:415–431.

Chifari R, Guerrini R, Pierluigi M, et al. 2002. Mild generalized epilepsy and developmental disorder associated with large inv dup(15). *Epilepsia* 43:1096–1100.

Chiron C, Raynaud C, Tzourio N, et al. 1989. Regional cerebral blood flow by SPECT imaging in Sturge-Weber disease: an aid for diagnosis. *J Neurol Neurosurg Psychiatry* 52:1402–1409.

Chiron C, Dulac O, Luna D, et al. 1990. Vigabatrin in infantile spasms. *Lancet* 335:363–364.

Chiron C, Dulac O, Beaumont D, et al. 1991a. Therapeutic trial of vigabatrin in refractory infantile spasms. *J Child Neurol* 6:S52–S59.

Chiron C, Raynaud C, Jambaqué J, et al. 1991b. A serial study of regional cerebral blood flow before and after hemispherectomy in a child. *Epilepsy Res* 8:232–240.

Chiron C, Dulac O, Bulteau C, et al. 1993. Study of regional cerebral blood flow in West syndrome. *Epilepsia* 34: 707–715.

Chiron C, Dumas C, Jambaque I, et al. 1997. Randomised trial comparing vigabatrin and hydrocortisone in infantile spasms due to tuberous sclerosis. *Epilepsy Res* 26:389–395.

Chiron C, Marchand MC, Tran A, et al. 2000. Stiripentol in severe myoclonic epilepsy in infancy: a randomised placebo-controlled syndrome-dedicated trial. STICLO study group. *Lancet* 356:1638–1642.

Chiron C, Véra P, Hollo A, et al. 2001. Ictal SPECT in temporal lobe seizures in children. In: Avanzini G, Beaumanoir A, Mira L, eds. *Limbic seizures in children.* Paris: John Libbey, 217–223.

Chodkiewicz JP, Vignal JP, Mann M, et al. 1988. Surgery for frontal lobe seizures. Sainte Anne Series [Abstract]. *Epilepsia* 29:219.

Chong SS, Pack SD, Roschke AV, et al. 1997. A revision of the lissencephaly and Miller-Dieker syndrome critical regions in chromosome 17p13.3. *Hum Mol Genet* 6: 147–155.

Christiansen C, Rodbro P, Nielsen CT. 1975. Iatrogenic osteomalacia in epileptic children. A controlled therapeutic trial. *Acta Paediatr Scand* 64:219–224.

Christie S, Guberman A, Tansley BW, et al. 1988. Primary reading epilepsy: investigation of critical seizure-provoking stimuli. *Epilepsia* 29:288–293.

Chugani HT, Conti JR. 1996. Etiologic classification of infantile spasms in 140 cases: role of positron emission tomography. *J Child Neurol* 11:44–48.

Chugani HT, Pinard JM. 1994. Surgical treatment. In: Dulac O, Chugani HT, Dalla Bernardina B, eds. *Infantile spasms and West syndrome.* Philadelphia: WB Saunders, 257–264.

Chugani HT, Mazziota JC, Engel J Jr, Phelps ME. 1987. The Lennox-Gastaut syndrome: metabolic subtypes determined by 2-dioxy-2-[^{18}F]fluoro-D-glucose positron emission tomography. *Ann Neurol* 21:4–13.

Chugani HT, Shewmon DA, Peacock WJ, et al. 1988. Surgical treatment of intractable neonatal onset seizures: the role of positron emission tomography. *Neurology* 38: 1178–1188.

Chugani HT, Mazziotta JC, Phelps ME. 1989. Sturge-Weber syndrome: a study of cerebral glucose utilization with positron emission tomography. *J Pediatr* 114:244–253.

Chugani HT, Shields WD, Shewmon DA, et al. 1990. Infantile spasms. I: PET identifies focal cortical dysgenesis in cryptogenic cases for surgical treatment. *Ann Neurol* 27:406–413.

Chugani HT, Shewmon A, Sankar R, et al. 1992. Infantile spasms. II: Lenticular nuclei and brain stem activation on positron emission tomography. *Ann Neurol* 31: 212–219.

Chugani HT, Shewmon DA, Shields WD, et al. 1993. Surgery for intractable infantile spasms: neuroimaging perspectives. *Epilepsia* 34:764–771.

Chugani HT, Da Silva E, Chugani DC. 1996. Infantile spasms. III: Prognostic implications of bitemporal hypometabolism on positron emission tomography. *Ann Neurol* 39:643–649.

Chugani HT, Da Silva E, Chugani DC, et al. 1997. PET in the diagnostic evaluation of children with focal epilepsy. In: Tuxhorn I, Holthausen H, Boenigk H, eds. *Pediatric epilepsy syndromes and their surgical treatment*. London: John Libbey, 592–606.

Chugani DC, Chugani HT, Muzik O, et al. 1998. Imaging epileptogenic tubers in children with tuberous sclerosis complex using α-[^{11}C]methyl-L-tryptophan positron emission tomography. *Ann Neurol* 44:858–866.

Chung S, Ahn C. 1994. Effects of anti-epileptic drug therapy on bone mineral density in ambulatory epileptic children. *Brain Dev* 16:382–385.

Chung MY, Walczak TS, Lewis DV, et al. 1991. Temporal lobectomy and independent bitemporal interictal activity: what degree of lateralization is sufficient? *Epilepsia* 32:195–201.

Ciardo F, Zamponi N, Specchio N, et al. 2001. Autosomal recessive polymicrogyria with infantile spasms and limb deformities. *Neuropediatrics* 32:325–329.

Cirignotta F, Lugaresi E. 1991. Partial motor epilepsy with "negative myoclonus." *Epilepsia* 32:54–58.

Cirignotta F, Cigogna P, Lugaresi E. 1980. Epileptic seizures during card games and draughts. *Epilepsia* 21:137–140.

Cirignotta F, Zucconi M, Mondini S, et al. 1986. Writing epilepsy. *Clin Electroencephalogr* 17:21–23.

Cirignotta F, Baldini MI, Mondini S, et al. 1990. Recurring coma and abnormal behavior-case report. In: Home J, ed. *Sleep '90*. Bochum, The Netherlands: Pontenagel Press, 1–3.

Claes S, Devriendt K, Lagae L, et al. 1997. The X-linked infantile spasms syndrome (MIM 308350) maps to Xp11.4-Xpter in two pedigrees. *Ann Neurol* 42:360–364.

Claes L, Del-Favero J, Ceulemans B, et al. 2001. De novo mutations in the sodium-channel gene *SCN1A* cause severe myoclonic epilepsy of infancy. *Am J Hum Genet* 68:1327–1332.

Clancy RR. 1983. Sharp electroencephalographic transients in neonates with seizures. *Ann Neurol* 14:377–378.

Clancy RR. 1989. Interictal sharp EEG transients in neonatal seizures. *J Child Neurol* 4:30–38.

Clancy RR, Legido A. 1987a. Neurologic outcome after EEG-proven neonatal seizures [Abstract]. *Pediatr Res* 21:489A.

Clancy RR, Legido A. 1987b. The exact ictal and interictal duration of electroencephalographic neonatal seizures. *Epilepsia* 28:537–541.

Clancy RR, Legido A. 1991. Postnatal epilepsy after EEG confirmed neonatal seizures. *Epilepsia* 32:69–76.

Clancy RR, Tharp BR. 1984. Positive rolandic sharp waves in the electroencephalograms of premature neonates with intraventricular hemorrhage. *Electroencephalogr Clin Neurophysiol* 57:395–404.

Clancy RR, Tharp BR, Enzman D. 1984. EEG in premature infants with intraventricular hemorrhage. *Neurology* 34:583–590.

Clancy RR, Malin S, Laraque D, et al. 1985. Focal motor seizures heralding strokes in full-term neonates. *Am J Dis Child* 139:601–606.

Clancy RR, Legido A, Lewis D. 1986. The effect of mental status and ictal duration on the clinical visibility of EEG-proved neonatal seizures [Abstract]. *Ann Neurol* 20:411.

Clancy RR, Legido A, Lewis D. 1988. Occult neonatal seizures. *Epilepsia* 29:256–261.

Clark CR, Geffen GM. 1989. Corpus callosum surgery and recent memory. *Brain* 112:165–175.

Clarke M, Gill J, Noronha M, et al. 1987. Early infantile epileptic encephalopathy with suppression-burst: Ohtahara syndrome. *Dev Med Child Neurol* 29: 520–528.

Clatterbuck RE, Eberhart CG, Crain BJ, et al. 2001. Ultrastructural and immunocytochemical evidence that an incompetent blood-brain barrier is related to the pathophysiology of cavernous malformations. *J Neurol Neurosurg Psychiatry* 71:188–192.

Cleland PG, Mosquera I, Steward WP, Foster JB. 1981. Prognosis of isolated seizures in adult life. *Br Med J (Clin Res Ed)* 283:1364.

Clemens B. 1988. Dopamine agonist treatment of self-induced pattern-sensitive epilepsy: a case report. *Epilepsy Res* 2:340–343.

Cloyd J. 1991. Pharmacokinetic pitfalls of present antiepileptic medications. *Epilepsia* 32:S53–S65.

Cobos JE. 1987. High-dose phenytoin in the treatment of refractory epilepsy. *Epilepsia* 28:111–114.

Cocito L, Maffini M, Perfumo P, et al. 1989. Vigabatrin in complex partial seizures: a long-term study. *Epilepsy Res* 3:160–166.

Cock HR, Shorvon SD. 2002. The spectrum of epilepsy and movement disorders in EPC. In: Guerrini R, Aicardi J, Andermann F, et al., eds. *Epilepsy and movement disorders*. Cambridge: Cambridge University Press, 211–227.

Cockerell OC, Johnson AL, Sander JW, et al. 1994. Mortality from epilepsy: results from a prospective population-based study. *Lancet* 344:918–921.

Cockerell OC, Johnson AL, Sander JW, et al. 1997. Prognosis of epilepsy: a review and further analysis of the first nine years of the British National General Practice Study of Epilepsy, a prospective population-based study. *Epilepsia* 38:31–46.

Cohen RJ, Suter C. 1982. Hysterical seizures: suggestion as a provocative EEG test. *Ann Neurol* 11:391–395.

Cohen BH, Bucy E, Packer RJ, et al. 1989a. Gadolinium-DTPH-enhanced magnetic resonance imaging in childhood brain tumors. *Neurology* 39:1178–1183.

Cohen M, Campbell R, Yaghmai F. 1989b. Neuropathological abnormalities in developmental dysphasia. *Ann Neurol* 25:567–570.

Coker SB. 1986. The use of phenacemide for intractable partial complex epilepsy in children. *Pediatr Neurol* 2: 230–232.

Colamaria V, Plouin P, Dulac O, et al. 1988. Kojewnikow's epilepsia partialis continua: two cases associated with striatal necrosis. *Neurophysiol Clin* 18:535–539.

Colamaria V, Sgro V, Caraballo R, et al. 1991. Status epilepticus in benign rolandic epilepsy manifesting as anterior opercular syndrome. *Epilepsia* 32:329–334.

Cole AJ, Andermann F, Taylor L, et al. 1988. The Landau-Kleffner syndrome of acquired epileptic aphasia: unusual clinical outcome, surgical experience and absence of encephalitis. *Neurology* 38:31–38.

Coleman M. 1971. Infantile spasms associated with 5-hydroxytryptophan administration in patients with Down's syndrome. *Neurology* 21:911–914.

Coleman M, Hart PN, Randall J, et al. 1977. Serotonin levels in the blood and central nervous system of a patient with sudanophilic leukodystrophy. *Neuropédiatrie* 8: 459–466.

Collaborative Group for the Study of Epilepsy. 1992. Prognosis of epilepsy in newly referred patients: a multicenter prospective study of the effects of monotherapy on the long-term course of epilepsy. *Epilepsia* 33:45–51.

Collings JA. 1990. Psychosocial well-being and epilepsy: an empirical study. *Epilepsia* 31:418–426.

Collins RC, Lothman EW, Olney JW. 1983. Status epilepticus in the limbic system: biochemical and pathological changes. In: Delgado-Escueta AV, Wasterlain CG, Treiman DM, Porter RJ, eds. *Status epilepticus: mechanisms of brain damage and treatment*. Advances in neurology, Vol. 34. New York: Raven Press, 277–287.

Commander M, Green SH, Prendergast M. 1991. Behavioural disturbances in children treated with clonazepam. *Dev Med Child Neurol* 33:362–363.

Commission on Classification and Terminology of the International League Against Epilepsy. 1981. Proposal for revised clinical and electroencephalographic classification of epileptic seizures. *Epilepsia* 22:489–501.

Commission on Classification and Terminology of the International League Against Epilepsy. 1985. Proposal for classification of epilepsies and epileptic syndromes. *Epilepsia* 26:268–278.

Commission on Classification and Terminology of the International League Against Epilepsy. 1989. Proposal for revised classification of epilepsy and epileptic syndromes. *Epilepsia* 30:389–399.

Commission on Neuroimaging of the International League Against Epilepsy. 1997. Recommendations for neuroimaging of patients with epilepsy. *Epilepsia* 38: 1255–1266.

Committee on Obstetric Practice and American Academy of Pediatrics: Committee on Fetus and Newborn. 1996. ACOG committee opinion. Use and abuse of Apgar score. Number 174-July 1996. American College of Obstetricians and Gynecologists. *Int J Gynaecol Obstet* 54:303–305.

Commission on Pediatric Epilepsy of the International League of Epilepsy. 1992. Workshop on infantile spasms. *Epilepsia* 33:195.

Congdon P, Forsythe W. 1980. Intravenous clonazepam in treatment of status epilepticus in children. *Epilepsia* 21:97–102.

Connell JA, Oozier R, de Vries L, et al. 1989. Continuous EEG monitoring of neonatal seizures: diagnostic and prognostic considerations. *Arch Dis Child* 64:452–458.

Connelly A, Jackson GD, Frackowiak RS, et al. 1993. Functional mapping of activated human primary cortex with a clinical MR imaging system. *Radiology* 188:125–130.

Connolly MB, Jan JE, Junker AK. 1991. Intravenous immunoglobulin and pyridoxine-dependent seizures. *Neurology* 41:1524.

Consensus Development Panel. 1980. Febrile seizures: long-term management of children with fever-associated seizures. *Pediatrics* 66:1009–1012.

Constantinou JE, Gillis J, Ouvrier RA, Rahilly PM. 1989. Hypoxic-ischaemic encephalopathy after near-miss sudden infant death syndrome. *Arch Dis Child.* 64:703–708.

Cook M, Stevens JM. 1995. Imaging in epilepsy. In: Hopkins A, Shorvon S, Cascino G, eds. *Epilepsy*. London: Chapman and Hall, 143–169.

Cook MJ, Fish DR, Shorvon SD, et al. 1992. Hippocampal volumetric and morphometric studies in frontal and temporal lobe epilepsy. *Brain* 115:1001–1016.

Cooper GW, Lee SI. 1991. Reactive occipital epileptiform activity: is it benign? *Epilepsia* 32:63–68.

Copeland GP, Foy PM, Shaw MD. 1982. The incidence of epilepsy after ventricular shunting operations. *Surg Neurol* 17:279–281.

Coppola G, Plouin P, Chiron C, et al. 1995. Migrating partial seizures in infancy: a malignant disorder with developmental arrest. *Epilepsia* 36:1017–1024.

Corbett JA. 1991. Epilepsy and mental retardation. In: Dam M, Gram L, eds. *Comprehensive epileptology*. New York: Raven Press, 271–280.

Corda D, Gélisse P, Genton P, et al. 2001. Incidence of drug-induced aggravation in benign epilepsy with centrotemporal spikes. *Epilepsia* 42:754–759.

Corey LA, Berg K, Pellock JM, et al. 1991. The occurrence of epilepsy and febrile seizures in Virginian and Norwegian twins. *Neurology* 41:1433–1436.

Cornblath M, Schwartz R. 1967. *Disorders of carbohydrate metabolism in infancy*. Philadelphia: WB Saunders.

Cornford ME, McCormick G. 1997. Adult onset temporal lobe epilepsy associated with smoldering herpes simplex 2 infection. *Neurology* 48:425–430.

Correa S. 1987. Locus of control in children with epilepsy. *Psychol Rep* 60:9–10.

Corsellis JAN, Bruton CJ. 1983. Neuropathology of status epilepticus in humans. In: Delgado-Escueta AV, Wasterlain CG, Treiman DM, Porter RJ, eds. *Status epilepticus: mechanisms of brain damage and treatment*. Advances in neurology, Vol. 34. New York: Raven Press, 129–139.

Cosgrove M, Pople S, Wallace SJ. 1990. Rapid anti-epileptic drug assay. *Dev Med Child Neurol* 32:796–799.

Cossette P, Riviello JJ, Carmant L. 1999. ACTH versus vigabatrin therapy in infantile spasms: a retrospective study. *Neurology* 52:1691–1694.

Cossette P, Liu L, Brisebois K, et al. 2002. Mutation of GABRA1 in an autosomal dominant form of juvenile myoclonic epilepsy. *Nat Genet* 31:184–189.

Costeff H, Avni A. 1982. Reported seizures in early childhood. A 14-year follow-up. *Dev Med Child Neurol* 24: 472–478.

Coulter DL. 1984. Partial seizures with apnea and bradycardia. *Arch Neurol* 41:173–174.

Coulter DL. 1986. Continuous infantile spasms as a form of status epilepticus. *J Child Neurol* 1:215–217.

Coulter DL. 1991. Carnitine, valproate and toxicity. *J Child Neurol* 6:7–14.

Coulter DA. 1995. Neurophysiological studies in animal models of absences. In: Duncan JS, Panayiotopoulos CP, eds. *Typical absences and related syndromes*. London: Churchill Communication Europe, 19–28.

Coulter DA, Huguenard JR, Prince DA. 1990. Differential effects of petit mal anticonvulsants on thalamic neurones: calcium current reduction. *Br J Pharmacol* 100:800–806.

Courjon J, Mauguière F. 1982. L'EEG dans les épilepsies post-traumatiques. *Bolletino Lega Italiana contre l'Epilepsia* 39:19–22.

Covanis A, Jeavons PM. 1980. Once daily sodium valproate in the treatment of epilepsy. *Dev Med Child Neurol* 22: 202–204.

Covanis A, Gupta AK, Jeavons PM. 1982. Sodium valproate: monotherapy and polytherapy. *Epilepsia* 23:693–720.

Cowan LD, Hudson LS. 1991. The epidemiology and natural history of infantile spasms. *J Child Neurol* 6:355–364.

Craig WS. 1960. Convulsive movements occurring in the first ten days of life. *Arch Dis Child* 35:336–344.

Craig HD, Gunel M, Cepeda O, et al. 1998. Multilocus linkage identifies two new loci for a mendelian form of stroke, cerebral cavernous malformation, at 7p15-13 and 3q25.2-27. *Hum Mol Genet* 7:1851–1858.

Crandall PH. 1982. Recent developments in the diagnosis and therapy of epilepsy: alternate therapy. Surgery for epilepsy. *Ann Intern Med* 97:590–591.

Crandall PH, Engel J Jr, Rausch R. 1983. Indications for depth electrode recordings in complex partial epilepsy and subsequent surgical results. In: Rose CF, ed. *Research progress in epilepsy*. London: Pitman, 507–526.

Cranford RE, Leppik IE, Patrick B, et al. 1979. Intravenous phenytoin in acute treatment of seizures. *Neurology* 29: 1474–1479.

Crawford P, Chadwick D. 1986. A comparative study of progabide, valproate and placebo as add-on therapy in patients with refractory epilepsy. *J Neurol Neurosurg Psychiatry* 49:1251–1257.

Crawford TO, Mitchell WG, Fishman LS, et al. 1988. Very high-dose phenobarbital for refractory status epilepticus in children. *Neurology* 38:1035–1040.

Crichton JU. 1966. Infantile spasms and skin anomalies. *Dev Med Child Neurol* 8:273–275.

Crichton J. 1969. Infantile spasms in children of low birth weight. *Dev Med Child Neurol* 10:36–41.

Critchley M. 1951. Types of visual perseveration: "palinopsia" and "illusory visual spread." *Brain* 74:267–299.

Critchley M. 1966. *The parietal lobes*. New York: Hafner.

Critchley M. 1977. Musicogenic epilepsy. In: Critchley M, Henson RA, eds. *Music and the brain*. London: Heineman, 344–353.

Croft RD, Jervis M. 1989. Munchausen syndrome in a 4-year old. *Arch Dis Child* 64:740–741.

Croona C, Kihlgren M, Lundberg S, et al. 1999. Neuropsychological findings in children with benign childhood epilepsy with centrotemporal spikes. *Dev Med Child Neurol* 41:813–818.

Cross JH, Gordon I, Jackson GD, et al. 1995. Children with intractable focal epilepsy: ictal and interictal 99TcM HMPAO single photon emission computed tomography. *Dev Med Child Neurol* 37:673–681.

Cross JH, Boyd SG, Gordon N, et al. 1997. Ictal cerebral perfusion related to EEG in intractable focal epilepsy of childhood. *J Neurol Neurosurg Psychiatry* 62:377–384.

Crumrine PK. 2000. Vagal nerve stimulation in children. *Semin Pediatr Neurol* 7:216–223.

Cukier F, André M, Monod N, Dreyfus-Brisac C. 1972. Apport de l'EEG au diagnostic des hémorragies intraventriculaires du prématuré. *Rev Electroencephalogr Neurophysiol Clin* 2:318–322.

Cukier F, Sfaello Z, Dreyfus-Brisac C. 1976. Les états de mal du nouveau-né à terme et du prématuré dans un centre de réanimation néonatale. Aspects cliniques, électroencéphalographiques et évolution. *Gaslini* 8: 100–106.

Curatolo P. 1996. Tuberous sclerosis: relationships between clinical and EEG findings and magnetic resonance imaging. In: Guerrini R, Andermann F, Canapicchi R, et al., eds. *Dysplasias of cerebral cortex and epilepsy*. Philadelphia: Lippincott-Raven, 191–198.

Curatolo P, Cusmai R. 1988. MRI in Bourneville disease: relationship with EEG findings. *Neurophysiol Clin* 18: 149–157.

Curatolo P, Cusmai R, Finocchi G, Boscherini B. 1984. Gelastic epilepsy and true precocious puberty due to hypothalamic hamartoma. *Dev Med Child Neurol* 26: 509–514.

Curatolo P, Cusmai R, Cortesi F, et al. 1987. Neuropsychiatric aspects of tuberous sclerosis. *Ann N Y Acad Sci* 615:8–16.

Curatolo P, Seri S, Verdecchia M, et al. 2001. Infantile spasms in tuberous sclerosis complex. *Brain Dev* 23: 502–507.

Curless RG, Holzman BH, Ramsay R. 1983. Paraldehyde therapy in childhood status epilepticus. *Arch Neurol* 40:477–480.

Currie S, Heathfield K, Henson R, et al. 1971. Clinical course and prognosis of temporal lobe epilepsy. *Brain* 94:173–190.

Currier RD, Kooi KA, Sandman LJ. 1963. Prognosis of pure petit mal: a follow-up study. *Neurology* 13:959–967.

Curtis PD, Matthews TG, Clarke TA, et al. 1988. Neonatal seizures: the Dublin Collaborative Study. *Arch Dis Child* 63:1065–1068.

Cusmai R, Dulac O, Diebler C. 1988. Lésions focales dans les spasmes infantiles. *Neurophysiol Clin* 18:235–241.

Czochauska J, Langer-Tyszka B, Losiowski Z, et al. 1994. Children who develop epilepsy in the first year of life: a prospective study. *Dev Med Child Neurol* 26:425–437.

D'Alessandro R, Ferrara R, Benassi G, et al. 1988. Computed tomographic scans in post-traumatic epilepsy. *Arch Neurol* 45:42–43.

D'Alessandro R, Piccirilli M, Tracci C, et al. 1990. Neuropsychological features of benign partial epilepsy of children. *Italian Journal of Neurologic Science* 11: 265–269.

Da Silva M, McArdle B, McGowan M, et al. 1989. Monotherapy for newly diagnosed childhood epilepsy: a comparative trial and prognostic evaluation [Abstract]. *Epilepsia* 30:662A.

Dabora SL, Jozwiak S, Franz DN, et al. 2001. Mutational analysis in a cohort of 224 tuberous sclerosis patients indicates increased severity of TSC2, compared with TSC1, disease in multiple organs. *Am J Hum Genet* 68: 64–80.

Dahl J, Melin L, Brorson L, et al. 1985. Effects of a broad-spectrum behavior modification treatment program on children with refractory epileptic seizures. *Epilepsia* 26:303–309.

Dahl J, Melin L, Leissner P. 1988. Effects of a behavioural intervention on epileptic seizure behaviour and paroxysmal activity: a systematic replication of three cases of children with intractable epilepsy. *Epilepsia* 29: 172–183.

Dalby MA. 1969. Epilepsy and 3 per second spike and wave rhythms, a clinical, EEG and prognostic analysis of 346 patients. *Acta Neurol Scand Suppl* 40:1–183.

Dalla Bernardina B, Beghini G. 1976. Rolandic spikes in children with and without epilepsy (20 subjects polygraphically studied during sleep). *Epilepsia* 17: 161–167.

Dalla Bernardina B, Tassinari CA. 1975. EEG of a nocturnal seizure in a patient with benign epilepsy of childhood with rolandic spikes. *Epilepsia* 16:497–501.

Dalla Bernardina B, Watanabe K. 1994. Interictal EEG: variations and pitfalls. In: Dulac O, Chugani HT, Dalla Bernardina B, eds. *Infantile spasms and West syndrome*. Philadelphia: WB Saunders, 63–81.

Dalla Bernardina B, Plouin P, Lerique A, et al. 1978a. Aspects électrocliniques des crises survenant dans les deux premières années de la vie. *Boll Lego It Epil* 22/ 23:137–144.

Dalla Bernardina B, Tassinari CA, Bureau M, et al. 1978b. Epilepsie partielle et état de mal électroencéphalographique pendant le sommeil. *Rev Electroencephalogr Neurophysiol Clin* 8:350–353.

Dalla Bernardina B, Bureau M, Dravet C, et al. 1980. Epilepsie bénigne de l'enfant avec crises à Séméiologie affective. *Rev Electroencephalogr Neurophysiol Clin* 10:8–18.

Dalla Bernardina B, Capovilla G, Gattoni MB, et al. 1982. Epilepsie myoclonique grave de la première année. *Rev Electroencephalogr Neurophysiol Clin* 12:21–25.

Dalla Bernardina B, Colamaria V, Capovilla G, et al. 1983a. Nosological classification of epilepsies in the first three years of life. In: Nistico G, Di Perri R, Meinardi H, eds. *Epilepsy: an update on research and therapy*. New York: Alan R. Liss,165–183.

Dalla Bernardina B, Dulac O, Fejerman N, et al. 1983b. Early myoclonic epileptic encephalopathy (EMEE). *Eur J Pediatr* 140:248–252.

Dalla Bernardina B, Chiamenti C, Capovilla G, et al. 1985a. Benign partial epilepsy with affective symptoms (benign psychomotor epilepsy). In: Roger J, Dravet C, Bureau M, et al., eds. *Epileptic syndromes in infancy, childhood and adolescence*. London: John Libbey, 171–175.

Dalla Bernardina B, Colamaria V, Capovilla G, et al. 1985b. Sleep and benign partial epilepsies of childhood. In: Degen R, Niedermeyer E, eds. *Epilepsy: sleep and sleep deprivation*. Amsterdam: Elsevier Science, 119–123.

Dalla Bernardina B, Capovilla G, Chiamenti C, et al. 1987. Cryptogenic myoclonic epilepsies of infancy and early childhood: nosological and prognostic approach. In: Wolf P, Dam M, Janz D, Dreifuss FE, eds. *Advances in epileptology*, Vol. 16. New York: Raven Press, 175–179.

Dalla Bernardina B, Fontana E, Sgro V, et al. 1990. Generalized or partial atonic seizures—inhibitory seizures in children with partial epilepsies. *Electroencephalogr Clin Neurophysiol* 75:S31–S32.

Dalla Bernardina B, Colamaria V, Chiamenti C, et al. 1992a. Benign partial epilepsy with affective symptoms (benign psychomotor epilepsy). In: Roger J, Bureau M, Dravet C, et al., eds. *Epileptic syndromes in infancy,* *childhood and adolescence*, 2nd ed. London: John Libbey, 219–223.

Dalla Bernardina B, Fontana E, Sgro V, et al. 1992b. Myoclonic epilepsy ('myoclonic status') in non-progressive encephalopathies. In: Roger J, Bureau M, Dravet C, et al., eds. *Epileptic syndromes in infancy, childhood and adolescence*, 2nd ed. London: John Libbey, 89–96.

Dalla Bernardina B, Sgro V, Fontana E, et al. 1992c. Idiopathic partial epilepsies in children. In: Roger J, Bureau M, Dravet C, et al., eds. *Epileptic syndromes in infancy, childhood and adolescence*, 2nd ed. London: John Libbey, 173–188.

Dalla Bernardina B, Zullini E, Fontana E, et al. 1992d. Sindrome di Angelman: studio EEG-poligrafico di 8 casi. *Bolletino Lega Italiana contre l'Epilepsia* 79/80: 257–259.

Dalla Bernardina B, Fontana E, Darra F. 2002. Myoclonic epilepsy ('myoclonic status') in non-progressive encephalopathies. In: Roger J, Bureau M, Dravet C, et al., eds. *Epileptic syndromes in infancy, childhood and adolescence,* 3rd ed. London: John Libbey, 137–144.

Daly DD. 1982. Complex partial seizures. In: Laidlaw J, Richens A, eds. *A textbook of epilepsy*, 2nd ed. Edinburgh: Churchill Livingstone, 131–144.

Daly DD, Markand ON. 1990. Focal brain lesions. In: Daly DD, Pedley JP, eds. *Current practice of clinical electroencephalography*, 2nd ed. New York: Raven Press, 335–370.

Daly DD, Pedley TA, eds. 1990. *Current practice of clinical electroencephalography*, 2nd ed. New York: Raven Press.

Dan NG, Wade MJ. 1986. The incidence of epilepsy after ventricular shunting procedures. *J Neurosurg* 65:19–21.

Daniele O, Mattaliano A, Natale E. 1987. Bimodal sensory stimulation-induced seizures. *Acta Neurol Scand* 76: 297–301.

Darby CE, De Korte RA, Binnie CD, Wilkins AJ. 1980. The self-induction of epileptic seizures by eye-closure. *Epilepsia* 21:31–41.

Dasheiff RM, McNamara D, Dickinson L. 1986. Efficacy of second line antiepileptic drugs in the treatment of patients with medically refractive complex partial seizures. *Epilepsia* 27:124–127.

Datta AN, Wirrell EC. 2000. Prognosis of seizures occurring in the first year. *Pediatr Neurol* 22:386–391.

Daumas-Duport C, Scheithauer BW, Chodkiewicz JP, et al. 1988. Dysembryoplastic neuroepithelial tumor: a surgically curable tumor of young patients with intractable partial seizures. Report of thirty-nine cases. *Neurosurgery* 23:545–556.

Davenport WJ, Siegel AM, Dichgans J, et al. 2001. CCM1 gene mutations in families segregating cerebral cavernous malformations. *Neurology* 56:540–543.

Davidoff RA, Johnson LC. 1963. Photic activation and photoconvulsive responses in a nonepileptic subject. *Neurology* 13:617–621.

Davidson S, Falloner MA. 1975. Outcome of surgery in 40 children with temporal lobe epilepsy. *Lancet* 1: 1260–1263.

Davidson S, Watson CW. 1956. Hereditary light sensitive epilepsy. *Neurology* 6:235–261.

Davies AG, Mutchie KD, Thompson JA, et al. 1981. Once daily dosing with phenobarbital in children with seizure disorders. *Pediatrics* 68:824–826.

Davis JM, Metrakos K, Apanda JV. 1986. Apnoea and seizures. *Arch Dis Child* 61:791–806.

De Falco FA, Majello L, Santangelo R, et al. 2001. Epileptic phenotypes associated with mitochondrial disorders. *Neurology* 56:1340–1446.

De Feo MR, Mecarelli O, Ricci G, et al. 1991. The utility of ambulatory EEG monitoring in typical absence seizures. *Brain Dev* 13:223–227.

De Fusco M, Becchetti A, Patrignani A, et al. 2000. The nicotinic receptor a2 subunit is mutated in nocturnal frontal lobe epilepsy. *Nat Genet* 26:275–276.

De Giorgio CM, Tomiyasu J, Gott PS, et al. 1992. Hippocampal pyramidal cell loss in human status epilepticus. *Epilepsia* 33:23–27.

De Lanerolle NC, Brines ML, Kim JH. 1992. Neurochemical remodeling of the hippocampus in human temporal lobe epilepsy. *Epilepsy Res Suppl* 9:205–220.

De Marco P, Lorenzin G. 1990. Growing bilateral occipital calcifications and epilepsy. *Brain Dev* 12:342–344.

De Marco P, Tassinari CA. 1981. Extreme somatosensory evoked potential (ESEP): an EEG sign forecasting the possible occurrence of seizures in children. *Epilepsia* 22:569–575.

de Menezes MA, Rho JM. 2002. Clinical and electrographic features of epileptic spasms persisting beyond the second year of life. *Epilepsia* 43:623–630.

De Negri M. 1993. Landau-Kleffner syndrome: some suggestions. *Arch Neurol* 50:896.

De Negri M, Baglietto MG, Biancheri R. 1993. Electrical status epilepticus in childhood: treatment with short cycles of high dosage benzodiazepine (preliminary note). *Brain Dev* 15:311–312.

De Negri M, Baglietto MG, Battaglia FM, et al. 1995. Treatment of electrical status epilepticus by short diazepam (DZP) cycles after DZP rectal bolus test. *Brain Dev* 17:330–333.

De Negri M, Baglietto MG, Gaggero R. 1997. Benzodiazepine (BDZ) treatment of benign childhood epilepsy with centrotemporal spikes (BECCT). *Brain Dev* 19:506.

De Rijk-van Andel JF, Arts WF, Hofman A, et al. 1991. Epidemiology of lissencephaly type I. *Neuroepidemiology* 10:200–204.

De Saint Martin A, Petiau C, Massa R, et al. 1999. Idiopathic rolandic epilepsy with "interictal" facial myoclonia and oromotor deficit: a longitudinal EEG and PET study. *Epilepsia* 40:614–620.

De Saint Martin A, Carcangiu R, Arzimanoglou A, et al. 2001. Semiology of typical and atypical rolandic epilepsy: a video-EEG analysis. *Epileptic Disord* 3:173–182.

De Toffol B. 2001. *Syndromes épileptiques et troubles psychotiques.* Paris: John Libbey Eurotext.

De Vivo DC. 1983. How to use other drugs (steroids) and the ketogenic diet. In: Morselli PL, Pippenger CE, Penry JK, eds. *Antiepileptic drugs in pediatrics.* New York: Raven Press, 283–291.

De Vivo DC, Trifiletti RR, Jacobson RI, et al. 1991. Defective glucose across the blood-brain barrier as a cause of persistent hypoglycorrhachia, seizures and developmental delay. *N Engl J Med* 325:703–709.

De Vivo DC, Burke C, Trifiletti RR, et al. 1994. Glucose transporter protein deficiency: an emerging syndrome with therapeutic implications [Abstract]. *Ann Neurol* 36:491.

De Vivo DC, Garcia Alvarez M, Ronen G. 1995. Glucose transporter protein deficiency: an emerging syndrome with therapeutic implications. *Inf Pediatr* 10:51–56.

De Weerdt CJ, Hooghwinkel GJ. 1976. Congenital retarded

myelination in a newborn child with infantile spasms. *Clin Neurol Neurosurg* 79:143–150.

Dean JC, Penry JK. 1988a. Carbamazepine/valproate therapy in 100 patients with partial seizures failing carbamazepine monotherapy: long-term follow-up [Abstract]. *Epilepsia* 29:687.

Dean JC, Penry JK. 1988b. Valproate monotherapy in 30 patients with partial seizures. *Epilepsia* 29:140–144.

Degen R. 1978. Epilepsy in children. An etiological study based on their obstetrical records. *J Neurol* 217:145–158.

Degen R, Degen HE. 1984. Sleep and sleep deprivation in epileptology. In: Degen R, Niedermeyer E, eds. *Epilepsy: sleep and sleep deprivation.* Amsterdam: Elsevier, 273–286.

Degen R, Degen HE. 1990. Some genetic aspects of rolandic epilepsy: waking and sleep EEGs in siblings. *Epilepsia* 31:795–801.

Degen R, Degen HE, Roth CH. 1990. Some genetic aspects of idiopathic and symptomatic absence seizures: waking and sleep EEGs in siblings. *Epilepsia* 31:784–794.

Degen R, Degen HE, Hans R. 1991. A contribution to the genetics of febrile seizures: waking and sleep EEG in siblings. *Epilepsia* 32:515–522.

Degen R, Ebner A, Lahl R, et al. 2002. Various findings in surgically treated epilepsy patients with dysembryoplastic neuroepithelial tumors in comparison with those of patients with other low-grade brain tumors and other neuronal migration disorders. *Epilepsia* 43:1379–1384.

Dehan M, Quilleron D, Navelet Y, et al. 1977. Les convulsions du cinquième jour de vie: un nouveau syndrome? *Arch Fr Pediatr* 34:730–742.

Del Giudice E, Aicardi J. 1979. Hypertensive encephalopathy in children. *Neuropadiatrie* 10:150–157.

Delabar JM, Theophile D, Rahmani Z, et al. 1993. Molecular mapping of twenty-four features of Down syndrome on chromosome 21. *Eur J Hum Genet* 1:114–124.

Delalande O, Pinard JM, Basdevant C, et al. 1992. Hemispherotomy: a new procedure for central disconnection [Abstract]. *Epilepsia* 33(Suppl. 3):99–100.

Delgado MR, Riela AR, Mills J, et al. 1996. Discontinuation of antiepileptic drug treatment after two seizure-free years in children with cerebral palsy. *Pediatrics* 97:192–197.

Delgado-Escueta AV. 1979. Epileptogenic paroxysms: modern approaches and clinical correlations. *Neurology* 29:1014–1022.

Delgado-Escueta AV, Enrile-Bacsal F. 1984. Juvenile myoclonic epilepsy of Janz. *Neurology* 34:285–294.

Delgado-Escueta AV, Walsh GO. 1983. The selection process for surgery of intractable complex partial seizures: surface EEG and depth electrography. In: Ward AA Jr, Penry JK, Purpura D, eds. *Epilepsy.* New York: Raven Press, 295–326.

Delgado-Escueta AV, Walsh GO. 1985. Type I complex partial seizures of hippocampal origin: excellent results of anterior temporal lobectomy. *Neurology* 35:143–154.

Delgado-Escueta AV, Kunze U, Waddell G, et al. 1977. Lapse of consciousness and automatisms in temporal lobe epilepsy: a videotape analysis. *Neurology* 27:144–155.

Delgado-Escueta AV, Enrile-Bacsal F, Treiman DM. 1982a. Complex partial seizures on closed-circuit television and EEG: a study of 691 attacks in 79 patients. *Ann Neurol* 11:292–300.

Delgado-Escueta AV, Treiman DM, Enrile-Bacsal F. 1982b. Phenotypic variations of seizures in adolescents and adults. In: Anderson VE, Hause WA, Penry JK, et al., eds. *Genetic basis of the epilepsies*. New York: Raven Press, 49–81.

Delgado-Escueta AV, Treiman DM, Walsh GO. 1983a. The treatable epilepsies. *N Engl J Med* 308:1508–1514.

Delgado-Escueta AV, Wasterlain CG, Treiman DM, Porter RJ. 1983b. *Status epilepticus: mechanisms of brain damage and treatment*. Advances in neurology, Vol. 34. New York: Raven Press.

Delgado-Escueta AV, Swartz BE, Maldonado HM, et al. 1987. Complex partial seizures of frontal lobe origin. In: Wieser HG, Elger CE, eds. *Presurgical evaluation of epileptics*. Berlin: Springer-Verlag, 267–299.

Delgado-Escueta AV, Greenberg D, Weissbecker K, et al. 1990a. Gene mapping in the idiopathic generalized epilepsies: juvenile myoclonic epilepsy, childhood absence epilepsy, epilepsy with grand mal seizures and early childhood myoclonic epilepsy. *Epilepsia* 31:S19–S29.

Delgado-Escueta AV, Greenberg D, Weissbecker K, et al. 1990b. Gene mapping in the idiopathic generalized epilepsies: juvenile myoclonic epilepsy, childhood absence epilepsy, epilepsy with grand mal seizures, and early childhood myoclonic epilepsy. *Epilepsia* 31:S19–S29.

Delgado-Escueta AV, Greenberg DA, Treiman L, et al. 1990c. Mapping the gene for juvenile myoclonic epilepsy. *Epilepsia* 30:S8–S18.

Delgado-Escueta AV, Alonso ME, Medina MT, et al. 2000. The search for epilepsy genes in juvenile myoclonus epilepsy: discoveries along the way. In: Schmitz B, Sander T, eds. *Juvenile myoclonic epilepsy: the Janz syndrome*. Petersfield: Wrightson Biomedical Publishing, 145–171.

Delgado-Escueta AV, Ganesh S, Yamakawa K. 2001. Advances in the genetics of progressive myoclonus epilepsy. *Am J Med Genet* 106:129–138.

Delgado-Escueta AV, Ganesh S, Suzuki T, et al. 2002. Lafora's progressive myoclonus epilepsy: clinical and genetic advances. *Brain Dev* 24:355–356.

Delivoria-Papadopoulos M, Younkin DP, Chance B. 1990. Cerebral metabolic studies during neonatal seizures with 31-P NMR spectroscopy. In: Wasterlain CG, Vert P, eds. *Neonatal seizures*. New York: Raven Press, 181–189.

DeLong GR, Heinz ER. 1997. The clinical syndrome of early-life bilateral hippocampal sclerosis. *Ann Neurol* 42:11–17.

DeLorenzo RJ, Pellock JM, Towne R, et al. 1995. Epidemiology of status epilepticus. *J Clin Neurophysiol* 12:316–325.

DeLorenzo RJ, Hauser WA, Towner AR, et al. 1996. A prospective, population-based epidemiologic study of status epilepticus in Richmond, Virginia. *Neurology* 46:1029–1035.

Demierre B, Stichnoth FA, Hori A, et al. 1986. Intracerebral ganglioglioma. *J Neurosurg* 65:177–182.

Dennis J. 1978. Neonatal convulsions: aetiology, late neonatal status and long-term outcome. *Dev Med Child Neurol* 20:143–158.

Deonna T. 1983. Rectal diazepam in the management of febrile convulsions. *Dev Med Child Neurol* 25:256–257.

Deonna T. 1991. Acquired epileptiform aphasia in children (Landau-Kleffner syndrome). *J Clin Neurophysiol* 8:288–298.

Deonna T. 1996. Epilepsies with cognitive symptomatology. In: Wallace S, ed. *Epilepsy in children*. London: Chapman Medical, 315–322.

Deonna T. 2000. Rolandic epilepsy: neuropsychology of the active epilepsy phase. *Epileptic Disord* 2:S59–S62.

Deonna T, Despland PA. 1989. Sensory-evoked (touch) idiopathic myoclonic epilepsy of infancy. In: Beaumanoir A, Gastaut H, Naquet R, eds. *Reflex seizures and reflex epilepsies*. Genève: Médecine et Hygiène, 99–102.

Deonna T, Martin D. 1981. Benign paroxysmal torticollis in infancy. *Arch Dis Child* 56:956–959.

Deonna T, Prod'hom LS. 1980. Temporal lobe epilepsy and hemianopsia in childhood of perinatal origin. An overlooked and potentially treatable disease? Report of two cases, one with a demonstrable etiology. *Neuropédiatrie* 11:85–90.

Deonna T, Roulet E. 1991. Treatment of acquired aphasia and epilepsy. *Dev Med Child Neurol* 33:834–835.

Deonna T, Ziegler AL. 2000. Hypothalamic hamartoma, precocious puberty and gelastic seizures: a special model of "epileptic" developmental disorders. *Epileptic Disord* 2:33–37.

Deonna T, Beaumanoir A, Gaillard F, et al. 1977. Acquired aphasia in childhood with seizure disorder: a heterogeneous syndrome. *Neuropédiatrie* 8:263–273.

Deonna T, Fletcher P, Voumard C. 1982. Temporary regression during language acquisition: a linguistic analysis of a 2½-year old child with epileptic aphasia. *Dev Med Child Neurol* 24:156–163.

Deonna T, Ziegler AL, Despland PA. 1984. Paroxysmal visual disturbances of epileptic origin and occipital epilepsy in children. *Neuropediatrics* 15:131–135.

Deonna T, Ziegler AL, Despland PA. 1986a. Combined myoclonic-astatic and "benign" focal epilepsy of childhood ("atypical benign partial epilepsy of childhood"). A separate syndrome? *Neuropediatrics* 17:144–151.

Deonna T, Ziegler AL, Despland PA, et al. 1986b. Partial epilepsy in neurologically normal children: clinical syndromes and prognosis. *Epilepsia* 27:241–247.

Deonna T, Peter C, Ziegler AL. 1989. Adult follow-up of the acquired aphasia-epilepsy syndrome in childhood. Report of 7 cases. *Neuropediatrics* 20:132–138.

Deonna T, Ziegler AL, Mouna-Serra J, et al. 1993. Autistic regression in relation to limbic pathology and epilepsy: report of two cases. *Dev Med Child Neurol* 33:166–176.

Deonna T, Zediger P, Davidoff V, et al. 2000a. Benign partial epilepsy of childhood: a longitudinal neuropsychological and EEG study of cognitive function. *Dev Med Child Neurol* 42:595–603.

Deonna T, Fohler M, Jalin C, et al. 2001. Epileptic stereotypies in children. In: Guerrini R, Aicardi J, Andermann F, Hallett M, eds. *Epilepsy and movement disorders*. Cambridge: Cambridge University Press, 319–332.

Des Portes V, Pinard JM, Billuart P, et al. 1998. A novel CNS gene required for neuronal migration and involved in X-linked subcortical laminar heterotopia and lissencephaly syndrome. *Cell* 92:51–61.

Desbiens R, Berkovic SF, Dubeau F, et al. 1993. Life-threatening focal status epilepticus due to occult cortical dysplasia. *Arch Neurol* 50:695–700.

Deshmukh A, Wittert W, Schnitzler E, et al. 1986. Lorazepam in the treatment of refractory neonatal seizures: a pilot study. *Am J Dis Child* 140:1042–1044.

Desmond MM, Schwanecke RP, Wilson GS, et al. 1972. Maternal barbiturate utilization and neonatal withdrawal symptomatology. *J Pediatr* 80:190–197.

DeToledo JC, Toledo C, DeCerce J, Ramsey RE. 1997. Changes in body weight with chronic, high-dose, gabapentin therapy. *Ther Drug Monit* 19:394–396.

Deuel RK, Lenn NJ. 1997. Treatment of acquired epileptic aphasia. *J Pediatr* 90:959–961.

Devinsky O. 1998. Nonepileptic psychogenic seizures: quagmires of pathophysiology, diagnosis and treatment. *Epilepsia* 39:458–462.

Devinsky O, Kelley K, Porter RS, et al. 1988. Clinical and electroencephalographic features of simple partial seizures. *Neurology* 38:1347–1352.

Devinsky O, Sato S, Kufta CV, et al. 1989. Electroencephalographic studies of simple partial seizures with subdural electrode recordings. *Neurology* 39:527–533.

Devinsky O, Honigfeld G, Patin J. 1991. Clozapine-related seizures. *Neurology* 41:369–371.

Devinsky O, Kelley K, Yacubian EM, et al. 1994. Postictal behavior. A clinical and subdural electroencephalographic study. *Arch Neurol* 51:254–259.

Devinsky O, Frasca J, Pacia SV, et al. 1995. Ictus emeticus: further evidence of nondominant temporal involvement. *Neurology* 45:1158–1160.

Devlin AM, Cross JH, Harkness W, et al. 2003. Clinical outcomes of hemispherectomy for epilepsy in childhood and adolescence. *Brain* 126:556–566.

Dhillon S, Ngwane E, Richens A. 1982. Rectal absorption of diazepam in epileptic children. *Arch Dis Child* 57: 264–267.

Di Capua M, Fusco L, Ricci S, et al. 1993. Benign neonatal sleep myoclonus: clinical features and video-polygraphic recordings. *Mov Disord* 8:191–194.

Di Rocco C. 1996. Surgical treatment of hemimeganencephaly. In: Guerrini R, Andermann F, Canapicchi R, et al., eds. *Dysplasias of cerebral cortex and epilepsy.* Philadelphia: Lippincott-Raven, 295–304.

Di Rocco C, Lanelli A, Pallini R, et al. 1985. Epilepsy and its correlation with cerebral ventricular shunting procedures in infantile hydrocephalus. *J Pediatr Neurosci* 1:255–263.

Diamantopoulos N, Crumrine PK. 1986. The effect of puberty on the course of epilepsy. *Arch Neurol* 43: 873–876.

Dianese G. 1979. Prophylactic diazepam in febrile convulsions. *Arch Dis Child* 54:244–245.

Diebler C, Ponsot G. 1983. Hamartomas of the tuber cinereum. *Neuroradiology* 25:93–101.

Diebold K. 1973. *Der erblichen myoklonisch-epileptisch dementiellen Kern Syndrome.* Berlin: Springer.

Dieterich E, Baier WK, Doose H, et al. 1985a. Long-term follow-up of childhood epilepsy with absences. I: Epilepsy with absences at onset. *Neuropediatrics* 16:149–154.

Dieterich E, Doose H, Baier WK, et al. 1985b. Long-term follow-up of childhood epilepsy with absences. II: Absence-epilepsy with initial grand mal. *Neuropediatrics* 16:155–158.

Dillon W, Brandt-Zawadki M, Sherry RG. 1984. Transient computed tomographic abnormalities after focal seizures. *Am J Neuroradiol* 5:107–109.

Dimario FJ, Clancy RR. 1988. Paradoxical precipitation of tonic seizures by lorazepam in a child with atypical absence seizures. *Pediatr Neurol* 4:249–251.

DiMario F Jr, Emery ES 3rd. 1987. The natural history of night terrors. *Clin Pediatr (Phila)* 26:505–511.

Dinesen H, Gram L, Andersen T, et al. 1984. Weight gain during treatment with valproate. *Acta Neurol Scand* 70:65–69.

Dinner DS, Lüders H, Rothner AD, Erenberg G. 1984. Complex partial seizures of childhood onset: a clinical and electroencephalographic study. *Cleve Clin Q* 51: 287–291.

Doberczak TM, Shanzer S, Cutler R, et al. 1988. One-year follow-up of infants with abstinence associated seizures. *Arch Neurol* 45:649–653.

Dobyns WB. 1987. Developmental aspects of lissencephaly and the lissencephaly syndromes. *Birth Defects* 23: 225–241.

Dobyns WB, Stratton RF, Greenberg F. 1984. Syndromes with lissencephaly. I: Miller-Dieker and Norman-Roberts syndromes and isolated lissencephaly. *Am J Med Genet* 18:509–526.

Dobyns WB, Michels VV, Groover RV, et al. 1987. Familial cavernous malformations of the central nervous system and retina. *Ann Neurol* 21:578–583.

Dobyns WB, Curry CJ, Hoyme HE, et al. 1991. Clinical and molecular diagnosis of Miller-Dieker syndrome. *Am J Hum Genet* 48:584–594.

Dobyns WB, Reiner O, Carrozzo R, et al. 1993. Lissencephaly: a human brain malformation associated with deletion of the LIS1 gene located at chromosome 17p13. *JAMA* 270:2838–2842.

Dobyns WB, Andermann E, Andermann F, et al. 1996. X-linked malformations of neuronal migration. *Neurology* 47:331–339.

Dobyns WB, Guerrini R, Czapansky-Beilman DK, et al. 1997. Bilateral periventricular nodular heterotopia (BPNH) with mental retardation and syndactyly in boys: a new X-linked mental retardation syndrome. *Neurology* 49:1042–1047.

Dobyns WB, Berry-Kravis E, Havernick NJ, et al. 1999a. X-linked lissencephaly with absent corpus callosum and ambiguous genitalia. *Am J Med Genet* 86: 331–337.

Dobyns WB, Truwit CL, Ross ME, et al. 1999b. Differences in the gyral pattern distinguish chromosome 17-linked and X-linked lissencephaly. *Neurology* 53:270–277.

Dodrill CB. 1986. Correlates of generalized tonic-clonic seizures with intellectual, neuropsychological, emotional and social function in patients with epilepsy. *Epilepsia* 27:399–410.

Dodrill CB, Wilensky AJ. 1992. Neuropsychological abilities before and after 5 years of stable antiepileptic drug therapy. *Epilepsia* 33:327–334.

Dodrill CB, Hermann BP, Rausch R, et al. 1993. Neuropsychological testing for assessing prognosis following surgery for epilepsy. In: Engle J, ed. *Surgical treatment of the epilepsies.* New York: Raven Press, 263–271.

Dodson WE. 1983. Antiepileptic drug use in newborns and infants. In: Pedley TA, Meldrum BS, eds. *Recent advances in epilepsy*, Vol. 1. Edinburgh: Churchill Livingstone, 231–248.

Dodson WE. 1987a. Carbamazepine efficacy and utilization in children. *Epilepsia* 28:S17–S24.

Dodson WE. 1987b. Special pharmacokinetic considerations in children. *Epilepsia* 28:S56–S70.

Donat JF. 1992. The age-dependent epileptic encephalopathies. *J Child Neurol* 7:7–21.

Donat JF, Wright FS. 1990. Episodic symptoms mistaken for seizures in the neurologically impaired child. *Neurology* 40:156–157.

Donat JF, Wright FS. 1991a. Seizures in series: similarities between seizures of the West and Lennox-Gastaut syndromes. *Epilepsia* 32:504–509.

Donat JF, Wright FS. 1991b. Simultaneous infantile spasms and partial seizures. *J Child Neurol* 6:246–250.

Donat JF, Wright FS. 1991c. Unusual variants of infantile spasms. *J Child Neurol* 6:313–318.

Dongier S. 1959. Statistical study of clinical and electroencephalographic manifestations of 536 psychotic episodes occurring in 516 epileptics between clinical seizures. *Epilepsia* 1:117–142.

Dongier S. 1977. Temporal lobe seizures. Behavioral aspects. In: Blaw ME, Rapin I, Kinsbourne K, eds. *Topics in child neurology*, Vol. 1. New York: Spectrum, 127–141.

Dooley J, Camfield P, Gordon K, et al. 1996. Lamotrigine-induced rash in children. *Neurology* 38:68–73.

Doose H. 1964. Zur Nosologie der Blitz-Nick-Salaam-Krämpfe. *Arch Psychiatr Nervenkr* 206:28–48.

Doose H. 1979. Photosensitivity: genetics and significance in the pathogenesis of epilepsy. In: Anderson VE, Hauser WA, Penry JK, et al., eds. *Genetic basis of the epilepsies*. New York: Raven Press, 113–121.

Doose H. 1983. Nonconvulsive status epilepticus in childhood: clinical aspects and classification. In: Delgado-Escueta AV, Wasterlain CG, Treiman DM, Porter RJ, eds. *Status epilepticus: mechanisms of brain damage and treatment*. Advances in neurology, Vol. 34. New York: Raven Press, 83–92.

Doose H. 1992. Myoclonic astatic epilepsy of early childhood. In: Roger J, Bureau M, Dravet C, et al., eds. *Epileptic syndromes in infancy, childhood and adolescence*, 2nd ed. London: John Libbey, 103–114.

Doose H, Baier WK. 1987. Genetic factors in epilepsies with primary generalized minor seizures. *Neuropediatrics* 18(Suppl. 1):1–64.

Doose H, Baier WK. 1988. Theta rhythms in the EEG: a genetic trait in childhood epilepsy. *Brain Dev* 10:347–354.

Doose H, Baier WK. 1989. Benign partial epilepsy and related conditions: multifactorial pathogenesis with hereditary impairment of brain maturation. *Eur J Pediatr* 149:152–158.

Doose H, Gerken H. 1973. On the genetics of EEG anomalies. IV: Photoconvulsive reaction. *Neuropädiatrie* 4:162–171.

Doose H, Völzke E. 1979. Petit mal status in early childhood and dementia. *Neuropédiatrie* 10:10–14.

Doose H, Völzke E, Scheffner D. 1965. Verlaufsformen kindlicher Epilepsien mit Spike wave-Absencen. *Arch Psychiatr Nervenkr* 207:394–415.

Doose H, Gerken H, Hien-Volpel KF, Völzke E. 1969. Genetics of photosensitive epilepsy. *Neuropédiatrie* 1:56–73.

Doose H, Gerken H, Leonhardt R, et al. 1970. Centrencephalic myoclonic-astatic petit mal. *Neuropédiatrie* 2:59–78.

Doose H, Gerken H, Horstmann T, et al. 1973. Genetic factors in spike-wave absences. *Epilepsia* 14:57–75.

Doose H, Spranger J, Warner M. 1975. EEG in mucolipidosis I. *Neuropédiatrie* 6:98–101.

Doose H, Ritter K, Völzke E. 1983. EEG longitudinal studies in febrile convulsions. Genetic aspects. *Neuropediatrics* 14:81–87.

Doose H, Baier W, Reinsberg E. 1984. Genetic heterogeneity of spike-wave epilepsies. In: *Advances in epileptology*, XVth International Symposium. New York: Raven Press, 513–519.

Doose H, Lunau H, Castiglione E, Waltz S. 1998. Severe idiopathic generalized epilepsy of infancy with generalized tonic-clonic seizures. *Neuropediatrics* 29:229–238.

Doose H, Hahn A, Pistohl J, et al. 2001. Atypical "benign" partial epilepsy or pseudo-Lennox syndrome. Part II: Family study. *Neuropediatrics* 32:9–13.

Drake ME, Jackson RD, Miller CA. 1986. Paroxysmal choreoathetosis after head injury. *J Neurol Neurosurg Psychiatry* 49:837–838.

Drake J, Hoffman HJ, Kobayashi J, et al. 1987. Surgical management of children with temporal lobe epilepsy and mass lesions. *Neurosurgery* 8:161–172.

Dravet C. 1992a. Comments on an epileptic syndrome with unilateral seizures. In: Roger J, Dravet C, Bureau M, et al., eds. *Epileptic syndromes in infancy, childhood and adolescence*, 2nd ed. London: John Libbey, 273–277.

Dravet C. 1992b. Myoclonic-astatic epilepsy. Presented at the Marseille Meeting on Myoclonic Epilepsies, Marseille, June 1992.

Dravet C. 1996. Le syndrome de Lennox-Gastaut et ses frontières. *Epilepsies* 8:73–88.

Dravet C, Bureau M. 1981. L'épilepsie myoclonique bénigne du nourrisson. *Revue d'Électroencéphalographie et de Neurophysiologie Clinique* 11:438–444.

Dravet C, Roger J. 1988. The Lennox-Gastaut syndrome: historical aspects from 1966 to 1987. In: Niedermeyer E, Degen R, eds. *The Lennox-Gastaut syndrome*. New York: Alan R. Liss, 9–23.

Dravet C, Munari C, Roger J. 1973. Evolution de 39 cas de syndrome de West en relation avec l'épilepsie ultérieure. In: Lugaresi E, Pazzaglia P, Tassinari CA, eds. *Evolution and prognosis of epilepsies*. Bologna: Aulo Gaggi, 119.

Dravet C, Dalla Bernardina B, Mesdjian E, et al. 1980. Dyskinésies paroxystiques au cours des traitements par la diphénylhydantoine. *Rev Neurol (Paris)* 136:1–14.

Dravet C, Roger J, Bureau M, Dalla Bernardina B. 1982. Myoclonic epilepsies in childhood. In: Akimoto H, Kazamatsuri H, Seino M, et al., eds. *Advances in epileptology*, XIIIth Epilepsy International Symposium. New York: Raven Press, 135–140.

Dravet C, Natale O, Magaudda A, et al. 1985. Les états de mal dans le syndrome de Lennox-Gastaut. *Rev Electroencephalogr Neurophysiol Clin* 15:361–368.

Dravet C, Giraud N, Bureau M, et al. 1986. Benign myoclonus of early infancy or benign non-epileptic spasms. *Neuropediatrics* 17:33–38.

Dravet C, Catani C, Bureau, et al. 1989. Partial epilepsies in infancy: a study of 40 cases. *Epilepsia* 30:807–812.

Dravet C, Bureau M, Guerrini R, et al. 1992a. Severe myoclonic epilepsy in infants. In: Roger J, Bureau M, Dravet C, et al., eds. *Epileptic syndromes in infancy, childhood and adolescence*, 2nd ed. London: John Libbey, 75–88.

Dravet C, Bureau M, Roger J. 1992b. Benign myoclonic epilepsy in infants. In: *Epileptic syndromes in infancy, childhood and adolescence*, 2nd ed. London: John Libbey, 67–74.

Dravet C, Guerrini R, Bureau M. 1997. Epileptic syndromes with drop seizures in children. In: Beaumanoir A, Andermann F, Avanzini G, et al., eds. *Falls in epileptic and non-epileptic seizures during childhood*. London: John Libbey, 95–111.

Dravet C, Bureau M, Oguni H, et al. 2002. Severe myoclonic epilepsy in infancy (Dravet syndrome). In: Roger J, Bureau M, Dravet C, et al., eds. *Epileptic syndromes in infancy, childhood and adolescence*, 3rd ed. London: John Libbey, 81–103.

Dreifuss FE. 1983. Treatment of the nonconvulsive epilepsies. *Epilepsia* 24:S45–S54.

Dreifuss FE. 1985. Discussion of absence and photosensitive epilepsy. In: Roger J, Dravet C, Bureau M, et al., eds. *Epileptic syndromes in infancy, childhood and adolescence*. London: John Libbey, 237–241.

Dreifuss FE, Holmes GL, Sackellares JC. 1981. Epilepsy and pseudoseizures in childhood. In: Dam M, Gram, L, Penry JK, eds. *Advances in epileptology*, XIIth Epilepsy International Symposium. New York: Raven Press, 323–327.

Dreifuss F, Farwell J, Holmes G, et al. 1986. Infantile spasms. Comparative trial of nitrazepam and corticotropin. *Arch Neurol* 43:1107–1110.

Dreifuss FE, Santilli N, Langer OH, et al. 1987. Valproic acid hepatic fatalities: a retrospective review. *Neurology* 37:379–385.

Dreyfus-Brisac C. 1979. Neonatal electroencephalography. In: Scarpelli EM, Cosmi EV, eds. *Reviews of perinatal medicine*, Vol. 3. New York: Raven Press, 397–472.

Dreyfus-Brisac C, Curzi-Dascalova L. 1979. The EEG during the first year of life. In: Remond A, ed. *Handbook of electroencephalography and clinical neurophysiology*, Vol. 6B. Amsterdam: Elsevier, 24–30.

Dreyfus-Brisac C, Monod N. 1972. Neonatal status epilepticus. *Electroencephalogr Clin Neurophysiol* 15:38–52.

Dreyfus-Brisac C, Monod N. 1977. Neonatal status epilepticus. In: Remond A, ed. *Handbook of electroencephalography and clinical neurophysiology*, Vol. 15B. Amsterdam: Elsevier, 39–52.

Dreyfus-Brisac C, Peschanski N, Radvanyi MF, et al. 1981. Convulsions du nouveau-né. Aspects clinique, électroencéphalographique, étiopathogénique et pronostique. *Rev Electroencephalogr Neurophysiol Clin* 11: 367–378.

Drinkenburg WH, Coenen AM, Vossen JM, Van Luijtelaar EL. 1991. Spike-wave discharges and sleep-wake states in rats with absence epilepsy. *Epilepsy Res* 9:218–224.

Drobitch RK, Svensson CK. 1992. Therapeutic drug monitoring in saliva: an update. *Clin Pharmacokinet* 23: 365–379.

Druckman R, Chao D. 1955. Massive spasms in infancy and childhood. *Epilepsia* 4:61–72.

Drury I, Beydoun A. 1991. Benign partial epilepsy of childhood with monomorphic sharp waves in centrotemporal and other locations. *Epilepsia* 32:662–667.

Du Plessis AJ, Kaufmann WE, Kupsky WJ. 1993. Intrauterine-onset myoclonic encephalopathy associated with cerebral cortical dysgenesis. *J Child Neurol* 8:164–170.

Dubeau F, Tampieri D, Lee N, et al. 1995. Periventricular and subcortical nodular heterotopia: a study of 33 patients. *Brain* 18:1273–1287.

Duchowny MS. 1987. Complex partial seizures of infancy. *Arch Neurol* 44:911–914.

Duchowny MS. 1988. Intensive monitoring in the epileptic child. *J Clin Neurophysiol* 2:203–219.

Duchowny MS. 1989. Surgery for intractable epilepsy: issues and outcome. *Pediatrics* 84:886–894.

Duchowny MS. 1992. The syndrome of partial seizures in infancy. *Arch Neurol* 44:911–914.

Duchowny M. 1999. Pediatric epilepsy surgery: the widening spectrum of surgical candidacy. *Epileptic Disord* 1: 143–151.

Duchowny M, Resnick TJ, Deray MJ, et al. 1988. Video EEG diagnosis of repetitive behavior in early childhood and its relationship to seizures. *Pediatr Neurol* 4: 162–164.

Duchowny M, Resnick TJ, Alvarez L. 1989. Dysplastic gangliocytoma and intractable partial seizures in childhood. *Neurology* 39:602–604.

Duchowny MS, Resnick TJ, Alvarez LA, et al. 1990. Focal resection for malignant partial seizures in infancy. *Neurology* 40:980–984.

Duchowny M, Levin B, Jayakar P, et al. 1992. Temporal lobectomy in early childhood. *Epilepsia* 33:298–303.

Duchowny MS, Shewmon DA, Wyllie E, et al. 1993. Special considerations for preoperative evaluation in childhood. In: Engel J, ed. *Surgical treatment of the epilepsies*, 2nd ed. New York: Raven Press, 415–427.

Duchowny M, Jayakar P, Resnick T, et al. 1994. Posterior temporal epilepsy: electroclinical features. *Ann Neurol* 35:427–431.

Duchowny MS, Altman N, Bruce J. 1996. Dysplastic gangliocytoma of the cerebral hemisphere. In: Guerrini R, Andremann F, Canapicchi R, eds. *Dysplasia of cerebral cortex and epilepsy*. Philadelphia: Lippincott-Raven, 93–100.

Duchowny MS, Harvey SA, Sperling MR, Williamson PD. 1997. Indications and criteria for surgical intervention. In: Engel J, Pedley TA, Aicardi J, et al., eds. *Epilepsy: a comprehensive textbook*, Vol. 2. Philadelphia: Lippincott-Raven, 1677–1685.

Duchowny M, Jayakar P, Resnick T, et al. 1998. Epilepsy surgery in the first three years of life. *Epilepsia* 39: 737–743.

Duchowny MS, Pellock JM, Graf WD, et al. 1999. A placebo-controlled trial of lamotrigine add-on therapy for partial seizures in children. Lamictal Pediatric Partial Seizure Study Group. *Neurology* 53:1724–1731.

Duffner PK, Cohen ME. 1975. Infantile spasms associated with histidinemia. *Neurology* 25:195–197.

Duffy FH, Lombroso CT. 1978. Treatment of status epilepticus. In: Klawans HL, ed. *Clinical neuropharmacology*, Vol. 3. New York: Raven Press, 41–56.

Dugas M, Masson M, Leheuzey MF, et al. 1982. Aphasie "acquise" de l'enfant avec épilepsie (syndrome de Landau et Kleffner), et propos de 12 observations personnelles. *Rev Neurol (Paris)* 138:755–780.

Dugas M, Gerard CL, Franc S, et al. 1995. Late onset acquired epileptic aphasia. In: Beaumanoir A, Bureau M, Deonna T, et al., eds. *Continuous spikes and waves during slow sleep: electrical status epilepticus during slow sleep*. London: John Libbey, 143–147.

Dulac O. 1992. Myoclonic-astatic epilepsy. Presented at the *Marseilles Meeting on Myoclonic Epilepsies in Children*, Marseilles, France, June 1992.

Dulac O. 1997. Infantile spasms and West syndrome. In: Engel J Jr, Pedley T, eds. *Epilepsy: a comprehensive textbook*. Philadelphia: Lippincott-Raven, 2277–2283.

Dulac O. 2001. What is West syndrome? *Brain Dev* 23: 447–452.

Dulac O, Arthuis M. 1980. Epilepsie "psychomotrice" bénigne de l'enfance. In: *Journées Parisiennes de Pédiatrie*. Paris: Flammarion, 211–220.

Dulac O, Arthuis M. 1982. L'épilepsie myoclonique sévère de l'enfant. In: *Journées Parisiennes de Pédiatrie.* Paris: Flammarion, 259–268.

Dulac O, Roger J. 1980. Sémiologie de la maladie de Sturge-Weber pendant les deux premières années de la vie. In: Gastaut H, ed. *Pathologie cérébrale du nourrisson, XXIVème Colloque de Marseille.* Marseille: Pinsard N. Lamy, 203–209.

Dulac O, Aicardi J, Rey E, et al. 1978. Blood levels of diazepam after single rectal administration to infants and children. *J Pediatr* 93:1039–1041.

Dulac O, Billard C, Arthuis M. 1983a. Aspects électrocliniques et évolutifs de l'épilepsie dans le syndrome aphasie-épilepsie. *Arch Fr Pediatr* 40:299–308.

Dulac O, Dravet C, Plouin P, et al. 1983b. Aspects nosologiques des épilepsies partielles continues chez l'enfant. *Arch Fr Pediatr* 40:697–704.

Dulac O, Plouin P, Perulli L, et al. 1983c. Aspects électroencéphalographiques de l'agyrie-pachygyrie classique. *Rev Electroencephalogr Neurophysiol Clin* 13:232–239.

Dulac O, Lemaitre A, Plouin P. 1984. Maladie de Bourneville: aspects cliniques et électroencéphalographiques de l'épilepsie dans la première année. *Bolletino Lega Italiana contre l'Epilepsia* 45/46:39–42.

Dulac O, Aubourg P, Checonry A. 1985. Etats de mal confritorfs de nourrisson. *Rev Electroencephalogr Neurophysiol Clin* 14:255–262.

Dulac O, Plouin P, Jambaqué I, et al. 1986a. Spasmes infantiles épileptiques bénins. *Rev Electroencephalogr Neurophysiol Clin* 16:371–382.

Dulac O, Steru D, Rey E, et al. 1986b. Sodium valproate monotherapy in childhood epilepsy. *Brain Dev* 8:47–52.

Dulac O, Raynaud C, Chiron C. 1987. Etude du débit sanguin cérébral dans le syndrome de West idiopathique: corrélation avec les données électroencéphalographiques. *Rev Electroencephalogr Neurophysiol Clin* 17:169–182.

Dulac O, Cusmai R, De Oliveira K. 1989. Is there a partial benign epilepsy of infancy? *Epilepsia* 30:79–81.

Dulac O, Chiron C, Luna D, et al. 1991a. Vigabatrin in childhood epilepsies. *J Child Neurol* 6:S30–S37.

Dulac O, Robain O, Chiron C, et al. 1991b. High-dose steroid treatment of epilepsia partialis continua due to chronic focal encephalitis. In: Andermann F, ed. *Chronic encephalitis and epilepsy: Rasmussen's syndrome.* Boston: Butterworth-Heinemann, 193–199.

Dulac O, Chugani T, Dalla Bernardina B. 1994. Overview. In: Dulac O, Chugani T, Dalla Bernardina B, eds. *Infantile spasms and West syndrome.* London: WB Saunders, 1–5.

Dulac O, Pinard JM, Plouin P. 1996. Infantile spasms associated with cortical dysplasia and tuberous sclerosis. In: Guerrini R, Andermann F, Canapicchi R, eds. *Dysplasias of cerebral cortex and epilepsy.* Philadelphia: Lippincott-Raven, 217–226.

Duncan JS. 1995. Treatment strategies for typical absences and related epileptic syndromes. In: Duncan JS, Panayiotopoulos CP, eds. *Typical absences and related syndromes.* London: Churchill Communication Europe, 354–360.

Duncan R. 2001. Infantile spasms: the original description of Dr. West (1841). *Epileptic Disord* 3:47–48.

Duncan JS, Koepp MJ. 2000. PET: central benzodiazepine neuroreceptor mapping in localization related epilepsies. *Adv Neurol* 83:131–136.

Duncan JS, Panayiotopoulos CP, eds. 1995a. *Typical ab-*

sences and related epileptic syndromes. London: Churchill Communication Europe.

Duncan JS, Panayiotopoulos CP. 1995b. Juvenile absence epilepsy: an alternative view. In: Duncan JS, Panayiotopoulos CP, eds. *Typical absences and related syndromes.* London: Churchill Communication Europe, 167–173.

Duncan JS, Sagar HJ. 1987. Seizure characteristics, pathology and outcome after temporal lobectomy. *Neurology* 37:405–409.

Duncan JS, Shorvon SD. 1987. Rates of antiepileptic drug reduction in active epilepsy—current practice. *Epilepsy Res* 1:357–364.

Duncan JS, Smith SJ, Forster A, et al. 1989. The effects of the removal of phenytoin, carbamazepine and sodium valproate on the electroencephalogram. *Epilepsia* 30:590–596.

Duncan JS, Shorvon SD, Trimble MR. 1990. Discontinuation of phenytoin, carbamazepine and valproate in patients with active epilepsy. *Epilepsia* 31:324–333.

Dunn DW. 1988. Status epilepticus in children: etiology, clinical features and outcome. *J Child Neurol* 3:167–173.

Dunn DW, Parekh HU. 1991. Theophylline and status epilepticus in children. *Neuropediatrics* 22:24–26.

Durner M, Sander T, Greenberg DA, et al. 1991. Localization of idiopathic generalized epilepsy on chromosome 6p in families of juvenile myoclonic epilepsy patients. *Neurology* 41:1651–1655.

Durner M, Zhou G, Fu D, et al. 1999. Evidence for linkage of adolescent-onset idiopathic generalized epilepsies to chromosome 8 and genetic heterogeneity. *Am J Hum Genet* 64:1411–1419.

Durner M, Keddache MA, Tomasini M, et al. 2001. Genome scan of idiopathic generalized epilepsy: evidence for major susceptibility gene and modifying genes influencing the seizure type. *Ann Neurol* 49:328–335.

Dwyer BE, Wasterlain CG. 1985. Neonatal seizures in monkeys and rabbits: brain glucose depletion in the face of normoglycemia, prevention by glucose load. *Pediatr Res* 19:992–995.

Eadie MJ. 1980. Unwanted effects of anticonvulsant drugs. In: Tyrer JH, ed. *The treatment of epilepsy.* Lancaster, United Kingdom: NIT Press, 129–160.

Eadie MJ, Bladin PF. 2001. *A disease once sacred: a history of the medical understanding of epilepsy.* London: John Libbey.

Eadie MJ, Tyrer JH. 1989. *Anticonvulsant therapy: pharmacological basis and practice*, 3rd ed. Edinburgh: Churchill Livingstone.

Eaton DM, Connell J, Dubowitz V, et al. 1992. Monitoring of the electroencephalogram during intensive care. In: Eyre JA, ed. *The neurophysiological examination of the newborn infant.* London: MacKeith.

Ebersole JS. 1992. Equivalent dipole modelling: a new EEG method for epileptogenic focus localization. In: Pedley TA, Meldrum BS, eds. *Recent advances in epilepsy*, Vol. 5. Edinburgh: Churchill Livingstone, 51–71.

Ebersole JS. 1998. EEG and MEG dipole source modeling. In: Engel J Jr, Pedley TA, eds. *Epilepsy: a comprehensive textbook.* Philadelphia: Lippincott-Raven, 919–935.

Ebersole JS, Bridgers SL. 1986. Ambulatory EEG monitoring. In: Pedley TA, Meldrum BS, eds. *Recent advances in epilepsy*, Vol. 3. Edinburgh: Churchill Livingstone, 111–135.

Ebersole JS, Leroy RF. 1983. An evaluation of ambulatory cassette monitoring. II: Detection of interictal abnormalities. *Neurology* 33:8–18.

Ebersole JS, Pacia SV. 1996. Localization of temporal lobe foci by ictal EEG patterns. *Epilepsia* 37:386–393.

Ebersole JS, Wade PB. 1990. Intracranial EEG validation of single versus dual bipolar sources for temporal spikes in presurgical candidates. [Abstract] *Epilepsia* 31:621.

Ebersole JS, Wade PB. 1991. Spike voltage topography identifies two types of frontotemporal epileptic foci. *Neurology* 41:1425–1433.

Ebner A, Kerdar MS. 2000. Olfactory and gustatory auras. In: Lüders HO, Noachtar S, eds. *Epileptic seizures: pathophysiology and clinical semiology.* Philadelphia: Churchill Livingstone, 313–319.

Echenne B, Dulac O, Parayre-Chanez MJ, et al. 1991. Treatment of infantile spasms with intravenous gamma-globulins. *Brain Dev* 13:313–319.

Edwards K, Schmidley JW, Simon RP. 1982. How often does CSF pleocytosis occur after generalized seizures? *Ann Neurol* 12:92–93.

Eeg-Olofsson O, Petersén I, Selldén U. 1971. The development of the electroencephalogram in normal children from the age of 1 through 15 years. Paroxysmal activity. *Neuropadiatrie* 2:375–404.

Efron R. 1961. Post-epileptic paralysis: theoretical critique and report of a case. *Brain* 84:381–394.

Egger J, Brett EM. 1981. Effects of sodium valproate in 100 children with special reference to weight. *BMJ* 283:577–581.

Egli M, Mothersill I, O'Kane M, et al. 1985. The axial spasm—the predominant type of drop seizure in patients with secondary generalized epilepsy. *Epilepsia* 26:401–415.

Ehrhardt P, Forsythe WI. 1989. Prognosis after grand mal seizures: a study of 187 children with three-year remission. *Dev Med Child Neurol* 31:633–639.

Eiberg H, Gardiner RM, Mohr J. 1989. Batten disease (Spielmeyer-Vogt disease) and haptoglobins (HP): indication of linkage and assignment to chromosome 16. *Clin Genet* 36:217–218.

Eke T, Talbot JF, Lawden MC. 1997. Severe persistent visual field constriction associated with vigabatrin. *BMJ* 314:180–181.

Eldridge R, Livanainen M, Stem R, et al. 1983. "Baltic" myoclonus epilepsy: hereditary disorder of childhood made worse by phenytoin. *Lancet* 2:838–842.

Elger CE, Wieser HG. 1987. Foramen ovale electrode recordings. In: Wieser HG, Elger CE, eds. *Presurgical evaluation of epileptics.* Berlin: Springer-Verlag, 177–182.

Elia M, Musumeci SA, Ferri R, et al. 1995. Seizures in Klinefelter's syndrome: a clinical and EEG study of five patients. *Ital J Neurol Sci* 16:231–238.

Elia M, Guerrini R, Musumeci SA, et al. 1998. Myoclonic absence-like seizures and chromosome abnormality syndromes. *Epilepsia* 39:660–663.

Ellenberg JH, Nelson KB. 1978. Febrile seizures and later intellectual performance. *Arch Neurol* 35:17–21.

Ellenberg JH, Hirtz DG, Nelson KB. 1984. Age of onset of seizures in young children. *Ann Neurol* 15:127–134.

Elliott FA. 1984. The episodic dyscontrol syndrome and aggression. *Neurol Clin* 2:113–125.

Ellison PH, Horn JL, Franklin S, et al. 1986. The results of checking a scoring system for neonatal seizures. *Neuropediatrics* 17:152–157.

Elmslie FV, Rees M, Williamson MP, et al. 1997. Genetic mapping of a major susceptibility locus for juvenile myoclonic epilepsy on chromosome 15q. *Hum Mol Genet* 6:1329–1334.

Elmslie FV, Wilson J, Rossiter MA. 1996. Familial rectal pain: is it underdiagnosed? *J R Soc Med* 89:290P–291P.

El-Radhi AS, Withana K, Banajeh S. 1986. Recurrence rate of febrile convulsion related to the degree of pyrexia during the first attack. *Clin Ped* 25:311–313.

Elster AD, Chen MY. 1990. MR imaging of Sturge-Weber syndrome: role of gadopentetate dimeglumine and gradient-echo techniques. *AJNR Am J Neuroradiol* 11:685–689.

Elterman RD, Glauser TA, Wyllie E, et al. 1999. A double-blind, randomized trial of topiramate as adjunctive therapy for partial-onset seizures in children. Topiramate YP Study Group. *Neurology* 52:1338–1344.

Elterman RD, Shields WD, Mansfield KA, et al. 2001. Randomized trial of vigabatrin in patients with infantile spasms. US Infantile Spasms Vigabatrin Study Group. *Neurology* 57:1416–1421.

Elwes RD, Reynolds EH. 1981. The early prognosis of epilepsy. In: Dam M, Gram L, eds. *Comprehensive epileptology.* New York: Raven Press, 715–727.

Elwes RD, Johnson AL, Shorvon SD, et al. 1984. The prognosis of seizure control in newly diagnosed epilepsy. *N Engl J Med* 311:944–947.

Elwes RD, Chesterman P, Reynolds EH. 1985. Prognosis after a first untreated tonic-clonic seizure. *Lancet* 2:752–753.

Elwes RD, Dunn G, Binnie CD, et al. 1991. Outcome following resective surgery for temporal lobe epilepsy: a prospective follow-up study of 102 consecutive cases. *J Neurol Neurosurg Psychiatry* 54:949–952.

Emerson R, D'Souza BJ, Vining EP, et al. 1981. Stopping medication in children with epilepsy: predictors of outcome. *N Engl J Med* 304:1125–1129.

Emery ES. 1990. Status epilepticus secondary to breath-holding and pallid syncopal spells. *Neurology* 40:859.

Engel J Jr. 1984. The use of positron emission tomography in epilepsy. *Ann Neurol* 15:S180–S191.

Engel J Jr. 1987. *Surgical treatment of the epilepsies.* New York: Raven Press.

Engel J Jr. 1989. *Seizures and epilepsies.* Philadelphia: FA Davis.

Engel J. 1992. Recent advances in surgical treatment of temporal lobe epilepsy. *Acta Neurol Scand* 86(Suppl. 140):71–80.

Engel J. 1993. *Surgical treatment of the epilepsies*, 2nd ed. New York: Raven Press.

Engel J Jr. 2001. A proposed diagnostic scheme for people with epileptic seizures and with epilepsy: report of the ILAE Task Force on Classification and Terminology. International League Against Epilepsy (ILAE). *Epilepsia* 42:796–803.

Engel J Jr, Pedley TA. 1997. Introduction: what is epilepsy? In: Engel J Jr, Pedley TA, eds. *Epilepsy: a comprehensive textbook*, Vol.1. Philadelphia: Lippincott-Raven, 1–7.

Engel J, Shewmon DA. 1992. Overview: who should be considered a surgical candidate? In: Engel J Jr, ed. *Surgical treatment of the epilepsies*, 2nd ed. New York: Raven Press, 23–34.

Engel J Jr, Driver MV, Falconer MA. 1975. Electrophysiological correlates of pathology and surgical results in temporal lobe epilepsy. *Brain* 98:129–156.

Engel J Jr, Rapin I, Giblin DR. 1977. Electrophysiological

studies in two patients with cherry-red spot-myoclonus syndrome. *Epilepsia* 18:73–87.

Engel J Jr, Ludwig BI, Fetell M. 1978. Prolonged partial complex status epilepticus: EEG and behavioral observations. *Neurology* 28:863–869.

Engel J Jr, Rausch R, Lieb JP, et al. 1981. Correlation of criteria used for localizing epileptic foci in patients considered for surgical therapy of epilepsy. *Ann Neurol* 9:215–224.

Engel J Jr, Brown J, Kuhl DE, et al. 1982a. Pathological findings underlying focal temporal lobe hypometabolism in partial epilepsy. *Ann Neurol* 12:518–528.

Engel J Jr, Kuhl DE, Phelps ME, et al. 1982b. Comparative localization of epileptic foci in partial epilepsy by PET and EEG. *Ann Neurol* 12:529–537.

Engel J Jr, Henry TR, Risinger MW, et al. 1990. Presurgical evaluation for partial epilepsy: relative contributions of chronic depth-electrode recording versus FDG-PET and scalp-sphenoidal ictal EEG. *Neurology* 40:1670–1677.

Engel J, Wieser HG, Spencer D. 1997. Overview: surgical therapy. In: Engel J Jr, Pedley TA, Aicardi J, et al., eds. *Epilepsy: a comprehensive textbook*, Vol. 2. Philadelphia: Lippincott Williams & Wilkins, 1673–1676.

Enoki H, Akiyama T, Hattori J, et al. 1998. Photosensitive fits elicited by TV animation: an electroencephalographic study. *Acta Paediatrica Japonica* 40:626–630.

Epstein AW. 1967. Body image alternations during seizures and dreams of epileptics. *Arch Neurol* 16:613–619.

Epstein MA, Duchowny M, Jayakar P, et al. 1994. Altered responsiveness during hyperventilation-induced EEG slowing: a non-epileptic phenomenon in normal children. *Epilepsia* 35:1204–1207.

Erba G, Browne TR. 1983. Atypical absence, myoclonic, atonic, and tonic seizures and the "Lennox-Gastaut syndrome." In: Browne TR, Feldman RG, eds. *Epilepsy: diagnosis and management*. Boston: Little, Brown and Company, 75–94.

Erba G, Cavazzuti V. 1977. Ictal and interictal response latency in Lennox-Gastaut syndrome [Abstract]. *Electroencephalogr Clin Neurophysiol* 42:717.

Erba G, Cavazzuti V. 1981. Tonic seizures with arousal: report of a case [Abstract]. *Sleep Research* 10:245.

Erba G, Cavazzuti V. 1990. Sturge-Weber syndrome: natural history and indications for surgery. *J Epilepsy* 3 (Suppl.):287–291.

Erba G, Duchowny MS. 1990. Partial epilepsy and tuberous sclerosis: indications for surgery in disseminated disease. *J Epilepsy* 3(Suppl.):315–319.

Erba G, Lombroso CT. 1973. La sindrome de Lennox-Gastaut. *Prospeltive in Paediatria* 3:145–165.

Erba G, Moschen K, Ferber R. 1981. Sleep-related changes in EEG discharge activity and seizure risk in patients with Lennox-Gastaut syndrome [Abstract]. *Sleep Research* 10:247.

Eriksson SH, Rugg-Gunn FJ, Symms MR, et al. 2001. Diffusion tensor imaging in patients with epilepsy and malformation of cortical development. *Brain* 124:617–626.

Ernst JP, Doose H, Baier WK. 1988. Bromides were effective in intractable epilepsy with generalized tonic-clonic seizures and onset in early childhood. *Brain Dev* 10: 385–388.

Escayg A, MacDonald BT, Meisler MH, et al. 2000. Mutations of *SCN1A*, encoding a neuronal sodium channel, in two families with GEFS+2. *Nat Genet* 24:343–345.

Escayg A, Heils A, MacDonald BT, et al. 2001. A novel

SNC1A mutation associated with generalized epilepsy with febrile seizures plus—and prevalence of variants in patients with epilepsy. *Am J Hum Genet* 68:866–873.

Estivill E, Sanmarti F, Fernandez-Alvarez E. 1983. Morphologie électroencéphalographique des crises du nouveau-né à terme. *Rev Electroencephalogr Neurophysiol Clin* 13:145–152.

Etzioni A, Jaffe M, Pollack S, et al. 1991. High dose intravenous gamma-globulin in intractable epilepsy in childhood. *Eur J Pediatr* 150:681–683.

Eunson LH, Rea R, Zuberi SM, et al. 2000. Clinical, genetic and expression studies of mutations in the potassium channel gene *KCNA 1* reveal new phenotypic variability. *Ann Neurol* 48:647–656.

European Chromosome 16 Tuberous Sclerosis Consortium. 1993. Identification and characterization of the tuberous sclerosis gene on chromosome 16. *Cell* 75: 1305–1315.

Evans DJ, Levene MI. 2000. Anticonvulsants for preventing mortality and morbidity in full term newborns with perinatal asphyxia. *Cochrane Database Syst Rev* 2: CD001240.

Evans OB, Gay H, Swisher A, et al. 1989. Hematologic monitoring in children with epilepsy treated with carbamazepine. *J Child Neurol* 4:286–290.

Eyre JA, Oozer RC, Wilkinson AR. 1983. Diagnosis of neonatal seizure by continuous recording and rapid analysis of the electroencephalogram. *Arch Dis Child* 58:785–790.

Faero O, Kastrup KW, Lykkegaard Nielsen E, et al. 1972. Successful prophylaxis of febrile convulsions with phenobarbital. *Epilesia* 13:279–285.

Faden AI, Demedijk P, Panter S. 1989. The role of excitatory aminoacids and NMDA receptors in traumatic brain injury. *Science* 244:798–800.

Fagan KJ, Lee SI. 1990. Prolonged confusion following convulsions due to generalized nonconvulsive status epilepticus. *Neurology* 40:1689–1694.

Fahn S. 1994. The paroxysmal dyskinesias. In: Marsden CD, Fahn S, eds. *Movement disorders*, 3rd ed. Oxford: Butterworth-Heinemann, 310–345.

Faingold CL, Browning RA. 1987. Mechanisms of anticonvulsant drug action. I: Drugs primarily used for generalized tonic-clonic and partial epilepsies. II. Drugs primarily used for absence epilepsy. *Eur J Pediatr* 146: 2–7;146:8–14.

Falconer MA. 1976. Surgical treatment of sequelae of severe febrile convulsions. In: Brazier MA, Coceani FA, eds. *Brain dysfunction in infantile febrile convulsions*. New York: Raven Press, 307–326.

Falconer MA, Cavanagh JB. 1959. Clinico-pathological considerations of temporal lobe epilepsy due to small focal lesions. *Brain* 82:483–504.

Falconer MA, Serafetinides EA, Corsellis JAN. 1964. Etiology and pathogenesis of temporal lobe epilepsy. *Arch Neurol* 19:353–361.

Fariello RG, Doro JM, Forster FM. 1974. Generalized cortical electrodecremental event: clinical and neurophysiological observations in patients with dystonic seizures. *Arch Neurol* 36:285–291.

Farmer JP, Cosgrove GR, Villemure JG, et al. 1988. Intracerebral cavernous angiomas. *Neurology* 38: 1699–1704.

Farnarier G, Kouna P, Genton P. 1995. Amplitude EEG mapping in three cases of CSWS. In: Beaumanoir A, Bureau

M, Deonna T, et al., eds. *Continuous spikes and waves during slow sleep: electrical status epilepticus during slow sleep.* London: John Libbey, 91–98.

Farrell K. 1993. Secondary generalized epilepsy and Lennox-Gastaut syndrome. In: Wyllie E, ed. *The treatment of epilepsy: principles and practice.* Philadelphia, Lea and Febiger, 604–613.

Farrell K. 2001. Benzodiazepines. In: Pellock JM, Dodson WE, Bourgeois BFD, eds. *Pediatric epilepsy: diagnosis and therapy,* 2nd ed. New York: Demos, 373–384.

Farrell MA, Derosa MJ, Curran JG, et al. 1992. Neuropathologic findings in cortical resections (including hemispherectomies) performed for the treatment of intractable childhood epilepsy. *Acta Neuropathol* 83: 246–259.

Farwell JR, Stuntz JT. 1984. Frontoparietal astrocytoma causing absence seizures and bilaterally synchronous epileptiform discharges. *Epilepsia* 25:695–698.

Farwell J, Milstein J, Opheim K, et al. 1984. Adrenocorticotropic hormone controls infantile spasms independently of cortisol stimulation. *Epilepsia* 25:605–608.

Farwell J, Lee YJ, Hirtz DG, et al. 1990. Phenobarbital for febrile seizures—effects on intelligence and on seizure recurrence. *N Engl J Med* 322:364–369.

Fayad MN, Chawiri R, Mikati M. 1997. Landau-Kleffner syndrome: consistent response to repeated intravenous gamma-globulin doses. A case report. *Pediatrics* 99: 560–566.

Fedio FR, Mirsky AF. 1969. Selective intellectual deficits in children with temporal lobe or centrencephalic epilepsy. *Neuropsychologia* 7:287–300.

Feely M, Callaghan M, Duggan B, et al. 1980. Phenobarbitone in previously untreated epilepsy. *J Neurol Neurosurg Psychiatry* 43:365–368.

Feinberg AP, Leahy WR. 1977. Infantile spasms: case report of sex-linked inheritance. *Dev Med Child Neurol* 19: 524–526.

Feindel W, Penfield W. 1954. Localization of discharge in temporal lobe automatism. *Arch Neurol Psychiatry* 72:603–630.

Fejerman N, Caraballo R. 2002. Appendix to shuddering and benign myoclonus of early infancy. In: Guerrini R, Aicardi F, Andermann F, et al., eds. *Epilepsy and movement disorders.* Cambridge: Cambridge University Press, 349–351.

Fejerman N, Di Blasi AM. 1987. Status epilepticus of benign partial epilepsies in children: report of two cases. *Epilepsia* 28:351–358.

Fejerman N, Medina CS. 1986. *Convulsiones en la infancia,* 2nd ed. Buenos Aires: El Ateneo.

Fejerman N, Caraballo R, Tenembaum S. 2000a. Atypical evolutions of benign localization-related epilepsies in children: are they predictable? *Epilepsia* 41:380–390.

Fejerman N, Cerosimo R, Caraballo R, et al. 2000b. Vigabatrin as a first-choice drug in the treatment of West syndrome. *J Child Neurol* 15:161–165.

Felbamate Study in Lennox-Gastaut Syndrome. 1993. Efficacy of felbamate in childhood epileptic encephalopathy (Lennox-Gastaut syndrome). *N Engl J Med* 328: 29–33.

Feldman RG. 1976. Clorazepate in temporal lobe epilepsy. *JAMA* 236:2603–2605.

Feldman RG. 1983a. Borderline areas. In: Browne TR, Feldman RG, eds. *Epilepsy: diagnosis and management.* Boston: Little, Brown and Company, 109–116.

Feldman RG. 1983b. Complex partial seizures (psychomotor or temporal lobe seizures). In: Browne TR, Feldman RG, eds. *Epilepsy: diagnosis and management.* Boston: Little, Brown and Company, 39–50.

Feldman RG, Ricks NL, Orren MM. 1983. Behavioral methods of seizure control. In: Browne TR, Feldman RG, eds. *Epilepsy: diagnosis and management.* Boston: Little, Brown and Company, 269–279.

Fenichel GM. 1982. Neurological complications of immunization. *Ann Neurol* 12:119–128.

Fenichel GM. 1983. Hypoxic-ischemic encephalopathy in the newborn. *Arch Neurol* 40:261–266.

Fenichel GM. 1985. Seizure in newborns. In: *Neonatal neurology.* Edinburgh: Churchill Livingstone, 25–52.

Fenichel GM, Olson BJ, Fitzpatrick JE. 1980a. Heart rate changes in convulsive and nonconvulsive neonatal apnea. *Ann Neurol* 7:577–582.

Fenichel GM, Olson BJ, Fitzpatrick JE. 1980b. Neonatal seizures. In: Lüders HL, Lesser RP, eds. *Epilepsy: electroclinical syndromes.* Berlin: Springer-Verlag, 13–47.

Fenichel GM, Webster DL, Wong WK. 1984. Intracranial hemorrhage in the term newborn. *Arch Neurol* 41: 30–34.

Fenwick PB. 1983. EEG epileptic waveforms, their genesis and clinical correlates. In: Rose CF, ed. *Research progress in epilepsy.* London: Pitman, 103–114.

Fenwick P. 1992. Behavioural therapy of epilepsy. In: Pedley TA, Meldrum BS, eds. *Recent advances in epilepsy,* 5th ed. Edinburgh: Churchill Livingstone, 223–235.

Fenwick P. 1994. The behavioral treatment of epilepsy generation and inhibition of seizures. *Neurol Clin* 12:175–202.

Fernandez G, Effenberger O, Vinz B, et al. 1998. Hippocampal malformation as a cause of familial febrile convulsions and subsequent hippocampal sclerosis. *Neurology* 50:909–917.

Fernandez-Alvarez E, Aicardi J. 2001. *Movement disorders in children.* London: MacKeith Press.

Fernandez-Calvo C, Olascoaga J, Resano A, et al. 2000. Lyell syndrome associated with lamotrigine. *Rev Neurol* 31:1162–1164.

Ferrendelli JA. 1987. Pharmacology of antiepileptic drugs. *Epilepsia* 28:S14–S16.

Ferrer I. 1984. A Golgi analysis of unlayered polymicrogyria. *Acta Neuropathol* 65:69–76.

Ferrer I, Catala I. 1991. Unlayered polymicrogyria: structural and developmental aspects. *Anat Embryol (Berl)* 184:517–528.

Ferrer I, Cusi MV, Liarte A, et al. 1986. A Golgi study of the polymicrogyric cortex in Aicardi syndrome. *Brain Dev* 8:518–525.

Ferrer I, Pineda M, Tallada M, et al. 1992. Abnormal local circuit neurons in epilepsia partialis continua associated with focal cortical dysplasia. *Acta Neuropathol* 83: 647–652.

Ferrie CD, De Marco P, Grunewald RA, et al. 1994. Video game induced seizures. *J Neurol Neurosurg Psychiatry* 57:925–931.

Ferrie CD, Giannakodimos S., Robinson RO, et al. 1995. Symptomatic typical absence seizures. In: Duncan JS, Panayiotopoulos CP, eds. *Typical absences and related syndromes.* London: Churchill Communication Europe, 241–252.

Ferrie CD, Beaumanoir A, Guerrini R, et al. 1997. Early-onset benign occipital seizure susceptibility syndrome. *Epilepsia* 38:285–293.

Feucht M, Brantner-Inthaler S. 1994. Gamma-vinyl-GABA (vigabatrin) in the therapy of Lennox-Gastaut syndrome: an open study. *Epilepsia* 35:993–998.

Finelli PF, Pueschel SM, Padre-Mendoza T, O'Brien MM. 1985. Neurological findings in patients with the fragile-X syndrome. *J Neurol Neurosurg Psychiatry* 48:150–153.

Fink JM, Dobyns WB, Guerrini R, et al. 1997. Identification of a duplication of Xq28 associated with bilateral periventricular nodular heterotopia (BPNH). *Am J Hum Genet* 61:379–387.

Finlayson RE, Lucas AR. 1979. Pseudoepileptic seizures in children and adolescents. *Mayo Clin Proc* 54:83–87.

Fiol ME, Leppik IE, Pretzel K. 1986. Eating epilepsy: EEG and clinical study. *Epilepsia* 27:441–445.

Fiol ME, Leppik IE, Mireles R, et al. 1988. Ictus emeticus and the insular cortex. *Epilepsy Res* 2:127–131.

Fischler E. 1962. Convulsions as a complication of shigellosis in children. *Helv Paediatr Acta* 17:389–394.

Fisgin T, Gurer Y, Tezic T, et al. 2002. Effects of intranasal midazolam and rectal diazepam on acute convulsions in children: prospective randomized study. *J Child Neurol* 17:123–126.

Fish DR. 1995. Blank spells that are not typical absences. In: Duncan JS, Panayiotopoulos CP, eds. *Typical absences and related syndromes*. London: Churchill Communication Europe, 253–262.

Fish DR, Espir ML. 1988. Convulsions associated with prophylactic antimalarial drugs: implications for people with epilepsy. *BMJ* 297:526–527.

Fish DR, Quesney LF, Rasmussen T. 1989. Preoperative evaluation of children with drug-resistant partial seizures: the importance of agreement between different investigative modalities. *Epilepsia* 30:636–639.

Fish DR, Andermann F, Olivier A. 1991. Complex partial seizures and small posterior temporal or extratemporal structural lesions: surgical management. *Neurology* 41:1781–1784.

Fish DR, Gloor P, Quesney FL, et al. 1993. Clinical responses to electrical brain stimulation of the temporal and frontal lobes in patients with epilepsy. Pathophysiological implications. *Brain* 116:397–414.

Fisher CM. 1978. Transient paralytic attacks of obscure nature: the question of non-convulsive seizure paralysis. *Can J Neurol Sci* 5:267–273.

Fisher RA, Clancy RC. 1987. Midline foci of epileptiform activity in children and neonates. *J Child Neurol* 2:224–228.

Fisher C, Kahn E, Edwards A, et al. 1974. A psychophysiological study of nightmares and night terrors. *J Nerv Ment Dis* 158:174–188.

Fisher J, Lockman L, Zaske D, et al. 1981. Phenobarbital maintenance dose requirements in treating neonatal seizures. *Neurology* 31:1042–1044.

Fisher RS, Chan DW, Bare M, et al. 1991. Capillary prolactin measurement for diagnosis of seizures. *Ann Neurol* 29:187–190.

Fisher E, Siemes H, Pund R, et al. 1992. Valproate metabolism in serum and urine during antiepileptic therapy in children with infantile spasms: abnormal metabolite pattern associated with reversible hepatotoxicity. *Epilepsia* 33:165–171.

Fisher RS, Mirski M, Krauss GL. 1997. Brain stimulation. In: Engel J, Pedley TA, Aicardi J, et al., eds. *Epilepsy: a comprehensive textbook*. Philadelphia: Lippincott-Raven, 1867–1875.

Fittipaldi F, Curra A, Fusco L, et al. 2001. EEG discharges on awakening: a marker of idiopathic generalized epilepsy. *Neurology* 56:123–126.

Fitzhardinge PM, Eisen A, Lejtenyl C. 1974. Sequelae of early steroid administration to the newborn infant. *Pediatrics* 53:877–883.

Flanigin H, King D, Gallagher B. 1985. Surgical treatment of epilepsy. In: Pedley TA, Meldrum BS, eds. *Recent advances in epilepsy*. Edinburgh: Churchill Livingstone, 297–339.

Fleiszar KA, Daniel WL, Imrey PB. 1977. Genetic study of infantile spasms with hypsarrhythmia. *Epilepsia* 18:55–62.

Fletcher WA, Hoyt WF, Narahara MH. 1988. Congenital quadrantanopsia with occipital lobe ganglioglioma. *Neurology* 38:1892–1894.

Fogli A, Guerrini R, Moro F, et al. 1999. Intracellular levels of the LIS1 protein correlate with clinical and neuroradiological findings in patients with classical lissencephaly. *Ann Neurol* 45:154–161.

Fois A, Malandrini F, Balestri P, et al. 1984. Infantile spasms—long term results of ACTH treatment. *Eur J Pediatr* 142:51–55.

Fois A, Malandrini F, Tonaccini D. 1988a. Clinical findings in children with occipital paroxysmal discharges. *Epilepsia* 29:620–625.

Fois A, Tomaccini D, Balestri P, et al. 1988b. Intractable epilepsy: etiology, risk factors and treatment. *Clin Electroencephalogr* 19:68–73.

Foldvary N, Acharya V, Lüders HO. 2000. Auditory auras. In: Lüders HO, Noachter S, eds. *Epileptic seizures*. Philadelphia: Churchill Livingstone, 25:304–311.

Foley CM, Polinsky MS, Gruskin AB, et al. 1981. Encephalopathy in infants and children with chronic renal disease. *Arch Neurol* 38:656–658.

Foley CM, Legido A, Miles DK, et al. 1995. Diagnostic value of pediatric outpatient video-EEG. *Pediatr Neurol* 12:120–124.

Foley CM, Legido A, Miles DK, et al. 2000. Long-term computer-assisted outpatient electroencephalogram monitoring in children and adolescents. *J Child Neurol* 15:49–55.

Folgarasi A, Jokeit H, Faveret E, et al. 2002. The effect of age on seizure semiology in childhood temporal lobe epilepsy. *Epilepsia* 43:638–643.

Fontan JP, Helot GP, Heyman MB, et al. 1984. Esophageal spasm associated with apnea and bradycardia in an infant. *Pediatrics* 73:52–55.

Forsgren L, Edvinsson SO, Blomquist HK, et al. 1990a. Epilepsy in a population of mentally retarded children and adults. *Epilepsy Res* 6:234–248.

Forsgren L, Sidenvall R, Blomquist HK, et al. 1990b. A prospective incidence study of febrile convulsions. *Acta Paediatr Scand* 79:550–557.

Forsgren L, Sidenvall R, Blomquist HK, et al. 1991. Pre- and perinatal factors in febrile convulsions. *Acta Paediatr Scand* 80:218–225.

Forster FM. 1977. *Reflex epilepsy, behavioral therapy and conditional reflexes*. Springfield, IL: Charles C Thomas Publisher.

Forsythe WI, Sills M. 1984. One drug for childhood grand mal: medical audit for three-year remissions. *Dev Med Child Neurol* 26:742–748.

Forsythe WI, Owens JR, Toothill C. 1981. Effectiveness of acetazolamide in the treatment of carbamazepine-resistant epilepsy in children. *Dev Med Child Neurol* 27: 743–748.

Forsythe I, Butler R, Breg I., et al. 1991. Cognitive impairment in new cases of epilepsy randomly assigned to carbamazepine, phenytoin and sodium valproate. *Dev Med Child Neurol* 33:524–536.

Foulon M, Noel P. 1977. Epilepsie post-traumatique précoce dans l'enfance. Signification et pronostic à court terme. *Acta Neurol Belg* 77:276–284.

Fox JW, Lamperti ED, Eksioglu YZ, et al. 1998. Mutations in filamen 1 prevent migration of cerebral cortical ceurons in human periventricular heterotopia. *Neuron* 21:1315–1325.

Frank LM, Enlow T, Holmes GL, et al. 1999. Lamictal (lamotrigine) monotherapy for typical absence seizures in children. *Epilepsia* 40:973–979.

Frantzen E, Lennox-Buchtal MA, Nygaard A. 1968. Longitudinal EEG and clinical study of children with febrile convulsions. *Electroencephalogr Clin Neurophysiol* 24:197–212.

Frantzen E, Lennox-Buchtal MA, Nygaard A. 1969. Febrile convulsions—a follow-up genetic study [Abstract]. In: Drake CG, Duvoisin R, eds. *Proceedings of Fourth International Congress of Neurological Surgery, Ninth International Congress of Neurology, New York*. Amsterdam: Excerpta Medica, 7.

Frantzen E, Lennox-Buchtal MA, Nygaard A, et al. 1970. A genetic study of febrile convulsions. *Neurology* 20: 909–917.

Franzoni E, Carboni C, Lambertini A. 1983. Rectal diazepam: a clinical and EEG study after a single dose in children. *Epilepsia* 24:35–41.

Fraser RT, Clemmons DC. 1989. Vocational and psychosocial interventions for youth with seizure disorders. In: Herman BP, Seidenberg M, eds. *Childhood epilepsies: neuropsychological, psychosocial and intervention aspects*. Chichester: John Wiley.

Freeman JM. 1983. Neonatal seizures. In: Dreifuss FE, ed. *Pediatric epileptology: classificiation and management of seizures in the child*. Boston: John Wright-PSG Inc., 159–172.

Freeman JM, Tibbles J, Camfield C, et al. 1987. Benign epilepsy of childhood: a speculation and its ramifications. *Pediatrics* 79:864–868.

Freeman JM, Vining EP, Pillas DJ, et al. 1997. Seizure outcome after hemispherectomy: the Johns Hopkins experience. In: Tuxhorn I, Holthausen H, Boenigk H, eds. *Paediatric epilepsy syndromes and their surgical treatment*. London: John Libbey, 743–748.

Freeman JM, Vining EP, Pillas DJ, et al. 1998. The efficacy of the ketogenic diet—1998: a prospective evaluation of intervention in 150 children. *Pediatrics* 102:1358–1363.

French JA, Williamson PD, Thadani M, et al. 1993. Characteristics of medial temporal lobe epilepsy. I: Results of history and physical examination. *Ann Neurol* 34: 774–780.

Friderichsen C, Melchior J. 1954. Febrile convulsions in children, their frequency and prognosis. *Acta Paediatr Scand* 43(Suppl. 100):307–317.

Fried I, Kim JH, Spencer DD. 1994. Limbic and neocortical gliomas associated with intractable seizures: a distinct clinicopathological group. *Neurosurgery* 34:815–823.

Friede RL. 1989. *Developmental neuropathology*, 2nd ed. Berlin: Springer-Verlag.

Friedman F, Pampiglione G. 1971. Prognostic implications of electroencephalographic findings in hypsarrhythmia in the first year of life. *BMJ* 4:323–325.

Friis ML. 1990. Stress convulsions. In: Dam M, Gram L, eds. *Comprehensive epileptology*. New York: Raven Press, 247–250.

Fritsch G, Ebner F, Schneider G. 1988. Computed tomography in partial epilepsies in childhood. *Eur Neurol* 28:306–310.

Fromm GH. 1985. Effects of different classes of antiepileptic drugs in brain-stem pathways. *Federation Proceedings* 44:2432–2435.

Fromm GH, Crumrine P. 1986. Ethosuximide: an update. In: Pedley TA, Meldrum BS, eds. *Recent advances in epilepsy*, Vol. 3. Edinburgh: Churchill Livingstone, 279–294.

Fröscher W. 1979. *Treatment of status epilepticus*. Baltimore: University Park Press.

Frost JD Jr, Hrachovy RA, Kellaway P, et al. 1978. Quantitative analysis and characterization of infantile spasms. *Epilepsia* 19:273–282.

Frost JD, Hrachovy RA, Glaze DG. 1992. Spike morphology in childhood focal epilepsy: relationship to syndromic classification. *Epilepsia* 33:531–536.

Fryns JP. 1997. The X-linked infantile spasms syndrome (MIM 308350) maps to Xp11.4-Xpter in two pedigrees. *Ann Neurol* 42:360–364.

Fu YH, Kuhl DP, Pizzuti A, et al. 1991. Variation of the CGG repeat at the fragile X site results in genetic instability: resolution of the Sherman paradox. *Cell* 67:1047–1059.

Fuji T, Okuno T, Go T, et al. 1987. Clorazepate therapy for intractable epilepsy. *Brain Dev* 9:288–291.

Fujiwara T, Ishida S, Miyakoshi M, et al. 1979. Status epilepticus in childhood: a retrospective study of initial status and subsequent epilepsies. *Folia Psychiatr Neurol Jpn* 33:337–344.

Fujiwara T, Nakamura H, Watanabe M, et al. 1990. Clinicoelectrographic concordance between monozygotic twins with severe myoclonic epilepsy in infancy. *Epilepsia* 31:281–286.

Fujiwara T, Sugawara T, Mazaki-Miyazaki E, et al. 2003. Mutations of sodium channel alpha subunit type 1 (SCN1A) in intractable childhood epilepsies with frequent generalized tonic-clonic seizures. *Brain* 126:531–546.

Fukuhara N, Tokiguchi S, Shirakawa K, et al. 1980. Myoclonus epilepsy associated with ragged-red fibres (mitochondrial abnormalities): disease entity or a syndrome? Light- and electron-microscopic studies of two cases and review of literature. *J Neurol Sci* 47: 117–133.

Fukuyama Y. 1960. Studies on the etiology and pathogenesis of flexor spasms in infancy. *Adv Neurol Sci (Tokyo)* 4:861.

Fukuyama Y. 1963. Borderland of childhood epilepsy—special reference to febrile convulsions and so-called infantile convulsions. *Seishin Igaku* 5:211–223.

Fukuyama Y. 1991. 13th Annual Conference on Febrile Convulsions, Tokyo, December 15, 1990. Abstracts. *Brain Dev* 13:203–211.

Fukuyama Y, Tsuchiya S. 1979. A study on Sturge-Weber syndrome. Report of a case associated with infantile spasms and electroencephalographic evolution in five cases. *Eur Neurol* 18:194–209.

Fukuyama Y, Tomori N, Sugitate M. 1977. Critical evaluation of the role of immunization as an etiological factor of infantile spasms. *Neuropédiatrie* 8:224–237.

Fukuyama Y, Kagawa K, Tanaka K. 1979. A genetic study of febrile convulsions. *Eur Neurol* 18:166–182.

Furman JM, Crumrine PK, Reinmuth OM. 1990. Epileptic nystagmus. *Ann Neurol* 27:686–688.

Furune S, Watanabe K, Negoro T, et al. 1986. Long-term prognosis and clinico-electroencephalographic evolution of Lennox-Gastaut syndrome. *Brain Dysfunction* 1: 146–153.

Fusco L, Vigevano F. 1993. Ictal clinical electroencephalographic findings of spasms in West syndrome. *Epilepsia* 34:671–678.

Fusco L, Lani C, Faedda MT, et al. 1990. Mesial frontal lobe epilepsy: a clinical entity not sufficiently described. *J Epilepsy* 3:123–135.

Fusco L, Ferracuti S, Fariello G, et al. 1992. Hemimeganencephaly and normal intellectual development. *J Neurol Neurosurg Psychiatry* 55:720–722.

Fusco L, Pachatz C, Cusmai R, et al. 1999. Repetitive sleep starts in neurologically impaired children: an unusual non-epileptic manifestation in otherwise epileptic subjects. *Epileptic Disord* 1:63–67.

Gabor AJ. 1974. Focal seizures induced by movement without sensory feedback mechanisms. *Electroencephalogr Clin Neurophysiol* 36:403–408.

Gabr M, Lüders H, Dinner D, et al. 1989. Speech manifestations in lateralization of temporal lobe seizures. *Ann Neurol* 25:82–87.

Gabriel YH. 1980. Unilateral hemispheric ganglioglioma with infantile spasms. *Ann Neurol* 7:287–288.

Gaggero R, Caputo M, Florio P, et al. 1995. SPECT and epilepsy with continuous spike waves during slow-wave sleep. *Childs Nerv Syst* 11:154–160.

Gaillard WD. 2001. Metabolic and functional neuroimaging. In: Wyllie E, ed. *The treatment of epilepsy: principles and practice.* Philadelphia: Lippincott Williams & Wilkins, 1053–1066.

Gaillard WD, Kopylev L, Weinstein S, et al. 2002. Low incidence of abnormal ^{18}FDG-PET in children with new-onset partial epilepsy: a prospective study. *Neurology* 58:717–722.

Gaily EK, Shewmon DA, Chugani HT, et al. 1995. Asymmetric and asynchronous infantile spasms. *Epilepsia* 36:873–882.

Gaily E, Appelqvist K, Kantola-Sorsa E, et al. 1999. Cognitive deficits after cryptogenic infantile spasms with benign seizure evolution. *Dev Med Child Neurol* 41:660–664.

Gaily E, Liukkonen E, Paetau R, et al. 2001. Infantile spasms: diagnosis and assessment of treatment response by video-EEG. *Dev Med Child Neurol* 43:658–667.

Gal P, Boer HR. 1982. Early discontinuation of anticonvulsants after neonatal seizures: a preliminary report. *South Med J* 75:298–300.

Gal P, Roop C, Robinson H. 1980. Theophylline-induced seizures in accidentally overdosed neonates. *Pediatrics* 65:547–549.

Gal P, Toback J, Boer HR, et al. 1982. Efficacy of phenobarbital monotherapy in treatment of neonatal seizures—relationship to blood levels. *Neurology* 32:1401–1404.

Gal P, Sharpless MK, Boer HR. 1984. Outcome in neonates with seizures: are chronic anticonvulsants necessary? *Ann Neurol* 15:610–611.

Gal P, Oles KS, Gilman JT, et al. 1988. Valproic acid efficacy, toxicity and pharmacokinetics in neonates with intractable seizures. *Neurology* 38:467–471.

Galaburda AM, Sherman GF, Rosen GD, et al. 1985. Developmental dyslexia: four consecutive patients with cortical anomalies. *Ann Neurol* 18:222–233.

Galanopoulou AS, Bojko A, Lado F, et al. 2000. The spectrum of neuropsychiatric abnormalities associated with electrical status epilepticus in sleep. *Brain Dev* 21: 279–285.

Gallucci M, Bozzao A, Curatolo P, et al. 1991. MR imaging of incomplete band heterotopia. *Am J Neuroradiol* 12: 701–702.

Gambardella A, Reutens DC, Andermann F, et al. 1994. Late-onset drop attacks in temporal lobe epilepsy: a reevaluation of the concept of temporal lobe syncope. *Neurology* 44:1074–1078.

Gambardella A, Gotman J, Cendes F, et al. 1995a. Focal intermittent delta activity in patients with mesiotemporal atrophy: a reliable marker of the epileptogenic focus. *Epilepsia* 36:122–129.

Gambardella A, Gotman J, Cendes F, et al. 1995b. The relation of spike foci and clinical seizure characteristics to different patterns of mesial temporal atrophy. *Arch Neurol* 52:287–293.

Gambardella A, Palmini A, Andermann F, et al. 1996. Usefulness of focal rhythmic discharges on scalp EEG of patients with focal cortical dysplasia and intractable epilepsy. *Electroencephalogr Clin Neurophysiol* 98: 243–249.

Gambardella A, Annesi G, De Fusco M, et al. 2000. A new locus for autosomal dominant nocturnal frontal lobe epilepsy maps to chromosome 1. *Neurology* 55: 1467–1471.

Gamstorp I. 1976. Carbamazepine in the treatment of epileptic disorders in infancy and childhood. In: Birkmayer W, ed. *Epileptic seizures, behaviour, pain.* Bern: Hans Huber.

Gamstorp I. 1983. Partial seizures. In: Morselli PL, Pippenger CE, Penry JK, eds. *Antiepileptic drug therapy in pediatrics.* New York: Raven Press, 163–171.

Gamstorp I, Sedin G. 1982. Neonatal convulsions treated with continuous intravenous infusion of diazepam. *Ups J Med Sci* 87:143–149.

Ganesh S, Agarwala KL, Ueda K, et al. 2000. Laforin, defective in progressive myoclonus epilepsy of Lafora type, is a dual specificity phosphatase associated with polyribosomes [Abstract]. *Hum Mol Genet* 65:A297.

Garcia PA, Laxer KD, Barbaro NM, et al. 1994. Prognostic value of qualitative MR imaging hippocampal abnormalities in patients undergoing temporal lobectomy for medically refractory seizures. *Epilepsia* 35:520–524.

Garcia Silva MT, Aicardi J, Goutières F, Chevrie JJ. 1987. The syndrome of myoclonic epilepsy with ragged-red fibers. Report of a case and review of the literature. *Neuropediatrics* 18:200–204.

Garcia-Flores E. 1987. Corpus callosum section for patients with intractable epilepsy. *Appl Neurophysiol* 50:390–397.

Gardiner M, Sandford A, Deadman M, et al. 1990. Batten disease (Spielmeyer-Vogt disease, juvenile onset ceroid-lipofuscinosis) gene (CLN3) maps to human chromosome 16. *Genomics* 8:387–390.

Gascon G, Barlow C. 1970. Juvenile migraine presenting as an acute confusional state. *Pediatrics* 45:628–635.

Gascon GG, Lombroso CT. 1971. Epileptic (gelastic) laughter. *Epilepsia* 12:63–76.

Gascon G, Victor D, Lombroso CT, et al. 1973. Language disorder, convulsive disorder, and electroencephalographic abnormalities. *Arch Neurol* 28:156–162.

Gastaut H. 1969a. Clinical and electroencephalographical classification of epileptic seizures. *Epilepsia* 11:102–113.

Gastaut H. 1969b. Introduction to the study of organic generalized epilepsies. In: Gastaut H, Jasper H, Bancaud A, et al., eds. *The physiopathogenesis of the epilepsies.* Springfield, IL: Charles C Thomas Publisher, 147–157.

Gastaut H. 1973. Part I: Definitions. *Dictionary of epilepsies.* Geneva: World Health Organization.

Gastaut H. 1974. Syncopes: generalized anoxic seizures. In: Vinken PJ, Bruyn GW, eds. *Handbook of clinical neurology,* Vol. 15. Amsterdam: North Holland, 815–835.

Gastaut H. 1981. The effects of benzodiazepines on chronic epilepsy in man (with particular reference to clobazam). In: Hindmarch I, Stonier PD, eds. *Clobazam.* The Royal Society of Medicine International Congress and Symposium Series, No. 43. London: Academic Press, 141–150.

Gastaut H. 1983. Classification of status epilepticus. In: Delgado-Escueta AV, Wasterlain CG, Treiman DM, Porter RJ. *Status epilepticus.* Advances in neurology, Vol. 34. New York: Raven Press, 75–81.

Gastaut H. 1985. Benign epilepsy of childhood with occipital paroxysms. In: Roger J, Dravet C, Bureau M, et al., eds. *Epileptic syndromes in infancy, childhood and adolescence.* London: John Libbey, 159–170.

Gastaut H. 1992. Benign epilepsy of childhood with occipital paroxysms. In: Roger J, Dravet C, Bureau M, et al., eds. *Epileptic syndromes in infancy, childhood and adolescence,* 2nd ed. London: John Libbey, 201–217.

Gastaut H, Broughton R. 1972. *Epileptic seizures.* Springfield, IL: Charles C Thomas Publisher.

Gastaut H, Gastaut Y. 1958. Etude électroencéphalographique et clinique des convulsions anoxiques de l'enfant. Leur situation dans le cadre des convulsions infantiles. *Rev Neurol (Paris)* 99:100–125.

Gastaut H, Gastaut JL. 1976. Computerized transverse axial tomography in epilepsies. *Epilepsia* 17:325–336.

Gastaut H, Lowe MD. 1979. Antiepileptic properties of clobazam, a 1,5 benzodiazepine, in man. *Epilepsia* 20:437–446.

Gastaut H, Pirovano E. 1949. Epilepsy induced with intermittent auditory stimulation. *Arch Psicol Neurol Psichiatr* 10:297–316.

Gastaut H, Regis H. 1961. On the subject of Lennox's akinetic petit mal. *Epilepsia* 2:298–305.

Gastaut H, Roger A. 1955. Origine et propagation des décharges épileptiques temporales provoquées. In: Alajouanine T, ed. *Les grandes activités du lobe temporal.* Paris: Masson, 83–133.

Gastaut H, Tassinari CA. 1975a. Ictal discharges in different types of seizures. In: Rémond A, ed. *Handbook of electroencephalography and clinical neurophysiology,* Vol. 13A. Amsterdam: Elsevier, 13–45.

Gastaut H, Tassinari CA. 1975b. Status epilepticus. In: Rémond A, ed. *Handbook of electroencephalography and clinical neurophysiology,* Vol. 13A. Amsterdam: Elsevier, 39–45.

Gastaut H, Zifkin BG. 1984. Ictal visual hallucinations of numerals. *Neurology* 34:950–953.

Gastaut H, Zifkin BG. 1985. Classification of the epilepsies. *J Clin Neurophysiol* 2:313–326.

Gastaut H, Zifkin BG. 1987. Benign epilepsy of childhood with occipital spike and wave complexes. In: Andermann F, Lugaresi E, eds. *Migraine and epilepsy* London: Butterworth-Heinemann, 47–81.

Gastaut H, Zifkin BG. 1988. Secondary bilateral synchrony and Lennox-Gastaut syndrome. In: Niedermeyer E, Degen R, eds. *The Lennox-Gastaut syndrome.* New York: Alan R. Liss, 221–242.

Gastaut H, Naquet R, Vigouroux R, et al. 1953. Etude électroencéphalographique chez l'homme et chez animal des décharges épileptiques dites psychomotrices. *Rev Neurol (Paris)* 88:310–354.

Gastaut H, Roger J, Roger A. 1956. Sur la signification de certaines fugues épileptiques. A propos d'une observation électroclinique "d'état de mal temporal". *Rev Neurol (Paris)* 94:298–301.

Gastaut H, Vigouroux M, Trevisan C, et al. 1957. Le syndrome hémiconvulsions-hémiplégie-épilepsie (syndrome HHE). *Rev Neurol (Paris)* 97:37–52.

Gastaut H, Poirier F, Payan H, et al. 1960. HHE syndrome: hemiconvulsion-hemiplegia-epilepsy. *Epilepsia* 1:418–447.

Gastaut H, Roger J, Soulayrol R, et al. 1962. Sur la nature et la signification des crises épileptiques hyperthermiques. A propos d'une observation familiale privilégiée. *Rev Neurol (Paris)* 107:235–241.

Gastaut H, Roger J, Ouachi S, et al. 1963. An electro-clinical study of generalized epileptic seizures of tonic expression. *Epilepsia* 4:15–44.

Gastaut H, Roger J, Soulayrol R, et al. 1964. *L'encéphalopathie myoclonique infantile avec hypsarythmie (syndrome de West).* Paris: Masson.

Gastaut H, Roger J, Soulayrol R, et al. 1966a. Childhood epileptic encephalopathy with diffuse spike-waves (otherwise known as "petit mal variant") or Lennox syndrome. *Epilepsia* 7:139–179.

Gastaut H, Tassinari CA, Bureau-Paillas M. 1966b. Etude polygraphique et clinique des "effondrements atoniques épileptiques." *Rivista di Neurologia (Napoli)* 36:3–8.

Gastaut H, Roger J, Lob H. 1967. *Les états de mal épileptiques.* Paris: Masson.

Gastaut H, Dravet C, Loubier D. 1973a. Evolution clinique et pronostic du syndrome de Lennox-Gastaut. In: Lugaresi E, Pazzaglia P, Tassinari CA, eds. *Evolution and prognosis of epilepsies.* Bologna: Aulo Gaggi, 133–154.

Gastaut H, Gastaut JA, Gastaut L, et al. 1973b. Epilepsie généralisée primaire grand mal. In: Lugaresi E, Pazzaglia P, Tassinari CA, eds. *Evolution and prognosis of epilepsies.* Bologna: Aulo Gaggi, 25–53.

Gastaut H, Broughton R, Roger J, et al. 1974a. Generalized convulsive seizures without local onset. In: Vinken PJ, Gruyn GW, eds. *The epilepsies.* Handbook of clinical neurology, Vol. 15. Amsterdam: Elsevier, 107–129.

Gastaut H, Broughton R, Roger J, et al. 1974b. Generalized non-convulsive seizures without local onset. In: Vinken PJ, Gruyn GW, eds. *The epilepsies.* Handbook of clinical neurology, Vol. 15. Amsterdam: Elsevier, 130–144.

Gastaut H, Broughton R, Tassinari CA, et al. 1974c. Unilateral epileptic seizures. In: Vinken PJ, Gruyn GW, eds. *The epilepsies.* Handbook of clinical neurology, Vol. 15. Amsterdam: Elsevier, 235–245.

Gastaut H, Gastaut JL, Goncalves e Silva GE, Fernandez Sanchez GR. 1975. Relative frequencies of different types of epilepsy: a study employing a classfication of the International League Against Epilepsy. *Epilepsia* 16:457–461.

Gastaut H, Pinsard N, Gastaut JL, et al. 1977. Etude tomod-ensitométrique des accidents cérébraux responsables des hémiplégies aiguës de l'enfant. *Rev Neurol (Paris)* 133:595–607.

Gastaut H, Gastaut JL, Régis H, et al. 1978. Computerized tomography in the study of West's syndrome. *Dev Med Child Neurol* 20:21–27.

Gastaut H, Santanelli P, Salinas Jara M. 1985. Une activité EEG intercritique spécifique d'une variété particulière d'épilepsie temporale. Le rythme theta temporal épileptique. *Rev Electroencephalogr Neurophysiol Clin* 15: 113–120.

Gastaut H, Aguglia V, Tinuper P. 1986a. Benign versive or circling epilepsy with bilateral 3-cps spike-and-wave discharges in late childhood. *Ann Neurol* 19:301–303.

Gastaut H, Zifkin BG, Mariani A, et al. 1986b. The long-term course of primary generalized epilepsy with persisting absences. *Neurology* 36:1021–1028.

Gastaut H, Pinsard N, Raybaud C, et al. 1987a. Lissencephaly (agyria-pachygyria): clinical findings and serial EEG studies. *Dev Med Child Neurol* 29: 167–180.

Gastaut H, Zifkin B, Maggauda A, et al. 1987b. Symptomatic partial epilepsies with secondary bilateral synchrony: differentiation from symptomatic generalized epilepsies of the Lennox-Gastaut type. In: Wieser HG, Elger CE, eds. *Presurgical evaluation of epileptics.* Berlin: Springer, 308–316.

Gastaut H, Zifkin B, Rufo M. 1987c. Compulsive respiratory stereotypes in children with autistic features: polygraphic recording and treatment with fenfluramine. *J Autism Dev Disord* 17:391–406.

Gates JR, Cruz-Rodriguez R. 1990. Mesial temporal sclerosis: pathogenesis, diagnosis, and management. *Epilepsia* 31:S55–S66.

Gates JR, Gumnit RJ. 1990. Partial seizures of temporal lobe origin. In: Dam M, Gram L, eds. *Comprehensive epileptology.* New York: Raven Press, 187–195.

Gates JR, Leppik IE, Yap J, et al. 1984. Corpus callosotomy: clinical and electroencephalographic effects. *Epilepsia* 25:308–316.

Gates JR, Rosenfeld WE, Maxwell RE, et al. 1987. Response of multiple seizure types to corpus callosum section. *Epilepsia* 28:28–34.

Geier S, Bancaud J, Talairach J, et al. 1973. Signification des correlations electro-cliniques au cours de crises visuelles enregistrées en tele-S.E.E.G. *Rev Electroencephalogr Neurophysiol Clin* 3:355–359.

Geier S, Bancaud J, Talairach J, et al. 1976. Automatisms during frontal lobe epileptic seizures. *Brain* 99:447–458.

Geier S, Bancaud J, Talairach J, et al. 1977. The seizures of frontal lobe epilepsy: a study of clinical manifestations. *Neurology* 27:951–958.

Geiger LR, Hanrer RN. 1978. EEG patterns at the time of focal seizure onset. *Arch Neurol* 35:276–286.

Gelisse P, Genton P, Thomas P, et al. 2001. Clinical factors of drug resistance in juvenile myoclonic epilepsy. *J Neurol Neurosurg Psychiatry* 70:240–243.

Genc BO, Genc E, Tastekin G, et al. 2001. Musicogenic epilepsy with ictal single photon emission computed tomography (SPECT): could these cases contribute to our knowledge of music processing? *Eur J Neurol* 8: 191–194.

Genton P. 1995a. Epilepsy with 3 Hz spike-and-waves without clinically evident absences. In: Duncan JS,

Panayiotopoulos CP, eds. *Typical absences and related syndromes.* London: Churchill Communication Europe, 231–238.

Genton P. 1995b. In discussion of Smith's paper. In: Duncan JS, Panayiotopoulos CP, eds. *Typical absences and related syndromes.* London: Churchill Communication Europe, 101.

Genton P, Dravet C. 1998. Lennox-Gastaut syndrome and other epileptic encephalopathies. In: Engel J Jr, Pedley TA, eds. *Childhood epilipsy: a comprehensive textbook.* Philadelphia: Lippincott-Raven, 2355–2365.

Genton P, Gelisse P. 2000. Atimyoclonic effect of levetiracetam. *Epileptic Disord* 2:209–212.

Genton P, Gelisse P. 2001. Premature death in juvenile myoclonic epilepsy. *Acta Neurol Scand* 104:125–129.

Genton P, Van Vleymen B. 2000. Piracetam and levetiracetam: close structural similarities but different pharmacological and clinical profiles. *Epileptic Disord* 2:99–105.

Genton P, McMenamin J. 1998. Summary. Aggravation of seizures by antiepileptic drugs: what to do in clinical practice. *Epilepsia* 39:S26–S29.

Genton P, Michelucci R, Tassinari CA, et al. 1990a. The Ramsay Hunt syndrome revisited: Mediterranean myoclonus vs. mitochondrial encephalomyopathy with ragged-red fibers and Baltic myoclonus. *Acta Neurol Scand* 81:8–15.

Genton P, Ogihara M, Samoggia G, et al. 1990b. Activation élective des paroxysmes temporaux à l'endormissement et pendant le sommeil dans un cas de syndrome de Landau-Kleffner. *Rev Electroencephalogr Neurophysiol Clin* 20:529.

Genton P, Medina MT, Roger J, et al. 1992. Syndrome de Klinefelter (dysgénésie gonadique avec caryotype 47, XXY) et épilepsie: 5 observations. *Bolletino Lega Italiana contre l'Epilepsia* 79/80:69–70.

Genton P, Salas Puig J, Tunon A, et al. 1994. Juvenile myoclonic epilepsy and related syndromes: clinical and neurophysiological aspects. In: Malafosse A, Genton P, Hirsch C, et al., eds. *Idiopathic generalized epilepsies: clinical, experimental and genetic aspects.* London: John Libbey, 253–265.

Genton P, Guerrini R, Bureau M, et al. 1995a. Continuous focal discharges in REM sleep in a case of Landau-Kleffner syndrome: a three-year follow up. In: Beaumanoir A, Bureau M, Deonna T, et al., eds. *Continous spikes and waves during slow sleep.* London: John Libbey, 155–159.

Genton P, Bartolomei F, Guerrini R. 1995b. Panic attacks mistaken for relapse of epilepsy. *Epilepsia* 36:48–51.

Genton P, Gelisse P, Thomas P. 2000a. Juvenile myoclonic epilepsy today: current definitions and limits. In: Schmitz B, Sander T, eds. *Juvenile myoclonic epilepsy: the Janz syndrome.* Petersfield: Wrightson Biomedical Publishing, 11–32.

Genton P, Gelisse P, Thomas P, Dravet C. 2000b. Do carbamazepine and phenytoin aggravate juvenile myoclonic epilepsy? *Neurology* 55:1106–1109.

Genton P, Guerrini R, Dravet C. 2000c. The Lennox-Gastaut syndrome. In: Meinardi, H, ed. *Handbook of Clinical Neurology: The Epilepsies, Part II.* Vol. 73 (29). Amsterdam: Elsevier Science, 211–222.

Genton P, Malafosse A, Moulard B, et al. 2002. Progressive myoclonus epilepsies. In: Roger J, Bureau M, Genton M, et al., eds. *Epileptic syndromes in infancy, childhood and adolescence*, 3rd ed. London: John Libbey 407–430.

Geoffroy G, Lassonde M, Delisle F, et al. 1983. Corpus callosotomy for control of intractable epilepsy in children. *Neurology* 33:891–897.

Gerber PE, Hamiwka L, Connolly MB, et al. 2000. Factors associated with behavioral and cognitive abnormalities in children receiving topiramate. *Pediatr Neurol* 22:200–203.

Gerken H, Doose H. 1973. On the genetics of EEG anomalies. III: Spikes and waves in the resting records and/or during hyperventilation. *Neuropédiatrie* 4:88–97.

Geshwind N. 1979. Behaviour changes in temporal lobe epilepsy. *Psychol Med* 9:217–219.

Geshwind N, Sherwin I. 1967. Language-induced epilepsy. *Arch Neurol* 16:25–31.

Gherpelli JL, Guerreiro MM, da Costa JC, et al. 1997. Vigabatrin in refractory childhood epilepsy. The Brazilian Multicentre Study. *Epilepsy Res* 29:1–6.

Ghilain S, Van Rijckevorsel-Harmant K, Harmant J, de Barsy TH. 1988. Midazolam in the treatment of epileptic seizures. *J Neurol Neurosurg Psychiatry* 51:732.

Gianelli M, Gentile S, Verzé L, et al. 1988. Free drug levels monitoring as a detector of false metabolic refractory epilepsy. *Eur Neurol* 28:349–353.

Giang DW, McBride MC. 1988. Lorazepam versus diazepam for the treatment of status epilepticus. *Pediatr Neurol* 4:358–361.

Gibberd FB. 1966. The prognosis of petit mal. *Brain* 89:531–538.

Gibberd FB, Park DM, Scott G, et al. 1982. A comparison of phenytoin and pheneturide in patients with epilepsy: a double-blind cross-over trial. *J Neurol Neurosurg Psychiatry* 45:1113–1118.

Gibbs FA, Gibbs EL. 1952. *Atlas of electroencephalography*, Vol. II. Cambridge, MA: Addison Wesley.

Gibbs FA, Gibbs EL, Lennox WG. 1937. Epilepsy: a paroxysmal cerebral dysrhythmia. *Brain* 60:377–388.

Gilchrist JM. 1985. Arrhythmogenic seizures: diagnosis by simultaneous EEG/ECG recording. *Neurology* 35:1503–1506.

Gilhus NE, Matte R. 1986. Carbamazepine effects on mononuclear blood cells in epileptic patients. *Acta Neurol Scand* 74:181–185.

Gillam GL. 1982. Convulsions following birth asphyxia/birth trauma: are long-term anticonvulsants necessary? *Aust Paediatr J* 18:90–91.

Gillberg C. 1992. Autism and autistic-like conditions. In: Aicardi J, ed. *Diseases of the nervous system in childhood*. London: MacKeith Press, 1295–1320.

Gillberg C. 1998. Autism and autistic-like conditions. In: Aicardi J, ed. *Diseases of the nervous system in childhood*, 2nd ed. London: MacKeith Press, 827–842.

Gillberg C, Schaumann H. 1983. Epilepsy presenting as infantile autism? Two case studies. *Neuropediatrics* 14:206–212.

Gillberg C, Uvebrant P, Carlson G, et al. 1996. Autism and epilepsy (and tuberous sclerosis?) in two preadolescent boys: neuropsychiatric aspects before and after surgery. *Journal of Intellectual Disability Research* 40:75–81.

Gilles FH, Sobel F, Leviton A, et al. 1992. Epidemiology of seizures in children with brain tumors. The Childhood Brain Tumor Consortium. *J Neurooncol* 13:336–344.

Gilliam F, Wyllie E. 1997. Functional outcome of children following corpus callosum section. In: Tuxhorn I,

Holthausen H, Pannek H, eds. *Paediatric epilepsy syndromes and their surgical treatment*. London: John Libbey, 850–853.

Gilly R, Lapras C, Tommasi M, et al. 1977. Maladie de Sturge-Weber-Krabbe. Réflexion à partir de 21 cas. *Pédiatrie* 32:45–64.

Gilman JT, Duchowny MS, Hershorin ER. 1988. Carbamazepine malabsorption: a case report. *Pediatrics* 82:518–519.

Gilman JT, Duchowny M, Jayakar P, et al. 1994. Medical intractability in children evaluated for epilepsy surgery. *Neurology* 44:1341–1343.

Gilsanz V, Stand R, Barnes P, et al. 1979. Results of presumed cryptogenic epilepsy in childhood by CT scanning. *Ann Radiol* 22:184–187.

Gimenez-Roldan S, Martin M. 1979. Effectiveness of clonazepam in startle-induced seizures. *Epilepsia* 20:255–261.

Gimenez-Roldan S, Martin M. 1980. Startle epilepsy complicating Down syndrome during adulthood. *Ann Neurol* 7:78–80.

Giovanardi Rossi P, Gobbi G, Melideo G, et al. 1988a. Myoclonic manifestations in the Lennox-Gastaut syndrome and other childhood epilepsies. In: Niedermeyer E, Degen R, eds. *The Lennox-Gastaut syndrome*. New York: Alan R. Liss, 137–158.

Giovanardi Rossi P, Ricciutello CD, Calaso E, et al. 1988b. Afasia acquisita con anomalie convulsive. Sindrome di Landau-Kleffner. In: *I. Corso di aggiornamento sulle epilessie dell'infanzia e dell'adolescenza*. Rome: Sigma-Tau, 218–224.

Giovanardi Rossi P, Santucci M, Gobbi G, et al. 1991. Long-term follow-up of severe myoclonic epilepsy in infancy. In: Fukuyama Y, Kamoshita S, Ohtsuka C, et al., eds. *Modern perspectives of child neurology*. Tokyo: Japanese Society of Child Neurology, 205–213.

Giovanardi Rossi P, Parmeggiani A, Posar A, et al. 1997. Benign myoclonic epilepsy: long-term follow-up of 11 new cases. *Brain Dev* 19:473–479.

Giovanardi Rossi P, Parmeggiani P, Posar A, et al. 1999. Landau-Kleffner syndrome (LKS): long term follow up and links with electrical status epilepticus during sleep (ESES). *Brain Dev* 21:90–98.

Giroud M, Borsotti JP, Michiels R, et al. 1990. Epilepsie et calcifications occipitales bilatérales: 3 cas. *Rev Neurol (Paris)* 146:288–292.

Giroud M, Gras D, Escousse A, et al. 1993. Use of injectable valproic acid in status epilepticus: a pilot study. *Drug Invest* 5:154–159.

Glaser GH. 1967. Limbic epilepsy in childhood. *J Nerv Ment Dis* 144:391–397.

Glaser GH. 1980. Treatment of intractable temporal lobe-limbic epilepsy (complex partial seizures) by temporal lobectomy. *Ann Neurol* 8:455–459.

Glaser GH. 1983. Medical complications of status epilepticus. In: Delgado-Escueta AV, Wasterlain CG, Treiman DM, Porter RJ, eds. *Status epilepticus*. Advances in neurology, Vol. 34. New York: Raven Press, 395–398.

Glaser GH, Dixon MS. 1956. Psychomotor seizures in childhood: a clinical study. *Neurology* 6:646–655.

Glauser TA, Clancy RR. 1992. Adequacy of routine EEG examination in neonates with clinically suspected seizures. *J Child Neurol* 7:215–220.

Glauser TA, Morita DA. 2001. Encephalopathic epilepsy after infancy. In: Pellock JM, Dodson WE, Bourgeois B, eds. *Pediatric epilepsy: diagnosis and therapy,* 2nd ed. New York: Demos, 201–218.

Glauser TA, Clark PO, Strawsburg R. 1998. A pilot study of topiramate in the treatment of infantile spasms. *Epilepsia* 39:1324–1328.

Glauser TA, Clark PO, McGee K. 2000a. Long-term response to topiramate in patients with West syndrome. *Epilepsia* 41:S91–S94.

Glauser TA, Nigro M, Sachdeo R, et al. 2000b. Adjunctive therapy with oxcarbazepine in children with partial seizures. The Oxcarbazepine Pediatric Study Group. *Neurology* 54:2237–2244.

Glauser TA, Pellock JM, Bebin EM, et al. 2002. Efficacy and safety of levetiracetam in children with partial seizures: an open-label trial. *Epilepsia* 43:518–524.

Glaze DG, Hrachovy RA, Frost JD Jr, et al. 1986. Computed tomography in infantile spasms: effects of hormonal therapy. *Pediatr Neurol* 2:23–27.

Glaze DG, Hrachovy RA, Frost JD Jr, et al. 1988. Prospective study of outcome of infants with infantile spasms treated during controlled studies of ACTH and prednisone. *J Pediatr* 112:389–396.

Gleeson JG, Allen KA, Fox JW, et al. 1998. Double cortin, a brain-specific gene mutated in human X-linked lissencephaly and double cortex syndrome, encodes a putative signaling protein. *Cell* 92:63–72.

Gleeson JG, Luo RF, Grant PE, et al. 2000a. Genetic and neuroradiological heterogeneity of double cortex syndrome. *Ann Neurol* 47:265–269.

Gleeson JG, Minnerath S, Kuzniecky RI, et al. 2000b. Somatic and germline mosaic mutations in the double cortin gene are associated with variable phenotypes. *Am J Hum Genet* 67:574–581.

Gleissner U, Sassen R, Lendt M, et al. 2002. Pre- and postoperative verbal memory in pediatric patients with temporal lobe epilepsy. *Epilepsy Res* 51:287–296.

Glista GG, Franck HG, Tracy FW. 1983. Video games and seizures. *Arch Neurol* 40:588.

Globus M, Lavi E, Fich A, et al. 1982. Ictal hemiparesis. *Eur Neurol* 21:165–168.

Gloor P. 1979. Generalized epilepsy with spike-and-wave discharge: a reinterpretation of its electroencephalographic and clinical manifestations. *Epilepsia* 20:571–588.

Gloor P. 1983. Electrophysiology of generalized epilepsy. In: Wheal H, Schwartzkroin P, eds. *Electrophysiology of epilepsy.* London: Academic Press.

Gloor P. 1986. Consciousness as a neurological concept in epileptology: a critical review. *Epilepsia* 27:S14–S26.

Gloor P. 1989. Epilepsy: relationship between electrophysiology and intracellular mechanisms involving second messengers and gene expression. *Can J Neurol Sci* 16:8–21.

Gloor P. 1990. Experiential phenomena of temporal lobe epilepsy: facts and hypotheses. *Brain* 113:1673–1694.

Gloor T. 1995. Feline generalised penicillin epilepsy: extrapolations to neurophysiological mechanisms in humans. In: Duncan JS, Panayiotopoulos CP, eds. *Typical absences and related syndromes.* London: Churchill Communication Europe, 74–82.

Gloor P, Rasmussen T, Altuzzara A, et al. 1976. Role of the intracarotid. Amobarbital-pentylenetetrazol EEG test in the diagnosis and surgical treatment of patients with complex seizure problems. *Epilepsia* 17:15–31.

Gloor P, Olivier A, Ives J. 1980. Loss of consciousness in temporal lobes seizures: observations obtained with stereotactic depth electrode recordings and stimulations. In: Canger R, Angeleri F, Penry, JK, eds. *Advances in epileptology.* XIth Epilepsy International Symposium. New York: Raven Press, 349–353.

Gloor P, Metrakos J, Metrakos K, et al. 1982a. Neurophysiological, genetic and biochemical nature of the epileptic diathesis. *Electroencephalogr Clin Neurophysiol* 55(Suppl. 35):45–56.

Gloor P, Olivier A, Quesney LF, et al. 1982b. The role of the limbic system in experiential phenomena of temporal lobe epilepsy. *Ann Neurol* 12:129–144.

Gloor P, Avoli M, Kostopoulos G. 1990. Thalamocortical relationships in generalized epilepsy with bilaterally synchronous spike-and-wave discharge. In: Avoli M, Gloor P, Kostopoulos G, Naquet R, eds. *Generalized epilepsy: neurobiological approaches.* Boston: Birkhauser, 190–212.

Gluckman MI, Stein L. 1978. Pharmacology of lorazepam. *J Clin Psychiatry* 39:3–10.

Glötzner FL. 1981. Antiepileptische Prophylaxe mit Carbamazepin bei Patienten mit schweren Schädel-Hirntraumen. In: Remschmidt H, Rentz R, Jungmann J, eds. *Epilepsie 1980.* Stuttgart: Thieme-Verlag, 144–147.

Glötzner FL, Haubitz I, Milner F, et al. 1983. Anfällsprophylaze mit Carbamazepin nach schweren Schädel-hirverletzungen. *Neurochirurgia* 26:66–79.

Gobbi G, Bruno L, Pini A, et al. 1987. Periodic spasms: an unclassified type of epileptic seizure in childhood. *Dev Med Child Neurol* 27:766–775.

Gobbi G, Sorrenti G, Santucci M, et al. 1988. Epilepsy with bilateral occipital calcifications: a benign onset with progressive severity. *Neurology* 38:913–920.

Gobbi G, Tassinari CA, Roger J, et al. 1989. Particularités électroencéphalographiques des épilepsies partielles symptomatiques sévères de l'enfant. *Neurophysiol Clin* 19:209–218.

Gobbi G, Ambrosetto G, Parmaggiani A, et al. 1991. The malignant variant of partial epilepsy with occipital spikes in childhood. *Epilepsia* 32(Suppl. 1):16–17.

Gobbi G, Bouquet F, Greco L, et al. 1992. Coeliac disease, epilepsy and cerebral calcifications. The Italian Working Group on Coeliac Disease and Epilepsy. *Lancet* 340:439–443.

Goddard GV, McIntyre DC, Leech CK. 1969. A permanent change in brain function resulting from daily electrical stimulation. *Exp Neurol* 25:295–330.

Goetting MG. 1986. Fatal pneumocystis pneumonia from ACTH therapy for infantile spasms. *Ann Neurol* 19:307–308.

Goitein KJ, Mussafi H, Melamed E. 1983. Treatment of status epilepticus with thiopentone sodium anaesthesia in a child. *Eur J Pediatr* 140:133–135.

Goldberg HJ. 1983. Neonatal convulsions—a 10 year review. *Arch Dis Child* 58:976–978.

Goldberg MA, McIntyre HB. 1983. Barbiturates in the treatment of status epilepticus. In: Delgado-Escueta AV, Wasterlain CG, Treiman DM, et al. *Status epilepticus.* Advances in neurology, Vol. 34. New York: Raven Press, 499–503.

Goldberg HJ. Sheehy EM. 1982. Fifth day fits: an acute zinc deficiency syndrome? *Arch Dis Child* 57:633–635.

Golden GS. 1979. The Alice in Wonderland syndrome in juvenile migraine. *Pediatrics* 63:517–519.

Golden GS, French JH. 1975. Basilar artery migraine in young children. *Pediatrics* 56:722–726.

Goldensohn E. 1983. Symptomatology of nonconvulsive seizures: ictal and postictal. *Epilepsia* 24:S5–S21.

Goldie L, Green JM. 1959. A study of psychological factors in a case of sensory reflex epilepsy: psychological factors in reflex epilepsy. *Brain* 82:505–524.

Goldring S, Gregorie EM. 1984. Surgical management of epilepsy using epidural recordings to localize the seizure focus: review of 100 cases. *J Neurosurg* 60:457–466.

Goldstein A, Aranow L, Kaplan SM. 1975. *Principles of drug action*, 2nd ed. New York: Wiley.

Gomez MR. 1988. *Tuberous sclerosis*, 2nd ed. New York: Raven Press.

Gomez MR, Bebin EM. 1987. Stürge-Weber syndrome. In: Gomez RM, ed. *Neurocutaneous diseases: a practical approach*. London: Butterworth-Heinemann, 356–367.

Gomori JM, Goldbreg HI, Hackney DB, et al. 1986. Occult cerebral vascular malformations: highfield MR imaging. *Radiology* 158:707–713.

Goode DJ, Penry JK, Dreifuss FE. 1970. Effects of paroxysmal spike-wave on continuous visual motor performance. *Epilepsia* 11:241–254.

Goodin DS, Aminoff MJ, Laxer KD. 1990. Detection of epileptiform activity by different noninvasive EEG methods in complex partial epilepsy. *Ann Neurol* 27:330–334.

Goodman R. 1986. Hemispherectomy and its alternatives in the treatment of intractable epilepsy in patients with infantile hemiplegia. *Dev Med Child Neurol* 28:251–258.

Goodman RN, Williamson PD, Reeves AG, et al. 1985. Interhemispheric commissurotomy for congenital hemiplegics with intractable epilepsy. *Neurology* 35:1351–1354.

Goodridge DM, Shorvon SD. 1983a. Epileptic seizures in a population of 6000. II: Treatment and prognosis. *Br Med J (Clin Res Ed)* 287:645–647.

Goodridge DM, Shorvon SD. 1983b. Epileptic seizures in a population of 6000. I: Demography, diagnosis and classification and the role of the hospital services. *Br Med J (Clin Res Ed)* 287:641–645.

Goossens LA, Andermann F, Andermann E, Remillard GM. 1990. Reflex seizures induced by calculation, card or board games, and spatial tasks: a review of 25 patients and delineation of the epileptic syndrome. *Neurology* 40:1171–1176.

Gordon N. 1977. Medium-chain triglycerides in a ketogenic diet. *Dev Med Child Neurol* 19:535–538.

Gordon N. 1979. Petit mal epilepsy and cortical epileptogenic foci. *Electroencephalogr Clin Neurophysiol* 11:151–153.

Gordon N. 1982. Duration of treatment for childhood epilepsy. *Dev Med Child Neurol* 24:84–88.

Gordon N. 1987. Breath holding spells. *Dev Med Child Neurol* 290:811–814.

Gordon N. 1992. Chronic progressive epilepsia partialis continua of childhood: Rasmussen syndrome. *Dev Med Child Neurol* 34:182–185.

Gordon N. 1997a. Pyridoxine dependency: an update. *Dev Med Child Neurol* 39:63–65.

Gordon N. 1997b. Rasmussen's encephalitis. *Dev Med Child Neurol* 39:133–136.

Gordon N. 1997c. The Landau-Kleffner syndrome: increased understanding. *Brain Dev* 19:311–316.

Gordon N. 1999. The long QT syndrome. *Brain Dev* 16:153–155.

Gordon N, Aird RB. 1991. Idiopathic childhood absences: a system disorder. Its diagnosis and differentiation. *Dev Med Child Neurol* 33:744–748.

Gorman DG, Shields D, Shewmon A, et al. 1992. Neurosur-gical treatment of refractory status epilepticus. *Epilepsia* 33:546–549.

Gospe SM, Choy M. 1989. Hereditary long Q-T syndrome presenting as epilepsy: electroencephalography laboratory diagnosis. *Ann Neurol* 25:514–516.

Gotman J, Ives JR, Gloor P. 1984. *Long-term monitoring of epilepsy*. Amsterdam: Elsevier.

Gottfried M, Lavine L, Roessmann U. 1981. Neuropathological findings in Wolf-Hirschhorn (4p-) syndrome. *Acta Neuropathol* 55:163–165.

Goulatia RK, Verma A, Mishra NK, et al. 1987. Disappearing CT lesions in epilepsy. *Epilepsia* 28:523–527.

Goulden KJ, Camfield P, Dooley JM, et al. 1986. Severe carbamazepine intoxication after coadministration of erythromycin. *J Pediatr* 109:135–138.

Goulden KJ, Shinnar S, Koller H, et al. 1991. Epilepsy in children with mental retardation: a cohort study. *Epilepsia* 32:690–697.

Goutières F. 1977. Convulsions néonatales familiales bénignes. In: *Neurologie infantile*. Marseille: Diffusion Générale de Librairie, 281–286.

Goutières F, Aicardi J. 1985. Atypical presentations of pyridoxine-dependent seizures: a treatable cause of intractable epilepsy in infants. *Ann Neurol* 17:117–120.

Goutières F, Challamel MJ, Aicardi J, Gilly R. 1972. Les hémiplégies congénitales. Sémiologie, étiologie et pronostic. *Arch Fr Pediatr* 29:839–851.

Gowers WR. 1901. *Epilepsy and other chronic convulsive diseases: their causes, symptoms and treatment*, 2nd ed. London: J & A Churchill.

Graff-Radford NB, Bosch EP, Stears JC, et al. 1986. Development Foix-Chavany-Marie syndrome in identical twins. *Ann Neurol* 20:632–635.

Gram L. 1988. Experimental studies and controlled clinical testing of valproate and vigabatrin. *Acta Neurol Scand* 78:241–270.

Gram L. 1989. Potential antiepileptic drugs: lamotrigine. In: Levy R, Mattson R, Meldrum B, et al., eds. *Antiepileptic drugs*, 3rd ed. New York: Raven Press, 947–953.

Gram L. 1990. Valproate. In: Dam M, Gram L, eds. *Comprehensive epileptology*. New York: Raven Press, 537–546.

Gram L. 1995. Acetazolamide, benzodiazepines and lamotrigine. In: Duncan JS, Panayiotopoulos CP, eds. *Typical absences and related syndromes*. London: Churchill Communication Europe, 368–375.

Gram L, Alving J, Sagild JC, et al. 1988. Juvenile myoclonic epilepsy in unexpected age groups. *Epilepsy Res* 2:137–140.

Granata T, Battaglia G, D'Incerti L, et al. 1996. Schizencephaly: clinical findings. In: Guerrini R, Andermann F, Canapicchi R, et al., eds. *Dysplasias of cerebral cortex and epilepsy*. Philadelphia: Lippincott-Raven, 407–415.

Granata T, Farina L, Faiella A, et al. 1997. Familial schizencephaly associated with EMX2 mutation. *Neurology* 48:1403–1406.

Grand W. 1974. The significance of post-traumatic status epilepticus in childhood. *J Neurol Neurosurg Psychiatry* 37:178–180.

Granieri E, Rosati G, Tola R, et al 1983. A descriptive study of epilepsy in the district of Copparo, Italy, 1964–1978. *Epilepsia* 24:502–514.

Granström ML, Gaily E, Liukkonen E. 1999. Treatment of infantile spasms: results of a population-based study with vigabatrin as the first drug for spasms. *Epilepsia* 40:950–957.

Grant R, Hadley DM, Condon B, et al. 1987. Magnetic resonance imaging in the management of resistant focal epilepsy: pathological case report and experience of 12 cases. *J Neurol Neurosurg Psychiatry* 50:1529–1532.

Grattan-Smith JD, Harvey AS, Desmond PM, et al. 1993. Hippocampal sclerosis in children with intractable temporal lobe epilepsy: detection by MR imaging. *Am J Radiol* 161:1045–1048.

Gray F, Serdaru M, Baron H, et al. 1987. Chronic localized encephalitis (Rasmussen's) in an adult with epilepsia partialis continua. *J Neurol Neurosurg Psychiatry* 50: 747–751.

Green JB. 1966. Self-induced seizures. *Arch Neurol* 15: 579–586.

Green JB. 1968. Seizures on closing the eyes. Electroencephalographic studies. *Neurology* 18:391–396.

Green S. 1985. Counseling the parent of the child with epilepsy. In: Ross EM, Reynolds EH, eds. *Paediatric perspectives on epilepsy*. London: John Wiley and Sons, 117–121.

Green JR, Troupin AS, Halpern LM, et al. 1974. Sulthiame: evaluation as an anticonvulsant. *Epilepsia* 15:329–349.

Green RC, Adler JR, Erba G. 1988. Epilepsy surgery in children. *J Child Neurol* 3:155–166.

Green CL, Rothrock SG, Clem KJ, et al. 1993. Can seizures be the sole manifestation of meningitis in febrile children? *Pediatrics* 92:527–534.

Greenberg DA, Delgado-Escueta A, Widelitz H, et al. 1988a. Juvenile myoclonic epilepsy (JME) may be linked to the BF and HLA loci on human chromosome 6. *Am J Med Genet* 31:185–192.

Greenberg DA, Delgado-Escueta AV, Maldonado HM, et al. 1988b. Segregation analysis of juvenile myoclonic epilepsy. *Genet Epidemiol* 51:81–94.

Greenberg D, Durner M, Sander T, et al. 1990. The implication of the linkage of juvenile myoclonic epilepsy for the understanding of the genetics of epilepsy. *Epilepsia* 31:815–816.

Greenberg DA, Durner M, Resor S, et al. 1995. The genetics of idiopathic generalized epilepsies of adolescent onset: differences between juvenile myoclonic epilepsy and epilepsy with random grand mal and with awakening grand mal. *Neurology* 45:942–946.

Greenberg DA, Durner M, Keddache M, et al. 2000. Reproducibility and complications in gene searches: linkage on chromosome 6, heterogeneity, association, and maternal inheritance in juvenile myoclonic epilepsy. *Am J Hum Genet* 66:508–516.

Gregory DL, Wong PK. 1992. Clinical relevance of a dipole field in rolandic spikes. *Epilepsia* 33:36–44.

Griffith PA, Karp HR. 1980. Lorazepam in therapy for status epilepticus. *Ann Neurol* 7:493.

Griffiths A, Hebdige S, Perucca E, Richens A. 1980. Quality control in drug measurement. *Ther Drug Monitor* 2: 51–59.

Griggs RC, Nutt JG. 1995. Episodic ataxias as channelopathies. *Ann Neurol* 37:285–287.

Groh C. 1975. Zur Frage der Heilbarkeit kindlisher Epilepsien. *Wien Klin Wochenschr Suppl* 40:1–23.

Gross-Selbeck G. 1995. Treatment of "benign" partial epilepsies of childhood including atypical forms. *Neuropediatrics* 26:45–50

Gross-Tsur V, Shinnar S. 1993. Discontinuing antiepileptic drug therapy in patients with epilepsy. In: Wyllie E, ed.

The treatment of epilepsy: principles and practice. Philadelphia: Lea and Febiger, 858–866.

Gross-Tsur V, Banin E, Shahar E, et al. 2000. Visual impairment in children with epilepsy treated with vigabatrin. *Ann Neurol* 48:60–64.

Grote CL, Van Slyke P, Hoeppner LA. 1999. Language outcome following multiple subpial transection for Landau-Kleffner syndrome. *Brain* 122:561–566.

Guberman A. 1982. Psychogenic pseudoseizures in nonepileptic patients. *Can J Psychiatry* 27:401–404.

Guberman A, Cantu-Reyna G, Stuss D, et al. 1986. Nonconvulsive generalized status epilepticus: clinical features, neuropsychological testing, and long-term follow-up. *Neurology* 36:1284–1291.

Guerreiro MM, Andermann E, Guerrini R, et al. 2000. Familial perisylvian polymicrogyria: a new familial syndrome of cortical maldevelopment. *Ann Neurol* 48:39–48.

Guerrini R. 1997. Clinical epilepsy syndromes in focal cortical dysplasias. In: Tuxhorn I, Holthausen H, Boenigk H, eds. *Pediatric epilepsy syndromes and their surgical treatment*. London: John Libbey, 170–184.

Guerrini R. 1999. Polymicrogyria and epilepsy. In: Avanzini G, Spreafico R, eds. *Abnormal cortical development and epilepsy*. London: John Libbey, 191–201.

Guerrini R. 2001. Idiopathic epilepsy and paroxysmal dyskinesia. *Epilepsia* 42(Suppl. 3):36–41.

Guerrini R, Carrozzo R. 2001a. Epilepsy and genetic malformations of the cerebral cortex. *Am J Med Genet* 106: 160–173.

Guerrini R, Carrozzo R. 2001b. Epileptogenic brain malformations: clinical presentation, malformative patterns and indications for genetic testing. *Seizure* 10:532–547.

Guerrini R, Dobyns WB. 1998. Bilateral periventricular nodular heterotopia with mental retardation and frontonasal malformation. *Neurology* 51:499–503.

Guerrini R, Dravet C. 1997. *Severe epileptic encephalopathies of infancy*. In: Engel J, Pedley TA, eds. *Epilepsy*, Vol. 2. Philadelphia: Lippincott-Raven, 2285–2302.

Guerrini R, Battaglia A, Stagi P, et al. 1989. Caratteristiche elettrocliniche dell'epilessia nella Sindrome di Down. *Bolletino Lega Italiana contre l'Epilepsia* 66/67:317–319.

Guerrini R, Bureau M, Mattei MG, et al. 1990a. Trisomy 12p syndrome: a chromosomal disorder associated with generalized 3-Hz spike and wave discharges. *Epilepsia* 31:557–566.

Guerrini R, Genton P, Bureau M, et al. 1990b. Reflex seizures are frequent in patients with Down syndrome and epilepsy. *Epilepsia* 31:406–417.

Guerrini R, Battaglia A, Mattei MG, et al. 1992a. Epilessia e crisi epilettiche nella sindrome del cromosoma X fragile. *Bolletino Lega Italiana contre l'Epilepsia* 79/80:73–74.

Guerrini R, Dravet C, Raybaud C, et al. 1992b. Neurological findings and seizure outcome in children with bilateral opercular macrogyric-like changes detected by magnetic resonance imaging. *Dev Med Child Neurol* 34:694–705.

Guerrini R, Dravet C, Raybaud C, et al. 1992c. Epilepsy and focal gyral anomalies detected by MRI: electroclinico-morphological correlations and follow-up. *Dev Med Child Neurol* 34:706–718.

Guerrini R, Genton P, Dravet C, et al. 1992d. Compulsive somatosensory self stimulation inducing epileptic seizures. *Epilepsia* 33:509–516.

Guerrini R, Dravet C, Ferrari AR, et al. 1993a. Evoluzione dell'epilessia nelle più frequenti forme genetiche con ritardo mentale. (sindrome di Down e sindrome dell'X fragile). *Pediatr Med Chir* 15:19–22.

Guerrini R, Dravet C, Genton P, et al. 1993b. Epileptic negative myoclonus. *Neurology* 43:1078–1083.

Guerrini R, Robain O, Dravet C, et al. 1993c. Clinical, electrographic and pathological findings in the gyral disorders. In: Fejerman N, Chamoles NA, eds. *New trends in pediatric neurology*. Elsevier, Amsterdam, 101–107.

Guerrini R, Dravet C, Gobbi G, et al. 1994a. Idiopathic generalized epilepsies with myoclonus in infancy and childhood. In: Malafosse A, Genton P, Hirsch E, et al., eds. *Idiopathic generalized epilepsies: clinical, experimental, and genetic aspects*. London: John Libbey, 267–280.

Guerrini R, Ferrari AR, Battaglia A, et al. 1994b. Occipitotemporal seizures with ictus emeticus induced by intermittent photic stimulation. *Neurology* 44:253–259.

Guerrini R, Dravet C, Genton P, et al. 1995. Idiopathic photosensitive occipital lobe epilepsy. *Epilepsia* 36: 883–891.

Guerrini R, Andermann F, Canapicchi R, et al., eds. 1996a. *Dysplasias of cerebral cortex and epilepsy*. Philadelphia: Lippincott-Raven.

Guerrini R, De Lorey T, Bonanni P, et al. 1996b. Cortical myoclonus in Angelman syndrome. *Ann Neurol* 40: 39–48.

Guerrini R, Dravet CH, Bureau M, et al. 1996c. Diffuse and localised dysplasias of cerebral cortex: clinical presentation, outcome and proposal for a morphologic MRI classification based on a study of 90 patients. In: Guerrini R, Andermann F, Canapicchi R, et al., eds. *Dysplasias of cerebral cortex and epilepsy*. Philadelphia: Lippincott-Raven, 255–269.

Guerrini R, Parmeggiani A, Bureau M, et al 1996d. Localized cortical dysplasia: good seizure outcome after sleep-related electrical status epilepticus. In: Guerrini R, Andermann F, Canapicchi R, et al., eds. *Dysplasia of the cerebral cortex and epilepsy*. New York: Lippincott-Raven, 329–335.

Guerrini R, Belmonte A, Veggiotti P, et al. 1997a. Delayed appearance of interictal EEG abnormalities in early onset childhood epilepsy with occipital paroxysms. *Brain Dev* 19:343–346.

Guerrini R, Bonanni P, Parmeggiani L, et al. 1997b. Adolescent onset of idiopathic photosensitive occipital epilepsy after remission of benign rolandic epilepsy. *Epilepsia* 38:777–781.

Guerrini R, Dubeau F, Dulac O, et al. 1997c. Bilateral parasagittal parietooccipital polymicrogyria and epilepsy. *Ann Neurol* 41:65–73.

Guerrini R, Gobbi G, Genton P, et al. 1997d. Chromosomal abnormalities. In: Engel J, Pedley TA, eds. *Epilepsy*, Vol. 3. Philadelphia: Lippincott- Raven, 2533–2546.

Guerrini R, Belmonte A, Carrozzo R. 1998a. Paroxysmal tonic upgaze of childhood with ataxia: a benign transient dystonia with autosomal dominant inheritance. *Brain Dev* 20:116–118.

Guerrini R, Belmonte A, Ferrari AR, et al. 1998b. Il panico come manifestazione parossistica nel bambino e nell'adolescente. In: Murri L, Iudice A, Cassano GB, eds. *Crisi, pseudocrisi e attacchi di panico*. Berlin: Springer-Verlag, 96–110.

Guerrini R, Belmonte A, Genton P. 1998c. Antiepileptic drug-induced worsening of seizures in children. *Epilepsia* 39:S2–S10.

Guerrini R, Bonanni P, Parmeggiani L, et al. 1998d. Induction of partial seizures by visual stimulation. In: Zifkin BG, Andermann F, Beaumanoir A, Rowan AJ, eds. *Reflex epilepsies and reflex seizures*. Advances in neurology, Vol. 75. Philadelphia: Lippincott-Raven, 159–178.

Guerrini R, Dravet C, Genton P, et al. 1998e. Lamotrigine and seizure aggravation in severe myoclonic epilepsy. *Epilepsia* 39:508–512.

Guerrini R, Genton P, Bureau M, et al. 1998f. Multilobar polymicrogyria, intractable drop attack seizures and sleep-related electrical status epilepticus. *Neurology* 51:504–512.

Guerrini R, Andermann E, Avoli M, Dobyns WB. 1999a. Cortical dysplasias, genetics and epileptogenesis. In: Delgado-Escueta AV, Wilson WA, Olsen RW, Porter RJ, eds. *Jasper's basic mechanisms of the epilepsies*, 3rd ed. Advances in neurology, Vol. 79. Philadelphia: Lippincott Williams & Wilkins, 95–121.

Guerrini R, Bonanni P, Nardocci N, et al. 1999b. Autosomal recessive rolandic epilepsy with paroxysmal exercise-induced dystonia and writer's cramp: delineation of the syndrome and gene mapping to chromosome 16p12-11.2. *Ann Neurol* 45:344–352.

Guerrini R, Dobyns WB, Dulac O, et al. 1999c. Genetically determined forms of partial symptomatic epilepsies: clinical phenotype, neuropathology and neurogenetic basis of seizures. In: Berkovic S, Genton P, Hirsch E, et al. *Genetics of focal epilepsies: clinical aspects and molecular biology*. London: John Libbey, 125–148.

Guerrini R, Barkovich AJ, Sztriha L, et al. 2000a. Bilateral frontal polymicrogyria: a newly recognized brain malformation syndrome. *Neurology* 54:909–913.

Guerrini R, Parmeggiani L, Berta E, et al. 2000b. Occipital lobe seizures. In: Oxbury JM, Polkey CE, Duchowny MS, eds. *Intractable focal epilepsy: medical and surgical treatment*. London: WB Saunders, 77–88.

Guerrini R, Shanahan JL, Carrozzo R, et al. 2000c. A nonsense mutation of the ATRX gene causing mild mental retardation and epilepsy. *Ann Neurol* 47:117–21.

Guerrini R, Battini R, Ferrari AR, et al. 2001a. The costs of childhood epilepsy in Italy: comparative findings from three health care settings. *Epilepsia* 42:641–646.

Guerrini R, Bonanni P, Patrignani A, et al. 2001b. Autosomal dominant cortical myoclonus and epilepsy (ADCME) with complex partial and generalized seizures: a newly recognized epilepsy syndrome with linkage to chromosome 2p11.1-q12.2. *Brain* 124:2459–2475.

Guerrini R, Arzimanoglou A, Brouwer O. 2002a. Rationale for treating epilepsy in children. *Epileptic Disord* 4: S9–S21.

Guerrini R, Bonanni P, Rothwell J, Hallet M. 2002b. Myoclonus and epilepsy. In: Guerrini R, Aicardi J, Andermann F, Hallett M, eds. *Epilepsy and movement disorders*. London: Cambridge University Press, 165–210.

Guerrini R, Holthausen H, Parmeggiani L, Chiron C. 2002c. Epilepsy and malformations of the cerebral cortex. In: Roger J, Bureau M, Dravet C, et al., eds. *Epileptic syndromes in infancy, childhood, and adolescence*, 3rd ed. London: John Libbey, 457–480.

Guerrini R, Parmeggiani L, Casari G. 2002d. Syndromes with epilepsy and paroxysmal dyskinesia. In: Guerrini

R, Aicardi J, Andermann F, et al., eds. *Epilepsy and movement disorders*. Cambridge: Cambridge University Press, 407–420.

Guerrini R, Parmeggiani L, Casari G. 2002e. Epilepsy and paroxysmal dyskinesia: co-occurrence and differential diagnosis. In: Fahn S, Frucht SJ, Hallett M, Truong DD, eds. *Myoclonus and paroxysmal dyskinesias*. Advances in neurology, Vol. 89. Philadelphia: Lippincott Williams & Wilkins, 433–441.

Guerrini R, Parmeggiani L, Kaminska A, Dulac O. 2002f. Epilepsy and malformations of the cerebral cortex. In: Roger J, Bureau M, Dravet C, et al., eds. *Epileptic syndromes in infancy, childhood and adolescence*, 3rd ed. London: John Libbey, 105–112.

Guerrini R, Parmeggiani L, Shewmon A, et al. 2002g. Motor dysfunction resulting from epileptic activity involving the sensori-motor cortex. In: Guerrini R, Aicardi J, Andermann F, et al. *Epilepsy and movement disorders*. Cambridge: Cambridge University Press, 77–96.

Guerrini R, Sanchez-Carpintero R, Deonna T, et al. 2002h. Early onset absence epilepsy and paroxysmal dyskinesia. *Epilepsia* 43:1224–1229.

Guerrini R, Carrozzo R, Rinaldi R, et al. 2003a. Angelman syndrome: etiology, clinical features, diagnosis and management of symptoms. *Paediatr Drugs* 5:647–661.

Guerrini R, Casari G, Marini C. 2003b. The genetic and molecular basis of epilepsy. *Trends in Molecular Medicine* 9:300–306.

Guerrini R, Moro F, Andermann E, et al. 2003c. Nonsyndromic mental retardation and cryptogenic epilepsy in women with DCX mutations. *Ann Neurol* 54:30–37.

Guey U, Tassinari CA, Charles C, et al. 1965. Variations du niveau d'efficience en relation avec des décharges épileptiques paroxystiques. *Rev Neurol (Paris)* 112:311–317.

Guey J, Bureau M, Dravet C, et al. 1969. A study of the rhythm of petit mal absences in children in relation to prevailing situations. *Epilepsia* 10:441–451.

Guilleminault C, Lugaresi E, eds. 1983. *Sleep-wake disorders: natural history, epidemiology, and long-term evolution*. New York: Raven Press.

Guilleminault C, Pelayo R. 1998. Narcolepsy in prepubertal children. *Ann Neurol* 43:135–142.

Guilleminault C, Billiard M, Montplaisir J, et al. 1975. Altered states of consciousness in disorders of daytime sleepiness. *J Neurol Sci* 26:377–393.

Guilleminault C, Elridge FL, Tilkian A, et al. 1977. Sleep apnea syndrome due to upper airway obstruction. *Arch Intern Med* 137:296–300.

Guilleminault C, McQuity J, Ariazno N, et al. 1982. Congenital central alveolar hypoventilation syndrome in six infants. *Pediatrics* 70:684–694.

Guipponi M, Rivier F, Vigevano F, et al. 1997. Linkage mapping of benign familial infantile convulsions (BFIC) to chromosome 19q. *Hum Mol Genet* 6:473–477.

Gulick TA, Spinks IP, King DW. 1982. Pseudoseizures: ictal phenomena. *Neurology* 32:24–30.

Gundel A, Doose H. 1986. Genetic EEG patterns in febrile convulsions. a multivariate analysis. *Neuropediatrics* 17:3–6.

Gundel A, Baier W, Doose H, Hoovey Z. 1981. Spectral analysis of EEG in the late course of primary generalized myoclonic-astatic epilepsy. I. EEG and clinical data. *Neuropediatrics* 12:62–74.

Gupta AK, Jeavons PM. 1985. Complex partial seizures: EEG foci and response to carbamazepine and sodium valproate. *J Neurol Neurosurg Psychiatry* 48: 1010–1014.

Gupta AK, Jeavons PM, Hugues RC, et al. 1983. Aura in temporal lobe epilepsy: clinical and electroencephalographic correlation. *J Neurol Neurosurg Psychiatry* 46: 1079–1083.

Gur R, Sussman N, Alavi A, et al. 1982. Positron emission tomography in two cases of childhood epileptic encephalopathy (Lennox-Gastaut syndrome). *Neurology* 32:1191–1194.

Gutierrez AR, Brick JF, Bodensteiner J. 1990. Dipole reversal: an ictal feature of benign partial epilepsy with centrotemporal spikes. *Epilepsia* 31:544–548.

Guzzetta F, Copp JA. 1997. Malformations. In: Graham DL, Lantos PL, eds. *Greenfield's neuropathology*, 6th ed. London: Arnold, 397–533.

Guzzetta F, Crisafulli A, Crinó MI. 1993. Cognitive assessment of infants with West syndrome: how useful is it for diagnosis and prognosis? *Epilepsia* 35:554–565.

Guzzetta F, Frisone MF, Ricci D, et al. 2002. Development of visual attention in West syndrome. *Epilepsia* 43:757–763.

Haan J, Kremer HP, Padberg GW. 1980. Paroxysmal choreoathetosis as presenting symptom of diabetes mellitus [Abstract]. *J Neurol Neurosurg Psychiatry* 52:133.

Haas DC, Ross GS. 1986. Transient global amnesia triggered by mild head trauma. *Brain* 109:251–257.

Hadjipanayis A, Hadjichristodoulou C, Youroukos S. 1997. Epilepsy in patients with cerebral palsy. *Dev Med Child Neurol* 39:659–663.

Haenggeli CA, Girardin E, Paunier L. 1991. Pyridoxine-dependent seizures, clinical and therapeutic aspects. *Eur J Pediatr* 150:452–455.

Haga Y, Watanabe K, Negoro T, et al. 1995. Do ictal, clinical, and electroencephalographic features predict outcome in West syndrome? *Pediatr Neurol* 13:226–229.

Hagberg B, Aicardi J, Dias K, et al. 1983. A progressive syndrome of autism, dementia, ataxia and loss of purposeful hand use in girls: Rett's syndrome. *Ann Neurol* 14: 471–479.

Hahn A. 2000. Atypical benign partial epilepsy/pseudo-Lennox syndrome. *Epileptic Dis* 2:S23–S28.

Hahn YS, Fuchs S, Flannery AM, et al. 1988. Factors influencing post-traumatic seizures in children. *Neurosurgery* 22:864–867.

Hahn A, Pistohl J, Neubauer BA, Stephani U. 2001. Atypical "benign" partial epilepsy or pseudo-Lennox syndrome. Part I: Symptomatology and long term prognosis. *Neuropediatrics* 32:1–8.

Hajek M, Antonini A, Leenders KL, et al. 1991. Epilepsia partialis continua studied by PET. *Epilepsy Res* 9: 44–48.

Hakamada S, Watanabe K, Hara K, et al. 1979. The evolution of electroencephalographic features in lissencephaly syndrome. *Brain Dev* 4:277–283.

Hakeen VF, Wallace SJ. 1990. EEG monitoring of therapy for neonatal seizures. *Dev Med Child Neurol* 32: 858–864.

Hakkarainen H. 1980. Carbamazepine vs. diphenylhydantoin vs. their combination in adult epilepsy [Abstract]. *Neurology* 30:354.

Hallett M. 1985. Myoclonus: relation to epilepsy. *Epilepsia* 26:S67–S77.

Hallett M, Chadwick D, Adams J. 1977. Reticular reflex myoclonus: a physiological type of human post-hypoxic myoclonus. *J Neurol Neurosurg Psychiatry* 40:253–264.

Hallett M, Chadwick D, Marsden CD. 1979. Cortical reflex myoclonus. *Neurology* 29:1107–1125.

Halliday AM. 1967. The electrophysiological study of myoclonus in man. *Brain* 90:241–284.

Hamer HM, Wyllie E, Lüders HO, et al. 1999. Symptomatology of epileptic seizures in the first three years of life. *Epilepsia* 40:837–844.

Hamer HM, Knake S, Schomburg U, et al. 2000. Valproate-induced hyperammonemic encephalopathy in the presence of topiramate. *Neurology* 54:230–232.

Hanai T. 1992. Quality of life in children with epilepsy. *Epilepsia* 33:S28–S32.

Hancock E, Osborne JP. 1999. Vigabatrin in the treatment of infantile spasms in tuberous sclerosis: literature review. *J Child Neurol* 14:71–74.

Hancock E, Osborne JP, Milner P. 2002. Treatment of infantile spasms. Cochrane Review. *Cochrane Database Syst Rev* CD001770.

Hankey GJ, Gubbay SS. 1988. Acquired aphasia of childhood with epilepsy: the Landau-Kleffner syndrome. In: Eadier MJ, Lander CM, eds. *Clinical and experimental neurology*. Sydney: Williams and Wilkins, 187–194.

Hanna JP, Ramundo ML. 1998. Rhabdomyolysis and hypoxia associated with prolonged propofol infusion in children. *Neurology* 50:301–303.

Hanson PA, Chodos R. 1978. Hemiparetic seizures. *Neurology* 28:920–923.

Harbaugh RE, Wilson DH, Reeves AG, et al. 1983. Forebrain commissurotomy for epilepsy: review of 20 consecutive cases. *Acta Neurochir (Wien)* 68:263–275.

Harbord MG, Manson JI. 1987. Temporal lobe epilepsy in childhood: reappraisal of etiology and outcome. *Pediatr Neurol* 3:263–268.

Harbord MG, Hwang PA, Robinson BH, et al. 1991. Infant-onset progressive myoclonus epilepsy. *J Child Neurol* 6:134–142.

Harden A, Pampiglione G. 1982. Neurophysiological studies (EEG/ERG/VEP/SEP) in 88 children with so-called neuronal ceroid lipofuscinosis. In: Armstrong D, Koppang N, Rider JA, eds. *Ceroid-lipofuscinosis (Batten's disease)*. Amsterdam: Elsevier, 61–70.

Harden CL, Tuchman A, Daras M. 1991. Infantile spasms in COFS syndrome. *Pediatr Neurol* 7:302–304.

Hardiman O, Burke T, Phillips J, et al. 1988. Microdysgenesis in resected temporal neocortex: incidence and clinical significance in focal epilepsy. *Neurology* 38: 1041–1047.

Harding BN. 1990. Progressive neuronal degeneration of childhood with liver disease (Alpers-Huttenlocher syndrome): a personal view. *J Child Neurol* 5:273–287.

Harding BN. 1997. Malformations. In: Graham DI, Lantos PL, eds. *Greenfield's neuropathology*, 6th ed. London: Arnold, 398–533.

Harding GFA. 1998. TV can be bad for your health. *Nat Med* 4:265–267.

Harding BN, Boyd SG. 1991. Intractable seizures from infancy can be associated with dentato-olivary dysplasia. *J Neurol Sci* 104:157–165.

Harding GFA, Jeavons PM. 1994. *Photosensitive epilepsy*, 2nd ed. London: MacKeith Press.

Harding GFA, Edson A, Jeavons PM. 1997. Persistence of photosensitivity. *Epilepsia* 38:663–669.

Harding GF, Spencer EL, Wild JM, et al. 2002. Field-specific visual-evoked potentials: identifying field defects in vigabatrin-treated children. *Neurology* 58:1261–1265.

Harkin LA, Bowser DN, Dibbens LM, et al. 2002. Truncation of the GABA$_A$-receptor γ_2 subunit in a family with generalized epilepsy with febrile seizures plus. *Am J Hum Genet* 70:530–536.

Harper JR. 1968. True myoclonic epilepsy in childhood. *Arch Dis Child* 43:28–35.

Harris R, Tizard JP. 1960. EEG in neonatal convulsions. *J Pediatr* 57:501–520.

Harris CM, Shawkat F, Russell-Eggitt I, et al. 1996. Intermittent horizontal saccade failure ('ocular motor apraxia') in children. *Br J Ophthalmol* 80:151–158.

Harrison RM, Taylor DC. 1976. Childhood seizures. A 25-year follow-up. *Lancet* 1:948–951.

Hart YM, Sander JW, Johnson AL, et al. 1990. National general practice study of epilepsy: recurrence after a first seizure. *Lancet* 336:1271–1274.

Hart YM, Cortez M, Andermann F, et al. 1994. Medical treatment of Rasmussen's syndrome (chronic encephalitis and epilepsy): effect of high-dose steroids or immunoglobulins in 19 patients. *Neurology* 44: 1030–1036.

Hartley LM, Gordon I, Harkness W, et al. 2002. Correlation of SPECT with pathology and seizure outcome in children undergoing epilepsy surgery. *Dev Med Child Neurol* 44:676–680.

Harvey AS, Berkovic SF. 1994. Functional neuroimaging with SPECT in children with partial epilepsy. *J Child Neurol* 9:S71–S81.

Harvey AS, Bowe JM, Hopkins IJ, et al. 1993a. Ictal 99mTc-HMPAO single photon emission computed tomography in children with temporal lobe epilepsy. *Epilepsia* 34: 869–877.

Harvey AS, Hopkins IJ, Bowe JM, et al. 1993b. Frontal lobe epilepsy: clinical seizure characteristics and localization with ictal 99mTc-HMPAO SPECT. *Neurology* 43: 1966–1980.

Harvey AS, Nolan T, Carlin JB. 1993c. Community-based study of mortality in children epilepsy. *Epilepsia* 34: 597–603.

Harvey AS, Grattan-Smith JD, Desmond PM, et al. 1995. Febrile seizures and hippocampal sclerosis: frequent and related findings in intractable temporal lobe epilepsy of childhood. *Pediatr Neurol* 12:201–206.

Harvey AS, Jayakar P, Duchowny M, et al. 1996. Hemifacial seizures and cerebellar ganglioglioma: an epilepsy syndrome of infancy with seizures of cerebellar origin. *Ann Neurol* 40:91–98.

Harvey AS, Berkovic SF, Wrennall JA, et al. 1997. Temporal lobe epilepsy in childhood: clinical, EEG, and neuroimaging findings and syndrome classification in a cohort with new-onset seizures. *Neurology* 49:960–968.

Harwood-Nash DC. 1983. Computed tomography and seizures in children. *J Neuroradiol* 10:130–136.

Hashimoto *T, Ohara K, Hiura K. 1978. Sleep polygraphic studies on infantile spasms.* Acta Paediatrica Japonica 20:1–7.

Hashimoto T, Hiura K, Suzue J, et al. 1981. Influence of ACTH therapy on overnight sleep polygrams in infantile spasms. *Brain Dev* 3:51–56.

Hashimoto K, Fujita T, Furuya M. 1989. Absence seizures following febrile seizures. *Brain Dev* 11:268.

Hauser WA. 1981. The natural history of febrile seizures. In: Nelson KB, Ellenberg JH, eds. *Febrile seizures*. New York: Raven Press, 5–17.

Hauser WA. 1983. Status epilepticus: frequency, etiology

and neurological sequelae. In: Delgado-Escueta AV, Wasterlain CG, Treiman DM, et al. *Status epilepticus. Advances in neurology*, vol. 34. New York: Raven Press, 3–14.

Hauser WA. 1986. Should people be treated after a first seizure? *Arch Neurol* 43:1287–1288.

Hauser WA. 1998. Incidence and prevalence. In: Engel J Jr, Pedley TA, eds. *Epilepsy: a comprehensive textbook*, Vol. 1. Philadelphia: Lippincott-Raven, 47–57.

Hauser WA, Anderson VE. 1986. Genetics of epilepsy. In: Pedley TA, Meldrum BS, eds. *Recent advances in epilepsy*, Vol. 3. Edinburgh: Churchill Livingstone, 21–36.

Hauser WA, Annegers JF. 1998. Epidemiology of acute symptomatic seizures. In: Engel J Jr, Pedley TA, eds. *Epilepsy: a comprehensive textbook*, Vol. 1. Philadelphia: Lippincott-Raven, 87–91.

Hauser WA, Hersdoffer DC. 1990. *Epilepsy: frequency, causes and consequences*. New York: Demos Publication.

Hauser WA, Kurland LT. 1975. The epidemiology of epilepsy in Rochester, Minnesota, 1935 through 1967. *Epilepsia* 16:1–66.

Hauser WA, Annegers JF, Elveback LR. 1980. Mortality in patients with epilepsy. *Epilepsia* 21:399–412.

Hauser WA, Annegers JF, Anderson VE, Kurland LT. 1985. The risk of seizure disorders among relatives of children with febrile convulsions. *Neurology* 35: 1268–1273.

Hauser WA, Devinsky O, De Bellis M, et al. 1989. Benzodiazepine withdrawal delirium with catatonic features: occurrence in patients with partial seizure disorders. *Arch Neurol* 46:699.

Hauser WA, Rich SS, Annegers JF, et al. 1990. Seizure recurrence after a first unprovoked seizure: an extended follow-up. *Neurology* 40:1163–1170.

Hauser WA, Annegers JF, Kurland LT. 1991. Prevalence of epilepsy in Rochester, Minnesota: 1940–1980. *Epilepsia* 32:429–445.

Hauser WA, Annegers JF, Kurland FT. 1993. Incidence of epilepsy and unprovoked seizures in Rochester, Minnesota, 1935–1984. *Epilepsia* 34:453–468.

Hayes WG, Shopfner CE. 1973. Plain skull roentgenographic findings in infants and children with convulsions. *Am J Dis Child* 126:785–787.

Hayman M, Scheffer IE, Chinvarun Y, et al. 1997. Autosomal dominant nocturnal frontal lobe epilepsy: demonstration of focal frontal onset and intrafamilial variation. *Neurology* 49:969–975.

Hecaen H, de Ajuriaguerra J. 1952. *Meconnaissances et hallucinations corporelles*. Paris: Masson et Cie, 170–217; 310–343.

Heckmatt J, Houston A, Clow D, et al. 1976. Failure of phenobarbitone to prevent febrile convulsions. *BMJ* 1: 559–561.

Hedström A, Olsson I. 1991. Epidemiology of absence epilepsy: EEG findings and their predictive value. *Pediatr Neurol* 7:100–104.

Heijbel J. 1980. Genetics of benign epilepsy in childhood. In: *Advances in epileptology*, the XIth Epilepsy International Symposium. New York: Raven Press, 319–322.

Heijbel J, Bohman M. 1975. Benign epilepsy of children with centrotemporal EEG foci: intelligence, behaviour and school adjustment. *Epilepsia* 16:679–687.

Heijbel J, Blom S, Bergfors PG. 1975a. Benign epilepsy of children with centrotemporal EEG foci. A study of incidence rate in outpatient care. *Epilepsia* 16: 657–664.

Heijbel J, Blom S, Rasmuson M. 1975b. Benign epilepsy of childhood with centrotemporal EEG foci. A genetic study. *Epilepsia* 16:285–293.

Heijbel J, Blom S, Bergfors PG. 1980. Simple febrile convulsions. A prospective incidence study and an evaluation of investigations initially needed. *Neuropediatrics* 11:45–51.

Heiskala H, Riikonen R, Santavuori P, et al. 1996. West syndrome: individualised ACTH therapy. *Brain Dev* 18. 456–460.

Heller AJ, Ring HA, Reynolds EH. 1988. Factors relating to dramatic response to clobazam therapy in refractory epilepsy. *Epilepsy Res* 2:276–280.

Heller AJ, Chesterman P, Elwes RD, et al. 1989. Monotherapy for newly diagnosed epilepsy: a comparative trial and prognostic evaluation. *Epilepsia* 30:648.

Hellström B, Barlach-Christoffersen M. 1980. Influence of phenobarbital on the psychomotor development and behaviour in preschool children with convulsions. *Neuropédiatrie* 2:151–160.

Hellström B, Oberger E. 1965. ACTH and corticosteroid treatment of infantile spasms with hypsarrhythmia. *Acta Paediatr Scand* 54:180–187.

Hellstrom-Westas L, Rosen I, Svenningsen SW. 1985. Silent seizures in sick children in early life. Diagnosis by continuous cerebral function monitoring. *Acta Paediatr Scand* 74:741–748.

Hendrick EB, Harris L. 1968. Post-traumatic epilepsy in children. *J Trauma* 8:547–555.

Hennessy MJ, Binnie CD. 2000. Photogenic partial seizures. *Epilepsia* 41:59–64.

Hennessy MJ, Elwes RD, Honavar M, et al. 2001. Predictors of outcome and pathological considerations in the surgical treatment of intractable epilepsy associated with temporal lobe lesions. *J Neurol Neurosurg Psychiatry* 70:450–458.

Henriksen O. 1980. Specific problems of children with epilepsy. *Epilepsia* 29:S6–S9.

Henriksen O. 1986. Absence seizures: multiple-drug therapy. In: Schmidt D, Morselli, PL, eds. *Intractable epilepsy: experimental and clinical aspects*. New York: Raven Press, 187–193.

Henriksen O. 1990. Education and epilepsy: assessment and remediation. *Epilepsia* 31:S21–S25.

Henriksen O, Johannessen SI. 1982. Clinical and pharmacokinetic observations on sodium valproate—a five-year follow-up study of 100 children with epilepsy. *Epilepsia* 23:435–439.

Henriksen O, Johanessen SI, Munthe-Kass AW. 1983. How to use carbamazepine. In: Morselle PL, Pippenger CE, Penry JK, eds. *Antiepileptic drug therapy in pediatrics*. New York: Raven Press, 237–243.

Henry TR, Chugani HT. 1997. Positron emission tomography. In: Engel J Jr, Pedley TA, eds. *Epilepsy: a comprehensive textbook*. Philadelphia: Lippincott-Raven, 947–968.

Henry TR, Sutherling WW, Engel J, et al. 1991. Interictal cerebral metabolism in partial epilepsies of neocortical origin. *Epilepsy Res* 10:174–182.

Henry TR, Chugani HT, Abou-Khalil BW, et al. 1992. Positron emission tomography. In: Engel J, ed. *Surgical treatment of the epilepsies*, 2nd ed. New York: Raven Press, 211–232.

Herlitz G. 1941. Studien über die sogennanten initialen FieberKrämpfe bei Kindern. *Acta Paediatr Scand* 29 (Suppl. 1):1–142.

Herman BP. 1982. Neuropsychological functioning and psychopathology in children with epilepsy. *Epilepsia* 23: 545–554.

Herman BP, Austin J. 1993. Psychosocial status of children with epilepsy and the effects of epilepsy surgery. In: Wyllie E, ed. *The treatment of epilepsy: principles and practice*. Philadelphia: Lea and Febiger, 141–1148.

Herman BP, Stickler GB, Lucas AR. 1981. Hyperventilation syndrome in children and adolescents: long-term follow-up. *Pediatrics* 67:183–187.

Herngren L, Nergardh A. 1988. Pharmacokinetics of free and total sodium valproate in adolescents and young adults during maintenance therapy. *J Neurol* 235:491–495.

Herngren L, Lundberg B, Nergardh A. 1991. Pharmacokinetics of total and free valproic acid during monotherapy in infants. *J Neurol* 238:315–319.

Herranz Tanarro FJ, Saenz Lope E, Cristobal Sassot S. 1984. La pointe-onde occipitale avec et sans épilepsie bénigne chez l'enfant. *Rev Electroencephalogr Neurophysiol Clin* 14:1–7.

Herranz JL, Armijo JA, Arteaga R. 1988. Clinical side effects of phenobarbital, primidone, phenytoin, carbamazepine, and valproate during monotherapy in children. *Epilepsia* 29:794–804.

Herranz JL, Arteaga R, Farr IN, et al. 1991. Dose-response study of vigabatrin in children with refractory epilepsy. *J Child Neurol* Suppl. 2:S45–S51.

Herskowitz J. 1986. Neurologic presentations of panic disorders in childhood and adolescence. *Dev Med Child Neurol* 28:617–623.

Herskowitz J, Rosman NP, Geschwind N. 1984. Seizures induced by singing and recitation: a unique form of reflex epilepsy in childhood. *Arch Neurol* 41: 1102–1103.

Hess R, Scollo-Lavizzari G, Wyss FE. 1971. Borderline cases of petit mal status. *Eur Neurol* 5:137–154.

Hill A, Volpe JJ. 1981. Seizures, hypoxic-ischemic brain injury and intraventricular hemorrhage in the newborn. *Ann Neurol* 10:109–121.

Hinchey J, Chaves C, Arpignani B, et al. 1996. A reversible posterior leukoencephalopathy syndrome. *N Engl J Med* 334:494–500.

Hirata K, Katayama S, Saito T, et al. 1991. Paroxysmal kinesigenic choreoathetosis with abnormal electroencephalogram during attacks. *Epilepsia* 32:492–494.

Hirose S, Iwata H, Akiyoshi H, et al. 1999. A novel mutation of CHRNA4 responsible for autosomal dominant nocturnal frontal lobe epilepsy. *Neurology* 53:1749–1753.

Hirose S, Okada M, Yamakawa K, et al. 2002. Genetic abnormalities underlying familial epilepsy syndromes. *Brain Dev* 24:211–222.

Hirsch JF, Sainte-Rose C, Pierre-Kahn A, et al. 1989. Benign astrocytic and oligodendrocytic tumors of the cerebral hemispheres in children. *J Neurosurg* 70:568–572.

Hirsch E, Marescaux C, Maquet P, et al. 1990. Landau-Kleffner syndrome: a clinical and EEG study of five cases. *Epilepsia* 31:756–767.

Hirsch LJ, Spencer SS, Spencer DD, et al. 1991a. Temporal lobectomy in patients with bitemporal epilepsy defined by depth electroencephalography. *Ann Neurol* 30:347–356.

Hirsch LJ, Spencer SS, Williamson PD, et al. 1991b. Comparison of bitemporal and unitemporal epilepsy defined by depth electroencephalography. *Ann Neurol* 30: 340–346.

Hirsch E, Velez A, Sellal F, et al. 1993. Electroclinical signs of benign neonatal familial convulsions. *Ann Neurol* 34:835–841.

Hirsch E, Blanc-Platier A, Marescaux C. 1994. What are the relevant criteria for a better classification of epileptic syndromes with typical absences? In: Malafosse A, Genton P, Hirsch C, et al., eds. *Idiopathic generalized epilepsies: clinical, experimental, and genetic aspects*. London: John Libbey, 87–93.

Hirsch E, Maquet P, Metz-Lutz MN, et al. 1995. The eponym "Landau-Kleffner syndrome" should not be restricted to childhood acquired aphasia with epilepsy. In: Beaumanoir M, Bureau T, Deonna L, et al., eds. *Continuous spike-and-waves during slow sleep: electrical status epilepticus during slow sleep, acquired aphasia and related conditions*. London: John Libbey, 57–62.

Hirsch E, de Saint-Martin A, Arzimanoglou A. 2000. New insights into the clinical management of partial epilepsies. *Epilepsia* 41:S13–S17.

Hirtz DG, Nelson KB. 1985. Cognitive effects of antiepileptic drugs. In: Pedley TA, Meldrum BS, eds. *Advances in epilepsy*, Vol. 2. Edinburgh: Churchill Livingstone, 161–181.

Hirtz DG, Nelson KB, Ellenberg JH. 1983. Seizures following childhood immunizations. *J Pediatr* 102: 14–18.

Hirtz DG, Ellenberg JH, Nelson KB. 1984. The risk of recurrence of nonfebrile seizures in children. *Neurology* 34:637–641.

Hirtz DG, Lee YJ, Ellenberg JH, et al. 1986. Survey on the management of febrile seizures. *Am J Dis Child* 140: 909–914.

Hirtz D, Ashwal S, Berg A, et al. 2000. Practice parameter: evaluating a first nonfebrile seizure in children. *Neurology* 55:616–623.

Hladky JP, Lejeune JP, Blond S, et al. 1994. Cerebral arteriovenous malformations in children: report on 62 cases. *Childs Nerv Syst* 10:328–333.

Ho SS, Kuzniecky RI, Gilliam F, et al. 1998. Temporal lobe developmental malformations and epilepsy: dual pathology and bilateral hippocampal abnormalities. *Neurology* 50:748–754.

Hoare P. 1984a. Psychiatric disturbances in the families of epileptic children. *Dev Med Child Neurol* 26:14–19.

Hoare P. 1984b. The development of psychiatric disorder among school children with epilepsy. *Dev Med Child Neurol* 26:3–13.

Hoare P, Russel M. 1995. The quality of life of children with chronic epilepsy and their families: preliminary findings with a new assessment measure. *Dev Med Child Neurol* 37:689–696.

Hockaday JM, Whitty CW. 1969. Factors determining the electroencephalogram in migraine. *Brain* 92:769–788.

Hodge S, Forsythe WI, Gillies D, et al. 1986. Bio-availability and dissolution of three phenytoin preparations for children. *Dev Med Child Neurol* 28:708–712.

Hodge SE, Greenberg DA, Durner M, et al. 1989. Is juvenile

myoclonic epilepsy polygenic? In: Beck-Mannagetta G, Anderson VE, Doose H, et al., eds. *Genetics of the epilepsies*. Berlin: Springer, 62–66.

Hodskins HB, Yakovlev PI. 1930. Anatomoclinical observations on myoclonus in epileptics and in related symptom complexes. *Am J Psychiatr* 9:827–838.

Hoeffer PF, Denapoli RA, Lesse S. 1963. Periodicity and hypsarrhythmia in the EEG. *Arch Neurol* 9:112–124.

Hoffman HJ. 1997. Benefits of early surgery in Sturge-Weber syndrome. In: Tuxhorn I, Holthausen H, Boenigk H, eds. *Paediatric epilepsy syndromes and their surgical treatment*. London: John Libbey, 364–370.

Hoffman HJ, Hendrick EB, Dennis M, Armstrong D. 1979. Hemispherectomy for Sturge-Weber syndrome. *Childs Brain* 5:233–248.

Hoffmann-Riem M, Diener W, Beninger C, et al. 2000. Nonconvulsive status epilepticus: a possible cause of mental retardation in patients with Lennox-Gastaut syndrome. *Neuropediatrics* 31:169–174.

Hogan GR, Dodge PR, Gill SR, et al. 1969. Pathogenesis of seizures occurring during restoration of plasma tonicity to normal in animals previously chronically hypernatremic. *Pediatrics* 43:54–64.

Hoikka V, Alhava EM, Karjalainen P, et al. 1984. Carbamazepine and bone mineral metabolism. *Acta Neurol Scand* 70:77–80.

Hojo H, Kataoka K, Nakona S. 1981. Reversible brain shrinkage following ACTH treatment. *Brain Dev* 3:153.

Holden KR, Freeman JM, Mellits ED. 1980. Outcomes of infants with neonatal seizures. In: Wada JA, Penry JK, eds. *Advances in epileptology*, The Xth Epilepsy International Symposium. New York: Raven Press, 155–158.

Holden KR, Mellits ED, Freeman JM. 1982. Neonatal seizures. I: Correlation of prenatal and perinatal events with the outcome. *Pediatrics* 70:165–176.

Holdsworth L, Whitmore K. 1974. A study of children with epilepsy attending ordinary schools. *Dev Med Child Neurol* 16:746–758.

Holmes GL. 1984. Partial complex seizures in children: an analysis of 69 seizures in 24 patients using EEG FM radiotelemetry and videotape record. *Electroencephalogr Clin Neurophysiol* 57:13–20.

Holmes GL. 1985. Neonatal seizures. In: Pedley TA, Meldrum BS, eds. *Recent advances in epilepsy*. Edinburgh: Churchill Livingstone, 207–237.

Holmes GL. 1986. Partial seizures in children. *Pediatrics* 77:725–731.

Holmes GL. 1987a. Genetics of epilepsy. In : *Diagnosis and management of seizures in children*. Philadelphia: WB Saunders, 56–71.

Holmes GL. 1987b. Pharmacology of antiepileptic drugs. In: *Diagnosis and management of seizures in children*, Vol. 30. Philadelphia: WB Saunders, 72–111.

Holmes GL. 1991a. Do seizures cause brain damage? *Epilepsia* 32:S14–S28.

Holmes GL. 1991b. The long-term effects of seizures on the developing brain: clinical and laboratory issues. *Brain Dev* 13:393–409.

Holmes GL. 1992. Rolandic epilepsy: clinical and electroencephalographic features. In: Degen R, eds. *The benign localized and generalized epilepsies of early childhood*. Amsterdam: Elsevier, 29–43.

Holmes GL. 1997. Epilepsy in the developing brain: lessons from the laboratory and clinic. *Epilepsia* 38:12–30.

Holmes GL. 2002. Overtreatment in children with epilepsy. *Epilepsy Res* 52:35–42.

Holmes GL, Russman BS. 1986. Shuddering attacks: evaluation using electroencephalographic frequency modulation radiotelemetry and videotape monitoring. *Am J Dis Child* 140:72–73.

Holmes GL, Stafström CE. 1997. Effects of seizures on the developing brain. In: Tuxhorn I, Holthausen H, Boenigk H, eds. *Pediatric epilepsy syndromes and their surgical treatment*. London: John Libbey, 489–504.

Holmes GL, Weber DA. 1986. Effect of ACTH on seizure susceptibility in the developing brain. *Ann Neurol* 20: 82–88.

Holmes GL, Sackellares JC, McKiernan J, et al. 1980. Evaluation of childhood pseudoseizures using EEG telemetry and videotape monitoring. *J Pediatr* 97:554–558.

Holmes GL, McKeever M, Saunders Z. 1981. Epileptiform activity in aphasia of childhood: an epiphenomenon? *Epilepsia* 22:631–639.

Holmes GL, McKeever M, Adamson M. 1987. Absence seizures in children: clinical and electroencephalographic features. *Ann Neurol* 21:268–273.

Holmes MD, Kelly K, Theodore WH. 1988. Complex partial seizures. Correlation of clinical and metabolic features. *Arch Neurol* 45:1191–1193.

Holmes GL, Sarkisian M, Ben-Ari Y, et al. 1999. Effects of recurrent seizures in the developing brain. In: Nehlig A, Motte J, Moshé SL, Plouin P, eds. *Childhood epilepsies and brain development*. Current problems in epilepsy, Vol. 14. London: John Libbey, 263–276.

Holmes LB, Harvey EA, Coull BA, et al. 2001. The teratogenicity of anticonvulsant drugs. *N Engl J Med* 344: 1132–1138.

Holowach J, Renda YA, Wapner I. 1961. Psychomotor seizures in childhood. A clinical study of 120 cases. *J. Pediatr* 59:339–346.

Holowach J, Thurston DL, O'Leary J. 1962. Petit mal epilepsy. *Pediatrics* 30:893–901.

Holowach J, Thurston DL, O'Leary J. 1972. Prognosis in childhood epilepsy. Follow-up study of 148 cases in which therapy had been suspended after prolonged anticonvulsant control. *N Engl J Med* 286:169–173.

Holowach-Thurston J, Thurston DL, Hixon BB, et al. 1982. Prognosis in childhood epilepsy. Additional follow-up of 148 children 15 to 23 years after withdrawal of anticonvulsant therapy. *N Engl J Med* 306: 831–836.

Holthausen H. 1994. Febrile convulsions, mesial temporal sclerosis and temporal lobe epilepsy. In: Wolf P, ed. *Epileptic seizures and syndromes*. London: John Libbey, 449–467.

Holthausen H, Hoppe M. 2000. Hypermotor seizures. In: Lüders HO, Noachtar S, eds. *Epileptic seizures: pathophysiology and clinical semiology*. Philadelphia: Churchill Livingstone, 439–448.

Holtmann M, Krause M, Opp J, et al. 2002. Oxcarbazepine-induced hyponatremia and the regulation of serum sodium after replacing carbamazepine with oxcarbazepine in children. *Neuropediatrics* 33:298–300.

Hommet C, Billard C, Motte J, et al. 2001. Cognitive function in adolescents and young adults in complete remission from benign childhood epilepsy with centrotemporal spikes. *Epileptic Disord* 3:207–216.

Honavar M, Janota I, Polkey CE. 1992. Rasmussen's encephalitis in surgery for epilepsy. *Dev Med Child Neurol* 34:3–14.

Honavar M, Janota I, Polkey CE. 1999. Histological heterogeneity of dysembryoplastic neuro-epithelial tumour: identification and differential diagnosis in a series of 74 cases. *Histopathology* 34:342–356.

Hook EB, Cross K. 1987. Extra structurally abnormal chromosomes (ESAC) detected at amniocentesis: frequency in approximately 75,000 prenatal cytogenic diagnoses and associations with maternal and paternal age. *Am J Hum Genet* 54: 748–756.

Hopkins IJ. 1972. Seizures in the first week of life: a study of aetiological factors. *Med J Aust* 2:647–651.

Hopkins IJ, Klug GL. 1991. Temporal lobectomy for the treatment of intractable complex partial seizures of temporal lobe origin in early childhood. *Dev Med Child Neurol* 33:26–31.

Hopkins A, Glarman A, Clarke C. 1988. The first seizure in adult life: value of clinical features, electroencephalography and computed tomographic scanning in prediction of seizure recurrence. *Lancet* 1:721–726.

Höppener RJ, Kuyer A, Meijer JW, Hulsman J. 1980. Correlation between fluctuations of carbamazepine serum levels and intermittent side-effects. *Epilepsia* 21: 341–350.

Hoppu K, Santavuori P. 1981. Diazepam rectal solution for home treatment of acute seizures in children. *Acta Paediatr Scand* 70:369–372.

Horita H, Hoashi E, Okuyama Y, et al. 1979. Overnight polygraphic studies of infantile spasms: influence of hormone therapy on sleep states, pulse respiration and seizure activities. *Folia Psychiatr Neurol Jpn* 33:269–277.

Horita H, Kumagai K, Maekawa K, et al. 1980. Overnight polygraphic study of agenesis of the corpus callosum with seizures resembling infantile spasms. *Brain Dev* 2:379–386.

Horn CA, Beckman RA, Dick M, et al. 1986a. The congenital long QT syndrome: an unusual cause of childhood seizures. *Am J Dis Child* 140:659–661.

Horn CS, Ater SB, Hurst DL. 1986b. Carbamazepine-exacerbated epilepsy in children and adolescents. *Pediatr Neurol* 2:340–345.

Hosain S, Nagarajan L, Carson D, et al. 1997. Felbamate for refractory infantile spasms. *J Child Neurol* 12:466–468.

Hosking GP. 1974. Fits in hydrocephalic children. *Arch Dis Child* 49:633–635.

Hosking G. 1989. The paediatric EPITEG trial: a comparative multicentre clinical trial of sodium valproate and carbamazepine in newly diagnosed childhood epilepsy. A preliminary communication. In: *Proceedings of Fourth International Symposium on Sodium Valproate and Epilepsy.* London: Royal Society of Medicine Services, 71–80.

Hosking GP, Cavanagh NP, Wilson J. 1978. Alternating hemiplegia: complicated migraine in infancy. *Arch Dis Child* 53:656–659.

Hosley MA, Abroms IF, Ragland RL. 1992. Schizencephaly: case report of familial incidence. *Pediatr Neurol* 8: 148–150.

Howe JG, Gibson JD. 1982. Uncinate seizures and tumors, a myth reexamined [Abstract]. *Ann Neurol* 12:227.

Howitz P, Platz P. 1978. Infantile spasms and HLA antigens. *Arch Dis Child* 53:680–682.

Hrachovy RA, Frost JD Jr. 1989. Infantile spasms. *Pediatr Clin North Am* 36:311–330.

Hrachovy RA, Frost JD, Kellaway P, et al. 1979. A controlled study of prednisone therapy in infantile spasms. *Epilepsia* 20:403–407.

Hrachovy RA, Frost JD Jr, Kellaway P. 1981. Sleep characteristics in infantile spasms. *Neurology* 31: 688–694.

Hrachovy RA, Frost JD, Kellaway P, et al. 1983. Double-blind study of ACTH vs. prednisone therapy in infantile spasms. *J Pediatr* 103:641–645.

Hrachovy RA, Frost JD Jr, Kellaway P. 1984. Hypsarrhythmia, variations on the theme. *Epilepsia* 25:317–325.

Hrachovy RA, Frost JD, Gospe SM Jr, et al. 1987. Infantile spasms following near-drowning: a report of two cases. *Epilepsia* 28:45–48.

Hrachovy RA, Mizrahi EM, Kellaway P. 1990. Electroencephalography of the newborn. In: Daly D, Pedley TA. eds. *Current practice of clinical electroencephalography,* 2nd ed. New York: Raven Press, 210–242.

Hrachovy RA, Gospe SM, Glaze DG. 1994. High-dose, long duration versus low-dose, short-duration corticotropin therapy for infantile spasms. *J Pediatr* 124:803–806.

Hudson LP, Munoz DG, Miller L, et al. 1993. Amygdaloid sclerosis in temporal lobe epilepsy. *Ann Neuol* 33: 622–631.

Huf R, Schain RS. 1980. Long-term experiences with carbamazepine (Tegretol) in children with seizures. *J Pediatr* 2:310–312.

Hughes JR, Cayaffa JJ. 1973. Is the "psychomotor variant" rhythmic mid-temporal discharge an ictal pattern? *Clin Electroencephalogr* 4:42–52.

Hughes JR, Zak S. 1987. EEG and clinical changes in patients with chronic seizures associated with slowly growing brain tumors. *Arch Neurol* 44:540–543.

Hughes JR, Fino J, Gagnon L. 1983. The use of the electroencephalogram in the confirmation of seizures in premature and neonatal infants. *Neuropediatrics* 14: 213–219.

Humphreys RP, Hoffman HJ, Drake JM, et al. 1996. Choices in the 1990s for the management of pediatric cerebral arteriovenous malformations. *Pediatr Neurosurg* 25: 277–285.

Hunt A, Dennis J. 1987. Psychiatric disorders among children with tuberous sclerosis. *Dev Med Child Neurol* 29: 190–198.

Huott AD, Madison DS, Niedermeyer E. 1974. Occipital lobe epilepsy: a clinical and electroencephalographic study. *Eur Neurol* 11:325–339.

Hurst DL. 1986. The use of imipramine in minor motor seizures. *Pediatr Neurol* 2:13–17.

Hurst DL. 1987a. Expanded therapeutic range of valproate. *Pediatr Neurol* 3:342–344.

Hurst DL. 1987b. Severe myoclonic epilepsy of infants. *Pediatr Neurol* 3:269–272.

Hurst DL. 1990. Epidemiology of severe myoclonic epilepsy of infancy. *Epilepsia* 31:397–400.

Hurst DL. 1996. Methsuximide therapy of juvenile myoclonic epilepsy. *Seizure* 5:47–50.

Hurst RW, Lee SI. 1986. Ictal tinnitus. *Epilepsia* 27: 769–772.

Husain AM, Foley CM, Legido A, et al. 2000. West syndrome in tuberous sclerosis complex. *Pediatr Neurol* 23:233–235.

Hussey EK, Dukes GE, Messenheimer JA, et al. 1990. Evaluation of the pharmacokinetic interaction between diazepam and ACC-9653 (a phenytoin prodrug) in healthy male volunteers. *Pharm Res* 7:1172–1176.

Huttenlocher PR. 1974. Dendritic development of neocortex of children with mental defect and infantile spasms. *Neurology* 24:203–210.

Huttenlocher PR. 1976. Ketonemia and seizures: metabolic and anticonvulsant effects of two ketogenic diets in childhood epilepsy. *Pediatr Res* 10:536–540.

Huttenlocher PR, Hapke RJ. 1990. A follow-up study of intractable seizures in childhood. *Ann Neurol* 28:699–705.

Huttenlocher PR, Taravath S, Mojtahedi S. 1994. Periventricular heterotopia and epilepsy. *Neurology* 44:51–55.

Hwang PA, Gilday DL, Spire JP, et al. 1991. Chronic focal encephalitis of Rasmussen: functional neuroimaging studies with positron emission tomography and single photon emission computed tomography scanning. In: Andermann F, ed. *Chronic encephalitis and epilepsy: Rasmussen's syndrome.* London: Butterworth-Heinemann, 61–72.

Hyland K, Buist NR, Powell BR, et al. 1995. Folinic acid responsive seizures: a new syndrome? *J Inherit Metab Dis* 18:177–181.

Hyson M, Andermann F, Olivier A, et al. 1984. Occult encephaloceles and temporal lobe epilepsy: developmental and acquired lesions in the middle fossa. *Neurology* 34:363–366.

Ianetti P, Fiorilli M, Sirianni MC, et al. 1982. Nonfebrile seizures after febrile convulsions: possible role of chronic cytomegalovirus infection. *J Pediatr* 101:27–31.

Igarashi M, Boehm RM, May WN, et al. 1988. Syncope associated with hair grooming. *Brain Dev* 10:249–251.

Iinuma K, Yanai K, Yanagisawa T, et al. 1987. Cerebral glucose metabolism in five patients with Lennox-Gastaut syndrome. *Pediatr Neurol* 3:12–18.

Iivanainen M, Leinikki P, Taskinen E, et al. 1981. CSF oligoclonal bands immunoglobulins, and viral antibodies in progressive myoclonus epilepsy. *Arch Neurol* 38:206–208.

Ikeno T, Shigematsu H, Miyakushi M, et al. 1985. An analytic study of epileptic falls. *Epilepsia* 26:612–621.

Illum N, Taudorf K, Heilmann C, et al. 1990. Intravenous immunoglobulin: a single-blind trial in children with Lennox-Gastaut syndrome. *Neuropediatrics* 21:87–90.

Ines DF, Markand ON. 1977. Epileptic seizures and abnormal electroencephalographic findings in hydrocephalus and their relation to the shunting procedures. *Eletroencephalogr Clin Neurophysiol* 42:761–763.

Ingram TT. 1966. The neurology of cerebral palsy. *Arch Dis Child* 41:337–357.

Ingvar M, Siesjö BK. 1983. Local blood flow and glucose consumption in the rat brain during sustained bicuculline-induced seizures. *Acta Neurol Scand* 68:129–144.

Inoue Y, Seino M, Kubota H, et al. 1994. Epilepsy with praxis-induced seizures. In: Wolf P, ed. *Epileptic seizures and syndromes.* London: John Libbey, Ltd., 81–91.

Inoue Y, Fujiwara T, Matsuda KS, et al. 1997. Ring chromosome 20 and nonconvulsive status epilepticus. A new epileptic syndrome. *Brain* 120:939–953.

Inthaler S, Donati F, Pavlincova E, et al. 1991. Partial complex epileptic seizures with ictal urogenital manifestations in a child. *Eur Neurol* 31:212–215.

Ishii K, Oguni H, Hayashi K, et al. 2002. Clinical study of catastrophic infantile epilepsy with focal seizures. *Pediatr Neurol* 27:369–377.

Isler W. 1971. *Acute hemiplegias and hemisyndromes in childhood.* London: Heinemann.

Isnard J, Fisher C, Bastuji H, et al. 1995. Auditory early (BAEP) and middle-latency (MLAEP) evoked potentials in patients with ESES and Landau-Kleffner syndrome. In: Beaumanoir A, Bureau M, Donna T, et al. eds. *Continuous spikes and waves during slow sleep.* London: John Libbey, 99–103.

Isnard J, Guenot M, Fischer C, et al. 1998. A stereoelectroencephalographic (SEEG) study of light-induced mesiotemporal epileptic seizures. *Epilepsia* 39:1098–1103.

Issakainen J, Bourgeois BF. 1987. Bioavailability of sodium valproate suppositories during repeated administration at steady-state in epileptic patients. *Eur J Pediatr* 146:404–407.

Italian League Against Epilepsy Genetic Collaborative Group. 1993. Concordance of clinical forms of epilepsy in families with several affected members. *Epilepsia* 34:819–826.

Ito M, Takao T, Okuno T, et al. 1983. Sequential CT studies of 24 children with infantile spasms on ACTH therapy. *Dev Med Child Neurol* 25:475–480.

Ito M, Sato K, Ohnuki A, et al. 1990. Sturge-Weber disease: operative indications and surgical results. *Brain Dev* 12:473–477.

Ito M, Okuno T, Hattori H, et al. 1991. Vitamin B6 and valproic acid in treatment of infantile spasms. *Pediatr Neurol* 7:91–96.

Ives JR, Warach S, Schmitt F, et al. 1993. Monitoring the patient's EEG during echo planar MRI. *Electroencephalogr Clin Neurophysiol* 87:417–420.

Jack CJ, Twomey CK, Zinsmeister AT, et al. 1989. Anterior temporal lobes and hippocampal formations: normative volumetric measurements from MR images in young adults. *Radiology* 172:549–554.

Jack CR, Sharbrough FW, Twomey CK. 1990. Temporal lobe seizures: lateralization with MR volume measurements of the hippocampal formation. *Radiology* 175:423–429.

Jack CR, Sharbrough FW, Cascino GD, et al. 1992. Magnetic resonance image-based hippocampal volumetry: correlation with outcome after temporal lobectomy. *Ann Neurol* 31:138–146.

Jackson JH. 1931. On a particular variety of epilepsy ("intellectual aura"): one case with symptoms of organic brain disease. In: Taylor J, ed. *Selected writings of J.H. Jackson,* Vol 1. London: Hodder and Stroughton, 1958: 400–405.

Jackson GD, Berkovic SE, Tress BM, et al. 1990. Hippocampal sclerosis can be reliably detected by magnetic resonance imaging. *Neurology* 40:1869–1875.

Jackson GD, Berkovic SF, Duncan JS, et al. 1993a. Optimising the diagnosis of hippocampal sclerosis using magnetic resonance imaging. *Am J Neuroradiol* 14:753–762.

Jackson GD, Connelly A, Duncan JS, et al. 1993b. Detection of hippocampal pathology in intractable partial epilepsy: increased sensitivity with quantitative magnetic resonance T2 relaxometry. *Neurology* 43:1793–1799.

Jackson GD, Kuzniecky RI, Cascino GD. 1994. Hippocampal sclerosis without detectable hippocampal atrophy. *Neurology* 44:42–46.

Jackson GD, McIntosh AM, Briellmann RS, et al. 1998. Hippocampal sclerosis studied in identical twins. *Neurology* 51:78–84.

Jacome DE, Fitzgerald R. 1982. Ictus emeticus. *Neurology* 32:209–212.

Jacome DE, Risko M. 1984. Pseudocataplexy: gelastic-atonic seizures. *Neurology* 34:1381–1383.

Jacome DE, McLain LW, Fitzgerald R. 1980. Postural reflex gelastic seizures. *Arch Neurol* 37:249–251.

Jalava M, Sillanpää M. 1997. Physical activity, health-related fitness, and health experience in adults with childhood-onset epilepsy: a controlled study. *Epilepsia* 38:424–429.

Jalava M, Sillanpää M. 1998. Concurrent illnesses in adults with childhood-onset epilepsy: a population-based 35-year follow-up study. *Epilepsia* 37:1155–1163.

Jalava M, Sillanpää M, Camfield C, Camfield P. 1997. Social adjustment and competence 35 years after onset of childhood epilepsy: a prospective controlled study. *Epilepsia* 38:708–715.

Jallon P. 2003. *Prognosis of the epilepsies.* Paris: John Libbey Eurotext.

Jambaqué I, Dulac O. 1989. Syndrome frontal réversible et épilepsie chez un enfant de 8 ans. *Arch Fr Pediatr* 46:525–529.

Jambaqué I, Cusmai R, Curatolo P, et al. 1991. Neuropsychological aspects of tuberous sclerosis in relation to epilepsy and MRI findings. *Dev Med Child Neurol* 33:698–705.

Jambaqué I, Chiron C, Dulac O, et al. 1993. Visual inattention in West syndrome: a neuropsychological and neurofunctional imaging study. *Epilepsia* 34:692–700.

Jambaqué I, Chiron C, Dumas C, et al. 2000. Mental and behavioural outcome of infantile epilepsy treated by vigabatrin in tuberous sclerosis patients. *Epilepsy Res* 38:151–160.

James MR, Marshall H, Carew-McColl M. 1991. Pulse oximetry during tonic-clonic seizures. *Lancet* 337:394–395.

Janota I, Polkey CE. 1992. Cortical dysplasia in epilepsy—a study of material from surgical resections for intractable epilepsy. In: Pedley TA, Meldrum, eds. *Recent advances in epilepsy*, 5th ed. Edinburgh: Churchill Livingstone, 37–49.

Janz D. 1962. The grand mal epilepsies and the sleeping-waking cycle. *Epilepsia* 3:69–109.

Janz D. 1969. *Die Epilepsien. Spezielle Pathologie und Therapie.* Stuttgart: Thieme.

Janz D. 1973. The natural history of primary generalized epilepsies: with sporadic myoclonias of the "impulsive petit mal" type. In: Lugaresi E, Pazzaglia P, Tassinari, CA, eds. *Evolution and prognosis of epilepsies.* Bologna: Aulo Gaggi, 55–61.

Janz D. 1974. Epilepsy and the sleep-waking cycle. In: Vinken PJ, Bruyn GW, eds. *The epilepsies.* Handbook of clinical neurology, Vol. 15. Amsterdam: Elsevier, 457–490.

Janz D. 1983. Prognosis and prophylaxis of traumatic epilepsy. In: Rose CF, ed. *Research progress in epilepsy.* London: Pitman, 161–174.

Janz D. 1991. Juvenile myoclonic epilepsy. In: Dam M, Gram L, eds. *Comprehensive epileptology.* New York: Raven Press, 171–185.

Janz D, Christian W. 1957. Impulsiv petit mal. *Dtsch Z Nervenheilkd* 176:346–386.

Janz D, Durner M. 1998. Juvenile myoclonic epilepsy. In:

Engel J Jr, Pedley TA, eds. *Epilepsy: a comprehensive textbook.* Philadelphia: Lippincott-Raven, 2389–2400.

Janz D, Waltz S. 1995. Juvenile myoclonic epilepsy with absences. In: Duncan JS, Panayiotopoulos CP, eds. *Typical absences and related syndromes.* London: Churchill Communication Europe, 174–183.

Janz D, Sommer-Burkhardt EM. 1976. Discontinuation of antiepileptic drugs in patients with epilepsy who have been seizure free for more than two years. In: Janz D, ed. *Epileptology.* Stuttgart: Thieme, 228–234.

Janz D, Dam M, Richens A, et al. 1982. *Epilepsy, pregnancy and the child.* New York: Raven Press.

Janz D, Beck-Manhagetta G, Sander T. 1992. Do idiopathic generalized epilepsies share a common susceptibility gene? *Neurology* 42(Suppl. 5):48–55.

Janz D, Beck-Mannagetta G, Spröder B, et al. 1994. Childhood absence epilepsy (pycnolepsy) and juvenile absence epilepsy: one or two syndromes. In: Wolf P, ed. *Epileptic seizures and syndromes.* London: John Libbey, 115–126.

Järvela I, Schleutker J, Hartaja L. 1991. Infantile form of neuronal ceroid lipofuscinosis (CLN 1) maps to the short arm of chromosome 1. *Genomics* 9:170–173.

Jasper H. 1954. Electroencephalography. In: Penfield W, Jasper H, eds. *Epilepsy and the functional anatomy of the human brain.* Boston: Little, Brown and Company, 569–666.

Jasper HH. 1964. Some physiological mechanisms involved in epileptic automatisms. *Epilepsia* 5:1–20.

Jawad S, Oxley J, Wilson J, et al. 1986. A pharmacologic evaluation of midazolam as an antiepileptic compound. *J Neurol Neurosurg Psychiatry* 49:1050–1054.

Jay V, Becker LE, Chan FW, Perry TL Sr. 1991. Puppet-like syndrome of Angelman: a pathologic and neurochemical study. *Neurology* 41:416–422.

Jayakar P, Chiappa KH. 1990. Clinical correlations of photoparoxysmal responses. *Electroencephalogr Clin Neurophysiol* 75:251–254.

Jayakar P, Duchowny MS. 1990. Complex partial seizures of temporal lobe origin in early childhood. *J Epilepsy* 3:41.

Jayakar P, Duchowny M. 1997. Invasive EEG and functional cortical mapping. In: Tuxhorn I, Holthausen H, Boenigk H, eds. *Paediatric epilepsy syndromes and their surgical treatment.* London: John Libbey, 547–556.

Jayakar PB, Seshia SS. 1991. Electrical status epilepticus during slow-wave sleep: a review. *J Clin Neurophysiol* 7:299–311.

Jayakar P, Duchowny M, Resnick T, et al. 1992. Ictal head deviation, lateralizing significance of the pattern of head movement. *Neurology* 42:1989–1992.

Jeavons PM. 1977. Nosological problems of myoclonic epilepsies in childhood and adolescence. *Dev Med Child Neurol* 19:3–8.

Jeavons PM. 1982. Myoclonic epilepsies: therapy and prognosis. In: Akimoto H, Kazamatsuri H, Seino M, et al., eds. *Advances in epileptology*, XIIIth Epilepsy International Symposium. New York: Raven Press, 141–144.

Jeavons PM. 1983a. Hepatotoxicity of antiepileptic drugs. In: Oxley J, Hebdiges S, Laidlaw J, et al., eds. *Antiepileptic therapy: chronic toxicity of antiepileptic drugs.* New York: Raven Press, 1–45.

Jeavons PM. 1983b. Non-epileptic attacks in childhood. In: Rose CF, ed. *Research progress in epilepsy.* London: Pitman, 224–230.

Jeavons P, Bower B. 1964. *Infantile spasms: a review of the literature and study of 112 cases.* Clinics in developmental medicine, No. 15. London: Heinemann.

Jeavons P, Bower B. 1974. Infantile spasms. In: Vinken PJ, Bruyn GW, eds. *The epilepsies.* Handbook of clinical neurology, Vol. 15. Amsterdam: Elsevier, 219–234.

Jeavons PM, Clark JE. 1974. Sodium valproate in treatment of epilepsy. *BMJ* 2:584–586.

Jeavons PM, Harding GF. 1970. Television epilepsy. *Lancet* 2:926–927.

Jeavons PM, Harding GF. 1975. *Photosensitive epilepsy: a review of the literature and a study of 460 patients.* London: Heinemann.

Jeavons PM, Livet MO. 1992. West syndrome: infantile spasms. In: Roger J, Bureau M, Dravet C, et al. *Epileptic syndromes in infancy, childhood and adolescence,* 2nd ed. London: John Libbey, 53–65.

Jeavons PM, Bower BD, Dimitrakoudi M. 1973. Long-term prognosis of 150 cases of "West syndrome." *Epilepsia* 14:153–164.

Jeavons PM, Clark JE, Maheshwary MC. 1977. Treatment of the generalized epilepsies of childhood and adolescence with sodium valproate (Epilim). *Dev Med Child Neurol* 19:9–25.

Jeavons PM, Bishop A, Harding GF. 1986. The prognosis of photosensitivity. *Epilepsia* 27:569–575.

Jellinger K. 1987. Neuropathological aspects of infantile spasms. *Brain Dev* 9:349–357.

Jennett B. 1973. Trauma as a cause of epilepsy in childhood. *Dev Med Child Neurol* 15:56–72.

Jennett B. 1974. Post-traumatic epilepsy. *Arch Neurol* 30:395–398.

Jennett B. 1975. Predicting outcome after head injury. *Journal of the Royal College of Physicians (Lond)* 9:231–237.

Jennett B, Teasdale G. 1981. *Management of head injuries.* Philadelphia: FA Davis.

Jennings MT, Bird TD. 1981. Genetic influences in the epilepsies. *Am J Dis Child* 135:450–457.

Jensen I. 1975. Temporal lobe surgery around the world: results, complications and mortality. *Acta Neurol Scand* 52:354–373.

Jensen I. 1976a. Temporal lobe epilepsy. Etiological factors and surgical results. *Acta Neurol Scand* 53:103–118.

Jensen I. 1976b. Temporal lobe epilepsy. Types of seizures, age and surgical results. *Acta Neurol Scand* 53:335–357.

Jensen I. 1977. Temporal lobe epilepsy: on whom to operate and when? In: Penry JK, ed. *Epilepsy,* VIIIth International Symposium. New York: Raven Press, 325–330.

Jensen PK, Dam M. 1990. Oxcarbazepine. In: Dam M, Gram L, eds. *Comprehensive epileptology.* New York: Raven Press, 621–629.

Jensen I, Larsen JK. 1979. Mental aspects of temporal lobe epilepsy: follow-up of 74 patients after resection of a temporal lobe. *J Neurol Neurosurg Psychiatry* 42:256–265.

Jensen I, Vaernet K. 1977. Temporal lobe epilepsy. Follow-up investigation of 74 temporal lobe resected patients. *Acta Neurochir (Wien)* 37:173–200.

Jervell A, Lange-Nielsen F. 1957. Congenital deaf, mutism, functional heart disease with prolongation of the QT interval, and sudden death. *Am Heart J* 54:59.

Jøhannessen SI, Tomson T. 2000. Laboratory monitoring of antiepileptic drugs. In: Levy RH, Mattson RH, Meldrum BS, et al., eds. *Antiepileptic drugs,* 5th ed. Philadelphia: Lippincott Williams & Wilkins, 103–111.

Jøhannessen SI, Morselli PL, Pippenger CE, et al. 1980. *Antiepileptic therapy: advances in drug monitoring.* New York: Raven Press,.

Jøhannessen SI, Løyning Y, Munthe-Kaas AW. 1991. Medical treatment. General aspects. In: Dam M, Gram L, eds. *Comprehensive epileptology.* New York: Raven Press, 505–524.

Johnsen SD, Tarby TJ, Sidell AD. 1984. Carbamazepine-induced seizures. *Ann Neurol* 16:392–393.

Johnson LC, DeBolt WL, Long MT, et al. 1972. Diagnostic factors in adult males following initial seizures: a three year follow-up. *Arch Neurol* 27:193–197.

Johnston MV. 1996. Developmental aspects of epileptogenesis. *Epilepsia* 37:S2–S9.

Jones KL. 1988. *Smith's recognizable patterns of human malformations,* 4th ed. Philadelphia: WB Saunders.

Jones CM, Dunn HG, Thomas EE, et al. 1994. Acute encephalopathy and status epilepticus associated with human herpes virus 6 infection. *Dev Med Child Neurol* 36:646–650.

Jones-Gotman M. 1991. Localization of lesions by neuropsychological testing. *Epilepsia* 32:S41–S52.

Jones-Gotman M, Smith ML, Wieser HG. 1997. Inter-arterial amobarbital procedures. In: Engel J, Pedley TA, Aicardi J, et al., eds. *Epilepsy: a comprehensive textbook.* Philadelphia: Lippincott Williams & Wilkins, 1767–1775.

Jooma R, Yeh H, Printera MD, et al. 1995. Lesionectomy versus electrophysiologically guided resection for temporal lobe tumors manifesting with complex partial seizures. *J Neurosurg* 83:231–236.

Joorabchi B. 1977. Expressions of the hyperventilation syndrome in children: studies in management, including an evaluation of the effectiveness of propanolol. *Clin Pediatr (Phila)* 16:1110–1115.

Jouvenceau A, Euson LH, Spauschus A, et al. 2001. Human epilepsy associated with dysfunction of the brain P/Q-type calcium channel. *Lancet* 358:801–807.

Joyce RP, Gunderson CH. 1978. Carbamazepine-induced orofacial dyskinesia. *Neurology* 30:1333–1334.

Juhász C, Chugani DC, Muzik O, et al. 2000a. Electroclinical correlates of flumazenil and fluorodeoxyglucose PET abnormalities in lesional epilepsy. *Neurology* 55:825–835.

Juhász C, Chugani DC, Muzik O, et al. 2000b. Is epileptogenic cortex truly hypometabolic on interictal positron emission tomography? *Ann Neurol* 48:88–96.

Juhász C, Chugani HT, Muzik O, et al. 2001a. Neuroradiological assessment of brain structure and function and its implication in the pathogenesis of West syndrome. *Brain Dev* 23:488–495.

Juhász C, Chugani DC, Muzik O, et al. 2001b. Relationship of flumazenil and glucose PET abnormalities to neocortical epilepsy surgery outcome. *Neurology* 56:1650–1658.

Juul-Jensen P. 1963. *Epilepsy: a clinical and social analysis of 1020 adult patients with epileptic seizures.* Copenhagen: Munskgaard.

Juul-Jensen P. 1964. Frequency of recurrence after discontinuance of anticonvulsant therapy in patients with epileptic seizures. *Epilepsia* 5:352–363.

Juul-Jensen P. 1968. Frequency of recurrence after discontinuance of anticonvulsant therapy in patients with epileptic seizures. A new follow-up study after 5 years. *Epilepsia* 9:11–16.

Juul-Jensen P, Foldspang A. 1983. Natural history of epileptic seizures. *Epilepsia* 24:297–312.

Kaga M. 1999. Language disorders in Landau-Kleffner syndrome. *J Child Neurol* 14:118–122.

Kahane P, Munari C, Minotti L, et al. 1997. The role of hypothalamic hamartoma in the genesis of gelastic and dacrystic seizures. In: Tuxhorn I, Holthausen H, Boenigk H, eds. *Paediatric epilepsy syndromes and their surgical treatment*. London: John Libbey, 447–461.

Kahane P, Hoffmann D, Francione S, et al. 1998. La stéréo-électro-encéphalographie chez l'enfant: outil diagnostique et préchirurgical. In: Bureau M, Kahane P, Munari C, eds. *Epilepsies partielles graves pharmaco-résistantes de l'enfant: stratégies diagnostiques et traitements chirurgicaux*. Paris: John Libbey Eurotext, 135–151.

Kahane P, Bureau M, Revol M, Roger J. 2002. Nonidiopathic partial epilepsies of childhood. In: Roger J, Bureau M, Dravet C, et al., eds. *Epileptic syndromes in infancy, childhood and adolescence,* 3rd ed. London: John Libbey, 229–246.

Kaibara M, Blume WT. 1988. The postictal electroencephalogram. *Electroencephalog Clin Neurophysiol* 70: 99–104.

Kairam R, De Vivo DC. 1981. Neurologic manifestations of congenital infections. *Clinics in Perinatology* 8: 445–465.

Kajitani T, Nakamura M, Ueoka K, et al. 1980. Three pairs of monozygotic twins with rolandic discharges. In: Wada JA, Penry JK, eds. *Advances in epileptology*, Xth Epilepsy International Symposium. New York: Raven Press, 171–175.

Kajitani T, Ueoka K, Nakamura M, et al. 1981. Febrile convulsions and rolandic discharges. *Brain Dev* 3:351–354.

Kalachikov S, Evgrafov O, Ross B, et al. 2002. Mutations in LGI1 cause autosomal-dominant partial epilepsy with auditory features. *Nat Genet* 30:335–341.

Kalviainen R, Nousiainen I, Mantyjarvi M, et al. 1999. Vigabatrin, a GABA-ergic antiepileptic drug, causes concentric visual field defects. *Neurology* 53:922–926.

Kameyama S, Fukuda M, Tomikawa M, et al. 2001. Surgical strategy and outcomes for epileptic patients with focal cortical dysplasia or dysembryoplastic neuroepithelial tumor. *Epilepsia* 42:37–41.

Kaminska A, Ickowicz A, Plouin P, et al. 1999. Delineation of cryptogenic Lennox-Gastaut syndrome and myoclonic astatic epilepsy using multiple correspondence analysis. *Epilepsy Res* 36:15–29.

Kaminska A, Chiron C, Ville D, et al. 2003. Ictal SPECT in children with epilepsy: comparison with intracranial EEG and relation to postsurgical outcome. *Brain* 126: 248–260.

Kammerman P. 1985. Alternate-day clonazepam treatment of intractable seizures. *Arch Neurol* 42:787–788.

Kamoshita S, Mizutani J, Fukuyama Y. 1970. Leigh's subacute necrotizing encephalomyelopathy in a child with infantile spasms and hypsarrhythmia. *Dev Med Child Neurol* 12:430–435.

Kananura C, Haug K, Sander T, et al. 2002. Splice-site mutation in *GABRG2* associated with childhood absence epilepsy and febrile convulsions. *Arch Neurol* 59: 1137–1141.

Kanayama M, Ishikawa T, Tauchi A, et al. 1989. ACTH-induced seizures in an infant with West syndrome. *Brain Dev* 11:329–331.

Kanazawa O. 1992. Medically intractable generalized tonic-clonic or clonic seizures in infancy. *J Epilepsy* 5:143–148.

Kanazawa O. 2001. Refractory grand mal seizures with onset during infancy including sever myoclonic epilepsy in infancy. *Brain Dev* 23:749–756.

Kanazawa O, Kawai I. 1990. Status epilepticus characterized by repetitive asymmetrical atonia: two cases accompanied by partial seizures. *Epilepsia* 31:536–543.

Kanazawa O, Sengoku A, Kawai I. 1989. Oculoclonic status epilepticus. *Epilepsia* 30:121–123.

Kandall SR, Gartner LM. 1974. Late presentation of drug withdrawal symptoms in newborn. *Am J Dis Child* 127:58–61.

Kaneko S, Otani K, Fukushima Y, et al. 1988. Teratogenicity of antiepileptic drugs: analysis of possible risk factors. *Epilepsia* 29:459–467.

Kanemoto K, Janz D. 1989. The temporal sequence of aura sensations in patients with complex focal seizures with particular attention to ictal aphasia. *J Neurol Neurosurg Psychiatry* 52:52–56.

Kanemoto K, Kawasaki J, Miyamoto T, et al. 2000. Interleukin (IL)1β, IL-1α, and IL-1 receptor and agonist gene polymorphisms in patients with temporal lobe epilepsy. *Ann Neurol* 47:571–574.

Kanner AM, Morris HH, Lüders H, et al. 1990. Supplementary motor seizures mimicking pseudoseizures: some clinical differences. *Neurology* 40:1404–1407.

Kanner AM, Morris HH, Lüders H, et al. 1993. Usefulness of unilateral interictal sharp waves of temporal lobe origin in prolonged video-EEG monitoring studies. *Epilepsia* 34:884–889.

Kaplan BJ. 1975. Biofeedback in epileptics: equivocal relationship of reinforced EEG frequency to seizure reduction. *Epilepsia* 16:477–485.

Kaplan PW. 2000. Prognosis in nonconvulsive status epilepticus. *Epileptic Disord* 2:185–193.

Kaplan BJ, Wilder BJ, Hammond ET, et al. 1982. Valproate tremors. *Neurology* 32:428–432.

Karbowski K. 1982. Vertigo und Epilepsie. *Schweiz Rundsch Med Prax* 71:1600–1604.

Karbowski K, Vassela F, Schneider H. 1970. Electro-encephalographic aspects of Lennox-syndrome. *Eur Neurol* 4:301–311.

Karenfort M, Krune B, Freitag H, et al. 2002. Epilepsy surgery outcome in children with focal epilepsy due to tuberous sclerosis complex. *Neuropediatrics* 33:255–261.

Kasteleijn-Nolst Trenité DG, Binnie CD, Meinardi H. 1987. Photosensitive patients: symptoms and signs during intermittent photic stimulation and their relation to seizures in daily life. *J Neurol Neurosurg Psychiatry* 50: 1546–1549.

Kasteleijn-Nolst Trenité DG, Bakker DJ, Binnie CD, et al. 1988. Psychological effects of subclinical EEG discharges in children. I: Scholastic skills. *Epilepsy Res* 2: 111–116.

Kasteleijn-Nolst Trenité DG, Siebelink BM, Berends SG, et al. 1990. Lateralized effects of subclinical epileptiform EEG discharges on scholastic performance in school children. *Epilepsia* 31:740–746.

Kasteleijn-Nolst Trenité DG, van Emde Boas W, Binnie CD. 1994. Photosensitive epilepsy as an age-related genetic disorder. In: Wolf P, ed. *Epileptic seizures and syndromes*. London: John Libbey, 41–48.

Kasteleijn-Nolst Trenité DG, Marescaux G, Stodieck S, et al. 1996. Photosensitive epilepsy: a model to study the effects of antiepileptic drugs. Evaluation of the piracetam analogue, levetiracetam. *Epilepsy Res* 25: 225–230.

Kasteleijn-Nolst Trenité DG, Binnie CD, Harding GF, et al. 1999. Medical technology assessment: photic stimulation—standardization of screening methods. *Neurophysiol Clin* 29:318–324.

Kasteleijn-Nolst Trenité DG, Guerrini R, Binnie CD, Genton P. 2001.Visual sensitivity and epilepsy: a proposed terminology and classification for clinical and EEG phenomenology. *Epilepsia* 42:692–701.

Kasteleijn-Nolst Trenité D, Hirsch E, Takahashi T. 2002a. Photosensitivity, visual induced seizures and syndromes. In: Roger J, Bureau M, Dravet C, et al., eds. *Epileptic syndromes in infancy, childhood and adolescence*, 3rd ed. London, Paris: John Libbey, 369–387.

Kasteleijn-Nolst Trenité DG, Martins da Silva A, Ricci S, et al. 2002b. Video games are exciting: a European study of video game-induced seizures and epilepsy. *Epileptic Disord* 4:121–128.

Kasteleijn-Nolst Trenité DG, Hirsch E. 2003. Levetiracetam: preliminary efficacy in generalized seizures. *Epileptic Disord* 5:S39–S44.

Kataoka K, Okuno T, Mikawa H, et al. 1988. Cranial computed tomographic and electroencephalographic abnormalities in children with post-convulsive hemiplegia. *Eur Neurol* 28:279–284.

Kattapong VJ, Hart BL, Davis LE. 1995. Familial cerebral cavernous angiomas: clinical and radiologic studies. *Neurology* 45:492–497.

Kaufman DW, Kelly JP, Anderson T, et al. 1997. Evaluation of case reports of aplastic anemia among patients treated with felbamate. *Epilepsia* 38:1265–1269.

Kawai I, Fujii S. 1979. Ictal body scheme disturbance induced by looking through a small opening. *Epilepsia* 20:535–540.

Kawazawa S, Nogaki H, Hara T, et al. 1985. Paroxysmal dystonic choreoathetosis in a case of pseudoidiopathic hypoparathyroidism. *Rinsho Shinkeigan* 25: 1152–1158.

Keen JH, Lee K. 1973. Sequelae of neonatal convulsions: study of 112 infants. *Arch Dis Child* 48:542–546.

Keeting JW, Knowles SA. 1989. Sudden death in childhood and adolescence. *J Pathol* 159:221–224.

Keidan I, Shif I, Keren G, Passwell JH. 1992. Rotavirus encephalopathy: evidence of central nervous system involvement during rotavirus infection. *Pediatr Infect Dis J* 11:773–775.

Kellaway P. 1959. Neurologic status of patients with hypsarrhythmia. In: Gibbs FA, ed. *Molecules and mental health*. Philadelphia: JB Lippincott, 134–149.

Kellaway P, Hrachovy RA. 1983. Status epilepticus in newborns: a perspective on neonatal seizures. In: Delgado-Escueta AV, Wasterlain CG, Treiman DM, Porter RJ, eds. *Status epilepticus*. Advances in neurology, Vol. 34. New York: Raven Press, 93–99.

Kellaway PM, Mizrahi EM. 1987. Neonatal seizures. In: Lüders H, Lesser RP, eds. *Epilepsy: electroclinical syndromes*. Berlin: Springer, 13–47.

Kellaway PM, Mizrahi EM. 1990. Clinical, electroencephalographic, therapeutic, and pathophysiologic studies of neonatal seizures. In: Wasterlain CG, Vert P, eds. *Neonatal seizures*. New York: Raven Press, 1–13.

Kellaway P, Hrachovy RA, Frost JD, et al. 1979. Precise characterization and quantification of infantile spasms. *Ann Neurol* 6:214–218.

Kellaway P, Frost JD, Hrachovy RA. 1983. Infantile spasms. In: Morselli PL, Pippenger CE, Penry JK, eds.

Antiepileptic drug therapy in pediatrics. New York: Raven Press, 115–136.

Kellaway et al., 1993 [cited in Chapter 3]

Kellerman K. 1978. Recurrent aphasia with subclinical bioelectric status epilepticus during sleep. *Eur J Pediatr* 128:207–212.

Kellett MW, Smith DF, Stockton PA, Chadwick DW. 1999. Topiramate in clinical practice: first year's post-licensing experience in a specialist epilepsy clinic. *J Neurol Neurosurg Psychiatry* 66:759–763.

Kelly JJ, Mellinger JF, Sundt TM. 1978. Intracranial arteriovenous malformations in childhood. *Ann Neurol* 3: 338–343.

Kelly PJ, Sharbrough FW, Kali BA, et al. 1987. Magnetic resonance imaging-based computer-assisted stereotactic resection of the hippocampus and amygdala in patients with temporal lobe epilepsy. *Mayo Clin Proc* 62: 103–108.

Kennett RP. 2000. Neurophysiologic investigation of adults. In: Oxbury JM, Polkey CE, Duchowny MS, eds. *Intractable focal epilepsy*. London: WB Saunders, 332–362.

Keränen T, Reinikainen K, Riekkinen PJ. 1984. Carbamazepine monotherapy versus polytherapy in chronic epilepsies. *Acta Neurol Scand* 69(Suppl. 98):87–88.

Kessler S, Guilleminault C, Dement W. 1974. A family study of 50 REM narcoleptics. *Acta Neurol Scand* 50: 503–512.

Kim WY, Pomerance JJ, Miller AA. 1979. Lidocaine intoxication following local anesthesia for episiotomy. *Pediatrics* 64:643–645.

Kimura S, Kobayashi T. 1996. Two patients with juvenile myoclonic epilepsy and nonconvulsive status epilepticus. *Epilepsia* 37:275–279.

Kinast M, Erenberg G, Rothner AD. 1980. Paroxysmal choreoathetosis. Report of five cases and review of the literature. *Pediatrics* 65:74–77.

Kinast M, Lüders H, Rothner AD, et al. 1982. Benign focal epileptiform discharges in childhood migraine. *Neurology* 32:1309–1311.

King D, Ajmone-Marsan C. 1977. Clinical features and ictal patterns in epileptic patients with EEG temporal lobe foci. *Ann Neurol* 2:138–147.

King M, Stephenson JB, Ziervogel M, et al. 1985. Hemimegalencephaly—a case for hemispherectomy? *Neuropediatrics* 16:46–55.

King DW, Flanigin HF, Gallagher BB, et al. 1986. Temporal lobectomy for partial complex partial seizures: evaluation, results, and 1-year follow-up. *Neurology* 36: 334–339.

King MA, Newton MR, Berkovic SF. 1999. Benign partial seizures of adolescence. *Epilepsia* 40:1244–1247.

Kinsman SL, Vining EP, Quaskey SA, et al. 1992. Efficacy of the ketogenic diet for intractable seizure disorders. Review of 58 cases. *Epilepsia* 33:1132–1136.

Kinton R, Johnson MR, Smith SJ, et al, et al. 2002. Partial epilepsy with pericentral spikes: a new familial syndrome with evidence of linkage to chromosome 14p 15. *Ann Neurol* 51:740–749.

Kiok MC, Terrence CF, Fromm GH, et al. 1986. Sinus arrest in epilepsy. *Neurology* 36:115–116.

Kirkpatrick PJ, Honavar M, Janota I, et al. 1993. Control of temporal lobe epilepsy following en bloc resection of low-grade tumors. *J Neurosurg* 78:19–25.

Kitamura K, Yanazawa M, Sugiyama M, et al. 2002. Mutation of ARX causes abnormal development of forebrain and testes in mice and X-linked lissencephaly with abnormal genitalia in humans. *Nat Genet* 32:359–369.

Kivity S, Lerman P. 1989. Benign partial epilepsy of childhood with occipital discharges. In: Manelis J, Bental E, Loeber JN, et al., eds. *Advances in epileptology*, XVIIth Epilepsy International Symposium. New York: Raven Press, 371–373.

Kivity S, Lerman P. 1992. Stormy onset with prolonged loss of consciousness in benign occipital childhood epilepsy with occipital paroxysms. *J Neurol Neurosurg Psychiatry* 55:45–48.

Klass DW, Westmoreland B. 1985. Nonepileptogenic epileptiform electroencephalographic activity. *Ann Neurol* 18: 627–635.

Klein B, Levin BE, Duchowny MS, et al. 2000. Cognitive outcome of children with epilepsy and malformations of cortical development. *Neurology* 55:230–235.

Kloss S, Pieper T, Pannek H, et al. 2002. Epilepsy surgery in children with focal cortical dysplasia (FCD): results of long-term seizure outcome. *Neuropediatrics* 33:21–26.

Knauss T, Marshall R. 1977. Seizures in a neonatal intensive care unit. *Dev Med Child Neurol* 19:719–728.

Knauss TA, Thomas A, Coldevin B, et al. 1978. Neonatal paroxysmal monorhythmic alpha activity. *Arch Neurol* 35:104–107.

Knott C. 1983. Measurement of saliva drug concentrations in the control of antiepileptic medication. In: Pedley TA, Meldrum BS, eds. *Recent advances in epilepsy*, Vol. 1. Edinburgh: Churchill Livingstone, 57–73.

Knudsen FU. 1977. Plasma diazepam in infants after rectal administration in solution and by suppositories. *Acta Paediatr Scand* 66:563–567.

Knudsen FU. 1979. Rectal administration of diazepam in solution in the acute treatment of convulsions in infants and children. *Arch Dis Child* 54:855–857.

Knudsen FU. 1985a. Effective short-term diazepam prophylaxis in febrile convulsions. *J Pediatr* 106:487–490.

Knudsen FU. 1985b. Recurrence risk after first febrile seizures and effect of short-term diazepam prophylaxis. *Arch Dis Child* 60:1045–1049.

Knudsen FU. 1988. Frequent febrile episodes and recurrent febrile convulsions. *Acta Neurol Scand* 78:414–417.

Knudsen FU. 1991. Intermittent diazepam prophylaxis in febrile convulsions. Pros and cons. *Acta Neurol Scand Suppl* S135:1–24.

Knudsen FU, Vestermark S. 1978. Prophylactic diazepam or phenobarbitone in febrile convulsions: a prospective controlled study. *Arch Dis Child* 53:660–663.

Ko TS, Holmes GL. 1999. EEG and clinical predictors of medically intractable childhood epilepsy. *Clin Neurophysiol* 110:1245–1251.

Kobayashi K, Murakami N, Yoshinaga H, et al. 1988. Nonconvulsive status epilepticus with continuous diffuse spike-and-wave discharges during sleep in childhood. *Japanese Journal of Psychiatry and Neurology* 42: 509–514.

Kobayashi K, Nishibayashi N, Ohtsuka Y, et al. 1994. Epilepsy with electrical status epilepticus during slow sleep and secondary bilateral synchrony. *Epilepsia* 35:1097–1103.

Koehn MA, Zupanc ML. 1999. Unusual presentation and MRI findings in Rasmussen's syndrome. *Pediatr Neurol* 21:839–842.

Koella WP. 1987. The role of limbic and related structures in

the "making" of behavior: the lessons from animal experimentation. In: Wieser HG, Elger CE, eds. *Presurgical evaluation of epilepsies*. Berlin: Springer, 15–22.

Koenigsberger M, Chutorian AM, Gold AP, et al. 1970. Benign paroxysmal vertigo of childhood. *Neurology* 20: 1108–1113.

Koepden D, Baruzzi A, Capozza M, et al. 1987. Clobazam in therapy-resistant patients with partial epilepsy: a double-blind placebo-controlled crossover study. *Epilepsia* 28:495–506.

Koepp MJ, Hansen ML, Pressler RM, et al. 1998. Comparison of EEG, MRI and PET in reading epilepsy: a case report. *Epilepsy Res* 29:251–257.

Kohno C, Terasaki T, Matsuda M. 1987. Epilepsies with seizure discharges induced by eye closure. In: Wolf P, Dam M, Janz D, et al., eds. *Advances in epileptology*, XVIth Epilepsy International Symposium. New York: Raven Press, 251–253.

Kollevold T. 1976. Immediate and early cerebral seizures after head injuries. *Journal of the Oslo City Hospital* 26: 99–114.

Konishi Y, Yasujima M, Kuriyama M, et al. 1992. Magnetic resonance imaging in infantile spasms: effects of hormonal therapy. *Epilepsia* 33:304–309.

Koo B. 1999. Vigabatrin in the treatment of infantile spasms. *Pediatr Neurol* 20:106–110.

Koo B, Hwang P. 1996. Localization of focal cortical lesions influences age of onset of infantile spasms. *Epilepsia* 37:1068–1071.

Koo B, Hwang PA, Logan WJ. 1993. Infantile spasms: outcome and prognostic factors of cryptogenic and symptomatic groups. *Neurology* 43:2322–2327.

Koren G, Butt W, Rajchgot P, et al. 1986. Intravenous paraldehyde for seizure control in newborn infants. *Neurology* 36:108–110.

Korobkin R. 1982. Neonatal stroke, a new clinical syndrome. Presented at the 3rd *International Child Neurology Congress*, Copenhagen, Denmark May 28.

Korten JJ, Notermans SL, Frenken CW, et al. 1974. Familial essential myoclonus. *Brain* 97:131–138.

Koskiniemi M, Donner M, Majuri H, et al. 1974. Progressive myoclonus epilepsy: a clinical and histopathological study. *Acta Neurol Scand* 50:333–359.

Koskiniemi M, van Vleymen B, Hakamies L, et al. 1998. Piracetam relieves symptoms of progressive myoclonus epilepsy: a multicentre, randomized, double blind, crossover study comparing the efficacy and safety of three dosages of oral piracetam with placebo. *J Neurol Neurosurg Psychiatry* 64:344–348.

Kossoff EH, Pyzik PL, McGrogan JR, et al. 2002. Efficacy of the ketogenic diet for infantile spasms. *Pediatrics* 109:780–783.

Kosteljanetz M, Christiansen J, Dam AM, et al. 1979. Carbamazepine vs phenytoin. A controlled clinical trial in focal motor and generalized epilepsy. *Arch Neurol* 36:22–24.

Kotagal P. 1991. Seizure symptomatology of temporal lobe epilepsy. In: Lüders HO, ed. *Epilepsy surgery*. New York: Raven Press, 143–156.

Kotagal P. 1997. The Wada test in children: do we really need it? In: Tuxhorn I, Holthausen H, Boenigk H, eds. *Paediatric epilepsy syndromes and their surgical treatment*. London: John Libbey, 681–683.

Kotagal P. 1999. Significance of dystonic posturing with unilateral automatisms. *Arch Neurol* 56:912–913.

Kotagal P. 2000. Automotor seizures. In: Lüders HO,

Noachtar S, eds. *Epileptic seizures.* Philadelphia: Churchill Livingstone, 449–457.

Kotagal P, Lüders H. 1992. Epilepsy surgery evaluation. In: Resor SR, Kutt H, eds. *The medical treatment of epilepsy.* New York: Marcel Dekker, 225–231.

Kotagal P, Lüders H. 1994. Recent advances in childhood epilepsy. *Brain Dev* 16:1–15.

Kotagal P, Rothner D. 1987. Complex partial seizures in children: diagnosis and management. *Int Pediatr* 2: 182–188.

Kotagal P, Rothner AD, Erenberg G, et al. 1987. Complex partial seizures of childhood onset: a five-year follow-up study. *Arch Neurol* 44:1177–1180.

Kotagal P, Lüders H, Morris HA, et al. 1989. Dystonic posturing in complex partial seizures of temporal lobe onset: a new lateralizing sign. *Neurology* 39:196–201.

Kotagal P, Cohen BH, Scheithauer BW. 1995a. Infantile spasms in a child with brain tumor: seizure-free outcome after resection. *J Epilepsy* 8:57–60.

Kotagal P, Lüders HO, Williams G, et al. 1995b. Psychomotor seizures of temporal lobe onset: analysis of symptom clusters and sequences. *Epilepsy Res* 20:49–67.

Kovisto M, Blanco-Sequeiros M, Krause U. 1972. Neonatal symptomatic and asymptomatic hypoglycaemia: a follow-up study of 151 children. *Dev Med Child Neurol* 14:603–614.

Kozhevnikov AY. 1992. A particular type of cortical epilepsy (epilepsia corticalis sive partialis continua). In: Andermann F, ed. *Chronic encephalitis and epilepsy: Rasmussen's syndrome.* Boston: Butterworth-Heinemann, 245–261.

Krägeloh I, Aicardi J. 1980. Alternating hemiplegia in infants. Report of five cases. *Dev Med Child Neurol* 22:784–791.

Krakow K, Woermann FG, Symms MR, et al. 1999. EEG-triggered functional MRI of interictal epileptiform activity in patients with partial seizures. *Brain* 122: 1679–1688.

Kral T, Kuczaty S, Blumcke I, et al. 2001. Postsurgical outcome of children and adolescents with medically refractory frontal lobe epilepsies. *Childs Nerv Syst* 17:595–601.

Kral T, Clusmann H, Blumcke I, et al. 2003. Outcome of epilepsy surgery in focal cortical dysplasia. *J Neurol Neurosurg Psychiatry* 74:183–188.

Kramer RE, Bracht KA. 2000. Abdominal auras. In: Lüders HO, Noachtar S, eds. *Epileptic seizures.* Philadelphia: Churchill Livingstone, 329–335.

Kramer RE, Dinner DS, Braun WE, et al. 1987a. HLA-DR2 and narcolepsy. *Arch Neurol* 44:853–855.

Kramer RE, Lüders H, Lesser RP, et al. 1987b. Transient focal abnormalities of neuroimaging studies during focal status epilepticus. *Epilepsia* 28:528–532.

Kramer RE, Lüders H, Goldstick LP, et al. 1988. Ictus emeticus: an electroclinical analysis. *Neurology* 38:1048–1052.

Kramer U, Sue WC, Mikati M. 1997. Focal features in West syndrome indicating candidacy for surgery. *Pediatr Neurol* 16:213–217.

Kramer U. 1999. Epilepsy in the first year of life: a review. *J Child Neurol* 14:485–489.

Kreindler A, Popescu U, Tismana GD. 1969. Interseizure activity in the EEG of patients with grand mal epilepsy. *Electroencephalogr Clin Neurophysiol* 27:655–658.

Kreisman NR, Rosenthal M, La Manna JC, et al. 1983. Cerebral oxygenation during recurrent seizures. In: Delgado-Escueta AV, Wasterlain CG, Treiman DM, Porter RJ, eds. *Status epilepticus.* Advances in neurology, Vol. 34. New York: Raven Press, 231–239.

Kriel RL, Cifuentes RF. 2001. Fosphenytoin in infants of extremely low birth weight. *Pediatr Neurol* 24:219–221.

Kriel RL, Fisher JA, Cloyd JC, et al. 1986. Valproic acid pharmacokinetics in children. III: Very high dosage requirements. *Pediatr Neurol* 2:202–208.

Kriel RL, Cloyd JC, Hadsall RS, et al. 1991. Home use of rectal diazepam for cluster and prolonged seizures: efficacy, adverse reactions, quality of life and cost analysis. *Pediatr Neurol* 7:13–17.

Krishnamoorthy KS. 1983. Pyridoxine-dependency seizure: report of a rare presentation. *Ann Neurol* 13:103–104.

Kristensen O, Klitgaard WA, Jönsson B, Sindrup S. 1983. Pharmacokinetics of 10-OH-carbamazepine, the main metabolite of the antiepileptic oxcarbazepine, from serum and saliva concentrations. *Acta Neurol Scand* 68: 145–150.

Kritzler R, Vining E, Plotnick L. 1983. Sodium valproate and corticotropin suppression in the child treated for seizures. *J Pediatr* 102:142–143.

Krohn W. 1963. Causes of death among epileptics. *Epilepsia* 4:315–321.

Kroll JS. 1985. Pyridoxine for neonatal seizures: an unexpected danger. *Dev Med Child Neurol* 27:377–379.

Kruse R. 1968. *Das myoklonisch-astatische Petit Mal.* Berlin: Springer.

Kubota H, Fujikawa Y, Fujiwara T, et al. 1990. Long-term outcomes of children with complex partial seizures. *Brain Dev* 12:631–636.

Kücük NÖ, Yigit A, Ibis E, et al. 1999. Functional imaging in reading epilepsy: a case report. *Ann Nucl Med* 13: 355–356.

Kuenzle CH, Steinlin M, Wohlrab G, et al. 1998. Adverse effects of vigabatrin in Angelman syndrome. *Epilepsia* 39:1213–1215.

Kuks JB, Cook MD, Fish DR, et al. 1993. Hippocampal sclerosis in epilepsy and childhood febrile seizures. *Lancet* 342:1391–1394.

Kumar A, Bleck TP. 1992. Intravenous midazolam for the treatment of refractory status epilepticus. *Crit Care Med* 20:438.

Kumps AH. 1982. Therapeutic drug monitoring: a comprehensive critical review of analytical methods for anticonvulsive drugs. *J Neurol* 228:1–16.

Kuo CC. 1998. A common anticonvulsant binding site for phenytoin, carbamazepine and lamotrigine in neuronal Na^+ channels. *Mol Pharmacol* 54:712–721.

Kurokawa T, Nagahide G, Fukuyama Y, et al. 1980. West syndrome and Lennox-Gastaut syndrome: a survey of natural history. *Pediatrics* 65:81–88.

Kurokawa T, Sasaki K, Hanai T, et al. 1981. Linear nevus sebaceus syndrome: report of a case with Lennox-Gastaut syndrome following infantile spasms. *Arch Neurol* 38:375–377.

Kurokawa T, Fung KC, Hanai T, et al. 1982. Mortality and clinical features in cases of death among epileptic children. *Brain Dev* 4:321–325.

Kusse MC, van Nieuwenhuizen O, van Huffelen AC, et al. 1993. The effect of non-depot ACTH $_{(1-24)}$ on infantile spasms. *Dev Med Child Neurol* 35:1067–1073.

Kutt H. 1984. Interactions between anticonvulsants and other commonly prescribed drugs. *Epilepsia* 25:S118–S131.

Kutt H. 1985. Therapeutic monitoring of antiepileptic drugs.

In: Pedley TA, Meldrum BS, eds. *Recent advances in epilepsy*, Vol. 2. Edinburgh: Churchill Livingstone, 183–205.

Kuwano A, Takakubo F, Morimoto Y, et al. 1996. Benign adult familial myoclonus epilepsy (BAFME): an autosomal dominant form not linked to the dentatorubral pallidoluysian atrophy (DRPLA) gene. *Journal of Medical Genetics* 33:80–81.

Kuzniecky RI. 1996. MRI in focal cortical dysplasia. In: Guerrini R, Andermann F, Canapicchi R, et al., eds. *Dysplasias of cerebral cortex and epilepsy*. Philadelphia: Lippincott-Raven, 145–150.

Kuzniecky RI, Jackson GD. 1995a. Disorders of cerebral hemispheres. In: *Magnetic resonance in epilepsy*. New York: Raven Press, 213–233.

Kuzniecky RI, Jackson GD. 1995b. *Magnetic resonance in epilepsy*. New York: Raven Press.

Kuzniecky R, Powers R. 1993. Epilepsia partialis continua due to cortical dysplasia. *J Child Neurol* 8:386–388.

Kuzniecky R, Rosenblatt B. 1987. Benign occipital epilepsy: a familial study. *Epilepsia* 28:346–350.

Kuzniecky R, De la Saillette V, Ethier R, et al. 1987. Magnetic resonance imaging in temporal lobe epilepsy: pathological correlations. *Ann Neurol* 22:341–347.

Kuzniecky R, Andermann F, Melanson D, et al. 1988. Focal cortical myoclonus and rolandic cortical dysplasia: clarification by magnetic resonance imaging. *Ann Neurol* 23:317–325.

Kuzniecky R, Andermann F, Tampieri D, et al. 1989. Bilateral central macrogyria: epilepsy, pseudobulbar palsy, and mental retardation. A recognizable neuronal migration disorder. *Ann Neurol* 25:547–554.

Kuzniecky R, Garcia JH, Faught E, et al. 1991. Cortical dysplasia in temporal lobe epilepsy: magnetic resonance imaging. *Ann Neurol* 29:293–298.

Kuzniecky R, Cascino GD, Palmini A, et al. 1992. Structural neuroimaging. In: Engel J, ed. *Surgical treatment of the epilepsies*, 2nd ed. New York: Raven Press, 197–209.

Kuzniecky R, Andermann F, Guerrini R, et al. 1993a. Congenital bilateral perisylvian syndrome. *Lancet* 341: 608–612.

Kuzniecky R, Murro A, King D, et al. 1993b. Magnetic resonance imaging in childhood intractable partial epilepsies: pathologic correlations. *Neurology* 43:681–687.

Kuzniecky R, Andermann F, Guerrini R. 1994a. Infantile spasms: an early epileptic manifestation in some patients with the congenital bilateral perisylvian syndrome. *J Child Neurol* 9:420–423.

Kuzniecky R, Andermann F, Guerrini R. 1994b. The epileptic spectrum in the congenital bilateral perysilvian syndrome. CBPS Multicenter Collaborative Study. *Neurology* 44:379–385.

Kuzniecky R, Guthrie R, Montz J, et al. 1997. Intrinsic epileptogenesis of hypothalamic hamartomas in gelastic epilepsy. *Ann Neurol* 42:60–67.

Kwan P, Brodie MJ. 2000. Early identification of refractory epilepsy. *N Engl J Med* 342:314–319.

Kwan P, Brodie MJ. 2001. Effectiveness of first antiepileptic drug. *Epilepsia* 42:1255–1260.

Kyllerman M. 1981. Dyskinetic cerebral palsy. Ph.D. Thesis. Department of Pediatrics, University of Göteborg, Gothenburg, Sweden.

Kyllerman M. 1995. On the prevalence of Angelman syndrome. *Am J Med Genet* 59:405

Kyllerman M, Sommerfeldt K, Hedström A, et al. 1991. Clinical and neurophysiological development of Unverricht-Lundborg disease in four Swedish siblings. *Epilepsia* 32:900–909.

Kyllerman M, Nyden A, Praquin N, et al. 1996. Transient psychosis in a girl with epilepsy and continuous spikes and waves during slow sleep. *Eur Child Adolesc Psychiatry* 5:216–221.

Kyriakides T, Hallam LA, Hockey A, et al. 1992. Angelman's syndrome: a neuropathological study. *Acta Neuropathol (Berl)* 83:675–678.

Laan LA, Renier WO, Arts WF, et al. 1997. Evolution of epilepsy and EEG findings in Angelman syndrome. *Epilepsia* 38:195–199.

Labauge P, Brunereau L, Coubes P, et al. 2001. Appearance of new lesions in two nonfamilial cerebral cavernoma patients. *Eur Neurol* 45:83–88.

Labauge P, Amer LO, Simonetta-Moreau M, et al. 2002. Absence of linkage to 8q24 in a European family with familial adult myoclonic epilepsy (FAME). *Neurology* 58:941–944.

Laberge-le Couteulx S, Jung HH, Labauge P, et al. 1999. Truncating mutations in CCM1, encoding KRIT1, cause hereditary cavernous angiomas. *Nat Genet* 23: 189–193.

Labrecque D, Gal P, Sharpless MK. 1984. Neonatal seizure recurrence following discontinuation of phenobarbital. *Clin Pharmacol* 3:649–652.

Lacey DJ, Singer WD, Horwitz SJ, Gilmore H. 1986. Lorazepam therapy of status epilepticus in children and adolescents. *J Pediatr* 108:771–774.

Lacy JR, Penry JK. 1976. *Infantile spasms*. New York: Raven Press.

Lado FA, Laureta EC, Moshé SL. 2002. Seizure-induced hippocampal damage in the mature and immature brain. *Epileptic Disord* 4:83–97.

Lagae LG, Silberstein J, Casaer P. 1998. Successful use of intravenous immunoglobulins in Landau-Kleffner syndrome. *Pediatr Neurol* 18:165–168.

Lagae L, Pauwels J, Monté CP, et al. 2001. Frontal absences in children. *Eur J Paediatr Neurol* 5:243–251.

Lagenstein I, Willig RP, Iffland E. 1978. Behandlung frühkindlicher Anfälle mit ACTH und Dexamethason unter standardisserten Bedingungen. I: Klinische Ergebnisse. II. Elektroencephalographische Beobachtungen. *Monatsschr Kinderheilkd* 126:492–499; 500–506.

Lagenstein I, Willig RP, Kühne D. 1979a. Cranial computed tomography (CCT) findings in children with ACTH and dexamethasone: first results. *Neuropédiatrie* 10: 370–384.

Lagenstein I, Willig RP, Kühne D. 1979b. Reversible cerebral atrophy caused by corticotrophin. *Lancet* 1: 1246–1247.

Lagenstein I, Sternowski H, Rothe M, et al. 1980. Cranial computerized tomography in different epilepsies with grand mal and focal seizures in 309 children: relation to clinical and electroencephalographic data. *Neuropediatrics* 11:323–338.

Lahat E, Katz Y, Bistritzer T, et al. 1990. Recurrent seizures in children with shigella-associated convulsions. *Ann Neurol* 28:393–395.

Lahat E, Goldman M, Barr J, et al. 2000. Comparison of intranasal midazolam with intravenous diazepam for treating febrile seizures in children: prospective randomised study. *BMJ* 321:83–86.

Lai CW, Ziegler DK. 1983. Repeated self-induced syncope and subsequent seizures. *Arch Neurol* 40:820–823.

Laidlaw J, Richens A, eds. 1982. *A textbook of epilepsy*, 2nd ed. Edinburgh: Churchill Livingstone.

Lake BD, Cavanagh NP. 1978. Early juvenile Batten's disease. A recognizable subgroup distinct from other forms of Batten's disease. *J Neurol Sci* 36:265–271.

Lalande J, De Paillerets F. 1978. Prevention of hyperthermic convulsions: utility of discontinuous treatment with clonazepam. In: Meinardi H, Rowans A, eds. *Advances in epileptology*, Ninth Symposium of the International Bureau for Epilepsy. Amsterdam: Swets and Zeitlinger, 313–317.

Lalioti M, Scott HS, Buresi C, et al. 1997. Dodecamer repeat in cystatin B in progressive myoclonus epilepsy (EPM1). *Nature* 356:847–851.

Lamarche M, Chauvel P. 1978. Movement epilepsy in the monkey with an experimental motor focus. *Electroencephalogr Clin Neurophysiol* 34:323–328.

Lance JW. 1977. Familial paroxysmal dystonic choreoathetosis and its differentiation from related syndromes. *Ann Neurol* 2:285–293.

Lancman ME, Morris HH. 1996. Epilepsy after central nervous infection: clinical characteristics and outcome after epilepsy surgery. *Epilepsy Res* 25:285–290.

Lancman ME, Penry JK, Asconape JJ, et al. 1993. Number 20 ring chromosome: a case with complete seizure control. *J Child Neurol* 8:186–187.

Lancman ME, Asconape JJ, Craven WJ, et al. 1994. Predictive value of induction of psychogenic seizures by suggestion. *Ann Neurol* 35:359–361.

Landau WM, Kleffner FR. 1957. Syndrome of acquired aphasia with convulsive disorder in children. *Neurology* 7:523–530.

Landrigan PJ, Witte JJ. 1973. Neurologic disorders following live measles-virus vaccination. *JAMA* 223:1459–1462.

Landy HJ, Khoury AN, Heyl PL. 1989. Antenatal ultrasonographic diagnosis of fetal seizure activity. *Am J Obstet Gynecol* 161:308.

Landy HJ, Curless RG, Ramsay RE, et al. 1993. Corpus callosotomy for seizures associated with band heterotopia. *Epilepsia* 34:79–83.

Langslet A, Meberg A, Bredesen JE, Lunde PK. 1978. Plasma concentrations of diazepam and *N*-desmethyldiazepam in newborn infants after intravenous, intramuscular, rectal and oral administration. *Acta Paediatr Scand* 67:699–704.

Lanska MJ, Lanska DJ, Baumann RJ, et al. 1995. A population-based study of neonatal seizures in Fayette County, Kentucky. *Neurology* 45:724–732.

Lapkin ML, Golden GS. 1978. Basilar artery migraine. A review of 30 cases. *Am J Dis Child* 132:278–281.

Lapkin ML, French JH, Golden GS, et al. 1977. The electroencephalogram in childhood basilar artery migraine. *Neurology* 27:580–583.

Laplante P, Saint-Hilaire JM, Bouvier G. 1983. Headache as an epileptic manifestation. *Neurology* 33:1493–1495.

Larner AJ, Anderson M. 1995. Rasmussen's syndrome: pathogenetic theories and therapeutic strategies. *J Neurol* 242:355–358.

Larrieu JL, Lagueny A, Julien J. 1985. Etat confusionnel sous acide valproique réversible après administration de clonazepam. *Rev Electroencephalogr Neurophysiol Clin* 15:179–184.

Larroche JC, Girard N, Narcy F, Fallet C. 1994. Abnormal cortical plate (polymicrogyria), heterotopias, and brain damage in monozygous twins. *Biol Neonate* 65:343–352.

Lascelles K, Dean AF, Robinson RO. 2002. Rasmussen's encephalitis followed by lupus erythematosus. *Dev Med Child Neurol* 44:572–574.

Laskowitz DT, Sperling MR, French JR, et al. 1995. The syndrome of frontal lobe epilepsy: characteristics and surgical management. *Neurology* 45:780–787.

Lassonde M, Sauerwein H, Chicoine AJ, Geoffroy G. 1991. Absence of disconnection syndrome in callosal agenesis and early callosotomy: brain reorganization or lack of structural specificity during ontogeny? *Neuropsychologia* 29:481–495.

Lathers CM, Schraeder PL. 1990. *Epilepsy and sudden death*. New York: Marcel Dekker.

Laucman ME, Graves S, Gibson PH. 1994. Psychogenic seizures in children: long-term analysis of 43 cases. *J Child Neurol* 9:404–407.

Lawden MC, Eke T, Degg C, et al. 1999. Visual field defects associated with vigabatrin therapy. *J Neurol Neurosurg Psychiatry* 67:716–722.

Laxer KD. 1991. Temporal lobe epilepsy with inflammatory pathologic changes. In: Andermann F, ed. *Chronic encephalitis and epilepsy: Rasmussen's syndrome*. Boston: Butterworth-Heinemann, 135–140.

Layton DD. 1962. Heterotopic gray matter as an epileptogenic focus. *J Neuropathol Exp Neurol* 21:244–281.

Leach JP, Girvan J, Paul A, et al. 1997. Gabapentin and cognition: a double blind, dose ranging, placebo controlled study in refractory epilepsy. *J Neurol Neurosurg Psychiatry* 62:372–376.

Leach MJ, Randall AD, Stefani A, et al. 2002. Lamotrigine: mechanisms of action. In: Levy RH, Mattson RH, Meldrum BS, et al., eds. *Antiepileptic drugs*, 5th ed. Philadelphia: Lippincott Williams & Wilkins, 363–369.

Leblanc R, Tampieri D, Robitaille Y, et al. 1991. Developmental anterobasal temporal encephalocele and temporal lobe epilepsy. *J Neurosurg* 74:933–939.

Leblanc R, Tampieri D, Robitaille Y, et al. 1996. Surgical treatment of focal epilepsy in patients with schizencephaly. In: Guerrini R, Andermann F, Canapicchi R, et al., eds. *Dysplasias of cerebral cortex and epilepsy*. Philadelphia: Lippincott-Raven, 417–426.

Ledoux JE. 1992. Emotion and the amygdala. In: Aggleton JP, ed. *The amygdala: neurobiological aspects of emotion, memory, and mental dysfunction*. New York: Wiley-Liss, 339–351.

Lee SI, Kirby D. 1988. Absence seizure with generalized rhythmic delta activity. *Epilepsia* 29:262–267.

Lee ST, Lui TN. 1992. Early seizures after mild closed head injury. *J Neurosurg* 76:435–439.

Lee K, Diaz M, Melchior JC. 1981. Temporal lobe epilepsy—not a consequence of childhood convulsions in Denmark. *Acta Neurol Scand* 63:231–236.

Lee BI, Lesser RP, Pippenger CE, et al. 1985. Familial paroxysmal hypnogenic dystonia. *Neurology* 35:1357–1360.

Lee BI, Markand ON, Siddiqui AR, et al. 1986a. Single photon emission computed tomography (SPECT) brain imaging (using N,N,N′-trimethyl-N′-(2 hydroxy-3-methyl-5-^{123}I-iodobenzyl)-1,3-propanediamine 2 HCl

(HIPDM): intractable complex partial seizures. *Neurology* 36:1471–1477.

Lee K, Taudorf K, Hvorslev V. 1986b. Prophylactic treatment with valproic acid or diazepam in children with febrile convulsions. *Acta Paediatr Scand* 75:593–597.

Lee BI, Markand ON, Wellman HN, et al. 1988. HIPDM-SPECT in patients with medically intractable complex partial seizures. Ictal study. *Arch Neurol* 45:397–402.

Lee WL, Low PS, Rajan V. 1993. Benign familial infantile epilepsy. *J Pediatr* 123:588–590.

Lee D, Steingard R, Cesena M, et al. 1996. Behavioral side effects of gabapentin in children. *Epilepsia* 37:87–90.

Lee WL, Tay A, Ong HT, et al. 1998. Association of infantile convulsions with paroxysmal dyskinesias (ICCA syndrome): confirmation of linkage to human chromosome 16p12-q12 in a Chinese family. *Hum Genet* 103: 608–612.

Lee WL, Bievert C, Hallman K, et al. 2000a. A *KCNQ2* splice site mutation causing benign neonatal convulsions in a Scottish family. *Neuropediatrics* 31:9–12.

Lee YC, Yen D, Lirng JF, Yiu CH. 2000b. Epileptic seizures in a patient by immersing his right hand into hot water. *Seizure* 9:605–607.

Leestma JE. 1990. Natural history of epilepsy. In: Lathers CM, Schraeder PL, eds. *Epilepsy and sudden death*. New York: Marcel Dekker Inc, 1–26.

Leestma JE, Kalelkar MB, Teas SS, et al. 1984. Unexpected death associated with seizures: analysis of 66 cases. *Epilepsia* 25:84–88.

Leestma JE, Annegers JF, Brodie MJ, et al. 1997. Sudden unexpected death in epilepsy: observations from a large clinical development program. *Epilepsia* 38:47–55.

Lefebre C, Koelmel HW. 1989. Palinopsia as an epileptic phenomenon. *Eur Neurol* 29:323–327.

Legarda S, Jayakar P, Duchowny M, et al. 1994. Benign rolandic epilepsy: high central and low central subgroups. *Epilepsia* 35:1125–1129.

Legido A, Clancy RR, Berman PH. 1988. Recent advances in the diagnosis, treatment and prognosis of neonatal seizures. *Pediatr Neurol* 4:79–86.

Legido A, Clancy RR, Berman PH. 1991. Neurologic outcome after electroencephalographically proven neonatal seizures. *Pediatrics* 88:583–596.

Lehesjoki AE, Koskiniemi M, Sistonen P. 1991. Localization of a gene for progressive myoclonus epilepsy to chromosome 21q22. *Proc Nat Acad Sci U S A* 88: 3696–3699.

Lehesjoki AE, Eldridge R, Eldridge J, et al. 1993. Progressive myoclonus epilepsy of Unverricht-Lundborg type: a clinical and molecular genetic study of a family from the United States with four affected sibs. *Neurology* 43:2384–2386.

Leijten FS, Dekker E, Spekreijse H, et al. 1998. Light diffusion in photosensitive epilepsy. *Electroencephalogr Clin Neurophysiol* 106:387–391.

Lemme-Plaghos L, Kucharczyk W, Brant-Zawadzki M, et al. 1986. MRI of angiographically occult vascular malformations. *AJR Am J Roentgenol* 146:1223–1228.

Lempert T, Bauer M, Schmidt D. 1994. Syncope: a videometric analysis of 56 episodes of transient cerebral hypoxia. *Ann Neurol* 36:233–237.

Lencz T, McCarthy G, Bronen RA, et al. 1992. Quantitative magnetic resonance imaging in temporal lobe epilepsy: relationship to neuropathology and neuropsychological function. *Ann Neurol* 31:629–637.

Lennox WG. 1947. The genetics of epilepsy. *Am J Psychiatry* 103:457–462.

Lennox WG. 1960. In: Lennox WG, Lennox MA, eds. *Epilepsy and related disorders*, Vol. 1. Boston: Little, Brown and Company, 532–574.

Lennox WG, Cobb S. 1933. Epilepsy: aura in epilepsy. A statistical review of 1,359 cases. Arch Neurol Psychiatry 374–387.

Lennox WG, Davis JP. 1950. Clinical correlates of the fast and slow spike-wave electroencephalogram. *Pediatrics* 5:626–644.

Lennox WG, Lennox MA, eds. 1960. *Epilepsy and related disorders*. Boston: Little, Brown and Company.

Lennox-Buchtal MA. 1971. Febrile and nocturnal convulsions in monozygotic twins. *Epilepsia* 12:147–156.

Lennox-Buchtal MA. 1972. Neutropenia in children with febrile convulsions: clinical correlations. *Dev Med Child Neurol* 14:21–30.

Lennox-Buchthal MA. 1973. Febrile convulsions. A reappraisal. *Electroencephalogr Clin Neurophysiol* 32:1–138.

Leppert M, Anderson VE, Quattlebaum T, et al. 1989. Benign familial neonatal convulsions linked to genetic markers on chromosome 20. *Nature* 337:647–648.

Leppik IE. 1990. Carbamazepine. In: Dam M, Gram L, eds. *Comprehensive epileptology*. New York: Raven Press, 525–535.

Leppik IE, Derivan AT, Homan RW. 1983a. Double-blind study of lorazepam and diazepam in status epilepticus. *JAMA* 249:1452–1454.

Leppik IE, Patrick BK, Cranford RE. 1983b. Treatment of acute seizures and status epilepticus with intravenous phenytoin. In: Delgado-Escueta AV, Wasterlain CG, Treiman DM, Porter RJ, eds. *Status epilepticus*. Advances in neurology, Vol. 34. New York: Raven Press, 447–451.

Leppik IE, Fisher J, Kriel R, et al. 1986. Altered phenytoin clearance with febrile illness. *Neurology* 36:1367–1370.

Leppik IE, Boucher BA, Wilder BJ, et al. 1990. Pharmacokinetics and safety of phenytoin prodrug given IV in patients. *Neurology* 40:456–460.

Lerche H, Jurkat-Rott K, Lehmann-Horn F. 2001. Ion channels and epilepsy. *Am J Med Genet* 106:146–159.

Lerique-Koechlin A, Sternberg B, Misès J, et al. 1973. Valeur pronostique de l'électroencéphalogramme dans les convulsions fébriles du jeune enfant. In: Lugaresi E, Pazzaglia P, Tassinari CA, eds. *Evolution and prognosis of epilepsies*. Bologna: Aulo Gaggi, 199–208.

Lerman P. 1986. Seizures induced or aggravated by anticonvulsants. *Epilepsia* 27:706–710.

Lerman P. 1992. Benign partial epilepsy with centro-temporal spikes. In: Roger J, Bureau M, Dravet CH, et al. *Epileptic syndromes in infancy, childhood and adolescence*, 2nd ed. London: John Libbey, 189–200.

Lerman P, Kivity S. 1975. Benign focal epilepsy of childhood. A follow-up study of 100 recovered patients. *Arch Neurol* 32:261–264.

Lerman P, Kivity S. 1982. The efficacy of corticotropin in primary infantile spasms. *J Pediatr* 101:294–296.

Lerman P, Kivity S. 1986. Benign focal epilepsies of childhood. In: Pedley TA, Meldrum BS, eds. *Recent advances in epilepsy*, Vol. 3. Edinburgh: Churchill Livingstone, 137–156.

Lerman P, Lerman-Sagie T. 1995. Sulthiame revisited. *J Child Neurol* 10:241–242.

Lerman P, Lerman-Sagie T, Kivity S. 1991. Effect of early

corticosteroid therapy for Landau-Kleffner syndrome. *Dev Med Child Neurol* 33:257–260.

Leroy RF, Ebersole JS. 1983. An evaluation of ambulatory, cassette EEG monitoring. I: Montage design. *Neurology* 33:1–7.

Lesser RP. 1985. Psychogenic seizures. In: Pedley TA, Meldrum BS, eds. *Recent advances in epilepsy*, Vol. 2. Edinburgh: Churchill Livingstone, 273–296.

Lesser RP. 1996. Psychogenic seizures. *Neurology* 46: 1499–1507.

Lesser RP, Lüders H, Dinner DS. 1983. Evidence for epilepsy is rare in patients with psychogenic seizures. *Neurology* 33:502–504.

Lesser RP, Pippenger CE, Lüders H, et al. 1984. High-dose monotherapy in treatment of intractable seizures. *Neurology* 34:707–711.

Lesser RP, Lüders H, Wyllie E, et al. 1986. Mental deterioration in epilepsy. *Epilepsia* 27:S105–S123.

Leszczyszyn DJ, Pellock JM. 2001. Status epilepticus. In: Pellock JM, Dodson WE, Bourgeois BFD, eds. *Pediatric epilepsy: diagnosis and therapy*, 2nd ed. New York: Demos Medical Publishing, 275–289.

Levene MI, Trounce JQ. 1986. Cause of neonatal convulsions: towards a more precise diagnosis. *Arch Dis Child* 61:78–87.

Levene MI, Chervenak FA, Whittle M, eds. 2001. *Fetal and neonatal neurology and neurosurgery*. London: Churchill Livingstone.

Leventer RJ, Cardoso C, Ledbetter DH, et al. 2001. LIS1 missense mutations cause milder lissencephaly phenotypes including a child with normal IQ. *Neurology* 57:416–422.

Levesque MF, Nakasato N, Vinters HV, et al. 1991. Surgical treatment of limbic epilepsy associated with extrahippocampal lesions: the problem of dual pathology. *J Neurosurg* 75:364–370.

Levey AI, Weiss H, Yu R, et al. 1988. Seizures following myelography with iopamidol. *Ann Neurol* 23:397–399.

Levin R, Banks S, Berg B. 1988. Psychosocial dimensions of epilepsy: a review of the literature. *Epilepsia* 29: 805–816.

Levitan M, Bruni J. 1986. Repetitive pseudoseizures incorrectly managed as status epilepticus. *Can Med Assn J* 134:1029–1031.

Leviton A, Cowan LD. 1982. Epidemiology of seizure disorders in children. *Neuroepidemiology* 1:40–83.

Leviton A, Nelson KB. 1992. Problems with definitions and classifications of newborn encephalopathy. *Pediatr Neurol* 8:85–90.

Levy RH, Krall RL. 1984. Treatment of status epilepticus with lorazepam. *Arch Neurol* 41:605–611.

Levy RL, Saunders RL. 1981. Citrobacter meningitis and cerebral abscesses in early infancy: cure by moxalactam. *Neurology* 31:1575–1577.

Levy RH, Schmidt D. 1985. Utility of free level monitoring of antiepileptic drugs. *Epilepsia* 26:199–205.

Levy RH, Cenraud B, Loiseau P, et al. 1980. Meal dependent absorption of enteric-coated sodium valproate. *Epilepsia* 21:273–280.

Levy RH, Moreland TA, Farwell JR. 1983. Drug interactions in epileptic children. In: Morselli PL, Pippenger CE, Penry JK, eds. *Antiepileptic drug therapy in pediatrics*. New York: Raven Press, 75–84.

Levy SR, Abroms IF, Marshall PC, et al. 1985. Seizures and cerebral infarction in the full-term newborn. *Ann Neurol* 17:366–370.

Levy RH, Dreifuss FE, Mattson RH, et al., eds. 1989. *Antiepileptic drugs*, 3rd ed. New York: Raven Press.

Levy RH, Mattson RH, Meldrum BS, Perucca E, eds. 2002. *Antiepileptic drugs*, 5th ed. Philadelphia: Lippincott Williams & Wilkins.

Lewis H, Wallace SJ. 2001. Vigabatrin. *Dev Med Child Neurol* 43:833–835.

Lewis HM, Parry JV, Parry RP, et al. 1979. Role of viruses in febrile convulsions. *Arch Dis Child* 54:869–876.

Lewis TB, Leach RJ, Ward K, et al. 1993. Genetic heterogeneity in benign familial neonatal convulsions: identification of a new locus on chromosome 8q. *Am J Hum Genet* 53:670–675.

Lewis TB, Shevell MI, Andermann E, et al. 1996. Evidence of a third locus for benign familial convulsions. *J Child Neurol* 11:211–214.

Lhatoo SD, Johnson AL, Goodridge DM, et al. 2001. Mortality in epilepsy in the first 11–14 years after diagnosis: multivariate analysis of a long-term prospective, population-based cohort. *Ann Neurol* 49:344–366.

Li LM, Dubeau F, Andermann F, et al. 1997. Periventricular nodular heterotopia and intractable temporal lobe epilepsy: poor outcome after temporal lobe resection. *Ann Neurol* 41:662–668.

Lieb JP, Walsh GO, Babb TL. 1976. A comparison of EEG seizure patterns recorded with surface and depth electrodes in patients with temporal lobe epilepsy. *Epilepsia* 12:137–160.

Lieb JP, Engel J Jr, Gevins A, et al. 1981. Surface and deep EEG correlates of surgical outcome in temporal lobe epilepsy. *Epilepsia* 22:515–538.

Lieb JP, Dasheiff RM, Engel J. 1991. Role of the frontal lobes in the propagation of mesial temporal lobe seizures. *Epilepsia* 32:822–837.

Lim J, Yagnik P, Schraeder P, et al. 1986. Ictal catatonia as a manifestation of nonconvulsive status epilepticus. *J Neurol Neurosurg Psychiatry* 49:833–836.

Lim SH, Dinner DS, Pillay PK, et al. 1994. Functional anatomy of the human supplementary sensorimotor area: results of extraoperative electrical stimulation. *Electroencephalogr Clin Neurophysiol* 91:179–193.

Lin JT, Ziegler DK, Lai CW, Bayer W. 1982. Convulsive syncope in blood donors. *Ann Neurol* 11:525–528.

Lin YP, Itomi K, Takada H, et al. 1998. Benign myoclonic epilepsy in infants: video-EEG features and long-term follow-up. *Neuropediatrics* 29:268–271.

Lin Y, Yoshiko K, Negoro T, et al. 2000. Cerebral oxygenation state in childhood moyamoya disease: a near-infrared spectroscopy study. *Pediatr Neurol* 22:365–370.

Lindsay J, Ounsted C, Richards P. 1979a. Long-term outcome in children with temporal lobe seizures. I: Social outcome and childhood factors. *Dev Med Child Neurol* 21:285–298.

Lindsay J, Ounsted C, Richards P. 1979b. Long-term outcome in children with temporal lobe seizures. II: Marriage, parenthood and sexual indifference. *Dev Med Child Neurol* 21:433–440.

Lindsay J, Ounsted C, Richards P. 1980a. Long-term outcome in children with temporal lobe seizures. III: Psychiatric aspects in childhood and adult life. *Dev Med Child Neurol* 21:630–636.

Lindsay J, Ounsted C, Richards P. 1980b. Long-term outcome in children with temporal lobe seizures. IV: Genetic factors, febrile convulsions and the remission of seizures. *Dev Med Child Neurol* 22:429–439.

Lindsay J, Ounsted C, Richards P. 1980c. Long-term outcome in children with temporal lobe seizures. V: Indications and contra-indications for neurosurgery. *Dev Med Child Neurol* 26:25–32.

Lindsay J, Glaser G, Richards P, et al. 1984. Developmental aspects of focal epilepsies of childhood treated by neurosurgery. *Dev Med Child Neurol* 26:574–587.

Lindsay J, Ounsted C, Richards P. 1987. Hemispherectomy for childhood epilepsy: a 36-year study. *Dev Med Child Neurol* 29:592–600.

Lippe BM, Sparkes RS. 1981. Ring 14 chromosome: association with seizures. *Am J Med Genet* 9:301–305.

Lipski S, Brunelle F, Aicardi J, et al. 1990. Gd-DOTA-enhanced MR imaging in two cases of Sturge-Weber syndrome. *Am J Neuroradiol* 11:690–692.

Lishman WA, Symonds CP, Whitty CW. 1962. Seizures induced by movement. *Brain* 85:93–108.

Liu AW, Delgado-Escueta AV, Serratosa JM, et al. 1995. Juvenile myoclonic epilepsy locus in chromosome 6p21.2-p11: linkage to convulsion and electroencephalographic trait. *Am J Hum Genet* 57:368–381.

Livet MO, Aicardi J, Plouin P, et al. 2002. Epilepsies in inborn errors of metabolism. In: Roger J, Bureau M, Dravet C, et al., eds. *Epileptic syndromes of infancy, childhood and adolescence*, 3rd ed. London: John Libbey, 389–405.

Livingston S. 1960. Management of the child with one epileptic seizure. *JAMA* 174:135–139.

Livingston S. 1972. *Comprehensive management of epilepsy in infancy, childhood and adolescence*. Springfield, IL: Charles C Thomas Publisher.

Livingston S. 1974. Diagnosis and treatment of childhood myoclonic seizures. *Pediatrics* 53:542–548.

Livingston JH. 1988. The Lennox-Gastaut syndrome. *Dev Med Child Neurol* 30:536–540.

Livingston J, Aicardi J. 1990. Unusual MRI appearance of diffuse subcortical heterotopia or "double cortex" in two children. *J Neurol Neurosurg Psychiatry* 53:617–620.

Livingston S, Eisner V, Pauli L. 1958. Minor motor epilepsy: diagnosis, treatment and prognosis. *Pediatrics* 21:916–928.

Livingston S, Torres I, Pauli LL, Rider RV. 1965. Petit mal epilepsy. Results of a prolonged follow-up study of 117 patients. *JAMA* 194:227–232.

Livingston JH, Beaumont D, Arzimanoglou A, Aicardi J. 1989. Vigabatrin in the treatment of epilepsy in children. *Br J Clin Pharmacol* 27:109S–112S.

Lockman LA, Kriel R, Zazke D, et al. 1979. Phenobarbital dosage for control of neonatal seizures. *Neurology* 29:1445–1449.

Logroscino G, Hesdorffer DC, Cascino GD, et al. 1997. Short-term mortality after incident status epilepticus. *Epilepsia* 38:1344–1349.

Logroscino G, Hesdorffer DC, Cascino GD, et al. 2002. Long-term mortality after a first episode of status epilepticus. *Neurology* 58:537–541.

Loiseau P. 1971. Epilepsies myocloniques. *Encéphale* 60:245–264.

Loiseau P. 1992. Absence epilepsy. In: Roger J, Dravet C, Bureau M, et al., eds. *Epileptic syndromes in infancy, childhood and adolescence*, 2nd ed. London: John Libbey, 106–120.

Loiseau P, Beaussart M. 1973. The seizures of benign childhood epilepsy with rolandic paroxysmal discharges. *Epilepsia* 14:381–389.

Loiseau P, Cohadon F. 1970. *Le petit mal et ses frontières*. Paris: Masson.

Loiseau P, Cohadon S. 1981. Les épilepsies à foyers EEG intercritiques multiples. *Rev Electroencephalogr Neurophysiol Clin* 11:259–266.

Loiseau P, Dartigues JF. 1981. Formes électrocliniques et évolutives des épilepsies de l'adolescence. *Rev Electroencephalogr Neurophysiol Clin* 11:493–501.

Loiseau P, Jallon P. 1972. *Les epilepsies*, 3rd ed. Paris: Masson.

Loiseau P, Orgogozo JM. 1978. An unrecognized syndrome of benign focal epileptic seizures in teenagers. *Lancet* 2:1070–1071.

Loiseau P, Geissmann P, Cohadon S, et al. 1962. Les paroxysmes rolandiques en dehors de l'épilepsie. *Rev Neurol (Paris)* 111:374–381.

Loiseau P, Cohadon F, Cohadon S. 1971. Gelastic epilepsy. A review and report of five cases. *Epilepsia* 12:313–323.

Loiseau P, Legroux M, Grimond P, et al. 1974. Taxometric classification of myoclonic epilepsies. *Epilepsia* 15:1–11.

Loiseau P, Cenraud B, Lévy RH, et al. 1982. Diurnal variations in steady-state plasma concentrations of valproic acid in epileptic patients. *Clin Pharmacokinet* 7:544–552.

Loiseau P, Dartigues JF, Pestre M. 1983a. Prognosis of partial epileptic seizures in the adolescent. *Epilepsia* 24:472–481.

Loiseau P, Pestre M, Dartigues JF, et al. 1983b. Long-term prognosis in two forms of childhood epilepsy: typical absence seizures and epilepsy with rolandic (centrotemporal) EEG foci. *Ann Neurol* 13:642–648.

Loiseau P, Strube E, Broustet D, et al. 1983c. Learning impairment in epileptic patients. *Epilepsia* 24:183–192.

Loiseau P, Cohadon S, Jogeix M, et al. 1984. Efficacité du valproate de sodium dans les épilepsies partielles: etude croisée valproate-carbamazépine. *Rev Neurol (Paris)* 140:434–437.

Loiseau P, Guyot M, Loiseau H, et al. 1986. Eating seizures. *Epilepsia* 27:161–163.

Loiseau P, Duché B, Cordova S, et al. 1988. Prognosis of benign childhood epilepsy with centrotemporal spikes: a follow-up study of 168 patients. *Epilepsia* 29:229–235.

Loiseau J, Loiseau P, Guyot M, et al. 1990. Survey of seizure disorders in the French southwest. I: Incidence of epileptic syndromes. *Epilepsia* 31:391–396.

Loiseau P, Duché B, Cohadon S. 1992. The prognosis of benign localized epilepsies in early childhood. In: Degen R, ed. *Localized and generalized epilepsies of early childhood*. Amsterdam: Elsevier, 75–81.

Lombroso CT. 1967. Sylvian seizures and midtemporal spike foci in children. *Arch Neurol* 17:52–59.

Lombroso CT. 1974. Seizures in the newborn period. In: Vinken PJ, Bruyn GW, eds. *The epilepsies*. Handbook of clinical neurology, Vol. 15. Amsterdam: North-Holland, 189–218.

Lombroso CT. 1978. Convulsive disorders in newborns. In: Thompson RA, Green JR, eds. *Pediatric neurology and neurosurgery*. New York: Spectrum, 205–239.

Lombroso CT. 1982. Neonatal electroencephalography. In: Niedermeyer E, Lopes de Silva F, eds. *Electroencephalography*. Baltimore: Urban and Schwarzenberg, 599–637.

Lombroso CT. 1983a. A prospective study of infantile

spasms: clinical and therapeutic correlations. *Epilepsia* 24:135–158.

Lombroso CT. 1983b. Differentiation of seizures in newborns and in early infancy. In: Morselli PL, Pippenger CE, Penry JK, eds. *Antiepileptic drug therapy in pediatrics.* New York: Raven Press, 85–102.

Lombroso CT. 1983c. Prognosis in neonatal seizures. In: Delgado-Escueta AV, Wasterlain CG, Treiman DM, Porter RJ. *Status epilepticus.* Advances in neurology, Vol. 34. New York: Raven Press, 101–113.

Lombroso CT. 1989. Intermittent home treatment of status and clusters of seizures. *Epilepsia* 30:S11–S14.

Lombroso CT. 1990. Early myoclonic encephalopathy, early infantile epileptic encephalopathy, and benign and severe infantile myoclonic epilepsies: a critical review and personal contributions. *J Clin Neurophysiol* 7: 380–408.

Lombroso CT. 1992. Neonatal seizures. In: Resor SR, Kutt H, eds. *The medical treatment of epilepsy.* New York: Marcel Dekker, 115–125.

Lombroso CT. 1995. Paroxysmal choreoathetosis: an epileptic or non-epileptic disorder? *Ital J Neurol Sci* 16: 271–277.

Lombroso CT. 1996. Neonatal seizures: a clinician's overview. *Brain Dev* 18:1–28.

Lombroso CT. 2000. Nocturnal paroxysmal dystonia due to subfrontal cortical dysplasia. *Epil Dis* 2:15–20.

Lombroso CT. 2002. Neonatal movement disorders: epileptic or non-epileptic. In: Guerrini R, Aicardi J, Andermann F, et al., eds. *Epilepsy and movement disorders.* Cambridge: Cambridge University Press, 279–305.

Lombroso CT, Erba G. 1982. Myoclonic seizures: considerations in toxonomy. In: Akimoto H, Kazamatsuri H, Seino M, et al., eds. *Advances in epileptology*, XIIIth Epilepsy International Symposium. New York: Raven Press, 129–134.

Lombroso CT, Fejerman N. 1977. Benign myoclonus in early infancy. *Ann Neurol* 1:138–143.

Lombroso CT, Forsythe I. 1960. A long-term follow-up of acetazolamide (Diamox) in the treatment of epilepsy. *Epilepsia* 1:493–500.

Lombroso CT, Lerman P. 1967. Breathholding spells (cyanotic and pallid infantile syncopes). *Pediatrics* 39:563–581.

Lombroso CT, Schwartz IH, Clark DM, et al. 1966. Ctenoids in healthy youth. Controlled study of 14- and 6-per-second positive spiking. *Neurology* 16: 1152–1156.

Long G, Moore JR. 1979. Parental expectations for their epileptic children. *J Child Psychol Psychiatry* 20: 299–312.

Loonen MC, van Dongen HR. 1990. Acquired childhood aphasia. Outcome 1 year after onset. *Arch Neurol* 47: 1324–1328.

Lopes-Cendes L, Scheffer IE, Berkovic SF, et al. 2000. A new locus for generalized epilepsy with febrile seizure plus maps to chromosome 2. *Am J Hum Genet* 66: 698–701.

Lorenz De Haas AM, Kullman M. 1964. Ethosuximide and grand mal. *Epilepsia* 5:90–96.

Loring DW, Lee GP, Meador KJ, et al. 1990. The intracarotid amobarbital procedure as a predictor of memory failure following unilateral temporal lobectomy. *Neurology* 40:605–610.

Lortie A, Chiron C, Dumas C, et al. 1997. Optimizing the in-

dication of vigabatrin in children with refractory epilepsy. *J Child Neurol* 12:253–259.

Lortie A, Chiron C, Mumford J, Dulac O. 1993. The potential for increasing seizure frequency, relapse, and appearance of new seizure types with vigabatrin. *Neurology* 43:S24–S27.

Lortie A, Plouin P, Chiron C, et al. 2002. Characteristics of epilepsy in focal cortical dysplasia in infancy. *Epilepsy Res* 51:133–145.

Lou HC, Friis-Hansen B. 1979. Arterial blood pressure elevations during motor activity and epileptic seizures in the newborn. *Acta Paediatr Scand* 68:803–806.

Lou HC, Brandt S, Bruhn P. 1977. Aphasia and epilepsy in children. *Acta Neurol Scand* 56:46–54.

Lowenstein DH, Alldredge BK. 1998. Status epilepticus. *N Engl J Med* 338:970–976.

Lowenstein DH, Bleck TP, MacDonald RL. 1999. It's time to revise the definition of status epilepticus. *Epilepsia* 40: 120–122.

Lucas M, Costa AF, Montori M, et al. 2001. Germline mutations in the CCM1 gene, encoding Krit1, cause cerebral cavernous malformations. *Ann Neurol* 49:529–532.

Lüders H, ed. 1992. *Epilepsy surgery.* New York: Raven Press.

Lüders HO. 1995. Cortical stimulation in humans: the negative motor area. *Adv Neurol* 67:115–119.

Lüders H, Comair YG. 2001. *Epilepsy surgery*, 2nd ed. Philadelphia: Lippincott Williams & Wilkins.

Lüders H, Noachtar S, eds. 1995. *Atlas und Video epileptische Anfälle und syndrome.* Wehr: Ciba-Geigy Verlag.

Lüders H, Lesser RP, Dinner DS, et al. 1985. The second sensory area in humans: evoked potential and electrical stimulation studies. *Ann Neurol* 17:177–184.

Lüders H, Lesser RP, Dinner DS, et al. 1987a. Language deficits elicited by electrical stimulation of the fusiform gyrus. In: Engel J Jr, Ojemann GA, Lüders HO, Williamson PD, eds. *Fundamental mechanisms of human brain function.* New York: Raven Press, 83–90.

Lüders H, Lesser RP, Dinner DS, et al. 1987b. Benign focal epilepsy of childhood. In: Lüders H, Lesser RP, eds. *Epilepsy: electroclinical syndromes.* Berlin: Springer, 303–346.

Lüders H, Dinner DS, Morris HH, et al. 1989a. EEG evaluation for epilepsy surgery in children. *Cleve Clin J Med* 56:S53–S61.

Lüders H, Hahn J, Lesser RP, et al. 1989b. Basal temporal subdural electrodes in the evaluation of patients with intractable epilepsy. *Epilepsia* 30:131–142.

Lüders HO, Burgess R, Noachtar S. 1993a. Expanding the international classification of seizures to provide localization information. *Neurology* 43:1650–1655.

Lüders HO, Engel J, Munari C. 1993b. General principles. In: Engel J, ed. *Surgical treatment of the epilepsies*, 2nd ed. New York: Raven Press, 137–153.

Lüders H, Acharya J, Baumgartner C, et al. 1998. Semiological seizure classification. *Epilepsia* 39:1006–1013.

Lüders HO, Noachtar S, Burgess RC. 2000. Semiologic classification of epileptic seizures. In: Luders HO, Noachtar S, eds. *Epileptic seizures: pathophysiology and clinical semiology.* Philadelphia: Churchill Livingstone, 263–285.

Ludwig B. 1987. Review: neuroradiological aspects of infantile spasms. *Brain Dev* 9:358–360.

Ludwig B, Ajmone-Marsan C. 1975. Clinical ictal patterns

in epileptic patients with occipital electroencephalographic foci. *Neurology* 25:463–471.

Ludwig BI, Ajmone-Marsan C, Van Bum JM. 1962. Seizures of probable orbitofrontal origin. *Epilepsia* 16:141–158.

Ludwig BI, Ajmone-Marsan C, Van Bum JM. 1976. Depth and direct cortical recording in seizure disorders of extra temporal origin. *Neurology* 26:1085–1099.

Lugaresi E, Cirignotta F. 1981. Hypnogenic paroxysmal dystonia: epileptic seizure or new syndrome? *Sleep* 4:129–136.

Lugaresi E, Pazzaglia P. 1975. Interictal electroencephalogram. In: *Epilepsies. handbook of electroencephalography and clinical neurophysiology*, Vol. 13A. Amsterdam: Elsevier, 13–19.

Lugaresi E, Pazzaglia P, Franck L. 1973. Evolution and prognosis of primary generalized epilepsies of the petit mal absence type. In: Lugaresi E, ed. *Evolution and prognosis of epilepsies*. Bologna: Aulo Gaggi, 3–22.

Lugaresi E, Pazzaglia P, Roger J, et al. 1974. Evolution and prognosis of petit mal. In: Harris P, Mawdsley C, eds. *Epilepsy: proceedings of the Hans Berger Centenary Symposium*. Edinburgh: Churchill Livingstone, 151–153.

Lugaresi E, Cirignotta F, Montagna P. 1984. Occipital lobe epilepsy with scotosensitive seizures: the role of central vision. *Epilepsia* 25:115–120.

Lugaresi E, Cirignotta F, Montagna P. 1986. Nocturnal paroxysmal dystonia. *J Neurol Neurosurg Psychiatry* 49:375–380.

Luna D, Chiron C, Dulac O, et al. 1988. Epidémiologie des épilepsies de l'enfant dans le département de l'Oise (France). In: Jallon P, ed. *Epidémiologie des Epilepsies, Journées d'étude de la Ligue Française contre l'épilepsie*. London: John Libbey, 41–53.

Luna D, Dulac O, Pajot N, et al. 1989a. Vigabatrin in the treatment of childhood epilepsies: a single-blood placebo-controlled study. *Epilepsia* 30:430–437.

Luna D, Dulac O, Plouin P. 1989b. Ictal characteristics of cryptogenic partial epilepsies in infancy. *Epilepsia* 30:827–832.

Lux AL, Edwards SW, Osborne JP, et al. 2001. Revised guideline for prescribing vigabatrin in children. Guideline's claim about infantile spasms is not based on appropriate evidence. *BMJ* 322:236–237.

Lynch BJ, Rust AS. 1994. Natural history of neonatal hypocalcemic and hypomagnesemic seizures. *Pediatric Neurology* 11:23–27.

Lyon G, Gastaut H. 1985. Considerations on the significance attributed to unusual cerebral histological findings recently described in eight patients with primary generalized epilepsy. *Epilepsia* 26:365–367.

Lyon G, Dodge PR, Adams RD. 1961. The acute encephalopathies of obscure origin in infants and children. *Brain* 84:680–708.

Ma X, Liporace J, O'Connor MJ, et al. 2001. Neurosurgical treatment of medically intractable status epilepticus. *Epilepsy Res* 46:33–38.

Maccario M, Hefferen SJ, Klebuser SJ, et al. 1982. Developmental dysphasia and electroencephalographic abnormalities. *Dev Med Child Neurol* 24:141–155.

MacDonald BK, Johnson AL, Sander JW, Shorvon SD. 1999. Febrile convulsions in 220 children—neurological sequelae at 12 years follow-up. *Eur Neurol* 41:179–186.

Mackay M, Weiss S, Snead OC 3rd. 2002. Treatment of infantile spasms: an evidence-based approach. *Int Rev Neurobiol* 49:157–184.

Mackenzie R, Klistorner A. 1998. Severe persistent visual field constriction associated with vigabatrin. Asymptomatic as well as symptomatic defects occur with vigabatrin. *BMJ* 316:233.

Mackintosh TF. 1970. Studies on prophylactic treatment of febrile convulsions in children. *Clin Pediatr* 9:283–286.

Mackintosh DA, Baird-Lampert J, Buchanan N. 1987. Is carbamazepine an alternative maintenance therapy for neonatal seizures? *Dev Pharmacol Ther* 10:49–54.

Madsen JA, Bray PF. 1966. The coincidence of diffuse electroencephalographic spikewave paroxysms and brain tumors. *Neurology* 16:546–555.

Maeda N, Watanabe K, Negoro T, et al. 1994. Evolutional changes of cortical hypometabolism in West's syndrome. *Lancet* 343:1620–1623.

Maekawa K, Ohta H, Tamai I. 1980. Transient brain shrinkage in infantile spasms after ACTH treatment. Report of two cases. *Neuropédiatrie* 11:80–84.

Magarian GJ. 1982. Hyperventilation syndromes: infrequently recognized common expressions of anxiety and stress. *Medicine* 61:219–236.

Magarian GJ, Olney RK. 1984. Absence spells, hyperventilation syndrome as a previously unrecognized cause. *Am J Med* 76:906–909.

Magaudda A. 1991. The syndrome of bilateral occipital calcifications (BOC), epilepsy and celiac disease: clinical and neuroimaging features in 13 patients [Abstract]. *Epilepsia* 32(Suppl. 1):119.

Maher J, McLachlan RS. 1995. Febrile convulsions. Is seizure duration the most important predictor of temporal lobe epilepsy? *Brain* 118:1521–1528.

Maheshwari MC, Jeavons PM. 1975. The prognostic implications of suppression-burst activity in the EEG in infancy. *Epilepsia* 16:127–131.

Maijkowski J, ed. 1977. *Post-traumatic epilepsy and pharmacological prophylaxis*. Warsaw: Polish Chapter of the ILAE.

Majoie HJ, Berfelo MW, Aldenkamp AP, et al. 2001. Vagus nerve stimulation in children with therapy-resistant epilepsy diagnosed as Lennox-Gastaut syndrome: clinical results, neuropsychological effects, and cost-effectiveness. *J Clin Neurophysiol* 18:419–428.

Mäkelä JP, Iivanaimen M, Pieninkeroinen IP, et al. 1993. Seizures associated with propofol anesthesia. *Epilepsia* 34:832–835.

Malafosse A, Dulac O, Leboyer M, et al. 1992. Confirmation of linkage studies of benign familial neonatal convulsions to P20S19 and D20S20. *Hum Genet* 89:54–58.

Malamud N. 1966. The epileptogenic focus in temporal lobe epilepsy from a pathological standpoint. *Arch Neurol* 14:190–195.

Maldonado HM, Delgado-Escueta AV, Walsh GO, et al. 1988. Complex partial seizures of hippocampal and amygdalar origin. *Epilepsia* 29:420–433.

Maldonado C, Castello J, Fuentes E. 1995. Vigabatrin in the management of Lennox-Gastaut syndrome [Abstract]. *Epilepsia* 36:S102.

Mamelle N, Mamelle JC, Plasse JC, et al. 1984. Prevention of recurrent febrile convulsions. A randomized therapeutic assay: sodium valproate, phenobarbital and placebo. *Neuropediatrics* 15:37–42.

Manaka S. 1992. Cooperative prospective study on post-traumatic epilepsy: risk factors and the effect of prophylactic anticonvulsants. *Jpn J Psychiatr Neurol* 46:311–315.

Manford M, Shorvon SD. 1992. Prolonged sensory or visceral symptoms: an underdiagnosed form of focal, nonconvulsive (simple partial) status epilepticus. *J Neurol Neurosurg Psychiat* 55:714–716.

Manford M, Fish DR, Shorvon SD. 1996a. An analysis of clinical seizure patterns and their localizing value in frontal and temporal lobe epilepsies. *Brain* 119:17–40.

Manford MR, Fish DR, Shorvon SD. 1996b. Startle provoked epileptic seizures: features in 19 patients. *J Neurol Neurosurg Psychiatry* 61:151–156.

Manganotti P, Miniussi C, Santorum E, et al. 1998. Influence of somatosensory input on paroxysmal activity in benign rolandic epilepsy with "extreme sensory potentials." *Brain* 121:647–658.

Mangin P, Krieger J, Kurtz D. 1982. Apnea following hyperventilation in man. *J Neurol Sci* 57:67–82.

Mani KS, Mani AJ, Ramesh CK, et al. 1974. Hot water epilepsy: clinical and electroencephalographic features. Study of 60 cases. *Neurology (Bombay)* 20:237–240.

Mannino FL, Trauner DA. 1983. Stroke in neonates. *J Pediatr* 102:605–609.

Manoumani V, Wallace SJ. 1994. Epilepsy with myoclonic absences. *Arch Dis Child* 70:288–290.

Mantovani JF, Gerger GJ. 1984. "Idiopathic" neonatal cerebral infarction. *Am J Dis Child* 138:359–362.

Mantovani JF, Landau WM. 1980. Acquired aphasia with convulsive disorder: course and prognosis. *Neurology* 30:524–529.

Manucheri K. 2000. Visual field defect associated with vigabatrin. Method of estimating prevalence was inappropriate. *BMJ* 320:1403–1404.

Maquet P, Hirsch E, Dive D, et al. 1990. Cerebral glucose utilization during sleep in Landau-Kleffner syndrome: a PET study. *Epilepsia* 31:778–783.

Marchuk DA, Gallione CJ, Morrison LA, et al. 1995. A locus for cerebral cavernous malformations maps to chromosome 7q in two families. *Genomics* 28:311–314.

Marciani MG, Gotman J, Andermann F, et al. 1985. Patterns of seizure activation after withdrawal of antiepileptic medication. *Neurology* 35:1537–1543.

Marcus EM, Watson CW. 1966. Bilateral synchronous spike-wave electroencephalographic patterns in the cat. Interaction of bilateral cortical foci in the intact, the bilateral cortical-callosal, and a diencephalic preparation. *Arch Neurol* 14:601–610.

Marescaux C, Warier JM, Laroye M, et al. 1983. Le valproate de sodium: une drogue hyperammonémiante (étude chez l'épileptique et chez le volontaire sain). *J Neurol Sci* 58:195–209.

Marescaux C, Hirsch E, Finck S, et al. 1990. Landau-Kleffner syndrome: a pharmacologic study of five cases. *Epilepsia* 31:768–777.

Margerison J, Corsellis JAN. 1966. Epilepsy and the temporal lobes. A clinical, electroencephalographic and neuropathological study of the brain in epilepsy, with particular reference to the temporal lobes. *Brain* 89:499–530.

Mariani E, Ferini-Strambi L, Sala M, et al. 1993. Epilepsy in institutionalized patients with encephalopathy: clinical aspects and nosological considerations. *Am J Ment Retard* 98(Suppl.):27–33.

Markand ON. 1977. Slow spike-wave activity in EEG and associated clinical features: often called "Lennox" or "Lennox-Gastaut" syndrome. *Neurology* 27:746–757.

Markand ON, Wheeler GL, Pollack SL. 1978. Complex partial status epilepticus (psychomotor status). *Electroencephalogr Clin Neurophysiol* 44:125–126.

Markand ON, Garg BP, Weaver DD. 1984. Familial startle disease (hyperexplexia). Electrophysiologic studies. *Arch Neurol* 41:71–74.

Marks DA, Katz A, Scheyer R, et al. 1991. Clinical and electrographic effects of acute anticonvulsant withdrawal in epileptic patients. *Neurology* 41:508–512.

Marks DA, Katz A, Hoffer P, et al. 1992a. Localization of extratemporal epileptic foci during ictal single photon emission computed tomography. *Ann Neurol* 31:250–255.

Marks DA, Kim J, Spencer DD, et al. 1992b. Characteristics of intractable seizures following meningitis and encephalitis. *Neurology* 42:1513–1518.

Marret S, Parain D, Ménard JF, et al. 1997. Prognostic value of neonatal electroencephalography in premature newborns less than 33 weeks of gestational age. *Electroencephalogr Clin Neurophysiol* 102:178–185.

Marseille Consensus Group. 1990. Classification of progressive myoclonus epilepsies and related disorders. *Ann Neurol* 28:113–116.

Marshall DW, Westmoreland BF, Sharbrough FW. 1983. Ictal tachycardia during temporal lobe seizures. *Mayo Clin Proc* 58:443–446.

Marson AG, Kadir ZA, Chadwick DW. 1996. New antiepileptic drugs: a systematic review of their efficacy and tolerability. *BMJ* 313:1169–1174.

Marson AG, Williamson PR, Hutton JL, et al. 2000. Carbamazepine versus valproate monotherapy for epilepsy. *Cochrane Database Syst Rev* CD001030.

Marson AG, Hutton JL, Leach JP, et al. 2001. Levetiracetam, oxcarbazepine, remacemide and zonisamide for drug resistant localization-related epilepsy: a systematic review. *Epilepsy Res* 46:259–270.

Marson AG, Williamson PR, Clough H, et al. 2002. Carbamazepine versus valproate monotherapy for epilepsy: a meta-analysis. *Epilepsia* 43:505–513.

Martin JH. 1985. Anatomical substrate for somatic sensation. In: Kandel ER, Schwartz JH, eds. *Principles of neural science*, 2nd ed. New York: Elsevier, 301–315.

Martin R, Kuznieckiy R, Ho S, et al. 1999. Cognitive effects of topiramate, gabapentin and lamotrigine in healthy young adults. *Neurology* 52:321–326.

Masland RL. 1974 The classification of the epilepsies. In: Vinken PJ, Bruyn GW, eds. *The epilepsies*. Handbook of clinical neurology, Vol. 15. Amsterdam: North-Holland, 1–29.

Massa R, de Saint-Martin A, Hirsch E, et al. 2000. Landau-Kleffner syndrome: sleep EEG characteristics at onset. *Clin Neurophysiol* 111:S87–S93.

Massa R, de Saint-Martin A, Carcangiu R, et al. 2001. EEG criteria predictive of cognitive complications in idiopathic focal epilepsy with rolandic spikes. *Neurology* 57:1071–1079.

Matalon R, Supple P, Wyandt H, et al. 1990. Transmission of ring 14 chromosome from mother to two sons. *Am J Med Genet* 36:381–385.

Mathai KV, Dunn OP, Kurland LT, et al. 1968. Convulsive disorders in the Marianna Islands. *Epilepsia* 9:77–85.

Mathieson G. 1975. Pathology of temporal lobe foci. In:

Penry JK, Daly DD, eds. *Complex partial seizures and their treatment*. Advances in neurology, Vol. 11. New York: Raven Press, 163–185.

Matricardi M, Brinciotti M, Benedetti P. 1989. Outcome after discontinuation of AED therapy in children with epilepsy. *Epilepsia* 30:582–589.

Matsuishi T, Yoshino M, Tokunaga O, et al. 1985. Subacute necrotizing encephalomyelopathy (Leigh disease): report of a case with Lennox-Gastaut syndrome. *Brain Dev* 7:500–504.

Matsumoto A, Watanabe K, Negoro T, et al. 1981a. Infantile spasms: etiologic factors, clinical aspects, and long term prognosis in 200 cases. *Eur J Pediatr* 135:239–244.

Matsumoto A, Watanabe K, Negoro T, et al. 1981b. Long-term prognosis after infantile spasms: a statistical study of prognostic factors in 200 cases. *Dev Med Child Neurol* 23:51–65.

Matsumoto A, Watanabe K, Negoro T, et al. 1981c. Prognostic factors of infantile spasms from the etiological viewpoint. *Brain Dev* 3:361–364.

Matsumoto A, Watanabe K, Sugiura M, et al. 1983a. Long-term prognosis of convulsive disorders in the first year of life: mental and physical development and seizure persistence. *Epilepsia* 24:321–329.

Matsumoto A, Watanabe K, Sugiura M, et al. 1983b. Prognostic factors of convulsive disorders in the first year of life. *Brain Dev* 5:469–473.

Matsumoto A, Kumagai T, Takeuchi T, et al. 1987. Clinical effects of thyrotropin-releasing hormone for severe epilepsy in childhood: a comparative study with ACTH therapy. *Epilepsia* 28:49–55.

Matsumoto A, Kumagai T, Miura K, et al. 1992. Epilepsy in Angelman syndrome associated with chromosome 15q deletion. *Epilepsia* 33:1083–1090.

Matsumoto R, Ikeda A, Ohara S, et al. 2000. Nonconvulsive focal inhibitory seizure: subdural recording from motor cortex. *Neurology* 55:429–431.

Matsumoto N, Leventer RJ, Kuc JA, et al. 2001. Mutation analysis of the DCX gene and genotype/phenotype correlation in subcortical band heterotopia. *Eur J Hum Genet* 9:5–12.

Matsuo T. 1983. Biochemical aspects of pathophysiology and treatment of intractable epilepsy in children. *Brain Dev* 5:100–106.

Matsuo A, Matsuzaka T, Tsuru A, et al. 2001. Epidemiological and clinical studies of West syndrome in Nagasaki Prefecture, Japan. *Brain Dev* 23:575–579.

Matsuoka H, Okuma T, Ueno T, et al. 1986. Impairment of parietal cortical functions associated with episodic prolonged spike-and-wave discharges. *Epilepsia* 27:432–436.

Matsuoka H, Takahashi T, Sasaki M, et al. 2000. Neuropsychological EEG activation in patients with epilepsy. *Brain* 123:318–330.

Matthes A. 1961. Die psychomotorische Epilepsie im Kindesalter. *Z Kinderheilk* 85:455–472.

Matthes A. 1977. *Epilepsie: diagnostik and therapie für klinik und praxis*. Stuttgart: Thieme.

Mattia D, Olivier A, Avoli M. 1995. Seizure-like discharges recorded in the human dysplastic neocortex maintained in vitro. *Neurology* 45:1391–1395.

Mattson RH. 1992. Drug treatment of uncontrolled seizures. In: Theodore WH, ed. *Surgical treatment of epilepsy*. Amsterdam: Elsevier, 29–35.

Mattson RH, Cramer JA, Caldwell BV, et al. 1981. Seizure frequency and the menstrual cycle: a clinical study. *Epilepsia* 22:242–247.

Mattson RH, Cramer JA, Collins JF, et al. 1985. Comparison of carbamazepine, phenobarbital, phenytoin and primidone in partial and secondarily generalized tonic clonic seizure. *N Engl J Med* 313:145–151.

Mattson RH, Cramer JA, Darny PD, et al. 1986. Use of oral contraceptives by women with epilepsy. *JAMA* 258:238–240.

Mattson RH, Cramer JA, Collins JF. 1992. A comparison of valproate with carbamazepine for the treatment of complex partial seizures and secondarily generalized seizures in adults. The Department of Veterans Affairs Epilepsy Cooperative Study No. 264 Group. *N Engl J Med* 327:765–771.

Matustik MC, Eisenberg HM, Meyer WJ III. 1981. Gelastic (laughing) seizures and precocious puberty. *Am J Dis Child* 135:837–838.

Mauguière F, Courjon J. 1978. Somatosensory epilepsy: a review of 127 cases. *Brain* 101:307–332.

Maulsby RL. 1979. EEG patterns of uncertain diagnostic significance. In: Klass DH, Daly DD, eds. *Current practice journal of clinical electroencephalography*. New York: Raven Press, 411–419.

Mayeux R, Lüders H. 1978. Complex partial status epilepticus: case report and proposal for diagnostic criteria. *Neurology* 28:957–961.

Mayeux R, Brandt J, Rosen J, et al. 1980. Interictal memory and language impairment in temporal lobe epilepsy. *Neurology* 30:120–125.

Maynard R, Garrel S. 1983. Les crises du nouveau-né; intérêt de la polygraphie. *Rev Electroencephalogr Neurophysiol Clin* 13:219–223.

Mayr N, Wimberger D, Dichler H, et al. 1987. Influence of television on photosensitive epileptics. *Eur Neurol* 27:201–208.

Maytal J, Shinnar S. 1990. Febrile status epilepticus. *Pediatrics* 86:611–616.

Maytal J, Novak GP, King KC. 1991. Lorazepam in the treatment of refractory neonatal seizures. *J Child Neurol* 6:319–323.

McBride MC, Dooling EC, Oppeheimer EY. 1981. Complex partial status epilepticus in young children. *Ann Neurol* 9:526–530.

McBride MC, Laroia N, Guillet R. 2000. Electrographic seizures in neonates correlate with poor neurodevelopmental outcome. *Neurology* 55:506–513.

McCown TJ, Breese GR. 1992. The developmental profile of seizure genesis in the inferior colliculus cortex of the rat: relevance to human neonatal seizures. *Epilepsia* 33:2–10.

McDonald BK, Johnson AL, Goodridge DM, et al. 2000. Factors predicting prognosis of epilepsy after presentation with seizures. *Ann Neurol* 48:833–841.

McGowan ME, Neville BG, Reynolds EH. 1983. Comparative monotherapy trial in children with epilepsy. *Br J Clin Pract* 27:115–119.

McIntyre I. 1976. Epilepsy and employment. *Community Health (Bristol)* 7:195–204.

McIntyre P, Kennedy R, Harris F. 1983. Occult pneumococcal bacteremia and febrile convulsions. *BMJ* 286:203–206.

McKinlay I, Newton R. 1989. Intention to treat febrile convulsions with rectal diazepam, valproate or phenobarbitone. *Dev Med Child Neurol* 31:617–625.

McKinney W, McGreal DA. 1974. An aphasic syndrome in children. *Can Med Assoc J* 110:637–639.

McLachlan RS. 1987. Pseudoatrophy of the brain with valproic acid monotherapy. *Can J Neurol Sci* 14:294–296.

McLachlan RS, Blume WT. 1980. Isolated fear in complex partial status epilepticus. *Ann Neurol* 8:639–641.

McLeod CM, Dekaban AS, Hunt E. 1978. Memory impairment in epileptic patients: selective effects of phenobarbital concentration. *Science* 202:1102–1104.

McMillan TM, Powell GE, Janota I, et al. 1987. Relationships between neuropathology and cognitive functioning in temporal lobectomy patients. *J Neurol Neurosurg Psychiatry* 50:167–176.

McNamara JO. 1999. Emerging insights into the genesis of epilepsy. *Nature* 399:A15–A22.

McNaughton FL, Rasmussen T. 1975. Criteria for selection of patients for neurosurgical treatment. In: Purpura DP, Penry JK, Walter RD, eds. *Neurosurgical management of the epilepsies*. Advances in neurology, Vol. 8. New York: Raven Press, 37–48.

McQueen JK, Blackwood DH, Harris P, et al. 1983. Low risk of late post-traumatic seizures following severe head injury: implications for clinical trials of prophylaxis. *J Neurol Neurosurg Psychiatry* 46:899–904.

McShane NA, Finn JP, Hall-Craggs MA, et al. 1990. Neonatal hemangiomatosis presenting as infantile spasms. *Neuropediatrics* 21:211–212.

Meador KJ. 1994. Cognitive side effects of antiepileptic drugs. *Can J Neurol Sci* 21:S12–S16.

Meador KJ. 2001. Cognitive effects of epilepsy and of antiepileptic medications. In: Wyllie E, ed. *The treatment of epilepsy*, 3rd ed. Philadelphia: Lippincott Williams & Wilkins, 1215–1225.

Meador KJ, Loring DW, Ray PG, et al. 1999. Differential cognitive effects of carbamazepine and gabapentin. *Epilepsia* 40:1279–1285.

Meador KJ, Loring DW, Ray PG, et al. 2001. Differential cognitive and behavioral effects of carbamazepine and lamotrigine. *Neurology* 56:1177–1182.

Meadow R. 1984. Fictitious epilepsy. *Lancet* 2:25–28.

Meadow R. 1991. Neurological and developmental variants of Munchausen syndrome by proxy. *Dev Med Child Neurol* 33:270–272.

Medical Research Council Antiepileptic Drug Withdrawal Study Group. 1991. Randomised study of antiepileptic drug withdrawal in patients in remission. *Lancet* 337:1175–1180.

Meencke HJ. 1985. Neuronal density in the molecular layer of the frontal cortex in primary generalized epilepsy. *Epilepsia* 26:450–454.

Meencke HJ. 1989. Pathology of childhood epilepsies. *Cleve Clin J Med* 56:S111–S120.

Meencke HJ, Gerhard C. 1985. Morphological aspects of aetiology and the course of infantile spasms (West syndrome). *Neuropediatrics* 16:59–66.

Meencke HJ, Janz D. 1984. Neuropathological findings in primary generalized epilepsy: a study of 8 cases. *Epilepsia* 25:8–21.

Meencke HJ, Janz D. 1985. The significance of microdysgenesis in primary generalized epilepsy: an answer to the considerations of Lyon and Gastaut. *Epilepsia* 26: 368–371.

Meierkord H, Will B, Fish D, et al. 1991. The clinical features and prognosis of pseudoseizures, diagnosed using video-EEG telemetry. *Neurology* 41:1643–1646.

Meijer JW. 1991. Knowledge, attitude and practice in antiepileptic drug monitoring. *Acta Neurol Scand Suppl* 134:1–128.

Meisler MH, Kearney J, Ottman R, et al. 2001. Identification of epilepsy genes in human and mouse. *Annu Rev Genet* 35:567–588.

Melchior JC. 1977. Infantile spasms and early immunization against whooping cough. Danish survey from 1970 to 1975. *Arch Dis Child* 52:134–137.

Melchior JC, Buchthal F, Lennox-Buchthal M. 1971. The ineffectiveness of diphenylhydantoin in preventing febrile convulsions in the age of greatest risk, under three years. *Epilepsia* 12:55–62.

Meldrum BS. 1978. Physiological changes during prolonged seizures and epileptic brain damage. *Neuropédiatrie* 9:203–212.

Meldrum B. 1983a. Pharmacological considerations in the search for new anticonvulsant drugs. In: Pedley TA, Meldrum BS, eds. *Recent advances in epilepsy*, Vol. 1. Edinburgh: Churchill Livingstone, 75–92.

Meldrum BS. 1983b. Metabolic factors during prolonged seizures and their relation to nerve cell death. In: Delgado-Escueta AV, Wasterlain CG, Treiman DM, Porter RJ, eds. *Status epilepticus*. Advances in neurology, Vol. 34. New York: Raven Press, 261–275.

Meldrum BS. 1990. Anatomy, physiology and pathology of epilepsy. *Lancet* 336:221–234.

Meldrum BS. 1991. Excitatory amino-acid transmitters in epilepsy. *Epilepsia* 32. S1–S3.

Meldrum BS, Porter RJ. 1986. *New anticonvulsant drugs*. Current problems in epilepsy, Vol. 4. London: John Libbey.

Mélékian R, Laplane R, Debray P. 1962. Considérations cliniques et statistiques sur les convulsions au cours des déshydratations aiguës. *Ann Pediatr* 9:290–302.

Mellits ED, Holden KR, Freeman JM. 1981. Neonatal seizures. II: Multivariate analysis of factors associated with outcome. *Pediatrics* 70:177–185.

Menini C, Meldrum BS, Riche D, et al. 1980. Sustained limbic seizures induced by intramygdaloid kainic acid in the baboon: symptomatology and neuropathological consequences. *Ann Neurol* 8:501–509.

Menkes J, Kinsbourne M. 1990. Workshop on neurologic complications of pertussis and pertussis vaccination. *Neuropediatrics* 21:171–176.

Ment LR, Duncan CC, Ehrenkranz RA. 1984. Perinatal cerebral infarction. *Ann Neurol* 16:559–568.

Merlis JK. 1974. Reflex epilepsy. In: Vinken PJ, Bruyn GW, eds. *The epilepsies*. Handbook of clinical neurology, Vol 15. Amsterdam: Elsevier, 440–456.

Mesdjian E, Dravet C, Cenraud B, et al. 1980. Carbamazepine intoxication due to triacetyloleandomycin administration in epileptic patients. *Epilepsia* 21:489–496.

Mesri JC, Pagano RA. 1987. Reading epilepsy. *Epilepsia* 28:301–304.

Messenheimer JA. 1998. Rash in adult and pediatric patients treated with lamotrigine. *Can J Neurol Sci* 25:S14–S18.

Messenheimer JA, Giorgi L, Risner M. 2000. The tolerability of lamotrigine in children. *Drug Saf* 22:303–312.

Messing RO, Closson RG, Simon RP. 1984. Drug-induced seizures: a 10-year experience. *Neurology* 34: 1582–1586.

Methahonkala L, Gaily E, Rantala H, et al. 2002. Focal and

global cortical hypometabolism in patients with newly diagnosed infantile spasms. *Neurology* 58:1646–1651.

Metrakos JD, Metrakos K. 1966. Childhood epilepsy of subcortical ("centrencephalic") origin. *Clin Pediatr* 5: 536–542.

Metrakos JD, Metrakos K. 1970. Genetic factors in epilepsy. In: Niedermeyer E, ed. *Epilepsy: modern problems in pharmacopsychiatry*, Vol 4. Basel: Karger, 71–86.

Metrick ME, Ritter FS, Gates JR, et al. 1991. Nonepileptic events in childhood. *Epilepsia* 32:322–328.

Meyer FB, Marsh WR, Laws ER, et al. 1986. Temporal lobectomy in children with epilepsy. *J Neurosurg* 64: 371–376.

Michon PE, Wallace SJ. 1984. Febrile convulsions: electroencephalographic changes related to rectal temperature. *Arch Dis Child* 59:371–373.

Mikami M, Yasuda T, Terao A, et al. 1999. Localization of a gene for benign adult familial myoclonic epilepsy to chromosome 8q23.3-q24.1. *Am J Hum Genet* 65: 745–751.

Mikati MA, Browne TR. 1988. Comparative efficacy of antiepileptic drugs. *Clinical Neuropharmacol* 11: 130–140.

Mikati M, Saab R. 2000. Use of intravenous immunoglobulins as initial monotherapy in Laudau-Kleffner syndrome. *Epilepsia* 41:880–886.

Mikati MA, Lee WL, Delong GR. 1985. Protracted epileptiform encephalopathy: an unusual form of partial complex status epilepticus. *Epilepsia* 26:563–571.

Mikati MA, Travathan E, Krishnamoorthy KS, Lombroso CT. 1991. Pyridoxine-dependent epilepsy: EEG investigations and long-term follow-up. *Electroencephalogr Clin Neurophysiol* 78:215–221.

Mikati M, Maguire H, Barlow CF, et al. 1992. A syndrome of autosomal dominant alternating hemiplegia. *Neurology* 42:2251–2257.

Mikkelsen B, Berggreen P, Joensen P, et al. 1981. Clonazepam and carbamazepine in psychomotor epilepsy: a randomized multicenter trial. *Epilepsia* 22:415–420.

Millichap JC. 1968. *Febrile convulsions*. New York: Macmillan.

Millichap JG, Colliver JA. 1991. Management of febrile seizures: survey of current practice and phenobarbital usage. *Pediatr Neurol* 7:243–248.

Millichap JG, Bickford RC, Klass DW, et al. 1962. Infantile spasms, hypsarrhythmia, and mental retardation: a study of etiologic factors in 61 patients. *Epilepsia* 3: 188–197.

Milligan N, Dhillon S, Oxley J, et al. 1982. Absorption of diazepam from the rectum and its effect on interictal spikes in the EEG. *Epilepsia* 23:323–331.

Milligan NM, Dhillon S, Griffiths A, et al. 1984. A clinical trial of single dose rectal and oral administration of diazepam for the prevention of serial seizures in adult epileptic patients. *J Neurol Neurosurg Psychiatry* 47: 235–240.

Mimaki T, Ono J, Yabuuchi H. 1983. Temporal lobe astrocytoma with infantile spasms. *Ann Neurol* 14:695–696.

Minagawa K, Miura H. 1981. Phenobarbital, primidone and sodium valproate in the prophylaxis of febrile convulsions. *Brain Dev* 3:385–393.

Minagawa K, Miura H, Mizuno S, et al. 1986. Pharmacokinetics of rectal diazepam in the prevention of recurrent febrile convulsions. *Brain Dev* 8:53–59.

Minassian BA. 2001. Lafora's disease; towards a clinical, pathologic, and molecular synthesis. *Pediat Neurol* 25: 21–29.

Minassian B, DeLorey T, Olsen RW, et al. 1998a. The epilepsy of Angelman syndrome due to deletion, disomy, imprinting center and UB3A mutations. *Ann Neurol* 43:485–493.

Minassian BA, Lee JR, Herbrick JA, et al. 1998b. Mutations in a gene encoding a novel protein tyrosine phosphatase cause progressive myoclonus epilepsy. *Nat Genet* 20: 171–174.

Minassian BA, Andrade DM, Ianzano L, et al. 2001. Laforin is a cell membrane and reticulum-associated protein tyrosine phosphatase. *Ann Neurol* 49:271–275.

Minchon P, Niswander K, Chalmers I, et al. 1987. Antecedents and outcome of very early neonatal seizures in infants born at or near term. *Br J Obstet Gynaecol* 94:431–439.

Minotti L, Kahane P, Tassi L, et al. 1998. Peut-on simplifier les investigations préchirurgicales chez l'enfant? In: Bureau M, Kahane P, Munari C, eds. *Epilepsies partielles graves pharmaco-résistantes de l'enfant: stratégies diagnostiques et traitements chirurgicaux*. Paris, John Libbey Eurotext, 181–192.

Mireles R, Leppik E. 1985. Valproate and clonazepam comedication in patients with intractable epilepsy. *Epilepsia* 26:122–126.

Mirsky AF, Van Buren JM. 1965. On the nature of the "absence" in centrencephalic epilepsy: a study of some behavioral, EEG and autonomic factors. *Electroencephalogr Clin Neurophysiol* 18:334–348.

Mischel PS, Nguyen LP, Vinters HV. 1995. Cerebral cortical dysplasia associated with pediatric epilepsy. Review of neuropathologic features and proposal for a grading system. *J Neuropathol Exp Neurol* 54:137–153.

Mitchell WG. 1996. Status epilepticus and acute repetitive seizures in children, adolescents, and young adults: etiology, outcome, and treatment. *Epilepsia* 37:S74–S80.

Mitchell WG, Greenwood RS, Messenheimer JA. 1983. Abdominal epilepsy: cyclic vomiting as the major symptom of simple partial seizures. *Arch Neurol* 40:251–252.

Mitchison HM, Taschner PE, Kremmidiotis G, et al. 1997. Structure of the CLN3 gene and predicted nature, location and function of CLN3 protein. *Neuropediatrics* 28: 12–14.

Mittan RJ, Wasterlain CG, Locke GE. 1982. Fear of seizures. In: Akimoto H, ed. *Advances in epileptology*, XIIIth Epilepsy International Symposium. New York: Raven Press, 459–461.

Miyazaki M, Hashimoto T, Fujii E, et al. 1994. Infantile spasms: localized cerebral lesions on SPECT. *Epilepsia* 35:988–992.

Mizrahi EM. 1984. Electroencephalographic/polygraphic/video-monitoring in childhood epilepsy. *J Pediatr* 105:1–9.

Mizrahi EM. 1987. Neonatal seizures: problems in diagnosis and classification. *Epilepsia* 28:S46–S55.

Mizrahi EM. 1999. Pediatric electroencephalographic video monitoring. *J Clin Neurophysiol* 16:100–110.

Mizrahi EM, Kellaway P. 1987. Characterization and classification of neonatal seizures. *Neurology* 37:1837–1844.

Mizrahi EM, Kellaway P. 1998. *Diagnosis and management of neonatal seizures*. Philadelphia: Lippincott-Raven.

Mizrahi EM, Kellaway P. 2001. Neonatal seizures. In: Pellock JM, Dodson WE, Bourgeois B, eds. *Pediatric epilepsy: diagnosis and therapy.* New York: Demos Medical Publishing, 145–161.

Mizrahi EM, Tharp BR. 1982. The neonatal EEG: statistical studies and prognostic value in full-term and pre-term babies. *Electroencephalogr Clin Neurophysiol* 32: 1215–1220.

Mizrahi EM, Kellaway P, Grossman RG, et al. 1990. Anterior temporal lobectomy and medically refractory temporal lobe epilepsy of childhood. *Epilepsia* 31: 302–312.

Mohamed A, Wyllie E, Ruggieri P, et al. 2001. Temporal lobe epilepsy due to hippocampal sclerosis in pediatric candidates for epilepsy surgery. *Neurology* 56: 1643–1649

Mohnot D, Snead OC 3rd, Benton JW Jr. 1982. Burn encephalopathy in children. *Ann Neurol* 12:42–47.

Molaie M, Cruz A, Culebras A. 1988. The effect of epileptiform discharges on neurohormonal release in epileptic patients with complex partial seizures. *Neurology* 38: 759–762.

Molina JA, Mateos F, Merino M, et al. 1989. Aicardi syndrome in two sisters. *J Pediatr* 115:282–283.

Molyneux A, Anslow P, Easterbrook P, et al. 1986. The radiologic investigation of temporal lobe epilepsy. *Acta Radiol Suppl* 369:400–402.

Molyneux ME, Taylor TE, Wirima JJ, Borgstein A. 1989. Clinical features and prognostic indicators in paediatric cerebral malaria: a study of 131 comatose Malawian children. *Q J Med* 71:441–459.

Monaco F, Piredda S, Mastropaolo C, et al. 1981. Diphenylhydantoin and primidone in tears. *Epilepsia* 22: 185–188.

Monaco F, Mele G, Meloni T, et al. 1984. A longitudinal study of valproate free fraction in the specific age group at greatest risk for febrile convulsions (children below 3 years). *Epilepsia* 25:240–243.

Monaco F, Sechi GP, Russo A, et al. 1985. Brain distribution of carbamazepine and phenobarbital given in combination in experimental epilepsy. *Epilepsia* 26:103–108.

Monod N, Dreyfus-Brisac C, Sfaello Z. 1969. Presentation et pronostic de l'état de mal épileptique néonatal: étude clinique et EEG de 150 cas. *Arch Fr Pediatr* 26: 1085–1102.

Monod N, Pajot N, Guidasci S. 1972. The neonatal EEG: statistical studies and prognostic value in full-term and pre-term babies. *Electroencephalogr Clin Neurophysiol* 32:529–544.

Monod N, Peirano P, Plouin P, et al. 1988. Seizure-induced apnea. *Ann N Y Acad Sci* 533:411–420.

Montagna P, Gallassi R, Medori R, et al. 1988. MELAS syndrome: characteristic migrainous and epileptic features and maternal transmission. *Neurology* 38:751–754.

Montagna P, Sforza E, Tinuper P, et al. 1990. Paroxysmal arousals during sleep. *Neurology* 40:1063–1066.

Montes JL, Rosenblatt B, Farmer JP, et al. 1995. Lesionectomy of MRI-detected lesions in children with epilepsy. *Pediatr Neurosurg* 22:167–173.

Moore T, Hecquet S, McLellan A, et al. 2001. Polymorphism analysis of JRK/JH8, the human homologue of mouse jerky, and description of a rare mutation in a case of CAE evolving to JME. *Epilepsy Res* 46:157–167.

Moran O, Conti F. 2001. Skeletal muscle sodium channel is affected by an epileptogenic β1 subunit mutation. *Biochem Biophys Res Commun* 282:55–59.

Moran NF, Fish DR, Kitchen N, et al. 1999. Supratentorial cavernous haemangiomas and epilepsy: a review of the literature and case series. *J Neurol Neurosurg Psychiatry* 66:561–568.

Morante-Redolat JM, Gorostidi-Pagola A, Piquer-Sirerol S, et al. 2002. Mutations in the LGI1/Epitempin gene on 10q24 cause autosomal dominant lateral temporal epilepsy. *Hum Mol Genet* 11:1119–1128.

Morikawa T. 2000. Rolandic discharges in BECTS and in other forms of epilepsy. *Epileptic Disord* 2:S11–S13.

Morikawa T, Osawa T, Ishihara O, et al. 1979. A reappraisal of "benign epilepsy" of children with centrotemporal foci. *Brain Dev* 4:257–265.

Morikawa T, Seino M, Osawa T, et al. 1985. Five children with continuous spikewave discharges during sleep. In: Roger J, Dravet C, Bureau M, et al., eds. *Epileptic syndromes in infancy, childhood and adolescence.* London: John Libbey, 205–212.

Morikawa T, Seino M, Watanabe Y, et al. 1989. Clinical relevance of continuous spike-waves during slow wave sleep. In: Manelis J, Bental E, Loeber JN, Dreifuss FE, eds. *Advances in epileptology*, XVII Epilepsy International Symposium. New York: Raven Press, 359–363.

Morikawa T, Seino M, Yagi K. 1992. Long-term outcome of four children with continuous spike-waves during sleep. In: Roger J, Bureau H, Dravet C, et al., eds. *Epileptic syndromes in infancy, childhood and adolescence*, 2nd ed. London: John Libbey, 257–265.

Morikawa T, Seino M, Watanabe K. 1995. Long-term outcome of ESES syndrome. In: Beaumanoir A, Bureau M, Deonna T, et al., eds. *Continuous spikes and waves in slow sleep.* London: John Libbey, 27–36.

Morimoto T, Hayakawa T, Sugie H, et al. 1985. Epileptic seizures precipitated by constant light, movement in daily life, and hot water immersion. *Epilepsia* 26: 237–242.

Moro F, Carrozzo R, Veggiotti P, et al. 2002. Familial periventricular heterotopia: missense and distal truncating mutations of the FLN1 gene. *Neurology* 58: 916–921.

Morrell F. 1985. Secondary epileptogenesis in man. *Arch Neurol* 42:318–335.

Morrell F. 1989. Varieties of human secondary epileptogenesis. *J Clin Neurophysiol* 6:227–275.

Morrell M. 2002. Antiepileptic drug use in women. In: Levy RH, Mattson RH, Meldrum BS, et al., eds. *Antiepileptic drugs*, 5th ed. Philadelphia: Lippincott Williams & Wilkins, 132–148.

Morrell F, Whisler WW, Bieck TP. 1989. Multiple subpial transection: a new approach to the surgical treatment of focal epilepsy. *J Neurosurg* 70:231–239.

Morrell F, Whisler WW, Hoeppner TJ, et al. 1992. Electrophysiology of heterotopic gray matter in the "double cortex" syndrome. *Epilepsia* 33(Suppl. 3):76.

Morrell F, Whisler WW, Smith MC, et al. 1995. Landau-Kleffner syndrome: treatment with subpial intracortical transection. *Brain* 118:1529–1546.

Morrell F, Kanner AM, Whisler WW. 1997. Multiple subpial transection: application to paediatric epilepsy surgery. In: Tuxhorn I, Holthausen H, Boenigk H, eds. *Paediatric epilepsy syndromes and their surgical treatment.* London: John Libbey, 865–875.

Morris HH III, Estes M, Lüders H, et al. 1987. Electrophysiologic pathologic correlations in patients with complex partial seizures. *Arch Neurol* 44:703–708.

Morris HH III, Dinner DS, Lüders H, et al. 1988. Supplementary motor seizures: clinical and electroencephalographic findings. *Neurology* 38:1075–1082.

Morselli PL. 1977. Pharmacokinetics of antiepileptic drugs during development. In: Gardner-Thorpe C, Janz D, Meinardi H, Pippenger CE, eds. *Antiepileptic drug monitoring*. Tunbridge Wells: Pitman, 57–72.

Morselli PL, Baruzzi A, Bossi L, et al. 1980. Intensive long-term monitoring in "resistant" epileptic patients: results of a two-year study. In: Wada J, Penry JK, eds. *Advances in epileptology*, Xth Epilepsy International Symposium. New York: Raven Press, 99–107.

Morselli PL, Pippenger CE, Penry JK. 1983. *Antiepileptic drug therapy in pediatrics*. New York: Raven Press.

Moshé SL. 1987. Epileptogenesis and the immature brain. *Epilepsia* 28:S3–S15.

Moshé SL. 1993. Seizures in the developing brain. *Neurology* 43:S3–S7.

Moshé SL, Albala BJ. 1983. Maturational changes in postictal refractoriness and seizure susceptibility in developing rats. *Ann Neurol* 13:552–557.

Moshé S, Shinnar S. 1993. Early intervention. In: Engel J, ed. *Surgical treatment of the epilepsies*, 2nd ed. New York: Raven Press, 123–132.

Mostofsky DI, Balaschak BH. 1977. Psychobiological control of seizures. *Psychol Bull* 84:723–759.

Motte J, Billard C, Fejerman N, et al. 1993. Neurofibromatosis type one and West syndrome: a relatively benign association. *Epilepsia* 34:723–726.

Moulard B, Guipponi M, Chaigne D, et al. 1999. Identification of a new locus for generalized epilepsy with febrile seizures plus (GEFS+) on chromosome 2q24-33. *Am J Hum Genet* 65:1396–1400.

Mount LA, Reback S. 1940. Familial paroxysmal choreoathetosis: preliminary report on a hitherto undescribed clinical syndrome. *Arch Neurol Psychiatry* 44:841–847.

Mouritzen A, Dam M. 1990. Neuropathology. In: Dam M, Gram L, eds. *Comprehensive epileptology*. New York: Raven Press, 43–55.

Moussali-Salefranque F, Misès J, Plouin P, et al. 1981. Les crises convulsives dans les maladies métaboliques à révélation néonatale. *Rev Electroencephalogr Neurophysiol Clin* 11:379–384.

Mukahira K, Oguni H, Awaya Y, et al. 1998. Study on surgical treatment of intractable childhood epilepsy. *Brain Dev* 20:154–164.

Munari C, Bancaud J. 1985. The role of stereoelectroencephalography (SEEG) in the evaluation of partial epileptic seizures. In: Porter RJ, Morselli PL, eds. *The epilepsies*. London: Butterworth-Heinemann, 267–306.

Munari C, Bancaud J. 1992. Electroclinical symptomatology of partial seizures of orbital frontal origin. In: Chauvel P, Delgado-Escueta AV, Halgren E, Bancaud J, eds. *Frontal lobe seizures and epilepsies*. Advances in neurology, Vol. 57. New York: Raven Press, 257–265.

Munari C, Bancaud J, Bonis A, et al. 1979. Rôle du noyau amygdalien dans la survenue de manifestations oro-alimentaires au cours des crises épileptiques chez l'homme. *Rev Electroencephalogr Neurophysiol Clin* 9:226–240.

Munari C, Bancaud J, Bonis A, et al. 1980a. Impairment of consciousness in temporal lobe seizures: a stereoelectroencephalographic study. In: Canger R, Angeleri F, Penry JK, eds. *Advances in epileptology*, XIth Epilepsy International Symposium. New York: Raven Press, 111–114.

Munari C, Talairach J, Bonis A, et al. 1980b. Differential diagnosis between temporal and "perisylvian" epilepsy in a surgical perspective. *Acta Neurochir Suppl (Wien)* 30:97–101.

Munari C, Stoffels C, Bossi L, et al. 1981. Automatic activities during frontal and temporal lobe seizures: are they the same? In: Dam H, Gram L, Penry JK, eds. *Advances in epileptology*, XIIth Epilepsy International Symposium. New York: Raven Press, 287–291.

Munari C, Bossi L, Stoffels C, et al. 1982a. Concentrations cérébrales des médicaments anti-comitiaux chez les malades ayant une epilepsie tumorale. *Rev Electroencephalogr Neurophysiol Clin* 12:38–43.

Munari C, Stoffels C, Bossi L, et al. 1982b. Partial seizures with elementary or complex symptomatology: a valid classification for temporal lobe seizures? In: Akimoto H, Kazamatsuri H, Seino M, et al., eds. *Advances in Epileptology*, XIIIth Epilepsy International Symposium. New York: Raven Press, 25–27.

Munari C, Bonis A, Koehen S, et al. 1984. Eye movements and occipital seizures in man. *Acta Neurochir* 33(Suppl.):47–52.

Munari C, Tassi L, Francione S, et al. 1993. Occipital seizures with childhood onset in severe partial epilepsy: a surgical perspective. In: Andermann F, Beaumanoir A, Mira L, et al., eds. *Occipital seizures and epilepsies in children*. London-Paris: John Libbey Eurotext, 203–211.

Munari C, Hoffmann D, Francione S, et al. 1994. Stereoelectroencephalography methodology: advantages and limits. *Acta Neurol Scand Suppl* 152:56–67.

Munari C, Kahane P, Francione S, et al. 1995. Role of the hypothalamic hamartoma in the genesis of epileptic fits. *Elecroencephogr Clin Neurophysiol* 95:154–160.

Munari C, Francione S, Kahane P, et al. 1996. Usefulness of stereo EEG investigations in partial epilepsy associated with cortical dysplastic lesions and gray matter heterotopia. In: Guerrini R, Andermann F, Canapicchi R, et al., eds. *Dysplasias of cerebral cortex and epilepsy*. Philadelphia: Lippincott-Raven, 383–394.

Munari C, Minotti L, Russo GL, et al. 1997. Indications and results of surgical treatment (excluding callosotomy) in children with epileptic 'falls'. In: Beaumanoir A, Andermann F, Avanzini G, et al., eds. *Falls in epileptic and non-epileptic seizures during childhood*. London: John Libbey, 159–173.

Munari C, Lo Russo G, Minotti L, et al. 1999a. Presurgical strategies and epilepsy surgery in children: comparison of literature and personal experiences. *Childs Nerv Syst* 15:149–157.

Munari C, Minotti L, Tassi L, et al. 1999b. Surgical management of severe partial epilepsy symptomatic of neuronal migration disorders. In: Spreafico R, Avanzini G, Andermann F, eds. *Abnormal cortical development and epilepsy*. London: John Libbey, 303–318.

Munari C, Tassi L, Lo Russo G, et al. 1999c. Research perspectives in cortical dysplasia and associated epilepsies. *Epileptic Disord* 1:255–259.

Munari T, Berta E, Francione S, et al. 2000. Clinical ictal symptomatology and anatomical lesions: their relationships in severe partial epilepsy. *Epilepsia* 41:S18–S36.

Murakami JW, Weinberger E, Shaw DW. 1999. Normal myelination of the pediatric brain imaged with fluid-attenuated inversion-recovery (FLAIR) MR imaging. *Am J Neuroradiol* 20:1406–1411.

Murphy MJ. 1985. Long-term follow-up of seizures associated with cerebral arteriovenous malformations: results of therapy. *Arch Neurol* 42:477–479.

Murphy JV, Sawasky F, Marquardt KM, et al. 1987. Deaths in young children receiving nitrazepam. *J Pediatr* 111: 145–147.

Murro AM, Flanigin HF, Gallagher BB, et al. 1988. Corpus callosotomy for the treatment of intractable epilepsy. *Epilepsy Res* 2:44–50.

Musico M, Beghi E, Solari A, Viani F. 1997. Treatment of the first tonic-clonic seizure does not improve the prognosis of epilepsy. First Seizure Trial Group (FIRST Group). *Neurology* 49:991–998.

Musumeci SA, Colognola RM, Ferri R. 1988. Fragile X syndrome: a particular epileptogenic EEG pattern. *Epilepsia* 29:41–47.

Musumeci SA, Ferri R, Elia M, et al. 1991. Epilepsy and fragile X syndrome: a follow-up study. *Am J Med Genet* 38:511–513.

Mutani R. 1980. The role of the corpus callosum in the interaction of multiple epileptogenic areas on neocortex. In: Canger R, Angeleri F, Penry JK, eds. *Advances in epileptology*, XIth Epilepsy International Symposium. New York: Raven Press, 1–7.

Muzik O, da Silva EA, Juhasz C, et al. 2000. Intracranial EEG versus flumazenil and glucose PET in children with extratemporal lobe epilepsy. *Neurology* 54: 171–179

Nabbout R. 2001. A risk-benefit assessment of treatments for infantile spasms. *Drug Saf* 24:813–828.

Nabbout RC, Chiron C, Mumford J, et al. 1997. Vigabatrin in partial seizures in children. *J Child Neurol* 12: 172–177.

Nabbout R, Melki I, Gerbaka B, et al. 2001. Infantile spasms in Down syndrome: good response to a short course of vigabatrin. *Epilepsia* 42:1580–1583.

Nabbout R, Gennaro E, Dalla Bernardina B, et al. 2003. Spectrum of *SCN1A* mutations in severe myoclonic epilepsy of infancy. *Neurology* 60:1961–1967.

Naidu S, Gruener G, Brazis D. 1986. Excellent results with chlorazepate in recalcitrant childhood epilepsies. *Pediatr Neurol* 2:18–22.

Najm IM, Janigro D, Babb TL. 2001. Mechanisms of epileptogenesis and experimental models of seizures. In: Wyllie E, ed. *The treatment of epilepsy*, 3rd ed. Philadelphia: Lippincott Williams & Wilkins, 33–44.

Nakano S, Okuno T, Mikawa H. 1989. Landau-Kleffner syndrome: EEG topographic studies. *Brain Dev* 11:43–50.

Nakken KO. 1999. Physical exercise in outpatients with epilepsy. *Epilepsia* 40:643–651.

Nanda RN, Johnson RH, Keogh HJ, et al. 1977. Treatment of epilepsy with clonazepam and the effect on other anticonvulsants. *J Neurol Neurosurg Psychiatry* 40: 538–543.

Naquet R, Fegersten L, Bert J. 1960. Seizure discharges localized to the posterior cerebral regions in man, provoked by intermittent photic stimulation. *Electroencephogr Clin Neurophysiol* 12:305–316.

Naquet R, Menini C, Riche D, et al. 1987. Photic epilepsy problems raised in man and animals. *Ital J Neurol Sci* 8:437–447.

Nashef L, Fish DR, Garner S, et al. 1995a. Sudden death in epilepsy: a study of incidence in a young cohort with epilepsy and learning difficulty. *Epilepsia* 36: 1187–1194.

Nashef L, Fish DR, Sander JW, et al. 1995b. Incidence of sudden unexpected death in an outpatient cohort with epilepsy at a tertiary referral centre. *J Neurol Neurosurg Psychiatry* 58:462–464.

National Institutes of Health Consensus Conference. 1990. Surgery for epilepsy. *JAMA* 264:729–733.

Navelet Y, D'Allest AM, Dehan M, et al. 1981. A propos du syndrome des convulsions néonatales du 5 ème jour. *Rev Electroencephalogr Neurophysiol Clin* 11: 390–396.

Navelet Y, Wood RC, Robieux C, et al. 1989. Seizures presenting as apnoea. *Arch Dis Child* 64:357–359.

Nealis JG. 1981. Management of febrile seizures by pediatricians in the United States. In: Nelson KB, Ellenberg JH, eds. *Febrile seizures*. New York: Raven Press, 81–86.

Nehlig A, Motte J, Moshé SL, et al, eds. 1999. *Childhood epilepsies and brain development*. London: John Libbey.

Neill JC. 1990. Pseudoseizures in impaired children. *Neurology* 40:1146.

Nelen W, Van Eil A, Sonnen AE. 1988. Is epilepsy a dangerous condition? In: Canger R, Loeber JN, Castellano F, eds. *Epilepsy and society*. Amsterdam: Excerpta Medica, 169–173.

Nelson KB. 1972. Discussion. In: Alter M, Hauser WA, eds. *The epidemiology of epilepsy: a workshop*. NINDS Monograph No. 14. Washington, D.C.: United States. Government Printing Office, 78.

Nelson KB. 1981. Can treatment of febrile seizures prevent subsequent epilepsy? In: Nelson KB, Ellenberg JH, eds. *Febrile seizures*. New York: Raven Press, 143–145.

Nelson KB, Broman SA. 1977. Perinatal risk factors in children with serious motor and mental handicaps. *Ann Neurol* 2:371–377.

Nelson KB, Ellenberg JH. 1976. Predictors of epilepsy in children who have experienced febrile seizures. *N Engl J Med* 295:1029–1033.

Nelson KB, Ellenberg JH. 1978. Prognosis in children with febrile seizures. *Pediatrics* 61:720–727.

Nelson KB, Ellenberg JH. 1981a. Apgar scores as predictors of chronic neurologic disability. *Pediatrics* 68:36–44.

Nelson KB, Ellenberg JH, eds. 1981b. *Febrile seizures*. New York: Raven Press.

Nelson KB, Ellenberg JH. 1982. Maternal seizure disorder, outcome of pregnancy and neurologic abnormalities in the children. *Neurology* 32:1247–1254.

Nelson KB, Ellenberg JH. 1983. Febrile seizures. In: Dreifuss F, ed. *Pediatric epileptology*. Boston: John Wright, 173–198.

Nelson KB, Ellenberg JH. 1986. Antecedents of seizure disorders in early childhood. *Am J Dis Child* 140:1053–1061.

Nelson KB, Ellenberg JH. 1990. Prenatal and perinatal antecedents of febrile seizures. *Ann Neurol* 27:127–131.

Nelson KB, Leviton A. 1991. How much of neonatal encephalopathy is due to birth asphyxia ? *Am J Dis Child* 145:1325–1331.

Nelson DA, Ray CD. 1968. Respiratory arrest from seizure discharges in limbic system. *Arch Neurol* 19:199–207.

Nespeca M, Wyllie E, Lüders H. 1990. EEG recording and functional localization studies with subdural electrodes in infants and young children. *J Epilepsy* 3(Suppl.): 103–107.

Neubauer BA, Fiedler B, Himmelein B, et al. 1998. Centrotemporal spikes in families with rolandic epilepsy:

linkage to chromosome 15q14. *Neurology* 51: 1608–1612.

Neubauer BA, Oguni H, Fejerman N. 2002. Papers presented at the Workshop on Myoclonic Epilepsies, December 5–6, 2002, Seattle, Washington.

Nevander A, Ingvar M, Aver R, et al. 1985. Status epilepticus in well-oxygenated rats causes neuronal necrosis. *Ann Neurol* 18:281–290.

Neville BG. 1972. The origin of infantile spasms: evidence from a case of hydranencephaly. *Dev Med Child Neurol* 14:644–647.

Neville BG, Harkness WF, Cross JH, et al. 1997. Surgical treatment of severe autistic regression in childhood epilepsy. *Pediatr Neurol* 16:137–140.

Neville B, Burch V, Cass H, et al. 1998. Motor disorders in Landau-Kleffner syndrome (LKS) [Abstract]. *Epilepsia* 39(Suppl. 6):123.

Newman P, Saunders M. 1980. A unique case of musicogenic epilepsy. *Arch Neurol* 37:244–245.

Newmark ME. 1983. Sensory evoked seizures. In: Dreifuss F, ed. *Pediatric epileptology*. New York: Raven Press.

Newmark ME, Penry JK. 1979. *Photosensitivity and epilepsy: a review*. New York: Raven Press.

Newmark ME, Penry JK. 1980. Catamenial epilepsy: a review. *Epilepsia* 21:281–300.

Newton RW. 1988. Randomized controlled trials of phenobarbitone and valproate in febrile convulsions. *Arch Dis Child* 63:1189–1191.

Newton R, Aicardi J. 1983. Clinical findings in children with occipital spike-wave complexes suppressed by eyeopening. *Neurology* 33:1526–1529.

Newton RW, McKinlay I. 1988. Subsequent management of children with febrile convulsions. *Dev Med Child Neurol* 30:402–406.

Newton C, Warrell D. 1998. Neurological manifestations of falciparum malaria. *Ann Neurol* 43:695–702.

Newton MR, Berkovic SF, Austin MC, et al. 1992. Dystonia, clinical lateralization and regional blood flow changes in temporal lobe seizures. *Neurology* 42:371–377.

Ng T. 1997. Role of the proton MR spectroscopy in the localization of childhood epilepsy. In: Tuxhorn I, Holthausen H, Boenigk H, eds. *Pediatric epilepsy syndromes and their surgical treatment*. London: John Libbey, 620–633.

Ngwane E, Bower B. 1980. Continuous sodium valproate or phenobarbitone in the prevention of "simple" febrile convulsions. *Arch Dis Child* 55:171–174.

Niedermeyer E. 1969. The Lennox-Gastaut syndrome: a severe type of childhood epilepsy. *Dtsch Z Nervenheilkd* 195:263–282.

Niedermeyer E. 1972a. *The generalized epilepsies*. Springfield, IL: Charles C Thomas Publisher.

Niedermeyer E. 1972b. Post-traumatic epilepsy with slow spike-wave complexes. In: *The generalized epilepsies*. Springfield, IL: Charles C Thomas Publisher, 74–86.

Niedermeyer E, Da Silva FL. 1993. *Electroencephalography: basic principles, clinical applications and related fields*, 3rd ed. Baltimore: Williams & Wilkins.

Niedermeyer E, Khalifeh R. 1965. Petit mal status ("spikewave stupor"). An electro-clinical appraisal. *Epilepsia* 6:250–262.

Niedermeyer E, Walker AE, Burton C. 1970. The slow spike-wave complex as a correlate of frontal and frontotemporal post-traumatic epilepsy. *Eur Neurol* 3: 330–346.

Niedermeyer E, Fineyre F, Riley T. 1979a. Absence status (petit mal status) with focal characteristics. *Arch Neurol* 38:417–421.

Niedermeyer E, Fineyre F, Riley T, et al. 1979b. Myoclonus and the electroencephalogram: a review. *Clin Electroencephogr* 10:75–96.

Niedermeyer E, Rett A, Renner H, et al. 1986. Rett syndrome and electroencephalogram. *Am J Med Genet* 24: 195–199.

Nielsen J, Vetner M, Holm V, et al. 1977. A newborn child with karyotype 47,XX,+der(12 (12pter leads to 12q12::9q24 leads to 8qter),t(8;12) (q24;q12)pat. *Hum Genet* 35:357–362.

Nieto-Sampedro M. 1988. Astrocyte mitogen inhibitor related to epidermal growth factor receptor. *Science* 240: 1784–1786.

Niijima SI, Wallace SJ. 1989. Effects of puberty on seizure frequency. *Dev Med Child Neurol* 31:174–180.

Nilsson L, Thompson T, Farahmand BY, et al. 1997. Cause specific mortality in epilepsy: a cohort study of more than 9000 patients once hospitalized for epilepsy. *Epilepsia* 38:1062–1068.

Nishino S, Ripley B, Overeem S, et al. 2000. Hypocretin (Orexin) deficiency in human narcolepsy. *Lancet* 355: 39–40.

Noachtar S, Arnold S. 2000. Clonic seizures. In: Lüders HO, Noachtar S, eds. *Epileptic seizures: pathophysiology and clinical semiology*. Philadelphia: Churchill Livingstone, 412–432.

Noachtar S, Lüders HO. 1999. Focal akinetic seizures as documented by electroencephalography and videorecordings. *Neurology* 53:427–429.

Noachtar S, Lüders HO. 2000. Akinetic seizures. In: Lüders HO, Noachtar S, eds. *Epileptic seizures: pathophysiology and clinical semiology*. Philadelphia: Churchill Livingstone, 489–500.

Noachtar S, Desudchit T, Lüders HO. 2000. Dialeptic seizures. In: Lüders HO, Noachtar S, eds. *Epileptic seizures: pathophysiology and clinical semiology*. Philadelphia: Churchill Livingstone, 361–376.

Nobre AC, Rao A. 2000. Functional imaging of epilepsy. In: Oxbury J, Polkey C, Duchowny M, eds. *Intractable focal epilepsy*. London: WB Saunders, 637–647.

Nohria V, Lee N, Tien RD, et al. 1994. Magnetic resonance imaging evidence of hippocampal sclerosis in progression: a case report. *Epilepsia* 35:1332–1336.

Nolte R. 1989. Neonatal sleep myoclonus followed by myoclonic astatic epilepsy: a case report. *Epilepsia* 30: 844–850.

Nordberg C, Sourander P, Silfvenius H. 1987. Mild cortical dysplasia in patients with intractable partial seizures: a histological study. In: Wolf P, Dam M, Janz D, Dreifuss FE, eds. *Advances in epileptology*, XVIth Epilepsy International Symposium. New York: Raven Press, 29–33.

Nordgren RE, Reeves AG, Viguera AC, et al. 1991. Corpus callosotomy for intractable seizures in the pediatric age group. *Arch Neurol* 48:364–372.

Nordli DR, De Vivo DC. 2001. The ketogenic diet. In: Wyllie E, ed. *The treatment of epilepsy*, 3rd ed. Philadelphia: Lippincott Williams & Wilkins, 1001–1006.

Nordli DR Jr, Bazil CW, Scheuer ML, et al. 1997. Recognition and classification of seizures in infants. *Epilepsia* 38:553–560.

Noriega-Sanchez A, Markand ON. 1976. Clinical and electroencephalographic correlation of independent multiple spike discharges. *Neurology* 26:667–672.

Norio R, Koskiniemi M. 1979. Progressive myoclonus epilepsy: genetic and nosological aspects with special reference to 107 Finnish patients. *Clin Genet* 15:382–398.

Norman RM. 1962. Neuropathological findings in acute hemiplegia in childhood with special reference to epilepsy as a pathogenic factor. In: Bax M, Mitchell RG, eds. *Acute hemiplegia in childhood.* London: Heinemann.

Norman RM. 1964. The neuropathology of status epilepticus. *Med Sci Law* 4:46–51.

Norrenmolle A, Nielson JE, Sorensen SA, et al. 1995. Elongated CAG repeats of the B37 gene in a Danish family with dentato-rubro-pallido-luysian atrophy (DRPLA). *Hum Genet* 95:313–318.

North KN, Ouvrier RA, Nugent M. 1990. Pseudoseizures caused by hyperventilation resembling absence epilepsy. *J Child Neurol* 5:288–294.

Nousiainen U, Mervaala E, Uusitupa M, et al. 1989. Cardiac arrhythmias in the differential diagnosis of epilepsy. *J Neurol* 286:93–96.

Novely RA, Augustine EA, Mattson RH, et al. 1984. Selective memory improvement and impairment in temporal lobectomy for epilepsy. *Ann Neurol* 15:64–67.

O'Brien JL, Goldensohn ES, Hoefer PF. 1959. EEG abnormalities in addition to bilateral 3 per second spike and wave activity in petit mal. *Electroencephalogr Clin Neurophysiol* 11:747–761.

O'Donoghue MF, Sander JW. 1997. The mortality associated with epilepsy with particular reference to sudden unexpected death: a review. *Epilepsia* 38:31–46.

O'Donohoe NV. 1985. *Epilepsies of childhood*, 2nd ed. London: Butterworth-Heinemann.

O'Donovan CA, Burgess RC, Lüders HO. 2000. Autonomic auras. In: Lüders HO, Noachter S, eds. *Epileptic seizures*. Philadelphia: Churchill Livingstone, 320–327.

O'Leary DS, Seidenberg M, Berent S, et al. 1981. Effects of age of onset of tonic clonic seizures on neuropsychological performance in children. *Epilepsia* 22:197–204.

O'Leary DS, Lowell MR, Sackellares C, et al. 1983. Effects of age of onset of partial and generalized seizures on neuropsychological performance in children. *J Nerv Ment Dis* 171:624–628.

O'Neil D, Byrne E, Roberts L, et al. 1991. Hemitonic seizures: etiological and diagnostic considerations. *Acta Neurol Scand* 84:59–64.

O'Rawe A, Mitchinson HM, Williams R, et al. 1997. Genetic linkage of a variant of juvenile onset with granular osmiophilic deposits. *Neuropediatrics* 28:21–22.

Obeid T, Panayatopoulos CP. 1988. Juvenile myoclonic epilepsy. a study in Saudi Arabia. *Epilepsia* 29:280–282.

Ochs R, Gloor P, Quesney F, et al. 1984. Does head-turning during a seizure have lateralizing or localizing significance? *Neurology* 34:884–890.

Ochs RF, Gloor P, Tyler JL, et al. 1987. Effects of generalized spike-and-wave discharge on glucose metabolism measured by positron emission tomography. *Ann Neurol* 21:458–464.

Offen ML, Davidoff RA, Troost RT, et al. 1976. Dacrystic epilepsy. *J Neurol Neurosurg Psychiatry* 34:829–834.

Offerman G, Pinto V, Kruse R. 1979. Antiepileptic drugs and vitamin D supplementation. *Epilepsia* 20:3–15.

Offringa M, Derksen-Lubsen G, Bossuyt PM, Lubsen J. 1992.

Seizure recurrence after a first febrile seizure: a multivariate approach. *Dev Med Child Neurol* 34:15–24.

Offringa M, Bossuyt PM, Lubsen J, et al. 1994. Risk factors for seizure recurrence in children with febrile seizures: a pooled analysis of individual data from studies. *J Pediatr* 124:574–584.

Ogier H, Aicardi J. 1998. Metabolic diseases. In: Aicardi J, ed. *Diseases of the nervous system in childhood*, 2nd ed. London: MacKeith Press, 245–323.

Ogino T, Ohtsuka Y, Yamatogi Y, et al. 1986. Severe myoclonic epilepsy in infancy: clinicoelectroencephalographic and long-term follow-up studies. *Brain Dev* 8:162–165.

Ogino T, Ohtsuka Y, Amano R, et al. 1988. An investigation in the borderland of severe myoclonic epilepsy in infancy. *Jpn J Psychiatr Neurol* 42:554–555.

Ogino T, Ohtsuka Y, Yamatogi Y, et al. 1989. The epileptic syndromes sharing common characteristics during early childhood with severe myoclonic epilepsy in infancy. *Jpn J Psychiatry Neurol* 43:479–481.

Oguni H, Andermann F, Rasmussen T. 1991a. The natural history of the syndrome of chronic encephalitis and epilepsy: a study of the MNI series of forty-eight cases. In: Andermann F, ed. *Chronic encephalitis and epilepsy: Rasmussen's syndrome.* Boston: Butterworth-Heinemann, 7–35.

Oguni H, Olivier H, Andermann F, et al. 1991b. Anterior callosotomy in the treatment of medically intractable epilepsies: a study of 43 patients with a mean follow-up of 39 months. *Ann Neurol* 30:357–364.

Oguni H, Andermann F, Rasmussen TB. 1992a. The syndrome of chronic encephalitis and epilepsy: a study based on the MNI study of 48 cases. In: Chauvel P, Delgado-Escueta AV, Halgren E, Bancaud J, eds. *Frontal lobe seizures and epilepsies.* Advances in neurology, Vol. 57. New York: Raven Press, 419–433.

Oguni H, Fukuyama Y, Imaizumi Y, et al. 1992b. Video-EEG analysis of drop seizures in myoclonic epilepsy of early childhood (Doose syndrome). *Epilepsia* 33:805–813.

Oguni H, Sato F, Hayashi K, et al. 1992c. A study of unilateral brief focal antonia in childhood partial epilepsy. *Epilepsia* 33:75–83.

Oguni H, Fukuyama Y, Imaizumi Y, Uehara T. 1993. Video analysis of drop seizures in myoclonic-astatic epilepsy of early childhood (Doose syndrome). *Epilepsia* 33:805–813.

Oguni H, Hayashi K, Oguni M, et al. 1994. Treatment of severe myoclonic epilepsy in infants with bromide and its borderline variant. *Epilepsia* 35:1140–1145.

Oguni H, Hayashi K, Awaya Y, et al. 2001. Severe myoclonic epilepsy in infants—a review based on the Tokyo Women's Medical University series of 84 cases. *Brain Dev* 23:736–748.

Oguni H, Tanaka T, Hayashi K, et al. 2002. Treatment and long-term prognosis of myoclonic-astatic epilepsy of early childhood. *Neuropediatrics* 33:122–132.

Ogunmekan AO, Hwang PA, Hoffman HJ. 1989. Sturge-Weber-Dimitri disease: role of hemispherectomy in prognosis. *Can J Neurol Sci* 16:78–80.

Ogunyemi AO, Gomez MR, Klass DW. 1988. Seizures induced by exercise. *Neurology* 38:633–634.

Ohmori I, Ouchida M, Ohtsuka Y, et al. 2002. Significant correlation of the SCN1A mutations and severe myoclonic epilepsy in infancy. *Biochem Biophys Res Commun* 295:17–23.

Ohtahara S. 1984. Seizure disorders in infancy and childhood. *Brain Dev* 6:509–519.

Ohtahara S. 1988. Lennox-Gestaut syndrome: considerations in its concept and categorization. *Jpn J Psychiatr Neurol* 42:535–542.

Ohtahara S, Yamatogi Y. 1990. Evolution of seizures and EEG abnormalities in childhood onset epilepsy. In: Wada JA, Ellingson RJ, eds. *Clinical neurophysiology of epilepsy*. Handbook of electroencephalography and clinical neurophysiology, revised series, Vol 4. Amsterdam: Elsevier, 457–477.

Ohtahara S, Yamatogi Y, Ohtsuka Y, et al. 1977. Prognosis in childhood epilepsy: a prospective follow-up study. *Folia Psychiatr Neurol Jpn* 31:301–313.

Ohtahara S, Oka E, Yamatogi Y, et al. 1979. Non-convulsive status epilepticus in childhood. *Folia Psychiatr Neurol Jpn* 33:345–351.

Ohtahara S, Yamatogi Y, Ohtsuka Y, et al. 1980. Prognosis of West syndrome with special reference to Lennox syndrome: a developmental study. In: Wada J, Penry JK, eds. *Advances in epileptology*, Xth Epilepsy International Symposium. New York: Raven Press, 149–154.

Ohtahara S, Ohtsuka Y, Yamatogi Y, et al. 1987. The early infantile epileptic encephalopathy with suppression burst: developmental aspects. *Brain Dev* 9:371–376.

Ohtahara S, Ohtsuka Y, Yoshinaga H, et al. 1988. Lennox-Gastaut syndrome: etiological considerations. In: Niedermeyer E, Degen R, eds. *Lennox-Gastaut syndrome*. New York: Alan R. Liss, 47–63.

Ohtahara S, Ohtsuka Y, Yamatogi Y, et al. 1992. Early infantile epileptic encephalopathy with suppression-bursts. In: Roger J, Bureau M, Dravet C, et al., eds. *Epileptic syndromes in infancy, childhood and adolescence*, 2nd ed. London: John Libbey, 25–34.

Ohtsuka Y, Ohtahara S. 1992. Treatment of intractable childhood epilepsy with high-dose valproate. *Epilepsia* 33:158–164.

Ohtsuka Y, Yoshida H, Miyake S, et al. 1982. Induced micoseizures: a clinical and electroencephalographic study. In: Akimoto H, Karamatsuri H, Seino M, et al., eds. *Advances in epileptology*, XIIIth Epilepsy International Symposium. New York: Raven Press, 33–35.

Ohtsuka Y, Matsuda M, Ogino T, et al. 1987. Treatment of West syndrome with high-dose pyridoxal phosphate. *Brain Dev* 9:418–421.

Ohtsuka Y, Ogino T, Amano R, et al. 1988. Rational treatment of refractory epilepsy in childhood. *Jpn J Psychiatr Neurol* 42:443–447.

Ohtsuka Y, Amano R, Mizukawa M, Ohtahara S. 1990. Long-term prognosis of the Lennox-Gastaut syndrome. *Jpn J Psychiatr Neurol* 44:257–264.

Ohtsuka Y, Ohno S, Oka E, Ohtahara S. 1993. Classification of epilepsies and epileptic syndromes of childhood according to the 1989 ILAE classification. *J Epilepsy* 6:272–276.

Ohtsuka Y, Murashima I, Oka E, et al. 1994. Treatment and prognosis of West syndrome. *J Epilepsy* 7:279–284.

Ohtsuka Y, Murashima I, Asano T, et al. 1996. Partial seizures in West syndrome. *Epilepsia* 37:1060–1067.

Ojemann GA, Ward AA. 1975. Stereotactic and other procedures for epilepsy. In: Purpura DP, Penry JK, Walter RD, eds. *Neurosurgical management of epilepsies*. Advances in neurology, Vol 8. New York: Raven Press, 241–263.

Oka H, Kako M, Matsushima M, Ando K. 1977. Traumatic spreading depression syndrome. Review of a particular type of head injury in 37 patients. *Brain* 100:287–298.

Oka E, Yamatogi Y, Ohtsuka Y, et al. 1989. Clinical course and prognosis of childhood epilepsy. *Acta Paediatr Jpn* 31:259–266.

Oka E, Ishida S, Ohtsuka Y, Ohtahara S. 1995. Neuroepidemiological study of childhood epilepsy by application of international classification of epilepsies and epileptic syndromes (ILAE, 1989). *Epilepsia* 36:658–661.

Oki J, Takedatsu M, Itoh J, et al. 1991. Hypocalcemic focal seizures in a one month old infant of a mother with a low circulating level of vitamin D. *Brain Dev* 13:132–134.

Okino S. 1997. Familial benign myoclonus epilepsy of adult onset: a previously unrecognized myoclonic disorder. *J Neurol Sci* 145:113–118.

Okuma T, Kumashiro H. 1981. Natural history and prognosis of epilepsy: report of a multiinstitutional study in Japan. *Epilepsia* 22:35–53.

Okuma Y, Shimo Y, Shimura H, et al. 1998. Familial cortical tremor with epilepsy: an under-recognized familial tremor. *Clinical Neurology and Neurosurgery* 100:75–78.

Okumura A, Watanabe K, Negoro T, et al. 1998. Evolutional changes and outcome of West syndrome: correlation with magnetic resonance imaging findings. *Epilepsia* 39(Suppl. 5):46–49.

Okumura A, Hayakawa F, Kato T, et al. 1999. Positive rolandic sharp waves in preterm infants with periventricular leukomalacia: their relation to background electroencephalographic abnormalities. *Neuropediatrics* 30:278–282.

Oldani A, Zucconi M, Ferini-Strambi R. 1996. Autosomal dominant frontal lobe epilepsy: electroclinical picture. *Epilepsia* 37:964–976.

Oldani A, Zucconi M, Asselta R, et al. 1998. Autosomal dominant nocturnal frontal lobe epilepsy. A videopolysmomnographic and genetic appraisal of 40 patients and delineations of the epileptic syndrome. *Brain* 121:205–223.

Oles KS, Penry JK, Cole DL, Howard G. 1989. Use of acetazolamide as an adjunct to carbamazepine in refractory partial seizures. *Epilepsia* 30:74–78.

Olivier A, Gloor P, Andermann F, Ives J. 1982. Occipitotemporal epilepsy studied with stereotaxically implanted depth electrodes and successfully treated by temporal resection. *Ann Neurol* 11:428–432.

Olivier A, Andermann F, Palmini A, et al. 1996. Surgical treatment of the cortical dysplasias. In: Guerrini R, Andermann F, Canapicchi R, et al., eds. *Dysplasias of cerebral cortex and epilepsy*. Philadelphia: Lippincott-Raven, 351–366.

Oller-Daurella L. 1970. A special type of attack observed in the Lennox-Gestaut syndrome in adults. *Electroencephalogr Clin Neurophysiol* 29:529.

Oller-Daurella L. 1973. Evolution et pronostic du syndrome de Lennox-Gastaut. In: Lugaresi E, Pazzaglia P, Tassinari CA, eds. *Evolution and prognosis of epilepsies*. Bologna: Aulo Gaggi, 155–164.

Oller-Daurella L, Dini J. 1970. Las crisis epilépticas desencadenadas por movimientos voluntarios. *Med Clin* 54:189–198.

Oller-Dauella L, Marquez J. 1972. Survey of 100 epileptics who have not had seizures for 10 years or more. *Epilepsia* 13:161–170.

Oller-Daurella LO, Oller LF. 1989. Partial epilepsy with seizures appearing in the first three years of life. *Epilepsia* 30:820–826.

Oller-Daurella L, Oller LF. 1992. Epilepsies with generalized tonic-clonic seizures in childhood: does a childhood "grand mal" syndrome exist? In: Roger J, Bureau M, Dravet C, et al., eds. *Epileptic syndromes in infancy, childhood and adolescence*, 2nd ed. London: John Libbey, 161–171.

Oller-Daurella L, Sanchez ME. 1981. Evolución de las ausencias típicas. *Rev Neurol (Barcelona)* 9:87–102.

Oller-Daurella L, Pamies R, Oller FV. 1976. Reduction or discontinuance of antiepileptic drugs in patients seizure-free for more than 5 years. In: Janz D, ed. *Epileptology*. Stuttgart: Thieme, 218–227.

Olson DM, Chugani DA, Shewmon A, et al. 1990. Electrocorticographic confirmation of focal positron emission tomographic abnormalities in children with intractable epilepsy. *Epilepsia* 31:731–739.

Olsson I. 1988. Epidemiology of absence epilepsy. I: Concept and incidence. *Acta Paediatr Scand* 77:860–866.

Olsson I. 1990. Absence epilepsy in Swedish children. M.D. thesis. University of Göteborg, Göteborg, Sweden.

Olsson I, Hedström A. 1991. Epidemiology of absence epilepsy. II: Typical absences in children with encephalopathies. *Acta Paediatr Scand* 80:235–242.

Olsson I, Campenhausen G. 1993. Social adjustment in young adults with absence epilepsy. *Epilepsia* 34:846–851.

Omtzigt JG, Los FJ, Grobee DE, et al. 1992. The risk of spina bifida aperta after first-trimester exposure to valproate in a prenatal cohort. *Neurology* 42(Suppl. 5):119–125.

Online Mendelian Inheritance in Man, OMIM 2002. From the McKusick-Nathans Institute for Genetic Medicine (Baltimore, MD); Johns Hopkins University (Baltimore, MD), National Center for Biotechnology Information (Bethesda, MD); National Library of Medicine (Bethesda, MD). 2002. Available at: http://www.ncbi.nlm.nih.gov/omim/. Accessed July, 2003.

Ono J, Nishiike K, Imai K, et al. 1999. Ring chromosome 14 complicated with complex partial seizures and hypoplastic corpus callosum. *Pediatr Neurol* 20:70–72.

Opitz A, Marschall M, Degen R, Koch D. 1983. General anesthesia in patients with epilepsy and status epilepticus. In: Delgado-Escueta AV, Wasterlain CG, Treiman DM, Porter RJ, eds. *Status epilepticus*. Advances in neurology, Vol. 34. New York: Raven Press, 531–535.

Orlowski JP, Rothner D, Lüders H. 1982. Submersion accidents in children with epilepsy. *Am J Dis Child* 136:777–780.

Ormson MJ, Kispert DB, Sharbrough FW, et al. 1986. Cryptic structural lesions in refractory partial epilepsy: MR imaging and CT studies. *Radiology* 160:215–219.

Opeskin K, Kalnins RM, Halliday G, et al. 2000. Idiopathic generalized epilepsy: lack of significant microdysgenesis. *Neurology* 55:1101–1106.

Ortibus EL, Sum JM, Hahn JS. 1996. Predictive value of EEG for outcome and epilepsy following neonatal seizures. *Electroencephalogr Clin Neurophysiol* 98:175–185.

Osorio I, Reed RC. 1989. Treatment of refractory generalized tonic-clonic status epilepticus with phenobarbital anesthesia after high dose phenytoin. *Epilepsia* 30:464–471.

Osorio I, Burnstine TH, Remler B, et al. 1989. Phenytoin-induced seizures: a paradoxical effect of toxic concentrations in epileptic patients. *Epilepsia* 30:230–234.

Otani K, Abe J, Futagi Y, et al. 1989. Clinical and electroencephalographic follow-up study of early myoclonic encephalopathy. *Brain Dev* 11:332–337.

Otani K, Tagawa T, Futagi Y, et al. 1991. Induced microseizures in West syndrome. *Brain Dev* 13:196–199.

Otero E, Cordova S, Diaz F, et al. 1989. Acquired epileptic aphasia (the Landau-Kleffner syndrome) due to neurocysticercosis. *Epilepsia* 30:569–572.

Ottman R. 1989. Genetics of the partial epilepsies: a review. *Epilepsia* 30:107–111.

Ottman R. 1997. Family studies. In: Engel J, Pedley TA, eds. *Epilepsy*, Vol. 3. Philadelphia: Lippincott-Raven, 177–183.

Ottman R, Annegers JF, Hauser WA, Kurland LT. 1989. Seizure risk in offspring of parents with generalized versus partial epilepsy. *Epilepsia* 30:157–161.

Ottman R, Risch N, Hauser WA, et al. 1995. Localization of a gene for partial epilepsy to chromosome q10. *Nat Genet* 10:56–60.

Ouellet D, Bockbrader HN, Wesche DL, et al. 2001. Population pharmacokinetics of gabapentin in infants and children. *Epilepsy Res* 47:229–241.

Ouelette EM. 1974. The child who convulses with fever. *Pediatr Clin North Am* 21:467–481.

Ounsted C. 1969. Aggression and epilepsy rage in children with temporal lobe epilepsy. *J Psychosom Res* 13:237–242.

Ounsted C, Lindsey JT, Norman RM. 1966. *Biological factors in temporal lobe epilepsy*. Clinics in Developmental Medicine, No. 22. London: Heinemann Medical.

Ounsted C, Glaser G, Lindsay J, et al. 1985. Focal epilepsy with mesial temporal sclerosis after purulent meningitis. *Arch Neurol* 42:1058–1060.

Ounsted C, Lindsay J, Richards P. 1987. *Temporal lobe epilepsy: a biographical study, 1948–1986*. London: MacKeith Press.

Ouvrier RA, Billsou F. 1988. Benign paroxysmal tonic upgaze of childhood. *J Child Neurol* 3:177–180.

Ouvrier RA, Goldsmith R. 1982. Phenobarbitone dosage in neonatal convulsions. *Arch Dis Child* 57:653–657.

Overweg J, Binnie CD, Oosting J, et al. 1987. Clinical and EEG prediction of seizure recurrence following antiepileptic drug withdrawal. *Epilepsy Res* 1:272–283.

Oxbury SM. 2000. Preoperative neuropsychologic assessment. In: Oxbury J, Polkey C, Duchowny H, eds. *Intractable focal epilepsy*. London: WB Saunders, 617–625.

Oxbury JM, Polkey CE. 2000. Seizure reduction. In: Oxbury J, Polkey C, Duchowny M, eds. *Intractable focal epilepsy*. London: WB Saunders, 771–781.

Oxbury JM, Whitty CW. 1971. Causes and consequences of status epilepticus in adults: a study of 86 cases. *Brain* 94:733–744.

Oxbury J, Polkey C, Duchowny M, eds. 2000. *Intractable focal epilepsy*. London: WB Saunders.

Oxley J, Hebdiges S, Laidlaw J, et al. 1980. A comparative study of phenobarbitone and primidone in the treatment of epilepsy. In: Johannessen S, Morselli PL, Pippenger CE, et al., eds. *Antiepileptic therapy: advances in drug monitoring*. New York: Raven Press, 237–245.

Oxley J, Janz D, Meinardi H, eds. 1983. *Chronic toxicity of antiepileptic drugs*. New York: Raven Press.

Ozek E, Ozek MM, Caliskan M, et al. 1995. Multiple pineal cysts associated with an ependymal cyst presenting with infantile spasms. *Childs Nerv Syst* 11:246–249.

Pachatz C, Fusco L, Vigevano F. 1999. Benign myoclonus of early infancy. *Epileptic Disord* 1:57–61.

Pachatz C, Fusco L, Vigevano F. 2002. Shuddering and benign myoclonus of early infancy. In: Guerrini R, Aicardi J, Andermann F, Hallett M, eds. *Epilepsy and Movement Disorders*. Cambridge University Press, 343–353.

Pacia SV, Ebersole JS. 1997. Intracranial EEG substrates of scalp ictal patterns from temporal lobe foci. *Epilepsia* 38:399–407.

Pacia SW, Devinsky O, Luciano DJ, et al. 1994. The prolonged QT syndrome presenting as epilepsy: a report of three cases and literature review. *Neurology* 44: 1408–1410.

Pacifici GM, Viani A. 1992. Methods of determining plasma and tissue binding of drug: pharmacokinetic consequences. *Clin Pharmacokinet* 23:449–468.

Pacquier et al. (1992) [cited in Chapter 11]

Paetau R, Kajola M, Korkman M, et al. 1991. Landau-Kleffner syndrome: epileptic activity in the auditory cortex. *Neuroreport* 2:201–204.

Paetau R, Granström ML, Blomstedt G, et al. 1999. Magnetoencephalography in presurgical evaluation of children with the Landau-Kleffner syndrome. *Epilepsia* 40: 326–335.

Page LK, Lombroso CT, Matson DD. 1969. Childhood epilepsy with late detection of cerebral glioma. *J Neurosurg* 31:253–261.

Paillas JE, Bureau M. 1982. Aspects cliniques de l'épilepsie post-traumatique: étude d'une série de 333 observations. *Bolletino Lega Italiana contre l'Epilepsia* 39:11–17.

Paillas JE, Vigouroux G, Darcourt G, et al. 1959. Considérations sur l'épilepsie occipitale (a propos de 12 observations de lésions occipitales opérées). *Neurochirurgie* 5:3–16.

Painter MJ. 1983. How to use primidone. In: Morselli PL, Pippenger CE, Penry JK, eds. *Antiepileptic drug therapy in pediatrics*. New York: Raven Press, 263–270.

Painter MJ. 1988. Neonatal seizures. *Int Pediatr* 3:97–103.

Painter MJ, Pippenger CE, McDonald H, et al. 1978. Phenobarbital and diphenylhydantoin levels in neonates with seizures. *J Pediatr* 92:315–319.

Painter MJ, Pippenger C, Wasterlain C, et al. 1981. Phenobarbital and phenytoin in neonatal seizures: metabolism and tissue distribution. *Neurology* 31:1107–1112.

Painter MJ, Bergman I, Crumrine P. 1986. Neonatal seizures. *Pediatr Clin North Am* 33:91–109.

Painter MJ, Scher MS, Stein AD, et al. 1999. Phenobarbital compared with phenytoin for the treatment of neonatal seizures. *N Engl J Med* 341:485–489.

Pakalnis A, Drake ME, John K, et al. 1987. Forced normalization: acute psychosis after seizure control in seven patients. *Arch Neurol* 44:289–292.

Pakalnis A, Drake ME, Phillips B. 1991. Neuropsychiatric aspects of psychogenic status epilepticus. *Neurology* 41:1104–1106.

Paladin F, Chiron C, Dulac O, et al. 1989. Electroencephalographic aspects of hemimegalencephaly. *Dev Med Child Neurol* 31:377–383.

Palcoux JB, Carla H, Tardieu M, et al. 1997. Plasma exchange in Rasmussen's encephalitis. *Ther Apher* 1: 79–82.

Palm L, Blennow G, Brun A. 1986. Infantile spasms and neuronal heterotopias: a report of six cases. *Acta Paediatr Scand* 75:855–859.

Palm DG, Brandt M, Korithenberg R. 1988. West syndrome on Lennox-Gastaut syndrome in children with porencephalic cysts. In: Niedermeyer E, Degen R, eds. *The Lennox-Gastaut syndrome*. New York: Alan R. Liss, 419–426.

Palmini A, Andermann F, Aicardi J, et al. 1991a. Diffuse cortical dysplasia or the 'double cortex' syndrome: the clinical and epileptic spectrum in 10 patients. *Neurology* 41:1656–1662.

Palmini A, Andermann F, Olivier A, et al. 1991b. Focal neuronal migration disorders and intractable partial epilepsy: results of surgical treatment. *Ann Neurol* 30:750–757.

Palmini A, Andermann F, Olivier A, et al. 1991c. Focal neuronal migration disorders and intractable partial epilepsy: a study of 30 patients. *Ann Neurol* 30:741–749.

Palmini A, Andermann F, Tampieri D. 1991d. Neuronal migration disorders: a contribution of modern neuroimaging to the etiologic diagnosis of epilepsy. *Can J Neurol Sci* 18:580–587.

Palmini A, Gambardella A, Andermann F, et al. 1995. Intrinsic epileptogenicity of human dysplastic cortex as suggested by corticography and surgical results. *Ann Neurol* 37:476–487.

Pampiglione G, Harden A. 1973. Neurophysiological identification of a late infantile form of neuronal lipoidosis. *J Neurol Neurosurg Psychiatry* 36:68–74.

Pampiglione G, Pugh E. 1975. Infantile spasms and subsequent appearance of tuberous sclerosis syndrome [Letter]. *Lancet* 2:1046.

Panayiotopoulos CP. 1974. Effectiveness of photic stimulation on various eye-states in photosensitive epilepsy. *J Neurol Sci* 23:165–173.

Panayiotopoulos CP. 1979. Conversion of photosensitive to scotosensitive epilepsy. *Neurology* 29:1550–1554.

Panayiotopoulos CP. 1980. Basilar migraine? Seizures and severe epileptic EEG abnormalities. *Neurology* 31: 1330–1333.

Panayiotopoulos CP. 1981. Inhibitory effect of central vision on occipital lobe seizures. *Neurology* 30:1122–1125.

Panayiotopoulos CP. 1987. Fixation-off-sensitive epilepsy in eyelid myoclonia with absence seizures. *Ann Neurol* 22: 87–89.

Panayiotopoulos CP. 1988. Vomiting as an ictal manifestation of epileptic seizures and syndromes. *J Neurol Neurosurg Psychiatry* 51:1448–1451.

Panayiotopoulos CP. 1988a. Absence epilepsy. In: Engel J, Pedley T, eds: *Epilepsy: a comprehensive textbook*. Philadelphia: Lippincott-Raven, 2327–2346.

Panayiotopoulos CP. 1989a. Benign childhood epilepsy with occipital paroxysms: a 15 year prospective study. *Ann Neurol* 26:51–56.

Panayiotopoulos CP. 1989b. Benign nocturnal childhood occipital epilepsy: a new syndrome with nocturnal seizures, tonic deviation of the eyes and vomiting. *J Child Neurol* 4:43–48.

Panayiotopoulos CP. 1994a. Elementary visual hallucinations in migraine and epilepsy. *J Neurol Neurosurg Psychiatry* 57:1371–1374.

Panayiotopoulos CP. 1994b. The clinical spectrum of typical absence seizures and absence epilepsies. In: Malafosse A, Genton P, Hirsch E, et al., eds. *Idiopathic generalized epilepsies: clinical and experimental aspects*. London: John Libbey, 75–85.

Panayiotopoulos CP. 1998. Absence epilepsies. In: Engel J Jr, Pedley TA, eds. *Epilepsy: a comprehensive textbook.* Philadelphia: Lippincott-Raven, 2327–2346.

Panayiotopoulos CP. 1999. *Benign childhood partial seizures and related epileptic syndromes.* London: John Libbey.

Panayiotopoulos CP. 2001. Panayiotopoulos syndrome. *Lancet* 358:68–69.

Panayiotopoulos CP. 2002. *Panayiotopoulos syndrome: a common and benign childhood epileptic syndrome.* London: John Libbey.

Panayiotopoulos CP, Igoe DM. 1992. Cerebral insult like partial status epilepticus in the early-onset variant of benign childhood epilepsy with occipital paroxysms. *Seizure* 1:99–102.

Panayiotopoulos CT, Obeid T. 1989. Juvenile myoclonic epilepsy: an autosomal recessive disease. *Ann Neurol* 25:440–443.

Panayiotopoulos CP, Obeid T, Waheed G. 1989a. Absences in juvenile myoclonic epilepsy: a clinical and video-electroencephalographic study. *Ann Neurol* 25: 391–397.

Panayiotopoulos CP, Obeid T, Waheed G. 1989b. Differentiation of typical absence seizures in epileptic syndromes—video EEG study of 224 seizures in 20 patients. *Brain* 112:1039–1056.

Panayiotopoulos CP, Tahan R, Obeid T. 1991. Juvenile myoclonic epilepsy: factors of error involved in the diagnosis and treatment. *Epilepsia* 32:672–676.

Panayiotopoulos CP, Ferrie CD, Knott C, Robinson RO. 1993. Interaction of lamotrigine with sodium valproate. *Lancet* 341:445.

Panayiotopoulos CP, Ferrie CD, Giannakodimos S, et al. 1995. Perioral myoclonia with absences. In: Duncan JS, Panayiotopoulos CP, eds. *Typical absences and related syndromes.* London: Churchill Communication Europe, 221–230.

Panayiotopoulos CP, Koutroumanidis M, Giannakodimos S, Agathonikou S. 1997. Idiopathic generalised epilepsy in adults manifested with phantom absences, generalised tonic-clonic seizures and frequent absence status. *J Neurol Neurosurg Psychiatry* 63:622–627.

Panayiotopoulos CP, Ferrie CD, Koutoumanidis M, et al. 2001. Idiopathic generalised epilepsy with phantom absences and absence status in a child. *Epileptic Disord* 3:63–66.

Pandya DN, Yeterian EH. 1987. Hodology of limbic and related structures: cortical and commissural connections. In: Wieser HG, Elger CE, eds. *Presurgical evaluation of epilepsies.* Berlin: Springer, 3–14.

Paneth N. 1993. The causes of cerebral palsy. Recent evidence. *Clin Invest Med* 16:95–102.

Paolicchi JM, Jayakar P, Dean P, et al. 2000. Predictors of outcome in pediatric epilepsy surgery. *Neurology* 54: 642–647.

Papatheopailou R, Jeavons PM, Disney ME. 1972. Recurrent abdominal pain: a clinical and electroencephalographic study. *Dev Med Child Neurol* 14:31–44.

Papini M, Pasquinelli A, Armellini M, et al. 1984. Alertness and incidence of seizures in patients with Lennox-Gastaut syndrome. *Epilepsia* 25:161–167.

Paquier PF, Van Dongen HR, Loonen CB. 1992. The Landau-Kleffner syndrome or 'acquired aphasia with convulsive disorder.' Long-term follow-up of six children and a review of the recent literature. *Arch Neurol* 49: 354–359.

Parent JM, Lowenstein DH. 1994. Treatment of refractory generalized status epilepticus with continuous infusion of midazolam. *Neurology* 44:1837–1840.

Park K, Buchhalter J, McClelland R, et al. 2002. Frequency and significance of acute postoperative seizures following epilepsy surgery in children and adolescents. *Epilepsia* 43:874–881.

Parke TJ, Stevens JE, Rice AS, et al. 1992. Metabolic acidosis and fatal myocardial failure after propofol infusion in children: five case reports. *BMJ* 305:613–616.

Parker S, Zuckerman B, Bauchner, et al. 1990. Jitteriness in full-term neonates: prevalence and correlates. *Pediatrics* 85:17–23.

Parker AP, Polkey CE, Robinson RO. 2001. Vagal nerve stimulation in the epileptic encephalopathies: 3-year follow-up. *Pediatrics* 108:221.

Parkes JD, Baraitser M, Marsden CD, et al. 1975. Natural history, symptoms and treatment of the narcoleptic syndrome. *Acta Neurol Scand* 52:337–353.

Parmeggiani A, Plouin P, Dulac O. 1990. Quantification of diffuse and focal activity in hypsarrhythmia. *Brain Dev* 12:310–315.

Parra J, Iriarte J, Kanner AM, et al. 1998. De novo psychogenic nonepileptic seizures after epilepsy surgery. *Epilepsia* 39:474–477.

Parsonage M. 1983. The classification of epileptic seizures (ILAE). In: Rose CF, ed. *Research progress in epilepsy.* London: Pitman, 22–38.

Parsonage M, Moran JH, Exley KA. 1976. So-called water immersion epilepsy. In: Janz D, ed. *Epileptology.* Stuttgart: Thieme, 55–60.

Pascual L, Sedano MJ, Polo JM, et al. 1988. Intravenous lidocaine for status epilepticus. *Epilepsia* 29:584–589.

Pascual-Castroviejo I, Lopez Martin L, Martinez Bermejo A, Perez Higueras A. 1992. Is cerebral arteritis the cause of the Landau-Kleffner syndrome? Four cases in childhood with angiographic study. *Can J Neurol Sci* 19:46–52.

Pasquier B, Péoc'H M, Fabre-Bocquentin B, et al. 2002. Surgical pathology of drug-resistant partial epilepsy. *Epileptic Disord* 4:99–119.

Patel VM, Jankovic J. 1988. Myoclonus. *Curr Neurol* 8: 109–156.

Patel H, Garg BP, Markand ON. 1994. Bathing epilepsy: video-EEG recording and literature review. *J Epilepsy* 7:290–294.

Patry G, Lyagoubi S, Tassinari CA. 1971. Subclinical 'electrical status epilepticus' induced by sleep in children: a clinical and EEG study of six cases. *Arch Neurol* 24:242–252.

Patsalos PN, Lascelles PT. 1982. Effect of sodium valproate and ethosuximide on phenobarbital plasma protein binding. *Neurology* 32:1052–1053.

Pavone L, Mollica F, Incorpora G, et al. 1980. Infantile spasms syndrome in monozygotic twins. *Arch Dis Child* 55:870–872.

Pavone L, Incorpora G, La Rosa M, et al. 1981. Treatment of infantile spasms with sodium dipropylacetic acid. *Dev Med Child Neurol* 23:454–461.

Paxton JW, Aman MG, Werry JS. 1983. Fluctuations in salivary carbamazepine and carbamazepine-10,11-epoxide concentrations during the day in epileptic children. *Epilepsia* 24:716–724.

Payne T, Bleck TP. 1996. Status epilepticus. *Crit Care Clin* 13:17–38.

Pazzaglia P, Pazzaglia L. 1976. Record in grade school of pupils with epilepsy: an epidemiological study. *Epilepsia* 17:361–366.

Pazzaglia P, Franck L, Orioli G, et al. 1969. L'evoluzione elettro-clinica del piccolo malo tipico. *Rev Neurol* 39:557–566.

Pazzaglia P, D'Alessandro R, Lozito A, et al. 1982. Classification of partial epilepsy according to the symptomatology of seizures: practical value and prognostic implications. *Epilepsia* 23:343–350.

Pazzaglia P, D'Alessandro R, Ambrosetto G, et al. 1985. Drop attacks: an ominous change in the evolution of partial epilepsy. *Neurology* 35:1725–1730.

Pearn J, Batt R, Yamaoka R. 1978. Drowning risks to epileptic children: a study from Hawaii. *Br Med J* 2: 1284–1285.

PeBenito R, Cracco JB. 1979. Periodic localized epileptiform discharges in children. *Ann Neurol* 37:47–50.

Pedersen SB, Petersen KA. 1998. Juvenile myoclonic epilepsy: clinical and EEG features. *Acta Neurol Scand* 97:160–163.

Pedley TA. 1988. Discontinuing antiepileptic drugs. *N Engl J Med* 318:982–984.

Pedley TA, Guilleminault C. 1977. Episodic nocturnal wanderings responsive to anticonvulsant drug therapy. *Ann Neurol* 2:30–35.

Pedley TA, Tharp BR, Herman K. 1981. Clinical and electroencephalographic characteristics of midline parasagittal foci. *Ann Neurol* 9:142–149.

Peiffer A, Thompson J, Charlier C, et al. 1999. A locus for febrile seizures (FEB3) maps to chromosome 2q23-24. *Ann Neurol* 46:671–678.

Peled R, Lavie P. 1986. Paroxysmal awakenings from sleep associated with excessive daytime somnolence: a form of nocturnal epilepsy. *Neurology* 36:95–98.

Pellock JM. 1987. Carbamazepine side effects in children and adults. *Epilepsia* 28:S64–S70.

Pellock JM. 1996. Fosphenytoin use in children. *Neurology* 46:S14–S16.

Pellock JM. 1998. Use of midazolam for refractory status epilepticus in pediatric patients. *J Child Neurol* 13: 581–587.

Pellock JM 1999. Felbamate. *Epilepsia* 40:S57–S62.

Pellock JM, Brodie MJ. 1997. Felbamate: 1997 update. *Epilepsia* 38:1261–1264.

Pellock JM, Hunt PA. 1996. A decade of modern epilepsy therapy in institutionalized mentally retarded patients. *Epilepsy Res* 25:263–268.

Pellock JM, Wilmore LJ. 1991. A rational guide to routine blood monitoring in patients receiving antiepileptic drugs. *Neurology* 41:961–964.

Peloekanos JT, Dooley JM, Camfield PR, et al. 1990. Stretch syncope in adolescence. *Neurology* 40:715–716.

Penfield W, Boldrey E. 1937. Somatic motor and sensory representation in the cerebral cortex of man as studied by electrical stimulation. *Brain* 60:389–443.

Penfield W, Gage L. 1933. Cerebral localisation of epileptic manifestations. *Arch Neurol Psychiatry* 30:709–727.

Penfield W, Jasper H. 1954. *Epilepsy and the functional anatomy of the human brain.* Boston: Little Brown.

Penfield W, Kristiansen K. 1951 *Epileptic seizure patterns.* Springfield, IL: Charles C Thomas Publisher.

Penfield W, Perot P. 1963. The brain's record of auditory and visual experience: a final summary and discussion. *Brain* 86:595–616.

Penfield W, Rasmussen T. 1951. Epileptic seizure patterns. In: *The cerebral cortex of man: a clinical study of localization of function.* New York: Macmillan.

Pennachio LA, Lehesjoki AE, Stone NE, et al. 1996. Mutations in the gene encoding cystatin B in progressive myoclonus epilepsy (EMP1). *Science* 271: 1731–1734.

Penry JK 1975. Perspectives in complex partial seizures. In: Penry JK, Daly DD, eds. *Complex partial seizures and their treatment.* Advances in neurology, Vol. 11. New York: Raven Press, 1–14.

Penry JK, Dreifuss FE. 1969. Automatisms associated with the absence of petit mal epilepsy. *Arch Neurol* 21:142–149.

Penry JK, Porter RJ. 1977. Intensive monitoring of patients with intractable seizures. In: Penry JK, ed. *Epilepsy,* VIIth International Symposium. New York: Raven Press, 98–101.

Penry JK, So E. 1981. Refractoriness of absence seizures and phenobarbital [Abstract]. *Neurology* 31(Suppl.):158.

Penry JK, Porter RJ, Dreifuss FE. 1975. Simultaneous recording of absence seizures with video tape and electroencephalography. A study of 37 seizures in 48 patients. *Brain* 98:427–440.

Penry JK, White BG, Brackett CE. 1979. A controlled prospective study of the pharmacological prophylaxis of post-traumatic epilepsy. *Neurology* 29:600–601.

Penry JK, Dean JC, Riela AR. 1989. Juvenile myoclonic epilepsy: long-term response to therapy. *Epilepsia* 20: S19–S23.

Pentella K, Bachman DS, Sandman CA. 1982. Trial of an ACTH 4-9 analogue (ORG 2766) in children with intractable seizures. *Neuropediatrics* 13:59–62.

Peretti P, Raybaud C, Dravet C, et al. 1989. Magnetic resonance imaging in partial epilepsy of childhood: seventy-nine cases. *J Neuroradiol* 16:308–316.

Perez J, Chiron C, Musial C, et al. 1999. Stiripentol: efficacy and tolerability in children with epilepsy. *Epilepsia* 40: 1618–1626.

Perez-Jimenez A, Villarejo FJ, Fourmier del Castillo MC, et al. 2003. Continuous giggling and autistic disorder associated with hypothalamic hamartoma. *Epileptic Disord* 5:31–37.

Perheentupa J, Riikonen R, Dunkel L, et al. 1986. Adrenocortical hyporesponsiveness after treatment with ACTH of infantile spasms. *Arch Dis Child* 61:750–753.

Perlman MJ. 1997. Intrapartum hypoxic-ischemic cerebral injury and subsequent cerebral palsy: medicolegal issues. *Pediatrics* 99:851–859.

Perucca E. 1996. The new generation of antiepileptic drugs: advantages and disadvantages. *Br J Clin Pharmacol* 42: 531–543

Perucca E. 2000. Is there a role for therapeutic drug monitoring of the new anticonvulsants? *Clin Pharmacokinet* 38:191–204.

Perucca E, Levy RH. 2002. Combination therapy and drug interactions. In: Levy RH, Mattson RH, Meldrum BS, Perucca E, eds. *Antiepileptic drugs,* 5th ed. Philadelphia: Lippincott Williams & Wilkins, 96–102.

Perucca E, Richens A. 1980. Anticonvulsant drug interactions. In: Tyrer JH, ed. *The treatment of epilepsy.* Lancaster, England: MTP Press, 95–128.

Perucca E, Gram L, Avanzini G, Dulac O. 1998. Antiepileptic drugs as a cause of worsening seizures. *Epilepsia* 39: 5–17.

Petit J, Roubertie A, Inoue Y, et al. 1999. Nonconvulsive status in the ring chromosome 20 syndrome: a video illustration of 3 cases. *Epileptic Disord* 1:237–241.

Pettit RE. 1987. Pyridoxine dependency seizures: report of a case with unusual features. *J Child Neurol* 2:38–40.

Pettit RE, Fenichel GM. 1980. Benign familial neonatal seizures. *Arch Neurol* 37:47–48.

Pfund Z, Chugani HT, Juhász C, et al. 2000. Lissencephaly: fetal pattern of glucose metabolism on positron emission tomography? *Neurology* 55:1683–1688.

Phillips RE, Solomon T. 1990. Cerebral malaria in children. *Lancet* 336:1355–1360.

Phillips SA, Shanahan RJ. 1989. Etiology and mortality of status epilepticus in children—a recent update. *Arch Neurol* 46:74–76.

Phillips HA, Scheffer IE, Berkovic SF, et al. 1995. Localization of a gene for autosomal dominant nocturnal frontal lobe epilepsy to chromosome 20q 13.2. *Nat Genet* 10:117–118.

Phillips HA, Scheffer IE, Crossland KM, et al. 1998. Autosomal dominant nocturnal frontal-lobe epilepsy: genetic heterogeneity and evidence for a second locus at 15q24. *Am J Hum Genet* 63:1108–1116.

Phillips HA, Marini C, Scheffer IE, et al. 2000. A de novo mutation in sporadic nocturnal frontal lobe epilepsy. *Ann Neurol* 48:264–267.

Phillips HA, Favre I, Kirkpatrick M, et al. 2001. CHRNB2 is the second acetylcholine receptor subunit associated with autosomal dominant nocturnal frontal lobe epilepsy. *Am J Hum Genet* 68:225–231.

Piao X, Basel-Vanagaite L, Straussberg R, et al. 2002. An autosomal recessive form of bilateral frontoparietal polymicrogyria maps to chromosome 16q12.2-21. *Am J Hum Genet* 70:1028–1033.

Piatt JH Jr, Hwang PA, Armstrong DC, et al. 1988. Chronic focal encephalitis (Rasmussen syndrome): six cases. *Epilepsia* 29:268–279.

Picard F, Bertrand S, Steinlein OK, Bertrand D. 1999. Mutated nicotinic receptors responsible for autosomal dominant nocturnal frontal lobe epilepsy are more sensitive to carbamazepine. *Epilepsia* 40:1198–1209.

Picard F, Baulac S, Kahane P, et al. 2000. Dominant partial epilepsies: a clinical, electrophysiological and genetic study of 19 European families. *Brain* 123:1247–1262.

Piccirilli M, D'Alessandro P, Tiacci C, et al. 1988. Language lateralization in children with benign partial epilepsy. *Epilepsia* 29:19–25.

Pierog S, Chandavasu D, Wexler I. 1977. Withdrawal symptoms in infants with the fetal alcohol syndrome. *J Pediatr* 90:630–633.

Pierson M, Swann J. 1999. The contribution of developmental plasticity to early-life seizures and chronic epilepsy. In: Nehlig A, Motte J, Moshé SL, Plouin P, eds. *Childhood epilepsies and brain development*. London: John Libbey, 25–38.

Pietz J, Benninger C, Schäfer H, et al. 1993. Treatment of infantile spasms with high-dosage vitamin B₆. *Epilepsia* 34:757–763.

Pignata C, Farina V, Andrian G, et al. 1983. Prolonged QT internal syndrome presenting as idiopathic epilepsy. *Neuropediatrics* 14:235–236.

Pilcher WH, Silbergeld DL, Berger MS, et al. 1993. Intraoperative electrocorticography during tumor resection: impact on seizure outcome in patients with gangliogliomas. *J Neurosurg* 78:891–912.

Pilz DT, Macha ME, Precht KS, et al. 1998. Fluorescence in situ hybridization analysis with LIS1 specific probes reveals a high deletion mutation rate in isolated lissencephaly sequence. *Genet Med* 1:29–33.

Pinard JM. 1991. Anterior and total callosotomy in epileptic children: prospective one-year follow-up study. *Epilepsia* 32(Suppl.):54.

Pinard JM, Delalande O, Chiron C, et al. 1999. Callosotomy for epilepsy after West syndrome. *Epilepsia* 40: 1727–1734.

Pineda M, Vilaseca MA, Artuch R, et al. 2000. 3-Phosphoglycerate dehydrogenase deficiency in a patient with West syndrome. *Dev Med Child Neurol* 42:629–633.

Pini A, Merlini L, Tome FM, et al. 1996. Merosin-negative congenital muscle dystrophy, occipital epilepsy with periodic spasms and focal cortical dysplasia. Report of three Italian cases in two families. *Brain Dev* 18: 316–322.

Pinsard N. 1980. Evolution a long terme du syndrome de West (à propos de 100 cas). *Gaslini* 12(Suppl. 1):24–26.

Pinsard N, Ferracci JP, Rufo M, et al. 1976. Aspects évolutifs du syndrome de West. A propos de 90 observations [Abstract]. *Pédiatrie* 31:92–93.

Pippenger CE. 1987. Clinically significant carbamazepine drug interactions: an overview. *Epilepsia* 28:S71–S76.

Pippenger CE, Rosen TV. 1975. Phenobarbital plasma levels in neonates. *Clin Perinatol* 2:111–115.

Pippenger CE, Penry JK, Kutt H, eds. 1978. *Antiepileptic drugs: quantitative analysis and interpretation*. New York: Raven Press.

Pisani F, Fazio A, Oteri G, et al. 1987. Differential interactions of valproic acid and valpromide with carbamazepine in humans. In: Wolf P, Dam M, Janz FE, et al., eds. *Advances in epileptology*, XVIth Epilepsy International Symposium. New York: Raven Press, 431–433.

Pisani F, Di Perri E, Perucca E, et al. 1993. Interaction of lamotrigine with sodium valproate. *Lancet* 341:1224.

Pisani F, Oteri G, Russo R, et al. 1999. The efficacy of valproate-lamotrigine co-medication in refractory complex partial seizures: evidence for a pharmacological interaction. *Epilepsia* 40:1141–1146.

Pitlick W, Painter M, Pippenger C. 1978. Phenobarbital pharmacokinetics in neonates. *Clin Pharmacol Ther* 23:346–358.

Plaster NM, Uyama E, Uchino M, et al. 1999. Genetic localization of the familial adult myoclonic epilepsy (FAME) gene to chromosome 8q24. *Neurology* 53: 1180–1183.

Plazzi G, Tinuper P, Montagna P, et al. 1995. Epileptic nocturnal wandering. *Sleep* 18:749–756.

Plouin P. 1990. Benign neonatal convulsions. In: Wasterlain CG, Vert P, eds. *Neonatal seizures*. New York: Raven Press, 51–59.

Plouin P. 1994. Benign idiopathic neonatal convulsions (familial and non-familial): open questions about these syndromes. In: Wolf P, ed. *Epileptic seizures and syndromes*. London: John Libbey, 193–202.

Plouin P, Dulac O, Dalla Bernardina B. 1979. Aspects électrocliniques des crises survenant au cours des troubles de l'équilibre hydrosodé chez le nourrisson. *Rev Electroencephalogr Neurophysiol Clin* 9:19–25.

Plouin P, Jalin C, Dulac O, et al. 1987. Enregistrement ambulatoire de l'EEG pendant 24 heures dans les spasmes infantiles épileptiques. *Rev Electroencephalogr Neurophysiol Clin* 17:309–318.

Poley JR, Dumermuth G. 1968. EEG findings in patients

with phenylketonuria before and during treatment with a low phenylalanine diet and in patients with some other inborn errors of metabolism. In: Holt KS, Coffey VP, eds. *Some recent advances in inborn errors of metabolism.* Edinburgh: Churchill Livingstone, 61–69.

Polkey CE. 1980. Selection of patients with intractable epilepsy for resective surgery. *Arch Dis Child* 55: 841–844.

Polkey CE. 1983. Effects of anterior temporal lobectomy apart from the relief of seizures: a study of 40 patients. *J R Soc Med* 76:354–358.

Polkey CE. 1989. Surgery for epilepsy. *Arch Dis Child* 64: 185–187.

Polkey C. 2000. Brain stimulation for epilepsy. In: Oxbury J, Polkey C, Duchowny M, eds. *Intractable focal epilepsy.* London: WB Saunders, 751–760.

Polkey CE. 2003. Alternative surgical procedures to help drug-resistant epilepsy—a review. *Epileptic Disord* 5:63–75.

Polkey CE, Binnie CD, Janota J. 1989. Acute hippocampal recording and pathology of temporal lobe resection and amygdalo-hippocampectomy for epilepsy. *J Neurol Neurosurg Psychiatry* 52:1050–1057.

Polkey CE, Chandler C, Doshi P, et al. 1997. Resection of hypothalamic hamartoma for intractable epilepsy [Abstract]. *Epilepsia* 38:S77.

Pollack MA, Golden GS, Schmidt R, et al. 1978. Infantile spasms in Down syndrome: a report of 5 cases and review of the literature. *Ann Neurol* 3:406–408.

Pollack MA, Zion TE, Kellaway P. 1979. Long-term prognosis of patients with infantile spasms following ACTH therapy. *Epilepsia* 20:255–260.

Porciatti V, Bonanni P, Fiorentini A, et al. 2000. Lack of cortical contrast gain control in human photosensitive epilepsy. *Nat Neurosci* 3:259–263.

Porfirio B, Valorani MG, Giannotti A, et al. 1987. Ring 20 chromosome phenotype. *J Med Genet* 24:375–377.

Porter RJ. 1981. Pharmacokinetic basis of intermittent and chronic anticonvulsant drug therapy in febrile seizures. In: Nelson KB, Ellenberg JH, eds. *Febrile seizures.* New York: Raven Press, 107–118.

Porter RJ. 1983a. International classification of epileptic seizures: 1981 revision. In: Rose CF, ed. *Research progress in epilepsy.* London: Pitman, 14–21.

Porter RJ. 1983b. Intractable seizures. In: Browne TR, Feldman RG, eds. *Epilepsy: diagnosis and management.* Boston: Little Brown, 355–361.

Porter RJ. 1987. How to initiate and maintain carbamazepine therapy in children and adults. *Epilepsia* 28: S59–S63.

Porter R. 1989. How to use antiepileptic drugs. In: Levy RH, Dreifuss FE, Mattson RH, et al., eds. *Antiepileptic drugs,* 3rd ed. New York: Raven Press, 117–132.

Porter RJ. 1992. Current medical therapy of epilepsy. *Acta Neurol Scand Suppl* 140:59–64.

Porter RJ, Penry JK. 1983. Petit mal status. In: Wasterlain CG, Treiman DM, Porter RJ, eds. *Status epilepticus: mechanisms of brain damage and treatment.* Advances in neurology, Vol. 34. New York: Raven Press, 61–67.

Porter RJ, Penry JK, Dreifuss FE. 1973. Responsiveness at the onset of spike-wave bursts. *Electroencephalogr Clin Neurophysiol* 34:239–245.

Poskanzer C, Brown E, Miller H. 1962. Musicogenic epilepsy caused only by a "discrete" frequency band of church bells. *Brain* 85:77–92.

Potter D, Edwards KR, Norton J. 1997. Sustained weight loss associated with 12-month topiramate therapy [Abstract]. *Epilepsia* 38(Suppl. 8):97.

Povey S, Burley MW, Attwood J, et al. 1994. Two loci for tuberous sclerosis: one on 9q34 and one on 16p13. *Ann Hum Genet* 58:107–127.

Powell C, Painter MJ, Pippenger CE. 1984. Primidone therapy in refractory neonatal seizures. *J Pediatr* 105:651–654.

Powell GE, Polkey CE, Canavan AG. 1987. Lateralization of memory function in epileptic patients by use of sodium amytal (Wada) technique. *J Neurol Neurosurg Psychiatry* 50:665–672.

Power C, Poland SD, Blume WT, et al. 1990. Cytomegalovirus and Rasmussen's encephalitis. *Lancet* 2: 1282–1284.

Poza JJ, Saenz A, Martinez-Gil A, et al. 1999. Autosomal dominant lateral temporal lobe epilepsy: clinical and genetic study of a large Basque pedigree linked to chromosome 10q. *Ann Neurol* 45:182–188.

Pranzatelli MR. 1996. Antidyskinetic drug therapy for pediatric movement disorders. *J Child Neurol* 11:355–359.

Pranzatelli MR, Pedley TA. 1991. Differential diagnosis in children. In: Dam M, Gram L, eds. *Comprehensive epileptology.* New York: Raven Press, 423–447.

Prasad AN, Stafstrom CE, Holmes GL. 1996. Alternative epilepsy therapies: the ketogenic diet, immunoglobulins, and steroids. *Epilepsia* 37:S81–S95.

Prats JM, Garaizar C, Rua MJ, et al. 1991. Infantile spasms treated with high doses of sodium valproate: initial response and follow-up. *Dev Med Child Neurol* 33: 617–625.

Prayson RA, Estes ML. 1995. Cortical dysplasia: a histopathologic study of 52 cases of partial lobectomy in patients presenting with seizures. *Hum Pathol* 26: 493–500.

Prayson RA, Estes ML, Morris HH. 1993. Coexistence of neoplasia and cortical dysplasia in patients presenting with seizures. *Epilepsia* 34:609–615.

Prevey ML, Delaney RC, Cramer JA, et al. 1996. Effect of valproate on cognitive functioning. Comparison with carbamazepine. The Department of Veterans Affairs Epilepsy Cooperative Study 264 Group. *Arch Neurol* 53:1008–1016.

Prince DA, Connors BW. 1986. Mechanisms of interictal epileptogenesis. In: Delgado-Escueta AV, Ward AA Jr, Woodbury DM, et al., eds. *Basic mechanisms of the epilepsies.* Advances in neurology, Vol. 44. New York: Raven Press, 275–299.

Pritchard PB 3rd, Lombroso CT, McIntyre M. 1980. Psychological complications of temporal lobe epilepsy. *Neurology* 30:227–232.

Pritchard PB 3rd, Holmstrom VL, Giacinto J. 1985. Self-abatement of complex partial seizures. *Ann Neurol* 18:265–267.

Provini F, Plazzi G, Tinuper P, et al. 1999. Nocturnal frontal lobe epilepsy. A clinical and polygraphic overview of 100 consecutive cases. *Brain* 122:1017–1031.

Pryor DS, Don N, Macourt DC. 1981. Fifth day fits: a syndrome of neonatal convulsions. *Arch Dis Child* 56: 753–758.

Pueschel SM, Louis S. 1993. Reflex seizures in Down syndrome. *Childs Nerv Syst* 9:23–24.

Pueschel SM, Louis S, McKnight P. 1991. Seizure disorders in Down syndrome. *Arch Neurol* 48:318–320.

Pupillo GT, Andermann F, Dubeau F, et al. 1996. Bilateral

sylvian parieto-occipital polymicrogyria [Abstract]. *Neurology* 46:A303.

Purvis RJ, McBarrie WJ, Mackay GS, et al. 1973. Enamel hypoplasia of the teeth associated with neonatal tetany: a manifestation of maternal vitamin D deficiency. *Lancet* 2:811–813.

Pynnönen S, Sillanpää M, Frey H, et al. 1977. Carbamazepine and its 10,11 epoxide in children and adults with epilepsy. *Eur J Clin Phamacol* 11:129–133.

Quan F, Zonana J, Gunter K, et al. 1995. An atypical case of fragile X syndrome caused by a deletion that includes the *FMR1* gene. *Am J Hum Genet* 56:1042–1051.

Quattelbaum TG. 1979. Benign familial convulsions in the neonatal period and early infancy. *J Pediatr* 95: 257–259.

Quesney LF. 1986. Seizures of frontal lobe origin. In: Pedley TA, Meldrum BS, eds. *Recent advances in epilepsy*, Vol. 3. Edinburgh: Churchill Livingstone, 81–110.

Quesney LF. 1987. Electroencephalographic and clinical manifestations of frontal and temporal lobe epilepsy. *Clin Neurol Neurosurg* 89(Suppl. 1):41–42.

Quesney LF. 1992. Extratemporal epilepsy: clinical presentation, pre-operative EEG localization and surgical outcome. *Acta Neurol Scand Suppl* 140:81–94.

Quesney LF, Gloor P. 1987. Special extracranial electrodes. In: Wieser HG, Elger CE, eds. *Presurgical evaluation of epileptics*. Berlin: Springer, 162–176.

Quesney LF, Olivier A. 1988. Pre-operative EEG evaluation in frontal lobe epilepsy. *Acta Neurol Scand Suppl* 117:61–72.

Quesney LF, Abou-Khalil B, Cole A, et al. 1988. Pre-operative extracranial and intracranial EEG investigation in patients with temporal lobe epilepsy: trends, results and review of pathophysiologic mechanisms. *Acta Neurol Scand Suppl* 117:52–60.

Quesney LF, Constain M, Fish DR, et al. 1990. The clinical differentiation of seizures arising in the parasagittal and anterolateral frontal convexities. *Arch Neurol* 47: 677–679.

Quesney LF, Risinger M, Shewmon DA. 1993. Extracranial EEG evaluation. In: Engel J, ed. *Surgical treatment of epilepsies*, 2nd ed. New York: Raven Press, 173–195.

Quirk JA, Kendall B, Kingsley DP, et al. 1993. EEG features of cortical dysplasia in children. *Neuropediatrics* 24: 193–199.

Radermecker J, Guazzi GC, Toga M, et al. 1967. Les Lésions cérébrales en rapport avec les crises épileptiques graves prolongées et notamment avec les états de mal chez l'homme. In: Gastaut H, Roger J, Lob H, eds. *Les etats de mal epileptique*. Paris: Masson, 287–325.

Radvanyi-Bouvet MF, Cukier-Hémeury F, Morel-Kahn F. 1981. Décharges critiques chez les prématurés et les nouveau-nés à terme. *Rev Electroencephalogr Neurophysiol Clin* 11:404–411.

Radvanyi-Bouvet MF, Vallecalle MH, Morel-Kahn F, et al. 1985. Seizures and electrical discharges in premature infants. *Neuropediatrics* 16:143–148.

Radvanyi-Bouvet MF, Torricelli A, Rey E, et al. 1990. Effects of lidocaine on seizures in the neonatal period: some electroclinical aspects. In: Wasterlain CG, Vert P, eds. *Neonatal seizures*. New York: Raven Press, 275–283.

Rafal RD, Laxer KD, Janowsky JS. 1986. Seizures triggered by blinking in a nonphotosensitive epileptic. *J Neurol Neurosurg Psychiatry* 49:445–447.

Raines A, Henderson TR, Swinyard E, et al. 1990. Comparison of midazolam and diazepam by the intramuscular route for the control of seizures in a mouse model of status epilepticus. *Epilepsia* 31:313–317.

Rajna P, Kundra O, Halasz P. 1983. Vigilance level-dependent tonic seizures—epilepsy or sleep disorder? A case report. *Epilepsia* 24:725–733.

Ramani V. 1983. Primary reading epilepsy. *Arch Neurol* 40:39–41.

Ramaratnam S, Baker GA, Goldstein L. 2001. Psychological treatments for epilepsy. *Cochrane Database Syst Rev* CD002029.

Ramsay RE, Pellock JM, Garnett WR, et al. 1991. Pharmacokinetics and safety of lamotrigine (Lamictal) in patients with epilepsy. *Epilepsy Res* 10:191–200.

Rao JK, Willis J. 1987. Hypothalamo-pituitary-adrenal function in infantile spasms: effects of ACTH therapy. *J Child Neurol* 2:220–223.

Rapin I. 1986. Myoclonus in neuronal storage and Lafora diseases. In: Fahn S, Marsden CD, Van Woert MH, eds. *Myoclonus*. Advances in neurology, Vol. 43. New York: Raven Press, 65–85.

Rapin I. 1995. Autistic regression and disintegrative disorder: how important the role of epilepsy? *Semin Pediatr Neurol* 2:278–285.

Rapin I, Mattis S, Rowan AJ, et al. 1977. Verbal auditory agnosia in children. *Dev Med Child Neurol* 19:192–207.

Rapin I, Goldfisher S, Katzman R, et al. 1978. The cherry-red spot myoclonus syndrome. *Ann Neurol* 3:234–242.

Rapin F, Astruc J, Echenne B, Rodiere M. 1988. Utilisation pédiatrique des immunoglobulines intraveineues en immunomodulation: a propos de 34 observations. *Ann Pediatr (Paris)* 35:481–488.

Rapola J, Santavuori P, Heiskala H. 1987. Diagnosis of infantile neuronal ceroid lipofuscinosis on placental villi. *Neuropediatrics* 18:120–121.

Rapport RL, Penry JK. 1970. A survey of attitudes toward the pharmacological prophylaxis of post-traumatic epilepsy. *Neurosurg* 38:159–166.

Rapport RI, Penry JK. 1972. Pharmacologic prophylaxis of post-traumatic epilepsy: a review. *Epilepsia* 13:295–304.

Rashkin MC, Youngs C, Penovich P. 1987. Phenobarbital treatment of refractory status epilepticus. *Neurology* 37: 500–503.

Rasmussen T. 1973. Postoperative superficial hemosiderosis of the brain, its diagnosis, treatment and prevention. *Trans Am Neurol Assoc* 98:133–137.

Rasmussen T. 1974. Seizures with local onset and elementary symptomatology. In: Vinken PJ, Bruyn GW, eds. *The epilepsies*. Handbook of clinical neurology, Vol. 15. Amsterdam: North Holland, 74–86.

Rasmussen T. 1975a. Cortical resection in the treatment of focal epilepsy. In: Purpura DP, Penry JK, Walter RD, eds. *Neurosurgical management of the epilepsies*. Advances in neurology, Vol. 8. New York: Raven Press, 139–154.

Rasmussen T. 1975b. Surgery for epilepsy arising in regions other than the temporal and frontal lobes. In: Purpura DP, Penry JK, Walter RD, eds. *Neurosurgical management of the epilepsies*. Advances in neurology, Vol. 8. New York: Raven Press, 207–226.

Rasmussen T. 1983a. Characteristics of a pure culture of frontal lobe epilepsy. *Epilepsia* 24:482–493.

Rasmussen T. 1983b. Hemispherectomy for seizures revisited. *Can J Neurol Sci* 10:71–78.

Rasmussen TB. 1983c. Surgical treatment of complex partial seizures: results, lessons and problems. *Epilepsia* 24:S65–S76.

Rasmussen T, Andermann F. 1989. Update on the syndrome of chronic encephalitis and epilepsy. *Cleve Clin J Med* 56(Suppl.):181–184.

Rasmussen T, Villemure JG. 1989. Cerebral hemispherectomy for seizures with hemiplegia. *Cleve Clin J Med* 56:S62–S68.

Rasmussen T, Olszewski J, Lloyd-Smith D. 1958. Focal seizures due to chronic localized encephalitides. *Neurology* 8:435–445.

Ratcliffe JC, Wolf SM. 1977. Febrile convulsions caused by meningitis in young children. *Ann Neurol* 1:285–286.

Rathgeb JP, Plouin P, Soufflet C, et al. 1998. Le cas particulier des crises partielles du nourrisson: sémiologie électroclinique. In: Bureau M, Kahane P, Munari C, eds. *Epilepsies partielles graves pharmaco-résistantes de l'enfant: stratégies diagnostiques et traitements chirurgicaux*. Paris: John Libbey Eurotext, 122–134.

Rating D. 2000. Treatment in typical and atypical rolandic epilepsy. *Epileptic Disord* 2:S69–S72.

Rating D, Seidel V, Grimm B, et al. 1987. The prognostic value of EEG patterns in epilepsies with infantile spasms. *Brain Dev* 9:361–364.

Rating D, Wolf C, Bast T. 2000. Sulthiame as monotherapy in children with benign childhood epilepsy with centrotemporal spikes: a 6-month randomized, double-blind, placebo-controlled study. Sulthiame Study Group. *Epilepsia* 41:1284–1288.

Rausch R. 1987. Psychological evaluation. In: Engel J, ed. *Surgical treatment of the epilepsies*, 2nd ed. New York: Raven Press, 181–195.

Raybaud CH, Girard N, Canto-Moreira N, et al. 1996. High definition magnetic resonance imaging identification of cortical dysplasias: micropolygyria versus lissencephaly. In: Guerrini R, Andermann F, Canapicchi R, et al., eds. *Dysplasias of cerebral cortex and epilepsy*. Philadelphia: Lippincott-Raven, 131–143.

Raymond AA, Fish DR, Stevens JM, et al. 1994a. Association of hippocampal sclerosis with cortical dysgenesis in patients with epilepsy. *Neurology* 44:1841–1845.

Raymond AA, Halpin SF, Alsanjari N, et al. 1994b. Dysembryoplastic neuroepithelial tumour. Features in 16 patients. *Brain* 117:461–475.

Raymond AA, Gilmore WV, Scott CA, et al. 1999. Video-EEG telemetry: apparent manifestation of both epileptic and non-epileptic attacks causing potential diagnostic pitfalls. *Epileptic Disord* 1:101–106.

Régis J. 2001. New techniques: gamma knife. In: Wyllie E, ed. *The treatment of epilepsy: principles and practice*, 3rd ed. Philadelphia: Lippincott Williams & Wilkins, 1185–1192.

Régis J, Bartolomei F, Hayashi M, et al. 2000a. The role of gamma knife surgery in the treatment of severe epilepsies. *Epileptic Disord* 2:113–122.

Régis J, Bartolomei F, Kida Y, et al. 2000b. Radiosurgery for epilepsy associated with cavernous malformation: retrospective study in 49 patients. *Neurosurgery* 47: 1091–1097.

Reife RA. 1996. Topiramate: a novel antiepileptic agent. In: Shorvon S, Dreifuss F, Fish D, et al., eds. *Treatment of epilepsy*. Oxford: Blackwell, 471–481.

Reife RA, Lim P, Pledger G. 1995. Topiramate: side-effect profile in double-blind studies [Abstract]. *Epilepsia* 36:S34.

Reiher J, Lebel M. 1977. Wicket spikes: clinical correlates of a previously undescribed EEG pattern. *Can J Neurol Sci* 4:39–47.

Reilly EL, Peters JF. 1973. Relationship of some varieties of electroencephalographic photosensitivity to clinical convulsive disorders. *Neurology* 23:1050–1057.

Reinikainen K, Keränen T, Halonen T, et al. 1987. Comparison of oxcarbazepine and carbamazepine: a double-blind study. *Epilepsy Res* 1:284–289.

Reisner T, Zeiler K, Wessely P. 1979. The value of CT and EEG in cases of posttraumatic epilepsy. *J Neurol* 221:93–100.

Reiter E, Tiefenthaler M, Freillinger M, et al. 2000. Familial idiopathic West syndrome. *J Child Neurol* 15:249–252.

Remillard GM, Ethier R, Andermann F. 1974. Temporal lobe epilepsy and perinatal occlusion of the posterior cerebral artery. A syndrome analogous to infantile hemiplegia and a demonstrable etiology in some patients with temporal lobe epilepsy. *Neurology* 24:1001–1009.

Renier WO. 1988. Neuromorphological and biochemical analysis of a brain biopsy in a second case of idiopathic Lennox-Gastaut syndrome. In: Niedermeyer E, Degen R, eds. *The Lennox-Gastaut syndrome*. New York: Alan R. Liss, 427–432.

Renier WO, Renkawek K. 1990. Clinical and neuropathological findings in a case of severe myoclonic epilepsy of infancy. *Epilepsia* 31:287–291.

Renier D, Flandin C, Hirsch E, Hirsch JF. 1988a. Brain abscess in neonates. A study of 30 cases. *J Neurosurg* 69: 877–882.

Renier WO, Gabreels FJ, Jaspar HH. 1988b. Morphological and biochemical analysis of a brain biopsy in a case of idiopathic Lennox-Gastaut syndrome. *Epilepsia* 29: 644–649.

Renkawek K, Renier WO, de Pont JJ, et al. 1992. Neonatal status convulsivus, spongiform encephalopathy and low activity of Na$^+$/K$^+$-ATPase in the brain. *Epilepsia* 33:58–64.

Requena I, Arias M, Lopez-Ibor L, et al. 1991. Cavernomas of the central nervous system: clinical and neuroimaging manifestations in 47 patients. *J Neurol Neurosurg Psychiatry* 54:590–594.

Resnick TJ, Moshé SL, Perotta L, Chambers HJ. 1986. Benign neonatal sleep myoclonus. Relationship to sleep states. *Arch Neurol* 43:266–268.

Resor SR, Resor LD. 1990. Chronic acetazolamide monotherapy in the treatment of juvenile myoclonic epilepsy. *Neurology* 40:1677–1681.

Rethore MO, Caille B, Huet de Barochez Y, et al. 1984. Ring chromosome 14. II: A case report of r(14) mosaicism. The r(14) phenotype. *Ann Genet* 27:91–95.

Rett A, Teubel R. 1964. Neugeborenen Krampfe im Rahmen einer epileptisch belasten Familie. *Wien Klin Wschr* 76:609–613.

Revol M. 1992. Non idiopathic partial epilepsies and epileptic syndromes in childhood. In: Roger J, Dravet C, Bureau M, et al., eds. *Epileptic syndromes in infancy, childhood and adolescence*, 2nd. London: John Libbey, 347–362.

Revol M, Gilly R, Challamel MJ, et al. 1984. Epilepsie et maladie de Sturge-Weber. *Bolletino Lega Italiana contre l'Epilepsia* 45/46:51–58.

Revol M, Isnard H, Beaumanoir A, et al. 1989. Touch evoked myoclonic seizure in infancy. In: Beaumanoir A, Gastaut H, Naquet R, eds. *Reflex seizures and reflex epilepsies*. Genève: Médecine et Hygiène, 103–105.

Rey E, D'Athis P, De Lauture D, et al. 1979. Pharmacokinetics of carbamazepine in the neonate and in the child. *Int J Clin Pharmacol Biopharm* 117:90–96.

Reynolds EH. 1975. Chronic antiepileptic toxicity: a review. *Epilepsia* 16:319–352.

Reynolds EH. 1983. Mental effects of antiepileptic medication: a review. *Epilepsia* 24:S85–S95.

Reynolds EH. 1988. The prevention of chronic epilepsy. *Epilepsia* 29:S25–S28.

Reynolds EH, Shorvon SD. 1981. Monotherapy or polytherapy for epilepsy. *Epilepsia* 22:1–10.

Reynolds EH, Shorvon SD, Galbraith AW, et al. 1981. Phenytoin monotherapy for epilepsy: a long-term prospective study, assisted by serum level monitoring, in previously untreated patients. *Epilepsia* 22: 475–488.

Reynolds EH, Elwes RD, Shorvon SD. 1983. Why does epilepsy become intractable? Prevention of chronic epilepsy. *Lancet* 2:952–954.

Ricci GB. 1990. Magnetoencephalography. In: Dam M, Gram L, eds. *Comprehensive epileptology*. New York: Raven Press, 405–421.

Ricci S, Vigevano F. 1993. Occipital seizures provoked by intermittent light stimulation: ictal and interictal findings. *J Clin Neurophysiol* 10:197–209.

Ricci GB, Vizzioli R. 1964. Bilateral spike and wave complexes and cortical focus [Abstract]. *Electroencephalogr Clin Neurophysiol* 6:534.

Ricci GF, Mecaelli O, De Feo MR. 1990. Ontogenesis of GABA-ergic and glutamatergic receptors in the developing brain. In: Westerlain CG, Vert P, eds. *Neonatal seizures*. New York: Raven Press, 209–220.

Ricci S, Cusmai R, Fariello G, et al. 1992. Double cortex. A neuronal migration disorder as a possible cause of Lennox-Gastaut syndrome. *Arch Neurol* 49:61–64.

Ricci S, Cusmai R, Fusco L, Vigevano F. 1995. Reflex myoclonic epilepsy: a new age-dependent idiopathic epileptic syndrome related to startle reaction. *Epilepsia* 36:342–348.

Ricci S, Vigevano F, Manfredi M, et al. 1998. Epilepsy provoked by television and video games: safety of 100 Hz screens. *Neurology* 50:790–793.

Rich KM, Goldring S, Gado M. 1985. Computed tomography in chronic seizure disorders caused by glioma. *Arch Neurol* 42:26–27.

Rich SS, Annegers IF, Hauser WA, et al. 1987. Complex segregation analysis of febrile convulsions. *Am J Hum Genet* 41:249–257.

Richards RI, Sutherland GR. 1992. Dynamic mutations: a new class of mutations causing human disease. *Cell* 70:709–712.

Richens A. 1982. Clinical pharmacology and medical treatment. In: Laidlaw J, Richens A, eds. *Textbook of epilepsy*, 2nd ed. Edinburgh: Churchill Livingstone, 292–348.

Richens A. 1991. Pharmacology and clinical pharmacology of vigabatrin. *J Child Neurol* Suppl. 2:S7–S10.

Richens A. 1992a. Lamotrigine. In: Pedley TA, Meldrum BS, eds. *Recent advances in epilepsy*, Vol. 5. Edinburgh: Churchill Livingstone, 197–210.

Richens A. 1992b. New drugs for epilepsy: a rapidly changing scene. *Acta Neurol Scand Suppl* 140:65–70.

Riela AR, Penry JK. 1990. Magnetic resonance imaging. In: Dam M, Gram L, eds. *Comprehensive epileptology*. New York: Raven Press, 359–374.

Rigamonti D, Hadley MN, Drayer BP, et al. 1988. Cerebral cavernous malformations: incidence and familial occurrence. *N Engl J Med* 319:343–347.

Riikonen R. 1978. Cytomegalovirus and infantile spasms. *Dev Med Child Neurol* 20:570–579.

Riikonen R. 1980. ACTH therapy in infantile spasms: side-effect. *Arch Dis Child* 55:664–672.

Riikonen R. 1982. A long-term follow-up study of 214 children with the syndrome of infantile spasms. *Neuropediatrics* 13:14–23.

Riikonen R. 1983. Infantile spasms: some new theoretical aspects. *Epilepsia* 24:159–168.

Riikonen R. 1984. Infantile spasms: modern practical aspects. *Acta Paediatr Scand* 73:1–12.

Riikonen R. 1996. Long-term outcome of West syndrome: a study of adults with a history of infantile spasms. *Epilepsia* 37:367–372.

Riikonen RS. 2000. Steroids or vigabatrin in the treatment of infantile spasms? *Pediatr Neurol* 23:403–408.

Riikonen R. 2001. Epidemiological data of West syndrome in Finland. *Brain Dev* 23:539–541.

Riikonen R, Amnell G. 1981. Psychiatric disorders in children with earlier infantile spasms. *Dev Med Child Neurol* 23:747–760.

Riikonen R, Donner M. 1972. Incidence and aetiology of infantile spasms from 1960 to 1976: a population study in Finland. *Dev Med Child Neurol* 1:333–343.

Riikonen R, Donner M. 1980. ACTH therapy in infantile spasms: side effects. *Arch Dis Child* 55:664–672.

Riikonen R, Perheentupa J. 1986. Serum steroids and success of corticotropin therapy in infantile spasms. *Acta Paediatr Scand* 75:598–600.

Riikonen R, Simell O. 1990. Tuberous sclerosis and infantile spasms. *Dev Med Child Neurol* 32:203–209.

Riikonen R, Santavuori P, Meretoja O, et al. 1988. Can barbiturate anaesthesia cure infantile spasms? *Brain Dev* 10:300–304.

Riley TL, Roy A. 1982. *Pseudoseizures*. Baltimore:Williams & Wilkins.

Rimmer EM, Milligan NM, Richens A. 1987. A comparison of the acute effect of single doses of vigabatrin and sodium valproate on photosensitivity in epileptic patients. *Epilepsy Res* 1:339–346.

Ring HA, Heller AJ, Far IN, et al. 1990. Vigabatrin: rational treatment for chronic epilepsy. *J Neurol Neurosurg Psychiatry* 53:1051–1055.

Rintahaka PJ, Chugani HT. 1997. Clinical role of positron emission topography in children with tuberous sclerosis complex. *J Child Neurol* 12:42–52.

Risinger MW. 2000. Noninvasive ictal electroencephalography in humans. In: Lüders HO, Noachtar S. eds. *Epileptic seizures*. Philadelphia: Churchill Livingstone, 32–48.

Riva R, Albani F, Ambrosetto G, et al. 1984. Diurnal fluctuations in free and total steady-state plasma levels of carbamazepine and correlation with intermittent side-effects. *Epilepsia* 25:476–481.

Roach ES, Kerr J, Mendelssohn D, et al. 1991. Detection of tuberous sclerosis by magnetic resonance imaging. *Neurology* 41:262–265.

Roach ES, Smith M, Huttenlocher P, et al. 1992. Diagnostic criteria: tuberous sclerosis complex. Report of the Diagnostic Criteria Committee of the National Tuberous Sclerosis Association. *J Child Neurol* 7:221–224.

Robain O. 1996. Introduction to the pathology of cerebral cortical dysplasia. In: Guerrini R, Andermann F,

Canapicchi R, et al., eds. *Dysplasias of cerebral cortex and epilepsy*. Philadelphia: Lippincott-Raven, 1–9.

Robain O, Dulac O. 1992. Early epileptic encephalopathy with suppression-bursts and olivary-dentate dysplasia. *Neuropediatrics* 23:162–164.

Robain O, Gelot A. 1996. Neuropathology of hemimegalencephaly. In: Guerrini R, Andermann F, Canapicchi R, et al., eds. *Dysplasias of cerebral cortex and epilepsy*. Philadelphia: Lippincott-Raven, 89–92.

Robain O, Vinters HV. 1994. Neuropathologic studies. In: Dulac O, Chugani HT, Dalla Bernardina B, eds. *Infantile spasms and West syndrome*. Philadelphia: WB Saunders, 99–117.

Robain O, Floquet C, Heldt H, Rozenberg F. 1988. Hemimegalencephaly: a clinicopathological study of four cases. *Neuropathol Appl Neurobiol* 14:125–135.

Roberts SA, Cohen MD, Forfar JO. 1973. Antenatal factors associated with neonatal hypocalcaemic convulsions. *Lancet* 2:809–811.

Robertson WC Jr, Fariello RG. 1979. Eating epilepsy associated with a deep forebrain glioma. *Ann Neurol* 6: 271–273.

Robillard A, Saint-Hilaire JM, Mercier M, et al. 1983. The lateralizing and localizing value of adversion in epileptic seizures. *Neurology* 33:1241–1242.

Robinson R. 1984. When to start and stop anticonvulsants. In: Meadow R, ed. *Recent advances in paediatrics*. Edinburgh: Churchill Livingstone, 155–174.

Robinson WP, Bernasconi F, Mutirangura A, et al. 1993. Nondisjunction of chromosome 15: origin and recombination. *Am J Hum Genet* 53:740–751.

Robinson RO, Baird G, Robinson G, Simonoff E. 2001. Landau-Kleffner syndrome: course and correlates with outcome. *Dev Med Child Neurol* 43:243–247.

Robitaille Y. 1987. Pathological changes relevant for seizure generation. In: Wieser HA, Elger CE, eds. *Presurgical evaluation of epileptics*. Berlin: Springer, 79–85.

Robitaille Y. 1991. Neuropathologic aspects of chronic encephalitis. In: Andermann F, ed. *Chronic encephalitis and epilepsy: Rasmussen syndrome*. London: Butterworth-Heineman, 79–110.

Rocca WA, Sharbrough FW, Hauser WA. 1987a. Risk factors for absence seizures: a population-based case-control study in Rochester, Minnesota. *Neurology* 37: 1309–1314.

Rocca WA, Sharbrough FW, Hauser WA. 1987b. Risk factors for generalized tonic-clonic seizures: a population-based case-control study in Rochester, Minnesota. *Neurology* 37:1315–1322.

Rocca WA, Sharbrough FW, Hauser WA, et al. 1987c. Risk factors for complex partial seizures: a population-based case-control study. *Ann Neurol* 21:22–31.

Rochat P, Hallas J, Gaist D, et al. 2001. Antiepileptic drug utilization: a Danish prescription database analysis. *Acta Neurol Scand* 104:6–11.

Rochkind S, Hoffman HJ, Hendrick EB. 1990. Sturge-Weber syndrome: natural history and prognosis. *J Epilepsy* (Suppl.):293–304.

Rodin EA. 1968. *The prognosis of patients with epilepsy*. Springfield, IL: Charles C Thomas Publishers.

Rodin E. 1989. Prognosis of cognitive functions in children with epilepsy. In: Hermann B, Seidenberg M, eds. *Childhood epilepsies: neuropsychological, psychosocial and intervention aspects*. Chichester, England: John Wiley and Sons, 25–33.

Rodin G, John G, Kobiljak J, et al. 1977. Discontinuation of anticonvulsant medication in remitted epileptic patients [Abstract]. *Electroencephalogr Clin Neurophysiol* 43: 905.

Rodin E, Klutke G, Chayasirisobohn S. 1982. Epileptic patients who are refractory to anticonvulsant medications. *Neurology* 32:1382–1384.

Rodin EA, Schmaltz S, Twitty G. 1986. Intellectual functions of patients with childhood-onset epilepsy. *Dev Med Child Neurol* 28:25–33.

Rodriguez I, Niedermeyer E. 1992. The aphasia-epilepsy syndrome in children: electroencephalographic aspects. *Clin Electroencephal* 13:23–35.

Rogawski MA. 2002. Principles of antiepileptic drug action. In: Levy RH, Mattson RH, Meldrum BS, et al., eds. *Antiepileptic drugs*, 5th ed. Philadelphia: Lippincott Williams & Wilkins, 3–22.

Roger J. 1974. Prognostic features of petit mal absences. *Epilepsia* 15:433.

Roger J, Gambarelli-Dubois D. 1988. Neuropathological studies of the Lennox-Gastaut syndrome. In: Niedermeyer E, Degen R, eds. *The Lennox-Gastaut Syndrome*. New York: Alan R. Liss, 73–93.

Roger J, Genton P. 1995. Definitions and ictal manifestations of typical absences. In: Duncan JS, Panayiotopoulos CP, eds. *Typical absences and related syndromes*. London: Churchill Communication Europe, 145–151.

Roger J, Tassinari CA. 1973. Epilepsie généralisée primaire grand mal. In: Lugaresi E, Pazzaglia P, Tassinari CA, eds. *Evolution and prognosis of epilepsies*. Bologna: Aulo Goggi, 42–48.

Roger J, Payan H, Toga M, et al. 1960. Manifestations cérébelleuses chez les épileptiques. *Rev Neurol (Paris)* 103: 410–414.

Roger J, Grangeon H, Guey J, et al. 1968. Incidences psychiatriques et psychologiques du traitement par l'ethosuccimide chez les épileptiques. *Encéphale* 57: 407–438.

Roger J, Lob H, Tassinari CA. 1974. Status epilepticus. In: Vinken PJ, Bruyn GW, eds. *The epilepsies*. Handbook of neurology, Vol. 15. Amsterdam: North Holland, 145–188.

Roger J, Gastaut JL, Dravet C, et al. 1977. Epilepsie partielle à sémiologie complexe et lésions atrophiques occipito-pariétales. Intérêt de l'examen tacoencéphalographique. *Rev Neurol (Paris)* 133:41–53.

Roger J, Dravet C, Bureau M. 1982. Unilateral seizures: hemiconvulsions-hemiplegia syndrome (HH) and hemiconvulsions-hemiplegia-epilepsy syndrome (HHE). *Electroencephalogr Clin Neurophysiol Suppl* 35: 211–221.

Roger J, Dravet CH, Boniver C, et al. 1984. L'épilepsie dans la sclérose tubéreuse de Bourneville. *Bolletino Lega Italiana contre l'Epilepsia* 45/46:33–38.

Roger J, Rémy C, Bureau M, et al. 1987. Le syndrome de Lennox-Gastaut chez l'adulte. *Rev Neurol (Paris)* 143: 401–405.

Roger J, Dravet C, Bureau M. 1989. The Lennox-Gastaut syndrome. *Cleve Clin J Med* 56:S172–S180.

Roger J, Bureau M, Genton P, Dravet C. 1990. Idiopathic partial epilepsies. In: Dam M, Gram L, eds. *Comprehensive epileptology*. New York: Raven Press, 155–170.

Roger J, Gobbi G, Bureau M, et al. 1991. Severe partial epilepsies in childhood. In: Fukuyama Y, Kamoshita S, Ohtsuka C, et al., eds. *Modern perspectives of child neurology*. Tokyo: Japanese Society of Child Neurology, 223–230.

Roger J, Genton P, Bureau M, Dravet C. 1992. Progressive myoclonus epilepsies of childhood and adolescence. In: Roger J, Dravet C, Bureau M, et al., eds. *Epileptic syndromes in infancy, childhood and adolescence,* 2nd ed. London: John Libbey, 381–400.

Rogers SW, Andrews PI, Gahring LC, et al. 1994. Autoantibodies to glutamate receptor GluR3 in Rasmussen encephalitis. *Science* 265:648–651.

Rohr-Le Floch J, Gauthier G, Beaumanoir A. 1988. Etats confusionnels d'origine épileptique. Intérêt de i'EEG fait en urgence. *Rev Neurol (Paris)* 144:425–436.

Rondouin G. 1990. GABA-ergic inhibition and convulsive seizures. In: Wasterlain CG, Vert P, eds. *Neonatal seizures*. New York: Raven Press, 221–230.

Ronen GM, Penney S. 1995. The epidemiology of clinical neonatal seizures in Newfoundland, Canada: a five year cohort. *Ann Neurol* 38:518–519.

Roos RA, van Dijk JG. 1988. Reflex-epilepsy induced by immersion in hot water: case report and review of the literature. *Eur Neurol* 28:6–10.

Roper SN, Gilmore RL. 1995. Orbitofrontal resections for intractable partial seizures. *J Epilepsy* 8:146.

Ropper AH, Kofke A, Bromfield EB, et al. 1986. Comparison of isoflurane, halothane, and nitrous oxide in status epilepticus. *Ann Neurol* 19:98–99.

Rosa FW. 1991. Spina bifida in infants of women treated with carbamazepine during pregnancy. *N Engl J Med* 324:674–677.

Rose AL, Lombroso CT. 1970. Neonatal seizure states: a study of clinical, pathological and electroencephalographic features in 137 full-term babies with a long-term follow-up. *Pediatrics* 45:404–425.

Rose DF, Sato S, Smith PD, et al. 1987. Localization of magnetic interictal discharges in temporal lobe epilepsy. *Ann Neurol* 22:348–354.

Rosen I, Salford L, Starck L. 1984. Sturge-Weber disease—neurophysiological evaluation of a case with secondary epileptogenesis, successfully treated with lobe-ectomy. *Neuropediatrics* 15:95–98.

Rosenfeld WE, Beniak TE, Lippmann SM, et al. 1987. Adverse behavioral response to clonazepam as a function of verbal IQ–performance IQ discrepancy. *Epilepsy Res* 1:347–356.

Rosenow F, Arzimanoglou A, Baulac M. 2003. Recent developments in treatment of status epilepticus: a review. *Epileptic Disord* 4:S41–S51.

Rosman NP. 1990. Management of febrile seizures. In: Fukuyama Y, Kamoshita S, Ohtsuka C, et al., eds. *Modern perspectives of child neurology*. Tokyo: Japanese Society of Child Neurology, 183–190.

Rosman NP, Colton T, Labazzo J, et al. 1993. A controlled trial of diazepam administered during febrile illnesses to prevent recurrences of febrile seizures. *N Engl J Med* 379:79–84.

Ross EM, Peckham CS. 1983. Seizure disorder in the national child development study. In: Rose CF, ed. *Research progress in epilepsy*. London: Pitman, 46–59.

Ross EM, West PB, Butler NR. 1980. Epilepsy in childhood: findings from the National Child Development Study. *BMJ* 1:207–210.

Rossi L, Brunelli G, Duzioni N, Rossi G. 1986. Lumbar puncture and febrile convulsions. *Helv Paediatr Acta* 41:19–24.

Rothner AD, Erenberg G. 1980. Status epilepticus. *Pediatr Clin North Am* 27:593–602.

Roubertie A, Petit J, Genton P. 2000. Chromosome 20 en anneau: un syndrome épileptique identifiable. *Rev Neurol* 156:149–153.

Rougier A, Loiseau P. 1988. Orbitofrontal epilepsy: a case report. *J Neurol Neurosurg Psychiatry* 51:146–157.

Rougier A, Loiseau P, Rivel J, et al. 1984. Epilepsies partielles de l'adolescence avec anomalies tomodensito-métriques, réaction astrocytaire localisée, évolution favorable. *Rev Neurol (Paris)* 140:171–178.

Roulet E, Deonna T, Despland PA. 1989. Prolonged intermittent drooling and oromotor dyspraxia in benign childhood epilepsy with centro-temporal spikes. *Epilepsia* 30:564–568.

Roulet E, Deonna T, Gaillard F, et al. 1991. Acquired aphasia, dementia, and behavior disorder with epilepsy and continuous spike and waves during sleep in a child. *Epilepsia* 32:495–503.

Roulet Perez E, Davidoff V, Despland PA, Deonna T. 1993. Mental and behavioural deterioration of children with epilepsy and ESES: acquired epileptic frontal syndrome. *Dev Med Child Neurol* 35:661–674.

Roulet Perez E, Seeck M, Mayer E. 1998. Childhood epilepsy with neuropsychological regression and continuous spike waves during sleep: epilepsy surgery in a young adult. *Eur J Paediatr Neurol* 2:303–311.

Rousselle C, Revol M. 1995. Relations between cognitive functions and continuous spikes and waves during slow sleep. In: Beaumanoir A, Bureau M, Donna T, et al., eds. *Continuous spikes and waves during slow sleep*. London: John Libbey, 123–133.

Rovit RL, Gloor P, Rasmussen T. 1961. Sphenoidal electrodes in the electroencephalographic study of patients with temporal lobe epilepsy. *J Neurosurg* 18:151–158.

Rowan AJ, Binnie CD, Warfield CA, et al. 1979. The delayed effect of sodium valproate on the photoconvulsive response in man. *Epilepsia* 20:61–68.

Rowan AJ, Overweg J, Sadikoglu S, et al. 1980. Seizure-prognosis in long-stay mentally subnormal epileptic patients: interrater EEG and clinical studies. *Epilepsia* 21:219–226.

Rowan AJ, Overweg J, Meijer JW. 1981. Monodose therapy with valproic acid: 24 hour telemetric EEG and serum level studies. In: Dam M, Gram F, Penry JK, eds. *Advances in epileptology*, XIIth Epilepsy International Symposium. New York: Raven Press, 533–539.

Rowan AJ, Meijer JW, de Beer-Pawlikowski N, et al. 1983. Valproate-ethosuximide combination therapy for refractory absence seizures. *Arch Neurol* 40:797–802.

Rowe JC, Holmes GL, Hafford J, et al. 1985. Prognostic value of the electroencephalogram in term and preterm infants following neonatal seizures. *Electroencephalogr Clin Neurophysiol* 60:183–196.

Rowe CC, Berkovic SF, Sia ST, et al. 1989. Localization of epileptic foci with postictal single photon emission computed tomography. *Ann Neurol* 26:660–668.

Rowe CC, Berkovic SF, Austin, MC, et al. 1991. Patterns of postictal cerebral blood flow in temporal lobe epilepsy: qualitative and quantitative analysis. *Neurology* 41: 1096–1103.

Rubboli G, Michelucci R, Valzania F, et al. 1997. Clinical and neurophysiological features of different forms of epileptic falls. In: Beaumanoir A, Andermann F, Avanzini G, et al., eds. *Falls in epileptic and non-*

epileptic seizures during childhood. London: John Libbey, 53–63.

Ruggieri V, Caraballo R, Fejerman N. 1989. Intracranial tumors and West syndrome. *Pediatr Neurol* 5:327–329.

Russell WR, Whitty CW. 1953. Studies in traumatic epilepsy. 2: Focal motor and somatic sensory fits: a study of 85 cases. *J Neurol Neurosurg Psychiatry* 16:73–97.

Russell-Jones DL, Shorvon SD. 1989. The frequency and consequences of head injury in epileptic seizures. *J Neurol Neurosurg Psychiatry* 52:659–662.

Rust R. 2001. Barbiturates and primidone. In: Pellock J, Dodson WE, Bourgeois BF, eds. *Pediatric epilepsy: diagnosis and therapy.* New York: Demos, 385– 404.

Rutledge SL, Snead OC III, Morawetz R, et al. 1987. Brain tumors presenting as a seizure disorder in infants. *J Child Neurol* 2:214–219.

Rutter N, Smales OR. 1977. Role of routine investigations in children presenting with their first febrile convulsions. *Arch Dis Child* 52:188–191.

Rutter M, Graham PJ, Yule W. 1970. *A neuropsychiatric study in childhood.* London: Spastics International Medical Publications.

Ryan SG, Wiznitzer M. 1990. Clinical heterogeneity in benign familial neonatal convulsions: a challenge for genetic analysis. *Epilepsia* 31:817.

Ryan SW, Forsythe I, Hartley R, et al. 1990. Slow release carbamazepine in treatment of poorly controlled seizures. *Arch Dis Child* 65:930–935.

Ryan SG, Wiznitzer M, Hollman C, et al. 1991. Benign familial neonatal convulsions: evidence for clinical and genetic heterogeneity. *Ann Neurol* 29:469–473.

Ryan SG, Sherman SL, Terry JC, et al. 1992. Startle disease or hyperekplexia: response to clonazepam and assignment of the gene (STHE) to chromosome 5q by linkage analysis. *Ann Neurol* 31:663–668.

Rylance GW, Moreland TA. 1981. Saliva carbamazepine and phenytoin level monitoring. *Arch Dis Child* 56:637–639.

Ryvlin P, Cinotti L, Froment JC, et al. 1991. Metabolic patterns associated with non-specific magnetic resonance imaging abnormalities in temporal lobe epilepsy. *Brain* 114:2363–2383.

Ryvlin P, Garcia-Larrea L, Philippon B, et al. 1992. High signal intensity of T2-weighted MRI correlates with hypoperfusion in temporal lobe epilepsy. *Epilepsia* 33:28–35.

Ryvlin P, Bouvard S, Le Bars D, et al. 1998. Clinical utility of flumazenil-PET versus [18F]fluorodeoxyglucose-PET and MRI in refractory partial epilepsy. A prospective study in 100 patients. *Brain* 121:2067–2081.

Ryvlin P, Coste S, Hermier M, et al. 2002. Temporal pole MRI abnormalities in temporal lobe epilepsy. *Epileptic Disord* 4:S33–S39.

Sachdeo RC, Glauser TA, Ritter F, et al. 1999. A double-blind, randomized trial of topiramate in Lennox-Gastaut syndrome. Topiramate YL Study Group. *Neurology* 52:1882–1887.

Sackellares JC, Dreifuss FE, Penry JK. 1981. Reduction of steady state valproate levels by other antiepileptic drugs. *Epilepsia* 22:437–441.

Sadler RM, Blume WT. 1989. Significance of bisynchronous spike-waves in patients with temporal lobe spikes. *Epilepsia* 20:143–146.

Sàenz-Lope E, Herranz FJ, Masdeu JC. 1984a. Startle epilepsy: a clinical study. *Ann Neurol* 16:78–81.

Sàenz-Lope E, Herranz-Tanarro FJ, Masdeu JC, et al. 1984b. Hyperexplexia: a syndrome of pathological startle responses. *Ann Neurol* 15:36–41.

Sàenz-Lope E, Herranz-Tanarro FJ, Masdeu JC. 1985. Primary reading epilepsy. *Epilepsia* 26:649–656.

Sagar HJ, Oxbury JM. 1987. Hippocampal neuron loss in temporal lobe epilepsy: correlation with early childhood convulsions. *Ann Neurol* 22:334–340.

Saint-Martin AD, Cazcangiu R, Arzimanoglou A, et al. 2001. Semiology of typical and atypical rolandic epilepsy: a video-EEG analysis. *Epileptic Disord* 3:173–182.

Saji M, Reis DS. 1987. Delayed transneuronal death of substanta migra neurons prevented by γ-aminobutyric acid agonist. *Science* 235:66–69.

Salanova V, Andermann F, Olivier A, et al. 1992. Occipital lobe epilepsy: electroclinical manifestations, electrocorticography, cortical stimulation and outcome in 42 patients treated between 1930 and 1991. *Brain* 115:1655–1680.

Salanova V, Morris HH, Van Ness PC, et al. 1993. Comparison of scalp electroencephalogram with subdural recordings and functional mapping in frontal lobe epilepsy. *Arch Neurol* 50:294–299.

Salanova V, Andermann F, Rasmussen T, et al. 1995a. Parietal lobe epilepsy. Clinical manifestations and outcome in 82 patients treated surgically between 1929 and 1988. *Brain* 118:607–627.

Salanova V, Morris HH, Van Ness P, et al. 1995b. Frontal lobe epilepsy: electroclinical syndromes. *Epilepsia* 36:16–24.

Salanova V, Markand O, Worth R. 2002. Temporal lobe epilepsy surgery: outcome, complications, and late mortality rate in 215 patients. *Epilepsia* 43:170–174.

Salas-Puig J, Ramos Polo E, Macarron Vincente J, Hernandez Lanos C. 1990a. Benign myoclonic epilepsy of infancy. Case report. *Acta Paediatr Scand* 79:1128–1130.

Salas-Puig X, Camara da Silva AM, Dravet C, Roger J. 1990b. L'épilepsie myoclonique juvénile dans la population du Centre Saint Paul. *Epilepsies* 2:108–113.

Sallustro C, Atwell F. 1978. Body rocking, head banging, and head rolling in normal children. *J Pediatr* 93:704–708.

Salomon GE, Kutt H, Plum F. 1983. *Clinical management of seizures.* New York: WB Saunders.

Salonen R, Somer M, Haltia M. 1991. Progressive encephalopathy with edema, hypsarrhythmia and optic atrophy. *Clin Genet* 39:287–293.

Saltik S, Kocer N, Dervent A. 2002. Informative value of magnetic resonance imaging and EEG in the prognosis of infantile spasms. *Epilepsia* 43:246–252.

Sammaritano M, Andermann F, Melanson D, et al. 1985. Prolonged focal cerebral edema associated with partial status epilepticus. *Epilepsia* 26:334–339.

Sammaritano M, de Lotbinière A, Andermann F, et al. 1987. False lateralization by surface EEG of seizure onset in patients with temporal lobe epilepsy and gross focal cerebral lesions. *Ann Neurol* 21:361–369.

Sammaritano M, Gigli GL, Gotman J. 1991. Interictal spiking during wakefulness and sleep and the localization of foci in temporal lobe epilepsy. *Neurology* 41:290–297.

Sander JW. 1993. Some aspects of prognosis of the epilepsies: a review. *Epilepsia* 34:1007–1016.

Sander JW. 1995. The epidemiology and prognosis of typical absence seizures. In: Duncan JS, Panayiotopoulos

CP, eds. *Typical absences and related syndromes*. London: Churchill Communication Europe, 135–144.

Sander JW, Shorvon SD. 1987. Remission periods in epilepsy and their relation to long-term prognosis. In: Wolf P, Dam M, Janz D, Dreifuss FE, eds. *Advances in epileptology, XVI Epilepsy International Symposium*. New York: Raven Press, 353–360.

Sander JW, Sillanpää M. 1998. Natural history and prognosis. In: Engel J Jr, Pedley TA, eds. *Epilepsy: a comprehensive textbook*, Vol. 1. Philadelphia: Lippincott-Raven, 69–86.

Sander JW, Patsalos PN, Oxley JR, et al. 1990a. A randomized double-blind placebo controlled add on trial of lamotrigine in patients with severe epilepsy. *Epilepsy Res* 6:221–226.

Sander JW, Trevisol-Bittencourt PC, Hart YM, et al. 1990b. The efficacy and long-term tolerability of lamotrigine in the treatment of severe epilepsy. *Epilepsy Res* 7: 226–229.

Sander JW, Hart YM, Patsalos PN, et al. 1991a. Lamotrigine in generalised seizures. *Epilepsia* 32(Suppl. 1):9–21.

Sander JW, Hart YM, Trimble MR, et al. 1991b. Vigabatrin and psychosis. *J Neurol Neurosurg Psychiatry* 54: 435–439.

Sander T, Bockenkamp B, Hildmann T, et al. 1997. Refined mapping of the epilepsy susceptibility locus EJM1 on chromosome 6. *Neurology* 49:842–847.

Sander T, Schulz H, Vieira-Saeker AM, et al. 1999. Evaluation of a putative major susceptibility locus for juvenile myoclonic epilepsy on chromosome 15q14. *Am J Med Genet* 88:182–187.

Sander T, Schultz H, Saar K, et al. 2000. Genome search for susceptibility loci of common idiopathic generalised epilepsies. *Hum Mol Genet* 9:1465–1472.

Sankar R, Curran JG, Kevill JW, et al. 1995. Microscopic cortical dysplasia in infantile spasms: evolution of white matter abnormalities. *AJNR Am J Neuroradiol* 16:1265–1272.

Santanelli P, Bureau M, Maggauda A, et al. 1989. Benign partial epilepsy with centrotemporal (or rolandic) spikes and brain lesion. *Epilepsia* 30:182–188.

Santavuori P, Haltia M, Rapola J. 1974. Infantile type of so-called neuronal ceroid lipofuscinosis. *Dev Med Child Neurol* 26:644–653.

Sapin JI, Riviello JJ, Grover WD. 1988. Efficacy of primidone for seizure control in neonates and young infants. *Pediatr Neurol* 4:292–295.

Sarisjulis N, Gamboni B, Plouin P, et al. 2000. Diagnosing idiopathic/cryptogenic epilepsy syndromes in infancy. *Arch Dis Child* 82:226–230.

Sarnat HB. 1992. *Cerebral dysgenesis: embryology and clinical expression*. New York: Oxford University Press.

Sass KJ, Spencer DD, Spencer SS, et al. 1988. Corpus callostomy for epilepsy. II: Neurologic and neurophysiological outcome. *Neurology* 38:24–28.

Sass KJ, Spencer DD, Kim JH, et al. 1990. Verbal memory impairment correlates with hippocampal pyramidal cell density. *Neurology* 40:1694–1697.

Sassover K, Duchowny M, Jayakar P, et al. 1994. EEG evaluation in children with Sturge-Weber syndrome and epilepsy. *J Epilepsy* 7:285–289.

Sato M. 1966. Clinical and electroencephalographical study of childhood epilepsy with special reference to the outcome due to treatment. *Psychiatr Neurol Jpn* 68: 1059–1064.

Sato S, Dreifuss FE, Penry JK. 1976. Prognostic factors in absence seizures. *Neurology* 26:788–796.

Sato H, Takeshi F, Hara H, et al. 1982a. Brain shrinkage and subdural effusion associated with ACTH administration. *Brain Dev* 4:13–20.

Sato W, White BG, Penry JK, et al. 1982b. Valproic acid versus ethosuximide in the treatment of absence seizures. *Neurology* 32:157–163.

Sato S, Dreifuss FE, Penry JK, et al. 1983. Long-term follow-up of absence seizures. *Neurology* 33:1590–1595.

Satoh J, Mizutani T, Morimatsu Y. 1986. Neuropathology of the brainstem in age-dependent epileptic encephalopathy—especially in cases with infantile spasms. *Brain Dev* 8:443–449.

Saunders M, Marschall C. 1975. Isolated seizures: an EEG and clinical assessment. *Epilepsia* 16:731–733.

Savard G, Andermann F, Remillard GM, et al. 1987. Postictal psychosis following partial complex seizures is analogous to Todd's paralysis. In: Wolf P, Dam M, Janz D, et al. *Advances in epileptology*, Vol. 16. New York: Raven Press, 603–605.

Sawhney IM, Suresh N, Dhand UK, Chopra JS. 1988. Acquired aphasia with epilepsy–Landau-Kleffner syndrome. *Epilepsia* 29:283–287.

Scampler G, Hopkins A. 1980. Social class, epileptic activity and disadvantage at work. *J Epidemiol Comm Health* 34:129–133.

Scarpa P, Carassini B. 1982. Partial epilepsy in childhood: clinical and EEG study of 261 cases. *Epilepsia* 23: 333–341.

Scarpa P, Chierici R, Tamisari L, et al. 1983. Criteria for discontinuing neonatal seizure therapy: a long-term appraisal. *Brain Dev* 5:541–548.

Schachter SC, Saper CB. 1998. Vagus nerve stimulation. *Epilepsia* 39:677–686.

Schain RJ, Ward JW, Guthrie D. 1977. Carbamazepine as an anticonvulsant in children. *Neurology* 27:476–480.

Schanzer S, April R, Atkin A. 1965. Seizures induced by eye deviation. *Arch Neurol* 13:621–626.

Scheel H, Tomiuk S, Hofman K. 2002. A common protein interaction domain links two recently identified epilepsy genes. *Hum Mol Genet* 11:1757–1762.

Scheffer IE. 2000. Autosomal dominant rolandic epilepsy with speech dyspraxia. *Epileptic Disord* 2:S19–S22.

Scheffer IE. 2003. Severe infantile epilepsies: molecular genetics. *Brain* 126:513–514.

Scheffer IE, Berkovic S. 1997. Generalized epilepsy with febrile seizures plus: a genetic disorder with heterogeneous clinical phenotypes. *Brain* 120:479–490.

Scheffer IE, Bhatia KP, Lopez Cendes I, et al. 1995a. Autosomal dominant frontal lobe epilepsy. A distinctive clinical disorder. *Brain* 118:61–73.

Scheffer IE, Jones L, Pozzebon M, et al. 1995b. Autosomal dominant rolandic epilepsy and speech dyspraxia: a new syndrome with anticipation. *Ann Neurol* 38: 633–642.

Scheffer IE, Phillips HA, O'Brien CE, et al. 1998. Familial partial epilepsy with variable foci: a new partial epilepsy syndrome with suggestion of linkage to chromosome 2. *Ann Neurol* 44:S90–S99.

Scheffner D, Weber R. 1981. Review on epilepsy and memory in children. *Acta Neurol Scand Suppl* 89:157–181.

Scheffner D, Konig S, Rautenberg-Ruland I. 1988. Fatal liver failure in 16 children with valproate therapy. *Epilepsia* 29:530–542.

Scheithauer BW, Forno LS, Dorfman LJ, et al. 1978. Neuroaxonal dystrophy (Seitelberger's disease with late onset, protracted course and myoclonic epilepsy). *J Neurol Sci* 36:247–258.

Schenk CH, Mahowald MW. 1992. Motor dyscontrol in narcolepsy: rapid eye movement (REM) sleep without atonia and REM sleep behavior disorder. *Ann Neurol* 32:3–10.

Scher MS. 2002. Controversies regarding neonatal seizure recognition. *Epileptic Disord* 4:138–158.

Scher MS. 2003. Prenatal contribution to epilepsy: lessons from the bedside. *Epileptic Disord* 5:77–91.

Scher MS, Beggarly M. 1989. Clinical significance of focal periodic discharges in neonates. *J Child Neurol* 4: 175–185.

Scher MS, Painter MJ. 1990. Electroencephalographic diagnosis of neonatal seizures: issues of diagnostic accuracy, clinical correlation and survival. In: Wasterlain CG, Vert P, eds. *Neonatal seizures.* New York: Raven Press, 15–25.

Scher MS, Aso K, Painter MJ. 1988. Comparisons between preterm and full-term neonates with seizures [Abstract]. *Ann Neurol* 24:344A.

Scher MS, Painter MJ, Bergman I, et al. 1989. EEG diagnosis of neonatal seizures: clinical correlations and outcome. *Pediatr Neurol* 5:17–24.

Scher MS, Aso K, Beggarly M, et al. 1993. Electrographic seizures in pre-term and full-term neonates: clinical correlates, associated brain lesions, and risk for neurologic sequelae. *Pediatrics* 91:128–134.

Scherzer E, Wessely P. 1978. EEG in posttraumatic epilepsy. *Eur Neurol* 17:38–42.

Scheuer ML. 1992. Medical aspects of managing seizures and epilepsy. In: Pedley TA, Meldrum BS, eds. *Recent advances in epilepsy,* 5th ed. Edinburgh: Churchill Livingstone, 127–157.

Scheyer RD. 2002. Valproic acid: drug interactions. In: Levy RH, Mattson RH, Meldrum BS, Perucca E, eds. *Antiepileptic drugs,* 5th ed. Philadelphia: Lippincott Williams & Wilkins, 801–807.

Schiottz-Christensen E. 1972. Genetic factors in febrile convulsions. *Acta Neurol Scand* 48:538–546.

Schiottz-Christensen E. 1973. Neurological finding in twins discordant for febrile convulsions. *Acta Neurol Scand* 49:368–378.

Schiottz-Christensen E, Bruhn P. 1973. Intelligence, behaviour and scholastic achievement subsequent to febrile convulsions: an analysis of discordant twin pairs. *Dev Med Child Neurol* 15:565–575.

Schlienger RG, Knowles SR, Shear NH. 1998. Lamotrigine-associated anticonvulsant hypersensitivity syndrome. *Neurology* 51:1172–1175.

Schlumberger E, Dulac O. 1994. A simple, effective and well-tolerated treatment regime for West syndrome. *Dev Med Child Neurol* 36:863–872

Schlumberger E, Chavew F, Dulac O. 1992a. Open study with lamotrigine (LTG) in child epilepsy. *Seizure* 1 (Suppl.):9–21.

Schlumberger E, Dulac O, Plouin P. 1992b. Early infantile epileptic syndrome(s) with suppression-burst: nosological considerations. In: Roger J, Bureau M, Dravet C, et al., eds. *Epileptic syndromes in infancy, childhood and adolescence,* 2nd ed. London: John Libbey, 35–42.

Schlumberger E, Chavez F, Palacios L, et al. 1994. Lamotrigine in treatment of 120 children with epilepsy. *Epilepsia* 35:359–367.

Schmidley JW, Simon RP. 1981. Postictal pleocytosis. *Ann Neurol* 9:81–84.

Schmidt D. 1981. Effect of antiepileptic drugs on estrogen and progesterone metabolism and on oral contraception. In: Dam M, Gram L, Penry JK, eds. *Advances in epileptology,* XIIth Epilepsy International Symposium. New York: Raven Press, 423–431.

Schmidt D. 1982. Two antiepileptic drugs for intractable epilepsy with complex-partial seizures. *J Neurol Neurosurg Psychiatry* 45:1119–1124.

Schmidt D. 1983a. Reduction of two-drug therapy in intractable epilepsy. *Epilepsia* 24:368–376.

Schmidt D. 1983b. Single drug therapy for intractable epilepsy. *J Neurol* 229:221–226.

Schmidt D. 1984. Prognosis of chronic epilepsy with complex partial seizures. *J Neurol Neurosurg Psychiatry* 47: 1274–1278.

Schmidt D. 1985. Benzodiazepines—an update. In: Pedley TA, Meldrum BS, eds. *Recent advances in epilepsy,* Vol. 2. Edinburgh: Churchill Livingstone, 125–135.

Schmidt D. 1986a. Diagnostic and therapeutic management of intractable epilepsy. In: Schmidt D, Morselli PL, eds. *Intractable epilepsy: experimental and clinical aspects.* New York: Raven Press, 237–257.

Schmidt D. 1986b. Toxicity of anti-epileptic drugs. In: Pedley TA, Meldrum BS, eds. *Recent advances in epilepsy,* Vol. 3. Edinburgh: Churchill Livingstone, 211–232.

Schmidt D. 1989. Adverse effects of antiepileptic drugs in children. *Cleve Clin J Med* 56:S132–S139.

Schmidt D, Haenel F. 1984. Therapeutic plasma levels of phenytoin, phenobarbital, and carbamazepine: individual variation in relation to seizure frequency and type. *Neurology* 34:1252–1255.

Schmidt D, Lampert T. 1990. Differential diagnosis in adults. In: Dam M, Gram L, eds. *Comprehensive epileptology.* New York: Raven Press, 449–471.

Schmidt D, Richter K. 1986. Alternative single anticonvulsant drug therapy for refractory epilepsy. *Ann Neurol* 19:85–87.

Schmidt D, Uteh K. 1986. Progabide for refractory partial epilepsy. *Neurology* 36:317–321.

Schmidt D, Tsai JJ, Janz D. 1983. Generalized tonic-clonic seizures in patients with complex-partial seizures: natural history and prognostic relevance. *Epilepsia* 24:43–48.

Schmidt R, Eviatar L, Nitowsky HM, et al. 1981. Ring chromosome 14: a distinct clinical entity. *J Med Genet* 18: 304–307.

Schmidt D, Tsai JJ, Janz D. 1985. Febrile seizures in patients with complex partial seizures. *Acta Neurol Scand* 72: 68–71

Schmidt D, Einicke I, Haenel F. 1986a. The influence of seizure type on the efficacy of plasma concentrations of phenytoin, phenobarbital and carbamazepine. *Arch Neurol* 43:263–265.

Schmidt D, Rohde M, Wolf P, et al. 1986b. Clobazam for refractory focal epilepsy: a controlled trial. *Arch Neurol* 3:824–826.

Schmitt B, Wohlrab G, Boltshauser E. 1994. Vigabatrin in newly diagnosed infantile spasms. *Neuropediatrics* 25:54.

Schneider H, Vassella F, Karbowski K. 1970. The Lennox syndrome. *Eur Neurol* 4:289–293.

Schoeman JF, Elyas AA, Brett EM, et al. 1984a. Altered ratio of carbamazepine-10,11-epoxide/carbamazepine in plasma of children: evidence of anticonvulsant drug interaction. *Dev Med Child Neurol* 26:749–755.

Schoeman JF, Elyas AA, Brett EM, et al. 1984b. Correlation between plasma carbamazepine-10,11-epoxide concentration and drug side-effects in children with epilepsy. *Dev Med Child Neurol* 26:756–764.

Schoenfeld J, Seidenberg M, Woodard A, et al. 1999. Neuropsychological and behavioural status of children with complex partial seizures. *Dev Med Child Neurol* 41: 724–731.

Schroeder BC, Kubisch C, Stein V, Jentsch TJ. 1998. Moderate loss of function of cyclic-AMP-modulated KCNQ2/KCNQ3 K$^+$ channels causes epilepsy. *Nature* 396:687–690.

Schubert R, Cracco JB. 1992. Familial rectal pain: a type of reflex epilepsy? *Ann Neurol* 32:824–826.

Schulte FJ. 1966. Neonatal convulsions and their relation to epilepsy in early childhood. *Dev Med Child Neurol* 8: 381–392.

Schwartz MS, Scott DF. 1974. Aminophylline-induced seizures. *Epilepsia* 54:501–505.

Schwartz RH, Eaton J, Ainsley-Green A, et al. 1983a. Ketogenic diets in the management of childhood epilepsy. In: Rose CF, ed. *Research progress in epilepsy*. London: Pitman, 326–332.

Schwartz RH, Eaton J, Bower BD, et al. 1983b. Ketogenic diets in the treatment of epilepsy: short-term clinical effects. *Dev Med Child Neurol* 31:145–151.

Schwartz RB, Bravo SM, Klufas RA, et al. 1995. Cyclosporine neurotoxicity and its relationship to hypertensive encephalopathy: CT and MR findings in 16 cases. *AJR Am J Roentgenol* 165:627–631.

Scott O, Macartney FJ, Deverall PB. 1976. Sick sinus syndrome in children. *Arch Dis Child* 51:100–105.

Scott RC, Gadian DG, King D, et al. 2002. Magnetic resonance imaging findings within five days of status epilepticus in children. *Brain* 125:1951–1959.

Seay AR, Bray PF. 1977. Significance of seizure in infants weighing less than 2500 g. *Arch Neurol* 34:381–382.

Sebire G, Devictor D, Huault G, et al. 1992. Coma associated with intense bursts of abnormal movements and long-lasting cognitive disturbances: an acute encephalopathy of obscure origin. *J Pediatr* 121:845–851.

See CC, Newman LJ, Berezin S, et al. 1989. Gastroesophageal reflux-induced hypoxemia in infants with apparent life-threatening events. *Am J Dis Child* 143: 951–954.

Seidenberg M, O'Leary DS, Berent S, et al. 1981. Changes in seizure frequency and test-retest scores on the Wechsler Adult Intelligence Scale. *Epilepsia* 2:75–83.

Seidenberg M, Beck N, Geisser M, et al. 1986. Academic achievement of children with epilepsy. *Epilepsia* 27: 717–723.

Seki T. 1990. Combination treatment of high-dose pyridoxal phosphate and low-dose ACTH in children with West syndrome and related disorders. *Jpn J Psychiatry Neurol* 44:219–237.

Seki Y, Kawahara Y, Hirose M. 1976. The long-term prognosis of infantile spasms followed in school age. *Folia Psychiatr Neurol Jpn* 30:297–306.

Semah F, Picot MC, Adam C, et al. 1996. Is the underlying cause of epilepsy a major prognostic factor for recurrence? *Neurology* 51:1256–1262.

Senanayake N. 1989. Epilepsia arithmetices revisited. *Epilepsy Res* 3:167–173.

Senanayake N. 1990. Familial eating epilepsy. *J Neurol* 237:386–391.

Seppäläinen AM, Similä S. 1971. Electroencephalographic findings in three patients with nonketotic hyperglycinemia. *Epilepsia* 12:101–107.

Seri S, Cerquiglini A, Pisani F. 1998. Spike-induced interference in auditory sensory processing in Landau-Kleffner syndrome. *Electroencephalog Clin Neurophysiol* 108:506–510.

Serratosa JM, Delgado-Escueta AV, Posada I, et al. 1995. The gene for progressive myoclonic epilepsy of the Lafora type maps to chromosome 6q. *Hum Mol Genet* 4:1657–1663.

Serratosa JM, Delgado-Escueta AV, Medina MT, et al. 1996. Clinical and genetic analysis of a large pedigree with juvenile myoclonic epilepsy. *Ann Neurol* 39:187–195.

Serratosa JM, Gomez-Garre P, Gallardo MA, et al. 1999. A novel protein tyrosine phosphatase gene is mutated in progressive myoclonus epilepsy of the Lafora type (EMP2). *Hum Mol Genet* 8:345–352.

Servit Z. 1977. Pharmacological prophylaxis of post-traumatic epilepsy—clinical results and theoretical interpretation. In: Majkowski J, ed. *Posttraumatic epilepsy and pharmacological prophylaxis*. Warsaw: Polish Chapter, International League Against Epilepsy, 183–191.

Servit Z, Musil F. 1981. Prophylactic treatment of post-traumatic epilepsy: results of a long-term follow-up in Czechoslovakia. *Epilepsia* 22:315–320.

Sfaello I, Castelnau P, Blanc N, et al. 2000. Infantile spasms and Menkes disease. *Epileptic Disord* 2:227–230.

Sgrò V, Riva E, Canevini MP, et al. 1995. 4p-syndrome: a chromosomal disorder associated with a particular EEG pattern. *Epilepsia* 36:1206–1214.

Shady JA, Black PM, Kupsky WJ, et al. 1994. Seizures in children with supratentorial astroglial neoplasms. *Pediatr Neurol* 21:23–30.

Shafrir Y, Prensky A. 1995. Acquired epileptiform opercular syndrome: a second case report, review of the literature and comparison to Landau-Kleffner syndrome. *Epilepsia* 36:1050–1057.

Shakir RA, Johnson RH, Lambie DG, et al. 1981. Comparison of sodium valproate and phenytoin as single drug treatment in epilepsy. *Epilepsia* 22:27–33.

Sharf B, Bental E. 1980. Eye closure seizures. In: Wada JA, Penry JK, eds. *Advances in epileptology*, Xth Epilepsy International Symposium. New York: Raven Press.

Sharp JD, Wheeler RB, Lake BD, et al. 1997. Loci for classical and a variant late infantile neuronal ceroid lipofuscinosis map to chromosomes 11p15 and 15q21-23. *Hum Mol Genet* 6:591–595.

Shaw MD, Foy PM. 1991. Epilepsy after craniotomy and the place of prophylactic anticonvulsant drugs: discussion paper. *J R Soc Med* 84:221–223.

Shaw NJ, Livingston JH, Minns RA, et al. 1988. Epilepsy precipitated by bathing. *Dev Med Child Neurol* 30: 108–111.

Sheen VL, Dixon PH, Fox JW, et al. 2001. Mutations in the X-linked filamin 1 gene cause periventricular nodular heterotopia in males as well as in females. *Hum Mol Genet* 10:1775–1783.

Shepherd CW, Stephenson JB. 1992. Seizures and intellectual disability associated with tuberous sclerosis in the west of Scotland. *Dev Med Child Neurol* 34:766–774.

Sherwin AL. 1983. Absence seizures. In: Morselli PL, Pippenger CE, Penry JK, eds. *Antiepileptic drug therapy in pediatrics*. New York: Raven Press, 153–161.

Sherwin AL, Eisen AA, Sokolowski CD. 1973. Anticonvulsant drugs in human brain—correlation of phenobarbital and phenytoin blood levels with plasma. *Arch Neurol* 29:73–77.

Sherwin I, Peron-Magnan P, Bancaud J, et al. 1982. Prevalence of psychosis in epilepsy as a function of the laterality of the epileptogenic lesion. *Arch Neurol* 39:621–625.

Sheth RD, Ronen GM, Goulden KJ, et al. 1995. Clobazam for intractable pediatric epilepsy. *J Child Neurol* 10:205–208.

Sheth RD, Buckley DJ, Gutierrez AR, et al. 1996. Midazolam in the treatment of refractory neonatal seizures. *Clin Neuropharmacol* 19:165–170.

Shewmon DA. 1983. Dissociation between cortical discharges and ictal movements in neonatal seizures. *Ann Neurol* 14:368.

Shewmon DA, Erwin RJ. 1988. Focal spike-induced cerebral dysfunction is related to the after-coming slow wave. *Ann Neurol* 23:131–137.

Shewmon DA, Shields WD, Chugani HT, et al. 1990. Contrasts between pediatric and adult epilepsy surgery: rationale and strategy for focal resection. *J Epilepsy* 3 (Suppl.):141–155.

Shewmon A, Shields WD, Sankar R, et al. 1997. Follow-up on infants with surgery for catastrophic epilepsy. In: Tuxhorn I, Holthausen H, Boenigk H, eds. *Paediatric epilepsy syndromes and their surgical treatment.* London: John Libbey, 513–525.

Shi VE, Efron ML, Mose HW. 1969. Hyperornithinemia, hyperammonemia and homocitrullinuria. A new disorder of amino acid metabolism associated with myoclonic seizures and mental retardation. *Am J Dis Child* 117:83–92.

Shibasaki H, Yamashita Y, Kuroiwa Y. 1978. Electroencephalographic study of myoclonus: myoclonus-related cortical spikes and high-amplitude somatosensory evoked potentials. *Brain* 101:447–460.

Shibasaki H, Ikeda A, Nagamine T, et al. 1994. Cortical reflex negative myoclonus. *Brain* 117:477–486.

Shields WD. 1997. Defining medical intractability: the differences in children compared to adults. In: Tuxhorn I, Holthausen H, Boenigk H, eds. *Paediatric epilepsy syndromes and their surgical treatment.* London: John Libbey, 93–98.

Shields WD, Saslow E. 1983. Myoclonic, atonic and absence seizures following institution of carbamazepine therapy in children. *Neurology* 33:487–1489.

Shields WD, Lake JL, Chugani HT. 1985. Amantadine in the treatment of refractory epilepsy: an open trial in 10 patients. *Neurology* 35:579–581.

Shields WD, Duchowny MS, Holmes GL. 1992a. Surgically remediable syndromes of infancy and early childhood. In: Engel J Jr, ed. *Surgical treatment of epilepsies*, 2nd ed. New York: Raven Press, 35–48.

Shields WD, Shewmon DA, Chugani HT, et al. 1992b. Treatment of infantile spasms: medical or surgical? *Epilepsia* 33:S26–S31.

Shields WD, Shewmon DA, Peacock WJ, et al. 1999. Surgery for the treatment of medically intractable infantile spasms: a cautionary case. *Epilepsia* 40:1305–1308.

Shimizu H, Abe J, Futagi Y, et al. 1982. Antiepileptic effects of clobazam in children. *Brain Dev* 4:57–62.

Shinnar S. 1998. Prolonged febrile seizures and mesial temporal sclerosis. *Ann Neurol* 43:411–412.

Shinnar S, Babb TL. 1997. Long-term sequelae of status epilepticus. In: Engel J Jr, Pedley JA, eds. *Epilepsy: a comprehensive textbook*, Vol. 1. Philadelphia: Lippincott-Raven, 755–763.

Shinnar S, Gross-Tsur V. 2001. Discontinuing antiepileptic drug therapy. In: Wyllie E, ed. *The treatment of epilepsy*, 3rd ed. Philadelphia: Lippincott Williams & Wilkins, 811–819.

Shinnar S, Pellock JM. 2002. Update on the epidemiology and prognosis of pediatric epilepsy. *J Child Neurol* 17:S4–S17.

Shinnar S, Vining EP, Mellits ED, et al. 1985. Discontinuing antiepileptic medication in children with epilepsy with two years without seizures. A prospective study. *N Engl J Med* 313:976–980.

Shinnar S, Berg AT, Moshé SL, et al. 1990. Risk of recurrence following a first unprovoked seizure in childhood: a prospective study. *Pediatrics* 85:1076–1085.

Shinnar S, Maytal J, Krasnoff L, et al. 1992. Recurrent status epilepticus in children. *Ann Neurol* 31:598–604.

Shinnar S, Berg AT, Ptachewich Y, et al. 1993. Sleep state and the risk of seizure recurrence following a first unprovoked seizure in childhood. *Neurology* 43:701–706.

Shinnar S, Berg AT, Moshé SL, et al. 1994. Discontinuing antiepileptic drugs in children with epilepsy: a prospective study. *Ann Neurol* 35:534–545.

Shinnar S, Pellock JM, Moshé SL, et al. 1997. In whom does status epilepticus occur: age-related differences in children. *Epilepsia* 38:907–914.

Shinnar S, Berg AT, O'Dell C, et al. 2000. Predictors of multiple seizures in a cohort of children prospectively followed from the time of their first unprovoked seizure. *Ann Neurol* 48:140–147.

Shoffner JM, Lott MT, Lezza AM, et al. 1990. Myoclonic epilepsy and ragged-red fiber disease (MERRF) is associated with a mitochondrial DNA tRNA(Lys) mutation. *Cell* 61:931–937.

Shorvon SD. 1984. The temporal aspects of prognosis in epilepsy. *J Neurol Neurosurg Psychiatry* 47:1157–1165.

Shorvon SD. 1987. Non-convulsive status epilepticus. *Lancet* 1:958–959.

Shorvon S. 1994. *Status epilepticus: its clinical features and treatment in children and adults.* Cambridge: Cambridge University Press.

Shorvon SD, Farmer PJ. 1988. Epilepsy in developing countries: a review of epidemiological, sociocultural and treatment aspects. *Epilepsia* 29:S36–S54.

Shorvon SD, Reynolds EH. 1980. Reduction in polypharmacy for epilepsy. In: Johanessen SI, Morselli CE, Pippenger CE, et al., eds. *Antiepileptic therapy: advances in drug monitoring.* New York: Raven Press, 203–209.

Shorvon SD, Reynolds EH. 1982a. Anticonvulsant peripheral neuropathy: a clinical and electrophysiological study of patients on single drug treatment with phenytoin, carbamazepine or barbiturates. *J Neurol Neurosurg Psychiatry* 45:620–626.

Shorvon SD, Reynolds EH. 1982b. Early prognosis of epilepsy. *BMJ* 285:1699–1701.

Shorvon SD, Chadwick D, Galbraith A, et al. 1978. One drug for epilepsy. *BMJ* 1:474–476.

Shoumaker RD, Bennett DR, Bray PF, Curless RG. 1974. Clinical and EEG manifestations of an unusual aphasic syndrome in children. *Neurology* 24:10–16.

Shuper A, Zalzberg J, Weitz R, et al. 1991. Jitteriness beyond the neonatal period: a benign pattern of movement in infancy. *J Child Neurol* 6:243–245.

Siebeling BM, Barker DJ, Binnie CD, et al. 1988. Psychological effects of subclinical EEG discharges in children. II: General intelligence tests. *Epilepsy Res* 2:117–121.

Siemes H, Spohr HL, Michael TH, et al. 1988. Therapy of infantile spasms with valproate: results of a prospective study. *Epilepsia* 29:553–560.

Siemes H, Brandl U, Spohr HL, et al. 1998. Long-term follow-up study of vigabatrin in pre-treated children with West Syndrome. *Seizure* 7:293–297.

Silfvenius H, Sâisä J, Olivecrona M, et al. 1997. The intracarotid amytal test in children: survey and experiences. In: Tuxhorn I, Holthausen H, Boenigk H, eds. *Paediatric epilepsy syndromes and their surgical treatment.* London: John Libbey, 672–680.

Sillanpää M. 1973. Medico-social prognosis of children with epilepsy: epidemiological study and analysis of 245 patients. *Acta Paediatr Scand* 237(Suppl.):1–104.

Sillanpää M. 1981. Carbamazepine. Pharmacology and clinical uses. *Acta Neurol Scand Suppl* 88:1–202.

Sillanpää M. 1983. Social functioning and seizure status of young adults with onset of epilepsy in childhood. An epidemiological 20-year follow-up study. *Acta Neurol Scand Suppl* 96:1–81.

Sillanpää M. 1990. Children with epilepsy as adults: outcome after 30 years of follow-up. *Acta Paediatr Scand Suppl* 368:1–78.

Sillanpää M. 2000. Long-term outcome of epilepsy. *Epileptic Disord* 2:79–88.

Sillanpää M, Shinnar S. 2002. Status epilepticus in a population-based cohort with childhood-onset epilepsy in Finland. *Ann Neurol* 52:303–310.

Sillanpää M, Pynnonen S, Laippala S, et al. 1979. Carbamazepine (Tegretol) in the treatment of partial epileptic seizures in infants and young children: a preliminary study. *Epilepsia* 20:563–569.

Sillanpää M, Jalava M, Kaleva O, et al. 1998a. Long-term prognosis of seizures with onset in childhood. *N Engl J Med* 338:1715–1722.

Sills GJ, Brodie MJ. 2001. Update on the mechanisms of action of antiepileptic drugs. *Epileptic Disord* 3:165–172.

Sills MA, Forsythe WI, Haidukewych D, et al. 1986. The medium chain triglyceride diet and intractable epilepsy. *Arch Dis Child* 61:1168–1172.

Silva ML, Cieuta C, Guerrini R, et al. 1996. Early clinical and EEG features of infantile spasms in Down syndrome. *Epilepsia* 37:977–982.

Silver JM, Shin C, McNamara JO. 1991. Antiepileptogenic effects of conventional anticonvulsants in the kindling model of epilepsy. *Ann Neurol* 29:356–363.

Silverstein F, Johnston MV. 1984. Cerebrospinal fluid monoamine metabolites in patients with infantile spasms. *Neurology* 34:102–105.

Silvestri R, De Domenico P, Musolino R, et al. 1989. Nocturnal complex partial seizures precipitated by REM sleep–a case report. *Eur Neurol* 29:80–85.

Simard JM, Garcia-Bengochea F, Ballinger WE, et al. 1986. Cavernous angioma: a review of 126 collected and 12 new clinical cases. *Neurosurgery* 18:162–172.

Simon RP. 1985. Management of status epilepticus. In: Pedley TA, Meldrum BS, eds. *Recent advances in epilepsy*, Vol. 2. Edinburgh: Churchill Livingstone, 137–160.

Simon D, Penry JK. 1975. Sodium di-*N*-propylacetate in the treatment of epilepsy. A review. *Epilepsia* 16:549–573.

Simonsen N, Mollgaard V, Lund M. 1976a. A controlled clinical and electroencephalographic study of myoclonic epilepsy (impulsive-petit mal): preliminary report. In: Janz D, ed. *Epileptology.* Stuttgart: Thieme, 41–48.

Simonsen N, Olsen PZ, Kulh V, et al. 1976b. A comparative study between carbamazepine and diphenylhydantoin in psychomotor epilepsy. *Epilepsia* 17:169–176.

Simonsson H. 1972. Incontinentia pigmenti, Bloch-Sulzbergers syndrome associated with infantile spasms. *Acta Paediatr Scand* 61:612–614.

Sindrup EH, Kristensen O. 1980. Psychosis and temporal lobe epilepsy. In: Kulig BM, Meinardi H, Stores G, eds. *Epilepsy and behavior '79.* Lisse, The Netherlands; Swets and Zeitlinger, 133–139.

Singer WD, Rabe EF, Haller JS. 1980. The effect of ACTH therapy upon infantile spasms. *J Pediatr* 96:485–489.

Singer WD, Haller JS, Sullivan LR, et al. 1982. The value of neuroradiology in infantile spasms. *J Pediatr* 100: 47–50.

Singh BJ, Strobos RJ. 1980. Epilepsia partialis continua associated with nonketotic hyperglycemia: clinical and biological profile in 21 patients. *Ann Neurol* 8:155–160.

Singh NA, Charlier C, Stauffer D, et al. 1998. A novel potassium channel gene, KCNQ2, is mutated in an inherited epilepsy of newborns. *Nat Genet* 18:25–29.

Singh R, Scheffer I, Crossland K, et al. 1999a. Generalized epilepsy with febrile seizures plus: a common childhood-onset genetic epilepsy syndrome. *Ann Neurol* 45: 75–81.

Singh R, Scheffer IE, Whitehouse W, et al. 1999b. Severe myoclonic epilepsy of infancy is part of the spectrum of generalized epilepsy with febrile seizures plus (GEFS+) [Abstract]. *Epilepsia* 40(Suppl. 2):175.

Singh R, Andermann E, Whitehouse WP, et al. 2001. Severe myoclonic epilepsy of infancy: extended spectrum of GEFS+? *Epilepsia* 42:837–844.

Singh R, Gardner RJ, Crossland KM, et al. 2002. Chromosomal abnormalities and epilepsy: a review for clinicians and gene hunters. *Epilepsia* 43:127–140.

Singhi S, Murthy A, Singhi P, et al. 2002. Continuous midazolam versus diazepam for refractory convulsive status epilepticus. *J Child Neurol* 17:106–110.

Sirven JI, Sperling MR, French JA, et al. 1996. Significance of simple partial seizures in temporal lobe epilepsy. *Epilepsia* 37:450–454.

Sisodiya SM, Free SL, Stevens JM, et al. 1995. Widespread cerebral structural changes in patients with cortical dysgenesis and epilepsy. *Brain* 118:1039–1050.

Sisodiya SM, Free S, Fish DR, et al. 1999. Novel magnetic resonance imaging methods for quantifying changes in the cortical ribbon in patients with epilepsy. *Adv Neurol* 81:81–87.

Sivelle G, Kahane P, de Saint-Martin A, et al. 1995. La multilocalité des lésions dans la sclérose tubéreuse de Bourneville contre-indique-t-elle une approche chirurgicale? *Epilepsies* 7:451–464.

Sivenius J, Kälviäinen R, Ylinen A, et al. 1991a. Double-blind study of gabapentin in the treatment of partial seizures. *Epilepsia* 32:539–542.

Sivenius J, Ylinen A, Murros K, et al. 1991b. Vigabatrin in drug-resistant partial epilepsy: a 5-year follow-up study. *Neurology* 41:562–565.

Slater R. 1979. Benign recurrent vertigo. *J Neurol Neurosurg Psychiatry* 42:363–367.

Slater E, Moran PA. 1969. The schizophrenia-like psychoses of epilepsy: relation between ages of onset. *Br J Psychiatry* 115:599–600.

Slatter KH. 1968. Some clinical and EEG findings in patients with migraine. *Brain* 91:85–98.

Sleat DE, Donnelly RJ, Lackland H, et al. 1997. Associations of mutations in a lysosomal protein with classical late-infantile neuronal ceroid lipofuscinosis. *Science* 277:1802–1805.

Sleat DE, Gin RM, Sohar I, et al. 1999. Mutational analysis of the defective protease in classic late-infantile neuronal ceroid-lipofuscinosis: a neurodegenerative lysosomal storage disorder. *Am J Hum Genet* 64:1511–1523.

Sloviter RS, Pedley TA. 1998. Subtle hippocampal malformation: importance in febrile seizures and development of epilepsy. *Neurology* 50:846–849.

Smaje JC, Davidson C, Teasdale GM. 1987. Sino-atrial arrest due to temporal lobe epilepsy. *J Neurol Neurosurg Psychiatry* 50:112–113.

Smith BH. 1960. Vestibular disturbances in epilepsy. *Neurology* 10:465–469.

Smith SJ. 1995. Clinical neurophysiology in humans. In: Duncan JS, Panayiotopoulos CP, eds. *Typical absences and related syndromes*. London: Churchill Communication Europe, 92–101.

Smith AJ, Wallace SJ. 1982. Febrile convulsions: intellectual progress in relation to anticonvulsant therapy and to recurrence of fits. *Arch Dis Child* 57:104–107.

Smith I, Clayton BF, Wolf OH. 1975. New variant of phenylketonuria with progressive neurological illness unresponsive to phenylalanine restriction. *Lancet* 1:1108–1112.

Smith DB, Mattson RH, Cramer JA, et al. 1987. Results of a nationwide Veterans Administration Cooperative study comparing the efficacy and toxicity of carbamazepine, phenobarbital, phenytoin and primidone. *Epilepsia* 28:S50–S58.

Smith PE, Howell SJ, Owen L, Blumhardt LD. 1989. Profiles of instant heart rate during partial seizures. *Electroencephalogr Clin Neurophysiol* 72:207–217.

Smith D, Baker G, Davies G, et al. 1993. Outcome with add-on treatment with lamotrigine in partial epilepsy. *Epilepsia* 34:312–322.

Snead OC III. 1990. Treatment of infantile spasms. *Pediatr Neurol* 6:147–150.

Snead OC, Chiron C. 1994. Medical treatment. In: Dulac O, Chugani HT, Dalla Bernardina B, eds. *Infantile spasms and West syndrome*. London: WB Saunders, 244–256.

Snead OC III, Hosey LC. 1985. Exacerbation of seizures in children by carbamazepine. *N Engl J Med* 313:916–921.

Snead OC, Martien KM. 2001. Adrenocorticotropin and steroids. In: Wyllie E, ed, *The treatment of epilepsy*, 3rd ed. Philadelphia: Lippincott Williams & Wilkins, 969–975.

Snead OC, Benton JW, Myers GJ. 1983. ACTH and prednisone in childhood seizure disorders. *Neurology* 33:966–970.

Snead OC, Benton JW, Hosey LC, et al. 1989. Treatment of infantile spasms with high-dose ACTH: efficacy and plasma levels of ACTH and cortisol. *Neurology* 39:1027–1031.

Snead OC III, Chen LS, Mitchell WG, et al. 1996. Usefulness of [18F]fluorodeoxyglucose positron emission tomography in pediatric epilepsy surgery. *Pediatr Neurol* 14:98–107.

Snoek JW, Minderhoud JM, Wilmink JT. 1984. Delayed deterioration following mild head injury in children. *Brain* 107:15–36.

Snyder RD. 1984. Seizures in childhood bacterial meningitis. *Ann Neurol* 16:395–396.

So N. 1993. Epileptic auras. In: Wyllie E, ed. *The treatment of epilepsy: principles and practices*. Baltimore: Williams & Wilkins, 1993.

So NK. 1995. Atonic phenomena and partial seizures: a reappraisal. In: Fahn S, Hallett M, Lüders HO, Marsden CD, eds. *Negative motor phenomena*. Advances in neurology, Vol. 67. Philadelphia: Lippincott-Raven, 29–39.

So NK, Andermann F. 1998. Rasmussen's syndrome. In: Engel J Jr, Pedley TA, eds. *Epilepsy: a comprehensive textbook*, Vol. 3. Philadelphia: Lippincott Raven, 2379–2388.

So NK, Gloor P. 1991. Electroencephalographic and electrocorticographic findings in chronic encephalitis of Rasmussen type. In: Andermann F, ed. *Chronic encephalitis and epilepsy: Rasmussen's syndrome*. Boston: Butterworth-Heinemann, 37–45.

So EL, King DW, Murvin AJ. 1984. Misdiagnosis of complex absence seizures. *Arch Neurol* 41:640–641.

So N, Gloor P, Quesney LF, et al. 1989a. Depth electrode investigations in patients with bitemporal epileptiform activity. *Ann Neurol* 25:423–431.

So N, Olivier A, Andermann F, et al. 1989b. Results of surgical treatment in patients with bitemporal epileptiform abnormalities. *Ann Neurol* 25:432–439.

So EL, Lai CW, Pellock J, et al. 1992. Safety and efficacy of valproate and carbamazepine in the treatment of complex partial seizures. *J Epilepsy* 5:149–152.

Soffer D, Melamed E, Assaf Y, et al. 1986. Hemispheric brain damage in unilateral status epilepticus. *Ann Neurol* 20:737–740.

Sofia RD, Kramer L, Perhach JL, et al. 1995. Felbamate. In: Lévy R, Mattson R, Meldrum B, et al., eds. *Antiepileptic drugs,* 4th ed. New York: Raven Press, 791–797.

Sofijanov NG. 1982. Clinical evolution and prognosis of childhood epilepsies. *Epilepsia* 23:61–69.

Sofijanov N, Emoto S, Kuturek M, et al. 1992. Febrile seizures: clinical characteristics and initial EEG. *Epilepsia* 33:52–57.

Somerville ER, Bruni J. 1983. Tonic status epilepticus presenting as confusional state. *Ann Neurol* 13:549–551.

Sonnen AE. 1980. Epilepsy and swimming. In: *Epilepsy, a clinical and experimental research monographs of neurological sciences*, Vol. 5. Basel: Karger, 265–270.

Sonnen AE. 1991. How to live with epilepsy. In: Dam M, Gram L, eds. *Comprehensive epileptology*. New York: Raven Press, 753–767.

Sorel L. 1964. L'épilepsie myokinétique grave de la première enfance avec pointe-onde lente (petit mal variant) et son traitement. *Rev Neurol (Paris)* 116:110–115

Sorel L. 1972. 196 cases of infantile myoclonic encephalopathy with hypsarrhythmia (IMEH: West syndrome) treated with ACTH. Danger of synthetic ACTH [Abstract]. *Electroencephalog Clin Neurophysiol* 32:576.

Sorel L, Rucquoi-Ponsar J. 1969. L'épilepsie fonctionnelle de maturation. *Rev Neurol (Paris)* 121:288–297.

Sossey-Alaoui K, Hartung AJ, Guerrini R, et al. 1998. Human double cortin (DCX) and the homologous gene in mouse encode a putative Ca^{2+}-dependent signaling protein which is mutated in human X-linked neuronal migration defects. *Hum Mol Genet* 7:1327–1332.

Souner R, Di Mascio A. 1978. Extrapyramidal syndromes and other neurological side effects of psychotropic drugs. In: Lipton MA, Di Mascio A, Killman AF, eds. *Psychopharmacology—a generation of progress.* New York: Raven Press.

Southall DP, Talbert DG, Johnson P, et al. 1985. Prolonged expiratory apnea: a disorder resulting in episodes of severe arterial hypoxaemia in infants and young children. *Lancet* 2:571–577.

Southall DP, Stephens V, Abraham N, et al. 1987. Prolonged apnoea with severe arterial hypoxaemia resulting from complex partial seizures. *Dev Med Child Neurol* 29:784–789.

Sowa MV, Pituck S. 1989. Prolonged spontaneous complex visual hallucinations and illusions as ictal phenomena. *Epilepsia* 30:524–526.

Sozuer DT, Atakli D, Atay T, et al. 1996. Evaluation of various antiepileptic drugs in juvenile myoclonic epilepsy [Abstract]. *Epilepsia* 37(Suppl. 4):128.

Specht U, Boenigk HE, Wolf P. 1989. Discontinuation of clonazepam after long-term treatment. *Epilepsia* 30:458–463.

Spencer SS. 1981. Depth electroencephalography in selection of refractory epilepsy for surgery. *Ann Neurol* 9:207–214.

Spencer SS. 1988. Corpus callosotomy in the treatment of intractable seizures. In: Pedley TA, Meldrum BS, eds. *Recent advances in epilepsy,* Vol. 4. Edinburgh: Churchill Livingstone, 181–204.

Spencer SS, Spencer DD. 1991. *Surgery for epilepsy.* Cambridge, MA: Blackwell Scientific Publications.

Spencer SS, Spencer DD, Williamson PD, et al. 1981. Ictal effects of anticonvulsant medication withdrawal in epileptic patients. *Epilepsia* 22:297–307.

Spencer SS, Spencer DD, Williamson PD, et al. 1982. The localizing value of depth electroencephalography in 32 patients with refractory epilepsy. *Ann Neurol* 12:248–253.

Spencer DD, Spencer SS, Mattson RH, et al. 1984a. Intracerebral masses in patients with intractable partial epilepsy. *Neurology* 34:432–436.

Spencer SS, Spencer DD, Glaser GH, et al. 1984b. More intense focal seizure types after callosal section: the role of inhibition. *Ann Neurol* 16:686–693.

Spencer SS, Spencer DD, Williamson PD, et al. 1985. Effects of corpus callosum section on secondary bilaterally synchronous interictal EEG discharges. *Neurology* 35:1689–1694.

Spencer SS, Spencer DD, Sass KJ, et al. 1987a. Partial versus total corpus callosotomy for epilepsy. In: Wolf P, Dam M, Janz D, et al., eds. *Advances in epileptology,* Vol. 16. New York: Raven Press, 323–325.

Spencer SS, Williamson PD, Spencer DD, et al. 1987b. Human hippocampal seizure spread studied by depth and subdural recording: the hippocampal commissure. *Epilepsia* 28:479–489.

Spencer SS, McCarthy G, Spencer DD. 1993. Diagnosis of medial temporal lobe seizure onset: relative specificity and sensitivity of quantitative MRI. *Neurology* 43:2117–2124.

Spencer SS, Sperling MR, Shewmon DA. 1997. Intracranial electrodes. In: Engel J Jr, Pedley TA, Aicardi J, et al., eds. *Epilepsy: a comprehensive textbook,* Vol. 2.

Philadelphia: Lippincott Williams & Wilkins, 1719–1748.

Spencer SS, Novotny E, de Lanerolle N, et al. 2001. Mesial temporal sclerosis: electroclinical and pathological correlations and applications to limbic epilepsy in childhood. In: Avanzini G, Beaumanoir A, Mira L, eds. *Limbic seizures in children.* Paris: John Libbey, 41–54.

Sperling MR, O'Connor MJ. 1989. Comparison of depth and subdural electrodes in recording temporal lobe seizures. *Neurology* 39:1497–1504.

Sperling MR, Mendius JR, Engel J Jr. 1986a. Mesial temporal spikes: a simultaneous comparison of sphenoidal, nasopharyngeal, and ear electrodes. *Epilepsia* 27:81–86.

Sperling MR, Pritchard PB, Engel J Jr, et al. 1986b. Prolactin in partial epilepsy: an indicator of limbic seizures. *Ann Neurol* 20:716–722.

Sperling MR, Feldman H, Kinman J, et al. 1999. Seizure control and mortality in epilepsy. *Ann Neurol* 46:45–50.

Sperner J, Schmauser I, Bitmer R, et al. 1990. MR-imaging findings in children with Sturge-Weber syndrome. *Neuropediatrics* 21:146–152.

Spitz MC. 1992. Severe burns as a consequence of seizures in patients with epilepsy. *Epilepsia* 33:103–107.

Spitzer AR, Boyle JT, Tuchman DN, et al. 1984. Awake apnea associated with gastroesophageal reflux: a specific clinical syndrome. *J Pediatr* 104:200–205.

Spreafico R, Battaglia G, Arcelli P, et al. 1998. Cortical dysplasia: an immunocytochemical study of three patients. *Neurology* 50:27–36.

Sprung C, Baerwald R, Henkes H, Schorner W. 1989. A comparative study of CT and MRI in midline tumors of childhood and adolescence. *Childs Nerv Syst* 5:102–106.

Sreenan C, Bhargava R, Robertson CM. 2000. Cerebral infarction in the term newborn: clinical presentation and long-term outcome. *J Pediatr* 137:351–355.

Staden UE, Isaacs E, Boyd SG, et al. 1998. Language dysfunction in children with rolandic epilepsy. *Neuropediatrics* 29:242–248.

Stafstrom CE, Konkol RJ. 1994. Infantile spasms in children with Down syndrome. *Dev Med Child Neurol* 36:576–585.

Stafstrom CE, Patxot OF, Gilmore HE, et al. 1991. Seizures in children with Down syndrome: etiology, characteristics and outcome. *Dev Med Child Neurol* 33:191–200.

Stagno SJ. 2001. Psychiatric aspects of epilepsy. In: Wyllie E, ed. *The treatment of epilepsy: principles and practice,* 3rd ed. Philadelphia: Lippincott Williams & Wilkins, 1227–1242.

Staudt F, Scholl M, Coen RW, et al. 1982. Phenobarbital therapy in neonatal seizures and the prognostic value of the EEG. *Neuropediatrics* 13:24–33.

Staunton T, Andermann F, Melançon D, et al. 1983. Focal macrogyria: a recognizable development disorder presenting with intractable focal seizures [Absract]. *Ann Neurol* 14:152A.

Stecker MM, Kramer TH, Raps EC, et al. 1998. Treatment of refractory status epilepticus with propofol: clinical and pharmacokinetic findings. *Epilepsia* 39:18–26.

Stefan H. 1987. Re-evaluation of the classification of epileptic seizures and epilepsies. *Clin Neurol Neurosurg* 89(Suppl. 1):39–40.

Stefan H, Burr W, Hidenbrand K, et al. 1982. Basic temporal structure of absence symptoms. In: Akimoto H, Kazamatsuri H, Seino M, et al., eds. *Advances in epileptology*, XIIIth Epilepsy International Symposium. New York: Raven Press, 55–60.

Stefan H, Buff W, Fichsel H, et al. 1984. Intensive follow-up monitoring in patients with once daily evening administration of sodium valproate. *Epilepsia* 25:152–160.

Stefan H, Schäfer H, Kuhnen C, et al. 1988. Clinical monitoring during carbamazepine slow-release, once-daily monotherapy. *Epilepsia* 29:571–577.

Stefan H, Bauer J, Feistel H, et al. 1990a. Regional cerebral blood flow during focal seizures of temporal and frontocentral onset. *Ann Neurol* 7:162–166.

Stefan H, Schneider S, Abraham-Fuchs K, et al. 1990b. Magnetic source localization in focal epilepsy. Multichannel magnetoencephalography correlated with magnetic resonance brain imaging. *Brain* 113:1347–1359.

Stefansson SD, Darby CE, Wilkins AJ, et al. 1977. Television epilepsy and pattern sensitivity. *BMJ* 2:88–90.

Steffenburg S, Gillberg CL, Steffenburg U, et al. 1996. Autism in Angelman syndrome: a population-based study. *Pediatr Neurol* 14:131–136.

Steffenburg U, Hedström A, Lindroth A, et al. 1998. Intractable epilepsy in a population-based study of mentally retarded children. *Epilepsia* 39:767–775.

Steinhoff BJ, Kruse R. 1992. Bromide treatment of pharmaco-resistant epilepsies with generalized tonic-clonic seizures: a clinical study. *Brain Dev* 14:144–149.

Steinhoff BJ, Neusüss K, Thegeder H, et al. 1996. Leisure time activity and physical fitness in patients with epilepsy. *Epilepsia* 37:1221–1227.

Steinlein OK. 2001. Genes and mutations in idiopathic epilepsy. *Am J Med Genet* 106:139–145.

Steinlein OK, Mulley J, Propping P, et al. 1995a. A missense mutation in the neuronal nicotinic acetylcholine receptor alpha 4 subunit is associated with autosomal dominant nocturnal frontal lobe epilepsy. *Nat Genet* 11:201–203.

Steinlein O, Schuster V, Fischer C, et al. 1995b. Benign familial neonatal convulsions: confirmation of genetic heterogeneity and further evidence for a second locus on chromosome 8q. *Hum Genet* 95:411–415.

Steinlein OK, Magnusson A, Stoodt J, et al. 1997. An insertion mutation of the CHRNA4 gene in a family with autosomal dominant nocturnal frontal lobe epilepsy. *Hum Mol Genet* 6:943–947.

Stengel-Rutkoswki S, Warkotsch A, Schimanek P, Stene J. 1984. Familial Wolf's syndrome with a hidden 4p deletion by translocation of an 8p segment. Unbalanced inheritance from a maternal translocation (4;8) (p15.3;p22). Case report, review and risk estimates. *Clin Genet* 25:500–521.

Stensman R, Ursing B. 1971. Epilepsy precipitated by hot-water immersion. *Neurology* 21:559–562.

Stephani U, ed. 2000. The sectrum of epileptic disorders. *Epileptic Disord* 2:S1–S66.

Stephenson JB. 1976. Two types of febrile seizures: anoxic (syncopal) and epileptic mechanisms differentiated by oculocardiac reflex. *BMJ* 2:726–728.

Stephenson JB. 1978a. Non-epileptic television syncope. *Br Med J* 1:1622.

Stephenson JB. 1978b. Reflex anoxic seizures ('white breath-holding'): nonepileptic vagal attacks. *Arch Dis Child* 53:193–200.

Stephenson JB. 1983. Febrile convulsions and reflex anoxic seizures. In: Rose FC, ed. *Research progress in epilepsy*. London: Pitman, 244–252.

Stephenson JB. 1990. *Fits and faints*. MacKeith, London.

Stephenson JB. 1996. Non-epileptic seizures, anoxic-epileptic seizures, and epileptic-anoxic seizures. In: Wallace SJ, ed. *Epilepsy in children*. London: Chapman and Hall, 5–26.

Stephenson JB. 1998. Cerebral palsy. In: Engel J Jr, Pedley TA, eds. *Epilepsy: a comprehensive textbook*, Vol. 3. Lippincott-Raven, Philadelphia, 2571–2577.

Stephenson JB. 2001. Anoxic seizures: self-terminating syncopes. *Epileptic Disord* 3:3–6.

Stephenson JB, Byrne KE. 1983. Pyridoxine responsive epilepsy: expanded pyridoxine dependency? *Arch Dis Child* 58:1034–1036.

Steriade M, McCormick DA, Sejnowski T. 1993. Thalamo-cortical oscillations in the sleeping and aroused brain. *Science* 262:679–685.

Stevens JR. 1959. Emotional activation of the electroencephalogram in patients with convulsive disorders. *J Nerv Ment Dis* 129:339–342.

Stevens JR. 1975. Interictal clinical manifestations of complex partial seizures. In: Penry JK, Daly D, eds. *Partial seizures and their treatment*. Advances in neurology, Vol. 11. New York: Raven Press, 85–112.

Stevens JR. 1983. Psychosis and epilepsy. *Ann Neurol* 14:347–348.

Stibler H, Westerberg B, Hanefeld F, Hagberg B. 1993. Carbohydrate-deficient glycoprotein (CDG) syndrome—a new variant, type III. *Neuropediatrics* 24:51–52.

Stodieck SR, Wieser HG. 1986. Autonomic phenomena in temporal lobe epilepsy. *J Auton Nerv Syst* (Suppl.): 611–621.

Stoffels C, Munari C, Brunie-Lozano E, et al. 1980. Manifestations automatiques dans les crises épileptiques partielles complexes d'origine frontale. *Bolletino Lega Italiana contre l'Epilepsia* 29/30:111–113.

Stokes MJ, Downham MA, Webb JK, et al. 1977. Viruses and febrile convulsions. *Arch Dis Child* 52:129–133.

Stone S, Lange LS. 1986. Syncope and sudden unexpected death attributed to carbamazepine in a 20-year-old epileptic. *J Neurol Neurosurg Psychiatry* 49:1460–1461.

Stores G. 1971. Cognitive functions in children with epilepsy. *Dev Med Child Neurol* 13:390–393.

Stores G. 1975. Behavioral effects of anti-epileptic drugs. *Dev Med Child Neurol* 17:647–658.

Stores G. 1978. School-children with epilepsy at risk for learning and behaviour problems. *Dev Med Child Neurol* 20:502–508.

Stores G. 1980. Children with epilepsy: psychosocial aspects. In: Herman B, ed. *A multidisciplinary handbook of epilepsy*. Springfield, IL: Charles C Thomas Publishers.

Stores G. 1981. Memory impairment in children with epilepsy. *Acta Neurol Scand Suppl* 89:21–29.

Stores G, Zaiwalla Z, Bergel N. 1991. Frontal lobe complex partial seizures in children: a form of epilepsy at particular risk of misdiagnosis. *Dev Med Child Neurol* 33: 998–1009.

Strandjord RE. 1984. Drug treatment of seizures in epilepsy. *Acta Neurol Scand* 69(Suppl.):67–76.

Strandjord RE, Gilhus NE. 1984. Single drug therapy with phenobarbital (PB) in patients with epilepsy: serum levels and clinical effect. *Acta Neurol Scand* 69(Suppl. 98):101–102.

Strandjord RE, Johannessen SI. 1980. Single drug therapy with carbamazepine in patients with epilepsy: serum levels and clinical effects. *Epilepsia* 21:655–662.

Striano S, Striano P, Cirillo S, et al. 2002. Small hypothalamic hamartomas and gelastic seizures. *Epileptic Disord* 4:129–133.

Stromme P, Sundet K, Mork C, et al. 1999. X linked mental retardation and infantile spasms in a family: new clinical data and linkage to Xp11.4-Xp22.11. *J Med Genet* 36:374–378.

Stromme P, Mangelsdorf ME, Shaw MA, et al. 2002. Mutations in the human ortholog of Aristaless cause X-linked mental retardation and epilepsy. *Nat Genet* 30:441–445.

Sugai K, Fukuyama Y, Yasuda K, et al. 2001. Clinical and pedigree study on familial cases of West syndrome in Japan. *Brain Dev* 123:558–564.

Sugama S, Kusano K. 1994. Monozygous twin with polymicrogyria and normal co-twin. *Pediatr Neurol* 11:62–63.

Sugama M, Oguni H, Fukuyama Y. 1987. Clinical and electroencephalographic study of severe myoclonic epilepsy in infancy. *Jpn J Psychiatr Neurol* 41:463–465.

Sugawara T, Tsurubuchi Y, Agarwala KL, et al. 2001. A missense mutation of the Na+ channel alpha II subunit gene Na(v)1.2 in a patient with febrile and afebrile seizures causes channel dysfunction. *Proc Natl Acad Sci U S A* 98:6384–6389.

Sugawara T, Mazaki-Miyazaki E, Fukushima K, et al. 2002. Frequent mutations of *SCN1A* in severe myoclonic epilepsy in infancy *Neurology* 58:1122 –1124.

Sugimoto T, Araki A, Yasuhara A, et al. 1994. Angelman syndrome in three siblings: genetic model of epilepsy associated with chromosomal DNA deletion of the GABA$_A$ receptor. *Jpn J Psychiatry Neurol* 42:271–273.

Sugimoto T, Otsubo H, Hwang P, et al. 1999. Outcome of epilepsy surgery in the first three years of life. *Epilepsia* 40:560–565.

Sujansky E, Conradi S. 1995. Sturge-Weber syndrome: age of onset of seizures and glaucoma and the prognosis for affected children. *J Child Neurol* 10:49–58.

Sutherling WW, Crandall PH, Engel J Jr, et al. 1987. The magnetic field of complex partial seizure agrees with intracranial localization. *Ann Neurol* 21:548–558.

Sutherling WW, Levesque MF, Crandall PH, et al. 1991. Localization of partial epilepsy using magnetic and electric measurements. *Epilepsia* 32:S29–S40.

Sutton GG, Mayer RF. 1974. Focal reflex myoclonus. *J Neurol Neurosurg Psychiatry* 7:207–217.

Sutton LN, Packer R, Rorke LB, et al. 1983. Cerebral gangliogliomas during childhood. *Neurosurgery* 13:124–128.

Sutula TP. 1990. Experimental models of temporal lobe epilepsy: new insights from the study of kindling and synaptic reorganization. *Epilepsia* 31:S49–S54.

Sutula TP, Sackellares JC, Miller JQ. 1981. Efficacy of prolonged hospitalization and intensive monitoring in refractory epilepsy. *Neurology* 31:243–247.

Sutula T, Cascino G, Cavazos J, et al. 1989. Mossy fiber synaptic reorganization in the epileptic human temporal lobe. *Ann Neurol* 26:321–330.

Suzuki Y, Nagai T, Ono J, et al. 1997. Zonisamide monotherapy in newly diagnosed infantile spasms. *Epilepsia* 38:1035–1038.

Suzuki Y, Imai K, Toribe Y, et al. 2002. Long-term response to zonisamide in patients with West syndrome. *Neurology* 58:1556–1559.

Sveinbjornsdottir S, Duncan JS. 1993. Parietal and occipital lobe epilepsy: a review. *Epilepsia* 34:493–521.

Swaiman KF, Franck Y. 1978. Seizure headaches in children. *Dev Med Child Neurol* 20:580–585.

Swanson PD. 1977. Neurological manifestations of hyper-

natremia. In: Vinken PJ, Bruyn GW, eds. *Handbook of clinical neurology*, Vol. 28. Amsterdam: North Holland, 443–459.

Swanson JW, Vick NA. 1978. Basilar artery migraine 12 patients, with an attack recorded electroencephalographically. *Neurology* 28:782–786.

Swartz BE, Halgren E, Delgado-Escueta E, et al. 1989. Neuroimaging in patients with seizures of probable frontal lobe origin. *Epilepsia* 30:547–558.

Swartz BE, Halgren E, Delgado-Escueta AV, et al. 1990. Multidisciplinary analysis of patients with extratemporal complex partial seizures. II: Predictive value of semiology. *Epilepsy Res* 5:146–154.

Swash M. 1983. Epileptic dizziness: a presenting feature of temporal lobe epilepsy. In: Rose CF, ed. *Recent progress in epilepsy*. London: Pitman, 144–150.

Symonds C. 1959. Excitation and inhibition in epilepsy. *Brain* 82:133–146.

Szepetowski P, Rochette J, Berquin P, et al. 1997. Familial infantile convulsions and paroxysmal choreoathetosis: a new neurological syndrome linked to the pericentromeric region of human chromosome 16. *Am J Hum Genet* 61:889–898.

Taft T, Cohen H. 1971. Hypsarrhythmia and infantile autism: a clinical report. *J Autism Child Schizophrenia* 1:327–336.

Takahashi T, Tsukahara Y. 1998. Pocket Monster incident and low luminance visual stimuli: special reference to deep red flicker stimulation. *Acta Paediatr Jpn* 40:631–637.

Takahashi I, Miura K, Nomura K, et al. 1990. Seizure prognosis and EEG evolution in complex partial seizures of childhood onset. *Brain Dev* 12:498–502.

Takahashi Y, Sato Y, Goto K, et al. 2001. Optical filters inhibiting television-induced photosensitive seizures. *Neurology* 57:1707–1773.

Takeda A, Bancaud J, Talairach J, et al. 1969. A propos des accès épileptiques d'origine occipitale. *Rev Neurol* 121:306–315.

Takeda Y, Baba A, Nakamura F, et al. 2000. Symptomatic generalized epilepsy associated with an inverted duplication of chromosome 15. *Seizure* 9:145–150.

Takeuchi Y, Takano T, Abe J, et al. 2001. Thyrotropin-releasing hormone: role in the treatment of West syndrome and related epileptic encephalopathies. *Brain Dev* 23:662–667.

Talairach J, Bancaud J. 1974. Stereotaxic exploration and therapy in epilepsy. In: Vinken PJ, Bruyn GW, eds. *The epilepsies*. Handbook of clinical neurology, Vol. 15. Amsterdam: North Holland, 758–782.

Talairach J, Szikla G. 1980. Application of stereotactic concepts to the surgery of epilepsy. *Acta Neurochir (Wien)* 30:35–54.

Talairach J, Tournoux P, Bancaud J. 1960. Chirurgie parietale de la doleur. *Acta Neurochir* 8:153–250.

Talairach J, Bancaud J, Szikla G, et al. 1974. Approche nouvelle de la neurochirurgie de l'épilepsie. *Neurochirurgie* 20:1–240.

Talwar D. 1990. Mechanisms of antiepileptic drug action. *Pediatr Neurol* 6:289–295.

Tampieri D, Melanson D, Romeo F. 1991. Imaging in chronic encephalitis. In: Andermann F, ed. *Chronic encephalitis and epilepsy: Rasmussen syndrome*. Boston: Butterworth-Heinemann, 47–60.

Tan N, Urich H. 1984. Postictal cerebral hemiatrophy with a contribution to the problem of crossed cerebellar atrophy. *Acta Neuropathol (Berlin)* 62:332–339.

Tanaka J, Mimaki T, Tagawa T, et al. 1990. Efficacy of bromide for intractable epilepsy of childhood. *Journal of the Japanese Epileptic Society* 8:105–109.

Tartara A, Manni R, Galimberti CA, et al. 1989. Vigabatrin in the treatment of epilepsy: a long-term follow-up study. *J Neurol Neurosurg Psychiatry* 52:467–471.

Tasker RC, Boyd SG, Harden A, et al. 1989. EEG monitoring of prolonged thiopentone administration for intractable seizures and status epilepticus in infants and young children. *Neuropediatrics* 20:147–153.

Tasker RC, Boyd SG, Harden A, et al. 1991. The clinical significance of seizures in critically ill young infants requiring intensive care. *Neuropediatrics* 22:129–138.

Tassi L, Colombo N, Garbelli R, et al. 2002. Focal cortical dysplasia: neuropathological subtypes, EEG, neuroimaging and surgical outcome. *Brain* 125:1719–1732.

Tassinari CA. 1976. Nosologie et frontières des syndromes avec respiration périodique au cours du sommeil (syndrome de Pickwick, syndrome d'Ondine, obstruction des voies aériennes supérieures, syndrome avec microsommeil, insomnie et narcolepsie). *Rev Electroencephalogr Neurophysiol Clin* 6:53–61.

Tassinari CA, Roger J. 1975. Prognosis and therapy of complex partial seizures with barbiturates, hydantoins and other drugs. In: Penry JK, Daly DD, eds. *Complex partial seizures and their treatment.* Advances in neurology, Vol. 11. New York: Raven Press, 201–219

Tassinari CA, Lyagoubi S, Santos V, et al. 1969. Etude des décharges de pointes ondes chez l'homme: les aspects cliniques. *Rev Neurol* 121:379–383.

Tassinari CA, Lyagoubi S, Gambarelli F, et al. 1971. Relationships between EEG discharge and neuromuscular phenomena. *Electroencephalogr Clin Neurophysiol* 31: 176–182.

Tassinari CA, Dravet C, Roger J, et al. 1972a. Tonic status epilepticus precipitated by intravenous benzodiazepine in five patients with Lennox-Gastaut syndrome. *Epilepsia* 13:431–435.

Tassinari CA, Mancia D, Dalla Bernardina B, et al. 1972b. Pavor nocturnus of nonepileptic nature in epileptic children. *Electroencephalogr Clin Neurophysiol* 33: 603–607.

Tassinari CA, Bureau-Paillas M, Dalla Bernardina B. 1976. Syndrome avec apnées centrales périodiques (syncopes par arrêt respiratoire). *Rev Electroencephalogr Neurophysiol Clin* 6:79–87.

Tassinari CA, Terzano G, Capocchi G, et al. 1977. Epileptic seizures during sleep in children. In: Penry JK, ed. *Epilepsy: the Eighth International Symposium.* New York: Raven Press, 345–354.

Tassinari CA, Bureau-Paillas M, Dalla Bernardina B, et al. 1978. La maladie de Lafora. *Rev Electroencephalogr Neurophysiol Clin* 8:107–122.

Tassinari CA, Daniele O, Michelucci R, et al. 1983. Benzodiazepines: efficacy in status epilepticus. In: Delgado-Escueta AV, Wasterlain CG, Treiman DM, Porter RJ, eds. *Status epilepticus: mechanisms of brain damage and treatment.* Advances in neurology, Vol. 34. New York: Raven Press, 465–475.

Tassinari CA, De Marco P, Plasmati R, et al. 1988. Extreme somatosensory evoked potentials (ESEP) elicited by tapping of hands or feet in children: a somatosensory cerebral evoked potentials study. *Neurophysiol Clin* 18: 123–128.

Tassinari CA, Michelucci R, Rubboli G. 1989a. Self-induced seizures. In: Beaumanoir A, Gastaut H, Naquet R, eds. *Reflex seizures and reflex epilepsies.* Genève: Editions Médecine and Hygiène, 363–368.

Tassinari CA, Rubboli G, Plasmati R, et al. 1989b. Television-induced epilepsy with occipital seizures. In: Beaumanoir A, Gastaut H, Naquet R, eds. *Reflex seizures and reflex epilepsies.* Genève: Éditions Médecine et Hygiène, 241–243.

Tassinari CA, Robboli G, Michelucci R. 1990. Reflex epilepsy. In: Dam M, Gram L, eds. *Comprehensive epileptology.* New York: Raven Press, 233–243.

Tassinari CA, Bureau M, Dravet C, et al. 1992a. Epilepsy with continuous spikes and waves during slow sleep—otherwise described as ESES (epilepsy with electrical status epilepticus during slow sleep). In: Roger J, Dravet C, Bureau M, et al., eds. *Epileptic syndromes in infancy, childhood and adolescence,* 2nd ed. London: John Libbey, 245–256.

Tassinari CA, Bureau M, Homas P. 1992b. Epilepsy with myoclonic absences. In: Roger J, Dravet C, Bureau M, et al., eds. *Epileptic syndromes in infancy, childhood and adolescence,* 2nd ed. London: John Libbey, 151–160.

Tassinari CA, Michelucci R, Rubboli G, et al. 1995. Myoclonic absence epilepsy. In: Duncan JS, Panayiotopoulos CP, eds. *Typical absences and related syndromes.* London: Churchill Communication Europe, 187–195.

Tassinari CA, Michelucci R, Shigematsu H, et al. 1997. Atonic and falling seizures. In: Engel J Jr, Pedley T, eds. *Epilepsy: a comprehensive textbook,* Vol. 1. Philadelphia: Lippincott-Raven, 605–615.

Tassinari CA, Riguzzi P, Rizzi R, et al. 1997a. Gelastic seizures. In: Tuxhorn I, Holthausen H, Boenigk H, eds. *Paediatric epilepsy syndromes and their surgical treatment.* London: John Libbey, 447–461.

Tassinari CA, Rubboli G, Shibasaki H. 1998. Neurophysiology of positive and negative myoclonus. *Electroencephalogr Clin Neurophysiol* 107:181–195.

Tassinari CA, Rubboli G, Volpi L, et al. 2002. Electrical status epilepticus during slow sleep (ESES or CSWS) including acquired epileptic aphasia (Landau-Kleffner syndrome). In: Roger J, Bureau M, Dravet C, et al., eds. *Epileptic syndromes in infancy, childhood and adolescence,* 3rd ed. London: John Libbey, 265–283.

Tateno A, Matsui A, Sakuragawa N, et al. 1985. Two siblings with multiple intracranial hemangiomatosis with calcifications. *J Neurol* 232:112–114.

Tatsuno M, Hayashi M, Iwamoto H, et al. 1984. Epilepsy in childhood Down syndrome. *Brain Dev* 6:37–44.

Tatum WO 4th, Passaro EA, Elia M, et al. 1998. Seizures in Klinefelter's syndrome. *Pediatr Neurol* 19:275–278.

Taylor J. 1931. *Selected writings of John Hughlings Jackson,* Vol. 1: On epilepsy and epileptiform convulsions. London: Hodder & Stoughton.

Taylor DC. 1972. Mental state and temporal lobe epilepsy. A correlative account of 100 patients treated surgically. *Epilepsia* 13:727–776.

Taylor DC. 1975. Factors influencing the occurrence of schizophrenia-like psychosis in patients with temporal lobe epilepsy. *Psychol Med* 5:249–254.

Taylor DC. 1993. Epilepsy as a chronic sickness: remediating its impact. In: Engel J, ed. *Surgical treatment of the epilepsies,* 2nd ed. New York: Raven Press, 11–22

Taylor DC, Bower BD. 1971. Prevention in epileptic disorders. *Lancet* 2:1136–1138.

Taylor DC, Lochery M. 1987. Temporal lobe epilepsy: origin and significance of simple and complex auras. *J Neurol Neurosurg Psychiatry* 50:673–681.

Taylor DC, Ounsted C. 1971. Biological mechanisms influencing the outcome of seizures in response to fever. *Epilepsia* 12:33–45.

Taylor DC, Falconer MA, Bruton DJ, et al. 1971. Focal dysplasia of the cerebral cortex in epilepsy. *J Neurol Neurosurg Psychiatry* 34:369–387.

Taylor S, Tudur S, Williamson PR, et al. 2001. Phenobarbitone versus phenytoin monotherapy for partial onset seizures and generalized onset tonic-clonic seizures. *Cochrane Database Syst Rev.* CD002217.

Temkin NR, Dikmen JS, Wilensky AJ. 1990. A randomized double-blind study of phenytoin for the prevention of post-traumatic seizures. *N Engl J Med* 323:497–502.

Temkin NR, Haglund MM, Winn HR. 1995. Causes, prevention and treatment of post-traumatic epilepsy. *New Horizons* 3:518–522.

Tennis P, Eldridge RR. 2002. Preliminary results on pregnancy outcomes in women using lamotrigine. *Epilepsia* 43:1161–1167.

Tennison MB, Greenwood RS, Miles MV. 1991. Methsuximide for intractable childhood seizures. *Pediatrics* 87:186–189.

Terada K, Ikeda A, Mima T. 1997. Familial cortical tremor as a unique form of cortical reflex myoclonus. *Movement Disorders* 12:370–377.

Terasaki T, Yamatogi Y, Ohtahara S. 1987. Electroclinical delineation of occipital lobe epilepsy of childhood. In: Andermann F, Lugaresi E, eds. *Migraine and epilepsy.* London: Butterworth-Heinemann, 125–137.

Terdjman P, Aicardi J, Sainte-Rose C, et al. 1991. Neuroradiological findings in Sturge-Weber syndrome (SWS) and isolated pial angiomatosis. *Neuropediatrics* 22:115–120.

Terzano MG, Parrino L, Manzoni GC, et al. 1983. Seizures triggered by blinking when beginning to speak. *Arch Neurol* 40:103–106.

Tettenborn B, Genton P, Polson D. 2002. Epilepsy and women's issues: an update. *Epileptic Disord* 4:S23–S31.

Tharp B. 1972. Orbital frontal seizures: a unique electroencephalographic and clinical syndrome. *Epilepsia* 13:627–642.

Tharp BR. 1981. Neonatal and pediatric electroencephalography. In: Aminoff MJ, ed. *Electrodiagnosis in clinical neurology.* Edinburgh: Churchill Livingstone, 67–117.

Tharp BR, Cukier F, Monod N. 1981. The prognostic value of the electroencephalogram in premature infants. *Electroencephalogr Clin Neurophysiol* 51:219–236.

Theodore WH, Porter RJ. 1983. Removal of sedative-hypnotic antiepileptic drug from the regimens of patients with intractable epilepsy. *Ann Neurol* 13:320–324.

Theodore WH, Newmark ME, Sato S, et al. 1983a. ^{18}F-Fluorodeoxyglucose positron emission tomography in refractory complex partial seizures. *Ann Neurol* 14:429–437.

Theodore WH, Porter RJ, Penry JK. 1983b. Complex partial seizures: clinical characteristics and differential diagnosis. *Neurology* 33:1115–1121.

Theodore WH, Schulman FA, Porter RJ. 1983c. Intractable seizures: long term follow-up after prolonged inpatient treatment in an epilepsy unit. *Epilepsia* 24:336–343.

Theodore WH, Brooks R, Sato S, et al. 1984a. The role of positron emission tomography in the evaluation of seizure disorders. *Ann Neurol* 15:S176–S179.

Theodore WH, Sato S, Porter RJ. 1984b. Serial EEG in intractable epilepsy. *Neurology* 34:863–867.

Theodore W, Porter RJ, Raubertas RF. 1987a. Seizures during barbiturate withdrawal: relation to blood level. *Ann Neurol* 22:644–647.

Theodore WH, Rose D, Patronas W, et al. 1987b. Cerebral glucose metabolism in the Lennox-Gastaut syndrome. *Ann Neurol* 21:14–21.

Theodore WH, Fishbein D, Dubinsky R. 1988. Patterns of cerebral glucose metabolism in patients with partial seizures. *Neurology* 38:1201–1206.

Theodore WH, Katz D, Kufta C, et al. 1990. Pathology of temporal lobe foci: correlation with CT, MRI, and PET. *Neurology* 40:797–803.

Theodore WH, Porter RJ, Albert P, et al. 1994. The secondarily generalized tonic-clonic seizure: a videotape analysis. *Neurology* 44:1403–1407.

Thirumalai S, Abou-Khalil B, Fakhoury T, et al. 2001. Video-EEG in the diagnosis of paroxysmal events in children with mental retardation and in children with normal intelligence. *Dev Med Child Neurol* 43:731–734.

Thomas P, Zifkin BG. 1999. Pure photosensitive ictus emeticus. *Epileptic Disord* 1:47–50.

Thomas JE, Reggan TJ, Klass DW. 1977. Epilepsia partialis continua. A review of 32 cases. *Arch Neurol* 34:266–275.

Thomas P, Picard F, Hirsch E, et al. 1998. Epilepsie frontale nocturne autosomique dominante. *Rev Neurol (Paris)* 154:228–235.

Thomas P, Genton P, Gelisse P, Wolf P. 2002. Juvenile myoclonic epilepsy. In: Roger J, Bureau M, Dravet C, et al., eds. *Epileptic syndromes in infancy, childhood, and adolescence,* 3rd ed. London: John Libbey, 335–356.

Thomas P, Arzimanoglou A, Aicardi J. 2003. Benign idiopathic occipital epilepsy: report of a case of the late (Gastaut) type. *Epileptic Disord* 5:57–59.

Thompson PJ. 1991. Memory function in patients with epilepsy. In: Smith DB, Treiman D, Trimble M, eds. *Neurobehavioral problems in epilepsy.* Advances in neurology, Vol. 55. New York: Raven Press, 369–384.

Thompson PJ, Trimble MR. 1981. Sodium valproate and cognitive functioning in normal volunteers. *Br J Clin Pharmacol* 12:819–824.

Thompson PJ, Trimble MR. 1982. Anticonvulsant drugs and cognitive functions. *Epilepsia* 23:531–544.

Thompson PJ, Trimble MR. 1983. Anticonvulsant serum levels: relationship to impairment of cognitive functioning. *J Neurol Neurosurg Psychiatry* 46:227–233.

Thompson PJ, Huppert FA, Trimble MR. 1981. Phenytoin and cognitive function: effects on normal volunteers and implications for epilepsy. *Br J Clin Psychol* 20:155–162.

Thompson PJ, Sander JW, Oxley J. 1987. Intellectual deterioration in severe epilepsy. In: Wolf P, Dam M, Janz D, et al., eds. *Advances in epileptology,* XVI Epilepsy International Symposium. New York: Raven Press, 611–614.

Thorn I. 1975. A controlled study of prophylactic long-term treatment of febrile convulsions with phenobarbital. *Acta Neurol Scand Suppl* 60:67–73.

Thorn I. 1981. Prevention of recurrent febrile seizures: intermittent prophylaxis with diazepam compared with continuous treatment with phenobarbital. In: Nelson KB, Ellenberg JH, eds. *Febrile seizures.* New York: Raven Press, 119–126.

Thorn I. 1982. The significance of electroencephalography in febrile convulsions. In: Akimoto H, Kazamatsun H, Seino M, et al., eds. *Advances in epileptology*, XIIIth Epilepsy International Symposium. New York: Raven Press, 93–95.

Thornton E, Pampiglione G. 1979. Psychiatric disorders following infantile spasms. *Lancet* 1:1297.

Thurston SE, Leigh RJ, Osorio I. 1985. Epileptic gaze deviation and nystagmus. *Neurology* 35:1518–1521.

Tibbles JA. 1980. Dominant benign neonatal seizures. *Dev Med Child Neurol* 22:664–667.

Tibbles JA, Prichard JS. 1965. The prognostic value of the electroencephalogram in neonatal convulsions. *Pediatrics* 35:778–786.

Tibbles JA, Camfield PR, Cron CC, et al. 1986. Dominant recurrent ataxia and vertigo of childhood. *Pediatr Neurol* 2:35–38.

Tiberge M, Calvet U, Soubiran C, et al. 1988. Landau-Kleffner syndrome with continuous sharp waves during REM sleep [Abstract]. *Electroencephalogr Clin Neurophysiol* 70:11.

Tijam AT, Stefanko S, Schenk VW, de Vlieger M. 1978. Infantile spasms associated with hemihypsarrhythmia and hemimegalencephaly. *Dev Med Child Neurol* 20:779–798.

Tinuper P, Aguglia U, Farnarier G, et al. 1983a. Le vomissement: un symptome critique épileptique. *Rev Electroencephalogr Neurophysiol Clin* 13:163–173.

Tinuper P, Aguglia U, Pellissier JF, et al. 1983b. Visual ictal phenomena in a case of Lafora disease proven by skin biopsy. *Epilepsia* 24:214–218.

Tinuper P, Aguglia U, Laudadio S, et al. 1987. Prolonged ictal paralysis: electroencephalographic confirmation of its epileptic nature. *Clin Electroencephalog* 18:12–14.

Tinuper P, Andermann F, Villemure MG, et al. 1988. Functional hemispherectomy for treatment of epilepsy associated with hemiplegia: rationale, indications, results, and comparison with callosotomy. *Ann Neurol* 24:27–34.

Tinuper P, Cerullo A, Cirignotta F, et al. 1990. Nocturnal paroxysmal dystonia with short-lasting attacks: three cases with evidence for an epileptic frontal origin of seizures. *Epilepsia* 31:549–556.

Tinuper P, Montagna P, Cortelli P, et al. 1992. Idiopathic recurring stupor: a case with possible involvement of the γ-aminobutyric acid (GABA)ergic system. *Ann Neurol* 31:503–506.

Tinuper P, Lugaresi E, Vigevano F, et al. 2001. Nocturnal frontal lobe epilepsy. In: Guerrini R, Aicardi J, Andermann F, et al., eds. *Epilepsy and movement disorders*. Cambridge: Cambridge University Press, 97–109.

Tirman PJ, Woody RC. 1988. Transient global amnesia precipitated by emotion in an adolescent. *J Child Neurol* 3:185–188.

Tizard B. 1962. The personality of epileptics. A discussion of the evidence. *Psychol Bull* 59:196–210.

Todorov AB, Lenn NJ, Gabor AJ. 1978. Exacerbation of generalized nonconvulsive seizures with ethosuximide therapy. *Arch Neurol* 35:389–391.

Todt H. 1984. The late prognosis of epilepsy in childhood: results of a prospective follow-up study. *Epilepsia* 25:137–144.

Todt H, Müller D. 1992. The therapy of benign myoclonic epilepsy in infants. In: Degen R, Dreifuss FE, eds. *The benign localized and generalized epilepsies in early childhood*. Epilepsy Research, suppl 6. Amsterdam: Elsevier, 137–139.

Tomson T, Forsgren L. 2003. Mortality studies in epilepsy. In: Jallon P, ed. *Prognosis of epilepsies*. Paris: John Libbey Eurotext, 12–20.

Tondi M, Carboni F, Deriu A, et al. 1987. Intermittent therapy with clobazam for simple febrile convulsions [Letter]. *Dev Child Neurol* 29:830–831.

Torbergsen T. 1991. Epilepsy in a mitochondrial disorder. *J Neurol Neurosurg Psychiatry* 54:1073–1076.

Toribe Y. 2001. High-dose vitamin B_6 treatment in West syndrome. *Brain Dev* 23:654–657.

Torrisi L, Sangiorgi E, Russo L, et al. 2001. Rearrangements of chromosome 15 in epilepsy. *Am J Med Genet* 106:125–128.

Touchon J. 1982. Effect of awakening on epileptic activity in primary generalized myoclonic epilepsy. In: Sterman MB, Shouse MN, Passouant P, eds. *Sleep and epilepsy*. New York: Academic Press, 239–248.

Towne AR, Pellock JM, Ko D, et al. 1994. Determinants of mortality in status epilepticus. *Epilepsia* 35:27–34.

Treiman DM. 1987. Efficacy and safety of antiepileptic drugs: a review of controlled trials. *Epilepsia* 28:S1–S8.

Treiman DM. 1989. Genetics of the partial epilepsies. In: Beck-Managetta G, Anderson VE, Doose H, Janz D, eds. *Genetics of the epilepsies*. Berlin: Springer-Verlag, 73–82.

Treiman DM, Delgado-Escueta AV. 1980. Status epilepticus. In: Thompson RA, Green JR, eds. *Critical care of neurological and neurosurgical emergencies*. New York: Raven Press, 55–99.

Treiman DM, Delgado-Escueta AV. 1983. Complex partial status epilepticus. In: Delgado-Escueta AV, Wasterlain CG, Treiman DM, Porter RJ, eds. *Status epilepticus: mechanisms of brain damage and treatment*. Advances in neurology, Vol. 34. New York: Raven Press, 69–81.

Treiman DM, Delgado-Escueta AV, Clark MA. 1981. Impairment of memory following partial complex status epilepticus. *Neurology* 31:109.

Treiman DM, Meyers PD, Walton NY, et al. 1998. A comparison of four treatments for generalized convulsive status epilepticus. Veterans Affairs Status Epilepticus Cooperative Study Group. *N Engl J Med* 339:792–798.

Trenerry MR, Jack CR Jr, Sharbrough FW, et al. 1993. Quantitative MRI hippocampal volumes: association with onset and duration of epilepsy, and febrile convulsions in temporal lobectomy patients. *Epilepsy Res* 15:247–252.

Trevathan E. 2002. Infantile spasms and Lennox-Gastaut syndrome. *J Child Neurol* 17:2S9–2S22.

Trevathan E, Cascino GD. 1988. Partial epilepsy presenting as focal paroxysmal pain. *Neurology* 38:329–330.

Trevathan E, Yeargin-Allsop M, Murphy CC, et al. 1988. Epilepsy among children with mental retardation [Abstract]. *Ann Neurol* 24:321.

Trevathan E, Murphy CC, Yeargin-Ilsopp M. 1997. Death among children with epilepsy in Atlanta. *Epilepsia* 38(Suppl.8):248–249.

Trevathan E, Murphy CC, Yeargin-Allsopp M. 1999. The descriptive epidemiology of infantile spasms among Atlanta children. *Epilepsia* 40:748–751.

Trimble MR. 1990a. Antiepileptic drugs, cognitive function, and behavior in children: evidence from recent studies. *Epilepsia* 31:S30–S34.

Trimble MR. 1990b. Neuropsychiatry. In: Dam M, Gram L,

eds. *Comprehensive epileptology*. New York: Raven Press, 485–494.

Trimble MR 1991. *The psychoses of epilepsy*. New York, Raven Press.

Trimble MR, Corbett JA. 1980. Behavioural and cognitive disturbances in epileptic children. *Ir Med J* 73(Suppl.): 21–28.

Trimble MR, Cull C. 1988. Children of school age: the influence of antiepileptic drugs on behavior and intellect. *Epilepsia* 29:S15–S19.

Trimble MR, Thompson PJ. 1983. Anticonvulsant drugs, cognitive function and behavior. *Epilepsia* 24:S55–S63.

Trinka E, Dubeau F, Andermann F, et al. 2000. Clinical findings, imaging characteristics and outcome of catastrophic post-encephalitic epilepsy. *Epileptic Dis* 2: 153–161.

Trojaborg W. 1968. Changes of spike foci in children. In: Kellaway P, Petersen I, eds. *Clinical electroencephalography of children*. New York: Grune and Stratton, 213–225.

Trostle JA, Hauser WA, Sharbrough FW. 1989. Psychologic and social adjustment to epilepsy in Rochester, Minnesota. *Neurology* 39:633–367.

Trounce JQ, Fawer CL, Punt J, et al. 1985. Primary thalamic haemorrhage in the newborn: a new clinical entity. *Lancet* 1:190–192.

Trounce JQ, Rutter N, Mellor DH. 1991. Hemimegalencephaly: diagnosis and treatment. *Dev Med Child Neurol* 33:257–266.

Troupin AS, Ojemann LM. 1975. Paradoxical intoxication—a complication of anticonvulsant medication. *Epilpesia* 16:753–758.

Tsai JJ, Beck-Mannagetta G, Janz D, et al. 1989. Photosensitivity in offspring of patients with epilepsy. In: Manelis J, Bental E, Loeber JN, et al., eds. *Advances in epileptology*, XVIIth Epilepsy International Symposium. New York: Raven Press, 379–382.

Tsairis P, Engel WK, Kark P. 1973. Familial myoclonic epileptic syndrome associated with skeletal muscle mitochondrial abnormalities. *Neurology* 23:408.

Tsuboi T. 1977a. Genetic aspects of febrile convulsions. *Hum Genet* 38:169–173.

Tsuboi T. 1977b. *Primary generalized epilepsy with sporadic myoclonus of myoclonic petit mal type*. Stuttgart: Thieme.

Tsuboi T. 1984. Epidemiology of febrile and afebrile convulsions in children in Japan. *Neurology* 34:175–181.

Tsuboi T. 1986. Seizures of childhood. A population-based and clinic-based study. *Acta Neurol Scand Suppl* 110: 1–237.

Tsuboi T, Christian W. 1973. On the genetics of the primary generalized epilepsy with sporadic myoclonias of impulsive petit mal type. A clinical and electroencephalographic study of 399 probands. *Humangenetik* 19: 155–182.

Tsuboi T, Endo S. 1977. Febrile convulsions followed by nonfebrile convulsions. A clinical electroencephalographic and follow-up study. *Neuropédiatrie* 8: 209–233.

Tsuboi T, Endo S, Lida N. 1991. Long-term follow-up of a febrile convulsion cohort. *Acta Neurol Scand* 84: 369–373.

Tsuchiya S, Kagawa K, Fukuyama Y. 1978. Critical evaluation of the role of immunization as an etiological factor in infantile spasms [Abstract]. *Brain Dev* 3:171.

Tsurui S, Oguni H, Fukuyama Y. 1989. Analysis of ictal EEG in benign familial infantile convulsions. *Teukan Kenkyu (Tokyo)* 7:160–168.

Tudur S, Marson AG, Williamson PR. 2001. Phenytoin versus valproate monotherapy for partial onset seizures and generalized onset tonic-clonic seizures. *Cochrane Database Syst Rev* CD001769.

Tudur S, Marson AG, Clough HE, et al. 2002. Carbamazepine versus phenytoin monotherapy for epilepsy. *Cochrane Database Syst Rev* CD001911.

Tuite GF, Polkey CE, Harkness W. 2000. Hemispherectomy. In: Oxbury J, Polkey C, Duchowny M, eds. *Intractable focal epilepsy*. London: WB Saunders, 715–733.

Tulinius MH, Hagne I. 1991. EEG findings in children and adolescents with mitochondrial encephalomyelopathies: a study of 25 cases. *Brain Dev* 13:167–173.

Turnbull DM, Rawlins MD, Weightman D, et al. 1982. A comparison of phenytoin and valproate in previously untreated adult epileptic patients. *J Neurol Neurosurg Psychiatry* 45:55–59.

Turnbull DM, Rawlins MD, Weightman D, et al. 1983. Plasma concentrations of sodium valproate: their clinical value. *Ann Neurol* 14:38–42.

Turnbull DM, Rawlins MD, Weightman D, et al. 1984. "Therapeutic" serum concentration of phenytoin: the influence of seizure type. *J Neurol Neurosurg Psychiatry* 47:231–234.

Tuxhorn I, Kerdar MS. 2000. Somatosensory auras. In: Lüders HO, Noachtar S, eds. *Epileptic seizures: pathophysiology and clinical semiology*. Philadelphia: Churchill Livingstone, 286–297.

Tuxhorn I, Holthausen H, Boenigk H, eds. 1997a. *Paediatric epilepsy syndromes and their surgical treatment*. London: John Libbey.

Tuxhorn I, Pieper T, Holthausen H, et al. 1997b. Seizure outcome after temporal lobectomy in childhood. In: Tuxhorn I, Holthausen H, Boenigk H, eds. *Paediatric epilepsy syndromes and their surgical treatment*. London: John Libbey, 334–344.

Uhari M, Rantala H, Vainionpää I, et al. 1995. Effect of acetaminophen and of low intermittent doses of diazepam on prevention of recurrences of febrile seizures. *J Pediatr* 126:991–995.

Uldall P, Alving J, Gram L, Beck S. 1991. Vigabatrin in pediatric epilepsy—an open study. *J Child Neurol* Suppl. 2:S38–S44.

Uldall P, Salholdt L, Alving J. 2000. Landau-Kleffner syndrome with onset at 18 months and an initial diagnosis of pervasive development disorder. *Eur J Paediatr Neurol* 4: 81–86.

Uthman BM, Reid SA, Wilder BJ, et al. 1991. Outcome for West syndrome following surgical treatment. *Epilepsia* 32:668–671.

Uthman B, Wilder BJ, Ramsay RE. 1996. Intramuscular use of fosphenytoin: an overview. *Neurology* 46(Suppl. 1):S24–S28.

Uvebrandt P. 1988. Hemiplegic cerebral palsy. Aetiology and outcome. *Acta Paediatr Scand Suppl* 345:1–100.

Vajda FJ, Aicardi J. 1983. Reassessment of the concept of a therapeutic range of anticonvulsant plasma levels. *Dev Med Child Neurol* 25:660–671.

Vajda FJ, Mihaly GW, Miles JL, et al. 1978. Rectal administration of sodium valproate in status epilepticus. *Neurology* 28:897–899.

Valente EM, Spacey SD, Wali GM, et al. 2000. A second

paroxysmal kinesigenic choreoathetosis locus (EKD2) mapping on 16q13-q22.1 indicates a family of genes which give rise to paroxysmal disorders on human chromosome 16. *Brain* 123:2040–2045.

Valmier J, Touchon J, Baldy-Moulinier M. 1989. Interictal regional cerebral blood flow during non specific activation test in partial epilepsy. *J Neurol Neurosurg Psychiatry* 52:364–371.

Van Bogaert P, Chiron C, Adamsbaum C, et al. 1993. Value of magnetic resonance imaging in West syndrome of unknown etiology. *Epilepsia* 34:701–706.

Van Bogaert P, Donner C, David P, et al. 1996. Congenital bilateral perisylvian syndrome in a monozygotic twin with intra-uterine death of the co-twin. *Dev Med Child Neurol* 38:166–171.

Van Buren JM, Ajmone Marsan C, Mutsuga N, et al. 1975. Surgery of temporal lobe epilepsy. In: Purpura DP, Penry JK, Walter RD, eds. *Neurosurgical management of the epilepsies*. Advances in neurology, Vol. 8. New York: Raven Press, 155–196.

Van den Berg BJ. 1972. Recurrence of febrile seizures in childhood. In: Alter M, Hauser WA, eds. *The epidemiology of epilepsy. A workshop*. NINDS Monograph No. 14. Washington, D.C.: United States Government Printing Office, 119–122.

Van den Berg BJ. 1974. Studies on convulsive disorders in young children. IV: Incidence of convulsions among siblings. *Dev Med Child Neurol* 16:457–464.

Van den Berg BJ, Yerushalmi J. 1969. Studies on convulsive disorders in young children. I: Incidence of febrile and nonfebrile convulsions by age and other factors. *Pediatr Res* 3:298–304.

Van den Berg BJ, Yerushalmi J. 1971. Studies on convulsive disorders in young children. II: Intermittent phenobarbital prophylaxis and recurrence of febrile convulsions. *J Pediatr* 78:1004–1012.

Van der Meij W, Van Huffelen AC, Wieneke GH, et al. 1992a. Sequential EEG mapping may differentiate "epileptic" from "non-epileptic" rolandic spikes. *Electroencephalogr Clin Neurophysiol* 82:408–414.

Van der Meij W, Van Huffelen AC, Willemse J, et al. 1992b. Rolandic spikes in the inter-ictal EEG of children: contribution to diagnosis, classification and prognosis. *Dev Med Child Neurol* 34:893–903.

Van der Meij W, Wieneke GH, Van Huffelen AC, et al. 1992c. Identical morphology of the rolandic spike-and-wave complex in different clinical entities. In: Van der Meij W, ed. *Rolandic epilepsy: clinical significance of quantitative spatial and temporal EEG analysis of rolandic spikes*. Den Hague, The Netherlands: Koniklijke Bibliotheek.

Van der Wens P, Binnie CD. 1987. Consistency of ictal signs in complex partial seizures. In: Wolf P, Dam M, Janz D, et al., ed. *Advances in epileptology*, XVI Epilepsy International Symposium. New York: Raven Press, 217–219.

Van Engelen BG, Renier WO, Weemaed CM, et al. 1994. High-dose intravenous immunoglobulin treatment in cryptogenic West and Lennox-Gastaut syndromes: an add-on study. *Eur J Paediatr* 153:762–769.

Van Huffelen AC. 1989. A tribute to Martinus Rulandus. *Arch Neurol* 46:445–447.

Van Landingham KE, Heinz ER, Cavazos JE, et al. 1998. Magnetic resonance imaging evidence of hippocampal injury after prolonged, focal febrile convulsions. *Ann Neurol* 43:413–426.

Van Lierde A, Mira L. 2001. Aetiological role of febrile convulsive attacks in limbic epilepsy. In: Avanzini G, Beaumanoir A, Mira L, eds. *Limbic seizures in children*. London: John Libbey, 159–165.

Van Ness PC. 1990. Pentobarbital and EEG burst-suppression in treatment of status epilepticus refractory to benzodiazepines and phenytoin. *Epilepsia* 31:61–67.

van Rijkevorsel-Harmant K, Delire M, Schmitz-Moorman W, Wieser HG. 1994. Treatment of refractory epilepsy with intravenous globulins. Results of the first double-blind/dose finding clinical study. *Int J Clin Lab Res* 24:162–166.

Van Slegtenhorst M, de Hoogt R, Hermans C, et al. 1997. Identification of the tuberous sclerosis gene *TSC1* on chromosome 9q34. *Science* 277:805–808.

Van Winter JT, Stickler GB. 1984. Panic attack syndrome. *J Pediatr* 105:661–665.

Vanasse M, Bédard M, Andermann F. 1976. Shuddering attacks in children: an early clinical manifestation of essential tremor. *Neurology* 26:1027–1030.

Vanasse M, Masson P, Geoffroy G, et al. 1984. Intermittent treatment of febrile convulsions with nitrazepam. *Can J Neurol Sci* 11:377–379.

Vanhatalo S, Paakkonen L, Nousiainen I. 1999. Visual field constriction in children treated with vigabatrin. *Neurology* 52:1713–1714.

Vanhatalo S, Nousiainen I, Eriksson K, et al. 2002. Visual field constriction in 91 Finnish children treated with vigabatrin. *Epilepsia* 43:748–756.

Vanucci RC. 1997. Hypoxia-ischemia: clinical aspects. In: Fanaroff A, Martin RJ, eds. *Neonatal-perinatal medicine*. St. Louis; CV Mosby, 877–891.

Varga-Khadem F, Mishkin M. 1997. Speech and language outcome after hemispherectomy in childhood: the John Hopkins experience. In: Tuxhorn I, Holthausen H, Boenigk H, eds. *Paediatric epilepsy syndromes and their surgical treatment*. London: John Libbey, 774–784.

Vargha-Khadem F, Isaacs EB, Papaleloudi H, et al. 1991. Development of language in six hemispherectomized patients. *Brain* 114:473–495.

Vargha-Khadem F, Isaacs E, Van der Werf S, et al. 1992a. Development of intelligence and memory in children with hemiplegic cerebral palsy. The deleterious consequences of early seizures. *Brain* 115:315–329.

Vargha-Khadem F, Isaacs EB, Watkins KE. 1992b. Medial temporal-lobe versus diencephalic amnesia in childhood. *J Clin Exp Neuropsychol* 14:371–372.

Varma RR, Crumrine PK, Bergman I, et al. 1983. Childhood oligodendrogliomas presenting with seizures and low-density lesions on computed tomography. *Neurology* 33:806–808.

Vassella F, Pavlincova E, Schneider HJ, et al. 1973. Treatment of infantile spasms and Lennox-Gastaut syndrome with clonazepam (Rivotril). *Epilepsia* 14:165–175.

Veall RM. 1974. The prevalence of epilepsy among mongols related to age. *J Ment Defic Res* 18:99–106.

Veelken N, Hagberg B, Hagberg G, et al. 1983. Diplegic cerebral palsy in Swedish term and preterm children. Differences in reduced optimality, relations to neurology and pathogenetic factors. *Neuropediatrics* 14:20–28.

Veggiotti P, Cieuta C, Rey E, et al. 1994. Lamotrigine in infantile spasms. *Lancet* 344:1375–1376.

Veggiotti P, Beccaria F, Papalia G, et al. 1998. Continuous

spikes and waves during sleep in children with shunted hydrocephalus. *Childs Nerv Syst* 14:188–194.

Veggiotti P, Cardinale E, Montalenti A, et al. 2001. Generalized epilepsy with febrile seizures plus and severe myoclonic epilepsy in infancy: a case report of two Italian families. *Epileptic Disord* 3:29–32.

Veggiotti P, Termine C, Granocchio E, et al. 2002. Long-term neuropsychological follow-up and nosological considerations in five patients with continuous spikes and waves during slow sleep. *Epileptic Disord* 4: 243–249.

Velasco F, Velasco M, Velasco AL, et al. 1995. Electrical stimulation of the centromedian thalamic nuclei in control of seizures patterns: long-term studies. *Epilepsia* 36:63–71.

Velez A, Dulac O, Plouin P. 1990. Prognosis for seizure control in infantile spasms preceded by other seizures. *Brain Dev* 12:306–309.

Veneselli E, Perrone MV, Di Rocco M, et al. 2001. Malignant migrating partial seizures in infancy. *Epilepsy Res* 46:27–32.

Ventura A, Basso T, Bortolan G, et al. 1982. Home treatment of seizures as a strategy for the long-term management of febrile convulsions in children. *Helv Paediat Acta* 37:581–588.

Ventura A, Bouquet F, Sartorelli C, et al. 1991. Coeliac disease, folic acid deficiency and epilepsy with cerebral calcifications. *Acta Paediatr Scand* 80:559–562.

Verdu A, Ruiz-Falco ML. 1991. Eating seizures associated with focal cortical dysplasia. *Brain Dev* 113:352–354.

Verduyn CM, Stores G, Missen A. 1988. A survey of mothers' impressions of seizure precipitants in children with epilepsy. *Epilepsia* 29:251–255.

Verity CM, Ross EU. 1985. Longitudinal studies of children's epilepsy. In: Ross E, Reynolds E, eds. *Paediatric perspectives on epilepsy*. Chichester: John Wiley and Sons, 133–139.

Verity CM, Golding J. 1991. Risk of epilepsy after febrile convulsion: a national cohort study. *BMJ* 303:1373–1376.

Verity CM, Strauss EM, Moyes PB, et al. 1982. Long-term follow-up after hemispherectomy: neurophysiological, radiologic and psychological findings. *Neurology* 32: 629–639.

Verity CM, Butler NR, Golding J. 1985a. Febrile convulsions in a national cohort followed up from birth. I: Prevalence and recurrence in the first five years of life. *BMJ* 290:1307–1310.

Verity CM, Butler NR, Golding J. 1985b. Febrile convulsions in a national cohort followed up from birth. II: Medical history and intellectual ability at 5 years of age. *BMJ* 290:1311–1315.

Verity CM, Hosking G, Easter DJ. 1995. A multicentre comparative trial of sodium valproate and carbamazepine in paediatric epilepsy. The Paediatric EPITEG Collaborative Group. *Dev Med Child Neurol* 37:97–108.

Verity CM, Greenwood R, Goldin J. 1998. Long-term intellectual and behavioral outcomes of children with febrile convulsions. *N Engl J Med* 338:1723–1728.

Vesa J, Hellsten E, Verkruyse IA, et al. 1995. Mutations of the palmitoyl protein thioesterase gene causing infantile neuronal ceroid lipofuscinosis. *Nature* 376:584–587.

Vestermark V, Vestermark S. 1991. Teratogenic effect of carbamazepine. *Arch Dis Child* 66:641–642.

Viani F, Avanzini G, Baruzzi A, et al. 1977. Long-term monitoring of antiepileptic drugs in patients with the Lennox-Gastaut syndrome. In: Penry JK, ed. *Epilepsy: the Eighth International Symposium*. New York: Raven Press, 131–138.

Viani F, Beghi E, Romeo A, et al. 1987. Infantile febrile status epilepticus: risk factors and outcome. *Dev Med Child Neurol* 29:495–501.

Viani F, Beghi E, Atza G, Gulotta MP. 1988. Classifications of epileptic syndromes: advantages and limitations for evaluation of childhood epileptic syndromes in clinical practice. *Epilepsia* 29:440–445.

Viani F, Romeo A, Viri M, et al. 1995. Seizure and EEG patterns in Angelman's syndrome. *J Child Neurol* 10: 467–471.

Viberg H, Blennow G, Polsky B. 1987. Epilepsy in adolescence: implications for the development of personality. *Epilepsia* 28:542–546.

Vickrey BG, Hays RD, Engel J Jr, et al. 1995. Outcome assessment for epilepsy surgery: the impact of measuring health-related quality of life. *Ann Neurol* 37:158–166

Vigabatrin Paediatric Advisory Group. 2000. Guideline for prescribing vigabatrin in children has been revised. *BMJ* 320:1404–1405.

Vigevano F. 1986. Status epilepticus in childhood. *Pediatr Med Chir* 8:779–785.

Vigevano F, Bureau M. 2002. Idiopathic and/or benign localization-related epilepsies in infants and young children. In: Roger J, Bureau M, Dravet C, et al., eds. *Epileptic syndromes in infancy, childhood and adolescence*, 3rd ed. London: John Libbey, 153–160.

Vigevano F, Cilio MR. 1997. Vigabatrin versus ACTH as first-line treatment for infantile spasms: a randomized prospective study. *Epilepsia* 38:270–274.

Vigevano F, Di Rocco C. 1990. Effectiveness of hemispherectomy in hemimegalencephaly with intractable seizures. *Neuropediatrics* 21:222–223.

Vigevano F, Fusco L. 1993. Hypnic tonic postural seizures in healthy children provide evidence for a partial epileptic syndrome of frontal origin. *Epilepsia* 34:110–119.

Vigevano F, Bosman C, Giscondi A, et al. 1981. Neonatal myoclonic epileptic encephalopathy without hyperglycinemia. *Electroencephalogr Clin Neurophysiol* 52: 52–53.

Vigevano F, Bertini E, Boldrini R, et al. 1989a. Hemimegalencephaly and intractable epilepsy: benefits of hemispherectomy. *Epilepsia* 30:833–843.

Vigevano F, Di Capna M, Dalla Bernardina B. 1989b. Startle disease: an avoidable cause of sudden infant death. *Lancet* 1:216.

Vigevano F, Fusco L, Di Capua M, et al. 1989c. A particular form of idiopathic partial epilepsy with hypnogenic tonic-automatic seizures in children. *Epilepsia* 30:692.

Vigevano F, Di Capua M, Fusco L, et al. 1992a. Sixth-month benign familial convulsions. *Epilepsia* 31:613.

Vigevano F, Fusco L, Di Capua M, et al. 1992b. Benign infantile familial convulsions. *Eur J Paediatr* 151: 608–612.

Vigevano F, Di Capua M, Cusmai R, et al. 1993. The idiopathic form of West syndrome. *Epilepsia* 34:743–746.

Vigevano F, Santanelli R, Fusco L, et al. 1994. Benign infantile familial convulsions. In: Malafosse A, Genton P, Hirsch E, et al., eds. *Idiopathic generalised epilepsies: clinical, experimental and genetic aspects*. London: John Libbey, 45–49.

Vigevano F, Fusco L, Granata T, et al. 1996. Hemimegalencephaly: clinical and EEG characteristics. In: Guerrini

R, Andermann F, Canapicchi R, et al., eds. *Dysplasias of cerebral cortex and epilepsy.* Philadelphia: Lippincott-Raven, 285–294.

Vigevano F, Fusco L, Pachatz C. 2001. Neurophysiology of spasms. *Brain Dev* 23:467–472.

Vigevano F, Fusco L, Lo Russo G, Broggi G, eds. 2003. Epilepsy and abnormalities of cortical development. *Epileptic Disord* 5(Suppl. 2).

Vignaendra V, Lim CL. 1978. Epileptic discharges triggered by eye convergence. *Neurology* 28:589–591.

Vignaendra V, Ng KK, Lim CL, et al. 1978. Clinical and electroencephalographic data indicative of brain tumours in a seizure population. *Postgrad Med* 54:1–5.

Vignal JP, Biraben A, Chauvel PY, et al. 1998. Reflex partial seizures of sensorimotor cortex (including cortical reflex myoclonus and startle epilepsy). In: Zifkin BG, Andermann F, Beaumanoir A, Rowan AJ, eds. *Reflex epilepsies and reflex seizures.* Advances in neurology, Vol. 75. Philadelphia: Lippincott-Raven, 207–226.

Villani F, Avanzini G. 2002. The use of immunoglobulins in the treatment of human epilepsy. *Neurol Sci* 23: S33–S37.

Villard L, Nguyen K, Cardoso C, et al. 2002. A locus for bilateral perisylvian polymicrogyria maps to Xq28. *Am J Hum Genet* 70:1003–1008.

Villemure JG, Mascott CR. 1995. Peri-insular hemispherotomy: surgical principles and anatomy. *Neurosurgery* 37:975–981.

Villemure JG, Andermann F, Rasmussen TB. 1991. Hemispherectomy for the treatment of epilepsy due to chronic encephalitis. In: Andermann F, ed. *Chronic encephalitis and epilepsy: Rasmussen's syndrome.* Boston: Butterworth-Heinemann, 235–242.

Villemure JG, Adams CB, Hoffman HJ, Peacock WJ. 1993. Hemispherectomy. In: Engel J Jr, ed. *Surgical treatment of the epilepsies,* 2nd ed. New York: Raven Press, 511–518.

Vining EP. 1987. Cognitive dysfunction associated with antiepileptic drug therapy. *Epilepsia* 28:S18–S22.

Vining E, Freeman J. 1985. Seizures which are not epilepsy. *Pediatr Ann* 14:716–719.

Vining EP, Freeman JM, Carso BS, et al. 1987a. "Bilateral" epileptic abnormalities: a unilateral cure [Abstract]. *Ann Neurol* 22:412.

Vining EP, Mellits ED, Dorsen MM, et al. 1987b. Psychologic and behavioral effects of antiepileptic drugs in children: a double-blind comparison between phenobarbital and valproic acid. *Pediatrics* 80:165–174.

Vining EP, Freeman JM, Brandt J, et al. 1993. Progressive unilateral encephalopathy of childhood (Rasmussen syndrome): a reappraisal. *Epilepsia* 34:639–650.

Vining EP, Freeman JM, Pillas DJ, et al. 1997. Why should we remove half a brain? The outcome of 58 children after hemispherectomy—The Johns Hopkins experience: 1968 to 1986. *Pediatrics* 100:163–171.

Vinters HV, Armstrong DL, Babb TL, et al. 1992a. The neuropathology of human symptomatic epilepsy. In: Engel J Jr, ed. *Surgical treatment of the epilepsies,* 2nd ed. New York: Raven Press, 593–608.

Vinters HV, Fisher RS, Cornford ME, et al. 1992b. Morphologic substrates of infantile spasms: studies based on surgically resected cerebral tissue. *Childs Nerv Syst* 8:8–17.

Vinters HV, De Ros MJ, Farrell MA. 1993. Neuropathologic study of resected cerebral tissue from patients with infantile spasms. *Epilepsia* 34:772–779.

Vles JS, Demandt E, Ceulemans B, et al. 1990. Single photon emission computed tomography (SPECT) in seizure disorders in childhood. *Brain Dev* 12:385–389.

Vohai D, Barnett SH. 1989. Absence and atonic seizures induced by piperazine. *Pediatr Neurol* 5:393–394.

Volpe JJ. 1987. *Neurology of the newborn,* 2nd ed. Philadelphia: WB Saunders.

Volpe JJ. 1989. Neonatal seizures: current concepts and classification. *Pediatrics* 84:422–428.

Volpe JJ. 1990. Neonatal seizures: clinical overview. In: Wasterlain CG, Vert P, eds. *Neonatal seizures.* New York: Raven Press, 27–39.

Volpe JJ. 2001. *Neonatal seizures. In Volpe JJ, ed.* Neurology of the newborn, 3rd ed. Philadelphia: WB Saunders, 172–207.

Wada JA. 1980a. New surgical treatments through experimental models. In: Wada JA, Penry JK, eds. *Advances in epileptology,* Xth Epilepsy International Symposium. New York: Raven Press, 195–204.

Wada JA. 1980b. Unilateral blinking as a lateralizing sign of partial complex seizure of temporal lobe origin. In: Wada JA, Penry JK, eds. *Advances in epileptology,* Xth Epilepsy International Symposium. New York: Raven Press.

Wada JA. 1989. Predominantly nocturnal recurrence of intensely affective vocal and facial expression associated with powerful bimanual, bipedal, and axial activity as ictal manifestations of mesial frontal lobe epilepsy. In: Manelis J, Behtal E, Loeber JN, et al., eds. *Advances in epileptology,* XVIIth Epilepsy International Symposium. New York: Raven Press.

Walker IA, Slovis CM. 1997. Lidocaine in the treatment of status epilepticus. *Acad Emerg Med* 4:918–922.

Walker JE, Homan RW, Vasko MR, et al. 1979. Lorazepam in status epilepticus. *Ann Neurol* 6:207–213.

Walker MC, Smith SJ, Sisodiya SM, Shorvon SD. 1995. Case of simple partial status epilepticus in occipital lobe epilepsy misdiagnosed as migraine: clinical, electrophysiological, and magnetic resonance imaging characteristics. *Epilepsia* 36:1233–1236.

Wallace SJ. 1972. Aetiological aspects of febrile convulsions. Pregnancy and perinatal factors. *Arch Dis Child* 47:171–178.

Wallace SJ. 1974. Recurrence of febrile convulsions. *Arch Dis Child* 49:763–775.

Wallace SJ. 1975. Continuous prophylactic anticonvulsants in selected children with febrile convulsions. *Acta Neurol Scand* (Suppl. 75):62–66.

Wallace SJ. 1976a. Factors predisposing to a complicated initial febrile convulsion. *Arch Dis Child* 50:943–947.

Wallace SJ. 1976b. Neurological and intellectual deficits: convulsions with fever viewed as acute indications of life-long developmental defects. In: Brazier MA, Coceani F, eds. *Brain dysfunction in infantile febrile convulsions.* New York: Raven Press, 259–277.

Wallace SJ. 1977. Spontaneous fits after convulsions with fever. *Arch Dis Child* 52:192–196.

Wallace SJ. 1978. Carbamazepine in childhood seizures. *Dev Med Child Neurol* 20:223–226.

Wallace SJ. 1982. Prognosis after prolonged unilateral febrile convulsions. In: Akimoto H, Kazamatsuri H, Seino M, et al., eds. *Advances in epileptology,* XIIIth Epilepsy International Symposium. New York: Raven Press, 97–99.

Wallace SJ. 1985. Convulsions and lumbar puncture. *Dev Med Child Neurol* 27:69–71.

Wallace SJ. 1988. *The child with febrile seizures.* Boston: John Wright.

Wallace SJ. 1990. Anti-epileptic drug monitoring: an overview. *Dev Med Child Neurol* 32:923–926.

Wallace SJ. 1991. Epileptic syndromes linked with previous history of febrile seizures. In: Fukuyama Y, Kamoshita S, Ohusuka C, et al., eds. *Modern perspectives of child neurology.* Tokyo: The Japanese Society of Child Neurology, 175–181.

Wallace SJ. 1992a. Drug management of epilepsy. *Dev Med Child Neurol* 34:1018–1021.

Wallace SJ. 1992b. Prenatal and perinatal risk factors for epilepsy. In: Pedley TA, Meldrum BS, eds. *Recent advances in epilepsy,* 5th ed. Edinburgh: Churchill Livingstone, 91–106.

Wallace SJ. 1998. Myoclonus and epilepsy in childhood: a review of treatment with valproate, ethosuximide, lamotrigine and zonisamide. *Epilepsy Res* 29:147–154.

Wallace SJ, Cull AM. 1979. Long-term psychological outlook for children w hose first fit occurs with fever. *Dev Med Child Neurol* 21:28–40.

Wallace SJ, Smith JA. 1980. Successful prophylaxis against febrile convulsions with valproic acid or phenobarbitone. *BMJ* 280:353–354.

Wallace SJ, Zealley H. 1970. Neurological, electroencephalographic and virological findings in febrile children. *Arch Dis Child* 45:611–623.

Wallace RH, Wang DW, Singh R, et al. 1998. Febrile seizures and generalized epilepsy associated with a mutation in the Na(+)-channel β-1 subunit gene *SCN1B. Nat Genet* 19:366–370.

Wallace RH, Marini C, Petrou S, et al. 2001a. Mutant GABA(A) receptor γ2-subunit in childhood absence epilepsy and febrile seizures. *Nat Genet* 28:49–52.

Wallace RH, Scheffer IE, Barnett S, et al. 2001b. Neuronal sodium-channel α1-subunit mutations in generalized epilepsy with febrile seizures plus. *Am J Hum Genet* 68:859–865.

Wallace RH, Scheffer IE, Parasivam G, et al. 2002. Generalized epilepsy with febrile seizures plus: mutation of the sodium channel subunit *SCN1B. Neurology* 58:1426–1429.

Walsh GO, Delgado-Escueta AV. 1984. Type II complex partial seizures: poor results of anterior temporal lobectomy. *Neurology* 34:1–13.

Walsh JT, Farrell MK, Keenan WJ, et al. 1981. Gastroesophageal reflux in infants: relation to apnea. *J Pediatr* 99:197–201.

Walson PD, Mimaki T, Curless R, et al. 1980. Once daily dose of phenobarbital in children. *J Pediatr* 97:303–305.

Walther B, Schmitt T, Reiter B. 1987. Identification of infants at risk for infantile spasms by neonatal polygraphy. *Brain Dev* 9:377–380.

Waltregny A, Roger J, Regis H, et al. 1969. Enregistrement polygraphique d'une crise atonique partielle clinique. *Rev Neurol (Paris)* 121:463–467.

Waltz S, Stephani U. 2000. Inheritance of photosensitivity. *Neuropediatrics* 31:82–85.

Wang PJ, Omori K, Utsumi H, et al. 1984. Partial inhibitory seizures: a report on two cases. *Brain Dev* 6:553–559.

Wannamaker BB. 1985. Autonomic nervous system and epilepsy [Review]. *Epilepsia* 26:S31–S39.

Ward AA Jr. 1983. Surgical management of epilepsy. In: Browne TR, Feldman RG, eds. *Epilepsy: diagnosis and management.* Boston: Little Brown, 281–296.

Ward AA Jr, Penry JK, Purpura D, eds. 1983. *Epilepsy.* New York: Raven Press.

Warner TT, Williams L, Harding AE. 1994. Autosomal dominant dentatorubro-pallidoluysian atrophy in the United Kingdom. *Mov Disord* 9:289–296.

Wassner E, Morris B, Fernando L, et al. 2001. Intranasal midazolam for treating febrile seizures in children: buccal midazolam for childhood seizures at home preferred to rectal diazepam. *BMJ* 322:108.

Wasterlain CG. 1976. Effects of neonatal status epilepticus on rat brain development. *Neurology* 26:975–986.

Wasterlain CG. 1978. Neonatal seizures and brain growth. *Neuropédiatrie* 9:213–228.

Wasterlain CG, Plum F. 1973. Vulnerability of developing rat brain to electro-convulsive seizures. *Arch Neurol* 29:38–45.

Watanabe K. 1996. Recent advances and some problems in the delineation of epileptic syndromes in children. *Brain Dev* 18:423–437.

Watanabe K, Okumara A. 2000. Benign partial epilepsies in infancy. *Brain Dev* 22:296–300.

Watanabe K, Iwase K, Hara K. 1973. The evolution of EEG features in infantile spasms: a prospective study. *Dev Med Child Neurol* 15:584–596.

Watanabe K, Hara K, Iwase K. 1976. The evolution of neurophysiological features in holoprosencephaly. *Neuropédiatrie* 7:19–41.

Watanabe K, Hara K, Miyazaki S, et al. 1982. Apneic seizures in the newborn. *Am J Dis Child* 15:584–596.

Watanabe K, Kuroiwa Y, Toyokura Y. 1984. Epilepsia partialis continua: epileptogenic focus in motor cortex and its participation in transcortical reflexes. *Arch Neurol* 41:1040–1044.

Watanabe K, Takeuchi T, Hakamada S, et al. 1987a. Neurophysiological and neuroradiological features preceding infantile spasms. *Brain Dev* 9:391–398.

Watanabe K, Yamamoto N, Negoro T. 1987b. Benign complex partial epilepsies in infancy. *Pediatr Neurol* 3:208–211.

Watanabe K, Kuroyanagi M, Hara K, et al. 1988. Neonatal seizures and subsequent epilepsy. *Brain Dev* 4:341–346.

Watanabe M, Fujiwara T, Terauchi N, et al. 1989a. Intractable grand mal epilepsy developed in the first year of life. In: Manelis J, Bental E, Loeber J, Dreifuss FE, eds. *Advances in epileptology,* XVII Epilepsy International Symposium. New York, Raven Press, 327–339.

Watanabe M, Fujiwara T, Yagi K, et al. 1989b. Intractable childhood epilepsy with generalized tonic-clonic seizures. *Journal of the Japanese Epileptic Society* 7: 96–105.

Watanabe K, Yamamoto N, Negoro T, et al. 1990. Benign infantile epilepsy with complex partial seizures. *J Clin Neurophysiol* 7:409–416.

Watanabe K, Negoro T, Aso K. 1993. Benign partial epilepsy with secondarily generalized seizures in infancy. *Epilepsia* 34:635–638.

Watanabe K, Yamamoto N, Negoro T, et al. 1994. Clinical, EEG and positron emission tomography features of childhood onset epilepsy with localized cortical dysplasia detected by magnetic resonance imaging. *J Epilepsy* 7:108–116.

Watanabe K, Negoro T, Okumura A. 2001. Symptomatology of infantile spasms. *Brain Dev* 23:453–466.

Watanabe K, Okumura A, Aso K, Duchowny M. 2002. Nonidiopathic localization-related epilepsies in infants and young children. In: Roger J, Bureau M, Dravet C, et al., eds. *Epileptic syndromes in infancy, childhood and adolescence*, 3rd ed. London: John Libbey, 161–177.

Waterman K, Wada JA. 1990. Frontal lobe epilepsy. In: Dam M, Gram L, eds. *Comprehensive epileptology*. New York: Raven Press, 197–213.

Waterman K, Purves SJ, Kosaka B, et al. 1987. An epileptic syndrome caused by mesial frontal lobe seizure foci. *Neurology* 37:577–582.

Watkins A, Szymonowicz W, Jin X, et al. 1988. Significance of seizures in very low-birthweight infants. *Dev Med Child Neurol* 30:162–169.

Weaver DF, Camfield P, Fraser A. 1988. Massive carbamazepine overdose: clinical and pharmacologic observations in five episodes. *Neurology* 38:755–759.

Weglage J, Densky A, Pietsch M, et al. 1997. Neuropsychological, intellectual and behavioral findings in patients with centrotemporal spikes with and without seizures. *Dev Med Child Neurol* 39:646–651.

Weig SG, Pollack P. 1993. Carbamazepine-induced heart block in a child. *Ann Neurol* 34:617–619.

Weiner SP, Painter MJ, Geva D, et al. 1991. Neonatal seizures: electroclinical dissociation. *Pediatr Neurol* 7: 363–368.

Weinman HM. 1988. Lennox-Gastaut syndrome and its relationship to infantile spasms (West syndrome). In: Niedermeyer E, Degen R, eds. *The Lennox-Gastaut syndrome*. New York: Alan R. Liss, 301–317.

Weiss GH, Feeney DM, Caveness WF. 1983. Prognostic factors for the occurrence of post-traumatic epilepsy. *Arch Neurol* 40:7–10.

Weiss GH, Salazar AM, Vance SC. 1986. Predicting post-traumatic epilepsy in penetrating head injury. *Arch Neurol* 43:771–773.

Weissbecker KA, Durner M, Janz D. 1991. Confirmation of linkage between juvenile myoclonic epilepsy locus and the HLA region of chromosome 6. *Am J Med Genet* 38:32–36.

Wells CR, Labar DR, Solomon GE. 1992. Aphasia as the sole manifestation of simple partial status epilepticus. *Epilepsia* 33:84–87.

Wennberg R, Arruda F, Quesney LF, et al. 2002. Preeminence of extrahippocampal structures in the generation of mesial temporal seizures: evidence from human depth electrode recordings. *Epilepsia* 43:716–726.

Westbrock E, Devinsky O, Geocadin R. 1998. Nonepileptic seizures after head injury. *Epilepsia* 39:978–982.

Westerveld M, Sass KJ, Chelune GJ, et al. 2000. Temporal lobectomy in children: cognitive outcome. *J Neurosurg* 92:24–30.

Westmoreland BF. 1979. EEG in the evaluation of headache. In: Klass DW, Daly DD, eds. *Current practice of clinical electroencephalography*. New York: Raven Press, 381–394.

Wheeler RB, Sharp JD, Mitchell WA, et al. 1999. A new locus for variant late infantile neuronal ceroid lipofuscinosis—CLN7. *Mol Genet Metab* 66:337–338.

Whelan HT, Hendeles L, Haberkern CM, et al. 1983. High intravenous phenytoin dosage requirement in a newborn infant. *Neurology* 33:106–108.

Wheless JW, Constantinou JE. 1997. Lennox-Gastaut syndrome. *Pediatr Neurol* 17:203–211.

Wheless JW, Maggio V. 2002. Vagus nerve stimulation therapy in patients younger than 18 years. *Neurology* 59:521–525.

Whilmhurst JM, Appleton DB, Gratten-Smith PJ. 2000. Migrating partial seizures in infancy: two new cases. *J Child Neurol* 15:717–722.

White JC. 1971. Epileptic nystagmus. *Epilepsia* 12:157–164.

White HS. 2002. Topiramate: mechanisms of action. In: Levy RH, Mattson RH, Meldrum BS, et al., eds. *Antiepileptic drugs*, 5th ed. Philadelphia: Lippincott Williams & Wilkins, 719–726.

White JC, Langston JW, Pedley TA. 1977. Benign epileptiform transients of sleep. Clarification of the small sharp spike controversy. *Neurology* 27:1061–1068.

Whitehouse WP, Rees M, Curtis D, et al. 1993. Linkage analysis of idiopathic generalized epilepsy (IGE) and marker loci on chromosome 6p in families of patients with juvenile myoclonic epilepsy: no evidence for an epilepsy locus in the HLA region. *Am J Hum Genet* 53: 652–662.

Whitty CW. 1953. Causalgic pain as an epileptic aura. *Epilepsia* 2:37–41.

Wieser HG. 1980. Temporal lobe or psychomotor status epilepticus: a case report. *Electroencephalogr Clin Neurophysiol* 48:558–572.

Wieser HG. 1983a. Depth recorded limbic seizures and psychopathology. *Neurosci Biobehav Rev* 7:427–440.

Wieser HG. 1983b. *Electroclinical features of the psychomotor seizure: a stereoelectroencephalographic study of ictal symptoms and chronotopographical seizure patterns including clinical effects of intracerebral stimulation*. Stuttgart: Gustav Fisher.

Wieser HG. 1986. Psychomotor seizure of hippocampal-amygdalar origin. In: Pedley TA, Meldrum BS, eds. *Recent advances in epilepsy*, Vol. 3. Edinburgh: Churchill Livingstone, 57–79.

Wieser HG. 1987. The phenomenology of limbic seizures. In: Wieser H, Speckman E, Engel J, eds. *The epileptic focus*. London: John Libbey, 113–136.

Wieser HG. 1988. Selective amygdalohippocampectomy for temporal lobe epilepsy. *Epilepsia* 29:S100–S113.

Wieser HG. 1991. Ictal manifestations of temporal lobe seizures. In: Smith DB, Treiman D, Trimble M, eds. *Neurobehavioral problems in epilepsy*. Advances in neurology, Vol. 55. New York: Raven Press, 301–315.

Wieser HG, Elger CE, eds. 1987. *Presurgical evaluation of epileptics*. Berlin: Springer.

Wieser HG, Kausel W. 1987. Limbic seizures. In: Wieser HG, Elger CE, eds. *Presurgical evaluation of epilepsies*. Berlin: Springer, 227–248.

Wieser HG, Metes HP. 1980. Limbic seizures: intracortical EEG activity and clinical signs. In: Girgis M, Kiloh LG, eds. *Limbic epilepsy and the dyscontrol syndrome*. Amsterdam: Elsevier, 195–206.

Wieser HG, Morris H. 1997. Foramen ovale and peg electrodes. In: Engel J Jr, Pedley TA, Aicardi J, et al., eds. *Epilepsy: a comprehensive textbook*, Vol. 2. Philadelphia: Lippincott Williams & Wilkins, 1707–1718.

Wieser HG, Müller RV. 1987. Neocortical temporal seizures. In: Wieser HG, Elger CE, eds. *Presurgical evaluation of epileptics*. Berlin: Springer, 252–266.

Wieser HG, Siegel AM. 1991. Analysis of foramen ovale electrode-recorded seizures and correlation with outcome following amygdalohippocampectomy. *Epilepsia* 32:838–850.

Wieser HG, Williamson PD. 1993. Ictal semiology. In: Engel J, ed. *Surgical treatment of the epilepsies*, 2nd ed. New York: Raven Press, 161–171.

Wieser HG, Yasargil G. 1987. Selective amgydalohip-pocampectomy: follow-up study of 103 patients. In: Wolf P, Dam M, Janz D, et al., eds. *Advances in epileptology*, XVI Epilepsy International Symposium. New York: Raven Press, 331–335.

Wieser HG, Bancaud J, Talairach J, et al. 1979. Comparative value of spontaneous and chemically and electrically induced seizures in establishing the lateralization of temporal lobe seizures. *Epilepsia* 20:47–59.

Wieser HG, Hailemariam S, Regard M, et al. 1985. Unilateral limbic status activity: stereo EEG, behavioral and cognitive data. *Epilepsia* 26:19–29.

Wieser HG, Swartz BE, Delgado-Escueta AV, et al. 1992. Differentiating frontal lobe seizures from temporal lobe seizures. *Adv Neurol* 57:267–285.

Wieser HG, Engel J, Williamson PD, et al. 1993. Surgically remediable temporal lobe syndromes. In: Engel J Jr, ed. *Surgical treatment of the epilepsies*, 2nd ed. New York: Raven Press, 49–62.

Wieser HG, Hajek M, Gooss A, Aguzzi A. 2000. Mesial temporal lobe epilepsy syndrome with hippocampal and amygdala sclerosis. In: Oxbury J, Polkey C, Duchowny M, eds. *Intractable focal epilepsy*. London: WB Saunders, 131–153.

Wild JM, Martinez C, Reinshagen G, et al. 1999. Characteristics of a unique visual field defect attributed to vigabatrin. *Epilepsia* 40:1784–1794.

Wilden JN, Kelly PJ. 1987. CT computerized stereotactic biopsy for low density CT lesions presenting with epilepsy. *J Neurol Neurosurg Psychiatry* 50:1302–1305.

Wilder BJ. 1983. Efficacy of phenytoin in treatment of status epilepticus. In: Delgado-Escueta AV, Wasterlain CG, Treiman DM, Porter RJ, eds. *Status epilepticus: mechanisms of brain damage and treatment*. Advances in neurology, Vol. 34. New York: Raven Press, 441–446.

Wilder BJ, Bruni J. 1981. *Seizure disorders: a pharmacological approach to treatment*. New York: Raven Press.

Wilder BJ, Ramsay E, Wilmore LJ, et al. 1977. Efficacy of intravenous phenytoin in the treatment of status epilepticus. *Ann Neurol* 1:511–518.

Wilder BJ, Ramsay RE, Murphy JV, et al. 1983. Comparison of valproic acid and phenytoin in newly diagnosed tonic-clonic seizures. *Neurology* 33:1474–1476.

Wilensky AJ, Ojemann LM, Temkin NR, et al. 1981. Chlorazepate and phenobarbital as antiepileptic drugs: a double-blind study. *Neurology* 31:1271–1276.

Wiles CM, Brown P, Chapel H, et al. 2002. Intravenous immunoglobulin in neurological disease: a specialist review. *J Neurol Neurosurg Psychiatry* 72:440–448.

Wilkins A, Lindsay J. 1985. Common forms of reflex epilepsy: physiological mechanisms and techniques for treatment. In: Pedley TA, Meldrum BS, eds. *Recent advances in epilepsy*, Vol. 2. Edinburgh: Churchill Livingstone, 239–271.

Wilkins AJ, Darby CE, Binnie CD. 1979a. Neurophysiological aspects of pattern-sensitive epilepsy. *Brain* 102:1–25.

Wilkins AJ, Darby CE, Binnie CD, et al. 1979b. Television epilepsy: the role of pattern. *Electroencephalogr Clin Neurophysiol* 47:163–171.

Wilkins AJ, Zifkin B, Andermann F, et al. 1982. Seizures induced by thinking. *Ann Neurol* 11:608–612.

Wilkus RJ, Dodrill CB, Thompson PM. 1984. Intensive EEG monitoring and psychological studies of patients with pseudoepileptic seizures. *Epilepsia* 25:100–107.

Williamson PD, Spencer S. 1986. Clinical and EEG features of complex partial seizures of extratemporal origin. *Epilepsia* 27:S46–S63.

Williamson PD, Spencer DD, Spencer SS, et al. 1985. Complex partial seizures of frontal lobe origin. *Ann Neurol* 18:497–504.

Williamson PD, Boon PA, Thadani VM, et al. 1992a. Parietal lobe epilepsy: diagnostic considerations and results of surgery. *Ann Neurol* 31:193–201.

Williamson PD, Thadani VM, Darcey TM, et al. 1992b. Occipital lobe epilepsy: clinical characteristics, seizure spread patterns, and results of surgery. *Ann Neurol* 31: 3–13.

Williamson PD, Van Ness PC, Wieser HG, et al. 1993. Surgically remediable extratemporal syndromes. In: Engel J Jr, ed. *Surgical treatment of the epilepsies*, 2nd ed. New York: Raven Press, 65–76.

Williamson PD, Engel J, Munari C. 1997. Anatomic classification of localization-related epilepsies. In: Engel J Jr, Pedley TA, eds. *Epilepsy: a comprehensive textbook*. Philadelphia: Lippincott-Raven, 2405–2416.

Willig RP, Lagenstein I. 1982. Use of ACTH fragments in children with infantile spasms. *Neuropediatrics* 13:55–58.

Willis J, Gould JB. 1980. Periodic alpha seizures with apnea in the newborn. *Dev Med Child Neurol* 22:214–222.

Willmore LJ. 1992. Post-traumatic epilepsy: mechanisms and prevention. In: Pedley TA, Meldrum BS, eds. *Advances in epilepsy*, 5th ed. Edinburgh: Churchill Livingstone, 107–117.

Wilson PJ. 1970. Cerebral hemispherectomy for infantile hemiplegia. A report of 50 cases. *Brain* 93:147–180.

Wilson JT. 1981. Observed and potential risks of anticonvulsant medications in children. In: Nelson KB, Ellenberg JH, eds. *Febrile seizures*. New York: Raven Press, 153–167.

Wilson DH, Reeves A, Gazzaniga M. 1980. Corpus callosotomy for the control of intractable seizures. In: Wada JA, Penry JK, eds. *Advances in epileptology*, Xth Epilepsy International Symposium. New York: Raven Press, 205–213.

Wilson DH, Reeves AG, Gazzaniga MS. 1982. "Central" commissurotomy for intractable generalized epilepsy: series two. *Neurology* 32:687–697.

Winawer MR, Ottman R, Hauser WA, et al. 2000. Autosomal dominant partial epilepsy with auditory features: defining the phenotype. *Neurology* 54:2173–2176.

Wingkun EC, Awad IA, Lüders H, et al. 1991. Natural history of recurrent seizures after resective surgery for epilepsy. *Epilepsia* 32:851–856.

Wirrel EC, Camfield PR, Gordon KE, et al. 1995. Benign rolandic epilepsy: atypical features are very common. *J Child Neurol* 10:455–458.

Wirrell E, Camfield P, Camfield S, et al. 1996. Accidental injury in a serious risk in children with typical absence epilepsy. *Arch Neurol* 53:929–932.

Wise MS, Rutledge SL, Kuznizecky RI. 1996. Rasmussen syndrome and long-term response to gamma-globulins. *Pediatr Neurol* 14:149–152.

Wisniewski KE. 2001. Pheno/genotypic correlations of neuronal ceroid lipofuscinoses. *Neurology* 57:576–581.

Wisniewski KE, Segan SM, Miezejesji EA, et al. 1991. The Fra(X) syndrome: neurological, electrophysiological, and neuropathological abnormalities. *Am J Med Genet* 38:476–480.

Woermann FG, Free SL, Koepp MJ, et al. 1999. Abnormal cerebral structure in juvenile myoclonic epilepsy demonstrated with voxel-based analysis of MRI. *Brain* 122:2101–2108.

Wohlrab G, Boltshauser E, Schmitt B. 1998. Vigabatrin as a first-line drug in West Syndrome: clinical and electroencephalographic outcome. *Neuropediatrics* 29: 133–136.

Wolf SM. 1981. Prevention of recurrent febrile seizures with continuous drug therapy: efficacy and problems of phenobarbital and phenytoin therapy. In: Nelson KB, Ellenberg JH, eds. *Febrile seizures.* New York: Raven Press, 127–134.

Wolf P. 1992a. Epilepsy with grand mal on awakening. In: Roger J, Dravet C, Bureau M, et al., eds. *Epileptic syndromes in infancy, childhood and adolescence.* London: John Libbey, 329–341.

Wolf P. 1992b. Juvenile absence epilepsy. In: Roger J, Dravet C, Bureau M, et al., eds. *Epileptic syndromes in infancy, childhood and adolescence.* London: John Libbey, 307–312.

Wolf P. 1992c. Juvenile myoclonic epilepsy. In: Roger J, Dravet C, Bureau M, et al., eds. *Epileptic syndromes in infancy, childhood and adolescence.* London: John Libbey, 313–327.

Wolf P. 1992d. Reading epilepsy. In: Roger J, Dravet C, Bureau M, et al., eds. *Epileptic syndromes in infancy, childhood and adolescence.* London: John Libbey, 281–298.

Wolf P. 1995a. Juvenile absence epilepsy. In: Duncan JS, Panayiotopoulos CP, eds. *Typical absences and related syndromes.* London: Churchill Communication Europe, 161–173.

Wolf P. 1995b. Nonmedical treatment of first epileptic seizures in adolescence and adulthood. *Seizure* 4:87–94.

Wolf P. 1998. Isolated seizures. In: Engel J Jr, Pedley TA, eds. *Epilepsy: a comprehensive textbook.* Philadelphia: Lippincott-Raven, 2475–2481.

Wolf SM, Forsythe AB. 1978. Behavior disturbances, phenobarbital and febrile seizures. *Pediatrics* 61:728–731.

Wolf P, Gooses R. 1986. Relation of photosensitivity to epileptic syndromes. *J Neurol Neurosurg Psychiatry* 49: 1386–1391.

Wolf P, Inoue Y. 2002. Complex reflex epilepsies: reading epilepsy and praxis induction. In: Roger J, Bureau M, Dravet C, et al., eds. *Epileptic syndromes in infancy, childhood and adolescence,* 3rd ed. London: John Libbey Ltd, 315–326.

Wolf P, Mayer T. 2000. Juvenile myoclonic epilepsy: a syndrome challenging syndromic concepts? In: Schmitz B, Sander T, eds. *Juvenile myoclonic epilepsy: the Janz syndrome.* Petersfield: Wrightson Biomedical Publishing, 33–39.

Wolf SM, Carr A, Davis DC, et al. 1977. The value of phenobarbital in the child who has had a single febrile seizure: a controlled prospective study. *Pediatrics* 59: 378–385.

Wolf SM, Forsythe A, Stunden AA, et al. 1981. Long-term effect of phenobarbital on cognitive function in children with febrile convulsions. *Pediatrics* 68:820–823.

Wolf B, Grier RE, Allen RJ, et al. 1983. Phenotypic variation in biotinidase deficiency. *J Pediatr* 103:233–237.

Wolf HK, Campos MG, Zentner J, et al. 1993. Surgical pathology of temporal lobe epilepsy. Experience with 216 cases. *J Neuropathol Exp Neurol* 52:499–506.

Wolf P, Schöndienst, Gülich E. 2000. Experiential auras. In: Lüders HO, Noachtar S, eds. *Epileptic seizures.* Philadelphia: Churchill Livingstone, 336–348.

Wong M, Trevathan E. 2001. Infantile spasms. *Pediatr Neurol* 24:89–98.

Woo E, Chan YM, Yu YL, et al. 1988. If a well stabilized epileptic patient has a subtherapeutic antiepileptic drug level, should the dose be increased? A randomized prospective study. *Epilepsia* 29:129–139.

Woodbury DM, Penry JK, Pippenger CE, eds. 1982. *Antiepileptic drugs,* 2nd ed. New York: Raven Press.

Woody RC. 1990. Bromide therapy for pediatric seizure disorder intractable to other antiepileptic drugs. *J Child Neurol* 5:65–67.

Woody RC, Brodie M, Hampton DK, et al. 1988a. Corn oil ketogenic diet for children with intractable seizures. *J Child Neurol* 3:21–24.

Woody RC, Yam A, Uchi T, et al. 1988b. Cerebrospinal fluid cell counts in childhood idiopathic status epilepticus. *Pediatr Infect Dis J* 7:298–299.

Worster-Drought C. 1971. An unusual form of acquired aphasia in children. *Dev Med Child Neurol* 13:563–571.

Wyler AR, Ojemann GA, Lettichi E, et al. 1984. Subdural strip electrodes for localizing epileptogenic foci. *J Neurosurg* 60:1195–1200.

Wyllie E. 1994. Children with seizures: when can treatment be deferred? *J Child Neurol* 9:S8–S13.

Wyllie E. 1995. Developmental aspects of seizure semiology: problems in identifying localised-onset seizures in infants and children. *Epilepsia* 36:1170–1172.

Wyllie E. 1996. Surgery for catastrophic localization-related epilepsy in infants. *Epilepsia* 37:S22–S25.

Wyllie E. 1997. Presurgical evaluation for infants with catastrophic epilepsy. In: Tuxhorn I, Holthausen H, Boenigk K, eds. *Pediatric epilepsy syndromes and their surgical treatment.* London: John Libbey, 505–512.

Wyllie E. 1998. Surgical treatment of epilepsy in children. *Pediatr Neurol* 19:179–188.

Wyllie E. 2000. Surgical treatment of epilepsy in pediatric patients. *Can J Neurol Sci* 27:106–110.

Wyllie E, ed. 2001. *The treatment of epilepsy: principles and practice.* 3rd ed. Philadelphia: Lippincott Williams & Wilkins.

Wyllie E, Bingaman WE. 2001. Epilepsy surgery in infants and children. In: Wyllie E, ed. *The treatment of epilepsy: principles and practice.* Philadelphia: Lippincott Williams & Wilkins, 1161–1173.

Wyllie E, Lüders H. 1989. Complex partial seizures in children. Clinical manifestations and identification of surgical candidates. *Cleve Clin J Med* 56:S43–S52.

Wyllie E, Lüders H, Pippenger C, et al. 1985. Postictal serum creatine kinase in the diagnosis of seizure disorders. *Arch Neurol* 42:123–126.

Wyllie E, Lüders H, Morris HH, et al. 1986a. Ipsilateral forced head and eye turning at the end of the generalized tonic-clonic phase of versive seizures. *Neurology* 36:1212–1217.

Wyllie E, Lüders H, Morris HH, et al. 1986b. The lateralizing significance of versive head and eye movements during epileptic seizures. *Neurology* 36:606–611.

Wyllie E, Lüders H, Morris HH III. 1987a. Clinical outcome after complete or partial cortical resection for intractable epilepsy. *Neurology* 37:1634–1641.

Wyllie E, Pippinger CE, Rothner AD. 1987b. Increased seizure frequency with generic primidone. *JAMA* 258:1216–1217.

Wyllie E, Lüders H, Morris HH, et al. 1988a. Subdural electrodes in the evaluation for epilepsy surgery in children and adults. *Neuropediatrics* 19:80–86.

Wyllie E, Wyllie R, Kanner A, et al. 1988b. A technique for comfortable insertion of sphenoidal electrodes in children and adolescents [Abstract]. *Epilepsia* 29: 656.

Wyllie E, Rothner AD, Lüders H. 1989. Partial seizures in children and surgical consideration. *Pediatr Clin North Am* 36:343–364.

Wyllie E, Friedman D, Lüders H, et al. 1991. Outcome of psychogenic seizures in children and adolescents compared with adults. *Neurology* 41:742–744.

Wyllie E, Chee M, Granstrom ML, et al. 1993. Temporal lobe epilepsy in early childhood. *Epilepsia* 34:859–868.

Wyllie E, Comair YG, Kotagal P, et al. 1996. Epilepsy surgery in infants. *Epilepsia* 37:625–637.

Wyllie E, Comair YG, Kotagal P, et al. 1998. Seizure outcome after epilepsy surgery in children and adolescents. *Ann Neurol* 44:740–748.

Wyllie E, Comair YG, Kotagal P, et al. 1999. Seizure outcome after epilepsy surgery in children and adolescents [Abstract]. *Ann Neurol* 45:547.

Xiong L, Labuda M, Li DS, et al. 1999. Mapping of a gene determining familial partial epilepsy with variable foci to chromosome 22q11-q12. *Am J Hum Genet* 65: 1698–1710.

Yacubian EM, Marie SK, Valerio RM, et al. 1997. Neuroimaging findings in Rasmussen's syndrome. *J Neuroimaging* 7:16–22.

Yaffe K, Ferriero D, Barkovich AJ, et al. 1995. Reversible MRI abnormalities following seizures. *Neurology* 45: 104–108.

Yakoub M, Dulac O, Jambaqué I, et al. 1992. Early diagnosis of severe motor epilepsy in infancy. *Brain Dev* 14: 299–303.

Yakovlev PI. 1962. Maturation of cortical substrata of epileptic events. *World Neurol* 3:299–315.

Yakovlev PI, Lecours AR. 1967. The myelogenetic cycles of regional maturation of the brain. In: Minkowski A, ed. *Regional development of the brain in early life.* Philadelphia: FA Davis, 3–70.

Yamamoto N, Watanabe K, Negoro T, et al. 1987a. Long-term prognosis of tuberous sclerosis with epilepsy in children. *Brain Dev* 9:292–295.

Yamamoto N, Watanabe K, Negoro T, et al. 1987b. Complex partial seizures in children: ictal manifestations and their relation to clinical course. *Neurology* 37: 1979–1982.

Yamamoto N, Watanabe K, Negoro T. 1988. Partial seizures evolving to infantile spasms. *Epilepsia* 29:34–40.

Yamatogi Y, Ohtahara S. 1981. Age-dependent epileptic encephalopathy: a longitudinal study. *Folia Psychiatr Neurol Jpn* 35:321–332.

Yamatogi Y, Ohtsuka Y, Ishida T, et al. 1979. Treatment of the Lennox syndrome with ACTH: a clinical and electroencephalographic study. *Brain Dev* 1:267–276.

Yanai S, Hanai T, Narazaki O. 1999. Treatment of infantile spasms with zonisamide. *Brain Dev* 21:157–161.

Yang PJ, Berger PE, Cohen ME, et al. 1979. Computed tomography and childhood seizure disorders. *Neurology* 29:1084–1088.

Yaqub BA. 1993. Electroclinical seizures in Lennox-Gastaut syndrome. *Epilepsia* 34:120–127.

Yarnell PR, Chu NS. 1975. Focal seizures and aminophylline. *Neurology* 25:819–822.

Yasargil MG, Teddy PJ, Roth P. 1985. Selective amygdalohippocampectomy: operative anatomy and surgical technique. In: Symon L, Bonhaye L, Guidetti B, et al., eds. *Advances and technical standards in neurosurgery.* Berlin: Springer, 93–123.

Yasawa I, Nukina N, Hashida H, et al. 1995. Abnormal gene product identified in hereditary dentatorubral-pallidoluysian atrophy (DRPLA) brain. *Nat Genet* 19: 99–103.

Yashura A, Yoshida H, Hatanaka T, et al. 1991. Epilepsy with continuous spike-waves during slow sleep and its treatment. *Epilepsia* 32:59–62.

Yates P, Stockdill G, McIntyre M. 1986. Hypersensitivity to carbamazepine presenting as pseudolymphoma. *J Clin Pathol* 39:1224–1228.

Yeh HW, Privitera MD. 1991. Secondary epileptogenesis in cerebral arteriovenous malformations. *Arch Neurol* 48: 1122–1124.

Yerbi MS. 1991. Pregnancy and epilepsy. *Epilepsia* 32: S51–S59.

Yoshimura K, Hamada F, Tomoda T, et al. 1998. Focal pachypolymicrogyria in three siblings. *Pediatr Neurol* 18:435–438.

Yoshioka H, Ishikawa A, Seki T, et al. 2001. Clinical and pedigree study on familial cases of West syndrome in Japan. *Brain Dev* 23:558–564.

Young GB, Blume WT. 1983. Painful epileptic seizures. *Brain* 106:537–554.

Young B, Rapp RP, Norton JA, et al. 1983. Failure of prophylactically administered phenytoin to prevent early post-traumatic seizures. *J Neurosurg* 58:231–235.

Young GB, Barr HW, Blume WT. 1986. Painful epileptic seizures involving the second sensory area [Letter]. *Ann Neurol* 19:412.

Young RS, Cowan BE, Petroff OA, et al. 1987. In vivo ^{31}P and in vitro ^{1}H nuclear magnetic resonance study of hypoglycemia during neonatal seizures. *Ann Neurol* 22: 622–628.

Younkin DP, Delivoria-Papadopoulos M, Maris J, et al. 1986. Cerebral metabolic effects of neonatal seizures measured in vivo ^{31}P NMR spectroscopy. *Ann Neurol* 20:513–519.

Youroukos S, Lazopoulou D, Michelakou D, Karagianni T. 2003. Acute psychosis associated with levetiracetam. *Epileptic Disord* 5:117–119.

Zara F, Gennaro E, Stabile M, et al. 2000. Mapping a locus for familial autosomal recessive idiopathic myoclonic epilepsy of infancy to chromosome 16p13. *Am J Hum Genet* 66:1552–1557.

Zareba W, Moss AJ, Schwartz PS, et al. 1998. Influence of the genotype in the clinical course of the long QT syndrome. *N Engl J Med* 339:960–965.

Zaret BS, Cohen RA. 1986. Reversible valproic-acid induced dementia: a case report. *Epilepsia* 27: 234–240.

Zarrelli MM, Beghi E, Rocca WA, Hauser WA. 1999. Incidence of epileptic syndromes in Rochester, Minnesota: 1980–1984. *Epilepsia* 40:1708–1714.

Zee DS, Yee RD, Singer HS. 1977. Congenital ocular/motor apraxia. *Brain* 100:581–599.

Zelante L, Torricelli F, Calvano S, et al. 1991. Ring chromosome 14 syndrome: report of two cases, including extended evaluation of a previously reported patient and review. *Ann Genet* 34:93–97.

Zelnik N, Nir A, Amit S, et al. 1990. Autonomic seizures in an infant: unusual cutaneous and cardiac manifestations. *Dev Med Child Neurol* 32:74–78.

Zeman W, Donahue S, Dyken P, et al. 1970. The neuronal ceroid-lipofuscinoses (Batten-Vogt syndrome). In: Vinken PJ, Bruyn GW, eds. *Leukodystrophies and poliodystrophies*. Handbook of clinical neurology, Vol. 10. Amsterdam: North-Holland, 588–679.

Zeutner J, Wolf HK, Ostertun B, et al. 1994. Gangliogliomas: clinical, radiological and histopathological findings in 51 patients. *J Neurol Neurosurg Psychiatry* 57:1497–1502.

Ziegler AL. 1990. Le rôle de l'autisme dans le spasmes infantiles. Presented to the Swiss Association of Child Neurology meeting, La Chaux de Fond, Switzerland.

Ziegler AL, Calame A, Marchand C, et al. 1976. Cerebral distress in full-term newborns and its prognostic value. A follow-up study of 90 infants. *Helv Paediatr Acta* 31:299–317.

Ziegler AL, Van Melle G, Calame A, et al. 1981. Détresse cérébrale du nouveau-né à terme: méthode de pronostic précoce quant à la qualité de la survie long terme. *Helvet Paediatr Acta* 36:341–358.

Zielinski JJ. 1975. Epilepsy and mortality rate and cause of death. *Epilepsia* 15:191–201.

Zifkin B, Andermann F, Beaumanoir A, et al., eds. 1998. *Reflex epilepsies and reflex seizures*. Philadelphia: Lippincott-Raven.

Zimmerman AW, Niedermeyer E, Hodges FJ. 1977. Lennox-Gastaut syndrome and computerized axial tomography findings. *Epilepsia* 18:463–464.

Zimmerman RS, Spetzler RF, Lee KS, et al. 1991. Cavernous malformations of the brain stem. *J Neurosurg* 75:32–39.

Zori RT, Hendrickson J, Woolven S, et al. 1992. Angelman syndrome: clinical profile. *J Child Neurol* 7:270–280.

Zuberi SM, Eunson LH, Spanschus A, et al. 1999. A novel mutation in the human voltage gated potassium channel gene associates with episodic ataxia type 1 and sometimes with partial epilepsy. *Brain* 122:817–825.

Zupanc ML, Handler EG, Levine RL, et al. 1990. Rasmussen encephalitis: epilepsia partialis continua secondary to chronic encephalitis. *Pediatr Neurol* 6:397–401.

Subject Index

Note: Page numbers followed by an *f* indicate figures; those followed by a *t* indicate tables.